ACUTE & CHRONIC WOUNDS

CURRENT MANAGEMENT CONCEPTS

THIRD EDITION

Ruth A. Bryant, RN, MS, CWOCN
Partner, Bryant Rolstad Consultants, LLC
Program Director, webWOC Nursing Education Program
Roseville, Minnesota

Denise P. Nix, RN, MS, CWOCN
President, Nix Consulting Inc.
Associate Director webWOC Nursing Education Program
Edina, Minnesota

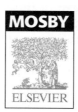

MOSBY

ELSEVIER

11830 Westline Industrial Drive
St. Louis, Missouri 63146

Notice

Knowledge and best practice in this field are constantly changing. As new research and experience broaden our knowledge, changes in practice, treatment and drug therapy may become necessary or appropriate. Readers are advised to check the most current information provided (i) on procedures featured or (ii) by the manufacturer of each product to be administered, to verify the recommended dose or formula, the method and duration of administration, and contraindications. It is the responsibility of the practitioner, relying on their own experience and knowledge of the patient, to make diagnoses, to determine dosages and the best treatment for each individual patient, and to take all appropriate safety precautions. To the fullest extent of the law, neither the Publisher nor the Authors assumes any liability for any injury and/or damage to persons or property arising out or related to any use of the material contained in this book.

The Publisher

ISBN-13: 978-0-323-03074-8
ISBN-10: 0-323-03074-2

Executive Publisher: N. Darlene Como
Developmental Editor: Barbara Watts
Publishing Services Manager: John Rogers
Senior Project Manager: Kathleen L. Teal
Design Direction: Amy Buxton

Printed in the United States of America

Last digit is the print number: 9 8 7 6 5 4 3 2 1

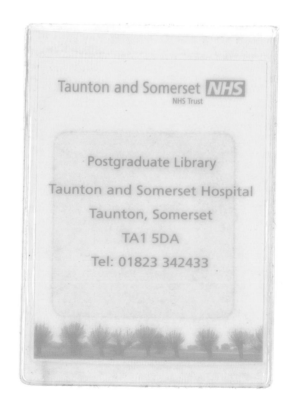

To my brothers and sisters:
Margie, Sarah and Charlie, you are still alive in my heart and I miss you every day.
Dorna, Steve and Liz, I cherish our bond, our laughs and our memories.

To my Mom:
You are my ever-present inspiration.

To my husband, Dennis, and sons, Michael Edward Confer and Charles Orman Confer:
You give my life meaning.

Ruth

To my husband and boys
John Joseph Nix, Ian Lee Nix, Adam Henry Nix

Denise

Contributors

Tara L. Beuscher, MSN, RN, APRN, BC, CWOCN, CFCN, APNP
Nurse Practitioner
Marshfield Clinic – Lakeland Center
Minocqua, Wisconsin

Joyce M. Black, PhD, RN, CWCN, CPSN
Associate Professor
University of Nebraska Medical Center
Omaha, Nebraska

Steven B. Black, MD, FACS
Director, Wound Care Services
Nebraska Medical Center
Omaha, Nebraska

Craig L. Broussard, PhD, RN, CNS, CHRNC, CWCN, CWS, FCCWS
Consultant
Clinical Consultants
Port Arthur, Texas

Susan Gallagher Camden, RN, CWOCN, MSN, MA, PhD
Clinical Affairs Coordinator
Sizewise Rentals
Ellis, Kansas

Richard A. F. Clark, MD
Professor of Biomedical Engineering, Dermatology, and Medicine
Director of the Center for Tissue Engineering
SUNY Stony Brook
Stony Brook, New York

Renee Cordrey, PT, PhD(c), MSPT, MPH, CWS
Wound Care Clinical Specialist
St. Francis Medical Center
Lynwood, California;

Associated Faculty
Mount St. Mary's College
Los Angeles, California

Dorothy B. Doughty, MN, RN, FAAN, CWOCN
Director, Wound Ostomy Continence Nursing Education Center
Emory University
Atlanta, Georgia

Vickie R. Driver, DPM, MS, FACFAS
Chief, Limb Preservation Center
Advocate Lutheran General Hospital
Park Ridge, Illinois;

Director, Clinical Research
Center for Lower Extremity Ambulatory Research
Dr. William M. Scholl College of Podiatric Medicine
Rosalind Franklin University of Medicine
North Chicago, Illinois

Jill Evans, RN, MSN
Coordinator, Pediatric Burn Services
Medical University of South Carolina Children's Hospital
Charlestown, South Carolina

Rita A. Frantz, PhD, RN, CWCN, FAAN
Professor & Chair
Systems & Practice Nursing
College of Nursing
University of Iowa
Iowa City, Iowa

Margaret T. Goldberg, RN, MSN, CWOCN
Wound Care Consultant
Wound Treatment Center
Delray Beach, Florida

Finn Gottrup, MD, DMSci
Professor
University of Southern Denmark
Odense, Denmark

Rhonda Holbrook, BSN, RN, CWOCN
Clinician/Instructor
Emory University
Atlanta, Georgia

Harriet W. Hopf, MD
Professor
Department of Surgery
Department of Anesthesia and Perioperative Care
University of California-San Francisco
San Francisco, California

Diane L. Krasner, PhD, RN, CWCN, CWS, FAAN
WOC Nurse
St. Agnes Hospital
Baltimore, Maryland

Mary Anne Landowski, RN, MSN, CWOCN, CFCN
Director, Wound Care Clinic
Madigan Army Medical Center
Tacoma, Washington

J.L. Madsen, MS, CRC
Madigan Army Medical Center
Tacoma, Washington

Margaret McGinn-Byer, RN, CWOCN, OCN
Outreach Service Coordinator
WOC Nurse
Fox Chase Cancer Center
Philadelphia, Pennsylvania

Susan Mendez-Eastman, RN, CWCN, CPSN
Wound Care Nurse
Wound Ostomy Department
Nebraska Medical Center
Omaha, Nebraska

Liza G. Ovington, PhD, FCCCWS
Associate Medical Director
Johnson & Johnson Wound Management
Ethicon, Inc.
Somerville, New Jersey

Ben Peirce, BA, RN, CWOCN
Manager of Wound Care
Gentiva ® Health Services
Ft. Lauderdale, Florida

Barbara Pieper, PhD, RN, CS, CWOCN, FAAN
Professor/Nurse Practitioner
College of Nursing
Wayne State University
Detroit, Michigan

Janet M. Ramundo, MSN, RN, CWOCN, FNP
Emory University Wound Ostomy Continence
    Nursing Education Center
Atlanta, Georgia

Bonnie Sue Rolstad, RN, MS, CWOCN
Administrative Director
webWOC Nursing Education Program
Minneapolis, Minnesota;

Community Faculty Member
School of Nursing
Metropolitan State University
St. Paul, Minnesota

Kathleen D. Schaum, MS
President
Kathleen D. Schaum & Associates, Inc.
Lake Worth, Florida

Gregory Schultz, PhD
Professor, Department of Obstetrics and Gynecology
Director, Institute for Wound Research
University of Florida
Gainesville, Florida

Dag Shapshak, MD
Fellow of Hyperbaric Medicine and Wound Care
Doctor's Medical Center
San Pablo, California

Bonnie Sparks-DeFriese, PT, RN, CWS, CWOCN
Emory WOC Nurse Clinician/Instructor
Emory Wound Ostomy Continence Nursing
    Education Center
Atlanta, Georgia

Nancy A. Stotts, RN, EdD, FAAN
Professor of Nursing
University of California-San Francisco
San Francisco, California

JoAnne D. Whitney, PhD, RN, CWCN, FAAN
Professor
University of Washington
Biobehavioral Nursing and Health Systems;

Nurse Research Scientist
Harborview Medical Center
Seattle, Washington

Annette B. Wysocki, PhD, RN, FAAN
Professor
School of Nursing
School of Medicine
University of Mississippi Medical Center
Jackson, Mississippi

Reviewers

Karen Huskey, RN, BSN, CWCN, COCN
Memorial Hospital
Chattanooga, Tennessee

Dianne Mackey, BSN, RN, PHN, CWOCN
Wound/Skin Coordinator
Kaiser Permanente
San Diego, California

Debra S. Netsch, RN, MSN, CNP, CWOCN
WOC Nurse and Family Nurse Practitioner
Mankato Clinic
Mankato, Minnesota;
WebWOC Nurse Education Program
Associate Director and Ostomy Faculty
Minneapolis, Minnesota

Linda Schiech, RN, MSN, AOCN
Clinical Nurse Specialist
Fox Chase Cancer Center
Philadelphia, Pennsylvania

Kristy Wright, MBA, RN, FAAN, CWOCN
Visiting Nurse's Association Western Pennsylvania
Butler, Pennsylvania

Colorplate Credits

Plate 6 Modified from Thompson JM, Wilson SF: Health assessment for nursing practice, St Louis, 1996, Mosby. In Seidel Henry M, Ball JW, Dains JE, Benedict GW: *Mosby's guide to physical examination*, 6th edition, St Louis, 2006, Mosby.

Plate 7 Modified from Wilson SF, Giddens JF: Health assessment for nursing practice, ed 3, St Louis, Mosby. In Seidel Henry M, Ball JW, Dains JE, Benedict GW: *Mosby's guide to physical examination*, 6th edition, St Louis, 2006, Mosby.

Plate 9 From Jarvis C: *Physical examination & health assessment*, ed 4, St Louis, 2004, Saunders.

Plate 33 Courtesy Judith L. Gates.

Plates 41, 44, 47, 49, 52, 55, 58 Courtesy Bonnie Sue Rolstad.

Plate 59 Courtesy Julie Freyberg.

Preface

The 1992 first edition of *Acute & Chronic Wounds* was published at a time when access to print information dedicated to the clinical care of the patient with a wound was extremely limited. Many health care providers were uninformed or skeptical of moist wound healing and few products were available. Today, many textbooks on wound care are available, wound clinics are commonplace and viewed as providing a "competitive edge," national wound care guidelines exist, the variety of wound dressings that populate the hospital formulary is vast, and many types of health care professionals study and specialize in wound care.

Acute & Chronic Wounds: Current Management Concepts (3rd edition) is intended for a wide audience of health care providers including the RN, Nurse Practitioner, Clinical Nurse Specialist, physical therapist, physician, physician's assistant, and others. The commitment to expand the intended audience stems from the recognition that effective and efficient evidence based wound care absolutely requires a multidisciplinary and transdisciplinary team. All health care providers have a role in risk assessment, skin assessment, skin health maintenance, and wound prevention, as well as timely interventions with the most appropriate goal directed treatments. Whether novice or expert in wound care, nurse, physical therapist, or physician, *Acute & Chronic Wounds: Current Management Concepts* (3rd edition) contains information that will deepen the reader's understanding of wound care, underscore the significance of multidisciplinary involvement and enhance an evidence based, outcome oriented practice.

Unique features have been maintained in each edition of the *Acute & Chronic Wounds* textbook. The progression of content gradually increases in complexity, thus facilitating the reader's ability to establish a solid foundation in core anatomy and wound healing physiology before diving into etiology and interventions. We have continued with that approach in this 3rd edition and incorporated the extensive advances that have occurred in the management of the patient with a wound. In addition, an extensive list of references is provided at the conclusion of each chapter to expedite the reader's ability to further explore specific topics of interest.

Recognizing that a "picture is worth a thousand words" the number of color plates in this edition has been increased to 59. In addition to the many tools for practice provided within the chapters of the text, the Appendix presents samples of policies, procedures, assessment, teaching and documentation tools designed to help bring evidence based practice to the bedside.

As in the previous editions, each chapter of *Acute & Chronic Wounds* begins with a set of behavioral objectives and ends with a self-assessment. The objectives are carefully crafted to address the key elements within the chapter so that readers can quickly identify gaps in their knowledge base and topics areas that would be personally beneficial to read. The Self-Assessment Exercises are provided to assist the reader to assess his or her level of comprehension and may be used as either a "pretest" or "posttest".

Finally, although there is the potential for considerable overlap in the content among the chapters, great care has been taken to streamline the content so as to avoid repetition by the chapter authors. For example, while the issue of ABI or lipodermatosclerosis is mentioned in the chapter on neuropathic foot ulcers, the reader will be referred back to the key chapter that presents this content in great detail. This feature expedites the reader's ability to access key content from the Index and thus use the textbook as a resource.

Organizationally, this textbook begins with two chapters that describe principles of practice essential for any wound care program, the justification for a multidisciplinary team approach to wound management and models for creating a multidisciplinary wound team in terms of structure and function. Within these chapters, difficult and sometimes confusing issues such as "who qualifies as a wound care clinician" and "what are the functions of the various members of the wound care team" are clarified. An attempt is also made to distinguish wound care from wound management. Of key interest to the reader will be the discussion addressing the relevance and purpose of national certification and the qualifications of certifying organizations.

Chapters 3 through 5 focus on creating a biologic basis in anatomy of the skin, physiology of wound healing, and the molecular regulation of the intact and the wounded skin. From this foundational content, the rationale for each aspect of managing the patient with, or at risk for developing, a wound can be built.

Chapters 6 through 9 focus on assessment of the patient with a wound and altered skin integrity. Terms are defined and a framework for classifying the various threats to skin integrity are provided with key distinctions in assessment parameters for each. The emphasis of the assessment chapter is an assessment of the patient as a whole, the wound specifically, and the ongoing assessments that provide the data needed for evaluation of the extent of healing. Specific chapters are dedicated to nutritional assessment and the assessment of contamination, colonization, critical colonization, and infection.

Chapters 10 and 11 explore the care of two specific situations: the necrotic wound and the acute surgical or traumatic wound. Strategies for debridement, advantages or disadvantages for each strategy, and contraindications for debridement are described. Interventions to actively support healing of the acute wound and factors that place the surgical incision, for example, at risk for impaired healing or dehiscence are discussed.

Chapters 12 through 18 address the various etiologies for the development of a wound, including risk factors, pathophysiology, assessment, and appropriate interventions. Within this section are several new additions. The use of support surfaces, skin care for the bariatric patient, and foot and nail care are addressed within a separate chapter for each.

With such a clear understanding of how the skin heals, assessment, and the causative factors for wound, Chapters 19-21 provide a framework for the management of the patient with a wound. The principles of wound management that were first introduced in the first edition of this textbook continue to be widely adopted in practice as the core directives guiding the holistic care of the patient with a wound. The eight objectives of local wound management remain valid and clinically useful in sorting through the maze of topical care options for these complex patient situations. The clinical relevance of these objectives is further apparent with the simplification of these objectives into the acronym TIME (described in Chapters 5 and 19). Complete with illustrations of each dressing, a formulary of wound care products (passive, active and skin care) is provided within Chapter 19 that can be adapted and implemented by the reader. Recognizing that treatments such as electrical stimulation and negative pressure wound therapy are no longer adjuvant therapies, this particular chapter is now entitled "Devices and Technology in Wound Care" and has been expanded to include interventions more commonly provided by physical therapy.

Chapters 22-24 address unique situations that pose a threat to skin integrity, such as oncology-related skin damage, draining wounds and fistulas, and gastrostomy tube management.

The final chapters of the 3rd edition of *Acute & Chronic Wounds: Current Management Concepts* are of particular value to all readers. Chapter 25 discusses managing wound pain and explores the pathology of pain, types of pain, and provides a systematic approach to managing wound pain, complete with recommended pharmacologic and nonpharmacologic interventions that can be readily adopted into practice. Chapter 26 is a new chapter in this edition and focuses on the approach of the health care provider to facilitate the patient's ability to establish a sustainable plan of care and thereby enhance consistency in self care. A case for omitting the concept of the "noncompliant patient" is advanced. Chapter 27 will also be of interest to all readers as the essentials of the interrelated issues of billing for services, coding, and reimbursement are explored. From this chapter, the reader will be better informed of the complexities and terms involved in billing and prepared to collaborate with the billing office personnel to further explore and improve upon the accuracy of the billing process.

It can be both exciting and overwhelming to stay abreast of all the advances in wound care that have evolved since the second edition of this textbook.

As experts in their fields with an active clinical practice, each author who has contributed to this textbook understands the pressures facing health care providers when caring for the patient with a wound. By sharing their knowledge (and their time) to create the third edition of *Acute & Chronic Wounds: Current* *Management Concepts,* each of us has the opportunity to expand our knowledge base and ultimately improve the quality of care for any patient with a wound or at risk for developing a wound!

Ruth A. Bryant

Acknowledgments

Life is so full of twists and turns. For me many of those twists and turns occurred during the editing of this third edition. This edition is a reality because of two extraordinary people: Barb Watts at Elsevier/Mosby and Denise Nix. Thank you, Barb for the compassion and support you provided that was above and beyond the call of duty of an editor. DeeDee, you are so much more than a co-editor in this project with me. The value of your contribution is beyond comprehension and words. Thank you for saying yes to co-editing this text with me. Thank you for sharing so much of your time, home, family, priorities and patience with me. Thank you for making me laugh so much and so often. And thank you for your deep commitment to quality patient care, love for the specialty of WOC nursing, and passion for education of future wound care providers!

Ruth

I would like to acknowledge Barb Watts at Elsevier/Mosby for your patience, encouragement and hard work during the production of this book. I am truly grateful to my incredibly supportive mom and dad, Barbara and Allan Henry, who teach by example and have touched and inspired so many, yet would never acknowledge or admit it. To my amazing colleagues at the webWOC Nursing Education Program; Bonnie, Deb, JoAnn, and Anne, thank you for your high standards and commitment to education, sisterhood and most importantly the patient. Finally, I want to thank Ruth, for the wonderful opportunity to work among the amazing contributors to this text. Ruth, it is an honor to be your colleague and friend.

Denise

Contents

1

Principles for Practice Development

RUTH A. BRYANT & DENISE P. NIX

OBJECTIVES

1. Describe the services the wound care specialist provides within the capacity of his or her role as expert clinician and as a provider of education, research, and leadership/management.
2. Compare and contrast the benefits of national certification as a wound care specialist.
3. Discriminate among prevalence, cumulative incidence, and incidence rate, addressing how each is calculated and the clinical utility of each measure.
4. Describe the essential elements of a time management database and how they can be used.
5. List at least three departments or groups the wound care specialist should approach specifically to describe the role of wound care specialist.
6. Cite three examples of how the wound care specialist can effect cost savings within an institution.

A comprehensive wound care program is essential to any organization, agency, or health care system offering a full scope of services to its clientele. The wound care specialist can provide a multitude of valuable services: state-of-the-art, evidence-based wound management; staff education; control of wound-related costs; quality improvement activities; protocol and formulary development; pressure ulcer risk reduction; and insight into efficient use of personnel and resources. The wound care specialist is instrumental in bringing together many departments to more fully appreciate and manage the condition of the patient with a wound. In addition, the wound care specialist can affect the quality of care in an organization or agency through administrative activities, collaboration with materials management personnel, establishing a skin/wound care team, direct patient care, and indirect patient care through consultation and education of the staff.

Many factors contribute to a successful practice as a wound care specialist. Obviously the specialist must have a strong knowledge base in wound care and in the relevant pathologies. In addition, the specialist must establish credibility, which is earned by demonstrating clinical competence, critical thinking, organization, self-confidence, and an eagerness to collaborate and share information with colleagues. However, a successful practice also requires the integration of business skills to develop goals that reflect the organization's mission and goals, effectively define services, identify benefits of services, outline a marketing approach to potential referral sources, and draft a conservative but realistic budget. Many decision-making tools and clinical resources will also be needed in a wound management program. The wound care specialist would be wise to assemble a business plan for new wound-related programs. Components of a business plan are listed in Box 1-1. In this chapter we will discuss the application of business skills in terms of educational qualifications, role development, time management, data collection, marketing, value-added services, and outcomes measurement.

QUALIFICATIONS OF A WOUND CARE SPECIALIST

When developing a wound management program, it is incumbent upon administration to expect appropriate educational preparation, qualifications, and credentialing of the health care professional who will function as the wound care specialist.

Definition of Terms

Much confusion exists among health care providers and administrators concerning the terms certified, certification, certificate of completion, and continuing education (CE). These terms describe either a process used to

BOX I-I Components of a Business Plan

- Executive summary
- Present situation/Background
- Goal Statement or Description of services
- Product and Service Description
- Market analysis
- Operations and Key assumptions
- Qualifications (staffing)
- Financial planning (budgeting)

attain education (certificate of completion and continuing education) or a process used to validate knowledge and expertise in a specific area (certified and certification). Most often, the wound care specialist is a graduate of an accredited, formal, wound education program; he or she is then eligible for a credentialing process (such as an examination) as a wound care specialist.

A wound care education program is a rigorous, formal curriculum provided by a nationally accredited provider that includes a structured clinical experience with a qualified preceptor who is an expert in wound management. The content in the formal wound care education program is comprehensive and addresses physical assessment, anatomy and physiology, pathophysiology, risk management, wound management interventions, evaluation, outcomes management, and program development. An academic setting or an established organization may conduct the wound management curriculum. Upon completion of the education program, the graduate is awarded a *certificate of completion*, is considered competent at an entry level in wound management, and is eligible for national certification.

Education can also be obtained in the less rigorous format of continuing education through a workshop or individual seminars. At the completion of these continuing education programs, the attendee will also receive a certificate of completion. In no way, however, should this certificate of completion be misconstrued as an indication of expertise, mastery, or competence. It simply denotes that the individual attended the educational event.

Certification, in contrast, is the formal recognition of an individual's knowledge and expertise in a defined functional or clinical area of care; it validates that individual's specialty knowledge, experience, and clinical judgment. A process for attaining certification in the subspecialty of wound care has been created by two different national organizations: the Wound Ostomy Continence Nursing Certification Board (WOCNCB) and American Academy of Wound Management (AAWM). The WOCNCB confers a "CWCN" (certified wound care nurse) certificate. The AAWM confers a "CWS" (certified wound specialist) certificate.

A key distinction between these two credentialing organizations is eligibility criteria. The WOCNCB certifies baccalaureate prepared nurses. In contrast the AAWM certifies multiple disciplines with various educational backgrounds. (i.e., physicians, physical therapist, occupational therapists, registered nurses, LPNs, dieticians) (WOCNCB, 2005; AAWM, 2006).

National standards exist concerning the operations and certification process used by credentialing organizations. Compliance of the credentialing organization with the national standards set by an independent national certifying group imparts "accreditation" status.

Value of National Certification

The process and techniques used by the organization providing the certification are variable. Key attributes of a national certifying organization include (1) use of psychometrically sound techniques for construction, administration, and evaluation of the certification process; (2) accreditation by an independent national certifying body; and (3) use of a legally defensible process for certification.

The national certification process typically requires a testing process to assess the candidate's knowledge base as well as an evaluation process to examine the accuracy and effectiveness of each test item. With a strong psychometric foundation underlying the certifying process, candidates can be assured of fairness in the testing process and accuracy of the content or process. Accreditation by an independent national certifying body denotes the certifying organization's compliance with national standards relevant to all aspects of the certifying process. A legally defensible certification process is valuable to the employer whenever there is a potential for a hiring decision to be

BOX 1-2   **Attributes of a Nationally Accredited Certifying Organization**

- Accredited by an independent national certifying body
- Conducts job analysis and role delineation studies
- Creates examination by using a committee of content experts
- Mission of the certifying organization is consistent with consumer goals
- Self-assessment opportunities are provided to prepare for certification (i.e., practice test that does not contain actual exam questions)
- Certifying organization requires that coursework from an outside accredited wound education program

made based on criteria such as certification, or a job description requires certification (Hess, 2005).

Box 1-2 provides additional attributes of a nationally accredited certifying agency. When the certifying body is compliant with these attributes, the patient and organization can expect the certified practitioner to have a current knowledge base and expertise; continued expertise is verified by requiring recertification at designated time intervals. National certification also raises the standard for wound care by validating a knowledge base within the specialty of wound management.

ROLES, FUNCTIONS, AND RESPONSIBILITIES OF A WOUND CARE SPECIALIST

Regardless of the health care setting in which the wound care specialist will practice, role implementation will share many common expectations: clinical expertise, consultation, education, research, and leadership/management.

Clinical Expertise

Clinical expertise requires clinical skills in physical assessment and wound assessment, appropriate use of interventions, a knowledge base of wound-related pathophysiology, and documentation and communication skills. The services provided as a wound care specialist are listed in Box 1-3.

The expert wound care specialist provides the assessment skills needed to establish an individual plan of care for the patient with actual or potential skin breakdown. Through ongoing assessment and evaluation of the effectiveness of interventions, the wound care specialist will modify the plan regularly. Many wound care specialists provide direct patient care for the most complex wounds.

As a clinical expert, the specialist must determine the parameters of his or her practice and what should be expected of staff members from other disciplines such as nursing, physical therapy, and dietary. This clear delineation of roles is important to foster an empowering environment, avoid duplication of efforts, and maximize the efficient use of resources, including personnel. Table 1-1 provides examples of role delineation.

Consultation

In most settings, the wound care specialist serves primarily as a consultant and is challenged to meet the majority of the patient's needs by creating a wound care program implemented by a multidisciplinary team of health care providers. The multidisciplinary approach to wound management is described in Chapter 2. A successful consultant must effectively communicate, collaborate, and educate. The consultant role builds on the foundations of the wound care specialist as a clinical expert; it expands the value of having the wound care specialist on the team by addressing cost effectiveness while increasing patient access to service (WOCN Society, 2005b). Clinical decision-making tools and resources such as protocols, formularies (support surface formulary and wound care product formulary), and standardized care plans pave the way for the wound care specialist to adopt a consultative approach within the organization.

Education

Knowledge about pressure ulcer prevention, appropriate wound care, and comprehensive, accurate documentation is essential to maintaining and restoring skin integrity. When the staff receives information about pressure ulcer prediction and prevention and wound care on a routine basis, they have more knowledge about these conditions, the incidence of pressure ulcers declines, costs of care decrease, and healing rates improve (Jones et al, 1993; Pieper and Mott, 1995; Specht, Bergquist, and Frantz, 1995).

BOX 1-3 Services Provided by the Expert Clinical Wound Care Specialist

Education
- Provides appropriate education to patient, caregiver, and staff regarding skin care, wound management, percutaneous tubes, and draining wound/fistula management
- Assists staff to maintain current knowledge and competence in the areas of skin and wound care through orientation and regularly scheduled in-service education programs
- Attends continuing education programs related to wound management

Leadership and Management
- Provides consultation and assistance to staff in developing and implementing protocols used in the identification and management of patient with potential or actual alteration in skin integrity
- Provides guidance to staff in implementation of protocols to identify, control, or eliminate etiologic factors for skin breakdown, including selection of appropriate support surface
- Establishes protocols and guidelines for appropriate and cost-effective use of therapeutic support surfaces
- Maintains records and statistics and submits reports to employer
- Analyzes inventory and recommends appropriate additions and deletions to ensure quality and cost-effectiveness of products used for skin and wound care
- Serves on agency-wide committees and participates in agency-wide projects as requested

Research
- Assists staff to maintain current state of the art practice by reviewing and revising policies and procedures to be consistent with national guidelines and other sources of evidence based literature
- Conducts prevalence and incidence studies
- Conducts product evaluations or contributes to research studies related to skin and wound care when indicated, and submits reports and recommendations based on results

Clinical Consultant/Expert
- Evaluates patient response to treatment and the progress of wound healing, making adjustments and modifications as indicated
- Where qualified and appropriate, provides conservative sharp debridement of devitalized tissue and applies silver nitrate to epibole of wound edges, hypertrophic granulation tissue, and areas with minor bleeding
- Provides follow-up for patients with draining or chronic wounds, fistulas, or percutaneous tubes through outpatient clinic visits and or phone consultations; initiates appropriate referrals for medical or surgical intervention
- Provides consultation and assistance to staff in developing a plan of care for patients with percutaneous tubes (i.e., tube stabilization, site care and appropriate drainage system)

Knowledge gaps among health care professionals concerning wound care are varied and unpredictable. Bostrom and Kenneth (1992) surveyed 245 staff registered nurses (RNs) from multiple health care settings about pressure ulcer prevention and found staff knowledge about pressure ulcer risk factors to be high (91% identified 9 out of 11 risk factors). Surprisingly, however, the staff did not consider promotion of skin integrity to be a priority, and only one third of the nurses had updated their knowledge regarding pressure ulcer treatment in the last 2 years. In a study of 75 experienced critical care nurses' knowledge of pressure ulcer prevention, staging, and description, Pieper and Mattern (1997) found that only a few had read the 1992 *AHCPR Guideline on Pressure Ulcer Prevention* (Bergstrom et al, 1994). This is of concern since critical care patients constitute a large proportion of hospitalized patients with pressure ulcers.

Beitz, Fey, and O'Brien (1999) surveyed a convenience sample of RNs, licensed practical nurses (LPNs), and nurse aides (NAs) (n = 86) and found their greatest knowledge deficits to be in the areas of etiologic factors generating pressure ulcers, support surfaces, staging, and treatment modalities. In a retrospective study of 167 patients using high or low air–loss beds and using documentation as a reflection of nursing

TABLE 1-1   Examples of Delineation of Roles: Wound Care Nurse and Staff Nurse

WOUND CARE NURSE	STAFF NURSE
1. Facilitate creation and implementation of pressure ulcer risk-assessment protocol.	Conduct risk assessment per protocol.
2. Establish protocol for prevention guidelines to correlate with risk assessment.	Implement appropriate risk-reduction interventions.
3. Establish protocol for management of minor skin lesions (candidiasis, skin tears, stages 1 and 2 pressure ulcers, etc.).	Implement appropriate care of minor skin lesions.
4. Formulate wound care formulary to specify indications and use parameters of wound dressings.	Use wound dressings as per formulary. Notify wound care nurse if product performs poorly or wound fails to respond.
5. Conduct comprehensive wound assessment, establish plan of care for complex ulcers (i.e., leg ulcers, stages III and IV pressure ulcers), and conduct regular reevaluation of wound.	Conduct focused wound assessment. Notify wound care nurse of complex wounds. Implement appropriate care as per wound care nurse direction.
6. Provide regular staff education opportunities for updates in procedures, products, assessment and so on.	Identify and recommend topics of interest for staff education and updates.
7. Identify quality-improvement activities concerning wound care and risk-assessment (e.g., documentation of interventions, reliability of assessments).	Participate in quality-improvement activities.

knowledge and abilities, Pieper et al (1990) reported that the nursing documentation was lacking critical wound descriptors such as location, stage, size, color, exudate, and odor. These knowledge gaps all underscore the importance of the role of the wound care specialist as educator.

By auditing chart documentation or surveying the staff's knowledge about specific areas of wound care, the wound care specialist can identify needs and target educational activities to satisfy those needs. Beitz, Fey, and O'Brien (1999) warn that "Professional staff who perceive little need for additional wound care education may disregard opportunities for increasing their knowledge base because they consider themselves competent."

Promoting Behavioral Change

Although education is an important role and tool for the wound care specialist, it does not guarantee behavioral change, or adoption of new practice patterns. The information could be viewed as a burden rather than an innovation that may decrease work time or improve patient outcomes (Landrum, 1998b). An individual's reaction to and decision about new information, ideas, or practice (i.e., innovations) is something that develops over time and is seldom spontaneous. The *Diffusion of Innovations* theory (Rogers, 1995) provides a framework for changing practices in a group, individual, or organization (Landrum, 1998a; Dobbins et al, 2005). This theory describes how people adopt innovations using five stages: knowledge, persuasion, decision, implementation, and confirmation. Whether the innovation is to implement a new product or improve upon an existing product, and whether the innovation is preventive or has immediate observable results, a failure to consider these stages can spell disaster and frustration. Table 1-2 outlines these stages and gives the definition of each stage and considerations relative to the specialty of wound care.

Innovation is more likely to be adopted and behaviors changed when the innovation is perceived as relevant and consistent with the individual's attitudes and perceived attitudes of colleagues within the organization (Hassinger, 1959; Dobbins et al, 2005). Generally, an individual will seek like-minded peers who have already embraced the innovation to discuss the consequences of adopting the innovation; motivation to embrace the innovation is increased when these

TABLE 1-2 Five Stages of Roger's Innovation-Decision Process

STAGE	DESCRIPTION
1. Knowledge stage	An individual becomes aware of an innovation and of how it functions. May occur with reading, reviewing posted flyers, attending lectures, and so on.
2. Persuasion stage	A favorable or unfavorable attitude toward an innovation forms. To form a favorable attitude, the individual must be convinced that the innovation has greater value than current practice (e.g., identify patients at risk for pressure ulcers or target appropriate interventions).
3. Decision stage	Individual receives enough information to form an opinion about innovation. The individual pursues activities that lead to adoption or rejection of the innovation.
4. Implementation stage	Once a decision to adopt the innovation has been made, barriers (structural, process, or psychic) to implementation must be overcome (e.g., adequate number of forms is available).
5. Confirmation stage	Individuals seek to reinforce their decision. Observable and positive results are critical at this stage to prevent a reversal in decision. Careful monitoring is required, and information validating positive effects is important (e.g., a decrease in the incidence of pressure ulcers after adoption of a new risk assessment tool).

Data from Landrum BJ: Marketing innovations to nurses, Part I. How people adopt innovations, JWOCN 25:194, 1998.

TABLE 1-3 Attributes that Influence Adoption of Innovation

ATTRIBUTES OF INNOVATION	DESCRIPTION
Relative advantage	Is this better than an existing practice (e.g., potential decrease in costs, decrease in staff time, ease of use)?
Compatibility	Is this consistent with the individual's existing values, experiences, and needs?
Complexity	Is this innovation difficult to understand or use? For example, when a protocol is developed that links risk-assessment scores with nursing interventions, the decision about which preventive nursing intervention to use may be perceived as less complex than before the protocol; therefore the protocol may be more likely to be adopted.
Trialability	Can the individual experiment with the innovation on a limited basis?
Observability	Are the results of an innovation visible to others? Subtle outcomes are harder to communicate to others, so the innovation is often slower to be adopted.

Adapted from Landrum BJ: Marketing innovations to nurses, Part I. How people adopt innovations. JWOCN 25:194, 1998.

colleagues are supportive and positive about the innovation. Five attributes of an innovation significantly influence the rate at which it is adopted: relative advantage, compatibility, complexity, trialability, and observability (Table 1-3). These attributes should be considered before the persuasion stage so that adjustments can be made to enhance the likelihood of success with the education efforts.

Research

The wound care specialist also serves as a researcher. The extent to which the specialist functions in this capacity can vary widely depending on his or her educational preparation, agency support, and general interests. However, three research-based activities are pertinent to all wound care specialists: "mini-studies" that support quality-improvement activities,

BOX 1-4 Formulas for Prevalence, Cumulative Incidence, and Incidence Density

$$\text{Prevalence} = \frac{\text{Number of persons with a condition (i.e., pressure ulcer)}}{\text{Number of persons in the target population at a particular point in time}} \times 100$$

$$\text{Cumulative Incidence} = \frac{\text{Number of persons who develop the condition (i.e., new pressure ulcer)}}{\text{Number of persons in the population at the beginning of the time period}} \times 100$$

$$\text{Incidence Density} = \frac{\text{Number of persons developing the condition (i.e., new pressure ulcer)}}{\text{Total time (patient days or years) they were free of the condition or observed}} \times 100$$

research utilization and evidence-based care, and data collection.

Quality Improvement Activities

Quality improvement activities are a high priority for the wound care specialist, and the ability to conduct such activities is a key benefit to the organization. Activities often consist of simple chart audits designed to ascertain adequacy of documentation of assessment parameters, interventions, and effects or outcomes. Quality improvement activities may also be used to identify quality care issues or to better define the characteristics of a clinical problem. Without a quality improvement plan, delays, inefficiencies, or harmful interventions may go undetected and thus contribute to staff dissatisfaction or frustration, delayed discharge, and increased costs of care. A quality improvement activity that should be central to all wound care programs is the prevalence and incidence study.

Prevalence and Incidence Studies. Prevalence, incidence, cumulative incidence, and incidence density are the primary epidemiologic measures of disease frequency used to express the rate of occurrence of a disease or disorder. These terms however are not interchangeable and are described in this section. Box 1-4 provides the formula for calculating each.

Prevalence. Prevalence is the number of individuals who have a specific condition at a particular moment in time. Expressed as a percentage or proportion (or a ratio, not a rate), prevalence is a cross-sectional measure. Essentially a snapshot in time, it reflects how many people in a target population (such as the orthopedic unit) have a condition (e.g., a pressure ulcer) at a point in time (e.g., during the month of July).

For example, the prevalence of pressure ulcers in the orthopedic unit for the month of July may be 5 out of a unit census of 50 (5/50, or 10%). The issue of whether the condition is "new" or ongoing is irrelevant when calculating prevalence; all patients with the condition are counted. Generally considered to be a stable measure, prevalence should not vary significantly over time unless changes in practice patterns, referral bases, or marketing have occurred or the average duration of the disease has changed. As a measure of disease frequency (or burden of disease), prevalence is a useful tool for health care planning (Gordis, 1996; Pieper et al, 1999). It provides a means of identifying workload needs, staff needs, or resource allocation needs to meet the demands of that disease burden or volume (Baumgarten, 1998). Prevalence should never be misconstrued as a measure of quality of care or a measure of risk. An institution or agency that specializes in wound care is expected to have a high volume or prevalence of wounds based on the fact that its marketing strategies are geared to the recruitment or enrollment of patients with wounds.

Incidence. Incidence is the proportion of patients who acquire the condition over a given period of time. In the case of pressure ulcers, for example, incidence is the number of patients in a defined population (i.e., patients in the Intensive Care Unit) who were ulcer-free initially but who developed a pressure ulcer within a particular time (e.g., during their hospital stay). Incidence is expressed as a percentage and is measured either as a cumulative incidence or an incidence density.

Cumulative incidence. Cumulative incidence is the more familiar technique. Cumulative incidence is the number of new patients in a group who develop a condition over a period of time. The denominator for cumulative incidence is the total number of people in the population being observed at the beginning of the designated time period (see Box 1-4). Cumulative incidence is a measure of risk and provides an estimate of the probability (risk) of developing a condition or disease over a specific period of time (Kelsey et al, 1996). Therefore, cumulative incidence can be used to gauge the effects of risk factors and prevention efforts. Characteristics of cumulative incidence include the following (Gordis, 1996):

1. Cumulative incidence is a measure of *new* cases (not existing cases) of a particular condition.
2. The denominator must include only those individuals *at risk* for developing the condition.
3. Cumulative incidence always refers to a specific time-period (e.g., 1 day, 1 week, 1 month, 1 year).
4. As with prevalence, cumulative incidence is a proportion (not a rate) and ranges from 0% to 100%.
5. All individuals in the group at risk (represented by the denominator) are followed or observed for the entire time-period specified.

To calculate cumulative incidence, consider the following situation. The number of patients with diabetes who have a major operation during July is 50 (the population at risk); 5 are admitted with an existing pressure ulcer, and 5 develop a pressure ulcer during that month. The cumulative incidence of pressure ulcers in the patient with diabetes after major surgery will be as follows: 50 patients minus the 5 patients with an existing pressure ulcer yields a total of 45 patients at risk (the denominator). Five of the 45 patients developed a pressure ulcer; so the cumulative incidence of pressure ulcers in patients with diabetes after a major operation during July is 5/45, or 11%.

Cumulative incidence is an accurate measure when a patients risk for a disease or condition is stable or unchanged for the same period of time. However, with regard to pressure ulcer formation, the patient is at risk for variable periods of time so an *incidence density* would be a more accurate measurement. (Baumgarten, 1998; Gordis, 1996; Hennekens and Buring, 1987; Oleske, 1995; WOCN Society, 2004b.)

Incidence density. This type of incidence measure differs from the cumulative incidence in that the denominator used to calculate incidence is time, rather than patients. For example, when calculating the incidence density of pressure ulcers in the postoperative patients with diabetes for the month of July, the length of time that each patient with diabetes remains in the hospital will vary. Some patients may be in the hospital 3 days before being discharged, whereas others may be in the hospital for 2 weeks after surgery. Consequently, these individuals will be observed (and at risk) for differing periods of time. The first patient is at risk of pressure ulcer formation for only 3 days, whereas the second patient is at risk for 2 weeks. If these two patients developed a pressure ulcer during their hospitalization, the incidence density would be 2 per 17 patient days.

An example of calculating incidence density is provided in Table 1-4.

Conducting Prevalence and Incidence Studies. Prevalence and incidence studies can be an onerous undertaking but yield considerable information if the objective is clear from the onset. Various methods have been described for conducting an incidence and prevalence study (Baumgarten, 1998; Gallagher, 1997; Lake, 1999). In *Prevalence and Incidence: A Toolkit for Clinicians*, the WOCN Society (2004b) outlines the specific steps required to prepare for and conduct a prevalence and incidence study; documentation forms generally required of such a process are also provided.

One of the key decisions in planning the study is to decide what population to study, or the at-risk population. The term *at risk* implies, from an epidemiologic standpoint, those who have the potential for developing a condition; *at risk* does NOT refer to the pressure ulcer risk assessment score obtained by using the Braden Scale, for example. With this broader interpretation of the concept of at risk, all patients in the hospital may be assumed to be at risk for pressure ulcer formation, for example. However, it is arguable whether the assumption holds that all patients who are hospitalized are at risk. When studies report incidence for hospital-wide populations, they typically exclude pediatrics, obstetrics, or mental health patient populations. For this reason, it may be more meaningful, as well as more feasible, to conduct incidence and prevalence studies on targeted patient populations (Aronovitch, 1999; Grous, Reilly, and Gift, 1997; Hammond et al, 1994; Jacksich, 1997).

For example, a study could examine all patients undergoing an operation lasting 3 hours or longer, all patients with a specific diagnosis such as hip fracture,

TABLE 1-4 Example of Calculation of Incidence Density

PATIENT	DEVELOPED A PRESSURE ULCER?	EVENT	NUMBER OF DAYS IN STUDY
1	No	Discharged on day 4	4
2	No	Discharged on day 15	15
3	Yes	Still in hospital day 30	30
4	No	Transferred to nursing home on day 22	22
5	Yes	Died on day 10	10
6	Yes	Transferred to different unit on day 12 and discharged from hospital on day 19	12
7	Yes	Discharged on day 5; readmitted 3 days later; discharged on day 7	5
8	No	Discharged on day 9	9

Totals:

8 new patients   4 new cases   107 patient days

Incidence (density) rate	=	4 new pressure ulcers per 107 patient days
	=	4 ÷ 107
	=	0.037 pressure ulcers per patient day, or 3.7 pressure ulcers per 100 patient days. A factor of 10 may be used to calculate the rate so that the decimal fraction created by dividing a large at-risk population (the denominator) into a small number of events (the numerator) can be eliminated. Generally, it is desirable to use the power of ten (i.e., 10, 100, 1000) that moves at least one digit to the left of the decimal point.

patients who have diabetes and are admitted to home care from Hospital Z, or all patients on a specific hospital unit. Allman and colleagues (1995) reported a 12.9% cumulative incidence of pressure ulcers after a median of 9 days from admission to final skin examination in a very specific patient population: patients were 55 years of age or older, had a hip fracture or were confined to bed or chair for at least 5 days, and did not have a stage 3 or greater pressure ulcer.

It is also possible to create an ongoing monthly record of incident cases by establishing a policy that all new pressure ulcers are reported to one central location, such as the wound care specialist (Kartes, 1996). In doing so, the incident pressure ulcer for 1 month must then be counted as a prevalent pressure ulcer in the subsequent months. Because this ongoing monthly record of incident cases relies on staff reports, some incident cases might be missed that would result in an underreporting of pressure ulcer incidence. Strategies such as comparing monthly reports with periodic audits could be conducted to assess reliability of this reporting method.

Generalizability of Incidence and Prevalence Measures. Benchmarking is a common practice for quality-improvement activities. However, comparing one setting's incidence and prevalence data with published incidence and prevalence data can lead to erroneous conclusions (Mark and Burleson, 1995). The key is to look at who was included in the incidence and prevalence study. For example, many studies do not include stage 1 pressure ulcers. This actually results in an underreporting of the frequency of pressure ulcers. Similarly, it is important to look at how incidence or prevalence was calculated; the choice of denominator will influence the resulting frequency. Patient populations should be similar to justify comparing incidence from different sources. It is also possible to calculate incidence and prevalence according to severity of risk as determined by the Braden Scale (Lake, 1999).

Although the incidence measures obtained from a narrow or specific at-risk patient population are unlikely to be appropriate to compare or benchmark against national incidence measures, repeated studies within the patient population of interest will provide a baseline and trends. The key advantages to conducting incidence studies on a defined at-risk patient population are twofold:

1. The study suddenly becomes much more feasible and less labor intensive. Implementation is vastly simplified by restricting the types of patient included.
2. Based on the results interventions can be targeted to the specific needs of that patient population.

Research Utilization and Evidence-Based Care

Integrating research results into practice (i.e., research utilization) is a fundamental expectation of the wound care specialist and a key component of an evidence-based practice. Evidence-based practice incorporates the collected results of research studies and other sources of evidence into the care of the patient. However, it is not only important for the wound care specialist to *apply* evidence to practice but also to *generate* evidence from practice (Ehrenberg et al, 2004). The value to the organization and the patient of research-based care is high: it has been demonstrated to offer patients better outcomes than routine procedural care based on the results of a meta-analysis of studies (Heater, Becker, and Olson, 1988).

Historically, there has been a gap in health care between what is known and what is practiced. The wound care specialist has a critical leadership role in making evidenced-based practice a reality. When leaders not only expect but also promote evidence-based practice with staff, research utilization is enhanced (Cummings, Mallidou, and Scott-Findlay, 2004). Caregivers are most effective in integrating research into practice when they are clinically based, have specific clinical expertise and knowledge, and express a positive attitude toward research (Ferguson, Milner, and Snelgrove-Clarke, 2004).

As a service that benefits the patient and organization, evidence-based care is defined as "the integration of best research evidence with clinical expertise and patient values to facilitate clinical decision making" (Sackett et al, 2000). Best research evidence is further defined as care decisions deriving from sources that are methodologically sound and clinically relevant (DiCenso, Ciliska, and Guyatt, 2005). In addition to the familiar issue of the effectiveness and safety of interventions, clinically relevant issues also include the accuracy and precision of assessment measures, the cost-effectiveness of interventions, the power of prognostic markers, and the strength of causal relationships.

There are many individual and organizational barriers to research utilization and evidence-based care (DiCenso, Ciliska, and Guyatt, 2005). One individual barrier is that the wound care specialist may feel inadequately prepared to evaluate the quality of research and without knowledgeable colleagues with whom to discuss research. In addition, access to the literature may be a hardship because of workload and time limitations. On an organizational level, barriers may arise from lack of interest, motivation, vision, and strategy on the part of managers. Organizational barriers may also exist related to library access, Internet access, and the extent of library holdings.

To embark on the path of evidence-based care, the wound care specialist must keep abreast of the relevant health care literature to "find the evidence." In the face of a constantly growing body of health care literature, remaining current in the literature may seem impossible or all-consuming. However, practical information sources, referred to as preprocessed resources, are available that will expedite access to evidence (Collins et al, 2005).

Preprocessed resources are products that have been developed by an individual or group who has reviewed the literature, filtered out the flawed studies, and included only the methodologically strongest studies. A hierarchy of preprocessed information sources with relevant examples is illustrated in Table 1-5. Such sources include practice guidelines, clinical pathways, evidence-based abstract journals, and systematic reviews. For example, guidelines pertinent to the wound care specialist have been published by the Wound, Ostomy and Continence Nurses Society (WOCN Society, 2002, 2003, 2004a, 2005a), the Wound Healing Society (WHS), the National Guideline Clearinghouse (at www.guideline.gov), the National Medical Directors Association, and the Cochrane Collaboration (www.cochrane.org).

When preprocessed information resources are not available relative to a particular clinical issue, unprocessed resources are necessary. Unprocessed resources are databases (CINAHL, MEDLINE, and EMBASE) that contain millions of primarily original study citations (Table 1-6).

The World Wide Web also constitutes an unprocessed resource, although the potential for inaccurate information is substantial. When using health care information on the Internet, seven criteria have been developed (Table 1-7) that can be used to assess the quality of the information (Health Summit Working Group, 1998; Holloway et al, 2000).

Because the methodological quality of studies obtained using unprocessed sources will vary, each study or report will require a critical appraisal to differentiate misleading research reports from valid reports. However, few care providers are completely comfortable with their research appraisal skills. To simplify the process, Cullum and Guyatt (2005) propose asking three discrete, sequential questions (Table 1-8):

1. "Are the results of the study valid?" The study must be designed and conducted in a valid manner so that the results are believable and credible. A study design that is less than rigorous and contains sources of bias will generate skewed and false conclusions. Only when the study methods are valid and rigorous should the reader continue on to further assess the study results.

2. "What are the results?" Any difference between the groups in the study will be expressed in terms of a risk measure such as risk reduction or benefit increase. The accuracy of the risk measure (the effect of the intervention) will be expressed in terms of a confidence interval or p-value. In general, a narrow confidence interval, that does not include zero, suggests more precision, therefore greater confidence, in the results.

3. "How can I apply these results to patient care?" The patients in the wound care specialist's practice should be similar to the patient population that participated in the study, if the research results are to be applied to them.

Hierarchy of Evidence. Evidence for an apparent relationship between health care events comes from many sources. Unsystematic clinical observations of an individual practitioner and the physiology-based

---

TABLE 1-5 **Hierarchy of Preprocessed Information Sources**

	HIERARCHY LEVELS	EXAMPLES
(Highest-Level Resource)	Systems	Clinical practice guidelines
		Evidence-based textbook summaries
		Clinical Evidence (published by BMJ Publishing Group)
	Synopses of syntheses	Evidence-based abstract journals (e.g., *Evidence-Based Nursing*)
		Systematic reviews
	Syntheses	Cochrane reviews
		Cochrane Library (www.cochrane.org)
	Synopses of single studies	Evidence-based abstract journals
(Lowest-Level Resource)	Single studies	PubMed clinical queries

TABLE 1-6 Features of Unprocessed Databases

DATABASE	MAINTAINED BY	UNIQUE FEATURES	CONTENTS
CINAHL	Information systems and updated quarterly	Largest bibliographic database specifically related to nursing, allied health disciplines, and consumer health	Full text articles Clinical practice guidelines Bibliographies of major articles Research instruments Government publications Comments Book reviews Evaluations of multimedia and computer software and systems Patient education materials
MEDLINE	United States National Library of Medicine	Readily accessible Searching effectively requires thorough knowledge of how database is structured and publications indexed	Comprehensive coverage of health care journals
EMBASE	Elsevier Science	Comprehensive bibliographic database of worldwide literature Requires thorough knowledge of how database is structured and publications are indexed	Biomedical and pharmaceutical literature fields Indexes large proportion of the European biomedical and science literature

TABLE 1-7 Seven Criteria for Evaluating Internet Health Information

CRITERIA	DESCRIPTION
Credibility	Includes the source, currency, relevance/utility, and editorial review process for the information
Content	Must be accurate and complete and provide an appropriate disclaimer
Disclosure	Includes informing the user of the purpose of the site, as well as any profiling or collection of information associated with using the site
Links	Evaluated according to selection, architecture, content, and back-linkages
Design	Encompasses accessibility, logical organization (navigability), and internal search capability
Interactivity	Includes feedback mechanisms and means for exchange of information among users
Caveats	Clarification of whether site function is to market products and services or is a primary information content provider

From Health Summit Working Group: Criteria for assessing the quality of health information on the Internet, Policy Paper, http://hitiweb.mitretek.org/docs/policy.pdf; Accessed March 14, 2006.

TABLE 1-8 Guide for Evaluating Intervention-Based Research

STEP	ISSUES TO CONSIDER
1. Are the results valid?	Did intervention and control groups begin the study with a similar prognosis?
	Were patients randomized?
	Was randomization concealed?
	Were patients analyzed in the groups to which they were randomized?
	Were groups shown to be similar in all known determinants of outcome, or were analyses adjusted for differences?
	Did intervention and control groups retain a similar prognosis after the study started?
	Were patients aware of group allocation?
	Were clinicians aware of group allocation?
	Were outcome assessors aware of group allocation?
	Was follow-up complete?
2. What are the results?	How large was the intervention effect?
	How precise was the estimate of the intervention effect?
3. How can results be applied to patient care?	Were the study patients similar to the patients in my clinical setting?
	Were all of the important outcomes considered?
	Are the likely intervention benefits worth the potential harm and costs?

Data from Cullum N, Guyatt G: Health Care Interventions and Harm: An introduction. In DiCenso A, Guyatt G, Chiliska D, editors: *Evidence-based nursing: a guide to clinical practice*, Philadelphia, 2005, Mosby.

TABLE 1-9 Hierarchy of Strength of Evidence

STRENGTH OF EVIDENCE	RATING	DEFINITION
(Highest Level)	Level 1	More than one randomized controlled trial (RCT) supports safety and efficacy or intervention (greatest strength)
↑	Level 2	Majority of RCT supports safety and efficacy or intervention, but others are equivocal or fail to support efficacy
	Level 3	Quasi-experimental studies (nonrandomized trials) support safety and efficacy
	Level 4	Case series or case studies suggest potential for safety and efficacy
(Lowest Level)	Level 5	Consensus or expert opinion (best practice)

opinion of the clinical expert constitute two sources of evidence. Systematic studies such as clinical trials, prospective studies, and case studies are additional sources of evidence. The more structured and systematic the source of evidence, the more reliable the conclusion and results will be. In general, unsystematic clinical observations and expert opinion (often referred to as best practice) provide important insights into further defining a clinical problem or an intervention from

which a systematic study can be designed. Therefore a hierarchy of evidence exists, largely defined by the source of the evidence and the process used to gather it (Table 1-9). Clinical observations, expert opinion, and generalizations from physiology form evidence; however, these sources constitute the weakest forms of evidence. The strongest evidence results from randomized clinical trials (RCT). However, not all clinical questions can be researched using a randomized clinical trial design (i.e. rare conditions and ethical concerns), therefore RCTs cannot be the expected standard applied to all research questions.

Data Collection

Data collection is a critical feature of any wound care program. This becomes the tool by which workload is measured, trends are identified, outcomes are quantified, and the valuable contribution of the wound care specialist is recorded so that it can be communicated. Data collection should be purposeful and outcomes oriented. In fact, data collection and practice improvement is inseparable because improvement requires measurement (Nelson et al, 1998). Box 1-5 illustrates ways in which data can be utilized. Data collection should be of two types: a time management program and a clinical practice database.

BOX I-5   Illustrations of Data Utilization

- Identify number and type of patients
- Document number of visits
- Identify trends
- Justify current and/or new position
- Determine utilization patterns
- Profile specific activities and scope of practice
- Evaluate use of time
- Demonstrate cost-effectiveness
- Conduct quality assurance activities
- Monitor patient follow-up
- Track referrals
- Monitor utilization of resources

Data from Wound, Ostomy and Continence Nurses Society (WOCN Society): *Professional practice manual*, ed 3, Mt. Laurel, NJ, 2005, Author.

Time Management Data Collection. When cost containment, efficient use of resources, and managed care dominate discussions, information concerning time use is invaluable. This type of data can validate any subjective perception of an increase or change in workload and communicates a strong objective message. Data should be recorded daily and tabulated weekly, monthly, quarterly, and annually (see Figures 1-1 through 1-4). Summary data (e.g., number of patient referrals, number of visits, average length of visits, average number of visits per patient or wound type, reason for referral, number of projects/activities, and time per project) should be submitted to the wound care specialist's supervisor on a monthly basis with trends highlighted. Plots can graphically display time or volume by month. Data collection can be maintained in paper format or entered into one of the many commercially available computer software packages for data management.

Clinical Practice Data Collection. The clinical practice data collection tool should serve as an information system within which demographic and clinical data can be stored and nursing interventions and outcomes documented (Jacobson, 1996). To be most useful, the clinical practice data collection tool should be integrated with the agency or institution information system and computerized. This reduces duplication of data entry, reduces the potential for errors in data entry, and expands the amount of information and the numbers of correlations and comparisons that can be extracted. Although several patient care-based data sets exist (e.g., Nursing Minimum Data Set, the OMAHA Intervention Classification Scheme, the Minimum Data Set Plus, and OASIS), no standardized

Rm #	Patient name	Adm date	Consult date	Adm diagnosis	Type of wound	MD	Mon	Tues	Wed	Thur	Fri	Total # visits	Total # units

Fig. I-I Sample weekly activity worksheet and patient demographics.

Date _____

	Monday		Tuesday		Wednesday		Thursday		Friday		Totals	
	Units	Visits	Units	Visits	Units	Visits	Units	Visits	Units	Visits	Units	Visits
Facility A (or unit)												
Facility B (or unit)												
Clinic												
Projects: Research committee												
Forms committee												
Quality improvement												
Activities: Administration												
Staff education												
Grand Totals												

Fig. 1-2 Sample weekly time summary form (unit = 15 min).

Month/Year _____

Patient name	Age	Facility			Type patient		Wound etiology*	Reason for consultation	Total # visits	Total # units
		Xyz	Abc	Tuv	New	Return				

*Wound etiology codes:

1 = Arterial ulcer	8 = Diabetic neuropathy	15 = Fistula
2 = Venous ulcer	9 = Mixed arterial/venous	16 = Other
3 = Pressure ulcer stage 1	10 = Epidermal stripping	
4 = Pressure ulcer stage 2	11 = Burn	
5 = Pressure ulcer stage 3	12 = Perianal denudation	
6 = Pressure ulcer stage 4	13 = Candidiasis	
7 = Pressure ulcer unstageable	14 = Pyoderma gangrenosum	

Fig. 1-3 Sample demographics record.

minimum database for wound care exists. However, the PUSH tool (NPUAP, 1999) and the PSST (Bates-Jensen, 1995) may evolve into such a function.

Leadership/Management

Many nonclinical functions typify the practice of the wound care specialist. Significant contributions by the wound care specialist include developing tools to guide decision making by the staff and to facilitate consistency in procedures. In addition, as a leader and manager, the wound care specialist will develop programs and projects that reflect the priorities of the corporation, are fiscally responsible, motivate colleagues to adopt evidence-based practice, and nurture the educational and professional development of staff.

(Week) Month/Year _____

Activity	Total number	# of Units	# of Visits
Patient Care			
Inpatients			
Clinic patients			
New referrals (inpatients)			
Reason for Referral			
Arterial ulcer			
Venous ulcer			
Mixed arterial/venous			
Pressure ulcer			
Projects			
Activities			

Fig. 1-4 Sample weekly/monthly activity summary.

Development of Policy, Procedure, and Documentation Tools. Fundamental activities of the clinical expert in any practice setting are the development and implementation of wound care policies, procedures, and decision support tools that incorporate standardized products (i.e., wound care formulary, specialty bed algorithms). Decision support tools enhance the clinician's decision-making capacity (Ehrenberg et al, 2004). Treatment protocols, for example, guide staff to (1) address critical assessment factors, (2) perform steps of assessment and treatment procedures in a proper sequence, (3) learn proper application and utilization of specific products, and (4) assess the effectiveness of interventions.

Policies and procedures are essential for guiding the delivery of care and meeting standards required by the Joint Commission on Accreditation of Healthcare Organization (JCAHO) and state health departments. Relative to wound care, each facility or health care organization should develop policies for prevention including pressure ulcer risk assessment, assessment of wounds, and treatment of wounds. In addition, a policy should exist to delineate appropriate interventions for different levels of pressure ulcer risk as well as for the referral of high-risk patients.

Incorporation of assessment data into the nursing admission form is critical to ensure that the data are collected. Such data can also be incorporated into the daily documentation flow sheets. Flow sheets that are dedicated to wound assessment and wound care interventions are particularly useful because they will best reflect changes in wound status over time. Documentation in multiple places increases the risk of error and should be avoided. A variety of clinical tool samples including policies, procedures, and documentation forms are in Appendix B and can be purchased from professional organizations (WOCN, 2005b).

Marketing and Communication

Visibility and role clarity are important in securing patient referrals, collaborating with colleagues, and avoiding costly duplication of services. A key factor to a successful wound care practice is effective communication with colleagues. Such communication is also a marketing strategy and serves to (1) clarify and describe the role of the wound care specialist and

(2) establish how to access the wound care specialist. Obviously the ultimate goal of a marketing plan in wound care is to become the provider of choice. Huffman (2005) identifies five key strategies essential to achieving this status:

- Identify your target population of patients
- Identify key physician referral sources
- Streamline wound referral processes and communication
- Implement essentials of advanced wound management
- Develop outcomes based wound care marketing tools

Before embarking on promotional efforts designed at marketing the wound care program, an essential step is to identify the recipient of the marketing activity: the customer. A customer can be of three types: decision maker, influencer, and end user. The decision maker is the individual who makes the decision to use the services and in most wound care scenarios, pays the provider's salary or consulting fee. This could be the manager who hires the wound care specialist, the physician who contracts for services, or the case manager for an HMO. The influencer is the customer who persuades or influences the decision maker and could be a patient's family, a staff nurse, or another physician. The end user is the customer who uses the service or product. This individual is typically the patient in the health care scenario.

Role Delineation. The wound care specialist is not responsible to conduct every wound assessment or dressing application Clarity in terms of expectations of the wound care specialist, staff nurse, and physical therapist is essential to promote collaboration and deliver comprehensive and effective wound care. Participation in staff orientation programs is a key strategy to communicate role, functions and responsibilities. This offers an opportunity to orient new staff members to their role in wound care and in pressure ulcer prevention, as well as demonstrate how the wound care specialist can be used and accessed. The nursing staff is often a key contact for obtaining appropriate referrals because they are so closely involved with the patient's entire plan of care. In contrast, the role of the wound care specialist will resemble that of a consultant and coordinator.

Key physicians should be approached, and the role of the wound care specialist discussed and clarified. As with all discussions, it is important to emphasize the benefits of wound care services to their practice. The support and confidence of key physicians is so critical that the extra effort and time it takes to nurture this relationship is time well spent. Ultimately, however, the wound care specialist will need to demonstrate competence and confidence in his or her practice. Allies within the nursing staff can be a source of positive influence with physicians.

Collaboration with multiple services and key stakeholder will maximize the effectiveness of a wound care specialist. A key stakeholder is someone who can positively or negatively effect outcomes. These services may include the diabetes educator, dietitian, physical therapist, occupational therapist, discharge planner, home health care staff, radiology/vascular laboratory, billing, materials management, and central supply.

BENEFITS AND OUTCOMES

The value of a wound care specialist is high and the benefits he or she confers numerous. And it is the responsibility of the wound care specialist to communicate these benefits to administration and other customers. Examples of the benefits of wound care services are listed in Box 1-6. Benefits of services to the organization become tangible and coherent when phrased in terms of outcomes. Outcomes should include specific patient population outcomes and organizational outcomes. Furthermore, potential outcomes should be relative to behaviors or physical conditions that

BOX 1-6 Benefits of Wound Care Services

- Prevent or reduce the incidence of nosocomial skin breakdown
- Appropriate management of support surfaces
- Collaborative consultation with case managers
- Oversight of required documentation
- Positive outcomes while minimizing visits and supplies
- Control of supply costs without compromising quality of care
- Oversight of support surface utilization
- Facilitate compliance with regulatory mandates

the wound care specialist is in the position to affect. For example, an outcome of shortened length of stay in the hospital may not be realistic, since many variables that are not under the control of the wound care specialist have an impact on that individual's length of stay. However, the outcome could be rephrased to more precisely define the patient population or type of wound for which length of stay will be decreased. Another outcome could address the control of wound care products; but to make this feasible to achieve, tools to assist the staff in appropriate product use such as protocols and a formulary would be required.

Increased Accountability

Another benefit of the services of a wound care specialist is increased accountability for standards of care and compliance with regulatory statutes. The Centers for Medicare and Medicaid Services (CMS) and JACHO are clear in their intent to encourage all facilities to adopt evidenced-based pressure ulcer protocols. The surveyor community has a common language that should be used in the medical record when referring to pressure ulcers. For example, the CMS recognition and definition of the *avoidable* and *unavoidable* pressure ulcer (Box 1-7) highlights the need for incorporation of regulatory updates into practice (van Rijswijk and Lyder, 2005). Wound care specialists are in a position to implement the requisite pressure ulcer prevention and treatment components. In addition to implementation, the wound care specialist can facilitate documentation that is clear, appropriate and accurately reflects appropriate prevention, assessment, and treatment of pressure ulcers.

Documentation by the wound care specialist should be in a consistent location in the chart. Preferably, documentation should be in the progress notes so that all physicians and ancillary services involved in the patient's care are kept informed. Documentation should be direct, concise, and objective. The documentation should include a thorough assessment, including pertinent quantitative information, interventions, education, and the plan for follow-up. A wound documentation form may also be used to record the initial consultation assessment and plan. A flowchart can also be developed to record wound assessments so that a trend in the status of the wound can be conveyed. The Pressure Ulcer Scale for Healing (PUSH) tool or the Pressure

---

BOX 1-7   CMS Terms Defined: Avoidable and Unavoidable Pressure Ulcer

Avoidable

The resident developed a pressure ulcer and the facility did not do one or more of the following:
- Evaluate the resident's clinical condition and pressure ulcer risk factors
- Define and implement interventions that are consistent with residents needs, residents goals, and recognized standards of practice
- Monitor and evaluate the impact of interventions
- Revise the interventions as appropriate

Unavoidable

The resident developed a pressure ulcer even though the facility did the following:
- Evaluated the resident's clinical condition and pressure ulcer risk factors
- Defined and implemented interventions that were consistent with residents needs, residents goals, and recognized standards of practice
- Monitored and evaluated the impact of interventions
- Revised the interventions as appropriate

Data from van Rijswijk L and Lyder CH: Pressure ulcer prevention and care: implementing the revised guidance to surveyors for long-term care facilities, *Ostomy Wound Manage*, Vol. 4, p. 57. 51, 4(Suppl):7, 2005.

Sore Status Tool (PSST) reflect changes in status over time and may be used instead of creating a flowchart (Bates-Jensen, 1995; NPUAP, 1999).

Improved Financial Outcomes

The wound care specialist has the opportunity and the ability to use resources more efficiently, and, in some situations, generate revenue. Through ongoing continuing education opportunities, the wound care specialist can foster state-of-the-art patient care and evidence-based practice by using products that have scientific evidence of their effectiveness. Again, not only do the patients benefit from this expertise, but the facility benefits financially by cutting expenditures. The wound care specialist can work with quality improvement team members to identify select aspects of care that could be monitored and tracked over time and thus obtain outcomes data and clinical effectiveness information.

Efficient Use of Resources. The wound care specialist must become cognizant of the implications of the efficient use of resources (both materials and personnel). Information concerning the cost implications of the wound care practice or cost savings that have been generated must be gathered and specifically communicated routinely to the supervisor. Wound management is costly; in most situations more costly than prevention (Lapsley and Vogels, 1996). Effective wound management reduces costs by allowing fewer supplies to be used and providing more efficient and effective use of dressings. In addition, cost savings can be realized when preventive interventions are linked to risk level (Richardson, Gardner, and Frantz, 1998). This could result in a significant decrease in annual expenditures for materials used. Cost-effectiveness is a positive way of acquiring the support of the nursing administration (Kuhn and Coulter, 1992), which is essential to obtain institutional support.

The wound care specialist should also get involved with the establishment of supply contracts to sort through the maze of different products and their indications. A successful means of proven cost-effectiveness is to limit the number of similar supplies stocked by the facility. By creating a formulary for wound care products and support surfaces, use of these products can be standardized and simplified. Furthermore, the wound care specialist can serve as a resource to materials management, providing clarification on product use. Collaboration with materials management can also increase the success of contractual arrangements with manufacturers and increase the ability to maintain compliance with the contract.

Another area that has potential for cost savings is standardizing the use of support surfaces. A policy should be developed that describes patient indicators for the use of specialty beds, and compliance with contracts for these specialty beds should be supported. It is also important to set up a procedure for "stepping down" from the specialty bed as the patient's condition warrants. In addition, units with a high prevalence of at-risk patient populations might benefit from the implementation of replacement mattresses. By standardizing the products and providing indicators or patient characteristics to guide their use, overuse can be reduced and appropriate use can be enhanced.

Finally, by virtue of incorporating appropriate use of wound care products and state-of-the-art wound care, the wound care specialist affects the use of personnel.

Decreased frequency of dressing changes, expedient access to the correct dressing supplies, and printed directions for dressing changes will reduce staff frustration and time required for wound care.

Revenue Services Generation. Reimbursement-related topics for the services of the wound care specialist are discussed in Chapter 27.

The wound care program, like all departments, must have a means to track productivity. With the assistance of the billing department, a mechanism to document visits and referrals could be formulated. One method could be to establish "charge codes" for the wound care services that are based on increments of time or services provided. This is an excellent way to track, document, and justify the value of a wound care specialist. However, it is important that the wound care specialist avoid providing services that are considered basic nursing care to inflate the number of charges. This charging system may also assist with the compilation of workload and time management data for the department. It is important to avoid focusing solely on the number of patients or charges, and to focus instead on the types of patients and services provided. Also to be considered is whether the wound care specialist's interventions are affecting outcomes.

Depending on payer sources, the services that are provided through the wound care program might be billable. If the services are classified as a therapy rather than a nursing service, the services may be billable. The availability of wound care services may also enable the institution to market itself for managed care contracts. This again defines the value of a wound care program. However, inpatient wound care services will seldom, if ever, be a revenue-producing area. Working closely with the billing department and fiscal intermediaries may be productive with regard to revenues.

The value of a wound care program is not limited to just providing care to inpatients. The wound care specialist can serve as a link to community programs and outreach programs and provide education that can draw attention to the wound care program and the facility. The wound care specialist can provide education within his or her facility in collaboration with colleagues, such as physical therapists and occupational therapists. Grants may be available from manufacturers to conduct some of these programs. The manufacturers often have established programs that have been approved by licensing boards for continuing education hours. These may be a cost-effective way to provide continuing education to staff. Continuing medical education programs may also be attractive. Well-recognized speakers can be invited to conduct an educational session at a dinner program.

When starting the wound care program, the wound care specialist may initially want to conduct a series of chart audits or perform a prevalence and incidence study. These activities will provide information that is helpful to determine if a certain problem (e.g., pressure ulcers, inadequate documentation) exists. From this information, the continuous improvement process can be initiated with involved departments and personnel so that problems can be discussed and possible solutions can be identified. As the wound care specialist begins an inpatient practice, it is essential to be visible. Being open to new ideas and opportunities will assist the wound care specialist in creating and maintaining a successful program. Maintaining visibility and an alliance with physicians and staff will reinforce the message that the wound care program is an indispensable service.

Staff Retention

A key role of the wound care specialist is to establish decision-making tools to expedite and standardize delivery of care. These tools help the staff to develop their comfort level in wound care, facilitate utilization of products, and implement appropriate preventive interventions. Recognition and rewards can be provided for program contributions or accomplishments. Establishing skill competencies in wound care can provide a professional objective for the staff to strive for, again targeting the individual's personal satisfaction.

SUMMARY

Establishing a wound care practice in any setting requires the skills of an entrepreneur and a strong foundation in pathophysiology and clinical management. The wound care specialist must determine how his or her role will be implemented, how his or her relationship with colleagues will be defined, what quality management processes can be implemented, and what type of data is needed. Data should describe how time is spent and what outcomes are being achieved.

The wound care specialist must also stay current in the art and science of wound management by adopting lifelong learning strategies such as regularly attending continuing education programs, critically reading journals, and monitoring select websites. The time and energy spent in initial and ongoing practice development is critical to a successful, satisfying, and effective wound care practice.

SELF-ASSESSMENT EXERCISE

1. Which of the following activities is reflective of a wound care specialist operating in a consultant capacity within an institution?
   a. Encourage referrals to the wound care specialist for patients with stages 1 and 2 pressure ulcers
   b. Conduct routine dressing changes for assessment purposes
   c. Establish protocols for pressure ulcer risk reduction based on level of risk
   d. Perform reassessment of pressure ulcer risk twice weekly
2. When implementing a new process for pressure ulcer risk reduction, you plan to meet with several staff nurses to discuss what is currently being done, discuss the current national standards, and present the advantages of the new process. According to Rogers' innovation-decision process, which stage does this reflect?
   a. Knowledge stage
   b. Persuasion stage
   c. Decision stage
   d. Confirmation stage
3. Which of the following statements is true of incidence density?
   a. Incidence density is a rate that describes how many people have a particular condition at a specific point in time
   b. Incidence density is a rate expressed in terms of person-time units
   c. Incidence density is a measure used to identify workload or staff needs
   d. Incidence density is calculated with a numerator that includes all the patients at risk for the condition
4. When a long-term care institution specializes in wound management, which of the following measures can be anticipated to be higher than the national average?
   a. Cumulative incidence
   b. Incidence density
   c. Prevalence
   d. Cumulative incidence and prevalence

REFERENCES

Allman RM et al: Pressure ulcer risk factors among hospitalized patients with activity limitation, *JAMA* 273(11):865, 1995.

American Academy of Wound Management (AAWM) Board Certification, http://www.aawm.org/certification.html accessed 2-5-06.

Aronovitch S: Intraoperatively acquired pressure ulcer prevalence: a national study, *J Wound Ostomy Continence Nurs* 26(3):130, 1999.

Bates-Jensen BM: Toward an intelligent wound assessment system, *Ostomy Wound Manage* 41(suppl 7A):80S, 1995.

Baumgarten M: Designing prevalence and incidence studies, *Adv Wound Care* 11:287, 1998.

Beitz JM, Fey J, O'Brien D: Perceived need for education vs actual knowledge of pressure ulcer care in a hospital nursing staff, *Dermatol Nurs* 11(2):125, 1999.

Bergstrom, N., et al for Agency for Health Care Policy and Research (AHCPR): Agency for Health Care Policy and Research. AHCPR Publication No. 95–052. *Treatment of pressure ulcers. Clinical practice guideline, No. 15.* Rockville, MD: U.S. Dept of Health and Human Services.

Bostrom J, Kenneth H: Staff nurse knowledge and perceptions about prevention of pressure sores, *Dermatol Nurs* 4(5):365, 1992.

Collins S et al: Finding the evidence. In DiCenso A, Guyatt G, Chiliska D, editors: *Evidence-based nursing. A guide to clinical practice*, Philadelphia, 2005, Mosby.

Cullum N, Guyatt G: Health Care Interventions and Harm: An introduction. In DiCenso A, Guyatt G, Chiliska D, editors: *Evidence-based nursing. A guide to clinical practice*, Philadelphia, 2005, Mosby.

Cummings GG, Mallidou AA, Scott-Findlay S. Does the workplace influence nurses' use of research? *J Wound Ostomy Continence Nurs* 31(3):106, 2004.

DiCenso A, Ciliska D, Guyatt G: Introduction to evidence-based nursing. In DiCenso A, Guyatt G, Chiliska D, editors: *Evidence-based nursing. A guide to clinical practice*, Philadelphia, 2005, Mosby.

Dobbins M et al: Changing nursing practice in an organization. In DiCenso A, Guyatt G, Chiliska D, editors: *Evidence-based nursing. A guide to clinical practice*, Philadelphia, 2005, Mosby.

Ehrenberg A, Fraser KD, Gunningberg L: Can decision support improve nurses' use of knowledge? *J Wound Ostomy Continence Nurs* 31(5):256, 2004.

Ferguson L, Milner M, Snelgrove-Clarke E: The role of intermediaries: getting evidence into practice, *J Wound Ostomy Continence Nurs* 31(6):325-327, 2004.

Gallagher SM: Outcomes in clinical practice: pressure ulcer prevalence and incidence studies, *Ostomy Wound Manage* 43(1):28, 1997.

Gordis L: *Epidemiology*, Philadelphia, 1996, W.B. Saunders.

Grous CA, Reilly NJ, Gift AG: Skin integrity in patients undergoing prolonged operations, *J Wound Ostomy Continence Nurs* 24:86, 1997.

Hammond MC et al: Pressure ulcer incidence on a spinal cord injury unit, *Adv Wound Care* 7(6):57, 1994.

Hassinger E: Stages in the adoption process, *Rural Sociology*, 24:52-53, 1959.

Health Summit Working Group: Criteria for assessing the quality of health information on the Internet, Policy Paper, http://hitiweb.mitretek.org/docs/policy.pdf; Accessed **2/2/06.**

Heater BS, Becker AM, Olson RK. Nursing interventions and patient outcomes: a meta-analysis of studies. *Nurs Res.* Sep-Oct;37(5):303-307, 1988.

Hennekens CH, Buring JE: *Epidemiology in medicine*, Boston, 1987, Little, Brown.

Hess, CT: WOC Credentials: a legally defensible process, http://www.wocncb.org/pdf/value_of_certification.pdf; Accessed August 25, 2005.

Holloway N et al: Evaluating health care information on the Internet. In Fitzpatrick JJ, Montgomery KS, editors: *Internet resources for nurses*, New York, 2000, Springer.

Huffman, M: Marketing wound care outcomes to physicians, *The Remington Report* 13(3):7-10, 2005.

Jacksich BB: Pressure ulcer prevalence and prevention of nosocomial development: one hospital's experience, *Ostomy Wound Manage* 43(3):32, 1997.

Jacobson T: Standardized ET nursing database: imagine the possibilities, *J Wound Ostomy Continence Nurs* 23:5, 1996.

Jones S et al: A pressure ulcer prevention program, *Ostomy Wound Manage* 39:33, 1993.

Kartes SK: A team approach for risk assessment, prevention, and treatment of pressure ulcers in nursing home patients, *J Nurse Care Qual* 10(3):34, 1996.

Kelsey JL et al: *Methods in observational epidemiology*, ed 2, New York, 1996, Oxford University Press.

Kuhn BA, Coulter SJ. Balancing the pressure ulcer cost and quality equation. *Nurs Econ.* 1992 Sep-Oct;10(5):353-359.

Lake NO: Measuring incidence and prevalence of pressure ulcers for intergroup comparison, *Adv Wound Care* 12:31, 1999.

Landrum BJ: Marketing innovations to nurses, Part 1. How people adopt innovations, *J Wound Ostomy Continence Nurs* 25:194, 1998a.

Landrum BJ: Marketing innovations to nurses, Part 2. Marketing's role in the adoption of innovations, *J Wound Ostomy Continence Nurs* 25:227, 1998b.

Lapsley HM, Vogels R: Cost and prevention of pressure ulcers in an acute teaching hospital. *Int J Qual Health Care.* Feb;8(1):61-6, 1996.

Mark BA, Burleson BL: Measurement of patient outcomes: data availability and consistency across hospitals, *J Nurs Adm* 25(4):52, 1995.

National Pressure Ulcer Advisory Panel (NPUAP): *PUSH tool*, August, 1999; www.npuap.org/pushins.htm.

Nelson EC et al: Building measurement and data collection in to medical practice, *Ann Intern Med* 128:460, 1998.

Oleske DM, editor: *Epidemiology and the delivery of health care services: methods and applications*, New York, 1995, Plenum Press.

Pieper B et al: Nurses' documentation about pressure ulcers, *Decubitus* 3:32, 1990.

Pieper B et al: Wound prevalence, types and treatment in home care, *Adv Wound Care* 12:117, 1999.

Pieper B, Mattern JC: Critical care nurses' knowledge of pressure ulcer prevention, staging, and description, *Ostomy Wound Manage* 43(2):22, 1997.

Pieper B, Mott M: Nurses' knowledge of pressure ulcer prevention, staging, and description, *Adv Wound Care* 8:34, 1995.

Richardson GM, Gardner S, Frantz RA. Nursing assessment: impact on type and cost of interventions to prevent pressure ulcers. *J Wound Ostomy Continence Nurs.* 1998 Nov;25(6):273-80.

Rogers EM: *Diffusion of innovations*, ed 4, New York, 1995, Free Press.

Rothman KJ, Greenland S: *Modern epidemiology*, ed 2, Philadelphia, 1998, Lippincott-Raven.

Sackett DL et al: *Evidence-based medicine: how to practice and teach EBM*, London, 2000, Churchill Livingstone.

Specht JP, Bergquist S, Frantz R: Adoption of research-based practice for treatment of pressure ulcers, *Nurs Clin North Am* 30:553, 1995.

van Rijswijk L, Lyder CH:. Pressure ulcer prevention and care: implementing the revised guidance to surveyors for long-term care facilities, *Ostomy Wound Manage* Apr Vol. 51, 4(Suppl):7, 2005.

Wound, Ostomy and Continence Nurses Society (WOCN): *Guideline for management of patients with lower extremity arterial disease*, WOCN clinical practice guideline series #1, Glenview IL, 2002, Author.

Wound, Ostomy and Continence Nurses Society (WOCN Society): *Guideline for management of pressure ulcers*, WOCN clinical practice guideline series #2, Glenview IL, 2003, Author.

Wound, Ostomy and Continence Nurses Society (WOCN Society): *Guideline for management of patients with lower extremity neuropathic disease*, WOCN clinical practice guideline series #1, Glenview IL, 2004a, Author.

Wound, Ostomy and Continence Nurses Society (WOCN Society): *Prevalence and Incidence: A toolkit for clinicians*, Glenview IL, 2004b, Author.

Wound, Ostomy and Continence Nurses Society (WOCN Society): *Guideline for management of patients with lower extremity venous disease*, WOCN clinical practice guideline series #1, Glenview IL, 2005a, Author.

Wound, Ostomy and Continence Nurses Society (WOCN Society): *Professional practice manual*, ed 3, Mt. Laurel, NJ, 2005b, Author.

Wound, Ostomy and Continence Nursing Certification Board (WOCNCB), 2005. Certification by Examination http://www.wocncb.org/cert/ accessed 2-5-06.

CHAPTER 2

The Multidisciplinary Team Approach to Wound Management

FINN GOTTRUP, DENISE P. NIX, & RUTH A. BRYANT

OBJECTIVES

1. Discriminate between wound management and wound care.
2. Explain the difference between multidisciplinary, inter-disciplinary, and transdisciplinary.
3. Identify six advantages to a centralized team of specialists for efficient management of the patient with a wound.
4. List five responsibilities of a multidisciplinary wound management committee or team.
5. List eight primary members and five consulting members of a wound management team.
6. Identify six elements of a multidisciplinary wound management program.

No single discipline can meet the multiplicity of needs that the patient with a wound presents. The best outcomes are generated by dedicated, well-educated personnel from multiple disciplines working together for the common goal of holistic patient care. This chapter will present the importance of the multidisciplinary team approach as well as factors to consider for establishing a successful multidisciplinary wound management program.

MAGNITUDE OF THE WOUND PROBLEM

Wound problems have been present as long as man has been on earth, and many different strategies and materials have been used to treat them. Although the known history of wound healing goes back to the Neolithic period (Steinbock, 1976), the oldest written documentation concerning wound management is from approximately 1500 BC and was found in the Edwin Smith Surgical Papyrus, the Papyrus Ebers, and the Estes' studies of ancient Egyptian medicine.

This documentation indicates that the Egyptians used oiled frog skins, honey, lint, and animal grease as wound coverage (Brown, 1992; Majno, 1975; Reiter, 1994).

Wounds are prevalent in nearly all aspects of health care. No health care specialty or subspecialty is exempt from the risk of having a patient develop a wound. Therefore, the need for access to wound management professionals touches all health care personnel in all health care settings. A chronic wound, as defined by the Wound Healing Society, is a wound that has not healed in a timely fashion (Lazarus, Cooper, Knighton et al, 1994).

The frequency of problem wounds varies according to the demographics of patient populations and the types of health care systems. In the industrialized world it is estimated that almost 1% to 1.5% of the population suffers from problem wounds, which accounts for 2% to 4% of health care expenses or even more (Anderson, Hansson, and Swanbeck, 1984; Dale, 1983; Gottrup, 1998; Gruen, Chang, and Maclellan, 1994; Lindholm, 1993; Liu, Eriksson, and Mustoe, 1991). In an acute hospital setting, the patient's risk for developing a pressure ulcer ranges from 14% to 20% of all patients (Allman et al, 1986; Elk and Boman, 1982). During hospitalization, 1.2% to 2.7% of all patients have a stage 2 or greater pressure ulcer (Anderson and Kvorning, 1982; Gerson, 1975; Gosnell, Johannsen, and Ayres, 1992), and about 5.4% of patients admitted without an ulcer will develop a stage 1 pressure ulcer. The frequency of problem wounds is not unique to the United States, however. In Denmark, wound problems occur in about 1% of the population of 5.2 million. Bergmark and colleagues (2004) reported that 34% of all patients had a pressure ulcer, and 14%

of the patients had stage II to IV pressure ulcers; and sadly, 58% of these ulcers were not documented in the medical or nurse's record. The prevalence of leg ulcers in the United States is similar to other countries (between 0.5% and 1%), and increases three- to four-fold for patients 65 years of age and older (Dale, 1983; Anderson, Hansson, and Swanbeck, 1984). The incidence of diabetic foot lesions in Scandinavia is around 3.6% for type 2 diabetes (Keyser, 1993), and the prevalence is 5.4%. These figures are expected to double in the next 20 years.

Total expense for the treatment of wounds is calculated to be approximately 2% to 3% of the total budget of the health care system in Denmark (Postnett, 2002). The treatment costs of a leg ulcer are calculated at approximately $3,000 to $6,000 per ulcer, each year (Lindholm, 1993; Gruen, Chang, and Maclellan, 1994). Expenses related to pressure ulcer care ranges from $22,000 to $30,000 per ulcer (Gottrup et al, 1995). When a major amputation is required, the cost will increase by a factor of 7 (Appelquist et al, 1994) as a consequence of the need to make home improvements to accommodate wheelchairs.

Clearly, the cost of treating problem wounds in most industrialized countries is very high. If patients at risk were identified and aggressive interventions put in place **before** the wound developed or progressed, morbidity and health care costs could be significantly decreased (Granick, McGowan, and Long, 1998; Long and Granick, 1998). These data underscore the point that regardless of the country and regardless of the etiology, problem wounds are a prevalent and very costly international health care concern.

TERMINOLOGY
Wound Management versus Wound Care

Problem wounds can be defined as wounds that have become chronic, more or less therapy-resistant, and especially risky for the patient (Gottrup et al, 2001). Problem wounds significantly reduce quality of life but do not necessarily decrease duration of life. Problem wounds require both wound management and wound care.

- *Wound management:* Wound management is conceived as being the comprehensive, holistic care of the patient in such a manner that all factors contributing to and affecting the wound and the patient are addressed. Typically a physician oversees this level of care. Many settings in the United States have a nationally certified wound care nurse or certified wound specialist work collaboratively with a designated physician or the patient's primary physician to collectively manage the patient with a wound.
- *Wound care:* Wound care is more focused on local or topical care of the wound. Skills that are required to provide wound care include wound-specific assessment (Chapter 7) and appropriate utilization of wound care products (Chapter 19). A certified wound care nurse or certified wound specialist can provide training to the professional who delivers wound care.

Multidisciplinary, Interdisciplinary, and Transdisciplinary Collaboration

The terms interdisciplinary and multidisciplinary are often used interchangeably. However, agencies such as the National Institutes of Health (NIH) and the National Science Foundation (NSF) are beginning to use specific definitions to distinguish these terms; the key distinction among them rests with expected interactions among the various caregivers, health care disciplines, and agencies.

- *Discipline:* A body of knowledge or branch of learning characterized by an accepted content and learning (Collins, 2003; Stokols et al, 2003)
- *Multidisciplinary:* Most collaboration among different disciplines starts as multidisciplinary. The collaboration is intended to produce outcomes that cannot be achieved without collaboration. A multidisciplinary approach brings together numerous experts from diverse disciplines to collectively address a complex problem. The nature of the problem makes it necessary for multiple disciplines to collaborate and share results. Contributions are, however, complementary rather than integrative (Collins, 2003; Stokols et al, 2003).
- *Interdisciplinary:* Interdisciplinary collaboration evolves from multidisciplinary collaboration. The integration of several disciplines creates a unified outcome that is sustained and substantial enough to enable a new discipline to develop over time.

TABLE 2-1 Factors that Affect the Work of the Multidisciplinary Wound Management Team

FACTOR	INHIBITS TEAMWORK	PROMOTES TEAMWORK
Team member attitude	Membership-mandated	Member has personal commitment or passion
Goal/vision	Discipline-related focus	Patient focus
Roles/communication	Members work in isolation and fail to recognize the value of other team members	Members recognize that the whole is greater than the sum of the parts, and responsibilities tend to overlap
Institutional support	Lack of resources allocated to complete committee activities	Adequate resources allocated to complete committee activities

Integration of multiple disciplines requires collaboration at the level of designing new approaches, and analysis that combines methods and concepts from different disciplines. While working jointly, members operate from each of their respective disciplinary perspectives (Collins, 2002; Stokols et al, 2003). Although skills specific to each discipline remain important, professional boundaries blur with interdisciplinary care. Interdisciplinary care requires trust, tolerance, and a willingness to share responsibility (Nolan, 1995).

- *Transdisciplinary:* Transdisciplinary care requires the highest degree of collaboration. The development and application of a shared, integrative conceptual framework transcends the respective disciplinary perspectives. Instead of working in parallel, members collaborate across levels of analysis and interventions to develop a comprehensive understanding of the problem (Collins, 2003; Stokols et al, 2003).

Ideally, a multidisciplinary team should become more than the sum of its parts and eventually evolve into interdisciplinary or transdisciplinary collaborators. Putting people together in groups representing many disciplines does not guarantee the development of a shared understanding and mutual respect. Table 2-1 identifies factors that encourage or inhibit multidisciplinary teamwork (Pirrie, Hamilton, and Wilson, 1999; Wilson and Pirrie, 1999). The remainder of this chapter will apply to multidisciplinary teams in various levels and degrees of *"multi-," "inter-"* and *"trans-"* disciplinary collaboration.

BUILDING A CASE FOR A MULTIDISCIPLINARY TEAM APPROACH

Most often, physician involvement in wound management has been dependent on the individual physician's level of interest. In the hospital, various physician specialists are involved in the treatment of the patient with a problem wound. For example, the dermatology specialist cares for the patient with a venous leg ulcer, a surgical specialist such as a plastic surgeon typically cares for the patient with a pressure ulcer, and an internist or a podiatrist may follow the patient with a diabetic foot ulcer. Unfortunately, this type of single discipline wound management is fraught with inefficiencies. In fact, no single discipline can meet the multiple needs that some patients with a wound have. Comparisons of single discipline versus interdisciplinary approaches to wound management are listed in Table 2-2.

An increased awareness of the difficulties and frustrations and the need for structure in the management of patients with problem wounds has led to the establishment of wound-healing groups and centers, as well as national and international societies. At the same time, health care systems around the world have restructured as they strive for increased efficiency, decreased costs, and improved patient outcomes. Together these events have substantiated the need for a multidisciplinary team approach.

TABLE 2-2 Comparison of Single Discipline vs. Interdisciplinary Approaches to Wound Management

	SINGLE DISCIPLINE	MULTIDISCIPLINARY
Assessments	Wounds-specific Discipline-specific	Holistic
Policies Procedures Treatment plans	Varies by discipline	Standardized
Research	Small patient volumes Limited wound types	Larger consolidated patient volumes Diverse wound types
Collaboration with other disciplines	Referrals "as needed," patient may require multiple appointments to multiple settings	Collaboration is standard through the continuum of care
Knowledge base of staff	Specific to discipline and wound type	Multiple wound types
Utilization of resources (i.e., diagnostic equipment)	Higher costs to allocate resources to multiple disciplines and areas	Lower costs to allocate resources to one area

In the United States, in a relatively brief period the health care industry and the structures that comprise it have changed more dramatically than during any time in the past (Souba, 1999). Today and in the future, the management of medicine will play an increasingly important role in enhancing performance (Drucker, 1998). Most notably in the United States, medicine has become more mercantile, and the nature of the relationship between patient and doctor has changed from one based on trust and commitment to one determined by market forces within managed care organizations (Drucker, 1998). In the future, medicine will be run even more like a business; cost of services will be compared with outcomes of services to arrive at efficient, effective, evidence-based, quality care. Providers (physicians) will negotiate for the patient, whereas the payers (employer, government, or insurance) will attempt to seek out the best caregivers for the lowest prices. This managed-care focus, along with the need for research-based, quantifiable data outcomes and standards, will result in a changed view of how to treat patients with problem wounds.

The lack of information about wound healing among general physician practitioners is another indicator of the need for multidisciplinary wound management teams. In a national cross-sectional investigation, 98% of general practitioners reported that wound healing significantly affected their patients. In contrast, only 16% of general practitioners understood basic wound-healing physiology (Baharestani, 1995).

The lack of standardized treatment and referral plans among primary health care providers further substantiates the need for a multidisciplinary team approach. In a study of the primary health care sector in the central part of Copenhagen, Vestergaard (1998) identified a number of problems in the care of patients with chronic wounds:

- 49% did not have appropriate diagnostic examinations
- 40% of those at risk for venous leg ulcers were not treated with compression
- 34% of patients with foot ulcers were not examined for diabetes mellitus
- 50% of patients with pressure ulcers did not receive pressure redistribution or off-loading

The two primary problems seem to be (1) a lack of organization and (2) care delivered by single disciplines, rather than by a team. This single discipline approach is not in the best interest of the patient (NPUAP, 1989). In 1996, Robson, a founding member of the Wound Healing Society and a wound-healing researcher, declared that it was time to integrate knowledge of wound healing, tissue repair, wound care, and long-term scarring and rehabilitation into routine clinical practice. This requires integration of the expertise of a team of disciplines into a comprehensive wound management approach. The team approach with collaboration between all health care professionals facilitates quality holistic care (Gray, 1996) and recognizes the talent and creativity of all employees (Reich, 1987). The team approach allows for the centralization of care and standardization of services that are clearly important in wound management (Gottrup, 1999; Gottrup, 2001). The ideal concept of wound management consists of interdisciplinary, well-educated personnel working full-time with patients with all types of wound problems throughout the entire course of treatment (Gottrup, 2002).

The establishment of multidisciplinary teams has been demonstrated to be beneficial for managing patients suffering from complicated wounds. The single most important reason for the increasing survival of patients with burns is related to the establishment of totally integrated multidisciplinary teams (Robson, 1985; Robson, Krizek, and Wray, 1979). Although it is generally acknowledged that wound management requires many specialists, no organized integration of multiple specialists in wound healing and care has existed until recently. During the last 10 years, different types of interdisciplinary and multidisciplinary concepts for managing patients with wounds have been created (Appelquist et al, 1994; Boulton Meneses, and Ennis, 1999; Edmonds et al, 1986; Frantz, Berquist, and Sprecht, 1995; Gottrup et al, 2001; Gottrup, 1998, 1999, 2000; Gray, 1996; Jaramillo et al, 1997). In the United States, commercial wound centers and wound care clinics in university settings have been organized (Ennis and Meneses, 1998; Keyser, 1993; Steed et al, 1993; Rees and Hirshberg, 1999). This approach to wound management has demonstrated a reduction in home visits and products used (Davey, Solomon, and Freeborn, 1994; Eagle, 1994). Furthermore, the standardizing of treatment plans has demonstrated improved healing of certain chronic wounds (Gottrup et al, 2001; Knighton et al, 1990; Steed, 1995).

WOUND MANAGEMENT MODELS

Optimally, one centralized, interdisciplinary team of specialists should manage patients with all types of wounds. The foundation for this concept culminates from the many advantages of such an approach, as previously described and listed in Table 2-2. For some years it has been discussed whether the wound management area should be a specialty comparable to classic medical specialties like dermatology, internal medicine, and subspecialties in surgery. However, the area of wound management involves too many disciplines to be classified as a specialty. It is much more suitable to consider it a type of interdisciplinary expert area similar to pain management or breast cancer management. It is vital for the existence and continuous development of an expert function in wound management that the area achieves status as an independent and integrated function of the health care system.

Wound Management Centers

In Denmark, the expert function in wound management has been conceptualized as "clinical wound healing," (2005) and incorporated into the relevant medical specialty societies (plastic surgery, orthopedics, vascular, general surgery, internal medicine, dermatology, and microbiology). The proposal has also been sent to the Danish National Board of Health (Gottrup, 2003).

Denmark is a small and well-organized country. Because the health care system is socialized, no patient pays for diagnostic or treatment procedures in the public hospitals. There are a few private hospitals covering only a small percentage of the total inpatient beds; the quality of care at the public hospitals is comparable to that of these private hospitals. Wound management in the primary health care sector has mainly been based on the work of district nurses, and partly carried out by private practice medical doctors. In the Danish health care system, the private practice physician is the referring person. Traditionally, however, the MD in the primary health care sector has little interest in or knowledge of wound management.

Several different specialists within the Danish hospitals (e.g., dermatology, vascular medicine, plastic surgery, orthopedic, internal medicine, and diabetology) are commonly involved in the treatment of the patient with a problem wound. The problem with this type of

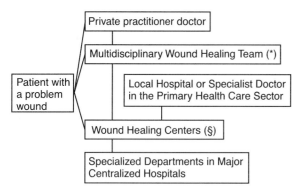

(*) One group for each geographic region in the Health Care System (in DK for each "Amt"). Consist of special educated doctors/nurses from both the primary and hospital sector.

(§) (e.g. University Center of Wound Healing and Copenhagen Wound Healing Center)

Fig. 2-1 Suggestion for organization of an expert function in wound healing and care: "Clinical Wound Healing." (Modified from Gottrup F et al: A new concept of a multidisciplinary wound healing center and a national expert function of wound healing, *Arch Surg* 136:765, 2001).

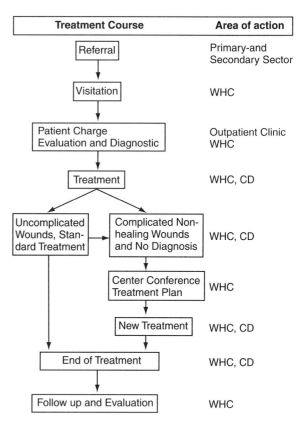

Fig. 2-2 Treatment course in a wound-healing center (WHC) and collaborating departments (CD). (Modified from Gottrup F: Optimizing wound treatment through health care structuring and professional education. *Wound Rep Reg* 12:129-133, 2004.)

approach is summarized in Table 2-2. The structure of Denmark's health care system makes the country an ideal setting for developing the concept of multidisciplinary wound management.

The clinical wound-healing model in Denmark (Figure 2-1) was generated in 1991 as a pilot. The concept included the establishment of a "multidisciplinary wound-healing team" in each of the 14 regions of the Danish health care system. The team consists of local staff and is the referral organ for wound patients within their region. This team organizes wound management for the patients in the primary sector as well as in the local hospitals. Patients needing more specialized treatment are seen at the centralized wound healing center. As of October 2004, two centralized wound healing centers were well-established. Figure 2-2 shows a structure for clinical wound healing.

Copenhagen Wound-Healing Center (CWHC).
The original model of the Copenhagen Wound-Healing Center (CWHC) was, from the author's point of view, close to the ideal model for a wound-healing center. The model was established in 1996 and housed in the Bispebjerg University Hospital in Copenhagen (Gottrup et al, 2001). It was an independent, clinical,

multidisciplinary department treating all types of problem wounds. The center consisted of an outpatient clinic and an inpatient ward. In the outpatient clinic, 30 to 35 patients were seen daily. Today, the center is connected to the dermatologic department of Bispebjerg University Hospital, with which it shares an inpatient department that has 15 beds for patients with wounds.

In the CWHC, a multidisciplinary staff of approximately 40 people work full-time with problem wounds. The staff consists of medical doctors, nurses, podiatrists, physiotherapists, secretaries, a hospital porter, and a doctor in education (i.e., residents). The center is surgery-oriented and has four types of specialized surgeons (vascular, orthopedic, gastrointestinal, and plastic surgery). The nursing staff includes clinical as well as research nurses with different levels of specialization. Nurses must complete an educational program to be eligible to work in the center.

University Center of Wound Healing (UCWH). The University Center of Wound Healing (UCWH) was established in 2003 and is housed in the Odense University Hospital, which is the largest hospital in Denmark. This center is part of the department of plastic and reconstructive surgery. Academic relationships have been established to include a professor in surgery, who is the specialist responsible for the center. The center consists of an outpatient clinic and an inpatient ward. At present the ward has 16 beds; it is in a structure belonging to the department but separate from the main plastic surgery department. The outpatient clinic includes all wound patients referred to the hospital, and 30 to 35 patients are seen daily.

With regard to categories of personnel, the multidisciplinary staff is similar to that of the CWHC, but not all are employed in the center full-time. Of the 40 caregivers, five are medical doctors. The additional staff is part-time in the center and represents collaborating departments such as orthopedics, vascular surgery, internal medicine, podiatry, and dermatology. Specialized medical doctors come to the wards daily and participate in multidisciplinary rounds. In the outpatient clinic, medical doctors from the center and the collaborating departments follow an agreed-upon schedule of participation. The nursing staff includes clinical as well as research nurses with different levels of specialty training. Currently, an educational program for nurses is being developed at the center.

Center Activities. In addition to the treatment of patients with problem wounds, the centers play a major role in education and research. Undergraduate and postgraduate education is conducted for doctors and nurses. A specific rotation at the wound-healing center has been accepted as a part of the specialty physician's training in dermatology. Similar arrangements are being discussed for specialty education in plastic surgery, orthopedics, and vascular surgery. Together with the Danish Nurse Association, since 1997 the center has since been performing a 6-month, four-module nursing course leading to a diploma.

A certain degree of research is vital to a specialty function. The centralization of patients with different types of problem wounds offers a unique opportunity for recruiting a sufficient number of patients for clinical research. Also, the possibility for research is of great value for the evolution of multidisciplinary wound care into an interdisciplinary wound care approach. In both centers a number of people are dedicated full-time to research activities.

Wound Care Teams

During the last decade, wound care committees and teams have become the model for comprehensive wound management in the United States. These committees and teams are multidisciplinary (Box 2-1), and members have specific responsibilities (Box 2-2). Through multidisciplinary collaboration, quality patient outcomes

---

BOX 2-1 Multidisciplinary Wound Management Team Representatives and Consultants

Members
- Medical director
- Certified wound care nurse/WOC nurse
- Physical therapist
- Nurse manager
- Dietician
- Social worker
- Utilization review specialist
- Occupational therapist
- Speech therapist

Consultants/Ad hoc Members*
- Infection control specialist
- Dermatologist
- Podiatrist
- Orthotics specialist
- Diabetologist
- Gerontologist
- Plastic surgeon
- Vascular surgeon
- Pharmacist
- Quality manager

*Some consultants may be needed as committee members, depending on the setting and patient population.
WOC, Wound, ostomy, and continence.

BOX 2-2 Multidisciplinary Wound Management Committee Responsibilities

Prevention
- Standardize protocols for risk assessment (Hunter et al, 1995; Kresevic and Naylor, 1995).
- Integrate risk assessment findings with appropriate preventive interventions
- Establish product formularies for the prevention of wounds
- Review and incorporate national prevention practice guidelines as appropriate for clinical setting and patient population

Treatment
- Establish product formularies for prevention and treatment of wounds
- Establish protocols for care of common clinical conditions
- Review and incorporate national treatment practice guidelines as appropriate for clinical setting and patient population

Documentation
- Standardized documentation for prevention, assessment and treatment
- Facilitate documentation methods that are accurate, efficient and accessible

Education
- Support development of patient education materials
- Conduct a staff wide assessment of education needs related to wound management
- Facilitate staff education and competency

Quality Management
- Review quality assurance findings and patient care outcomes
- Develop and implement strategies for quality improvement (Gates, 1996; Lessner, 1996).
- Evaluate and disseminate outcome analysis results (Tomaselli and Oxler, 1997).

Research
- Direct clinical trials of products using standard evaluation protocols (Turnbull, 1996)

Care Conferences
- Establish an individualized wound management plan for each patient
- Review, update and plan for follow-up for each patient at routine intervals

---

(AHCPR, 1992) are enhanced and opportunities are identified to reduce liability (Miller and Delozier, 1994). Such a format also fosters a consistent approach to the documentation and communication of clinical findings (Motta, Thimsen-Whitaker, and Demoor, 1995).

Members of the wound care team and their responsibilities are summarized in Boxes 2-1 and 2-2 and described later in this chapter. The appropriateness of membership and responsibilities will vary according to the needs of the patient population, community laws, and the regulating bodies of the various disciplines involved. Wound care committees fulfill many functions:

1. Formalize and standardize operations such as clinical, financial, and biomedical issues related to prevention and treatment of wounds (Granick et al, 1996)
2. Serve as the final reviewing body for wound care–related issues; provides recommendations to other committees as appropriate

3. Recommend changes and/or revisions to policies, procedures, and patient care standards (Baharestani, 1995)
4. Provide interface with clinical working groups such as housekeeping, materials management, specialty bed committee, practice and procedure committee, quality review committee, and a research committee
5. Meet periodically to review, develop, coordinate, and implement advisory group recommendations

Despite recommendations for a multidisciplinary approach in establishing national standards and guidelines for care, the quality and structure of wound management programs varies throughout the United States by community and practice setting. In terms of quality, there is a wide variance in the educational preparation of the wound care staff across all practice settings. In fact, some teams may be coordinated by a staff member who has no formal wound care education or certification but is considered a wound care specialist based on personal interest and motivation. Chapter 1 provides a discussion of the value of formal wound education and certification.

Similarly, the organization of wound management services varies greatly by care setting. Ideally, the wound management team would employ qualified professionals who are readily accessible to provide their input in the patient's care as needed. Unfortunately, within the acute care setting or the medical center, this care is typically fragmented. Specialty clinics such as plastic surgery, orthopedics, vascular surgery, and dermatology often care for the patient with a wound without benefit of the crucial input needed from other specialties. If consultation with another specialty does occur, it will be at another time; this lag further delays appropriate care, presents a hardship to the patient, and complicates the coordination of care. Some home care agencies use a multidisciplinary approach, and some do not. Most often, the home care patient with a wound is referred to a specialized department and experiences the limitations of a single discipline, fragmented approach. Furthermore, facilities providing wound management may be multidisciplinary—making use of the services of a nurse, a dietician, and a physical therapist, for example—but not inclusive of all of the appropriate disciplines. Consequently, input from additional disciplines is obtained through referrals and future appointments rather than by the synchronous collaboration of a true multidisciplinary team approach.

ESTABLISHING A MULTIDISCIPLINARY WOUND MANAGEMENT PROGRAM

In the process of developing a multidisciplinary wound management program, several steps must be planned (Box 2-3). Steps include characterization of the problem, aim, or goal; choosing a model or concept; achieving integration in the health care organization; and finally, establishing single elements of the concept such as the wound management center and team.

Characterize the Problem

Although we may recognize the limitations of current wound management models as described in Table 2-2, it is important to present a persuasive and compelling argument to administration. The problem(s) must be characterized in terms that are meaningful to the

---

BOX 2-3   Steps to Establishing a Multidisciplinary Wound Management Approach

1. Characterize the problem
2. Define goals
3. Select a model or concept
4. Integrate the concept into the over all health care system/setting
5. Create the single elements of the organization (teams/centers)

---

individual health care organization and draw from the organization's mission or vision statement.

Define Goals or Aim

Once the problem is established, the aim of a multidisciplinary wound management program should be identified. The common aim or goal for the concept should be to improve wound treatment and care in general. Thus an increase in healing rates should be realized in conjunction with reduced hospital time and enhanced, cost-effective outcomes. This is more likely to be attained through the use of standardized wound classifications, with standardized diagnostic and treatment plans that offer optimal management to patients with all types of problem wounds. Box 2-4 shows an example of a group of standardized wound classifications (Gottrup, 2001). Additional components that require standardization can be found in Box 2-5.

Select a Model

The health care provider's approach to the care of the patient with the wound must be such that the patient is placed in the middle of the team; or, as exemplified by Sir William Osler: "Care more for the individual than for the special features of the disease" (Osler, 1904; Robson, 1996). To obtain this goal, different models can be used. Wound treatment and care is based on the same principles all over the world. With a few modifications, most health care systems should be able to establish an effective model for their wound care program.

The leader of the wound care management program could be a single person, normally a medical doctor, but there could also be a combined leadership between

BOX 2-4 Standardized Wound Classifications

Wounds related to changes in vessels	• Arterial (ischemic) wounds • Venous wounds • Lymphatic wounds
Wounds related to neuropathy	• Diabetic wounds • Alcoholic wounds • Other neuropathic wounds
Wounds related to pressure/friction	• Pressure ulcers
Wounds related to trauma and surgery	• Originally contaminated wounds • Originally clean surgical wounds • Specialized surgical wounds
Other types of wounds	• Anorectal fistulas • Stoma-related wounds • Specific infection–related wounds (e.g., AIDS) • Neoplasmic wounds • Vasculitis wounds • Other inflammatory wounds • Wounds in the oral cavity • Self-inflicted wounds (self-mutilation) • Hypergranulating wounds and keloids

From Gottrup F: Recent development in wound healing and care, Hospital Healthcare Europe 2001/2002, Hope (Hospitals of the European Union) Reference Book, *Theatre and Surgery* T55, 2001; Gottrup F, Olsen L, editors: *Sår—Baggrund, diagnostik og behandling* (Wounds—background, diagnostics and treatment), Munksgaard, Copenhagen, 1996.

BOX 2-5 Standardized Components of a Multidisciplinary Wound Management Program

• Prevention
• Diagnostics/assessment
• Classification
• Policies and procedures
• Formularies
• Protocols
• Documentation of prevention, assessment, and treatment
• Follow-up
• Quality indicators
• Research
• Education

two disciplines—for example, a medical doctor and a certified wound care nurse. However, it is crucial that all specialties and disciplines are recognized (Neubauer and Redesign 1993) and considered equally important members of the team (Delamothe, 1988; Neubauer, 1995). The wound-healing area is a perfect example of a multidisciplinary area of expertise and should be classified in the health care system as such. The team concept should ultimately include all types of personnel who have a connection to wound management. The ideal team would provide scientific as well as clinical support.

Models for wound-healing centers range from those with a few part-time employees in an outpatient setting to full departmental structures with staff and resources dedicated solely to wound management. For example, in the Danish concept, a wound-healing center is defined as a multidisciplinary department (or part of a specialty department) with both an outpatient clinic and an inpatient ward, where the staff works exclusively with wound-healing problems.

The ideal concept has probably not yet been determined. Nonetheless, several attempts have been made to produce multidisciplinary wound-healing teams or centers. They operate as wound care teams connected to specialized hospital departments or as specialized units in the primary health care sector. These entities are subunits of larger organizations whose main purpose is different from wound healing and care. The personnel who carry out wound care functions only do so part-time, usually once or twice per week. In the case of the need for hospitalization, the patient is placed in a specialized department where wound care is a minor part of the clinical practice. Furthermore, geographic differences in the structure of the health care system can lead to the same type of wound being referred to different specialties and receiving different types of treatment. This lack of organization is the major problem when care is delivered by individuals instead of by a team; as previously stated, such care is not in the patient's best interest (NPUAP, 1989). Individual specialists may be more likely to recognize illness and the need for treatment, rather than seeing all aspects of the patient's situation (Friedson, 1971). This is especially relevant to wound healing and care. When medical specialists function as individuals, it has been shown that they believe there is little to add after the technical procedures have been accomplished (Robson, 1985). This contributes to the exclusion of the other members of a multidisciplinary team.

Integration into the Overall Health Care System or Setting

It is vital for the continuous development and existence of an expert function in wound management that the field achieves status as an independent and integrated subspecialty available within health care systems. Within a healthcare system, there should be system-wide wound management structure consisting of centers and teams, as well as systematic education to ensure the recruitment of new experts in the area.

Elements of the Wound Management Structure

Team composition. The membership and responsibilities of the wound management team will vary according to the needs of the patient population, community laws, and the regulating bodies of the various disciplines involved. Examples are listed in Boxes 2-1 and 2-2 and described below.

Certified wound care specialist. At least one member of the wound management team should be certified in wound care by an independent national certification organization that validates specialty knowledge, experience, and clinical judgement. This should not be mistaken with continuing education (CE) or a certificate of completion, which simply denotes that a course or activity has been completed. This is particularly important for the delivery of quality outcomes as well as the ability to legally defend the validity of the certification. The value of certification, as well as factors to consider when choosing a legally defensible certification process, is described in Chapter 1.

Medical director. The medical director of the wound management team is a physician. The medical director oversees ongoing treatment and overall management of patients with complex wounds. The medical director interacts as needed with primary and consulting physicians to facilitate consistent and effective wound management that is aligned with overall patient goals. Responsibilities include but are not limited to assisting the facility in the development and implementation of policies and procedures for prevention and treatment of skin breakdown that are consistent with national standards of care. Ideally, the medical director of a wound management program is a certified

wound specialist. However, when supported by qualified and competent team members, physicians without certification have been very effective as medical directors of wound management teams.

Nursing. The nurse directs the development and implementation of an individualized plan of care based on the needs and goals assessed for the patient. Nursing focuses on risk assessment, early problem identification, preventive measures to promote skin integrity, and responses to treatments. The nurse documents and reports condition changes and revises the plan of care as necessary. In the United States, there are several training pathways for nurses, ranging from licensed practical nurses to advanced practice and nurses with doctoral degrees.

The certified wound nurse or the wound, ostomy, and continence (WOC) nurse has been prepared at the baccalaureate level, and the WOC nurse who is a nurse practitioner has been prepared at the master's degree level. The WOC nurse often serves as wound care program coordinator by (1) organizing prevalence and incidence studies, (2) providing individualized holistic patient assessments, (3) making recommendation for wound care products, adjunctive therapies, and specialty beds or equipment, (4) performing debridement, if within the individual's skill level and scope of practice, (5) providing ongoing assessment and evaluation of healing for patients with complex wounds, and (6) educating staff in the prevention, assessment, and treatment of wounds.

Physical therapy. The physical therapist's (PT) role can differ widely among care settings and facilities. Physical therapists have educational preparations at the baccalaureate, master's degree, and doctorate levels. Master's- and doctoral-level programs include wound management in the curriculum. The role of the physical therapist who is involved in wound care may appear to overlap with that of the certified wound nurse or the WOC nurse. The PT may collaborate during evaluation and care planning, or may coordinate a team. Physical therapists are often involved throughout the process of care, from the prevention of breakdown to facilitation of healing. PT interventions address range of motion, strength training, seating and positioning, support surfaces, and functional mobility training. Physical therapists may offer therapeutic intervention for contractures, edema, motor control, muscle weakness, and pain. Other interventions such as electrical stimulation, pulsed lavage, and sharp debridement may be within the scope of practice for some physical therapists. As with nurses, it is important that physical therapists function within their scope of practice comply with accreditation and education regulations are regulated by accredited educational programs and curricula, and have certifications with sound practicum experience.

Occupational therapy. The occupational therapist (OT) plays a rehabilitative role, assessing cognitive and functional capabilities and then introducing patient-specific adaptive techniques and equipment. Patient-specific adaptive techniques and equipment promote optimal performance of activities of daily living, including the ability to take an active role in wound care. The patient with a slow-healing or nonhealing wound may benefit from the expertise of the OT to promote overall health maintenance and quality of life by incorporating wound care into the patient and family's daily routine.

Speech therapy. The speech therapist helps promote optimal nutrition by ensuring that the patient is able to safely swallow. Speech therapy may include strengthening oral and/or pharyngeal musculature, swallowing trials for diet advancement, and/or providing compensatory techniques with oral intake to improve the safety of the patient's swallowing and reduce aspiration risk. The speech therapist focuses on improving the patient's ability to effectively communicate to his or her maximum functional level. Cognitively, speech therapy works to improve cognitive-linguistic skills for safe and effective communication upon transition to the least restrictive environment possible.

Dietician or nutritionist. The dietician promotes optimal nutrition through nutritional assessment and intervention. The dietician monitors nutritionally-related laboratory values, anthropometric measurements, and food intake or nutrition support parameters. The dietician collaborates with the team to make recommendations that optimally meet the nutritional needs and goals of the patient.

Social services. The social worker is relied upon as a key member of the wound management team. The patient with a wound is often vulnerable and requires astute assessment of the home situation, particularly as it relates to safety, support, and the ability to realistically meet wound management goals. The social worker is knowledgeable about financial resources and the barriers to follow-up care that are unique to each individual situation. The social worker obtains prior authorization for supplies and other services needed upon discharge to avoid unexpected costs to the patient. As the key liaison between care settings, the social worker coordinates and leads discharge planning conferences, which include the patient, wound management team members, and families. Representatives from facilities and agencies responsible for future care are often included in discharge planning meetings for patients with complex management issues. This collaboration between the patient and families and health care team members from both settings helps to establish mutual goals and continuity in care.

Utilization review. In the United States, the utilization review (UR) specialist functions as a critical link between the patient, the physician, and the payer (insurance companies, health maintenance organizations, and state or federal providers). Both nurses and social workers have held utilization review positions. In many care settings, the UR responsibilities have become incorporated into the case management role. The UR specialist provides information to payers to ensure funding for the most appropriate and cost-effective care.

Wound Management Center. Elements of a wound management center are listed in Box 2-6 and described in the following sections.

Staff. The employees of the center should be recruited from relevant specialties to form a multidisciplinary staff (see Box 2-1). In the optimal set-up, all

BOX 2-6 Elements of a Multidisciplinary Wound Management Center
••

- Staff
- Departments
- Equipment
- Policies and procedures
- Documentation
- Database
- Research
- Education

members of the staff work full-time at the center. However, it is more realistic in most cases for the center to follow a model that mixes full-time with part-time personnel. The staff should be organized in a way that provides the most consistent patient care possible. In addition to clinical responsibilities, the employees of a wound-healing center should be prepared to be involved in research and education.

The nursing staff is the major group at this type of center. Nursing staff should include nurses with both a clinical and a scientific background. The center should include wound nurses certified by a nationally recognized accredited organization such as the WOCNCB. In the United States, advanced practice nurses who are certified in wound care may function most effectively in the coordinating role because of their educational preparation and prescriptive privileges.

Staff members should be clearly and accurately identified. Nurses need to consult with regulatory and professional agencies to ensure compliance in the use of titles and credentials. For example, a nurse may not be called a "wound specialist" or a "clinical nurse specialist" without the appropriate educational preparation and/or certification.

Departments. The center should be structured as a general clinical department consisting of an outpatient clinic and an inpatient ward. Both should focus on patients with problem wounds. The inpatient ward should have a significant number of beds. Ideally the wound ward comprises its own unit, where only the wound staff work. The number of beds established should be based on the expected number of referrals. To optimally serve patients, the outpatient clinic should be in daily operation. In the interdisciplinary team model, all or as many different specialties as possible should be present simultaneously. A sufficient number of examining rooms should be available, because outpatients with problem wounds require more clinic time than most other patients. A mean of 30 to 40 minutes should be allowed for each wound patient (Gottrup et al, 2001). There should also be rooms for performing patient procedures and, ideally, one room could be used for surgical procedures done under local anesthesia.

Equipment. The equipment needs are related to the condition of the patient population, who are commonly

TABLE 2-3   Distribution of Patients by Frequency

OUTPATIENT	INPATIENT
Venous leg ulcers	Diabetic leg/foot ulcers
Diabetic leg/foot ulcers	Venous leg ulcers
Pressure ulcers	Pressure ulcers
Acute wounds	Acute wounds
Other types of wounds	Other types of wounds

Ranked by frequency at the Copenhagen Wound-Healing Center (CWHC) and the University Center of Wound Healing (UCWH).
From Gottrup F. A specialized wound-healing center concept: importance: of a multidisciplinary department structure and surgical facilities in the treatment of chronic wounds. *Am J Surg* 187 (Suppl to May) 38S-43S, 2004.

elderly and have impaired mobility. Outpatients may have different needs from inpatients. For example, in Denmark the patient with a diabetic foot ulcer is more frequently an inpatient because of the acute nature of this problem. The distribution of patients in Danish centers in outpatient clinics as compared to inpatient departments is shown in Table 2-3.

The diagnostic armamentarium of a center or team must be sufficient, if it is to function well. Clinical examination may require a variety of diagnostic tests such as Doppler scans, ankle-brachial index, toe pressures, transcutaneous oxygen tension, and angiography. The equipment and personnel needed to conduct these procedures must be readily available.

Referral policy. Ideally, a referral policy should be based on the principle that all types of complex wounds should be referred to the wound management team. If the general staff is knowledgeable and competent in providing basic prevention, assessment, and treatment to patients with wounds, facility protocols and algorithms can be developed that prompt a wound management team referral for more complex or recalcitrant wounds. Typically, the type of setting will drive the referral policy. Table 2-4 shows an example of a referral policy. Many hospitals in the United States automatically treat each patient who has a complex wound with a holistic, multidisciplinary approach. Other hospitals have a referral policy that uses the less-than-ideal "pay per visit" approach if the wound specialist or consultant is employed outside of the hospital. Wound management centers

TABLE 2-4   Example of a Referral Policy

CONDITION	ACTION
Diabetic foot ulcer patients	Acute, subacute, priority evaluation (acute in 24 hours, subacute in a week)
Arteriosclerotic wound patients	Referred directly to vascular surgery department
Venous leg ulcer	Priority evaluation (related to the condition of the wound. Normally 2 to 4 weeks)
Trauma wound patients	Acute, subacute (as for diabetic foot)
Fistula and other acute wounds	Priority evaluation (related to condition of the wound. Normally 2 to 6 weeks)

CWHC, Copenhagen Wound-Healing Center; *UCWH*, University Center of Wound Healing.

and clinics in the United States must follow referral policies established by managed care and payer sources in order to receive reimbursement. Chapter 27 of this text discusses reimbursement and billing.

Standardized treatment plans. An accepted, standardized treatment plan for each type of problem wound is pivotal. Little evidence is available for the healing rate of the "standard" treated problem wounds because of the lack of specific standardized treatment plans and of the failure to register the different parameters involved in a course of treatment. This means that no base-line healing rate exists for the comparison of different types of problem wounds. In addition to the lack of treatment plans, wound assessment and documentation are rarely well-defined outside specialist units, and often do not appear in health care database systems. This makes it is almost impossible to produce any specific data related to wounds. The problem has been compounded by the lack of adequate wound diagnosis. Similarly, information on the treatment of wounds, including dressing materials and pharmaceuticals, has been lacking. The solution, a multidisciplinary wound management environment, provides an incredible opportunity to standardize care and allow

for record keeping and data collection; thus increasing the available evidence related to wound management and outcomes.

Database. A functional wound database offers the ability to collect and use all types of information about the patient and the patient's wound. Development of clinical data sets together with economic outcomes data will make it possible to evaluate different types of treatment with respect to both clinical outcomes and cost-effectiveness. With a database, it is feasible to conduct analyses of clinical trials, meta-analyses, and cost-effectiveness investigations. This has not been possible with the databases currently used for health care evaluation.

Ideally, the database should include the entire population of patients with wounds, in similar fashion to a registry. This registry for wound data would be invaluable in shaping the future of wound treatment (Coerper et al, 2004). Such a database has been initiated at the UCWH Denmark and by the European Wound Management Association (Franks and Gottrup, 2004).

Research and education. Research is vital for the continued evolution of the specialty of wound management from a multidisciplinary approach to a transdisciplinary one. The centralization of patients with different types of problem wounds offers a unique opportunity for recruiting patients for clinical research. In a center incorporating the concepts previously described, it is possible to recruit diverse and sufficient numbers of patients to satisfy specifications stipulated by research protocols.

Education of internal as well as external personnel is a critical, fundamental function of a wound management center. Further motivation for addressing education are the increasing expectations of regulatory bodies for improved staff education and competence as well as patient education and community outreach.

SUMMARY

Ideal wound management is greatly dependent on the evolution of multidisciplinary collaboration into an interdisciplinary approach. Successful multidisciplinary wound management teams and centers can improve outcomes through standardization, education, and research. All disciplines are valuable partners in the wound management program and provide unique and essential contributions that cumulatively create a successful environment for the consistent delivery of efficient, organized, and evidence-based patient care.

SELF-ASSESSMENT EXERCISE

1. Describe the difference between wound management and wound care.
2. Identify six advantages to a multidisciplinary centralized team of specialists.
3. List five responsibilities of a multidisciplinary wound management committee or team.
4. List four steps critical to establishing a multidisciplinary wound management approach.
5. Identify six elements of a multidisciplinary wound management program.

REFERENCES

Agency for Health Care Policy and Research (AHCPR): Pressure ulcers in adults: prediction and prevention, Rockville, Md, USDHHS, *AHCPR* Pub. No. 92-0047, 1992.

Allman R et al: Pressure sores among hospitalized patients, *Ann Intern Med* 105:337, 1986.

Anderson E, Hansson C, Swanbeck G: Leg and foot ulcers: an epidemiological survey, *Acta Derm Venereol (Stockh)* 64:227, 1984.

Anderson K, Kvorning S: Medical aspects of the decubitus ulcer, *Int J Dermatol* 21:265, 1982.

Appelquist J et al: Diabetic foot ulcers in a multidisciplinary setting. An economic analysis of primary healing and healing with amputation, *J Intern Med* 235:463-471, 1994.

Baharestani M: Clinical decision making in wound care management: the need for a paradigmatic shift, *Wounds Compendium Clin Res Pract* 7(suppl A):84A, 1995.

Bergmark S, Zimmerdahl V, Muller K: Prevalence investigation of pressure ulcers, *EWMA J* 4(1):7, 2004.

Boulton AJ, Meneses P, Ennis WJ: Diabetic foot ulcers: a framework for prevention and care, *Wound Rep Reg* 7:7, 1999.

Brown H: Wound healing research through the ages. In: Cohen I, Diegelmann R, Lindblad W, editors: *Wound healing, biological and clinical aspects*, Philadelphia, 1992, W.B. Saunders.

Coerper S et al: Documentation of 7051 chronic wounds using a new computerized system within a network of wound care centers, *Arch Surg* 139:251, 2004.

Collins J P: May You Live in Interesting Times: Using Multidisciplinary and Interdisciplinary Programs to Cope with Change in the Life Sciences. Issn: 0006-3568 Journal: BioScience Volume: 52 Issue: 1 Pages: 75-83, 2003.

Dale J: Chronic ulcers of the leg: a study of the prevalence in a Scottish Community, *Health Bulletin* 41:310, 1983.

Davey L, Solomon JM, Freeborn SF: A multidisciplinary approach to wound care, *J Wound Care* 3:249, 1994.

Delamothe T: Not a profession, not a career, *BMJ* 296:271, 1988.

Drucker PF: *Managing in a time of great changes*, New York, 1998, Truman Tally Books/Plume.

Eagle M: Education for nurses by nurses, *Proceedings of the 3rd European Conference on Advances in Wound Management*, London, 1994, McMillan.

Edmonds ME et al: Improved survival of the diabetic foot: the role of a specialized foot clinic, *Quart J Med* 60:763, 1986.

Elk A, Boman G: A descriptive study of pressure sores: the prevalence of pressure sores and the characteristics of patients, *J Adv Nurs* 7:51, 1982.

Ennis WJ, Meneses P: Managing wounds in a managed care environment: the integrated concept, *Ostomy, Wound Manage* 44:22, 28, 34, 1998.

Franks PJ, Gottrup F: Outcomes and structures of care: the European perspective, *Wounds* 16:173, 2004.

Frantz R, Berquist S, Sprecht J: The cost of treating pressure ulcers following implementation of a research-based skin care protocol in a long term care facility, *Adv Wound Care* 8:36, 1995.

Friedson E: Profession of medicine: a study of the sociology of applied knowledge, New York, 1971, Dodd, Mead.

Gates J: Total quality management: pressure ulcer prevention, *Nurs Manage* 27(4):48E, 1996.

Gerson LW: The incidence of pressure sores in active treatment hospitals, *Int J Nurs Stud* 12(4):201, 1975.

Gosnell D, Johannsen J, Ayres M: Pressure ulcer incidence and severity in a community hospital, *Decubitus* 5:56, 1992.

Gottrup F: Setting up a wound healing center in Copenhagen, *Primary Intention* 6:22, 1998.

Gottrup F: Wound treatment and care, Hospital Healthcare Europe 1999/2000, Hope (Hospitals of the European Union) Reference Book, *Theatre and Surgery* 47, 1999.

Gottrup F: Prevention of surgical-wound infections, *N Engl J Med* 342:202, 2000 (editorial).

Gottrup F: Recent development in wound healing and care, Hospital Healthcare Europe 2001/2002, Hope (Hospitals of the European Union) Reference Book, *Theatre and Surgery* T55, 2001.

Gottrup F: Interdisciplinary wound treatment and care. In Clark RAF, editor: *Textbook of wound care*, New York, 2002, W.B. Saunders (in press).

Gottrup F: Organization of wound healing services: the Danish experience and the importance of surgery, *Wound Rep Reg* 11:452, 2003.

Granick MS et al: Wound management and wound care. In Habal HB, editor: *Advances in plastic and reconstructive surgery*, vol 12, St Louis, 1996, Mosby.

Granick MS, McGowan E, Long CD: Outcome assessment of an in-hospital cross-functional wound care team, *Plast Reconstr Surg* 101(5):1243, 1998.

Gray BL: Developing a model for clinical practice, *J Wound Care* 5:428, 1996.

Gruen RL, Chang S, Maclellan DG: The real costs of leg ulcers: a hospital based audit, *Proc Austral Int Wound Manage Conf* 251, 1994.

Hunter SM et al: The effectiveness of skin care protocols for pressure ulcers, *Rehabil Nurs* 20(5):250, 1995.

Jaramillo O et al: Practical guidelines for developing a hospital-based wound and ostomy clinic, *Wounds* 9:94, 1997.

Keyser JE: Diabetic wound healing and limb salvage in an outpatient wound care program, *Southern Med J* 86:311, 1993.

Knighton DR et al: Simulation of repair in chronic nonhealing cutaneous ulcers using platelet-derived wound healing formula, *Surg Gynecol Obstet* 170:56, 1990.

Kresevic D, Naylor M: Preventing pressure ulcers through the use of protocols in a mentoring nursing model, *Geriatr Nurs* 16(5):225, 1995.

Lazarus GS, Cooper DM, Knighton DR, et al: Definitions and guidelines for assessment of wounds and evaluation of healing. *Arch Dermatol* 130:489-493, 1994.

Lessner W: Small but successful changes prepare MDs for advent of decubitus protocol, *Qual Improvement/Total Qual Manage* 6(1):1, 1996.

Lindholm C: Leg ulcer patients. Clinical studies from prevalence to prevention, Thesis, Lunds Universitet, Sweden, 1993.

Liu PY, Eriksson E, Mustoe TA: Wound healing: practical aspects. In: Russels RC, editor: PSEF Instructional Courses, St. Louis, 1991, Mosby.

Long C, Granick M: A multidisciplinary approach to wound care in the hospitalized patient, *Clin Plast Surg* 25(3):425, 1998.

Majno G: *The healing hand: man and wound in the ancient world*, Cambridge, MA, 1975, Harvard University Press.

Miller H, Delozier J: Cost implications of the pressure ulcer treatment guideline, Center for Health Policy Studies, Columbia, Md, sponsored by *AHCPR*, Contract No. 282-91-0070, 1994.

Motta GJ, Thimsen-Whitaker K, Demoor MA: Documenting outcomes of wound care, *Contin Care* 14(8):16, 1995.

National Pressure Ulcer Advisory Panel (NPUAP): Pressure ulcers prevalence, cost and risk assessment, Consensus Development Conference statement, *Decubitus* 2:24, 1989.

Neubauer JF: Redesign: Managing role changes and building new teams, *Semin Nurse Manage* 1:26, 1993.

Neubauer JF: The value of nursing, *J Nurse Manage* 3:301, 1995.

Nolan M: Towards an ethos of interdisciplinary practice, *BMJ* 11(5):305, 1995.

Osler W: *Aequanimatas*, Philadelphia, 1904, Blakiston.

Pirrie A, Hamilton V, Wilson V: Multidisciplinary education: some issues and concerns. *Educ Res* 41(3):301, 1999.

Postnett J: Workshop on Multidisciplinary Concepts in Wound Healing, *Danish Wound Healing Society*, Helsingør, Denmark, 2002.

Rees RS, Hirshberg JA: Wound care centers: cost, care and strategies, *Adv wound care* 12(Suppl 2):4, 1999.

Reich RB: Entrepreneurship reconsidered: the team as hero, *Harvard Business Rev* 65:77, 1987.

Reiter D: Methods and materials for wound management, *Otolaryngol Head Neck Surg* 110:550, 1994.

Robson MC: Communication in improving the work of the head and neck cancer team, *Plast Reconstr Surg* 76:611, 1985.

Robson MC: A time to integrate the complete wound team: from bench to bedside and beyond, *Wound Rep Reg* 4:187, 1996.

Robson MC, Krizek TJ, Wray RC: Care of the thermally injured patient. In: Zuidema GD, Rutherford RB, Ballinger WF, editors: *The management of trauma*, Philadelphia, 1979, W.B. Saunders.

Souba WW: Reinventing the academic medical center, *J Surg Res* Feb 81(2): 113-22, 1999.

Steed DL: Clinical evaluation of recombinant human platelet-derived growth factor for the treatment of lower extremity diabetic ulcers, *J Vasc Surg* 21:71, 1995.

Steed DL et al: Organization and development of a universal multidisciplinary wound care clinic, *Surgery* 114:775, 1993.

Steinbock R: *Paleopathological Diagnosis and Interpretation (Bone Disease in Ancient Human Populations)*, Springfield, Ill, 1976, CC Thomas.

Stokols D et al: Evaluating transdisciplinary science, *Nicotine Tob Res* 5(Suppl 1):S21, Dec 2003.

Tomaselli N, Oxler K: *Thomas Jefferson University Hospital comprehensive skin care program*, Philadelphia, 1997, Thomas Jefferson University Hospital.

Turnbull G: The international committee on wound management (ICWM) statement on cost-effective wound care: evaluating your supply use to prepare for managed care, *Ostomy Wound Manage* 42(2):72, 1996.

Vestergaard S et al: Sårbehandling i hjemmeplejen, *Sygeplejersken* 98:30, 1998.

Wilson V, Pirrie A: Developing professional competence: lessons from the emergency room, *Studies Higher Ed* 24(2):211, 1999.

3 *Anatomy and Physiology of Skin and Soft Tissue*

ANNETTE B. WYSOCKI

OBJECTIVES

1. Explain the importance of normal skin integrity.
2. Describe the size, thickness, function, vascular supply, and cellular composition of the major layers of the skin.
3. List the key structures and functions of the layers of the epidermis.
4. Discuss the significance of the following structures and cells: rete ridges, keratinocytes, melanocytes, basement membrane zone, and tropocollagen.
5. Distinguish between the composition of the papillary dermis and that of the reticular dermis.
6. Describe the six major functions of the skin.
7. Identify three ways in which the skin protects against pathogenic invasion.
8. Describe the role of the following cells in providing the skin immune system: Langerhans' cells, tissue macrophages, and mast cells.
9. Explain the relationship between skin pigmentation and protection against ultraviolet radiation.
10. Identify the two mechanisms by which the skin provides thermoregulation.
11. Compare and contrast the structural and cellular development of the skin in the premature infant (between 23 to 32 weeks' gestation), the full-term neonate, the adolescent, and the adult.
12. Describe at least two effects that the following have on the skin: hydration, sun, nutrition, soaps, and medications.

The skin is the one organ of the body that is constantly exposed to a changing environment. Maintaining its integrity is a complex process, and without appropriate treatment, assaults from surgical incisions, injuries, or burns can lead to life-threatening consequences.

Human skin is divided into two primary layers—epidermis (outermost layer) and dermis (innermost layer) (Figure 3-1). These two layers are separated by a structure called the basement membrane. Beneath the dermis is a layer of loose connective tissue called the hypodermis, or subcutis. Major functions of the skin are protection, immunity, thermoregulation, sensation, metabolism, and communication (Jacob, Francone, and Lossow, 1982; Millington and Wilkinson, 1983; Woodburne and Burkel, 1988).

The skin of the average adult covers approximately 3000 square inches, or an area almost equivalent to 2 square meters. From birth to maturity the skin covering will undergo a sevenfold expansion. It weighs about 6 pounds (or up to 15% of total adult body weight), is the largest organ, and receives one third of the body's circulating blood volume. The skin forms a protective barrier from the external environment while maintaining a homeostatic internal environment. Epidermal appendages—nails, hair follicles, and sweat or sebaceous glands—that are lined with epidermal cells are also present in the skin. During the healing of partial-thickness wounds, these epidermal cells migrate to resurface the wound. This organ is capable of self-regeneration and can withstand limited mechanical and chemical assaults. The skin varies in thickness from 0.5 mm in the tympanic membrane to 6 mm in the soles of the feet and the palms of the hands. Variations are attributable to differences in the thickness of the skin layers covering underlying organs, bones, muscle, and cartilage. Diseases of the skin can result from genetic causes, so-called genodermatoses, infection, immune dysfunction, and trauma. Skin diseases can involve some or all skin layers.

SKIN LAYERS
Epidermis

The epidermis, the outermost skin layer, is avascular and is derived from embryonic ectoderm. This layer is relatively uniform in thickness over the body and is

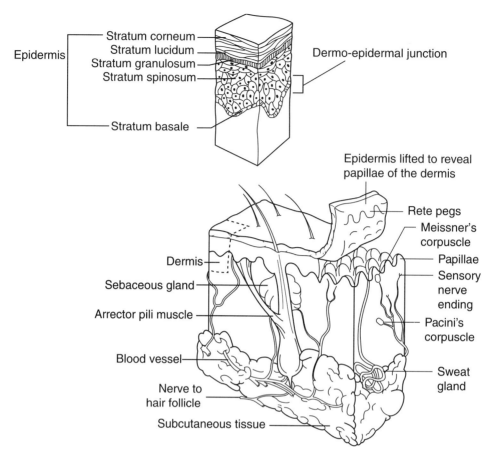

Fig. 3-1 Schema of anatomy of skin and subcutaneous tissue. (From Hooper BJ, Goldman MP: *Primary dermatologic care,* St. Louis, 1999, Mosby.)

between 75 and 150 μm except on the soles and palms, where thickness is between 0.4 and 0.6 mm. The epidermal layer is constantly being renewed; the turnover time ranges from 26 to 42 days. Complete epidermal renewal occurs over a period lasting between 45 and 75 days, or about every 2 months (Odland, 1991). The epidermal layer is composed of stratified squamous epithelial cells, or keratinocytes, and is divided into five layers (see Figure 3-1). These layers, beginning from the outermost to the innermost, are the stratum corneum, the stratum lucidum, the stratum granulosum, the stratum spinosum, and the stratum basale (stratum germinativum or, simply, the basal layer).

Stratum Corneum. The stratum corneum, or horny layer, is the top layer and is composed of dead keratinized cells. These squames, or corneocytes, are the cells that are abraded by the daily mechanical and chemical trauma of hand-washing, scratching, bathing, exercising, and the changing of clothes. The stratum corneum is composed of layers of thin, stacked, pancake-appearing, anucleate cells. About 80% of these cells are filled with keratin, a tough, fibrous, insoluble protein; hence they are called keratinocytes. Keratinocytes are initially formed in the basal layer and undergo the process of differentiation. The normal stratum corneum is composed of completely differentiated keratinocytes. Keratin is resistant to changes in temperature or pH and to chemical digestion by trypsin and pepsin. This same protein is found in hair and nails; in these structures, keratin is referred to as "hard" keratin compared with the "soft" keratin of the skin (Jacob, Francone, and Lossow, 1982; Solomons, 1983). Stratum corneum thickness varies with age, sex, and disease (Haake and Holbrook, 2001). The deeper layer of the stratum corneum is called the stratum compactum, and the keratin in these cells is more densely packed. These cells also have a diminished capacity to bind water (Haake, Scott, and Holbrook, 2001). Cells in the uppermost layer are partly shed as a result of the proteolytic degradation of the desmosomes, and this layer is also called the stratum dysjunctum.

Stratum Lucidum. The stratum lucidum is the layer directly below the stratum corneum. This layer is found in areas where the epidermis is thicker, such as the palms of the hands or the soles of the feet. The stratum lucidum is absent from thinner skin, such as the eyelids. This layer can be one to five cells thick and is transparent. Cell boundaries are often difficult to identify in histologic sections under a light microscope. The stratum lucidum is a transitional layer where active lysosomal enzymes degrade the nucleus and cellular organelles before moving into the stratum corneum (Jacob, Francone, and Lossow, 1982; Wysocki, 1995).

Stratum Granulosum. The stratum granulosum, or granular layer, is beneath the stratum lucidum when that is present; otherwise it lies beneath the stratum corneum. This layer is one to five cells thick and is so named because of the granules present in the keratinocytes of this layer. The cells of the stratum granulosum have not yet been compressed into a flattened layer and are diamond-shaped. The structures contained in these cells are keratohyalin granules, which become intensely stained with the appropriate acid and basic dyes. The proteins contained in these granules, profilaggrin, intermediate keratin filaments, and loricrin, help to organize the keratin filaments in the intracellular space. Cells in this layer still have active nuclei (Millington and Wilkinson, 1983; Wheater, Burkitt, and Daniels, 1987).

Stratum Spinosum. The stratum spinosum is the next layer, below the stratum granulosum. This layer is often described as the prickly layer because cytoplasmic structures in these cells take on this morphology. Generally the cells of this layer are polyhedral. A prominent feature of the prickle layer is the desmosome, a type of cell-cell junction. Cells in this layer begin to synthesize involucrin, a soluble precursor of the cornified envelopes (Millington and Wilkinson, 1983). The spinous cells contain large bundles of newly synthesized keratin filaments, K1/K10 in addition to K5/K14 still present from the basal layer (Haake, Scott, and Holbrook, 2001).

Stratum Basale or Stratum Germinativum. The stratum basale, or stratum germinativum, is the innermost epidermal layer. It is often referred to simply as the basal layer and can be seen in Figure 3-1. It is a single layer of mitotically active cells called basal keratinocytes, or basal cells. These active cells respond to several factors, such as extracellular matrix, growth factors, hormones, and vitamins. Skin metabolism is mediated by glucose. Glucose utilization in the skin is comparable to muscle. Glucose leaving the circulation crosses the basement membrane and forms a concentration gradient that decreases as it moves to the upper layers of the epidermis.

Once cells leave the basal layer they begin an upward migration, which can take 2 to 3 weeks. It takes approximately 14 days for a cell to move to the stratum corneum and another 14 days to move through the strateum corneum and desquamate (Haake, Scott, and Holbrook, 2001). After leaving the basal layer, the cells begin the process of differentiation. All layers of the epidermis consist of peaks and valleys. This arrangement is more dramatic in the basal layer. In fact, the epidermal protrusions of the basal layer that point downward into the dermis are called rete ridges, or rete pegs. Rete ridges are partly responsible for anchoring the epidermis, thus providing structural integrity. Basal cells in the base of the rete ridges have an increased proliferative capacity compared with cells at the top of the ridges (Briggamann, 1982).

Epidermal stem cells comprise about 10% of the basal cell population. These stem cells have a slow cell cycle and when labeled with a radiolabeled DNA precursor retain the label for long periods. These cells have been identified as the label-retaining cells (Bickenbach 1981). Once cell division occurs, the daughter cell that will undergo differentiation as it moves toward the stratum corneum is called the transient amplifying cell. These transient amplifying cells make up about 50% of the basal keratinocyte population. A portion of the stem cell population is found in the epidermal crypts of the rete pegs and in the bulge region of hair follicles. Dividing cells go through the cell cycle, and the G_1 phase is shortened in states such as wound healing.

The normal keratinocyte cell cycle time is 300 hours but may be as short as 36 hours when psoriasis is present. These stem cell compartments and the transient amplifying cells are both capable of limited or continuing cell division and thus are the cells most likely to reside long enough in the skin to undergo genetic modifications that lead to the development of skin cancers. The use of stem cells alone and in combination with tissue engineering approaches is an area of active research and development in wound care (Griffith and Naughton, 2002).

Also distributed in this layer are melanocytes, the cells responsible for skin pigmentation. These are dendritic cells arising from the neural crest that synthesize melanin. Melanocytes can be detected at 50 days gestation in fetal development (Holbrook, 1998). Under normal conditions, melanocytes rarely divide. In normal skin the number of melanocytes present is nearly the same, regardless of skin color. There is approximately one melanocyte for every 36 basal cells. Dendritic melanocyte structures are responsible for the transfer of pigment to a large number of keratinocytes. The primary difference between light- and dark-skinned individuals is the size and distribution of the melanosomes, the structures containing the melanin pigment, and the activity of the melanocytes. Carotene or carotenoids are responsible for imparting the yellow hue to the skin of some individuals (Jacob, Francone, and Lossow, 1982; Sams, 1990; Solomons, 1983).

Basement Membrane Zone

The basement membrane zone (BMZ), or dermal-epidermal junction (DEJ), is the area that separates the epidermis from the dermis. Closer examination of the BMZ in the past decade has revealed it to be more complex than previously believed. Basal keratinocytes use hemidesmosomes to structurally and functionally attach to the basement membrane zone. The BMZ is subdivided into two distinct zones—lamina lucida and lamina densa. The lamina lucida is so named because it is an electron-translucent zone compared with the electron-dense zone of the lamina densa. The major proteins found in the BMZ are fibronectin, an adhesive glycoprotein; laminin, also a glycoprotein; type IV collagen, a non–fiber-forming collagen; and heparan sulfate proteoglycan, a glycosaminoglycan. A lesser amount of type VII collagen has also been detected. The BMZ anchors the epidermis to the dermis and is the layer that is affected in blister formation. During wound healing the BMZ is disrupted and must be re-formed (Sams, 1990).

Dermis

The dermis, or corium, is the thickest tissue layer of the skin. Compared with the cellular epidermal layer, the dermis is sparsely populated primarily by fibroblast cells and is vascularized and innervated. The dermal layer is derived from the middle embryonic germ layer, the mesoderm. Dermal thickness ranges from 2 to 4 mm but on average is 2 mm. Variations in dermal thickness account for differences in total skin thickness that have been measured throughout the body. The dermis of the back is thicker than the dermis covering the scalp, forehead, abdomen, thigh, wrist, and palm.

The dermal vasculature consists of a network of papillary loops, supported by a deep horizontal plexus. The vasculature functions to provide nutritional support, immune surveillance, wound healing, thermal regulation, hemostasis, and the inflammatory response ion. The formation of the vascular system involves vasculogenesis and angiogenesis. Vasculogenesis is the process that occurs de novo during embryonic development. This process is mediated by antioblasts derived from the mesoderm. Angiogenesis is the process whereby new vessels are formed from preexisting vessels. Angiogeneis is the process involved in wound healing, tumor growth and metastasis, hemangiomas, telangectasia, psoriasis, and scleroderma. Vascular endothelial growth factor or vascular permeability factor (VEGF/VPF), secreted by keratinocytes in response to hypoxia, is responsible for the stimulation of angiogenesis. VEGF/VPF is known to be increased in wound healing. Other factors known to stimulate angiogenesis include acidic and basic fibroblast growth factor (FGF), interleukin-8, platelet-derived endothelial growth factor, placental growth factor, transforming growth factors α and β, oncostatin M, angiogenin, and heparin-binding epidermal growth factor. Inhibitors of angiogenesis include angiostatin, thrombospondin, endostatin, interferon-γ, interleukin-12, and platelet factor 4.

The major proteins found in the dermis are collagen and elastin. The other category of proteins found occupying the space between collagen and elastin fibers is referred to as the ground substance. This category of proteins is largely composed of proteoglycans (PGs) and glycosaminoglycans (GAGs). Included in this category of proteins are chondroitin sulfates and dermatan sulfate (versican, decorin, biglycan), heparan and heparan sulfate proteoglycans (syndecan, perlecan), and chondroitin-6 sulfate proteoglycans. Although these proteins only account for about 0.2% of the dry weight of the dermis, these large molecules are capable of binding up to 1000 times their volume. Thus PGs and GAGs play a role in regulating the water-binding capacity of the dermis that can determine dermal volume and compressibility. Hyaluronan is also found in the dermis and is higher abundance in fetal skin, where it forms a watery, less stable matrix that allows greater cell movement; and is also a factor in scarless healing (Longaker et al, 1990). This material can bind growth factors and provide cellular linkages with other matrix materials (Haake and Holbrook, 1999). Fibroblasts are the cells distributed in this layer that synthesize and secrete these proteins. The dermis is a matrix supporting the epidermis and can be divided into two areas—papillary dermis and reticular dermis (see Figure 3-1).

Papillary Dermis. The papillary dermis lies immediately below the BMZ and forms interdigitating structures with the rete ridges of the epidermis called dermal papillae. The dermal papillae contain papillary loops (Figure 3-2), which supply the necessary oxygen and nutrients to the overlying epidermis via the BMZ. The collagen fibers contained in the papillary dermis are much smaller in diameter and form smaller, wavy, cablelike structures compared with the reticular dermis. This portion of the dermis also contains small elastic fibers and has a greater proportion of ground substance than the reticular dermis.

Reticular Dermis. The reticular dermis is the area below the papillary dermis and forms the base of the dermis. The collagen fibers in this layer are thicker in diameter and form larger cablelike structures. There is no clear separation of papillary and reticular dermis, because the collagen fibers change in size gradually

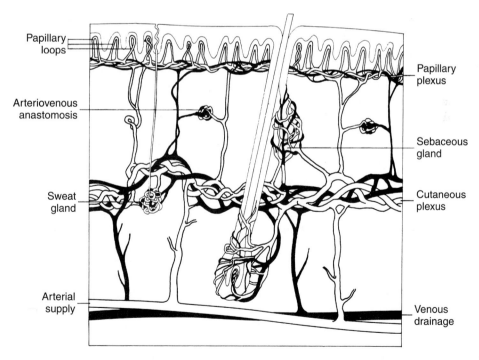

Fig. 3-2 Blood circulation in the skin with papillary loops, which supply oxygen and nutrients to the epidermis, and dermal cutaneous plexuses, which arise from the deeper blood supply located in the hypodermis. (From Wheater PR, Burkett HG, Daniels VG: *Functional histology: a text and colour atlas*, ed 2, Edinburgh, 1987, Churchill Livingstone.)

between the two layers. Thicker elastic fibers are found in the reticular dermis, but substantially less ground substance is present. A complex of cutaneous blood vessels is also found in this part of the dermis.

Dermal Proteins

Collagen. Collagen is the major structural protein found in the dermis and is secreted by dermal fibroblasts as tropocollagen. After additional extracellular processing, mature collagen fibers are formed. Normal human dermis is primarily composed of type I collagen, a fiber-forming collagen. Type I collagen represents about 77% to 85% of the collagen present, and type III collagen, also a fiber-forming collagen, represents the remaining 15% to 23% (Gay and Miller, 1978). Types V and VI collagen are also found in small amounts. Collagen is the protein that gives the skin its tensile strength. Chemically processed collagen from bovine sources leather handbags valued for their strength and long life. The primary constituents of collagen are proline, glycine, hydroxyproline, and hydroxylysine.

Elastin. Elastin, another protein found in the dermis, provides the skin's elastic recoil. This characteristic prevents the skin from being permanently reshaped. Elastin is a fiber-forming protein like collagen and has a high amount of proline and glycine. However, unlike collagen, elastin lacks large amounts of hydroxyproline. Elastin fibers form structures similar to a spring or coil that allow this protein to be stretched and, when released, to return to its inherent configuration. It accounts for less than 2% of the skin's dry weight (Millington and Wilkinson, 1983; Sams, 1990; Wysocki, 1995).

Other cells found in the dermis are mast cells, macrophages, and lymphocytes. All of these cells are involved with immune surveillance of the skin, often referred to as the skin immune system (SIS).

Hypodermis

Hypodermis, or superficial fascia, forms a subcutaneous layer below the dermis. This is an adipose layer containing a subdermal plexus of blood vessels giving rise to the cutaneous plexus in the dermis, which in turn gives rise to the papillary plexus and loops of the papillary dermis (see Figure 3-2). The hypodermis attaches the dermis to underlying structures. This layer provides insulation for the body, a ready reserve of energy, and additional cushioning, and it also adds to the mobility of the skin over underlying structures (Haake and Holbrook, 1999). In certain pathologic disease states such as Werner's syndrome and scleroderma, this layer is largely absent.

SKIN FUNCTIONS

Protection

The skin provides protection against aqueous, chemical, and mechanical assaults; bacterial and viral pathogens; and ultraviolet radiation (UVR). It also prevents excessive loss of fluids and electrolytes to maintain the homeostatic environment. The effectiveness of the skin in preventing excessive fluid loss can be seen in patients with burns; patients with burns involving 30% of their body can lose up to 4.1 liters of fluid compared with 710 ml for a normal adult (Rudowski, 1976). The skin maintains the internal milieu, and a progressive decrease in water content across the epidermal layers helps to prevent excessive transepidermal water loss under basal conditions. The basal layer is about 65% to 70% water, which decreases to 40% in the granular layer and some 15% in the stratum corneum (Warner, Myers, and Taylor, 1988). The skin's barrier function is so effective that percutaneous drug delivery is limited; in general compounds are restricted to those with a molecular mass of 500 daltons or less with a daily dose around 10 mg or less. Protection against mechanical assaults is mainly provided by the tough fibroelastic tissue of the dermis, collagen, and elastin. Collagen, the most abundant protein in mammals, represents 25% of the skin's total weight (Stryer, 1995) and provides tensile strength, which makes the skin resistant to tearing forces. Elastin is distributed with collagen but in smaller amounts. Large concentrations of elastin are present in blood vessels, especially the aortic arch near the heart.

Protection against Pathogens. Protection against aqueous, chemical, bacterial, and viral pathogens is provided by the stratum corneum, secretions from the sebaceous glands, and the skin immune system. The primary line of defense against all of these agents is an intact stratum corneum (Roth and James, 1988). As mentioned previously, the insoluble protein keratin found in the horny layer provides good resistance. In addition, the constant shedding of squames from the stratum corneum prevents the entrenchment of microorganisms.

Sebum, a lipid-rich, oily substance secreted by the sebaceous glands onto the skin surface, usually via hair follicles and shafts, provides an acidic coating with a pH ranging from 4 to 6.8 (Spince and Mason, 1987) and a mean pH of 5.5 (Roth and James, 1988). This acidity, together with natural antibacterial substances found in sebum, retards the growth of microorganisms. These glands are stimulated by sex hormones (androgens) and become very active during adolescence. Sebum, along with keratin, provides resistance to aqueous and chemical solutions. When sebaceous glands occur in association with hair follicles, they are called a pilosebaceous unit. Sebaceous glands are not found on palms or soles and occur in areas that lack hair, such as the lips. These glands are largest on the face and when associated with hair follicles. Sebaceous glands may increase in size by 100 to 150 times as the sebum accumulates. Maximum secretion occurs in the late teens to early twenties. Rates of secretion are higher in men and decline 32% per decade in females compared to 23% per decade in males.

Resistance to pathogenic microorganisms is also provided by normal skin flora through bacterial interference (Weinberg and Swartz, 1987). Conceptually, there are two categories of skin flora—resident (the bacteria normally found on a person) and transient (bacteria that are not normally found on a person and are usually shed by daily hygienic practices, such as bathing and hand washing). Resident bacteria are found on exposed skin; moist areas such as the axillae, perineum, and toe webs; and covered skin. Bacterial microcolonies are found in hair follicles and at the edges of squames as halos in the upper loose surface layers. The following species of bacteria are found in human skin: *Staphylococcus, Micrococcus, Peptococcus, Corynebacterium, Brevibacterium, Proprionibacterium, Streptococcus, Neisseria,* and *Acinetobacter*. The yeast *Pityrosporum* and the mite *Demodex* are also found. Not all species are found on any one individual, but most carry at least five of these genera. Normal viral flora are not known to exist (Noble, 1983). However, viruses have been detected in compromised skin and in individuals who are not immunocompetent.

There is an association between skin pH and bacteria, for example *Proprionibacterium acnes* grows well at pH values such as 6 and 6.5, but there is a marked decrease in growth at pH 5.5 (Korting and Braun-Falco, 1996).

However, it appears that this relationship can vary depending on pH, the specific bacterial species involved, and body location. More recently the formation of bacterial biofilms is being scrutinized (Wysocki, 2002). The role of normal skin flora on the formation of these biofilms is another area of active investigation. Biofilms are essentially an extracellular polysaccharide matrix, or glycocalyx, in which microorganisms are embedded. These biofilms are made up of mixed bacterial species living in their own microniche in a complex, metabolically cooperative microbial community that maintains its own form of homeostasis and rudimentary circulatory system (Costerton et al, 1995). Biofilms are resistant to host immune responses and are markedly more resistant to antibiotic and topical bacteriacidals (Xu, McFeter, and Stewart, 2000). Reports indicate that biofilm cells can be at least 500 times more resistant to antibacterial agents (Costerton et al, 1995). The formation of these biofilms is familiar to clinicians and can be identified on endotracheal tubes, Hickman catheters, central venous catheters, contact lenses, and orthopedic devices. *Pseudomonas aeruginosa* is known to form biofilms in conjunction with other bacterial species. Quorum sensing is a feature of the bacteria in biofilm formation. These biofilms complicate the eradication of infections because they give rise to sessile and planktonic bacteria. Planktonic bacteria can be cleared by phagocytosis, antibodies, and antibiotics (Costerton, Stewart, and Greenberg, 1999). The sessile bacteria in biofilms can evade antibiotics by giving rise to planktonic bacteria that respond to antibiotics and the host immune responses, while the sessile bacteria remain. Many times, cycles of antibiotic treatment are instituted to no avail, and the symptoms of infection recur. In these situations, biofilm formation should be suspected, and the surgical removal of the sessile population will most likely be required to eliminate the pathogenic bacteria. Moist skin areas such as the axillae, perineum, toe webs, hair follicles, nail beds, and sweat glands are especially prone to an increased presence of bacteria. Protection from bacterial invasion is in part mediated by proteins called defensins (Hoffman et al, 1999). Findings show that β-defensin is abundant in skin and may be important for wound healing. Defensins act in conjunction with phagocytosing neutrophils and the membrane attack complex of complement. Thus, optimal skin and wound care is a cornerstone of clinical practice to prevent the progression from bacterial colonization to infection (Wysocki, 2002).

Protection against Ultraviolet Radiation. Protection against ultraviolet radiation is provided by skin pigmentation, which results from synthesis of the pigment melanin. Harmful effects are primarily attributable to the long-wave form of UVR, or UVA, which ranges spectrally from 320 to 400 nm, and UVB, or short-wave ultraviolet, ranging from 290 to 320 nm (Council on Scientific Affairs, 1989). The shorter the waves, the more dangerous they become. UVC is effectively blocked by an intact ozone layer. With holes appearing in the ozone layer, there is concern over the effects that this may have on skin diseases caused by UVR. Because of the increased synthesis, amount, and distribution of melanin in dark skin, darker-skinned individuals are better protected against skin cancer. Melanin is distributed in all layers of the epidermis in dark skin in contrast to light skin (Spince and Mason, 1987). Exposure to UVR can lead to skin cancer, sunburn (first- or second-degree burns), compromised immunity, and long-term skin damage. Sun-exposed epidermal skin is thicker and rougher than unexposed skin. It is more prone to benign and malignant growths and to have a greater decrease in Langerhans' cells. Sun-exposed dermis has increased elastogenesis and a greater decrease in mature collagen with fragmented collagen fibrils, compared to unexposed dermis.

Skin Immune System (SIS)

The SIS also provides protection against invading microorganisms and antigens. The cells of the skin that provide immune protection are the Langerhans' cells, an antigen-presenting cell found in the epidermis; tissue macrophages, which ingest and digest bacteria and other substances; mast cells, which contain histamine (released in inflammatory reactions); and dendrocytes. Both macrophages and mast cells are found in the dermis (Auger, 1989; Benyon, 1989; Wolff and Stingl, 1983).

Langerhans' cells are responsible for the recognition, uptake, processing, and presentation of soluble antigens and haptens to sensitized T lymphocytes. This occurs through the binding of T cells to Langerhans' cells. Exposure to UVB light decreases the functional capability of the Langerhans' cells (Bergstresser, Toews, and Streilein, 1980).

Tissue macrophages are derived from monocytes, which are derived from bone marrow precursor cells. Macrophages are among the most important cells of the skin immune system because they are versatile. Once these monocytes migrate into the tissue, they differentiate and become macrophages. Cells in the dermis that are not completely differentiated are difficult to distinguish, and much effort has been made in the last decade to recognize the various cells in the dermis. Macrophages, in addition to their antibacterial activity, can process and present antigen to immunocompetent lymphoid cells, are tumoricidal, and can secrete growth factors, cytokines, and other immunomodulatory molecules. Macrophages are involved in coagulation, atherogenesis, wound healing, and tissue remodeling (Haake and Holbrook, 1999).

Mast cells are usually found distributed in the papillary dermis, around epidermal appendages, blood vessels, and nerves found in the subpapillary plexus, and in subcutaneous fat. These cells are distributed in connective tissue throughout the body in places where there is an interface of an organ with the environment. Mast cells contain or secrete on demand a host of proteins. Thus mast cells are the primary effector cells in an allergic reaction. They are also involved in the presence of subacute and chronic inflammatory disease. Increased numbers of mast cells have been detected in tissues affected by chronic eczema, psoriasis, scleroderma, porphyria cutanea tarda, lichen simplex chronicus, and lichen planus, and in healing wounds. As a part of the SIS, mast cells play a role in protection against parasites, stimulate chemotaxis, promote phagocytosis, are involved in the activation and proliferation of eosinophils, are capable of altering vasotension and vascular permeability, and can promote connective tissue repair and angiogenesis. Their role in tumor surveillance awaits further study (Haake and Holbrook, 1999).

Dermal dendrocytes are highly phagocytic cells found in the papillary and upper reticular dermis. They are also distributed near vessels in the subpapillary plexus, reticular dermis, and subcutaneous fat. These are immunologically competent cells that are highly phagocytic and can be recognized as melanophages. In fetal, infant, photoaged, and pathologic skin conditions such as psoriasis or eczema, their number is increased (Headington, 1986). In malignant fibrotic tumors and fibroproliferative lesions, such as keloids, scars, and scleroderma, their numbers are decreased (Headington and Cerio, 1990).

Thermoregulation

Thermoregulation of the body is provided by the skin, which acts as a barrier between the outside and inside environments to maintain body temperature. The two primary thermoregulatory mechanisms are circulation and sweating. Blood vessels can either dilate to dissipate heat or constrict to shunt heat to underlying body organs. When dilated, these vessels have an increased blood flow and release heat by conduction, convection, radiation, and evaporation. Vasoconstriction is often accompanied by actions of the arrector pili muscle attached to hair follicles, which results in the hair standing vertically. In mammals that depend on hair for warmth, this action fluffs up the fur to increase thermal capacity. The bulge around the hair shaft that is visible when this occurs is commonly referred to as goose bumps. In humans, shivering is more important for maintaining body temperature when the outside environment is cold than the vertical orientation of hair (Jacob, Francone, and Lossow, 1982; Sams, 1990). In cold weather the "core" body temperature encompasses a smaller zone, whereas in warm weather the "core" is expanded. Sensations of cold and warm are generally detected below 30° C and above 37° C. Clinically it has been estimated that for each 1° C (1.8° F) increase in fever there is a 13% increase in a patient's fluid and calorie needs. At rest the trunk, the viscera, and the brain account for 70% of heat production but comprise only 36% of body mass. However, during exercise, muscle and skin account for 90% of heat production while representing 56% of body mass (Wenger, 1999).

Hair follicles, unlike other skin structures, have a repeated cycle of growth and regression. Follicle development begins in the fourth month of gestation. The hair growth cycle consists of anagen (growth phase), catagen (follicle involution), and telogen phases (dormant or resting phase). Also, a population of epidermal stem cells are found in the bulge region of the hair follicle, and this cell population contributes to reepithelialization in partial-thickness wounds. Hair shape varies depending on ethnicity and location. Asians have the largest diameter scalp hair and Caucasians the smallest. In the scalp, about 85% of hair is in anagen phase and 15% in telogen phase, with the anagen phase lasting from 2 to 5 years. On the extremities, anagen lasts from 22 to 28 days (Freinkel, 2001).

Sweating occurs when there is an increase in the activity of the sweat glands. It has been estimated that there are about 2 to 5 million sweat glands. Sweat glands are of two types—eccrine and apocrine. Eccrine glands arise from epidermal invagination and are found abundantly on the palms of the hand and the soles of the feet. There are anywhere from 2 to 5 million glands, 0.05 to 0.1 mm in size. These glands are largely under the control of the nervous system, responding to temperature differences and emotional stimulation. Muscular activity also influences their secretory activity. The sweat glands, located in the dermis as a coil, secrete fluid that is 99% to 99.5% water, with the remainder consisting of sodium chloride, urea, sulfates, and phosphates (Solomons, 1983; Spince and Mason, 1987). The pH is slightly acidic. Thermoregulatory control occurs as a result of cooling when fluid is evaporated from the skin surface, since such evaporation requires heat. The odor associated with sweat is largely a result of bacterial action. Eccrine sweat glands are capable of producing 1 to 4 liters per hour, resulting in a 75% to 90% reduction in body heat. Man is capable of losing heat more rapidly and for longer periods than any other animal (Quinton, 1983).

Apocrine sweat glands are usually found in association with hair follicles but do not play a significant role in thermoregulation. These coiled, tubular glands are present in the axillae and the anogenital area; modifications of these glands are found in the ear and secrete ear wax, or cerumen (Spince and Mason, 1987). There are approximately 100,000 apocrine glands, each 2 to 3 mm in diameter. Secretions from these glands are small in amount, are turbid, and contain iron, carbohydrates, and lipids.

Sensation

Nerve receptors located in the skin are sensitive to pain, touch, temperature, and pressure. Nerve fibers are located in the dermis and throughout the epidermis. Nerve structures found in the skin originate from the neural crest and are detectable in the developing embryo at around 5 weeks' gestation. When stimulated, these receptors transmit impulses to the cerebral cortex where they are interpreted. Combinations of these four basic types of sensations result in burning, tickling, and itching (Jacob, Francone, and Lossow, 1982). These sensations are propagated by unmyelinated free nerve endings, Merkel cells, Meissner's corpuscles, Krause's end bulbs, Ruffini's terminals, and Pacini's corpuscles. Identification of particular responses with specific nerve structures has not been successful. In part, the reason is that some receptors seem to respond to a variety of stimuli. However, it is known that Meissner's corpuscles are involved in touch reception; Pacini's corpuscles (see Figure 3-1) respond to pressure, coarse touch, vibration, and tension; and free nerve endings respond to touch, pain, and temperature (Wheater, Burkitt, and Daniels, 1987).

Skin sensation is a part of the body's integrative response to protect itself from the surrounding environment. Sensation assists with the skins regulatory function and can signal sweating, shivering, weight shifts (Alterescu and Alterescu, 1988), laughter, and scratching.

Merkel cells function as mechanoreceptors, and in the epidermis these cells produce nerve growth factor, whereas in the dermis, Merkel cells express receptors for nerve growth factor (Narasawa et al, 1992). Merkel cells are found around the arrector pili muscle in the bulge region of hair follicles and contribute to the development of eccrine sweat glands, nails, and nerves of the skin (Kim and Holbrook, 1995; Narasawa, Hashimoto, and Kohda, 1996).

Sensation also moderates psychobiologic phenomena made famous by Harlow, who demonstrated the preference of young animals for warm objects and those that provided better tactile sensitivity. In addition, early studies by Spitz (1947) point to the importance of touch in mediating social interactions with children and infants. Deprivation of touch can lead to psychomotor retardation and an increased risk of death (Ottenbacher et al, 1987). Other studies on touch indicate that it may be a factor in the development of atherosclerotic lesions in animals. In studies examining the effect of stroking, handling, talking, and playing with rabbits, investigators (Nerem, Levesque, and Cornhill, 1980) found a 60% reduction in aortic atherosclerotic lesions in treated animals compared with controls, even though both groups were fed the same cholesterol-containing diet and had similar blood pressures, heart rates, and serum cholesterol levels.

In healing wounds, sensory nerves sprout abundantly for about the first 3 weeks, subsequently returning to their normal density. The role of neuropeptides to stimulate the growth of connective tissue is increasingly being recognized. This includes a role for these neuropeptides in modulating matrix production by fibroblasts and in acting as growth factors for keratinocytes (Metze and Luger, 2001; Baraniuk, 1997; Kiss et al, 1995).

Metabolism

Synthesis of vitamin D occurs in the skin in the presence of sunlight. Ultraviolet radiation converts a sterol (7-dehydrocholesterol) to cholecalciferol (vitamin D). Vitamin D participates in calcium and phosphate metabolism and is important in the mineralization of bone. Because vitamin D is synthesized in the skin but then transmitted to other parts of the body, it is considered an active hormone when converted to calcitriol (1,25-dihydroxycholecalciferol) (Lehninger, 1982; Stryer, 1995).

Communication

In addition to its biologic, structural, functional, and physiologic functions, human skin also functions as an organ of communication and identification. The skin over the face is especially important for identification of a person and plays a role in internal and external assessments of beauty. Injury to the skin can result in not only functional and physiologic consequences, but also changes in body image. Scarring from trauma, surgery, or incisions can lead to changes in clothing choices, avoidance of public exposure, and a decrease in self-esteem. Research (Shuster et al, 1978) indicates that with increased scarring from facial acne, the self-image is progressively reduced. Adolescents are especially sensitive to physical appearance (Bernstein, 1976). As an organ of communication, facial skin along with underlying muscles is capable of expressions such as smiling, frowning, and pouting. The sensation of touching can also convey feelings of comfort, concern, friendship, and love.

FACTORS ALTERING SKIN CHARACTERISTICS
Age

Age is an important factor in altering skin characteristics. More recently the scarless healing of fetal tissue has come under more intense investigation (Longaker et al, 1990; Siebert et al, 1990). It has been found that wounds heal without scarring in fetal lambs up until 120 days of gestation. Collagen deposition in fetal wounds occurs more rapidly and in a normal dermal pattern (Longaker et al, 1990). The ratio of type I and type III collagen is different in fetal skin, and about 30% to 60% of the collagen is type III, whereas in adult skin it comprises about 10% to 15% (Bullard, Longaker, and Lorenz, 2003). In addition, an important difference between fetal and adult skin is the amount of hyaluronic acid, a glycosaminoglycan. In the laboratory setting, topical application of hyaluronic acid has been associated with a reduction in scar formation in postnatal wounds. This glycosaminoglycan is associated with collagen, and it has been proposed that a hyaluronic acid-collagen-protein complex plays a role in fetal scarless healing (Siebert et al, 1990). Transforming growth factor beta-1 (TGF-β1) is the other modulator of scarless healing in fetal wounds. Fetal wounds usually contain less TGF-β1 compared with adult wounds (Roberts and Sporn, 1996). In addition, differential patterns of expression of the various isoforms of TGF- also affect the relative amount of scarring in fetal as opposed to adult wounds. Wounding in fetal skin also reveals differences in the cell responses, showing a decrease in inflammatory cells, particularly polymorphonuclear leukocytes and macrophages. Platelets do not aggregate in response to collagen or release the amount of TGF-β and platelet derived growth factor-AB (PDGF-AB) like that in adult cells. Fibroblasts are able to migrate at a faster rate and synthesize more total collagen. Differences in protease and inhibitor activity, level of growth factors, and expression of homeobox genes have also been detected (Bullard, Longaker, and Lorenz, 2003).

At birth the skin and nails are thinner than those in an adult, but with aging they will gradually increase in thickness. Formation of the epidermal and dermal layers occurs within the first 2 weeks of embryonic development. Epidermal development is complete by the end of the second trimester, and at birth, epidermal thickness is almost that of adult skin, although newborn skin is not as effective as adult skin in providing a barrier to transcutaneous water loss. On the other hand, development of the dermis lags behind and does not take on the characteristics of adult dermis until after birth.

The ratio of type I to type III collagen is similar to the fetal ratios. Soluble collagen is about 24%, compared with 1% in the adult. This persists until about 6 months of age. The newborn dermis is about 60% as thick as that found in an adult and, as expected, the dermal fibers are significantly finer. Newborn dermis contains a much higher cellular component compared with mature adult skin. The epidermal-dermal junction remains flat until the beginning of the third trimester, and at birth the rete ridges are only weakly developed, thus making premature and newborn skin prone to tearing or blistering. At birth the capillary beds do not have a mature adult pattern and are still disorganized. An adult pattern of capillary loops occurs at about 14 to 17 weeks, after skin growth slows (Holbrook, 1991).

Immature skin, or skin from premature infants between 23 or 24 weeks' and up to 32 weeks' gestation, requires special attention compared with that of infants beyond 32 weeks' gestation. In particular, before 28 weeks' gestation the skin is thin and poorly keratinized and functions weakly as a barrier. An article appearing in *Lancet* (Immature skin, 1989) has characterized the skin of infants born at the limits of viability as more suitable to an "aquatic environment" than to atmospheric conditions. Transepidermal water loss is high, and application of adhesives to the outer immature epidermal layer can leave behind raw, damaged skin prone to infection and occasional scarring. At 24 weeks' gestation, transepidermal water loss can be 10 times greater per unit area compared with an infant born at term (Rutter, 1988). Infants born between 22-25 weeks' gestation may require up to 4 weeks to develop a functional stratum corneum (Evans and Rutter, 1986; Harpin and Rutter, 1983; Kalia et al, 1998). In addition, premature infants have high evaporative heat losses, resulting in increased risk for hypothermia.

Because premature infants have a greater surface-area-to-volume ratio compared with full-term infants, they are at an increased risk for skin complications and systemic toxicity from topically applied agents. These infants may also have alterations in metabolism, excretion, distribution, and protein binding of chemical agents, placing them at increased risk for local or systemic toxicity from soaps, lotions, or other topical agents (Weston and Lane, 1999). Other dangers are percutaneous absorption of topical agents, including antiseptics. Hemorrhagic necrosis of the dermis from alcohol absorption has been reported, if the alcohol does not quickly evaporate, and is sometimes mistaken for bruising. The use of topical antibiotic sprays containing neomycin should be avoided since it is an ototoxic aminoglycoside. Thus water-based topical antiseptics are preferred but should be used sparingly. Cleaning should be done with care, using normal saline or water. Chlorhexidine, a commonly used antiseptic, is not known to have any adverse effects, but it is probably absorbed from the skin and should be used judiciously. Likewise iodine has been reported to be absorbed, leading to goiter and hypothyroidism (Rutter, 1988). If required, moisturizing creams or ointments may be applied to dry, flaking, or fissured skin, and the best agents appear to be those with few or no preservatives since these offer the greatest benefit with decreased risk (Weston and Lane, 1999).

Interestingly, exposure of the premature infant's skin to air seems to accelerate skin maturation; full maturation occurs in about 2 weeks after birth. Similar findings using an animal model support these observations. Interventions that seem to be helpful during this 2-week period are the avoiding of tape applications to the skin by means of the use of a self-adherent wrap (e.g., Coban, 3M Co.). Coban roll gauze or stockinette material (Bryant, 1988). Raising the humidity of the air close to the skin surface in the incubator or use of a waterproof blanket appears useful. The use of surface probes should be minimized, if possible. It has been reported that the use of polyurethane film dressings, such as Tegaderm or Opsite, have several advantages. This dressing material results in a 50% reduction in transepidermal water loss, allows the attachment of temperature and electrocardiogram (ECG) electrodes, resulting in the achievement of normal readings, and can provide a surface that can be taped. Polyurethane film dressings provide air exchange but prevent bacterial invasion, and they have good release characteristics that eliminate or minimize skin damage from stripping when removed. Karaya gum ECG electrodes also seem to be beneficial by reducing pain and epidermal damage when removed, and they can be repositioned for ultrasound or radiographic examinations. Polyurethane film dressings can hinder gas transfer, and PO_2 and PCO_2 readings are not accurate when they are in place. Skin sealants appear to eliminate this problem. Further studies of the use of polyurethane film dressings is warranted (Immature skin, 1989).

The next period of change occurs in adolescence, when hormonal stimulation results in increased activity of sebaceous glands and hair follicles. Sebaceous glands increase their secretory rate, and hair follicles become activated, giving rise to secondary sexual characteristics. From adolescence to adulthood there is a gradual change in skin characteristics. By the time the skin reaches mature adulthood, several changes become apparent. The dermis decreases in thickness by about 20%, whereas the epidermis remains relatively unchanged. Epidermal turnover time is increased; this means that wound healing may take longer. For instance, in young adults, epidermal turnover takes about 21 days, but by 35 years of age this turnover time is doubled. Barrier function is reduced, and such reduction may increase the risk of irritation. The number of active melanocytes per unit body surface area decreases with aging, which means that protection against UVR is diminished. Skin dryness is also associated with aging and an increase in wrinkles. Sensory receptors are diminished in capacity, meaning that the skin is more likely to be burned or traumatized without perception. Vitamin D production is decreased and may be a factor in osteomalacia.

With aging there is a decrease in the number of Langerhans' cells, which affects the immunocompetence of the skin and can lead to an increased risk of skin cancer and infection by invading microorganisms. The density of Langerhans' cells changes from 10 per 3 mm cross-section of unexposed skin in 22- to 26-year-old persons to 5.8 per 3 mm cross-section in 62- to 68-year-old persons (Gilchrest, Murphy, and Soter, 1982). There is also a decrease in the numbers of mast cells and melanocytes. The inflammatory response is decreased, and such a decrease may alter allergic reactions and healing. A decrease in the number of sweat glands, diminished vascularity, and a reduction in the amount of subcutaneous fat compromise the thermoregulatory capacity of the skin. Epidermal-dermal junction changes, such as the flattening of the prominent dermal papillae and of the rete ridges, alter junctional integrity. Consequently, the skin is more easily torn in response to mechanical trauma, especially shearing forces. Because the epidermal rete pegs flatten, the unique microenvironment of the basal keratinocytes changes; it is thought that this explains the decrease in epidermal proliferative capacity that occurs with aging (Lavker, Zheng, and Dong, 1986).

Skin elasticity decreases with age and is related to a combination of aging and solar damage. Microscopic analysis of collagen and elastin fibers reveals that these are more compact, with a loss of ground substance from the spaces between these cablelike structures. Collagen fibers appear to be unwinding whereas elastin fibers appear to be lysing. The degradation of elastin can be detected at about 30 years of age but becomes marked at 70 years of age (Braverman, 1986). Changes in dermal proteoglycans usually occur after 40 years of age (Yanagishita, 1994). By 70 years of age, most of the elastin network is affected. Changes in collagen content and structure are mediated by an under-expression of procollagen, an over-expression of collagenase (MMP-1), stromelysin (MMP-3), and gelatinase A (MMP-2), and a decreased expression of tissue inhibitors of matrix metalloproteinase-1 (TIMP-1). There is also a marked reduction in vascular beds in the vertical capillary loops in the dermal papillae. There is an approximately 35% decrease in the cross-sectional area of these loops in aged skin. It is thought that this leads to atrophy of the hair bulbs, the sweat glands, and the sebaceous glands. Because the hypodermis also becomes thinner, mature individuals are more prone to pressure necrosis (Gilchrest, 1989). With aging, a progressive loss of mechanoreceptors to one third of their average density occurs from the second to the ninth decade (Metze and Luger, 2001).

The density of skin melanocytes is relatively constant until about 40 years of age. By about 45 years of age, skin melanocytes have decreased in density to approximately half that seen between 30 and 39 years of age (Nordlund, 1986). Melanocytes decrease 6% to 8% each decade after age 30. It is thought that the loss of skin melanocytes contributes to an increase in the formation of skin cancers. Other overt changes are wrinkling and sagging, which occur as a result of the loss of underlying tissue, in addition to changes seen in collagen and elastin.

Changes in hair color and hair follicles also accompany aging. Age-related changes in active melanocytes result in gray hair. About 50% of the body's hair will be gray by the age of 50 in about 50% of the population. This change is accompanied by a reduction in the number of hair follicles and a decrease in the diameter of the hair. The rate of hair growth is also decreased (Silverberg and Silverberg, 1989). Nail growth rates also decrease by 40% to 50%.

Changes in thermoregulatory capacity occur with age, and older individuals are more prone to hypothermia and heat stroke. This has been attributed to changes in blood capillaries and eccrine sweat glands. In healthy older individuals, sweating may be decreased by up to 70% (Gilchrest, 1991). Sebum secretion also declines with age. Barrier function decreases with aging owing to the decreased level of all the major lipid species, especially ceramides. In addition, corneocytes are larger and less cohesive. In addition to these changes, pain perception is dulled, and there is reduced skin reactivity upon exposure to irritants. Cutaneous immune function also changes with aging, as seen by a reduction in Langerhans' cell density. Skin damaged by sun exposure, or actinically damaged skin, has been found to have a 50% reduction of Langerhans' cell density compared with sun-protected skin (Sauder, 1986). Reduction in immunocompetence of the skin is thought to contribute in part to skin cancer in the elderly.

Other factors that may contribute to the development of skin cancer in aged individuals are cumulative exposure to carcinogens, diminished DNA repair capacity, decreased melanocyte density, and alterations in dermal matrix (Lin and Carter, 1986). Not surprisingly, wound healing in older individuals is delayed compared with that of younger individuals.

Sun

Excessive exposure to UVR can have harmful effects that accelerate aging of the skin. For this reason the condition associated with UVR-damaged skin is referred to as photoaging. Dermatologically, it is called dermatoheliosis. Obvious clinical signs of photodamaged skin are dryness, tough and leathery texture, wrinkling (as a result of collagen and elastin degeneration), and irregular pigmentation (from changes in melanin distribution) (Silverberg and Silverberg, 1989). Excessive exposure to UVR increases the risk of developing skin cancers such as basal or squamous cell carcinoma and malignant melanoma. Damage to the DNA of skin cells leads to transformation of cells and cancer (Council on Scientific Affairs, 1989). Changes also occur in epidermal and dermal cells; epidermal cells become thickened, fibroblasts become more numerous, and dermal vessels become dilated and tortuous. Langerhans' cells are reduced in number by about 50%, thereby diminishing the immunocompetence of the skin (Lober and Fenske, 1990).

Exposure to UVR can lead to sunburn. Sunburn is partly the result of a vasodilatory response that increases blood volume. Whether an individual will become sunburned depends on the extent of skin pigmentation. Naturally, those with the least pigmentation are more prone to sunburn and the harmful, long-term effects of UVR. Severe short-term exposure of unprotected, lightly pigmented skin can lead to blistering (a second-degree burn).

There is an association between melanoma and sunburn: if a patient has had more than six serious sunburns, then he or she is at an increased risk for melanoma (Green et al, 1985). Exposure to UVR and the rise of malignant melanomas has led to the development of more effective sun-blocking agents. Over time the lifetime risk of malignant melanoma has increased from 1/1500 people in 1930 to 1/250 in 1980 to 1/62 in 2005. By the year 2010 the lifetime risk is expected to be 1/50 (Potts, 1990; Rigel et al, 2005). Sunscreens should be used on a regular basis, be applied at least 30 minutes before exposure, and have a sun protection factor (SPF) ranging from 15 to 30 (Pathak et al, 1999). Individuals with moderately pigmented skin require about 3 to 5 times more exposure to UVR to induce sunburn inflammation compared with Caucasians, and for individuals with darker skin, 10 times more exposure is required (McGregor and Hawk, 1999).

Hydration

Adequate skin hydration is normally provided by sebum secretion and an intact stratum corneum with its keratinized cells. Several factors can affect skin hydration. Among these are relative humidity, removal of sebum, and age. Each of these factors increase water loss from the skin, leading to dryness and scaling. Application of emollients to the skin replaces the barrier function of lost sebum or decreased evaporative water loss when the relative humidity is low. Retention of water in the epidermal layers after application of a lotion leads to swelling of the skin, which is perceived as smoothness and softness.

Often, various products are promoted with claims of superiority over others without adequate in vitro, in vivo, or clinical data. The superiority of oil baths over water baths was found to be only marginal (Stender, Blichmann, and Serup, 1990). Twenty minutes after both kinds of bath, skin hydration was increased when measured by water evaporation and electrical conductance and capacitance. A small but significantly greater amount of water was bound in the skin after the oil bath, whereas no change was seen in evaporation, conductance, or capacitance. Thus increases in water-holding capacity of the skin after an oil bath may not be of importance. On the other hand, a difference was found in skin-surface lipids, which lasted at least 3 hours. This effect is comparable with application of a traditional moisturizing lotion. The authors of this study conclude that because daily use of bath oil is not practical, application of moisturizing lotions may be more advantageous and that the beneficial effects of bath oils are related to lipidization of the skin surface (Stender, Blichmann, and Serup, 1990).

Soaps

Washing or bathing with an alkaline soap reduces the thickness and number of cell layers in the stratum corneum (White, Jenkinson, and Lloyd, 1987). Generally, soap emulsifies the lipid coating of the skin and removes it along with resident and transient bacteria. Excessive use of soap or detergents can interfere with the water-holding capacity of the skin and may impair bacterial resistance. Use of alkaline soaps increases skin pH, which may change bacterial resistance. The time for recovery to normal skin pH of 5.5 depends on the length of exposure. Ordinary washing requires 45 minutes to restore skin pH, whereas prolonged exposure can require 19 hours (Bettley, 1960). Other agents that can lead to delipidization or dehydration of skin are alcohol and acetone. Currently, acidic skin cleansers appear to be less irritating than neutral or alkaline ones, and there is some evidence to suggest that acidic cleansers decrease the number of acne lesions on the face (Korting and Braun-Falco, 1996).

Nutrition

Normal, healthy skin integrity can be maintained by an adequate dietary intake of protein, carbohydrate, fats, vitamins, and minerals. Under normal conditions in healthy persons, supplementary nutrition is not beneficial if there is adequate dietary intake. If the skin is damaged, increased dietary intake of some substances, such as vitamin C for collagen formation, may be beneficial. A healthy diet of protein breaks down to supply the necessary amino acids for protein synthesis. Fats are broken down into essential fatty acids, which can then be used by cells to form their lipid bilayer. Carbohydrates are digested to supply energy for cell metabolism. Needed to maintain a normal, healthy skin are vitamins C, D, and A; the B vitamins pyridoxine and riboflavin; the mineral elements iron, zinc, and copper; and many others. Adequate dietary intake can be ensured by ingestion of amounts consistent with the recommended daily allowances (RDA) (Roe, 1986).

Medications

Various medications affect the skin. Some of the best studied are the corticosteroids, which are known to interfere with epidermal regeneration and collagen synthesis (Ehrlich and Hunt, 1968; Pollack, 1982). Photosensitive and phototoxic reactions are also known to occur from medications. Some categories of medications that can affect the skin are antibacterials, antihypertensives, analgesics, tricyclic antidepressants, antihistamines, antineoplastic agents, antipsychotic drugs, diuretics, hypoglycemic agents, sunscreens, and oral contraceptives (Potts, 1990). Skin flora can be changed by the use of antibacterials, orally administered steroids, and hormones. Analgesics, antihistamines, and nonsteroidal antiinflammatory drugs (NSAIDs) can alter inflammatory reactions. Thus whenever drugs are prescribed and skin reactions occur, medications should always be checked to see whether they are responsible.

SUMMARY

As the body's largest organ, the skin serves several complex functions: protection, thermoregulation, sensation, metabolism, and communication. Numerous factors influence the skin's ability to adequately provide these functions such as age, UVR exposure, hydration, medications, nutrition, and soaps. The skin's integrity can also be jeopardized by many of these factors.

Wound management and skin care must be grounded in a comprehensive knowledge base of the structure and function of the skin. After reviewing this chapter, the care provider should closely scrutinize many of the skin-care practices and bathing routines that are subconsciously engrained in day-to-day patient care activities and that may compromise the function and integrity of the skin.

SELF-ASSESSMENT EXERCISE

1. Explain why maintenance of skin integrity is vital to health and life.
2. List the key layers of the skin.
3. Explain why the cells of the stratum corneum are also called keratinocytes.
4. Which of the following is known as the reproductive layer of the epidermis?
   a. Stratum lucidum
   b. Stratum granulosum
   c. Stratum germinativum, or basal layer
   d. Stratum spinosum, or prickly layer
5. Describe the significance of rete ridges.
6. From which of the following does the epidermis receive its vascular nourishment?
   a. Basement membrane
   b. Papillary dermis
   c. Reticular dermis
   d. Stratum germinativum
7. Describe the purpose and key constituents of the two dermal proteins.
8. List the six major functions of the skin.
9. Identify at least two mechanisms by which the skin protects against pathogenic invasion.
10. Which of the following components of the skin immune system are derived from bone marrow precursor cells?
    a. Mast cells
    b. Fibroblasts
    c. Macrophages
    d. Langerhans' cells
11. Which of the following can be synthesized in the skin?
    a. Vitamin E
    b. Vitamin K
    c. Vitamin D
    d. Vitamin A
12. List characteristics of premature skin and newborn skin.
13. Identify changes in the skin that occur in adolescence and in adulthood.
14. Excessive exposure to ultraviolet radiation creates all of the following skin changes EXCEPT:
    a. Irregular pigmentation
    b. Increased number of Langerhans' cells
    c. Malignant melanoma
    d. Wrinkling
15. True or False: Excessive use of soaps or detergents may impair the bacterial resistance of the skin.

16. Which of the following is known to interfere with epidermal regeneration and collagen synthesis?
   a. Antibiotics
   b. Oral contraceptives
   c. Steroids
   d. Antihypertensives

REFERENCES

Alterescu V, Alterescu K: Etiology and treatment of pressure ulcers, *Decubitus* 1(1):28, 1988.

Auger MJ: Mononuclear phagocytes, *BMJ* 298:546, 1989.

Baraniuk JN: Neuropeptides in the skin. In Bos JD, editor: *The skin immune system*, ed 2, Boca Raton, 1997, CRC Press.

Benyon RC: The human skin mast cell, *Clin Exp Allergy* 19:375, 1989.

Bergstresser PR, Toews GB, Streilein JW: Natural and perturbed distributions of Langerhans cells: responses to ultraviolet light, heterotopic skin grafting, and dinitrofluorobenzene sensitization, *J Invest Dermatol* 75:73, 1980.

Bernstein NR: Appearance: concepts of perception and disfigurement; Body and face images: personality and self-representation; Disfigurement and personality development. In Bernstein NR: *Emotional care of the facially burned and disfigured*, Boston, 1976, Little, Brown.

Bettley FR: Some effects of soap on the skin, *BMJ* 1:1675, 1960.

Bickenbach JR: Identification and behavior of label-retaining cells in oral mucosa and skin, *J Dent Res* 60:1611, 1981.

Braverman IM: Elastic fiber and microvascular abnormalities in aging skin. In Gilchrest BA, editor: The aging skin, *Dermatol Clin* 4:391, 1986.

Briggamann RA: Epidermal-dermal interaction in adult skin, *J Invest Dermatol* 88:569, 1982.

Bryant RA: Saving the skin from tape injuries, *Am J Nurs* 88(2):189, 1988.

Bullard KM, Longaker MT, Lorenz HP: Fetal wound healing: current biology, *World J Surg* 27:54, 2003.

Costerton JW et al: Microbial biofilms, *Annu Rev Microbiol* 49:711, 1995.

Costerton JW, Stewart PS, Greenberg EP: Bacterial biofilms: a common cause of persistent infections, *Science* 284:1318, 1999.

Council on Scientific Affairs: Harmful effects of ultraviolet radiation, *JAMA* 262:380, 1989.

Ehrlich HP, Hunt TK: Effects of cortisone and vitamin A on wound healing, *Ann Surg* 167:324, 1968.

Evans NJ, Rutter N: Development of the epidermis in the newborn, *Biol Neonate* 49:74, 1986.

Freinkel RK: Hair. In Freinkel RK, Woodley DT, editors: *The biology of the skin*, New York, 2001, Parthenon Publishing Group.

Gay S, Miller S: *Collagen in the physiology and pathology of connective tissue*, Stuttgart, Germany, 1978, Gustav Fischer Verlag.

Gilchrest BA: Physiology and pathophysiology of aging skin. In Goldsmith LA, editor: *Physiology, biochemistry, and molecular biology of the skin*, ed 2, New York, 1991, Oxford University Press.

Gilchrest BA: Skin aging and photoaging, *J Am Acad Dermatol* 21:610, 1989.

Gilchrest BA, Murphy G, Soter N: Effect of chronologic aging and the ultraviolet irradiation on Langerhans cells in human epidermis, *J Invest Dermtol* 79:85, 1982.

Green et al: Sunburn and malignant melanoma, *Br J Cancer* 51:393, 1985.

Griffith LG, Naughton G: Tissue engineering—current challenges and expanding opportunities, *Science* 295:1009, 2002.

Haake AR, Holbrook K: The structure and development of skin. In Freedberg IM et al, editors: *Fitzpatrick's dermatology in general medicine*, ed 5, New York, 1999, McGraw-Hill.

Haake A, Scott GA, Holbrook KA: Structure and function of the skin: overview of the epidermis and dermis. In Freinkel RK, Woodley DT, editors: *The biology of the skin*, New York, 2001, Parthenon Publishing Group.

Harpin VA, Rutter N: Barrier properties of the newborn infant's skin, *J Pediatr* 102:419, 1983.

Headington JT: The dermal dendrocyte, *Adv Dermatol* 1:159, 1986.

Headington JT, Cerio R: Dendritic cells and the dermis, *Am J Dermatopathol* 12:217, 1990.

Hoffman JA et al: Phylogenetic perspectives in innate immunity, *Science* 284:1313, 1999.

Holbrook KA: Structure and function of the developing human skin. In Goldsmith LA, editor: *Physiology, biochemistry, and molecular biology of the skin*, ed 2, New York, 1991, Oxford University Press.

Holbrook KA: Melanocytes in human embryonic and fetal skin: a review and new findings, *Pigment Cell Res* 1(Suppl):6, 1998.

Immature skin, *Lancet* 2(8672):1138, 1989.

Jacob SW, Francone CA, Lossow WJ: *Structure and function in man*, ed 5, Philadelphia, 1982, W.B. Saunders.

Kalia VN et al: Development of skin barrier function in premature infants, *J Invest Dermatol* 111:320, 1998.

Kim DK, Holbrook KA: The appearance, density and distribution of Merkel cells in human embryonic and fetal skin: their relation to sweat glands, and hair follicle development, *J Invest Dermatol* 104:411, 1995.

Kiss M et al: Alpha-melanocyte stimulating hormone induces collagenase/matrix metalloproteinase-1 in human dermal fibroblasts, *Biol Chem Hoppe Seyler* 376:425, 1995.

Korting HC, Braun-Falco O: The effect of detergents on skin pH and its consequences, *Clinics Dermatol* 14:23, 1996.

Lavker RM, Zheng P, Dong G: Morphology of aged skin. In Gilchrest BA, editor: The aging skin, *Dermatol Clin* 4:379, 1986.

Lehninger AL: *Principles of biochemistry*, New York, 1982, Worth Publishers.

Lin AN, Carter DM: Skin cancer in the elderly, *Dermatol Clin* 4(3):467, 1986.

Lober CW, Fenske NA: Photoaging and the skin: differentiation and clinical response, *Geriatrics* 45:36, 1990.

Longaker MT et al: Studies in fetal wound healing. VI. Second and early third trimester fetal wounds demonstrate rapid collagen deposition without scar formation, *J Pediatr Surg* 25:63, 1990.

Longaker MT et al: Studies in fetal wound healing. VII. Fetal wound healing may be modulated by hyaluronic acid and stimulating activity in amniotic fluid, *J Pediatr Surg* 25:430, 1990.

McGregor JM, Hawk JLM: Acute effects of ultraviolet radiation on the skin. In Freedberg IM et al, editors: *Fitzpatrick's dermatology in general medicine*, ed 5, New York, 1999, McGraw-Hill.

Metze D, Luger T: Nervous system in the skin. In Freinkel RK, Woodley DT, editors: *The biology of the skin*, New York, 2001, Parthenon Publishing Group.

Millington PF, Wilkinson R: *Skin*, Cambridge, England, 1983, Cambridge University Press.

Narasawa Y et al: Biological significance of dermal Merkel cells in development of cutaneous nevus in human fetal skin, *J Histochem Cytochem* 40:65, 1992.

Narasawa Y, Hashimoto K, Kohda H: Merkel cells participate in the induction and alignment of epidermal ends of arrector pili muscles of human fetal skin, *Br J Dermatol* 134:494, 1996.

Nerem RM, Levesque MJ, Cornhill JF: Social environment as a factor in diet-induced atherosclerosis, *Science* 208:1475, 1980.

Noble WC: *Microbial skin disease: its epidemiology*, London, 1983, Edward Arnold.

Nordlund JJ: The lives of pigment cells. In Gilchrest BA, editor: The aging skin, *Dermatol Clin* 4:407, 1986.

Odland GF: Structure of the skin. In Goldsmith LA, editor: *Physiology, biochemistry, and molecular biology of the skin*, ed 2, New York, 1991, Oxford University Press.

Ottenbacher KJ et al: The effectiveness of tactile stimulation as a form of early intervention: a quantitative evaluation, *J Dev Behav Pediatr* 8:68, 1987.

Pathak MA et al: Sun-protective agents: formulations, effects, and side effects. In Freedberg IM et al, editors: *Fitzpatrick's dermatology in general medicine*, ed 5, New York, 1999, McGraw-Hill.

Pollack SV: Systemic medications and wound healing, *Int J Dermatol* 21:489, 1982.

Potts JF: Sunlight, sunburn, and sunscreens, *Postgrad Med* 87:52, 1990.

Quinton PM: Sweating and its disorders, *Annu Rev Med* 34:429, 1983.

Rigel DS, Friedman RJ, Kopf AW, Polsky D: ABCDE-An evolving concept in the early detection of melanoma, *Arch Dermatol* 141:1032, 2005.

Roberts AB, Sporn MB: Transforming growth factor-β. In Clark RAF, editor: *The molecular and cellular biology of wound repair*, ed 2, New York, 1996, Plenum Press.

Roe DA: *Nutrition and the skin*, New York, 1986, Alan R. Liss.

Roth RR, James WD: Microbial ecology of the skin, *Annu Rev Microbiol* 42:441, 1988.

Rudowski W: *Burn therapy and research*, Baltimore, 1976, Johns Hopkins University Press.

Rutter N: The immature skin, *Br Med Bull* 44:957, 1988.

Sams WM: Structure and function of the skin. In Sams WM, Lynch PJ, editors: *Principles and practice of dermatology*, New York, 1990, Churchill Livingstone.

Sauder DN: Effect of age on epidermal immune function. In Gilchrest BA, editor: The aging skin, *Dermatol Clin* 4:447, 1986.

Shuster S et al: The effect of skin disease on self image, *Br J Dermatol* 90(Suppl 16):18, 1978.

Siebert JW et al: Fetal wound healing: a biochemical study of scarless healing, *Plast Reconstr Surg* 85:495, 1990.

Silverberg N, Silverberg L: Aging and the skin, *Postgrad Med* 86:131, 1989.

Solomons B: *Lecture notes on dermatology*, ed 5, Oxford, 1983, Blackwell Scientific.

Spince AP, Mason EB: *Human anatomy and physiology*, Menlo Park, Calif, 1987, Benjamin/Cummings.

Spitz R: An inquiry into the genesis of psychiatric conditions in early childhood. In Nagera H: *Psychoanalytical studies of the child*, vol 2, London, 1947, International.

Stender IM, Blichmann C, Serup J: Effects of oil and water baths on the hydration state of the epidermis, *Clin Exp Dermatol* 15:206, 1990.

Stryer L: *Biochemistry*, ed 4, New York, 1995, WH Freeman.

Warner RR, Myers MC, Taylor DA: Electron probe analysis of human skin: Determination of the water concentration profile, *J Invest Dermatol* 90:218, 1988.

Weinberg AN, Swartz MN: General considerations of bacterial diseases. In Fitzpatrick TB et al, editors: *Dermatology in general medicine: textbook and atlas*, New York, 1987, McGraw-Hill.

Wenger CB: Thermoregulation. In Freedberg IM et al, editors: *Fitzpatrick's dermatology in general medicine*, ed 5, New York, 1999, McGraw-Hill.

Weston WL, Lane AT: Neonatal dermatology. In Freedberg IM et al, editors: *Fitzpatrick's dermatology in general medicine*, ed 5, New York, 1999, McGraw-Hill.

Wheater PR, Burkitt HG, Daniels VG: *Functional histology*, ed 2, Edinburgh, 1987, Churchill Livingstone.

White MI, Jenkinson DM, Lloyd DH: The effect of washing on the thickness of the stratum corneum in normal and atopic individuals, *Br J Dermatol* 116:525, 1987.

Wolff K, Stingl G: The Langerhans' cell, *J Invest Dermatol* 80:17S, 1983.

Woodburne RT, Burkel WE: *Essentials of human anatomy*, New York, 1988, Oxford University Press.

Wysocki AB: A review of the skin and its appendages, *Adv Wound Care* 8:53, 1995.

Wysocki AB: Evaluating and managing open skin wounds: colonization versus infection, *AACN Clinical Issues*, 13(3):382, 2002.

Xu KD, McFeter FA, Stewart PS: Biofilm resistance to antimicrobial agents, *Microbiology* 146:547, 2000.

Yanagishita M: A brief history of proteoglycans, *EXS* 70:3, 1994.

4

Wound-Healing Physiology

···

DOROTHY B. DOUGHTY & BONNIE SPARKS-DEFRIESE

OBJECTIVES

1. Compare and contrast wound-healing processes for each type of closure: primary intention, secondary intention, and tertiary intention.
2. Distinguish between partial-thickness wound repair and full-thickness wound repair, addressing the key components, phases, usual time frames, and wound appearance.
3. Explain the difference between acute and chronic full-thickness wounds.
4. Describe four characteristics of a chronic wound.
5. Describe the role of the following cells in the wound repair process: platelets, polymorphonuclear leukocytes, macrophages, fibroblasts, endothelial cells, and keratinocytes.
6. Identify the roles of MMPs and TIMPs in regulating wound repair.
7. Describe features and characteristics of scarless healing.
8. Distinguish between keloid and hypertrophic scarring and the treatment for each.
9. Describe the effects of at least seven cofactors (conditions or treatments) on the wound-healing process.

Nurses play a vital role in wound management. They are responsible for dressing and monitoring acute wounds, such as surgical incisions, and are frequently asked to establish management protocols for chronic wounds, such as pressure ulcers or vascular ulcers. Nursing interventions can either enhance or delay the wound-healing process; thus nurses must be knowledgeable regarding the wound-healing process and the implications for wound management.

For centuries, wound healing was regarded as a mysterious process, with wound management based on practitioner preference as opposed to scientific principles. Research over the past 3 decades has contributed much information regarding the wound-healing process and the factors that facilitate this process. We now know that repair is an extremely complex process involving hundreds, possibly thousands, of overlapping and "linked" processes (Goldman, 2004). It is critical for all wound care clinicians to base their interventions and recommendations on current data and to remain abreast of new findings and their implications for care. In this chapter the process of wound healing is reviewed and the implications for wound management are discussed.

PHYSIOLOGY OF WOUND HEALING

The ability to repair tissue damage is an important survival tool for any living organism. Regardless of the type or severity of the injury, there are only two mechanisms by which repair occurs—regeneration, or replacement of the damaged or lost tissue with more of the same, and scar formation, in which the damaged or lost tissue is replaced by new connective tissue proteins. Regeneration is obviously the preferred mechanism of repair since it maintains normal function and appearance. Scar formation is a less satisfactory alternative and occurs only when the tissues involved are incapable of regeneration. Many invertebrate and amphibian species have the ability to regenerate entire limbs; however, humans have limited capacity for regeneration, and most wounds heal by scar formation (Calvin, 1998; Mast and Schultz, 1996).

In humans, the mechanism of repair for any specific wound is determined by the tissue layers involved and their capacity for regeneration. Wounds that are confined to the epidermal and superficial dermal layers heal by regeneration because epithelial, endothelial, and connective tissue can be reproduced. In contrast, the deep dermal structures (hair follicles, sebaceous glands, and sweat glands), subcutaneous tissue, muscle, tendons, ligaments, and bone lack the capacity to regenerate;

therefore loss of these structures is permanent, and wounds involving these structures must heal by scar formation (Martin, 1997; Mast and Schultz, 1996).

Whereas the standard repair mechanism for human soft tissue wounds is connective tissue (scar) formation, the early-gestation fetus represents an exception to this rule. Intrauterine surgical procedures performed during the second trimester result in scarless healing, a phenomenon that has been consistently reproduced in laboratory studies. Interestingly, the late-gestation fetus loses the ability to heal without scarring; repair during the third trimester and the postnatal period follows the "usual" rules for repair and results in scar formation. There are a number of differences in the molecular environment for repair in the early-gestation fetus that are thought to contribute to scarless repair, which will be discussed later in this chapter (Bullard, Longaker, and Lorenz, 2002; Dang et al, 2003; Samuels and Tan, 1999; Yang et al, 2003).

DEFINITIONS AND CLASSIFICATIONS

Wounds and wound healing are classified according to tissue layers involved (partial-thickness vs. full-thickness), onset and duration (acute versus chronic), and types of wound closure (primary, secondary, and tertiary intention).

Partial Thickness/Full Thickness

Partial-thickness wounds are those involving only partial loss of the skin layers, meaning they are confined to the epidermal and superficial dermal layers. Full-thickness wounds involve total loss of the skin layers (epidermis and dermis) and frequently involve loss of the deeper tissue layers as well (subcutaneous tissue, muscle, and bone). (See illustrations of skin and soft tissue layers in Chapter 3.) The time frame for repair and the repair process itself differ significantly for partial-thickness and full-thickness wounds.

Acute/Chronic

Acute wounds are typically traumatic or surgical in origin. These wounds occur suddenly, move rapidly and predictably through the repair process, and result in durable closure. Chronic wounds, in contrast, are wounds that fail to proceed normally through the repair process. Chronic wounds are frequently caused by vascular compromise, chronic inflammation, or

repetitive insults to the tissue, and either fail to close in a timely manner or fail to result in durable closure (Brissett and Hom, 2003; Clark, 2002).

Primary, Secondary, Tertiary

Classification of repair as primary-, secondary-, or tertiary-intention healing is based on the ideal of primary surgical closure for all wounds. Primary closure minimizes the volume of connective tissue deposition required for wound repair and restores the epithelial barrier to infection (Figure 4-1, *A*).

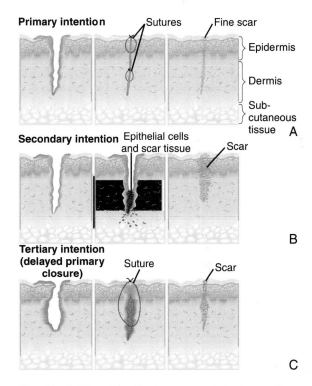

Fig. 4-1 A, Wound healing by primary intention, such as with a surgical incision. Wound edges are approximated and secured with sutures, staples, or adhesive tapes, and healing occurs by epithelialization and connective tissue deposition. **B,** Wound healing by secondary intention. Wound edges are not approximated, and healing occurs by granulation tissue formation, contraction of the wound edges, and epithelialization. **C,** Wound healing by tertiary (delayed primary) intention. Wound is kept open for several days. The superficial wound edges are then approximated, and the center of the wound heals by granulation tissue formation. (From Black JM, Hawks JH: *Medical surgical nursing, clinical management for positive outcomes,* ed 7, St Louis, 2005, WB Saunders.)

Approximated surgical incisions are therefore said to heal by *primary intention*; they usually heal quickly, with minimal scar formation, as long as infection and secondary breakdown are prevented. Wounds that are left open and allowed to heal by scar formation are classified as healing by *secondary intention* (Figure 4-1, *B*). These wounds heal more slowly because of the volume of connective tissue required to fill the defect and are more subject to infection because they lack the epidermal barrier to microorganisms. These wounds are characterized by prolonged phases of healing (inflammation, proliferation and maturation). Chronic wounds such as pressure ulcers and vascular ulcers typically heal by secondary intention. Wounds managed with delayed closure are classified as healing by *tertiary intention*, or delayed primary closure (Figure 4-1, *C*). This is an approach sometimes required for abdominal incisions complicated by significant infection (Rosenberg and de la Torre, 2003). Closure and/or approximation of the wound is delayed until the risk of infection is resolved and the wound is free of debris.

WOUND-HEALING PROCESS

Wound healing is best understood as a cascade of events. Injury sets into motion a series of physiologic responses that are coordinated and sequenced and that, under normal circumstances, invariably result in repair (Figure 4-2). Our current understanding of wound repair is based primarily on acute wound–healing models. Therefore, the processes for partial-thickness wound healing and full-thickness wounds healing by primary intention will be presented first followed by a discussion of the repair process for wounds healing by secondary intention.

Partial-Thickness Wound Repair

Partial-thickness wounds are shallow wounds involving epidermal loss and possibly partial loss of the dermal layer (Plate 1). These wounds are moist and painful because of the loss of the epidermal covering and the resultant exposure of the nerve endings. When the wound involves loss of the epidermis with exposure of the basement membrane, the wound base appears bright pink or red. In the presence of partial dermal loss, the wound base usually appears pale pink with distinct red "islets." These "islets" represent the basement membrane of the epidermis, which projects deep

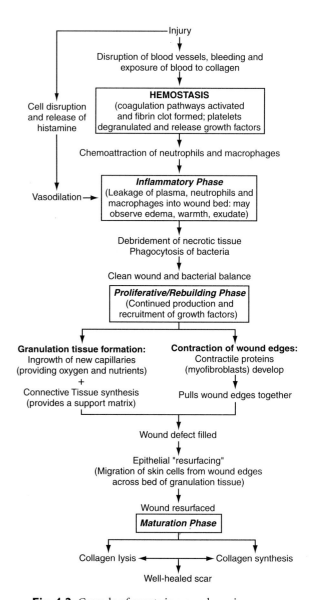

Fig. 4-2 Cascade of events in wound repair process.

into the dermis to line the epidermal appendages. These islands of epidermal basement membrane are important in partial-thickness wound healing, because all epidermal cells are capable of regeneration and each islet will serve as a source of new epithelium (Clark, 2002; Winter, 1979).

The major components of partial-thickness repair include an initial inflammatory response to injury,

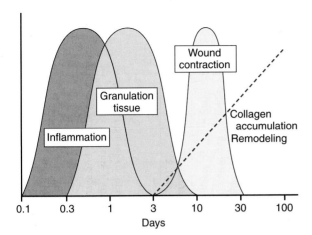

Fig. 4-3 Orderly phases of healing. Time line (in days) reflects healing trajectory of acute wound healing model. (Modified from Clark RA: In Goldsmith LA, editor: *Physiology, biochemistry and molecular biology of the skin,* ed 2, vol 1, New York, 1991, Oxford University Press, p. 577. In Kumar V, Cotran RS, Robbins ST: *Robbins basic pathology,* ed 7, Philadelphia, 2003, WB Saunders.

epithelial proliferation and migration (resurfacing), and reestablishment and differentiation of the epidermal layers to restore the barrier function of the skin (Monaco and Lawrence, 2003; Staiano-Coico et al, 2000; Winter, 1979). If the wound involves dermal loss, connective tissue repair (granulation tissue formation) will proceed concurrently with epithelial repair (Figure 4-3) (Jahoda and Reynolds, 2001).

Epidermal Repair. Tissue trauma triggers an acute inflammatory response, which produces erythema, edema, and a serous exudate containing leukocytes. When this exudate is allowed to dry on the wound surface, a dry crust commonly referred to as a "scab" is formed. In partial-thickness wounds the inflammatory response is limited, typically subsiding in less than 24 hours (Winter, 1979).

Epidermal resurfacing begins within hours of injury in response to cytokines and growth factors in wound fluid (e.g., interleukin-1, interleukin-6, interleukin-8, transforming growth factor-α (TGF-α) transforming growth factor-β (TGF-β), epidermal growth factor, and keratinocyte growth factor). The basal cells at the wound edge and throughout the wound bed respond to these substances by elongating and migrating laterally as a monolayer (Chen and Abatangelo, 1999; Frank et al, 2002; Henry and Garner, 2003;

Monaco and Lawrence, 2003; Staiano-Coico et al, 2000; Werner and Grose, 2003).

In order to migrate, the epidermal cells must acquire a migratory phenotype, which means they must break free of cellular attachments to one another and to the basement membrane (desmosomes and hemidesmosomes). They then undergo cytoskeletal alterations that support lateral movement. These alterations include flattening of the cells at the advancing edge of epithelium and formation of protrusions, known as lamellipods that attach to binding sites in the wound bed to help pull the cell across the wound surface. The epithelial cells within the wound bed continue this pattern of lateral migration until they contact epithelial cells migrating from the opposite direction. Once the epithelial cells meet, lateral migration ceases; a phenomenon known as contact inhibition (Staiano-Coico et al, 2000; Monaco and Lawrence, 2003).

Epithelial resurfacing is supported by increased production of basal cells throughout the wound bed, which peaks between 24 and 72 hours following injury. Low levels of nitric oxide and selected growth factors stimulate this proliferative "burst." Resurfacing is also supported by maintenance of a moist wound surface. Winter (1979) found that partial-thickness wounds left open to air required 6 to 7 days to resurface, whereas moist wounds reepithelialized in 4 days. This is because cells can migrate much more rapidly in a moist environment (Figure 4-4). In contrast, when the surface of the wound is covered with a "scab," migration is delayed while the epithelial cells secrete enzymes known as matrix metalloproteases (MMPs) to loosen the scab covering, and create a moist vascular pathway for the keratinocytes to migrate across (Clark, 2002; Monaco and Lawrence, 2003; Staiano-Coico et al, 2000; Winter, 1979). The newly resurfaced epithelium appears pale, pink, and dry in people of all races (see Plate 1). Because it is only a few cell layers thick, the new epithelium is very fragile and requires protection against mechanical forces such as shear and friction.

Once epithelial resurfacing is complete, the epithelial cells resume vertical migration and epidermal differentiation so that normal epidermal thickness and function is restored. The normal anchors to adjacent epidermal cells and to the basement membrane are reestablished. The "new" epidermis gradually repigments, matching the individual's normal skin tone (see Plate 1). This has

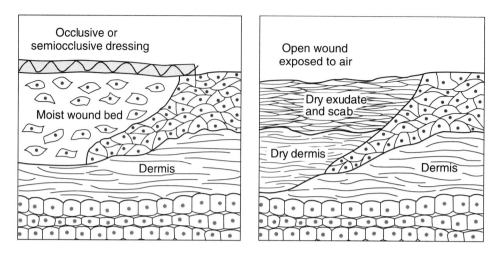

Fig. 4-4 Diagram of migration of epidermal cells in moist environment and dry environment.

clinical relevance in that the wound is not completely healed until repigmentation has occurred (Monaco and Lawrence, 2003).

The transition to vertical migration may be controlled partly by rising levels of nitric oxide. As the number of keratinocytes in the wound bed increases, the nitric oxide levels rise. This elevated nitric oxide level seems to eliminate the stimulus to keratinocyte proliferation and establishes a signal for vertical migration and epidermal differentiation (Goldman, 2004).

Dermal Repair. In wounds involving both dermal and epidermal loss, dermal repair proceeds concurrently with reepithelialization. By the fifth day after injury, a layer of fluid separates the epidermis from the dermal tissue. New blood vessels begin to sprout, and fibroblasts become plentiful by about the seventh day. Collagen fibers are visible in the wound bed by the ninth day. Collagen synthesis continues to produce new connective tissue until about 10 to 15 days after injury. This new connective tissue grows upward into the fluid layer. At the same time, the flat epidermis falls down around the new vessels and collagen fibers, recreating ridges at the dermal-epidermal junction. As the new connective tissue gradually contracts, the epidermis is drawn close to the dermis (Winter, 1979). The epithelial dermal cells in the sheath surrounding the hair follicles are thought to contribute significantly to dermal repair in partial-thickness wounds, a hypothesis supported by reports of faster healing in wounds involving "hairy"

areas, such as scalp donor sites (Jahoda and Reynolds, 2001; Winter, 1979).

Full-Thickness Wound Repair

Healing by Primary Intention. Full-thickness wounds, by definition, extend at least to the subcutaneous tissue layer and possibly as deep as the fascia-muscle layer or bone (see Plate 2). Full-thickness wounds may be either acute or chronic; this section will address the acute wound healing by primary intention, such as a surgical incision.

There are many steps involved in full-thickness repair, but they are commonly conceptualized as four major phases—hemostasis, inflammation, proliferation, and remodeling (Figure 4-5). There is considerable overlap among the phases, and the cells involved in one phase produce the chemical stimuli and substances that serve to move the wound into the next phase. Thus normal repair is a complex and well-orchestrated series of events (see Figure 4-3 and Table 4-1).

Hemostasis. Any acute injury extending beyond the epidermis causes bleeding, which activates a series of overlapping events that provide for hemostasis and a temporary barrier to bacterial invasion. Immediately upon injury, disruption of blood vessels exposes the subendothelial collagen to platelets, which triggers platelet activation and aggregation. Simultaneously, injured cells in the wound area release clotting factors that activate both the intrinsic and extrinsic

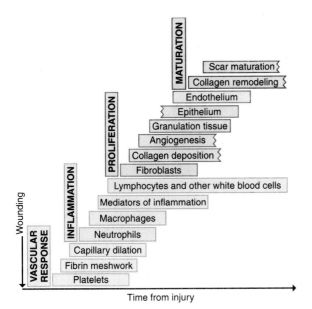

Fig. 4-5 Normal wound healing. The wound-healing proceeds through four phases: (1) the vascular response, (2) inflammation, (3) proliferation of cells to heal the wound, and (4) maturation of the wound. Each step has many components. The jagged edge depicts an ongoing process. (Modified from Cohen I et al, editors: *Wound healing*, 1992, Philadelphia, WB Saunders. In Black JM, Hawks JH: *Medical surgical nursing, clinical management for positive outcomes*, ed 7, St Louis, 2005, WB Saunders.)

TABLE 4-1 Key Cells and Substances in Each Phase of the Healing Process

PHASE	CELLS	SUBSTANCES
Hemostasis	Platelets	Growth factors
Inflammatory phase	Neutrophils Macrophages	Proteases
Proliferative phase	Macrophages Keratinocytes Endothelial cells Fibroblasts	Growth factors Collagen Glycosaminoglycans Proteoglycans (e.g., hyaluronic acid, fibronectin)
Maturation phase	Fibroblasts	Proteases Collagen

coagulation pathways. As part of the coagulation pathway, circulating prothrombin is converted to thrombin, which is used to convert fibrinogen to fibrin. The end result is formation of a *clot* composed of fibrin, aggregated platelets, and blood cells. Hemostasis is further accomplished by a brief period of vasoconstriction mediated by thromboxane A2 and prostaglandin 2-α, substances released by the damaged cells and activated platelets. Clot formation serves to seal the disrupted vessels so that blood loss is controlled. The clot also provides a temporary bacterial barrier, a reservoir of growth factors, and an interim matrix that serves as scaffolding for migrating cells (Brissett and Hom, 2003; Monaco and Lawrence, 2003; Phillips, 2000; Werner and Grose, 2003).

Clot formation, followed by fibrinolysis (clot breakdown), is a critical event in the sequence of wound healing (Figure 4-6). The activation and degranulation of

platelets causes the α-granules and dense bodies of the platelets to rupture, releasing a potent "cocktail" of energy-producing compounds and cytokines/growth factors (including complement factor C5a). These substances attract the cells needed to begin the repair process and also provide fuel for the energy-intensive process of wound healing. The platelet-derived substances thought to be most critical to repair include platelet-derived growth, transforming growth factor-β, and fibroblast growth factor-2. Thus hemostasis, which is the body's normal response to tissue injury, actually initiates the entire wound-healing cascade. The importance of hemostasis to wound healing is underscored by the finding that inadequate clot formation is associated with impaired wound healing and that the extrinsic coagulation pathway is critical to repair (Brissett and Hom, 2003; Frank et al, 2002; Monaco and Lawrence, 2003; Samuels and Tan, 1999; Staiano-Coico et al, 2000).

Inflammation. Once the bleeding is controlled, the focus becomes establishment of a clean wound bed. This can be compared to the repair of a damaged home or building; before the rebuilding can begin, the damaged components must be removed. Wound "cleanup" involves breakdown of any devitalized or damaged tissue and elimination of excess bacteria by a team of white blood cells.

Within 10 to 15 minutes following injury, vasoconstriction subsides, followed by vasodilation and

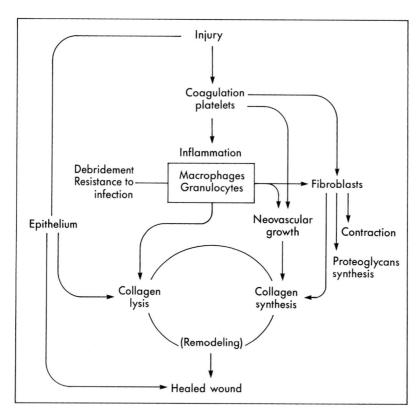

Fig. 4-6 Schema demonstrating that coagulation triggers the wound-healing cascade. (From Levenson S, Seiffer E, Van Winkle E Jr: Nutrition. In Hunt TK, Dunphy JE, editors: *Fundamentals of wound management*, New York, 1979, Appleton.)

increased capillary permeability. Vasoactive substances released by the damaged cells and by clot breakdown (histamine, prostaglandins, complement factor, and thrombin) mediate this response. The dilated capillaries permit plasma and blood cells to leak into the wound bed. Clinically, this is observed as edema, erythema, and exudate. At the same time, the cytokines and growth factors released by the platelets chemoattract or recruit leukocytes (neutrophils, macrophages, and lymphocytes) to the wound bed. The twin processes of chemoattraction and vasodilation result in the delivery of multiple phagocytic cells to the wound site within minutes of injury.

Leukocyte migration out of the vessels and into the wound bed occurs via margination and diapedesis (Figure 4-7). Margination involves adherence of the leukocytes to the endothelial cells lining the capillaries

in the wound bed. Integrins on the surface of the leukocytes attach to cell adhesion molecules on the surface of the endothelial cells, causing the leukocytes to "line up" against the vessel wall. Through a process known as diapedesis, the leukocytes then migrate through the dilated capillaries into the wound bed (Cross and Mustoe, 2003; Monaco and Lawrence, 2003).

The first leukocytes to arrive in the wound space, the neutrophils, are present in the wound bed within the first hour following injury and dominate the scene for the first 2 to 3 days. The primary function of neutrophils is phagocytosis of bacteria and foreign debris. Neutrophils first bind to the damaged tissue or target bacteria via cell adhesion molecules and then engulf and destroy the target molecules via intracellular enzymes and free oxygen radicals. Growth factors are also released by the neutrophils that will attract additional

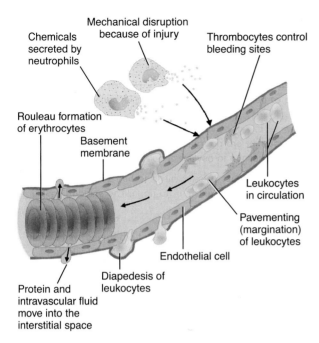

Chemicals
secreted by
neutrophils

Mechanical disruption
because of injury

Thrombocytes control
bleeding sites

Rouleau formation
of erythrocytes

Basement
membrane

Leukocytes
in circulation

Pavementing
(margination)
of leukocytes

Endothelial cell

Diapedesis of
leukocytes

Protein and
intravascular fluid
move into the
interstitial space

Fig. 4-7 Several changes occur in a capillary after injury. Neutrophils are attracted to the site of injury by chemotactic factors at the site. The neutrophil leaves the blood vessel by sliding through holes in the vessel wall (diapedesis). The leukocytes also line the vessel wall, and the erythrocytes stack like coins (rouleau formation) to slow blood flow. (From Black JM, Hawks JH: *Medical surgical nursing, clinical management for positive outcomes,* ed 7, St Louis, 2005, WB Saunders.)

TABLE 4-2 **Functions of the Macrophage**

PHAGOCYTIZE	SYNTHESIZE	RELEASE
Bacteria Damaged tissues	Nitric oxide Collagenase Elastase TIMPs	Growth factors • Platelet derived growth factors • Fibroblast growth factors • Insulin-like growth factors • Epidermal growth factors

leukocytes to the area (Cross and Mustoe, 2003; Goldman, 2004; Monaco and Lawrence, 2003; Schultz et al, 2003).

By about the third day after injury, the neutrophils begin to spontaneously disappear as a result of apoptosis and are replaced by macrophages (activated monocytes). The many functions the macrophage provides in the wound repair process have earned the macrophage the title of "regulator of wound repair" (Table 4-2) (Schultz et al, 2003). The macrophages continue to phagocytize bacteria and break down damaged tissues via the processes outlined above. Macrophages also synthesize nitric oxide, a substance that has antimicrobial effects, and enzymes (collagenase and elastase), which contribute to the break down of devitalized tissue. This enzymatic destruction of damaged tissue presents a potential threat to the healthy

tissue in the area. Under normal conditions, the macrophages also produce substances known as tissue inhibitors of matrix metalloproteases (TIMPs) which protect the healthy tissue by inhibiting enzymatic activity (Cross and Mustoe, 2003; Monaco and Lawrence, 2003; Schultz et al, 2003). In addition to these functions, the macrophages release a large number of potent growth factors that stimulate angiogenesis, fibroblast migration and proliferation, and connective tissue synthesis.

T lymphocytes are present in the wound tissue in peak quantities between days 5 and 7 after injury. T lymphocytes contribute to the inflammatory phase of wound healing by secreting additional wound-healing cytokines and by destroying viral organisms and foreign cells. The elimination of these cells can delay or compromise the repair process (Monaco and Lawrence, 2003).

While all leukocytes contribute to elimination of bacteria and devitalized tissue and establishment of a clean wound bed, it is the macrophage that actually controls the entire wound-repair process; only the macrophage is considered essential to repair. Studies indicate that wounds can heal without neutrophils, especially if there is no bacterial contamination. However, elimination of macrophages severely inhibits or even prevents wound repair (Cross and Mustoe, 2003; Rosenberg and de la Torre, 2003).

The result of the inflammatory phase of wound healing is a clean wound bed. In acute wounds healing by primary intention, the inflammatory phase lasts approximately 3 days. At this point, bacterial levels are usually controlled and any devitalized tissue has been removed. Elimination of these noxious stimuli allows the wound to transition to the "rebuilding" phase. During this transition, the cells in the wound bed begin to produce more growth factors that stimulate proliferation rather than inflammation (Goldman, 2004; Staiano-Coico et al, 2000). However, in wounds complicated by necrosis and/or infection, the inflammatory phase is prolonged and wound healing is delayed (Clark, 2002). A prolonged inflammatory phase increases the risk for wound dehiscence, because maintaining approximation of the incision is totally dependent upon the suture material until sufficient connective tissue is synthesized to provide tensile strength to the incision. (Tensile strength during the inflammatory phase is 0%.) An excessive or prolonged inflammatory phase is also thought to be a risk factor for hyperproliferative scarring, probably as a result of increased production of cytokines and growth factors that stimulate connective tissue synthesis (Dubay and Franz, 2003; Rahban and Garner, 2003; Robson, 2003b).

Proliferation. The third phase of acute full-thickness wound healing is the proliferative phase. During this phase, vascular integrity is restored, the incisional defect is mended with new connective tissue, and the wound surface is covered with new epithelium. The key components of the proliferative phase are epithelialization, neoangiogenesis, and matrix deposition/collagen synthesis. Limited contraction of the newly formed extracellular matrix may also occur.

Epithelialization. As with partial-thickness wound healing, epithelialization of a full-thickness wound healing by primary intention actually begins during the inflammatory phase and proceeds in the same fashion.

In a normally healing incision, epithelial resurfacing is typically complete within 24 to 48 hours. This "neoepithelium" is only a few cells thick but is sufficient to provide a closed wound surface and a bacterial barrier. This is the basis for the Centers for Disease Control recommendation that new surgical incisions be covered with a sterile dressing for the first 24 to 48 hours postoperatively. (Cross and Mustoe, 2003; Mangram et al, 1999; Monaco and Lawrence, 2003.) As with partial-thickness wound repair, the process of lateral migration, vertical migration, and differentiation continues throughout the proliferative phase and gradually reestablishes epidermal thickness and function. In full-thickness wounds, the new epidermis is slightly thinner than the original epidermis. Because the neoepidermis is covering scar tissue as opposed to normal dermis, the rete pegs that normally dip into the dermis are lacking (Monaco and Lawrence, 2003).

Granulation tissue formation. A hallmark outcome of the proliferative phase is the formation of granulation tissue. Granulation tissue is composed primarily of capillary loops and newly synthesized connective tissue proteins often referred to as extracellular matrix (ECM) (Figure 4-8). Fibroblasts and inflammatory cells are also present in this new matrix. Neoangiogenesis and connective tissue synthesis occur simultaneously in a codependent fashion to form the new extracellular matrix that will fill the wound defect. Through angiogenesis, new capillaries are formed and joined with existing severed capillaries, thus restoring the delivery of oxygen and nutrients to the wound bed. The newly formed ECM serves to provide support to these fragile new capillaries.

Neoangiogenesis. Neoangiogenesis is stimulated by angiogenic growth factors secreted by the keratinocytes at the wound edge (i.e., vascular endothelial growth factor or VEGF), and the hypoxic gradient that exists between the center of the wound and the vascularized tissue at the periphery. In response to these stimuli, endothelial cells in the vessels adjacent to the wound bed begin to multiply and produce enzymes that create pathways into the ECM. These pathways allow the newly formed endothelial cells to project "sprouts" into the wound bed that gradually develop into new capillary tubes (Frank et al, 2002; Goldman, 2004; Staiano-Coico et al, 2000; Werner and Grose, 2003). Capillary production is followed by reconnection to vascular channels in the surrounding tissue, thus achieving consistent perfusion of the wound bed. Finally, ECM components are deposited to create a new basement membrane within the capillaries. Angiogenesis is regulated by a complex interplay between the hypoxic environment, various growth factors, and additional factors such as nitric oxide. Nitric oxide is thought to "upregulate" the production of VEGF and thus stimulate endothelial proliferation (Goldman, 2004).

Matrix deposition/collagen synthesis. Fibroblasts are responsible for synthesis of collagen and other

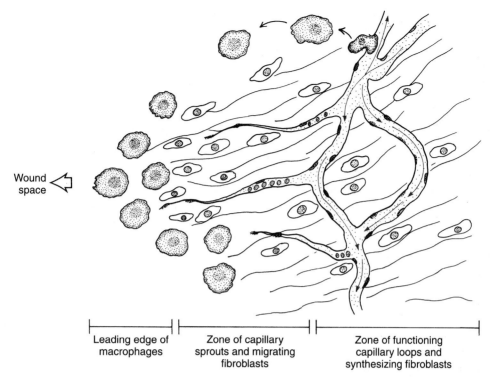

Wound
space

Leading edge of
macrophages

Zone of capillary
sprouts and migrating
fibroblasts

Zone of functioning
capillary loops and
synthesizing fibroblasts

Fig. 4-8 Advancing module of reparative tissue during proliferative and remodeling phases. (From Whalen GF, Zetter BR: Angiogenesis. In Cohen IK, Dieglemann RF, Lindbald WJ, editors: *Wound healing: biochemical and clinical aspects*, Philadelphia, 1992, WB Saunders.)

connective tissue substances and are therefore critical to the repair process. Fibroblasts migrate into the wound bed from the surrounding tissues in response to growth factors released by degranulating platelets and activated leukocytes (neutrophils and macrophages). Migration requires upregulation of binding sites (integrin receptors) on the cell wall, which is mediated by PDGF and TGF-β. This "upregulation" of binding sites is essential because fibroblasts migrate by maintaining attachment to one binding site while extending a lamellipod in search of another site. Once the fibroblast is able to bind to a new site, it releases the original attachment and "moves" in the direction of the wound bed (Monaco and Lawrence, 2003). Fibroblasts begin to appear in the wound bed toward the end of the inflammatory phase, that is, 2 to 3 days after injury. By day 4, fibroblasts are the predominant cell in the wound matrix (Dubay and Franz, 2003). Once fibroblasts arrive at

the wound site, growth factors bind to fibroblast receptor sites and trigger intracellular processes that move the fibroblast into the reproductive phase of the cell cycle, thus stimulating proliferation of the fibroblast. Finally, the fibroblasts are converted into "wound fibroblasts" by TGF-β, a growth factor secreted by macrophages. These wound fibroblasts differ from typical dermal fibroblasts in that they exhibit decreased proliferative behavior but increased collagen synthesis and wound contraction (Frank et al, 2003).

A new ECM gradually replaces the provisional fibrin matrix formed during the inflammatory phase to support cell migration. The development of the ECM, or "scar tissue," involves multiple phases and the synthesis of many connective tissue substances such as collagen, glycosaminoglycans (GAGs), and proteoglycans. As the ECM matures, collagen becomes the predominant protein, representing a little over 50% of the new ECM. Proteoglycans, such as hyaluronic acid are present in small amounts but serve critical functions. Hyaluronic acid facilitates cell migration, protects cells against free-radical and proteolytic damage, and contributes viscoelastic properties to the new matrix (Chen and Abatangelo, 1999; Monaco and Lawrence, 2003).

The early collagen is characterized by poorly organized collagen fibers with limited tensile strength. At 3 weeks after injury, the healing wound exhibits only 20% of the strength of intact dermis. As the collagen matures, type III collagen is converted to type I collagen, the type normally found in dermal tissue. However, even the final form of collagen does not exhibit the normal basket-weave pattern of the collagen in unwounded dermis. Rather, the fibers of "repair collagen" are aligned parallel to the stress lines of the wound. The new ECM also lacks elastin, which provides the uninjured skin with elasticity; thus scar tissue is "stiff" as compared to normal tissue (Monaco and Lawrence, 2003).

Collagen synthesis follows the established process for synthesis of any protein. The collagen molecule is characterized by a glycine-X-Y repeating sequence. After undergoing a series of intracellular modifications, the collagen molecule is then secreted into the extracellular environment as the triple helix procollagen. One of the most critical intracellular modifications of collagen is "cross-linking" of proline and lysine molecules, which is known as hydroxylation. These cross-links are required for the development of tensile strength.

Hydroxylation requires oxygen, ascorbic acid, iron, and copper in addition to specific enzymes. Enzymes required for hydroxylation are suppressed by corticosteroids. Thus vitamin C deficiency, copper deficiency, or high-dose corticosteroid administration during the proliferative phase may result in diminished cross-linking of the collagen and increased risk of incisional breakdown. Once the procollagen molecule is secreted into the extracellular environment, it undergoes additional steps that culminate in the formation of cross-linked fibrils. The enzyme lysyl oxidase is essential to these processes and to the development of stable collagen fibers. Over time, collagen fibers thicken, and the tensile strength of the wound increases (Monaco and Lawrence, 2003).

Wounds healing by primary intention, such as sutured incisions, require a limited amount of connective tissue to mend the defect. In these wounds, collagen synthesis usually peaks at about the fifth day, and ECM production is essentially complete within 14 to 21 days (Clark, 2002; Henry and Garner, 2003; Monaco and Lawrence, 2003). Although the granulation tissue is not visible in these wounds, by day 5 it is possible to palpate a "healing ridge" just under the intact suture line. This healing ridge is produced by the newly formed collagen. Absence of this healing ridge indicates impaired healing and increased risk for dehiscence (Hunt and Van Winkle, 1997).

Contraction. Contraction occurs when specialized fibroblasts known as myofibroblasts exert tractional forces on the ECM to reduce the size of the wound. In wounds healing by primary intention, contraction plays a very limited role, because the wound edges have been surgically approximated (Monaco and Lawrence, 2003).

Maturation/Remodeling. The final phase in full-thickness wound healing is the maturation, or remodeling phase, which begins around the twenty-first day after wounding and continues beyond 1 year. Remodeling involves the continuation of matrix breakdown and matrix synthesis. Fibroblasts continue to regulate these dual processes as they do in the proliferative phase. The new collagen that is formed is more orderly and strong, thus providing more tensile strength to the wound. However, the tensile strength of subsequent scar tissue is never more than 80% of the tensile strength in nonwounded tissue (Clark, 2002; Monaco and Lawrence, 2003).

An imbalance between the dual processes of matrix synthesis and matrix breakdown can complicate wound healing. For example, hypertrophic scarring and keloid formation are believed to be caused in part by an excess of matrix synthesis as compared with matrix degradation (Rahban and Garner, 2003). On the other hand, hypoxia, malnutrition, or excess levels of MMPs can interfere with synthesis and deposition of new matrix proteins, resulting in wound breakdown (Monaco and Lawrence, 2003).

CHARACTERISTICS OF FULL-THICKNESS WOUNDS HEALING BY SECONDARY INTENTION

Wounds healing by secondary intention include dehisced surgical wounds and wounds caused by underlying morbidities such as chronic venous insufficiency or pressure necrosis. While many wounds healing by secondary intention are chronic wounds refractory to healing, some are acute wounds that failed to achieve durable closure that then respond quickly to appropriate management. Table 4-3 provides a comparison of the key events in the healing process with the full-thickness wound healing by secondary intention, the primary-intention healing of a full-thickness wound, and the partial-thickness wound. Figure 4-2 further describes the process by which full-thickness secondary-intention wound healing occurs.

Absence of Hemostasis

Bleeding and hemostasis do not occur in wounds healing by secondary intention, this compromises the repair process because the wound-healing sequence of events is normally initiated by clot breakdown and the subsequent release of growth factors. The absence of hemostasis, therefore, has a tremendous impact on the healing trajectory for these wounds. One theorized benefit of surgical debridement is the fact that it causes bleeding, thus activating (or reactivating) the repair process.

TABLE 4-3 Comparison of Key Events in Healing Process

PROGRESSION OF KEY EVENTS	SECONDARY INTENTION FULL-THICKNESS WOUND HEALING	PRIMARY INTENTION FULL-THICKNESS WOUND HEALING	PARTIAL-THICKNESS WOUND HEALING
Nature of Injury	Chronic injury disease process or acute wound dehiscence	Acute injury	Acute or chronic injury limited to epidermis or dermis
Bleeding	No bleeding No coagulation Hemostasis ABSENT	Bleeding Hemostasis: platelets release growth factors Coagulation pathways (intrinsic and extrinsic) activated	Bleeding Coagulation LIMITED hemostasis
Inflammatory Phase	Necrotic tissue removed Bacterial balance restored Phase prolonged owing to presence of excess inflammatory proteases	Necrotic tissue removed Bacterial balance restored	Mild erythema, edema and pain Serous exudate (scab)
Proliferative Phase	Granulation tissue formation Neoangiogenesis Connective tissue Contraction of wound edges	Epithelialization Connective tissue synthesis Integrity of incision restored	Dermal repair if dermis involved Epithelium restored
Maturation (Remodeling) Phase	Epithelialization Continuation of granulation and contraction	Collagen synthesis and lysis Tensile strength re-established	Dermal repair continues Epithelium differentiates

Prolonged Inflammatory Phase

The inflammatory phase is frequently prolonged. Since the goal of this phase is to establish a clean wound bed and to obtain bacterial balance, the wound will remain in this phase until necrotic tissue has been eliminated and bacterial loads have been controlled. Wound healing by secondary intention may be complicated by large amounts of devitalized tissue and heavy bacterial loads. Thus the inflammatory phase generally lasts considerably longer than the 3 days that are typical of the approximated incision.

Prolonged Proliferative Phase

The proliferative phase is prolonged, and the sequence of events is different. In wounds healing by primary intention, epithelialization occurs first, followed by angiogenesis and a small amount of granulation tissue formation and contraction. These processes are usually complete within 14 to 21 days. In secondary-intention wound healing, the proliferative phase begins with granulation tissue formation (to fill in the soft tissue defect) followed by contraction (to minimize the defect); epithelialization is the final phase. In addition, hypoxia plays a more significant role in secondary-intention wound healing because it is a trigger for macrophage activity. Figure 4-8 illustrates the migration of macrophages into the hypoxic center of a wound.

The volume of granulation tissue required to fill in the defect (and the time required for this phase of repair) is determined by the size of the wound and by the degree to which contraction is able to reduce the size of the defect. Since the wound bed is visible, the clinician is able to assess progress in healing. Healthy granulation tissue presents as a red, vascular, granular wound bed, as a result of the numerous capillary loops in combination with the newly synthesized ECM proteins. (See Plate 3.)

Increased Amount of Contraction

Contraction is much more important in secondary-intention wound healing than in closed wounds, because it reduces the size of the soft tissue defect and thus reduces the amount of granulation tissue required. The rate of contraction for open wounds averages 0.6 to 0.7 mm per day (Gabbiani, 2003; Monaco and Lawrence, 2003). The degree to which a specific wound will contract is determined partly by

the mobility of the surrounding tissue. For example, the tissue surrounding sacral and abdominal wounds is quite mobile and can contract easily; in contrast, the tissue surrounding a wound on the extremity or overlying a bony prominence has limited potential for contraction. Contraction is considered undesirable in some wounds because it can cause cosmetic deformities or flexion contractures of joints (Gabbiani, 2003; Monaco and Lawrence, 2003).

Myofibroblasts, modified fibroblasts containing actin and myosin monofilaments and smooth muscle proteins, are thought to mediate contraction. A contractile force between intracellular actin filaments and extracellular fibronectin actually exerts a mechanical pull to "shrink" the ECM. The conversion of fibroblasts to myofibroblasts is most likely stimulated by mechanical stress exerted on the wound bed, and the production of actin filaments is mediated by TGF-β (Gabbiani, 2003).

Delayed Epithelialization

Because full-thickness wounds involve loss of the deep dermis and epidermal appendages (along with their epithelial lining), epithelialization in these wounds proceeds from the periphery of the wound inward in a centripetal fashion. Epithelial migration requires an open, proliferative wound edge.

Closed, nonproliferative wound edges, also known as epibole, are sometimes seen in open wounds healing by secondary intention, probably due to premature keratinization of the wound edges (Figure 4-9). (See Plate 4.) In these wounds, an open edge must be reestablished, either via surgical excision or chemical cauterization, before epithelial migration can occur (Cross and Mustoe, 2003; Monaco and Lawrence, 2003). It is theorized that high serum calcium levels cause premature keratinization and inhibit epithelial migration, therefore precipitating epibole (Lansdown, 2002).

Prolonged Remodeling

The remodeling process for wounds healing by secondary intention is essentially the same as that for those healing by primary intention. Clinicians and caregivers must remain acutely aware that newly "healed" wounds initially lack tensile strength, and measures should be initiated to minimize stress on the remodeling wound until tensile strength has developed, which

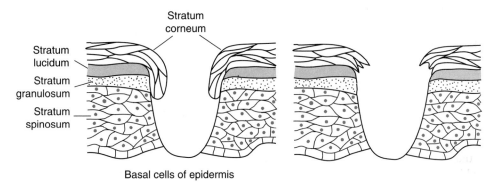

Fig. 4-9 Schematic depiction of closed wound edges *(left)* in which epidermis of wound edges has rolled under so that epithelial cells cannot migrate. Open wound edges *(right)* from which epithelial cells can migrate.

occurs 2 to 3 months after closure. (For example, the patient with a newly healed pressure ulcer should remain on a therapeutic support surface and should minimize time spent lying on the involved surface.)

WHAT MAKES A CHRONIC WOUND CHRONIC?

An acute wound in a relatively healthy host will heal fairly quickly because of a cascade of growth factors and cellular stimulants that tend to keep the acute wound on the "healing track." In clinical practice, however, chronic wounds such as pressure ulcers, vascular ulcers, and neuropathic wounds behave much differently and may be extremely slow to heal. In order to intervene effectively, the clinician must be knowledgeable regarding the various factors contributing to delayed healing.

Over the past decade, extensive research analyzing the cellular, biochemical, and molecular components of acute and chronic wounds has significantly expanded the understanding of the detailed complexities of normal wound healing and the pathophysiologic mechanisms of chronic wounds. Box 4-1 summarizes the characteristics of a chronic wound.

Underlying Pathology

The nature of the injury differs between acute and chronic wounds. Acute wounds usually begin with a sudden, solitary insult and proceed to heal in an orderly manner. In contrast, chronic wounds are commonly caused by an underlying pathologic process, such as

---

BOX 4-1 Characteristics of a Chronic Wound

Prolonged inflammatory phase
Cellular senescence
Deficiency of growth factor receptor sites
No initial bleeding event to trigger fibrin production and release of growth factors
High level of proteases

---

vascular insufficiency, that produces repeated and prolonged insults to the tissues. Failure to correct or control the underlying pathology can result in a persistent cycle of injury that causes repetitive tissue damage (Figure 4-10). In contrast, correction of the underlying pathology can frequently shift the wound to a healing pathway (Goldman, 2004).

Prolonged Inflammatory Phase

Chronic wounds are commonly complicated by impediments to healing such as local ischemia, necrotic tissue, and heavy bacterial loads. These factors prolong the inflammatory phase of wound healing by continuing to recruit macrophages and neutrophils into the wound bed, which will produce inflammatory proteases that degrade ECM (Goldman, 2004). Studies indicate that the level of inflammatory substances in chronic wounds is 100 times higher than the levels in acute wounds (Berg and Robson, 2003). Fortunately, this cycle can be interrupted by elimination of the noxious stimuli, that is, by the debridement of necrotic tissue and control of the bacterial burden (Goldman, 2004).

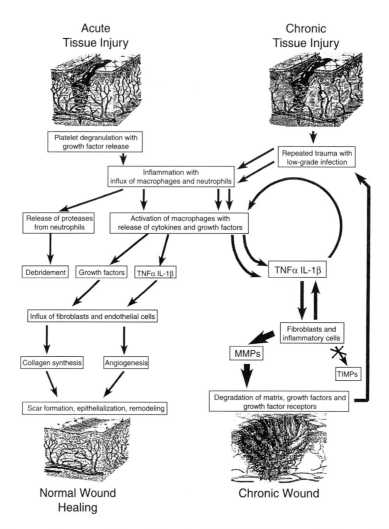

Fig. 4-10 Diagrammatic representation of the pathophysiologic "vicious cycle" characteristic of chronic wounds. Prolonged inflammation and elevated levels of proinflammatory cytokines stimulate protease synthesis, which degrades ECM and stimulates additional secretion of inflammatory cytokines. (From Mast BA, Schultz GS: Interactions of cytokines, growth factors and proteases in acute and chronic wounds, *Wound Rep Regen* 4(4):411, 1996.)

Low Levels of Growth Factors

In addition to high levels of inflammatory proteases, low levels of growth factors commonly characterize the environment of chronic wounds. Normal levels of growth factors are critical to repair, because a "threshold level" of growth factors is required to move target cells out of the quiescent G0 phase and into the reproductive cycle (Berg and Robson, 2003). The low levels of growth factors commonly found in chronic wounds may be the result of inadequate production by the cells of the wound bed (or insufficient numbers of the "producer" cells). Additional potential causes include rapid breakdown of growth factors by the high levels of proteases, or "binding" of the growth factors by the ECM (Berg and Robson, 2003; Henry and Garner, 2003; Steed, 2003). While this imbalance between inflammatory and proliferative cytokines is usually thought to be the **cause** of impaired healing, some authors suggest that the imbalance may instead be a **result** of chronicity. When the wound begins to heal, the ratio of inflammatory to proliferative cytokines normalizes (Goldman, 2004; Henry and Garner, 2003; Staiano-Coico et al, 2000).

A deficiency of growth factor receptor sites on host target cells and cellular senescence (a decrease in proliferation potential of dermal fibroblasts and inability of cells to respond to growth factors) have also been identified as characteristics of the chronic wound. In addition, cellular senescence is particularly common among elderly individuals (Berg and Robson, 2003). However, optimal wound management may result in successful "recruitment" of nonsenescent cells to the wound bed.

Miscellaneous Host Conditions

Additional "host factors" that trigger chronicity in a wound include ischemia, malnutrition, and comorbidities such as diabetes (Steed, 2003). Malnutrition is a particularly common contributor to wound chronicity. Fibroblasts cannot synthesize connective tissue proteins when they lack the requisite "raw ingredients." The importance of nutritional status is reflected in studies documenting consistently impaired wound healing in patients whose albumin levels were lower than 2.0 (Burns, Mancoll, and Phillips, 2003). In addition, in a study on wound fluid as a predictor of healing, the only constituents found to reliably predict healing were total protein and albumin, that is, albumin levels greater than 20 g/l (James et al, 2000; Schultz et al, 2003).

Pale pink tissue that is smooth rather than granular is indicative of delayed healing and a compromised ability to synthesize collagen and other connective tissue proteins. (See Plate 5.)

Denervation

Denervation is another potential cause for failure to heal. Sensory nerves secrete neuropeptides (e.g., substance P) that are highly chemotactic for inflammatory cells. Denervated wounds are therefore subject to impaired inflammation and compromised healing. Denervation may be one of the factors contributing to chronicity of pressure ulcers in spinal cord–injured patients and neuropathic ulcers in diabetic patients (Richards et al, 1997).

In summary, differences in the healing trajectory for acute and chronic wounds stem from the nature of the injury, the cellular events that follow, and miscellaneous host factors. In general, high mitotic activity, therapeutic levels of inflammatory cytokines, low levels of proteases, and mitotically competent cells characterize healing wounds. In contrast, chronic wounds exhibit low mitotic activity, excessive levels of inflammatory cytokines, high levels of proteases, and senescent or mitotically incompetent cells.

MEDIATORS OF WOUND HEALING

In order for healing to occur normally, the appropriate cells must be recruited to the wound bed (at the appropriate time), stimulated to reproduce and then, finally, directed to carry out specific components of the repair process such as connective tissue synthesis. This complex process is controlled and coordinated by an equally complex array of regulatory substances or mediators: chemical, environmental and molecular. Molecular mediators are the most significant and are discussed in detail in Chapter 5. Chemical and environmental factors thought to influence healing are briefly discussed the following sections. The effect of these regulatory factors is further influenced by "host" factors such as cell receptor sites, cellular senescence, availability of nutrients and cofactors required for phagocytosis and collagen synthesis, and status of the ECM.

Chemical Mediators

Chemical mediators that may affect the wound repair process include nitric oxide and calcium.

Nitric Oxide. Nitric oxide is one of the end results of the metabolism of L-arginine, an amino acid known to be essential to wound repair. Nitric oxide seems to be most important during the inflammatory phase, possibly because of its ability to combine with oxygen to produce reactive oxygen species, which contribute significantly to bacterial control. These reactive oxygen species (ROS) may also contribute to the regulation of repair, probably by activating specific cytokines (Sen, 2003). Nitric oxide levels also affect keratinocyte migration and differentiation and may be a stimulus to MMP production during the remodeling phase.

According to some studies, high levels of nitric oxide may actually inhibit collagen synthesis during the proliferative phase.

Patients who have impaired wound healing associated with antiinflammatory agents, corticosteroids, and diabetes may experience reduced nitric oxide production. The administration of nitric oxide has been shown in some studies to enhance collagen synthesis in subjects with diabetes and in subjects receiving nonsteroidal antiinflammatory drugs (NSAIDs). It seems clear that nitric oxide plays an important role in the regulation of repair, though additional study is needed to further delineate its specific impact (Frank et al, 2002; Reichner et al, 1999; Witte and Barbul, 2002; Witte and Barbul, 2003).

Calcium. The exact role of calcium as a potential mediator remains unclear. There is evidence that calcium may serve as an intracellular messenger and therefore affect cell proliferation, cell migration, and ECM deposition. Keratinocytes are highly responsive to variations in calcium level. Low levels seem to stimulate keratinocyte proliferation, whereas high levels support differentiation. These findings suggest that calcium channel blockers may interfere with keratinocyte differentiation; however, more studies are needed to clearly identify calcium's role in repair and the implications for wound management (Lansdown, 2002).

Environmental Mediators

The ECM may itself serve as a regulator of wound repair, by either facilitating or inhibiting cell migration and differentiation. For example, cell migration is dependent on the availability of fibronectin fragments within the ECM and is also affected by the orientation of connective tissue fibers within the wound bed (Dubay and Franz, 2003; Monaco and Lawrence, 2003). Another ECM factor potentially affecting repair is wound bed pH; an acidic pH stimulates platelet degranulation and release of PDGF (critical to the inflammatory phase of repair), while a neutral or alkaline pH increases the release of TGF-β (the dominant cytokine during the proliferative phase). This helps to explain why the pH of a normally healing wound is initially acidic, shifting to a neutral and finally an alkaline pH as the wound moves into the proliferative and remodeling phases (Liu et al, 2002).

Finally, wound repair may be regulated in part by direct communication between adjacent cells in the wound bed, via gap junctional intercellular communications.

Researchers have identified gated channels between cells that permit select molecules (e.g., sugar, amino acids, oxygen, calcium, and cAMP) to pass directly from one cell to another. It is thought that these channels may promote repair through the transfer of nutrients or other substances important to connective tissue synthesis. In studies done to date, disruption of these gated channels interferes with ECM production but supports cell proliferation. Again, more study is needed before the significance of these gated channels (and implications for wound management) can be clearly understood (Ehrlich and Diez, 2003).

INTERPLAY OF MEDIATORS

Cells involved in wound healing exhibit variable responses to regulatory substances. Factors such as the concentration and combination of the various regulatory substances, specificity of the cellular receptors, and effects of cell activation determine the specific response of the cell.

Concentration and Combination of Regulatory Substances

Cytokines and growth factors may affect the same target cell differently, depending on the concentration and combination of the regulatory factors and on the wound milieu. For example, PDGF acts as a chemoattractant for fibroblasts at low levels, whereas higher levels stimulate fibroblast proliferation (Cross and Mustoe, 2003; Martin, 1997; Monaco and Lawrence, 2003; Werner and Grose, 2003; Witte and Barbul, 1997). Similarly, fibroblasts cultured in a fibrin-fibronectin gel respond to PDGF by upregulating the integrin receptors that support diapedesis and cell migration, whereas fibroblasts cultured in a collagen gel respond to the same growth factor by synthesizing collagen. This is consistent with the wound milieu and fibroblast activity during the inflammatory and proliferative phases of wound repair. During the inflammatory phase the wound matrix is composed of fibrin and fibronectin and the release of PDGF serves as a chemoattractant to fibroblasts. In contrast, a collagen-based matrix and ongoing collagen synthesis by the fibroblasts characterize the proliferative phase (Monaco and Lawrence, 2003; Robson, 2003a; Schultz and Mast, 1998).

Specificity of Receptors

Although all cells within the wound bed are exposed to the same mix of regulatory substances, only select cells respond. In addition, different cells may exhibit different responses to the same regulatory substance because the regulatory substances exert their effects primarily through binding with cell receptors. Therefore only cells with the specific receptor sites respond to the regulatory substance, and the effects of receptor binding vary based on cell type. For example, PDGF stimulates migration of some cells and mitosis in others, whereas some cells are completely unaffected by PDGF (Martin, 1997; Witte and Barbul, 1997). Furthermore, studies indicate that the fibroblasts and keratinocytes in elderly individuals have a decreased number of receptor sites, which may explain why elderly patients tend to exhibit a diminished response to some regulatory substances (Ashcroft, Mills, and Ashworth, 2002).

Cell Activation

The effects of cell activation further affect the complexity of the response to regulatory substances. All cells involved in wound repair must undergo activation. A cell is "activated" when a regulatory substance binds to a specific receptor site and causes the cell to undergo a change in structure or function. For example, receptor binding may cause the cell to express a new surface antigen, which then alters the cell's activity and response to regulatory substances. Activated macrophages and fibroblasts commonly produce additional cytokines, further altering the wound environment (Witte and Barbul, 1997).

EXTREMES OF REPAIR: SCARLESS HEALING VERSUS EXCESSIVE SCARRING

This chapter has focused on what is currently considered "normal" repair for full-thickness wounds, that is, formation of granulation tissue (scar) to mend the defect, with a covering of new epithelium. This form of repair represents an intermediate point between "ideal" repair, also referred to as scarless healing, and "abnormal" repair. Hypertrophic and keloid scars are examples of abnormal repair or excessive scarring. As we learn

more about the factors that lead to "normal" and excessive scarring, we will hopefully be able to optimize repair and minimize scarring for all patients.

Scarless Healing

As mentioned earlier in this chapter, the early-gestation fetus typically heals without scarring, an ability that is lost during the third trimester. Features and characteristics of early gestation healing are listed in Box 4-2 and described below:

1. Platelet aggregation is diminished, resulting in a marked reduction in the level of growth factors released upon platelet degranulation, such as PDGF (Bullard, Longaker, and Lorenz, 2002; Dang et al, 2003; Samuels and Tan, 1999).

2. The inflammatory response is minimized; studies indicate a total absence of neutrophils and a significantly reduced number of monocytes/ macrophages. This is probably due in part to the immature fetal immune system, but the major factor is thought to be the significantly diminished level of inflammatory cytokines. A number of studies have confirmed a marked reduction in levels of "proinflammatory" and "profibrotic" substances, specifically TGF-β1 and TGF-β2. The result is fewer numbers of macrophages and minimal production of proteases. The lower levels of PDGF and TGF-β1 and TGF-β2 also reduce the chemoattraction for fibroblasts, which helps to modulate the proliferative response (Bullard et al, 2002; Dang et al, 2003; Samuels and Tan, 1999; Yang et al, 2003).

3. Early-gestation fetal wounds move very quickly through the inflammatory phase and into the proliferative phase. Fibroblasts, keratinocytes, and endothelial cells move rapidly into the wound bed

BOX 4-2 Features of Scarless Healing

- Decreased amount of PDGF
- Decreased amount of proinflammatory proteases and growth factors
- Increased levels of fibronectin and hyaluronic acid
- Balance of TIMP and MMP
- New collagen structure and function indistinguishable from native collagen

TIMP, tissue inhibitors of matrix metalloproteases; *MMP,* matrix metalloproteases.

in response to elevated levels of fibronectin, tenascin, and hyaluronic acid. Fibronectin is a chemoattractant, tenascin promotes rapid migration by limiting cell adhesion, and hyaluronic acid facilitates the influx of fibroblasts by creating spaces in the ECM (Bullard et al, 2002; Dang et al, 2003; Samuels and Tan, 1999; Yang et al, 2003). After migrating into the wound bed, fibroblasts simultaneously proliferate and synthesize connective tissue proteins, predominantly type III collagen (the type normally found in unwounded dermis). Contraction and the resulting scar formation do not occur in these fetal wounds because fibroblasts do not differentiate into myofibroblasts (Dang et al, 2003; Yang et al, 2003).

4. There is a balance between growth factors that stimulate connective tissue synthesis (e.g., TGF-β1 and TGF-β2), and those that promote ECM breakdown (TGF-β3), which is thought to play a major role in preventing the accumulation of excess connective tissue (Bullard et al, 2002).

5. The newly synthesized collagen is indistinguishable from native collagen. It is organized in a reticular pattern that matches the surrounding tissue and demonstrates normal "flexibility," probably due to reduced cross-linking. The differences in the collagen produced in early-gestation fetal repair and that produced in late gestation or postnatal repair are thought to be due to differences in cellular receptors that modulate collagen production (Bullard et al, 2002).

In summary, early-gestation fetal repair is characterized by a significantly reduced inflammatory response, and a rapid and balanced proliferative phase that restores the dermal architecture without scarring. (See Box 4-3.)

Excessive Scarring

Hypertrophic and keloid scars are two types of excessive scarring that represent fairly common complications of wound healing. Clinically, both types of scars are raised, erythematous, and pruritic (due to abnormally high levels of mast cells). On a histologic basis, both are composed of connective tissue with increased cell density and increased density of blood vessels. Differences between hypertrophic scars and keloids are listed in Table 4-4 (Rahban and Garner, 2003). (See Plates 7c and 7d.)

TABLE 4-4   Differences between Hypertrophic Scars and Keloids

HYPERTROPHIC SCARS	KELOID SCARS
Are confined to area of original injury	Extend beyond the borders of the original wound
Commonly occur over joints	Are more likely to occur on upper back, chest, deltoid, and earlobes
May regress spontaneously	Very rarely regress
Are associated with contractures	Keloids lack myofibroblasts so they do not shorten nor cause contractures

Risk factors for excessive scarring include darkly pigmented skin, age less than 30 years, familial history, and wound location in areas exposed to stretch or tension. Anecdotal evidence also supports puberty and pregnancy as potential risk factors, suggesting a hormonal influence (Rahban and Garner, 2003).

The pathology of hypertrophic scarring is in many ways the reverse of the process for scarless healing. Whereas scarless healing is associated with a minimal inflammatory response and muted proliferative response, hypertrophic scarring is associated with a prolonged or exaggerated inflammatory response followed by overproduction of new blood vessels and connective tissue. The stimulus for this exaggerated response is thought to be a prolonged inflammatory phase with a resultant increase in the production of "profibrotic" cytokines such as TGF-β1 and TGF-β2 (Rahban and Garner, 2003; Robson, 2003a). In addition, during the remodeling phase, collagen synthesis exceeds collagen lysis which is the reverse of normal. While it would seem that this excessive scar tissue would lend strength to the wound, the converse is true because the collagen in hypertrophic scars lacks the normal cross-links that provide tensile strength (Robson, 2003a).

Treatment options for hypertrophic and keloid scars range from topical pressure and dressings to injections to surgical excision (Table 4-5) (Rahban and Garner, 2003; Robson, 2003b). Animal studies support the value of antibodies to the profibrotic cytokines, but these are not yet clinically available (Robson, 2003a).

TABLE 4-5 Treatment Options for Excessive Scarring

TREATMENT OPTION	RATIONALE
Silicone sheeting	Reduces fibroblast activity and down-regulates TGF-β2 during the remodeling phase
Intralesional steroid injections	Provide antiproliferative effects
Tamoxifen	Reduces the production of proinflammatory cytokines and collagen synthesis
Pressure garments	Have value in the prevention and treatment of hypertrophic scars
Surgical excision	Used in combination with other modalities (intralesional steroids, silicone gel sheeting, radiation therapy, or pressure garments) to prevent recurrence of the hyperproliferative scarring

FACTORS AFFECTING THE REPAIR PROCESS

By observing a number of similar wounds and tracking their time to healing, it is possible to construct a curve that represents the healing "trajectory" for that type of wound. For example, it is well documented that epithelialization of a surgical wound healing by primary intention is typically complete within 48 hours, a healing ridge should be palpable by day 5, and initial collagen deposition should be complete by the twenty-first postoperative day. Interestingly, it is also possible to plot a "healing trajectory" for neuropathic ulcers, venous ulcers, and pressure ulcers. Studies indicate that the usual "time to healing" is similar for all patients with a particular type of wound (Steed, 2003). Knowledge regarding the normal healing trajectory for any wound allows the clinician to promptly identify wounds with impaired healing and to intervene accordingly. It also allows investigators to objectively determine the impact of various interventions or impediments on the repair process. For example, any deterrent to healing would shift the healing trajectory to the right, whereas interventions that enhanced healing would shift the trajectory to the left. At this point in time, it is not known whether or not "normal" healing can be "accelerated" via use of exogenous growth factors or other interventions, though accelerated healing would be tremendously beneficial to the many patients undergoing surgical procedures. Of course, we do know that there are a number of factors that can delay the healing process and shift the trajectory to the right; those factors are listed in Box 4-3 and are the focus of this section.

Tissue Perfusion and Oxygenation

Oxygen fuels the cellular functions essential to the repair process; therefore the ability to perfuse the tissues with adequate amounts of oxygenated blood is critical to wound healing. Although the negative effects of ischemia on wound repair are well known, the specific oxygen level required for the support of healing is not clear. Oxygen tension in normal tissue is approximately 40 mm Hg, and clinicians have used cut-off values between 20 and 40 mm Hg to predict the potential for wound healing in patients with arterial insufficiency (Waldorf and Fewkes, 1995). Current evidence suggests that tissue oxygen requirements vary based on the specific stage of repair. Oxygen requirements are highest during the inflammatory phase. Leukocyte migration and ingestion of bacteria requires

BOX 4-3 Factors that Impair Wound Healing

Hypovolemia
Hypotension
Vasoconstriction
Edema
Vascular disease
Cigarette smoking
Inadequate intake of protein, calories, vitamins A or C, zinc, magnesium, copper, iron, arginine and glutamine
Infection
Diabetes mellitus
Obesity
Chemotherapeutic agents
Antiinflammatory medications
Corticosteroids
Age
Stress
Hematopoietic processes
Malignancy
Sepsis
Irradiation
Renal disease
Pulmonary disease

oxygen tensions greater than 30 mm Hg. Bacterial killing requires even higher oxygen levels, with tissue pO_2 levels of at least 45 to 80 mm Hg (Whitney, 2003). The proliferative phase can proceed at somewhat lower oxygen levels. While fibroblast migration occurs best at oxygen tensions above 30 mm Hg, keratinocyte mitosis and collagen synthesis can proceed as long as the tissue oxygen levels are greater than 15 mm Hg (Wilson and Clark, 2003). However, recent evidence suggests that higher tissue oxygen levels may provide for better quality collagen and enhanced tensile strength. Some investigators have found a small but significant increase in tensile strength among postoperative patients with normal perfusion who were treated with supplemental oxygen at 30% to 80% (Whitney, 2003). The one potentially beneficial effect of moderate hypoxia is enhanced stimulus to neoangiogenesis (Wilson and Clark, 2003; Zamboni, Browder, and Martinez, 2003).

Obviously, tissue oxygen levels are dependent both on perfusion status and on oxygenation of the blood. However, because wounds remove only 1 ml of oxygen per each 100 ml of blood perfusing the tissues, compromised perfusion is more likely to jeopardize wound healing than compromised oxygenation secondary to pulmonary conditions (Waldorf and Fewkes, 1995). Therefore tissues that are adequately perfused are usually able to heal even if the blood is poorly oxygenated or the patient is anemic. In fact, anemia usually does not significantly affect repair unless the hematocrit drops below 20% (Stotts and Wipke-Tevis, 2001). Factors most likely to adversely affect perfusion to the wound bed include hypovolemia, hypotension, factors producing vasoconstriction (such as cold and sympathetic stimulation), vascular disease, and edema.

Cigarette smoking is particularly deleterious to wound repair because it affects both perfusion and oxygenation. The three byproducts of cigarette smoking are nicotine, carbon monoxide, and hydrogen cyanide. Nicotine is a potent vasoconstrictor and potentiates platelet aggregation, carbon monoxide lowers oxygen saturation, and hydrogen cyanide interferes with cellular transport of oxygen (Burns et al, 2003; Stotts and Wipke-Tevis, 2001). Studies indicate a higher incidence of wound infection, dehiscence, and delayed healing among smokers as compared to nonsmokers. Therefore patients should be counseled regarding the negative effect of smoking and should be offered a comprehensive program to assist them with smoking cessation (Burns et al, 2003; Manassa, Hertl, and Olbrisch, 2003; Sorensen, Karlsmark, and Gottrup, 2003; Stotts and Wipke-Tevis, 2001).

It is evident that supportive care for the patient with a wound must include measures to enhance perfusion. "Standard" interventions to enhance tissue perfusion include maintenance of warmth, hydration, and blood volume, pain control, and measures to eliminate edema. Investigational approaches include routine use of supplemental oxygen, use of epidural anesthetic blockade to increase blood flow in the microcirculation, and the use of angiogenic growth factors in the management of ischemic wounds (Clark, 2002; Quirina and Viidik, 1998; Veering and Cousins, 2000; Wu and Mustoe, 1995).

Nutritional Status

Nutritional status is another key factor in wound repair (MacKay and Miller, 2003; Williams and Barbul, 2003). Nutrients provide the raw materials needed for the multitude of cellular activities that constitute wound healing. Adequate nutrition is also essential to a competent immune system and prevention of infection. Protein, calories, vitamin C, vitamin A, zinc, magnesium, copper, and iron are all critical to collagen synthesis and development of normal tensile strength. Therefore nutritional monitoring should include these elements and supplementation should be provided when there is clear clinical or laboratory evidence of deficiency. For example, normal zinc levels (100 mcg/100 ml) are essential to healing, but because abnormally high zinc levels are deleterious, supplemental zinc should be administered only to patients with evidence of zinc deficiency and only on a short-term basis (Gray, 2003; Williams and Barbul, 2003).

When evaluating the adequacy of protein intake, the clinician should also ensure adequate intake of arginine and glutamine; these are two amino acids that have been found to play essential roles in wound healing. Glutamine is necessary for protein synthesis during acute stress states and has been found to promote lymphocyte production and macrophage function. Arginine is the sole dietary precursor to ornithine and nitric oxide, each of which play vital roles in the repair process. Although additional research is needed to more clearly define the role of these amino acids in wound repair, studies have shown that a diet supplemented with both glutamine and arginine increases collagen deposition in elderly patients. It has also been shown that arginine is not produced in sufficient amounts during periods of growth, metabolic stress, and illness; therefore, supplementation is frequently required for patients with chronic wounds (Burns et al, 2003; Clark, 2002; Flanigan, 1997; Kiy, 1997; Schaffer and Barbul, 1997; Ter Riet, Kessels, and Knipschild, 1995; Thomas, 1997; Williams and Barbul, 2003). Additional information concerning the role of the various nutrients in the wound healing process and the daily requirement levels are available in Chapter 8.

Infection

A third factor affecting wound repair is the presence of infection. Wound infection prolongs the inflammatory phase, delays collagen synthesis, prevents epithelialization, and increases the production of inflammatory cytokines, which may lead to additional tissue destruction. Infection is a common cause of wound chronicity and necessitates prompt, aggressive treatment. Specifically, treatment is indicated for osteomyelitis, cellulitis, or evidence of "critical colonization" (Campton-Johnson and Wilson, 2001; Carlson, 1997; Guttman, 2002; Robson, 1997; Schultz et al, 2003; Waldorf and Fewkes, 1995). While treatment is clearly indicated for infections involving the soft tissue or bone, systemic antibiotics are **not** indicated for bacterial control at the wound surface; this is an important distinction, given the increasing incidence of bacterial resistance (Schultz et al, 2003). Issues pertaining to infection are addressed further in Chapter 9.

Diabetes Mellitus

Impaired wound healing in patients with diabetes mellitus has been well established. Diabetes mellitus represents a significant problem in the United States since approximately 18 million Americans currently have diabetes (American Diabetes Association, 2004). Studies indicate that wound repair in patients with diabetes mellitus is characterized by reduced collagen synthesis and deposition and decreased tensile strength. A direct relationship between tensile strength and glycosylated hemoglobin levels has been described (Clark, 2002). These differences in wound repair may be partially explained by increased levels of proteases (e.g., gelatinase), decreased levels of proliferative cytokines (growth factors), and abnormal insulin levels (Bitar and Labbad, 1996). The impact of altered insulin levels and reduced growth factors is supported by studies that show increased collagen deposition and enhanced tensile strength in patients with diabetes who were treated with insulin therapy and exogenous growth factors (Bitar, 1997; Bitar, 1998; Bitar and Labbad, 1996; Greenhalgh, 2003; Waldorf and Fewkes, 1995).

Diabetes can also result in compromised perfusion. Patients with diabetes are at high risk for microvascular disease. Consequently the delivery of micronutrients at the capillary level is impaired and there is an increase in vascular permeability. The end result seems to be increased risk of infection and diminished support for healing (Greenhalgh, 2003; Niinikoski, 2003). In addition, hyperglycemia produces advanced glycosylation end products (AGEs), which are thought to cause increased oxidative stress and further hypoxia at the cellular level (Greenhalgh, 2003).

Patients with diabetes also experience impaired leukocyte chemotaxis, impaired phagocytosis, a decrease in the number of macrophages in the wound matrix, and increased infection rates (Bitar, 1997; Waldorf and Fewkes, 1995). Many of the adverse effects of diabetes are at least partially related to glycemic control; therefore, the management of diabetic patients with wounds should include strict glycemic control as well as measures to maximize tissue perfusion and reduce repetitive trauma. (A more detailed discussion of pathophysiologic changes in patients with diabetes is provided in Chapter 16.)

Obesity

Obesity as a risk factor for impaired healing is becoming increasingly relevant as the number of morbidly obese individuals in the United States continues to rise at an epidemic rate. Adipose tissue is poorly vascularized. In addition, cardiac function is frequently compromised in the obese patient, further diminishing tissue perfusion. As a result, infection, seroma formation, anastomotic leaks, and wound dehiscence are all more common among this patient population. Nursing measures to optimize healing for the obese patient include incisional support (e.g., careful use of binders), use of wound suction to prevent seroma formation, control of pain and nausea (to improve mobility and respiratory function and to prevent vomiting), and nutritional support to maintain positive nitrogen balance (Wilson and Clark, 2003). This topic is discussed in more detail in Chapter 14.

Medications

There are a number of medications that can negatively affect wound healing The two categories of medications most likely to compromise repair are chemotherapeutic agents and antiinflammatory medications. Chemotherapeutic drugs are the category of drugs most likely to interfere with repair, owing to their impact on rapidly dividing cells. The cells most profoundly affected are the fibroblasts and myofibroblasts, resulting in impaired collagen synthesis and wound contraction. These effects are greatest when chemotherapeutic agents are given preoperatively or within the first 2 weeks after surgery (Burns et al, 2003).

Administration of corticosteroids or the hypercortisolemia produced during periods of stress affects wound healing through several mechanisms: suppression of inflammation, antimitotic effects on keratinocytes and fibroblasts, decreased synthesis of ECM components, and delayed epithelialization (Anstead, 1998; Bitar, 1998; Waldorf and Fewkes, 1995). One way in which corticosteroids exert their powerful antiinflammatory effect is by stabilization of lysosomal membranes. Lysosomes are cellular structures that normally are activated to facilitate the breakdown of phagocytized material within the macrophage. Stabilization of lysosomal membranes by high levels of cortisol renders the lysosomes inactive, which severely compromises macrophage function. Dose equivalents of less than 10 mg of prednisone a day do not exert adverse effects; however, doses greater than 30 to 40 mg/day have definite deleterious effects on wound healing (Anstead, 1998; Waldorf and Fewkes, 1995). Long-term corticosteroid administration is also associated with zinc deficiency, further compromising the repair process (Williams and Barbul, 2003).

Vitamin A and anabolic steroids can partially counteract the effects of corticosteroids. Anabolic agents stimulate cellular proliferation and regulation of gene transcription. This tends to "offset" the negative effects of elevated cortisol levels on these processes (Anstead, 1998; Erlich and Hunt, 1968). While the mechanism by which vitamin A works is not fully understood, it is believed that vitamin A works by labilizing, or breaking down, lysosomal membranes so that the normal inflammatory response is restored (Ulland and Caldwell, 1997). Although vitamin A is effective in steroid-impaired wound healing, it does not enhance healing beyond the normal rate. Furthermore, there is inconclusive evidence of any beneficial effects in the absence of corticosteroids (Anstead, 1998; Erlich and Hunt, 1969).

Vitamin A can be taken systemically or applied topically. Topical preparations are generally preferred to systemic administration because there is less risk of reversing the desired therapeutic effect of the steroid therapy. A dose of 25,000 is recommended for oral administration and 25,000 to 100,000 international units for topical therapy. Vitamin A should be used with caution in patients with preexisting liver disease because of decreased toxicity thresholds (Anstead, 1998; Wicke et al, 2000).

NSAIDS in high doses have also been linked to delayed wound healing. However, NSAIDs may actually improve healing in ischemic wounds, owing to their ability to limit necrosis in these wounds (Burns et al, 2003).

Age

The aging process produces many changes in the skin and underlying tissues that render a person more susceptible to injury and less able to heal. Aging affects all phases of wound healing. The most significant changes include a diminished inflammatory response, reduced production of cytokines/growth factors, reduced cytokine receptors, and increased numbers of senescent cells (cells that are unable to respond to growth factors) (Ashcroft, Mills, and Ashworth, 2002; Harding, 2002). Aging is also associated with factors that may adversely affect healing such as concomitant medical conditions and polypharmaceutical use. Aging is inevitable, so it is critical to maximize healing in the older patient by providing optimal systemic and topical support and eliminating any correctable impediments.

Stress

Both psychologic and physiologic stress has been implicated as a potential cofactor in impaired wound healing. Specific ways in which stress negatively affects healing include elevated serum corticosteroid levels, which compromises immune function, and sympathetic stimulation, which compromises perfusion due to vasoconstriction (Padgett, Marucha, and Sheridan, 1998; Stotts and Wipke-Tevis, 1996). Both animal and human studies have confirmed that stress is positively related to hypercortisolemia and delayed wound healing as compared with controls. Cellular analysis has revealed a delayed onset of cellular infiltration into the wound bed, indicating a lag in the initiation of inflammation (Broadbent et al, 2003; Padgett, Marucha, and Sheridan, 1998). Most studies related to the effects of stress on wound repair were performed on acute wounds; further research is needed to replicate these findings in chronic wounds. However, it is evident that comprehensive wound management must include interventions to reduce physiologic or psychologic stress. Specific stress-reducing strategies include environmental control (e.g., noise reduction and temperature control), affirmations, pain control, guided imagery, music therapy, patient education, and counseling (Wientjes, 2002).

Immunosuppression

Any disease process or medication that suppresses the immune system can alter healing. This is attributable primarily to impairment of the inflammatory process. An impaired immune system is less able to initiate chemotaxis and the release of proinflammatory cytokines, such as lymphokines, from the T lymphocytes. Lymphokines are particularly important because they regulate chemoattraction of macrophages, destruction of target cells, and promotion of cellular proliferation (Schaffer and Barbul, 1998). Thus immunosuppression can retard wound healing and increase susceptibility to infection.

Other Factors Affecting Wound Repair

In addition to the specific conditions noted previously, any systemic condition that adversely affects health status can negatively affect wound healing. Renal and hepatic disease, malignancy, and sepsis are among these conditions. Hematopoietic abnormalities can impair wound healing because red blood cells are needed for oxygen transport and platelets are necessary for hemostasis and initiation of the wound-healing cascade. Since the late 1800s, radiation therapy has been known to delay healing because of damage to the keratinocytes and fibroblasts as well as the nutrient blood vessels (Phillips, 2000).

In addition to systemic factors, local factors such as wound bed desiccation, wound bed pH, hypothermia, excess wound fluid, and/or heavy bacterial colonization can affect the repair process; wound healing is best supported by a moist, clean wound surface that is maintained at a temperature of about 30°C (Phillips, 2000). Local factors are also discussed in Chapter 19.

SUMMARY

In summary, wound healing is a complex series of events. It is normally initiated by an injury that leads to clot formation and platelet degranulation, controlled by a myriad of cytokines and growth factors, and affected significantly by systemic factors such as perfusion, nutritional status, and steroid levels. Effective management of any wound requires an understanding of the normal repair process and the factors that may interfere with normal repair. This understanding provides the foundation for comprehensive assessment of the wound and the patient, and selection of interventions designed to optimize healing.

SELF-ASSESSMENT EXERCISE

1. Explain why wounds confined to the epidermal and dermal layers heal by regeneration, whereas wounds extending through the dermal layer into the subcutaneous tissue or fascia or muscle layer must heal by scar formation.
2. Explain what is meant by primary-, secondary-, and tertiary-intention wound healing.
3. Identify the major components of partial-thickness repair.
4. Explain why epidermal resurfacing and dermal repair proceed more rapidly when the wound surface is kept moist.
5. Summarize the activities that occur in the three key phases of repair for full-thickness wounds healing by primary intention (in order).
6. Which of the following cells are responsible for collagen synthesis?
   a. Macrophages
   b. Neutrophils
   c. Fibroblasts
   d. Platelets

7. The process of contraction is important for wound healing in which of the following?
 a. Wounds healing by primary intention
 b. Wounds healing by secondary intention
 c. Superficial abrasions
 d. Partial-thickness wounds

8. Explain why large wounds healing by secondary intention may require skin grafting, whereas large, partial-thickness wounds will epithelialize.

9. Summarize the differences between acute and chronic wound healing.

10. List at least six factors that affect wound healing.

11. Which of the following characterize the molecular environment of a chronic wound?
 a. High levels of growth factors
 b. Increased levels of proteases (MMPs)
 c. Increased levels of protease inhibitors (TIMPs)
 d. Excessive collagen synthesis

REFERENCES

American Diabetes Association: *Diabetes statistics*, http://www.diabetes.org/diabetes-statistics.jsp; Accessed May 16, 2004.

Anstead G: Steroids, retinoids, and wound healing, *Advances in Wound Care* 11:277, 1998.

Ashcroft GS, Mills SJ, Ashworth JJ: Aging and wound healing, *Biogerontology* 3(6):337, 2002.

Berg Vande JS, Robson MC: Arresting cell cycles and the effect on wound healing, *Surg Clin North Am* 83:509, 2003.

Bitar M: Glucocorticoid dynamics and impaired wound healing in diabetes mellitus, *Am J Pathol* 152:547, 1998.

Bitar M: Insulin-like growth factor-1 reverses diabetes-induced wound healing impairment in rats, *Horm Metab Res* 29:83, 1997.

Bitar M, Labbad Z: Transforming growth factor-β and insulin-like growth factor-1 in relation to diabetes-induced impairment of wound healing, *J Surg Res* 61(1):113, 1996.

Brissett AE, Hom DB: The effects of tissue sealants, platelet gels, and growth factors on wound healing, *Curr Opin Otolaryngol Head Neck Surg* 11(4):245, 2003.

Broadbent E et al: Psychological stress impairs early wound repair following surgery, *Psychosom Med* 65(5):865, 2003.

Bullard KM, Longaker MT, Lorenz HP: Fetal wound healing: current biology, *World J Surg* 27:54, 2002.

Burns JL, Mancoll JS, Phillips LG: Impairments to wound healing, *Clin Plast Surg* 30:47, 2003.

Calvin M: Cutaneous wound repair, *Wounds* 10(1):12, 1998.

Campton-Johnson SM, Wilson JA: Infected wound management: advanced technologies, moisture-retentive dressings, and die-hard methods, *Crit Care Nurs Q* 24(2):64, 2001.

Carlson M: Acute wound failure, *Surg Clin North Am* 77(3):607, 1997.

Chen WYJ, Abatangelo G: Functions of hyaluronan in wound repair, *Wound Rep Regen* 7:79, 1999.

Clark JJ: Wound repair and factors influencing healing, *Crit Care Nurs Q* 25(1):1, 2002.

Cross KJ, Mustoe TA: Growth factors in wound healing, *Surg Clin North America*, 83:531, 2003.

Dang C et al: Fetal wound healing: current perspectives, *Clin Plast Surg* 30:13, 2003.

Dubay KA, Franz MG: Acute wound healing: the biology of acute wound failure, *Surg Clin North Am* 83:463, 2003.

Ehrlich HP, Diez T: Role for gap junctional intercellular communications in wound repair, *Wound Rep Regen* 11(6):481, 2003.

Ehrlich P, Hunt T: Effects of cortisone and Vitamin A on wound healing, *Ann Surg* 167(3):324, 1968.

Ehrlich P, Hunt T: The effects of cortisone and anabolic steroids on the tensile strength of healing wounds, *Ann Surg* 170(2):203, 1969.

Flanigan K: Nutritional aspects of wound healing, *Adv Wound Care* 10(3):48, 1997.

Frank S et al: Nitric oxide drives skin repair: novel functions of an established mediator, *Kidney Int* 61:882, 2002.

Gabbiani G: The myofibroblast in wound healing and fibrocontractive diseases, *J Pathol* 200:500, 2003.

Goldman R: Growth factors and chronic wound healing: past, present, and future, *Adv Skin Wound Care* 17(1):24, 2004.

Gray M: Does oral zinc supplementation promote healing of chronic wounds? *J Wound Ostomy Continence Nurs* 30(6):295, 2003.

Greenhalgh DG: Wound healing and diabetes mellitus, *Clin Plast Surg* 30:37, 2003.

Guttman C: Effective wound care looks at bacterial balance, *Dermatol Times* 23(8):42, 2002.

Harding KG, Morris HL, Patel GK: Healing chronic wounds, *BMJ* 324(7330):160, 2002.

Henry G, Garner WL: Inflammatory mediators in wound healing, *Surg Clin North Am* 83:483, 2003.

Hunt TK, Van Winkle W Jr: Normal repair. In Hunt TK, Dunphy JE, editors: *Fundamentals of wound management*, New York 1997, Appleton-Century-Crofts.

Jahoda CAB, Reynolds AJ: Hair follicle dermal sheath cells: unsung participants in wound healing, *Lancet,* 358(9291):1445, 2001.

James TJ et al: Simple biochemical markers to assess chronic wounds, *Wound Rep Regen* 8:264, 2000.

Kiy A: Nutrition in wound healing: a biopsychosocial perspective, *Nurs Clin North Am,* 32(4):849, 1997.

Lansdown ABG: Calcium: a potential central regulator in wound healing in the skin, *Wound Rep Regen* 10:271, 2002.

Liu Y et al: Fibroblast proliferation due to exposure to a platelet concentrate in vitro is pH dependent, *Wound Rep Regen* 10:336, 2002.

MacKay D, Miller AL: Nutritional support for wound healing, *Altern Med Rev* 8(4):359, 2003.

Manassa EH, Hertl CH, Olbrisch RR: Wound healing problems in smokers and nonsmokers after 132 abdominoplasties, *Plast Reconstr Surg* 111(6):2082, 2003.

Mangram et al: Guideline for prevention of surgical site infection, *Infect Control Hosp Epidemiol* 20(1):247, 1999.

Martin P: Wound healing: aiming for perfect skin regeneration, *Science,* 276:75, 1997.

Mast BA, Schultz G: Interactions of cytokines, growth factors, and proteases in acute and chronic wounds, *Wound Rep Regen* 4:411, 1996.

Monaco JL, Lawrence WT: Acute wound healing: An overview, *Clin Plast Surg* 30:1, 2003.

Niinikoski J: Hyperbaric oxygen therapy of diabetic foot ulcers, transcutaneous oxymetry in clinical decision making, *Wound Rep Regen* 11(6):458, 2003.

Padgett D, Marucha P, Sheridan J: Restraint stress slows cutaneous wound healing in mice, *Brain Behav Immun* 12:64, 1998.

Phillips SJ: Physiology of wound healing and surgical wound care, *ASAIO Journal* 46(6):S2-S5, 2000.

Quirina A, Viiidik A: The effect of recombinant basic fibroblast growth factor (bFGF) in fibrin adhesive vehicle on the healing of ischaemic and normal incisional skin wounds, *Scand J Plast Reconstr Surg Hand Surg,* 32:9, 1998.

Rahban SR, Garner WL: Fibroproliferative scars, *Clin Plast Surg* 30:77, 2003.

Reichner JS et al: Molecular and metabolic evidence for the restricted expression of inducible nitric oxide synthase in healing wounds, *Am J Pathol* 145(4):1097, 1999.

Richards AM et al: Neural innervation and healing, *Lancet*, 350(9074):339, 1997.

Robson MC: Cytokine manipulation of the wound, *Clin Plast Surg* 30:57, 2003a.

Robson MC: Proliferative scarring, *Surg Clin North Am* 33:557, 2003b.

Robson M: Wound infection: a failure of wound healing caused by an imbalance of bacteria, *Surg Clin North Am* 77(3):637, 1997.

Rosenberg L, de la Torre J: Wound healing, growth factors, 2003, *Emedicine*, http://www.emedicine.com/plastic/topic457.htm; Accessed March 12, 2004.

Samuels P, Tan AKW: Fetal scarless wound healing, *J Otolaryngol* 28(5):296, 1999.

Schaffer M, Barbul A: Lymphocyte function in wound healing and following injury, *Br J Surg*, 85:444, 1998.

Schaffer M, Barbul A: Use of exogenous amino acids in wound healing. In Ziegler T, Pierce G, Herndon D, editors: *Growth factors and wound healing: basic science and clinical applications*, Norwell, Mass, 1997, Springer.

Schultz G, Mast B: Molecular analysis of the environment of healing and chronic wounds: Cytokines, proteases, and growth factors, *Wounds* 10(Suppl F):1F, 1998.

Schultz GS et al: Wound bed preparation: a systematic approach to wound management, *Wound Repair and Regeneration* 11(s1):1, 2003.

Sen CK: The general case for redox control of wound repair, *Wound Rep Regen* 11(6):431, 2003.

Sorensen LT, Karlsmark T, Gottrup F: Abstinence from smoking reduces incisional wound infection: a randomized controlled trial, *Ann Surg* 238(1):1, 2003.

Staiano-Coico L et al: Wound fluids: a reflection of the state of healing, *Ostomy Wound Manage* S46(1A):85, 2000.

Steed DL: Wound-healing trajectories, *Surg Clin North Am* 83:547, 2003.

Stotts N, Wipke-Tevis D: Co-factors in impaired wound healing, *Ostomy Wound Manage* 42:44, 1996.

Stotts NA, Wipke-Tevis DD: Co-factors in impaired wound healing. In Krasner D, Rodeheaver GT, Sibbald RG, editors: *Chronic wound care: a clinical source book for healthcare professionals*, ed 3, King of Prussia, Pennsylvania, 2001, HMP Communications.

Tarnuzzer R, Schultz G: Biochemical analysis of acute and chronic wound environments, *Wound Rep Regen* 4:321, 1996.

Ter Riet G, Kessels A, Knipschild P: Randomized clinical trial of ascorbic acid in the treatment of pressure ulcers, *J Clin Epidemiol* 48(12):453, 1995.

Thomas D: Specific nutritional factors in wound healing, *Adv Wound Care* 10(4):40, 1997.

Ulland A, Caldwell M: Vitamin A-growth factor interactions in wound healing. In Ziegler T, Pierce G, Herndon D, editors: *Growth factors and wound healing: basic science and clinical applications*, Norwell, Mass, 1997, Springer.

Veering BT, Cousins MJ: Cardiovascular and pulmonary effects of epidural anaesthesia, *Anaesth Intens Care* 28(6):620, 2000.

Waldorf H, Fewkes J: Wound healing, *Adv Dermatol* 10:77, 1995.

Werner S, Grose R: Regulation of wound healing by growth factors and cytokines, *Physiol Rev* 83:835, 2003.

Whitney JD: Supplemental perioperative oxygen and fluids to improve surgical wound outcomes: translating evidence into practice, *Wound Rep Regen* 11(6):462, 2003.

Wicke C et al: Effects of steroids and retinoids on wound healing, *Arch Surg* 135(11):1265, 2000.

Wientjes KA: Mind-body techniques in wound healing, *Ostomy Wound Manage* 48(11):62, 2002.

Williams JZ, Barbul A: Nutrition and wound healing, *Surg Clin North Am* 83:571, 2003.

Wilson JA, Clark JJ: Obesity: impediment to wound healing, *Crit Care Nurs Q* 26(2):119, 2003.

Winter G: Epidermal regeneration studied in the domestic pig. In Hunt T, Dunphy J, editors: *Fundamentals of wound management*, New York, 1979, Appleton-Century-Crofts.

Witte M, Barbul A: General principles of wound healing, *Surg Clin North Am* 77(3):509, 1997.

Witte MB, Barbul A: Role of nitric oxide in wound repair, *Am J Surg* 183(4):406, 2002.

Witte MB, Barbul A: Arginine physiology and its implication for wound healing, *Wound Rep Regen* 11(6):419, 2003.

Wu L, Mustoe T: Effect of ischemia on growth factor enhancement of incisional wound healing, *Surgery* 117(5):570, 1995.

Yang GP et al: From scarless fetal wounds to keloids: molecular studies in wound healing, *Wound Rep Regen* 11(6):411, 2003.

Zamboni WA, Browder LK, Martinez J: Hyperbaric oxygen and wound healing, *Clin Plast Surg* 30:67, 2003.

5

Molecular Regulation of Wound Healing

GREGORY SCHULTZ

OBJECTIVES

1. Describe the importance of adhesion and the migration of leukocytes in inflammation.
2. Identify important processes in wound healing that are regulated by growth factors, cytokines, proteases, or hormones.
3. Describe the molecular environment that growth factors need to promote wound healing.
4. List one member, a key target cell, and one main action for each of the six families of growth factors.
5. Describe the molecular differences between acute, healing wounds and chronic, nonhealing wounds and how applying the principles of wound bed preparation remove the barriers to healing.

Wound healing in the skin has been studied extensively in animal models and in humans, and much has been learned about the cells and the molecules that regulate this complex process. At the cellular level, healing of skin wounds involves platelets, leukocytes, epidermal cells, fibroblasts, and vascular endothelial cells. At the molecular level, results of cell culture studies, animal wound models, and human clinical trials have demonstrated that many growth factors, cytokines, proteases, and hormones regulate most of the key actions of cells during wound healing.

These actions include the directed movement of the cells into a wound (chemotactic migration), replacement of damaged epidermal and dermal cells (mitosis), growth of new blood vessels (neovascularization), formation of scar tissue (synthesis of extracellular matrix proteins), and remodeling of scar tissue (proteolytic turnover of extracellular matrix proteins) (Bennett and Schultz, 1993a, 1993b). Any condition that disrupts the normal actions of these molecular regulators in wounds will directly impair healing and promote the establishment and maintenance of chronic wounds (Mast and Schultz, 1996; Tarnuzzer and Schultz, 1996). If these two concepts are correct, then it should be possible to identify abnormalities in the actions of these molecules in chronic wounds and design therapies that reestablish an environment in chronic wounds that permits these molecular regulators to function normally and leads to the healing of chronic wounds.

BIOLOGIC ROLES OF CYTOKINES AND GROWTH FACTORS IN WOUND HEALING

General Phases of Wound Healing

The phases of wound healing are hemostasis, inflammation, proliferation and repair, and remodeling. There is considerable temporal overlap of these phases of healing, and the entire process lasts for several months. Immediately after injury the process of blood clotting is initiated by activation of a proteolytic cascade, which ultimately converts fibrinogen into fibrin. As the fibrin molecules self-associate into a weblike net, red blood cells (RBCs) and platelets become entrapped. The aggregate of fibrin, RBCs, and platelets quickly grows large enough to form a tampon that blocks an injured capillary and stops the flow of blood.

The process of blood clotting also induces platelet degranulation, which releases a burst of preformed growth factors stored in platelet granules. These include platelet-derived growth factor (PDGF), transforming growth factor (TGF-β), epidermal growth factor (EGF), and insulin-like growth factor-I (IGF-I). These growth factors initiate two major processes: inflammation and initiation of tissue repair. The growth factors released from platelets quickly diffuse from the wound into the surrounding tissues and attract leukocytes into the injured area (Bennett and Schultz, 1993a; Bennett and Schultz, 1993b).

Adhesion Molecules and Adhesion Receptors in Inflammation. Chemotactic attraction of leukocytes to a wound and their movement from the blood into wounded tissue (extravasation) involves expression and activation of adhesion molecules and adhesion receptors on leukocytes, platelets, and vascular endothelial cells. Cytokines and growth factors play key roles in these processes (Arai et al, 1990; Frenette and Wagner, 1996a, 1996b; Springer, 1990). Among the many types of adhesion molecules and receptors on the cell surface, four major families of transmembrane proteins stand out in the process of inflammation: integrins, selectins, cell adhesion molecules, and cadherins.

1. *Integrins* are glycoproteins composed of two different types of subunits, designated α and β. In simple terms, integrins are cellular receptors for extracellular matrix proteins, as shown with $\alpha 5 \beta 1$, which is a receptor for fibronectin. A short amino acid sequence, such as arginine-glycine-aspartate (RGD), is often the site of recognition by the integrin receptor. Integrins are important because they are capable of generating signals inside cells when the integrin receptor binds to a specific extracellular matrix protein, in much the same way the insulin receptor generates intracellular signals, which regulates glucose transport into a cell when insulin binds to its cellular receptor. Expression of $\beta 2$ integrins is limited to leukocytes, whereas $\beta 1$ integrins are expressed on most cell types. $\beta 1$ integrins primarily bind to extracellular matrix components such as fibronectin, laminin, and collagens. (These substances are discussed in more detail in Chapter 3 and 4.)

2. *Selectins* are proteins that have a unique structure called a lectin domain at the distal end, which can bind specific carbohydrate groups of glycoproteins or mucins on adjacent cells. So, unlike other adhesion proteins, which recognize specific protein structures, selectins recognize and bind to carbohydrate ligands on leukocytes and vascular endothelial cells. E-selectin appears on endothelial cells after they have been activated by inflammatory cytokines, and P-selectin is stored in α-granules of platelets and the storage granules of endothelial cells (Weible-Palade bodies).

3. *Cell adhesion molecules (CAMs)* are members of the immunoglobulin superfamily of proteins, and CAMs can bind to other CAMs or to integrins on cells. CAMs that are important in inflammation include the platelet–endothelial cell adhesion molecule (PECAM), vascular-cell adhesion molecule (VCAM), and intercellular adhesion molecule-1 (ICAM-1).

4. *Cadherins* are important in establishing molecular links between adjacent cells, especially during embryonic development. They form zipperlike structures of dimers at specialized regions of contact between neighboring cells called adherens junctions. Cadherins are linked to the cytoskeleton through molecules called catenins, which associate with actin microfilaments.

During the process of extravasation of inflammatory cells into a wound, important interactions occur between blood vessels and blood cells (Arai et al, 1990; Frenette and Wagner, 1996a; Frenette and Wagner, 1996b; Springer, 1990). Initially, circulating leukocytes begin rolling on endothelial cells through the binding of glycoproteins expressed on their cell surface to selectins, transiently expressed by activated endothelial cells of venules (Figure 5-1). The binding affinity of selectins is relatively low, but it is enough to serve as a biologic brake, making leukocytes quickly decelerate by rolling on endothelial cells. While rolling, leukocytes can become activated by chemoattractants (cytokines, growth factors, or bacterial products). After activation, leukocytes firmly adhere to endothelial cells as a result of the binding between their $\beta 2$ class of integrins and ligands, such as VCAM and ICAM expressed on activated endothelial cells. Chemotactic signals present outside the venule induce leukocytes to squeeze between endothelial cells of the venule and migrate into the inflammatory center by using their $\beta 1$ class of integrins to recognize and bind to extracellular matrix components.

Adhesion and degranulation of platelets at sites of vascular injury also use a system of adhesion molecules and adhesion receptor proteins. Vascular injury immediately induces endothelial cells to release the contents

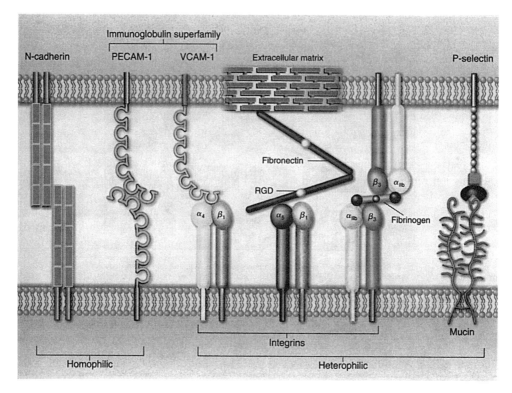

Fig. 5-1 Four major classes of adhesion proteins and adhesion receptors embedded in a theoretic plasma membrane (integrins, selectins, cell adhesion molecules [PECAM-1 and VCAM-1], and cadherins). (From Frenette PS, Wagner DD: Adhesion molecules. Part I, *N Engl J Med* 334:1526, 1996. Massachusetts Medical Society. All rights reserved.)

of their storage granules (Weible-Palade bodies), including the proteins P-selectin and von Willebrand factor. P-selectin promptly moves to the plasma membrane of endothelial cells, where it induces rolling of platelets on endothelial cells, and von Willebrand factor is quickly deposited on the exposed extracellular matrix, where it plays a crucial role in the adhesion of platelets to the damaged site.

Inflammatory Cell Proteases. When the inflammatory cascade is activated, neutrophils enter the wound initially, followed by macrophages. Neutrophils and macrophages become activated and engulf and destroy bacteria through their production of reactive oxygen species (super oxide anion, oxygen free radicals, or hydrogen peroxide). Activated neutrophils and macrophages also release several proteases, including

neutrophil elastase (a serine type of protease), neutrophil collagenase (a matrix metalloproteinase type of protease designated as MMP-8) and macrophage metalloelastase (MMP-12). These proteases play important, beneficial roles in initiating normal wound healing by removing (proteolytically degrading) damaged extracellular matrix components, which must be replaced by new, intact extracellular matrix molecules for wound healing to proceed. These proteases also are important for enabling inflammatory cells to move through the basement membrane that surrounds capillaries.

Inflammatory Cell Cytokines and Growth Factors in Proliferation and Repair. The growth factors released by platelets diffuse away from a wound within a few hours, but they are replaced by growth factors and cytokines that are produced by neutrophils, macrophages, activated fibroblasts, vascular endothelial cells, and epidermal cells that are drawn into the wound area. For example, activated macrophages secrete several important cytokines, including tumor necrosis factor alpha (TNFα) and interleukin-1beta (IL-1β), which have a variety of actions on different cells. TNF-α and IL-1β are potent inflammatory cytokines, which further stimulate inflammation. TNFα also induces macrophages to produce IL-1β, which is mitogenic for fibroblasts and upregulates expression of MMPs. Both TNF-α and IL-1β directly influence deposition of collagen in the wound by inducing synthesis of collagen by fibroblasts and by upregulating expression of MMPs. Additionally, these cytokines downregulate expression of the tissue inhibitors of metalloproteinases (TIMPs), which are the natural inhibitors of MMPs. Interferon gamma (IFN-γ), produced by lymphocytes attracted into the wound, inhibits fibroblast migration and downregulates collagen synthesis (see Table 5-1).

Inflammatory cells secrete other growth factors, including TGF-β, transforming growth factor alpha (TGF-α), heparin-binding epidermal growth factor (HB-EGF), and basic fibroblast growth factor (bFGF). The growth factors secreted by macrophages continue to stimulate migration of fibroblasts, epithelial cells, and vascular endothelial cells into the wound. As the fibroblasts, epithelial cells, and vascular endothelial cells migrate into the site of injury, they begin to proliferate, and the cellularity of the wound increases. This begins the proliferative and repair phase, which often lasts several weeks. If the wound is not infected, the number of inflammatory cells in a wound begins to decrease after a few days. Other types of cells drawn into the wound, such as fibroblasts, endothelial cells, and keratinocytes, begin to synthesize growth factors. Fibroblasts secrete IGF-I, bFGF, TGF-β, PDGF, and keratinocyte growth factor (KGF). Endothelial cells produce vascular endothelial cell growth factor (VEGF), bFGF, and PDGF. Keratinocytes synthesize TGF-α, TGF-β, and IL-1β. These growth factors continue to stimulate cell proliferation and synthesis of extracellular matrix proteins and to promote formation of new capillaries.

Remodeling Phase. After the initial scar forms, proliferation and neovascularization cease and the wound enters the remodeling phase, which can last for many months. During this last phase, a new balance is reached between the synthesis of extracellular matrix components in the scar and their degradation by metalloproteinases such as collagenase, gelatinase, and stromelysin. Fibroblasts synthesize a majority of the collagen, elastin, and proteoglycans that comprise the dermal scar matrix. Fibroblasts also are a major source of the MMPs that degrade the scar matrix as well as their inhibitors, the TIMPs. They also secrete lysyl oxidase, which is an enzyme that covalently cross-links components of the extracellular matrix such as collagen and elastin molecules, producing a stable extracellular matrix. Keratinocytes secrete much of the type 4 collagen that reforms the basement membrane, which separates the epidermal and dermal layers and forms the surface on which keratinocytes prefer to migrate. Angiogenesis ceases and the density of capillaries decreases in the wound site as a result of programmed cell death of the vascular endothelial cells (apoptosis). Eventually, remodeling of the scar tissue reaches equilibrium, although the mature scar is never as strong as uninjured skin.

GENERAL PROPERTIES OF GROWTH FACTORS AND THEIR RECEPTORS
Discovery, Purification, and Cloning of Growth Factors

Protein growth factors were initially discovered as a consequence of their ability to stimulate multiple cycles of cell growth (mitosis) when added to cultures of normal, quiescent cells. This distinguishes growth factors from essential nutrients such as vitamins, cofactors, and trace minerals (such as selenium), which are required for metabolic processes but are not sufficient to initiate cell division by themselves. Both nutrients and growth factors are necessary for mitosis, but only growth factors can initiate mitosis of quiescent cells.

Based on the ability of growth factors to stimulate continuous mitosis of cells in culture, it is not surprising that many growth factors initially were isolated from medium conditioned by tumor cells. Other sources of growth factors included platelets, macrophages, and normal tissues that can proliferate rapidly, such as ovarian follicles or placenta. Although growth factors were present in minute quantities from these natural sources, tiny amounts eventually were purified using traditional biochemical methods of column chromatography, ion-exchange chromatography, high-pressure liquid chromatography (HPLC), ultracentrifugation, and gel electrophoresis. The amino acid sequences of the proteins were determined, which permitted the growth factor genes to be cloned and sequenced. With the development of recombinant DNA technology, large amounts of synthetic human growth factors were produced from cultures of bacteria, yeast, or human cells that carried the gene for the growth factor. The availability of large amounts of the synthetic growth factors enabled research to be performed that led to a better understanding of the biologic roles of growth factors in wound healing and other physiologic processes such as fetal development, aging, and cancer. Ultimately, this led to experiments that evaluated the effects of the synthetic growth factors in animal wound healing models and eventually to clinical trials in patients.

Autocrine and Paracrine Action of Growth Factors

Growth factors are synthesized and secreted by many types of cells involved in wound healing including platelets, inflammatory cells, fibroblasts, epithelial cells, and vascular endothelial cells. Moreover, growth factors usually act either on the producer cell (autocrine stimulation) or on adjacent cells (paracrine stimulation). In contrast to classical endocrine hormones, growth factors generally do not enter the blood stream and act on cells at a great distance (Figure 5-2).

Receptors for Growth Factors

All peptide growth factors initiate their effects on target cells by binding to specific, high-affinity receptor proteins located in the plasma membrane of target cells (Fantl, Johnson, and Williams, 1993). Only cells that express the specific receptor protein can respond to the growth factor. Binding of the growth factor to its

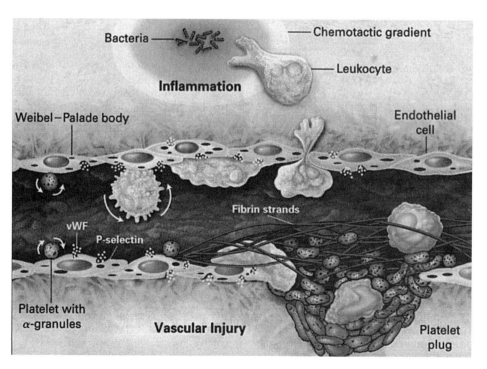

Fig. 5-2 Interactions between blood cells and a stimulated or injured venule. (From Frenette PS, Wagner DD: Adhesion molecules. Part II: Blood vessels and blood cells, *N Engl J Med* 335:43, 1996. Massachusetts Medical Society. All rights reserved.)

receptor usually initiates dimerization of two receptor proteins, which activates a region of receptor protein called a kinase domain that is located inside the cell (Figure 5-3). Kinase domains have the enzymatic ability to covalently transfer a phosphate group from the high-energy molecule (ATP) to an amino acid, such as tyrosine, serine, or threonine, in a protein. The activated receptor protein is the "first messenger" in the response system of a cell to a growth factor.

The activated receptor kinase domain then phosphorylates amino acids on a small number of specific cytoplasmic proteins. These cytoplasmic proteins become activated when phosphorylated and are the first in a series of second messenger proteins that eventually generate a response in the cell to the growth factor. Second messenger proteins also typically contain kinase domains that are activated when the proteins are phosphorylated. The activated cytoplasmic kinase proteins in turn phosphorylate other cytoplasmic proteins in a sequential cascade of phosphorylations and activations that eventually leads to the activation of special proteins called RNA transcription factors. Activated RNA transcription factors bind with selected regions of the DNA to help initiate transcription of genes into messenger RNAs (mRNAs), which are translated into proteins that ultimately alter the functions of the target cell.

Another system of cytoplasmic proteins acts to turn off the transcription of genes that are turned on by growth factors. These proteins are called phosphatases, and they remove the phosphate groups that were added to the amino acids of the second messenger kinase proteins and to the RNA transcription factors. Removal of the phosphate groups inactivates the second messenger proteins and the transcription factors. Thus the effects of growth factors on target cells require an integrated balance between receptor proteins, second messenger kinase proteins, RNA transcription factors, and phosphatases.

MAJOR FAMILIES OF GROWTH FACTORS

The first attempt to use growth factors to promote healing of human wounds was based on the concept that platelets contained numerous growth factors that were released at the time of injury. Furthermore, substantial amounts of activated platelet supernatant could be obtained either from individual patients with chronic skin ulcers or from apheresis donors. This would permit patients to be treated with their own activated platelet supernatant or from carefully screened platelet donors. To test this concept, an FDA-approved, randomized, controlled, multicenter, dose-response trial of topically applied activated platelet supernatant in chronic, nonhealing diabetic wounds was conducted (David et al, 1992; Holloway et al, 1993).

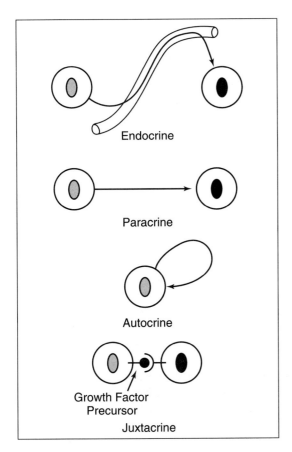

Fig. 5-3 Growth factor action. Secreted growth factors act predominately by autocrine (self-stimulation) or by paracrine (adjacent cells) pathways and not usually by classical endocrine pathways. Membrane-bound growth factors may also interact with adjacent cells by juxtacrine stimulation. (From Bennett NT, Schultz GS: Growth factors and wound healing: biochemical properties of growth factors and their receptors, *Am J Surg* 165:728, 1993. With permission, Excerpta Medica Inc.)

A total of 97 patients from four sites were randomized to receive either placebo or one of three dilutions of activated platelet supernatant (CT-102). The study population consisted of patients who had diabetes mellitus with at least one chronic, nonhealing diabetic ulcer of at least 8 weeks' duration with no signs of systemic wound infection and a supine periwound transcutaneous oxygen tension of at least 30 mm Hg. Before topical application of double-blind therapy, the wounds were debrided of all necrotic and infected soft and bony tissues. Wounds were treated daily until they healed or until a total of 20 weeks of treatment was achieved. The use of placebo treatment, combined with good basic wound care, reduced wound area 77% and reduced wound volume 83% from baseline to final visit, although only 29% of the placebo group healed completely. However, all healing parameters were significantly improved in patients treated with all doses of platelet releasate. For example, 63% of the patients treated with platelet releasate achieved complete healing ($p = 0.01$), with a 93% mean area reduction ($p = 0.002$) and a 95% mean volume reduction at the final visit ($p = 0.005$). The adverse experience profile of patients receiving platelet releasate was similar to that of patients receiving placebo. These results demonstrated the benefit of the treatment of chronic diabetic wounds with a mixture of growth factors and proteins released from platelets.

Table 5-1 presents an overview of the five major families of growth factors and includes those growth factors that have been shown to play roles in wound healing in animals or humans (not all known growth factors are included).

Epidermal Growth Factor (EGF) Family

EGF was the first growth factor to be purified and biochemically characterized (Carpenter and Cohen, 1990). Other members of the EGF family that influence wound healing are TGF-α (Massague, 1990) and HB-EGF (Shigeki et al, 1992). Members of the EGF family are small (about 6000 molecular weight), single-chain proteins that contain a characteristic triple-loop structure, which is required for biologic activity. They bind to a common receptor protein (EGF receptor) that has tyrosine kinase activity and is expressed on almost all types of cells. Members of the EGF family have similar, but not identical, biologic effects on target cells. They are chemoattractants and mitogens for epidermal cells, fibroblasts, and vascular endothelial cells but are most effective for epidermal cells.

EGF or TGF-α are synthesized as membrane-bound precursors that are released by proteolysis in a wide range of cells, including cells of the lacrimal and salivary glands. EGF and TGF-α are present in saliva and tears, and data from many different types of experiments strongly suggest that EGF and TGF-α play important roles in both the normal turnover of epithelial cells of the gut and cornea and in the healing of wounds in these tissues. Specifically, in the skin, epidermal cells synthesize large amounts of TGF-α, and mice that lack TGF-α or EGF receptor have abnormal hair and skin architecture. Levels of EGF receptor are elevated in the leading edge of epidermal cells in burn wounds (Nanney and King, 1996). Specific inhibition of the EGF receptor delays healing of partial-thickness skin injuries in animals. HB-EGF is produced by macrophages and presumably is retained in a wound for longer periods of time than EGF or TGF-α because of reversible binding to heparin.

Current models of skin wound healing propose that TGF-α is the growth factor that is primarily responsible for the normal maintenance and turnover of epidermal cells of the skin. When a skin injury occurs, epidermal cell proliferation and migration is stimulated by TGF-α produced by epidermal cells; EGF produced by epithelial cells lining the hair follicles, sweat glands, and sebaceous glands; and HB-EGF produced by macrophages that enter the wound. In addition, fibroblasts surrounding the wound secrete KGF, a member of the fibroblast growth factor system, which exclusively promotes migration and mitosis of keratinocytes.

Therapeutic Uses. EGF has been evaluated in burn care and venous ulcers. Early studies in normal animals showed accelerated healing of partial-thickness burns or excisional wounds when treated with EGF, TGF-α, or HB-EGF (Brown et al, 1986). In a prospective, double-blind, paired study of 12 patients with split-thickness skin donor sites, EGF treatment significantly decreased the average length of time to 25% healing and 50% healing by approximately 1 day and decreased time to 75% healing and 100% healing by approximately 1.5 days ($p < 0.02$) as compared with silver sulfadiazine

TABLE 5-1   **Growth Factors Involved in Skin Wound Healing**

MAJOR GROWTH FACTOR FAMILIES		
GROWTH FACTOR FAMILY	CELL SOURCE	ACTIONS
Transforming growth factor-β TGF-β1, TGF-β2 TGF-β3	Platelets Fibroblasts Macrophages	Fibroblast chemotaxis and activation ECM deposition Collagen synthesis TIMP synthesis MMP synthesis Reduces scarring Collagen Fibronectin
Platelet-derived growth factor PDGF-AA, PDGF-BB, VEGF	Platelets Macrophages Keratinocytes Fibroblasts	Activation of immune cells and fibroblasts ECM deposition Collagen synthesis TIMP synthesis MMP synthesis Angiogenesis
Fibroblast growth factor Acidic FGF, basic FGF, KGF	Macrophages Endothelial cells Fibroblasts	Angiogenesis Endothelial cell activation Keratinocyte proliferation and migration ECM deposition
Insulin-like growth factor IGF-I, IGF-II, insulin	Liver Skeletal muscle Fibroblasts Macrophages Neutrophils	Keratinocyte proliferation Fibroblast proliferation Endothelial cell activation Angiogenesis Collagen synthesis ECM deposition Cell metabolism
Epidermal growth factor EGF, HB-EGF, TGF-α, amphiregulin, betacellulin	Keratinocytes Macrophages	Keratinocyte proliferation and migration ECM deposition
Connective tissue growth factor CTGF	Fibroblasts Endothelial cells Epithelial cells	Mediates action of TGF-βs on collagen synthesis

cream (Brown et al, 1989). These results demonstrated that recombinant human growth factors could accelerate healing of acute skin wounds in patients and prompted the evaluation of EGF treatment for chronic skin ulcers.

Because epidermal regeneration is an important component of healing venous ulcers, a prospective, randomized, double-blind, placebo-controlled study was conducted evaluating topical use of recombinant human EGF for treatment of chronic venous ulcers (Falanga et al, 1992). Thirty-five patients with venous ulcers were randomly assigned to either a placebo group or treatment with an aqueous solution of EGF (10 mcg/ml). All patients applied a nonadherent dressing pad saturated with the EGF or placebo solution to the ulcer twice daily; a gauze bandage and a compression roll were also applied. At the end of the 10-week study, 6 of 17 ulcers treated with EGF had completely epithelialized compared with 2 of 18 ulcers treated with saline ($p = 0.01$). The mean (and median) percent reduction and ulcer size at the end of the study was 48% (73%) for EGF compared with 13% (33%) for placebo ($p = 0.32$). Although topical application of EGF in the dose and manner used in this study did not significantly enhance epithelialization of venous ulcers, a greater reduction in ulcer size and a larger number of healed ulcers occurred with the use of the EGF. Further investigations with EGF in venous ulcers seem warranted.

Platelet-Derived Growth Factor (PDGF) Family

The PDGF family comprises two major proteins, PDGF and VEGF, that influence wound healing (Heldin and Westermark, 1996). PDGF and VEGF share about 25% amino acid sequence homology, and both are composed of two subunits that are covalently linked by disulfide bonds. PDGF has two different subunits (designated types A and B). Human platelets contain high levels of PDGF, and many types of human cells important in skin wound healing can secrete PDGF including fibroblasts, vascular smooth muscle cells, and vascular endothelial cells.

PDGF and VEGF bind to different receptor proteins (both are tyrosine kinases) and stimulate different biologic actions. Two distinct PDGF receptors have been characterized. The PDGF-α receptor recognizes both α- and β-subunits of PDGF, whereas the PDGF-β receptor only recognizes the B-subunit of PDGF.

PDGF is a chemoattractant and mitogen primarily for fibroblasts, whereas VEGF is a chemoattractant and mitogen primarily for vascular endothelial cells. VEGF is one of the most effective angiogenic factors yet discovered, and synthesis of VEGF by vascular endothelial cells is increased by hypoxia.

Therapeutic Uses. PDGF, effective at stimulating formation of extracellular matrix and granulation tissue, has been evaluated clinically in pressure ulcers and diabetic ulcers. The PDGF-BB isoform was chosen for evaluation in clinical studies because it is able to bind to both PDGF-α and PDGF-β receptors.

Robson and colleagues (1992a) first studied PDGF-BB in 20 patients with pressure ulcers. Topical synthetic human PDGF-BB was applied daily to chronic pressure ulcers for 28 days. In this prospective, randomized, double-blind, placebo-controlled phase I/II trial, dosing solutions containing 1, 10, or 100 mcg/ml of PDGF-BB was evaluated. Patients treated with 100 mcg/ml of PDGF-BB had pronounced healing responses compared with patients treated with placebo, 1 mcg/ml, or 10 mcg/ml PDGF-BB. Although the results of this initial, small study did not achieve statistical significance at the 95% confidence level for both reduction of ulcer depth and reduction of ulcer volume, it strongly suggested that PDGF-BB improved healing of chronic pressure ulcers.

In a second major clinical study, PDGF-BB was evaluated for the treatment of noninfected, lower-extremity diabetic ulcers. All ulcers had a transcutaneous partial pressure of oxygen of 30 mm Hg or greater on the dorsum of the foot or at the ulcer margin (Steed and the Diabetic Ulcer Study Group, 1995). A total of 118 patients with chronic, full-thickness, lower-extremity diabetic ulcers were enrolled in this prospective, double-blind, placebo-controlled, multi-site clinical trial. PDGF-BB was formulated at 30 mcg/g in a gel. Ulcers were treated once a day at a dose equivalent to approximately 2.2 mcg PDGF-BB/cm^2 ulcer area for 20 weeks or until complete wound healing was achieved. The gel was spread evenly over the entire ulcer surface, a nonadherent saline-soaked gauze dressing was placed directly over the ulcer, and the foot was wrapped circumferentially with roll gauze. Patients were assessed weekly for the first month and thereafter every 2 weeks until completion of the study. The wound area was measured, and complete healing was defined as the achievement of 100% wound closure with no drainage present and no dressing required.

About 48% of the 61 patients randomized to the PDGF-BB treatment group achieved complete wound healing during the study compared with only 25% of 57 patients randomized to the placebo group ($p < 0.01$). The median reduction from initial wound area for the PDGF-BB group was 99% compared with 82% reduction for the placebo group ($p < 0.09$). These results demonstrated that once-daily topical application of PDGF-BB is safe and effective in stimulating the healing of chronic, full-thickness, lower-extremity diabetic neurotrophic ulcers. This study was the basis for approval of PDGF-BB (Regranex) by the U.S. Food and Drug Administration (FDA) for treatment of diabetic foot ulcers.

Another important result that emerged from the study of PDGF-BB–treated diabetic foot ulcers was the contribution of debridement (Steed et al, 1996). A lower rate of healing was observed in centers that performed less frequent debridement. Furthermore, the improved response rate associated with more frequent debridement occurred in both the PDGF-BB–treated group and the placebo group. These data indicate that wound debridement is a vital adjunct in the care of diabetic foot wounds.

Transforming Growth Factor-Beta (TGF-β) Family

The TGF-β family of proteins is the newest family to be discovered (Roberts and Sporn, 1996). Three distinct TGF-βs have been identified in humans: TGF-β1, TGF-β2, and TGF-β3. All three TGF-β isoforms are homodimers with covalently linked subunits of 12,500 molecular weight. They are synthesized as inactive proteins that must be activated by proteolytic removal of a segment of the proteins. The TGF-βs are synthesized by a variety of cell types including platelets, macrophages, lymphocytes, fibroblasts, bone cells, and keratinocytes, and nearly all nucleated cells have TGF-β receptors. Thus TGF-βs are probably the most broadly acting of all the families of growth factors.

Three different TGF-β receptor proteins have been identified and are designated type I, type II, and type III receptors. Although all three TGF-β isoforms bind to all three types of TGF-β receptors, they do not appear to have the same biologic effects on target cells. This may be due to differences in the ways the TGF-β isoforms interact with the three TGF-β receptor proteins. Two of the most important actions of TGF-βs in the context of skin wound healing are their ability to stimulate chemotaxis of inflammatory cells and to stimulate synthesis of extracellular matrix. Elevated, chronic production of TGF-β has been strongly implicated in nearly all fibrotic diseases including hepatic cirrhosis, pulmonary fibrosis, kidney glomerulonephritis, and pelvic adhesions (Border and Noble, 1994). This has stimulated research into methods to inhibit the action of TGF-β in vivo. For example, neutralizing antibodies to TGF-βs have been reported to reduce scar formation in rat skin incisions (Kurt et al, 1992; Shah, Foreman, and Ferguson, 1992; Shah, Foreman, and Ferguson, 1994).

Excessive scar formation is an important area for future research.

Therapeutic Uses. Although TGF-β has been reported to stimulate healing in a large number of animal models, it has been evaluated in only one clinical trial in patients with chronic skin ulcers (Robson et al, 1995). In a three-arm, prospective, randomized, observer-blinded, placebo-controlled study, 36 patients were randomly assigned to one of three treatment groups consisting of 12 patients each: conventional dressing only, placebo collagen vehicle group, and TGF-β group. Ulcers were located at or proximal to the malleolus and distal to the tibial tuberosity, had an ankle-brachial index (ABI) greater than 0.5, had no clinical signs of infection, and had a bacterial count less than 105 bacteria/g tissue. During the 6-week treatment period, the mean ulcer area expressed as a percentage of initial ulcer area decreased more rapidly for ulcers treated with TGF-β2 than for ulcers treated with placebo or conventional dressings. Three ulcers in the TGF-β group, three in the placebo group, and two in the standard dressing group healed completely during the treatment period. Overall, these differences favored treatment with TGF-β2 but were not statistically significant.

Connective Tissue Growth Factor (CTGF)

Recently, TGF-βs were shown to induce synthesis of another important protein, connective tissue growth factor (CTGF) (Bradham et al, 1991; Frazier et al, 1996). CTGF is a potent inducer of extracellular matrix synthesis, and much of the increase in extracellular matrix that occurs in the skin after treatment with TGF-β is probably due to the action of CTGF. Many human fibrotic diseases have been reported to contain elevated levels of CTGF protein, as indicated by immunohistochemical staining of tissue sections (Ito et al, 1998; Kucich et al, 2001). Macrophages and fibroblasts, as well as epithelial cells, secrete CTGF. The receptor for CTGF has not been conclusively identified, but it may bind to the low density lipoprotein (LDL)–like receptor protein (Segarini et al, 2001) or a 280,000 molecular weight membrane protein (Nishida et al, 1998). No clinical studies have been performed with CTGF, but adding exogenous CTGF to stimulate healing of chronic wounds is logical.

Conversely, inhibiting CTGF action by adding neutralizing antibodies or antisense oligonucleotides to wounds should reduce fibrosis.

Fibroblast Growth Factor (FGF) Family

Three proteins of the FGF family are thought to be important regulators of wound healing: acidic FGF (aFGF or FGF-1), basic FGF (bFGF or FGF-2), and keratinocyte growth factor (KGF or FGF-7) (Abraham and Klagsbrun, 1996). Over 30 synonyms have appeared in the literature to describe proteins that eventually were shown to be either aFGF or bFGF. As their names imply, aFGF and bFGF are potent mitogens for fibroblasts that share many similar biochemical and biologic properties. Both aFGF and bFGF are single-chain proteins that are proteolytically derived from precursor molecules to generate biologically active proteins of about 15,000 molecular weight. Their names reflect their different isoelectric points of pH 5.6 and 9.6. Neither aFGF nor bFGF have a conventional secretory peptide sequence at their amino-terminus that usually is necessary for secretion of proteins, and the mechanism of release for aFGF and bFGF from cells is not clear.

An important characteristic of FGFs is the ability to bind the glycosaminoglycan heparin and its protein-bound counterpart, the proteoglycan heparan sulfate. Immunohistochemical analysis of tissues for bFGF often reveals bFGF in association with the extracellular matrix and in basement membranes attached to heparan sulfate. The binding of bFGF to extracellular matrix constituents may serve several functions. Heparan sulfate protects bFGF from proteolytic degradation, and binding of aFGF to heparin or to heparan sulfate proteoglycans in the membranes of cells increases the affinity of FGF binding to its receptor, which results in a substantial increase in cell division. Release of matrix-degrading enzymes such as heparinase, cathepsin D, or collagenase after an injury to the skin may liberate bound FGF. These data imply that binding of FGFs by heparin-containing components of the extracellular matrix may regulate the activity of FGF by acting as a potential storage and release site and by potentiating its effects on receptors of target cells.

FGFs appear to play major roles in wound healing. FGFs stimulate proliferation of the major cell types involved in wound healing including fibroblasts, keratinocytes, and endothelial cells. FGFs and VEGF probably are the major angiogenic factors in wound healing. Many of the cells that respond to FGF also synthesize the peptide including fibroblasts, endothelial cells, and smooth muscle cells.

KGF has 37% sequence homology to bFGF and shares the ability to bind to heparin. KGF is a single-chain polypeptide of 28,000 molecular weight that is proteolytically derived from a larger precursor. In contrast to aFGF and bFGF, synthesis of KGF is restricted to fibroblasts, and KGF expression is rapidly upregulated in fibroblasts after an injury (Werner et al, 1992). More importantly, KGF only stimulates mitosis of keratinocytes and not fibroblasts, since the receptor for KGF is not expressed by fibroblasts. This has led to the concept that KGF is a paracrine effector of epithelial cell growth.

Four FGF receptors have been identified (FGFR1, FGFR2, FGFR3, and FGFR4), and they share about 60% sequence homology. All four of the FGF receptors can bind aFGF, but the receptors and their multiple splice variants (different mRNAs generated from a single gene) differ in their ability to bind bFGF and KGF. Expression of different FGF receptor variants by cells may provide another method to regulate the response of cells to FGFs.

Therapeutic Uses.   FGF has been studied in both pressure ulcers and burns. A prospective, randomized, blinded, placebo-controlled trial was performed on 50 patients with grades 3 and 4 pressure ulcers using three different concentrations of bFGF (Robson et al, 1992b). More patients treated with bFGF achieved >70% wound closure compared with patients treated with vehicle ($p = 0.05$). Histologically, bFGF treatment produced a marked increase in fibroblasts and capillaries compared with ulcers treated with vehicle. These data demonstrated that bFGF was an effective adjuvant treatment for chronic pressure ulcers.

A synthetic bovine bFGF has also been evaluated for treatment of second-degree burns (Fu et al, 1998). Compared with placebo treatment, bFGF treatment significantly reduced the time for complete healing of superficial second-degree burns from 12.4 ± 2.7 days to 9.9 ± 2.5 days ($p = 0.0008$) and reduced healing of deep second-degree burns from 21.2 ± 4.9 days to 17.4 to 4.6 days ($p = 0.0003$). Histologic evaluation of granulation tissue in biopsies of burns after 7 days of treatment also showed more capillary sprouts or tubes in bFGF-treated wounds than in placebo-treated wounds. After more than 1.5 years of follow-up since treatment has stopped, neoplasia at the burn site has not been observed.

Insulin-Like Growth Factor (IGF) Family

IGF-I and IGF-II have substantial amino acid sequence homology to proinsulin, and both are synthesized as precursor molecules that are proteolytically cleaved to generate active monomeric proteins of about 7000 molecular weight. IGF-II is synthesized more prominently during fetal development, whereas IGF-I synthesis persists at high levels in many adult tissues, especially in the liver in response to stimulation by pituitary-derived growth hormone. Many of the biologic actions originally attributed to growth hormone such as cartilage and bone growth are mediated in part by IGF-I. However, combinations of growth hormone and IGF-I are more effective than either hormone alone.

Unlike other growth factors, substantial levels of IGF-I are contained in plasma, which primarily reflects hepatic synthesis. High-affinity IGF-binding proteins reversibly bind almost all the IGF-I in plasma. Because the IGFs are inactive while bound to their binding proteins, the dynamic balance between free and bound IGFs has a substantial influence on the effects of IGF-I in wound healing. IGF-I also is found in high levels in platelets and is released during platelet degranulation. IGF-I is a potent chemotactic agent for vascular endothelial cells, and IGF-I released from platelets or produced by fibroblasts may promote migration of vascular endothelial cells into the wound area, resulting in increased neovascularization. IGF-I also stimulates mitosis of fibroblasts and may act synergistically with PDGF to enhance epidermal and dermal regeneration.

IGF-I and IGF-II each have distinct receptor proteins. The IGF-I receptor is similar in structure to the insulin receptor, and consists of two α subunits that contain the IGF-I binding site linked by disulfide bonds to the two β subunits that contain the transmembrane and cytoplasmic regions with the tyrosine kinase domain. The IGF-I receptor binds IGF-I with high affinity, binds IGF-II with lower affinity, and binds

insulin weakly. The IGF-II receptor is a monomeric protein that has no kinase activity but binds proteins that contain the sugar mannose-6-phosphate. The IGF-II receptor binds IGF-II with high affinity, binds IGF-I with low affinity, and does not bind insulin.

Therapeutic Uses. There are no published reports of clinical studies evaluating IGF-I treatment of wounds. However, IGF-I and growth hormone may act synergistically to promote wound healing. Topical growth hormone treatment of chronic leg ulcers was reported to improve healing (Rasmussen et al, 1991). In a prospective, double-blind, placebo-controlled trial, 37 patients with chronic leg ulceration were randomized to receive either topical synthetic human growth hormone or placebo in addition to a standard treatment of compression and hydrocolloid dressing. Patients receiving growth hormone treatment had a significantly faster rate of ulcer healing than the placebo group, and more patients treated with growth hormone achieved 50% reduction in initial ulcer size.

A prospective, randomized, double-blind, placebo-controlled study was conducted to test the efficacy of the systemic administration of synthetic human growth hormone on healing times of split-thickness skin graft donor sites in pediatric patients with severe burns. The total body surface area (TBSA) of burns was greater than 40%, and the TBSA of full-thickness burns was greater than 20% (Gilpin et al, 1994). Donor sites in patients receiving growth hormone healed at approximately 6.5 days, whereas donor sites in patients receiving placebo healed at 8.5 days ($p = 0.01$). These studies suggest that topical application of growth hormone to leg ulcers or systemic administration of growth hormone to severely burned patients may enhance healing.

DISTINGUISHING CYTOKINES FROM GROWTH FACTORS

Proliferation and differentiation of nonimmune system cells is regulated primarily by the proteins described in the five major families of growth factors. Although the term cytokine can be used broadly to include the classical growth factors, its more current use is restricted to describing molecules that primarily regulate the interactions between cells that participate in the immune response (Frenette and Wagner,

1996a; Frenette and Wagner, 1996b; Springer, 1990). These molecules could be further classified as lymphokines or monokines, depending on their major target cells. They are produced extensively by activated T cells and macrophages, although nonimmune system cells such as keratinocytes and vascular endothelial cells also produce some cytokines. Studies have revealed that cytokines generally induce multiple biologic activities (pleiotropic) and that a single cytokine can act both as a positive signal and a negative signal, depending on the type of the target cell. Cytokines such as IL-1, IL-2, IL-3, IL-4, IL-5, IL-6, IL-10, granulocyte-monocyte colony-stimulating factor (GM-CSF), granulocyte colony-stimulating factor (G-CSF), IFN-γ and TNF-α are key mediators of immune and inflammatory responses. Two cytokines in particular, TNF-α and IL-1β, have activities that substantially influence skin wound healing through their ability to increase production of MMPs and suppress production of TIMPs. Table 5-2 presents cytokines involved in wound healing along with cell source and biologic activity.

Therapeutic Uses

Cytokines have not been investigated extensively in human wound healing studies. IL-1β was evaluated in a prospective, randomized, double-blind, placebo-controlled trial performed on 26 patients with pressure ulcers of grades 3 and 4 (Robson et al, 1994). Measurements of the pressure ulcer area and volume as determined with alginate molds were made at weekly intervals. No statistically significant differences were seen in the percentage decreases of wound volumes between the treatment groups over the 4-week treatment evaluation.

POTENTIAL LIMITATIONS OF GROWTH FACTOR TECHNOLOGY

From practical and theoretic standpoints, growth factor therapy has certain limitations. One major limitation is the concept of "barren soil." If a growth factor or a mixture of growth factors is applied to a wound, the cells in or adjacent to the wound must be properly prepared so they can respond. This means the cells

TABLE 5-2 Cytokines Involved in Wound Healing

CYTOKINE	CELL SOURCE	BIOLOGIC ACTIVITY
Proinflammatory Cytokines		
TNF-α	Macrophages	PMN margination and cytotoxicity, collagen synthesis; provides metabolic substrate
IL-1	Macrophages Keratinocytes	Fibroblast and keratinocyte chemotaxis, collagen synthesis
IL-2	T lymphocytes	Increases fibroblast infiltration and metabolism
IL-6	Macrophages PMNs Fibroblasts	Fibroblast proliferation, hepatic acute-phase protein synthesis
IL-8	Macrophages Fibroblasts	Macrophage and PMN chemotaxis, keratinocyte maturation
IFN-γ	T lymphocytes Macrophages	Macrophage and PMN activation; retards collagen synthesis and cross-linking; stimulates collagenase activity
Antiinflammatory Cytokines		
IL-4	T lymphocytes Basophils Mast cells	Inhibition of TNF, IL-1, IL-6 production; fibroblast proliferation, collagen synthesis
IL-10	T lymphocytes Macrophages Keratinocytes	Inhibition of TNF, IL-1, IL-6 production; inhibits macrophage and PMN activation

must have adequate levels of oxygen, nutrients, and intact extracellular matrix components to be able to support cell mitosis, migration, and attachment. The underlying condition that caused the wound to become chronic must be corrected.

Because the molecular environment of chronic wounds is different from that of acute wounds (Figures 5-4 and 5-5), the imbalances in cytokines and proteases in chronic wounds also must be corrected as much as possible before exogenous growth factors are added. Three key differences in the molecular environment of chronic wounds have been identified:

1. Chronic wound fluid does not consistently stimulate growth (mitosis) of skin fibroblasts (Alper, Tibbetts, and Sarazen, 1985; Bucalo, Eaglstein, and Falanga, 1993; Katz et al, 1991).

2. Ratios of proinflammatory cytokines (TNF-α and IL-1β) and natural receptors are significantly increased (Harris et al, 1995; Mast and Schultz, 1996).

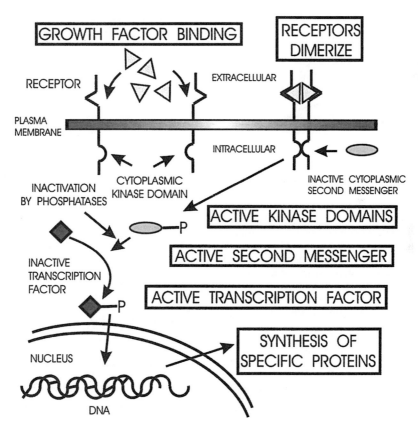

Fig. 5-4 Growth factor receptor signal generation. Growth factors typically affect cells by binding to specific, high-affinity receptor proteins located in the plasma membrane of target cells, which then dimerize and activate tyrosine or serine/threonine kinase domains located in the cytoplasmic region of the receptor. The activated receptor then phosphorylates second messenger proteins, which also are frequently kinases that participate in a cascade of phosphorylation/activation steps that ultimately activate an RNA transcription factor, which selectively initiates synthesis of proteins that alters the behavior of the target cell. The second messenger system is turned off by enzymes called phosphatases that remove phosphate groups from proteins.

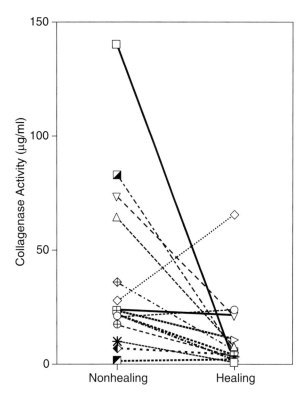

Fig. 5-5 Protease levels in fluids from chronic venous ulcers before and after initiating healing. Protease activity was measured in fluids collected from nonhealing venous leg ulcers of 15 patients at the start of hospitalization and 2 weeks later, after the ulcers had clinical evidence of healing. Lines connecting the protease levels measured in the two samples from each patient (nonhealing and healing) indicate that protease activity tends to decrease as ulcers begin to heal. (From Schultz GS, Mast BA: Molecular analysis of the environment of healing and chronic wounds: cytokines, proteases and growth factors, Wounds 10:1F, 1998. Health Management Publications, Inc., Wayne, Penn.)

3. Protease activity in chronic wounds is significantly elevated (Bullen et al, 1995; Harris et al, 1995; Mast and Schultz, 1996; Nwomeh et al, 1998; Rogers et al, 1995; Tarnuzzer and Schultz, 1996; Yager et al, 1996; Yager et al, 1997).

Protease activity and levels may be one of the most important factors preventing chronic wounds from healing because proteases can degrade proteins that are essential for healing such as growth factors, their receptors, and extracellular matrix proteins.

Experiments have shown that growth factors added to chronic wound fluids are quickly degraded by the proteases (MMPs and serine proteases such as neutrophil elastase) present in the fluid. Fortunately, levels of protease activity decrease in chronic wounds as they begin to heal (Figure 5-5). Frequent sharp debridement may be instrumental in converting the detrimental chronic wound environment into a pseudoacute wound molecular environment in which growth factors can function more effectively.

Another major limitation of growth factor therapy of chronic wounds may be the status of the wound cells themselves. Addition of exogenous growth factors may have little effect on cells in long-established chronic wounds if the cells are approaching senescence and are unable to respond (Agren, 1998). Healing would depend on repopulation of chronic wounds with healthy cells that migrate either from areas adjacent to the chronic wound or from artificial skin substitutes, such as Dermagraft-TC (Advanced Tissue Sciences) and Apligraf (Organogenesis, Novartis Pharmaceuticals Corp.), applied to the chronic wound.

A third consideration relates to the cost-effectiveness of growth factor therapy. For this high-priced technology to find broad application, it must ultimately be shown to have a significant positive effect (e.g., decreased duration of confinement, reduced cost of supplemental therapies, reduced amputation rate). The promise of growth factor therapy remains enormous but will require additional clinical investigations that are carefully conducted and properly designed.

WOUND BED PREPARATION

The identification of major differences in the molecular and cellular environments of acute and chronic wounds implies that they are barriers to healing that must be corrected before healing can progress or before advanced therapies can be effectively employed. This has led to the concept of "wound bed preparation," which draws heavily on clinical experience and laboratory data (Schultz et al, 2003). Wound bed preparation is an integrated approach that addresses four major concepts of wound care that are captured by the acronym of "TIME," which incorporates aspects of *t*issue, *i*nfection/inflammation, *m*oisture, and the *e*dge of the wound. The process of creating an optimum

TABLE 5-3   TIME* – Principles of Wound Bed Preparation (WBP)

CLINICAL OBSERVATIONS	PROPOSED PATHOPHYSIOLOGY	WBP CLINICAL ACTIONS	EFFECT OF WBP ACTIONS	CLINICAL OUTCOMES
Tissue nonviable or deficient	Defective matrix and cell debris impair healing	Debridement (episodic or continuous) • autolytic, sharp surgical, enzymatic, mechanical or biologic agents	Restoration of wound base and functional extracellular matrix proteins	Viable wound base
Infection or inflammation	High bacterial counts or prolonged inflammation ↑ inflammatory cytokines ↑ protease activity ↓ growth factor activity	• Remove infected foci • Implement topical/systemic • antimicrobials • antiinflammatories • protease inhibition	Low bacterial counts or controlled inflammation: ↓ inflammatory cytokines ↓ protease activity ↑ growth factor activity	Bacterial balance and reduced inflammation
Moisture imbalance	Desiccation slows epithelial cell migration Excessive fluid causes maceration of wound margin	Apply moisture balancing dressings Compression, negative pressure or other methods of removing fluid	Restored epithelial cell migration, desiccation avoided Edema, excessive fluid controlled, maceration avoided	Moisture balance
Edge of wound—non-advancing or undermined	Nonmigrating keratinocytes Nonresponsive wound cells and abnormalities in extracellular matrix or abnormal protease activity	Reassess cause or consider corrective therapies • debridement • skin grafts • biologic agents • adjunctive therapies	Migrating keratinocytes and responsive wound cells Restoration of appropriate protease profile	Advancing edge of wound

MOLECULAR ENVIRONMENT OF WOUNDS

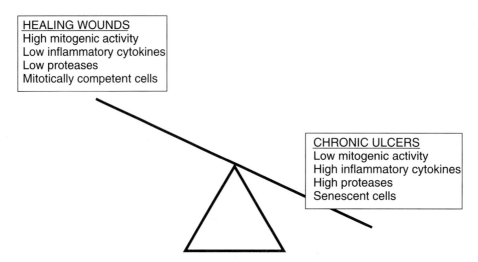

Fig. 5-6 Imbalanced activities in acute and chronic wounds. Healing wounds generally have high levels of mitogenic activity, low levels of inflammatory cytokines, low levels of proteases, high levels of growth factors, and mitotically competent fibroblasts. In contrast, chronic skin wounds tend to have low levels of mitotic activity, high levels of inflammatory cytokines, high levels of proteases, low levels of growth factors, and nearly senescent fibroblasts. (From Schultz GS, Mast BA: Molecular analysis of the environment of healing and chronic wounds: cytokines, proteases and growth factors, *Wounds* 10:1F, 1998. Health Management Publications, Inc., Wayne, Penn.)

wound environment, as implied by the acronym "TIME", is discussed in great detail in Chapter 19.

SUMMARY

The clinical management of skin wounds is entering a new phase because of the increased understanding of the roles that growth factors, adhesion molecules, extracellular matrix molecules, cytokines, and proteases play in healing of acute wounds and how these key molecules are altered in chronic wounds. New products, including recombinant growth factors (PDGF) and biologically active, engineered artificial skin substitutes, are a direct result of this increased understanding of the molecular regulation of wound healing. However, these new products only function optimally when properly applied to wounds that are able to respond to them. Thus the wound specialist must stay abreast of new discoveries in these areas of basic wound research to be able to effectively integrate these new advances into clinical practice.

SELF-ASSESSMENT EXERCISE

1. Name three types of adhesion molecules or adhesion receptors that participate in inflammation.
2. True or false: Growth factors are proteases.
3. All of the following growth factors have shown significant benefit in healing acute or chronic wounds in clinical trials EXCEPT which of the following?
   a. Fibroblast growth factor
   b. Epidermal growth factor
   c. Transforming growth factor-beta
   d. Insulin-like growth factor

REFERENCES

Abraham J, Klagsbrun M: Modulation of wound repair by members of the fibroblast growth factor family. In Clark RAF, editor: *The molecular and cellular biology of wound repair*, New York, 1996, Plenum Press.

Agren M: *Fibroblast growth in acute and chronic wounds*, European Tissue Repair Society Annual Meeting Abstract, abstract #33, 1998.

Alper JC, Tibbetts LL, Sarazen AAJ: The in vitro response of fibroblasts to the fluid that accumulates under a vapor-permeable membrane, *J Invest Derm* 84:513, 1985.

Arai K et al: Cytokines: coordinators of immune and inflammatory responses, *Annu Rev Biochem* 59:783, 1990.

Bennett NT, Schultz GS: Growth factors and wound healing: biochemical properties of growth factors and their receptors, *Am J Surg* 165:728, 1993a.

Bennett NT, Schultz GS: Growth factors and wound healing. II. Role in normal and chronic wound healing, *Am J Surg* 166:74, 1993b.

Border WA, Noble NA: Transforming growth factor-β in tissue fibrosis, *N Engl J Med* 10:1286, 1994.

Bradham DM et al: Connective tissue growth factor: a cysteine-rich mitogen secreted by human vascular endothelial cells is related to the SRC-induced immediate early gene product CEF-10, *J Cell Biol* 114(6):1285, 1991.

Brown GB et al: Enhancement of epidermal regeneration by biosynthetic epidermal growth factor, *J Exp Med* 163:1319, 1986.

Brown GL et al: Enhancement of wound healing by topical treatment with epidermal growth factor, *N Eng J Med* 321:76, 1989.

Bucalo B, Eaglstein WH, Falanga V: Inhibition of cell proliferation by chronic wound fluid, *Wound Rep Reg* 1:181, 1993.

Bullen EC et al: Tissue inhibitor of metalloproteinases-1 is decreased and activated gelatinases are increased in chronic wounds, *J Invest Dermatol* 104:236, 1995.

Carpenter G, Cohen S: Epidermal growth factor, *J Biol Chem* 265:7709, 1990.

David LS et al: Randomized prospective double-blind trial in healing chronic diabetic foot ulcers, *Diabetes Care* 11:1598, 1992.

Falanga V et al: Topical use of human recombinant epidermal growth factor (h-EGF) in venous ulcers, *Phlebology* 18:604, 1992.

Fantl WJ, Johnson DE, Williams LT: Signaling by receptor tyrosine kinases, *Annu Rev Biochem* 62:453, 1993.

Frazier K et al: Stimulation of fibroblast cell growth, matrix production, and granulation tissue formation by connective tissue growth factor, *J Invest Dermatol* 107:404, 1996.

Frenette PS, Wagner DD: Adhesion molecules, blood vessels and blood cells, *N Engl J Med* 335:43, 1996a.

Frenette PS, Wagner DD: Molecular medicine, adhesion molecules, *N Engl J Med* 334:1526, 1996b.

Fu X et al: Randomised placebo-controlled trial of use of topical recombinant bovine basic fibroblast growth factor for second-degree burns, *Lancet* 352:1661, 1998.

Gilpin DA et al: Recombinant human growth hormone accelerates wound healing in children with large cutaneous burns, *Ann Surg* 220:19, 1994.

Harris IR et al: Cytokine and protease levels in healing and non-healing chronic venous leg ulcers, *Exp Dermatol* 4:342, 1995.

Heldin C, Westermark B: Role of platelet derived growth factor in vivo. In Clark RAF, editor: *The molecular and cellular biology of wound repair*, New York, 1996, Plenum Press.

Holloway GA et al: A randomized, controlled, multicenter, dose response trial of activated platelet supernatant, topical CT-102 in chronic, nonhealing, diabetic wounds, *Wounds* 5:198, 1993.

Ito Y et al: Expression of connective tissue growth factor in human renal fibrosis, *Kidney Int* 53:853, 1998.

Katz MH et al: Human wound fluid from acute wounds stimulates fibroblast and endothelial cell growth, *J Am Acad Dermatol* 25:1054, 1991.

Kucich U et al: Signaling events required for transforming growth factor-β stimulation of connective tissue growth factor expression by cultured human lung fibroblasts, *Arch Biochem Biophys* 395:103, 2001.

Kurt S et al: Transforming growth factor-β acts as an autocrine growth factor in ovarian carcinoma cell lines, *Cancer Res* 52:341, 1992.

Massague J: Transforming growth factor-α, *J Biol Chem* 265:21393, 1990.

Mast BA, Schultz GS: Interactions of cytokines, growth factors, and proteases in acute and chronic wounds, *Wound Rep Regen* 4:411, 1996.

Nanney LB, King LE: Epidermal growth factor and transforming growth factor-α. In Clark RAF, editor: *The molecular and cellular biology of wound repair*, New York, 1996, Plenum Press.

Nishida T et al: Demonstration of receptors specific for connective tissue growth factor on a human chondrocytic cell line (HSC-2/8), *Biochem Biophys Res Commun* 247:905, 1998.

Nwomeh BC et al: Dynamics of the matrix metalloproteinases MMP-1 and MMP-8 in acute open human dermal wounds, *Wound Rep Regen* 6:127, 1998.

Rasmussen LH et al: Topical human growth hormone treatment of chronic leg ulcers, *Phlebology* 6:23, 1991.

Roberts AB, Sporn MB: Transforming growth factor-β. In Clark RAF, editor: *The molecular and cellular biology of wound repair*, New York, 1996, Plenum Press.

Robson MC et al: Recombinant human platelet-derived growth factor-BB for the treatment of chronic pressure ulcers, *Ann Plast Surg* 29:193, 1992a.

Robson MC et al: The safety and effect of topically applied recombinant basic fibroblast growth factor on the healing of chronic pressure sores, *Ann Surg* 216:401, 1992b.

Robson MC et al: Safety and effect of topical recombinant human interleukin-1β in the management of pressure sores, *Wound Rep Regen* 2:177, 1994.

Robson MC et al: Safety and effect of transforming growth factor-B2 for treatment of venous stasis ulcers, *Wound Rep Regen* 3:157, 1995.

Rogers AA et al: Involvement of proteolytic enzymes—plasminogen activators and matrix metalloproteinases—in the pathophysiology of pressure ulcers, *Wound Rep Regen* 3:273, 1995.

Schultz G et al: Wound bed preparation, a systemic approach to wound bed management, *Wound Rep Regen* 11(Suppl):1, 2003.

Segarini PR et al: The low density lipoprotein receptor-related protein/α$_2$ is a receptor for connective tissue growth factor, *J Biol Chem* 276:40659, 2001.

Shah M, Foreman DM, Ferguson MWJ: Control of scarring in adult wounds by neutralising antibody to transforming growth factor beta, *Lancet* 339:213, 1992.

Shah M, Foreman DM, Ferguson MWJ: Neutralising antibody to TGF-β1,2 reduces cutaneous scarring in adult rodents, *J Cell Sci* 107:1137, 1994.

Shigeki H et al: Structure of heparin-binding EGF-like growth factor, *J Biol Chem* 267:6205, 1992.

Springer TA: Adhesion receptors of the immune system, *Nature* 346:425, 1990.

Steed DL, Diabetic Ulcer Study Group: Clinical evaluation of recombinant human platelet-derived growth factor for the treatment of lower extremity diabetic ulcers, *J Vasc Surg* 21:71, 1995.

Steed DL et al: Effect of extensive debridement and treatment on the healing of diabetic foot ulcers, *J Am Coll Surg* 183:61, 1996.

Tarnuzzer RW, Schultz GS: Biochemical analysis of acute and chronic wound environments, *Wound Rep Regen* 4:321, 1996.

Werner S et al: Large induction of keratinocyte growth factor expression in the dermis during wound healing, *Proc Natl Acad Sci* 89:6896, 1992.

Yager DR et al: Ability of chronic wound fluids to degrade peptide growth factors is associated with increased levels of elastase activity and diminished levels of proteinase inhibitors, *Wound Rep Regen* 5:23, 1997.

Yager DR et al: Wound fluids from human pressure ulcers contain elevated matrix metalloproteinase levels and activity compared to surgical wound fluid, *J Invest Dermatol* 107:743, 1996.

6

Skin Pathology and Types of Damage

RUTH A. BRYANT & RICHARD A.F. CLARK

OBJECTIVES

1. Describe the process of at least five factors that contribute to skin damage.
2. Distinguish between the following lesions: macule, papule, plaque, nodule, wheal, pustule, vesicle, and bulla.
3. Differentiate between erosion and ulcer.
4. Describe four types of mechanical trauma by the extent of tissue damage associated with each.
5. Discuss at least three interventions to prevent each type of mechanical trauma.
6. For three common causes of chemical damage, describe three preventive interventions.
7. Describe the process of an allergic contact dermatitis.
8. Identify factors that predispose a patient to candidiasis.
9. Describe the types of lesions common to candidiasis, folliculitis, impetigo, and pyoderma gangrenosum.
10. Differentiate between herpes simplex and herpes zoster according to cause, onset, clinical presentation, and treatment.
11. Describe the process of tissue damage, treatment goals, and treatment options for vasculitis, calciphylaxis, epidermolysis bullosa (EB), calciphylaxis, graft-versus-host disease (GVHD), and toxic epidermal necrolysis (TEN).

Normal skin integrity can be jeopardized or compromised by a multitude of factors: mechanical, chemical, vascular, infectious, allergic, inflammatory, systemic disease–related, burn-related, and those deriving from miscellaneous assaults. Each type of injury creates a complex set of skin responses such as erythema, macules, papules, pustules, vesicles/bullae, erosion, or ulcers. Primary lesions of the skin are the first recognizable lesions in the skin. Plate 6 provides the definition and appearance of common primary lesions. Secondary skin lesions evolve from the primary lesion either because of the natural history of the disease or

as a result of scratching or infection. Common secondary lesions are depicted and defined in Plate 7. Because periwound skin can develop skin complications, the care provider for the patient with a wound must be familiar with these terms.

ASSESSMENT

A systematic assessment of skin lesions is essential to obtain an accurate description of the history and evolution of the skin complication. This assessment commonly will narrow the field of differential diagnoses. The components to be addressed are listed in Table 6-1.

Before a treatment plan for a chronic or acute wound is initiated, it is imperative that the underlying cause for the wound be determined. Clues to the cause can be found by assessment of the following parameters: location, characteristics, distribution, and the patient's subjective comments as enumerated in Table 6-2. These clues can be used to direct the subsequent tests that may be necessary to develop a definitive diagnosis. Once the cause of the wound is identified, realistic goals for the wound can be established and a comprehensive, multidisciplinary treatment plan devised. This chapter briefly describes the pathophysiologic process of key types of skin damage and appropriate interventions.

MECHANICAL DAMAGE

The forces that are applied externally to the skin such as pressure, shear, friction, and skin stripping (skin tears) create mechanical damage. Each may occur in isolation or in combination with other mechanical injuries. This section presents shear, friction, and skin stripping. (Pressure damage is discussed in detail in Chapter 12.) Morphologic characteristics of skin lesions are described in Table 6-1.

TABLE 6-1 Morphologic Characteristics of Skin Lesions

CHARACTERISTIC	DESCRIPTION	EXAMPLES
Distribution		
Localized	Lesion appears in one small area	Impetigo, herpes simplex (e.g., labialis), tinea corporis ("ringworm")
Regional	Lesions involve a specific region of the body	Acne vulgaris (pilosebaceous gland distribution), herpes zoster (nerve dermatomal distribution), psoriasis (flexural surfaces and skin folds)
		Urticaria, disseminated drug eruptions
Generalized	Lesions appear widely distributed or in numerous areas simultaneously	
Shape/Arrangement		
Round/discoid	Coin- or fine-shaped (no central clearing)	Nummular eczema
Oval	Ovoid shape	Pityriasis rosea
Annular	Round, active margins with central clearing	Tinea corporia, sarcoidosis
Zosteriform (dermatomal)	Following a nerve or segment of the body	Herpes zoster
Polycyclic	Interlocking or coalesced circles (formed by enlargement of annular lesions)	Psoriasis, urticaria
Linear	In a line	Contact dermatitis
Iris/target lesion	Pink macules with purple central papules	Erythema multiforme
Stellate	Star-shaped	Meningococcal septicemia
Serpiginous	Snakelike or wavy line track	Cutanea larva migrans
Reticulate	Netlike or lacy	Polyarteritis nodosa, lichen planus lesions of erythema infectiosum
Morbilliform	Measles-like: maculopapular lesions that become confluent on the face and body	Measles, roseola
Border/Margin		
Discrete	Well demarcated or defined, able to draw a line around it with confidence	Psoriasis
Indistinct	Poorly defined, have borders that merge into normal skin or outlying ill defined papules	Nummular eczema
Active	Margin of lesion shows greater activity than center	*Tinea* sp. eruptions
Irregular	Nonsmooth or notched margin	Malignant melanoma
Border raised above center	Center of lesion is depressed compared to the edge	Basal cell carcinoma
Advancing	Expanding at margins	Cellulitis
Associated Changes within Lesions		
Central clearing	An erythematous border surrounds lighter skin	Tinea eruptions
Desquamation	Peeling or sloughing of skin	Rash of toxic shock syndrome
Keratotic	Hypertrophic stratum corneum	Callouses, warts
Punctation	Central umbilication or dimpling	Basal cell carcinoma
Telangiectasias	Dilated blood vessels within lesion blanch completely, may be markers of systematic disease	Basal cell carcinoma, actinic keratosis

Continued

TABLE 6-1 Morphologic Characteristics of Skin Lesions—cont'd

CHARACTERISTIC	DESCRIPTION	EXAMPLES
Pigmentation		
Flesh	Same tone as the surrounding skin	Neurofibroma, some nevi
Pink	Light red undertones	Eczema, pityriasis rosea
Erythematous	Dark pink to red	Tinea eruptions, psoriasis
Salmon	Orange-pink	Psoriasis
Tan-brown	Light to dark brown	Most nevi, pityriasis versicolor
Black	Black or blue-black	Malignant melanoma
Pearly	Shiny white, almost iridescent	Basal cell carcinoma
Purple	Dark red-blue-violet	Purpura, Kaposi sarcoma
Violaceous	Light violet	Erysipelas
Yellow	Waxy	Lipoma
White	Absent of color	Lichen planus

From Seidel Henry M, Ball JW, Dains JE, Benedict GW: *Mosby's guide to physical examination*, ed 6, St Louis, 2006, Mosby.

TABLE 6-2 Common Clues to the Causes of Wounds

CAUSE	LOCATION	CHARACTERISTICS
Pressure	Bony prominence in mobility-restricted patient	Stages 1 to 4
Shear	Surfaces exposed to bed or chair surface in patient with reduced mobility or poor tissue turgor	May be superficial (limited to epidermis), or dermal-epidermal junction may separate May present as hematoma
Chemical (such as urine or stool from incontinence)	Areas exposed to urine, stool, or drainage	Superficial (epidermal, superficial dermal)
Moisture	Intertriginous areas	Maceration; superficial erosion of epidermis
Venous hypertension	Lower leg	Hyperpigmentation, edema, exudative wounds, varicose veins
Ischemia	All digits, lower extremities, areas of trauma	Surrounding tissue cool and pale Diminished or absent pulses Delayed capillary refill Pain
Neuropathy	Peripheral neuropathy most common Areas of sensory loss exposed to trauma or pressure (such as feet and heels)	Common in patients with diabetes Associated with abnormal gait; opening at skin level may be small, tunnels present; extensive subcutaneous tissue damage

Shear

Shearing force is created by the interaction of tangential forces and friction (resistance) against the surface of the skin. Friction is always present when shearing force is present. The classic example of shear is when a patient is in a semi-Fowler's position. While the torso slides downward to the foot of the bed, the bed surface generates enough resistance that the skin over the sacrum remains in the same location (Figure 6-1). Ultimately, the skin is held in place while the skeletal structures pull the body (by gravity) toward the foot of the bed. Consequently, blood vessels in the area are stretched and angulated, and such changes may create small vessel thrombosis and tissue death.

Shear may cause shallow or deep ulcers and extends the tissue damage of pressure ulcers. This extension is manifested in the pressure ulcer by the presence of undermining (dissection or separation of tissue parallel to the skin surface).

Shear injury is predominantly localized at the sacrum or coccyx and is most commonly a consequence of elevating the head of the bed or of improper transfer technique. Prevention requires an awareness of those situations in which the skin is subjected to shearing force. For example, the patient with pulmonary distress requires the head of the bed to be elevated to facilitate adequate ventilation; however, the patient is at great risk for shear injury. Likewise, the patient with a cerebrovascular accident may experience shear injury when being transferred from the bed to the wheelchair.

Strategies for prevention of shear are listed in Box 6-1. However, research to substantiate these preventive measures (particularly use of genuine sheepskin) is lacking. Because shear is an important contributing factor to pressure ulcer development, strategies to simultaneously prevent shear and pressure are warranted. Many support surfaces have a slick fabric covering,

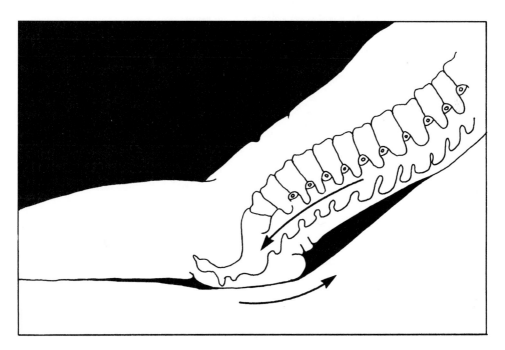

Fig. 6-1   Shearing force. (From Loeper JM et al: *Therapeutic positioning and skin care*, Minneapolis, 1986, Sister Kenny Institute.)

BOX 6-1 Prevention of Mechanical Skin Damage*

Pressure

1. Implement a level 1 support surface pressure if the patient is able to reposition or if the wound is on only one turning surface. (Redistributes weight over larger surface area.)
2. Implement a level 2 support surface if the patient is unable to reposition or if the wound is on more than one turning surface. (There are limited intact body surfaces that can be used to absorb and redistribute weight.)
3. Establish a turning schedule. (Consistency and continuity of care will be enhanced.)
4. Alternate patient position between supine and 30-degree lateral positions. (The 30-degree lateral position does not exert pressure on any bony prominence.)
5. Keep pressure off heels by using positioning aids and pillows. (Heel interface pressures often exceed capillary closing pressure regardless of support surface.)

Shear

1. Elevate head of bed to no more than 30 degrees and for limited times. (This reduces pull of gravity and sliding of tissues.)
2. Position feet against a footboard. (This prevents sliding down in bed.)
3. Use knee gatch when head of bed is elevated. (This prevents sliding down in bed.)
4. Use lift sheet to reposition patient. (This prevents dragging of patient's skin across bed.)

Friction (Superficial Shear)

1. Apply transparent dressing, thin hydrocolloid, or skin sealant to skin surface. (This provides a barrier to friction.)
2. Use sheepskin elbow or heel protectors. (This reduces exposure of skin to friction.)
3. Apply moisturizers to skin. (Adequately maintained epidermis is more resistant to stressors.)
4. Reduce shear. (Friction always occurs in combination with shear.)

Skin Stripping

1. Apply tape without tension. (This prevents blistering of skin under tape.)
2. Use porous tapes. (This allows moisture to evaporate.)
3. To remove tape, slowly peel tape away from anchored skin or pull one corner of tape at an angle parallel with skin. (This decreases trauma to the epidermis and dermal-epidermal junction.)
4. Secure dressings with roll gauze, tubular stockinette, or self-adhering tape. (This avoids unnecessary tapes on skin.)
5. Use skin sealants, thin hydrocolloids, low-adhesion foam dressings, or solid-wafer skin barriers under adhesives. (This provides a protective layer over the skin for adhering tapes.)
6. Secure dressings with Montgomery straps. (This prevents repeated tape applications.)

Note: When protective devices are used to protect the skin from mechanical trauma, the product should be removed at regular intervals to allow inspection and assessment of the area.
* The material in parentheses represents the rationale for each intervention.

which is believed to reduce shear. Unfortunately, there is no standardized method for measuring the ability of a support surface to reduce shear.

Fontaine, Risley, and Castellino (1998) proposed a calculated pressure/shear factor (PSF), which would quantify support surface efficiency for the combined effect of pressure and shear reduction. PSF is calculated by adding the rounded average interface pressure (mm Hg) to the rounded average gross shearing force (g)

multiplied by the impact factor of 4. The equation is as follows:

$$\text{Pressure} + (4 \times \text{shearing force}) = \text{PSF or}$$
$$\text{mm Hg} + (4 \times g) = \text{PSF}$$

A pressure sensor and a shear sensor are required to obtain the values to put into this PSF equation. Potentially, the PSF could become a supplement to current support surface measurements, which are strictly interface pressure measurements. In this way the PSF would provide additional objective information concerning the potential for the support surface to prevent ulceration. For example, Fontaine and colleagues (1998) studied the PSF for three support surfaces classified as group-2 devices according to the Medicare Part B policy. The PSF was calculated for a powered, alternating-pressure mattress overlay; a powered, zoned, air-filled mattress replacement device; and a nonpowered fluid overlay. The resulting PSFs were 939, 1043, and 331, respectively. The implication is that the nonpowered fluid overlay was more effective in reducing the pressure/shearing force. However, because PSF is a newly defined variable, further research is required to establish validity of the variable as well as its predictive value and clinical effectiveness.

The primary intervention to reduce shear is to use lift sheets when repositioning the patient; this method eliminates drag on the sacral skin. Elevation of the head of bed should be limited to short periods of time at no more than 30 degrees. Sheepskin may be used; however, it should not be confused with pressure-redistribution measures. Also, the knee gatch can be used to interrupt gravity's pull on the body toward the foot of the bed.

Friction (A Misnomer of Superficial Shear)

Skin injury by superficial shearing forces results from two surfaces rubbing together; it appears as an abrasion. As stated above, shearing force is created by the interaction of tangential forces and friction (resistance) against the surface of the skin. This type of injury is frequently seen on elbows or heels because the patient easily abrades these surfaces against sheets when repositioning. Injury is characteristically very shallow and limited to the epidermis. Tissue necrosis does not occur with superficial shear.

Interventions to prevent superficial shear are listed in Box 6-1. These involve the use of protective sheepskin over the elbows or heels and moisturizers applied to vulnerable areas to maintain proper hydration of the epidermis. Both maneuvers decrease friction and thereby decrease shear. Transparent adhesive dressings, thin hydrocolloids, low-adhesion foam dressings, and skin sealants are effective at reducing friction. Adhesive dressings are contraindicated if the shear is sufficient to loosen the dressing. Braces, splints, prosthetic devices,

and shoes should be assessed frequently for evidence of shear, and modifications should be implemented as needed.

Skin Stripping and Lacerations (Epidermal and Dermal)

Skin stripping is the inadvertent removal of the epidermis with or without the dermis by mechanical means. Trauma such as tape removal, and lacerations caused by blunt trauma such as bumping into furniture, can lead to skin tears (Bryant, 1988; Payne and Martin, 1990). A taxonomy for severity of skin tears is listed in Box 6-2. Distinguishing characteristics of a category I skin tear is that the resulting skin flap or the avulsed skin can cover the exposed wound. Category II wounds are distinguished by the degree of damage to the

---

BOX 6-2 Skin Tears: Definition and Payne-Martin Classification System

....

Category I: Skin tear can fully approximate wound

  A: *Linear skin tear.* Full-thickness wound that occurs in wrinkle or furrow of skin. Both epidermis and dermis are pulled apart as if an incision has been made, exposing tissue below.

  B: *Flap-type skin tear.* Partial-thickness wound in which the epidermal flap can be completely approximated or approximated so that no more than 1 millimeter of dermis is exposed.

Category II: Skin tear with partial-thickness loss

  A: *Scant tissue loss.* Partial-thickness wound in which 25% or less of the epidermal flap is lost and at least 75% or more of the dermis is covered by the flap.

  B: *Moderate to large tissue loss.* Partial-thickness wound in which more than 25% of the epidermal flap is lost and more than 25% of the dermis is exposed.

Category III: Skin tears with complete tissue loss

  A partial-thickness wound in which an epidermal flap is absent.

From Payne RL, Martin ML: Defining and classifying skin tears: need for a common language, *Ostomy Wound Manage* 39(5):16, 1993.

epidermal avulsed skin. Category III lesions have no epidermal flap. Only category IA lesions are full thickness (involve the dermis). Typically, these lesions are irregularly shaped and shallow, involving only the epidermis. The most frequent location of skin-stripping injuries is the upper extremities (73% to 80%), although they have been observed on the legs and feet (20%), head (3% to 4%), and torso (3%) (Malone et al, 1991; McGough-Csarny and Kopac, 1998; Payne and Martin, 1990).

Risk factors for a skin tear include advanced age, compromised nutrition, history of previous skin tears, cognitive impairment, dependency, poor locomotion, and presence of ecchymosis (McGough-Csarny and Kopac, 1998). However, it is important to remember that even independent, ambulatory patients are at risk for this injury; they experience the second highest number of skin tears (Baranoski, 2001). This patient population often has edema, purpura (Plate 30), or ecchymosis, and the skin tears occur primarily on the lower extremities.

Daily care activities such as bathing, dressing, transfers, and toileting all require frequent handling of the patient with vulnerable skin. Therefore their potential for inducing a skin tear increases. Use of equipment (e.g., mechanical lifts, wheelchairs, and geri-chairs) also increases the patient's exposure to potential trauma, which may precipitate a skin tear. However, almost half of all skin tears have no clear cause (McGough-Csarny and Kopac, 1988).

Elderly skin and immature skin are both vulnerable to skin tears because the dermal-epidermal junction is not optimally functional. The interlocking dermal papillae and epidermal rete pegs at the dermal-epidermal junction are critical to providing resiliency and the ability to withstand mechanical forces. In the premature infant's skin, the dermal-epidermal junction is undeveloped and weak. As the skin ages the epidermis thins, the dermal-epidermal junction flattens, and cohesion is diminished. In addition, the amount of collagen and elastin present in the aging skin decreases so that the skin becomes wrinkled, thin, and less compliant. Furthermore, similar connective tissue changes around blood vessels increase the fragility of capillaries. Therefore mechanical stresses can trigger a subcutaneous hemorrhage (e.g., senile purpura) between the skin layers, which results in further separation of the dermis and epidermis. Disease management regimens can also alter the skin's vitality. For example, corticosteroids reduce tissue collagen strength and elasticity and thereby increase the patient's risk of skin tears. Radiation therapy in the long-term causes epidermal atrophy, microvascular occlusions, reduced fibroblast proliferation, and tissue fibrosis.

A key component to the prevention of skin tears is to recognize fragile, thin, vulnerable skin, particularly when associated with ecchymotic skin. Extreme care and a gentle touch are critical when touching the patient or performing patient care, since most skin tears occur in the course of providing routine patient care activities (e.g., bathing, dressing, transferring) (Malone et al, 1991; McGough-Csarny and Kopac, 1998; White, Karam, and Cowell, 1994).

Beyond these measures, the current focus of prevention is on the application of products to the skin to serve as a barrier between the skin and causes of traumatic events. Skin tears resulting from adhesives can be prevented by (1) appropriate application and removal of tape; (2) use of solid-wafer skin barriers, thin hydrocolloids, low-adhesion foam dressings, or skin sealants under adhesives; (3) use of porous tapes; and (4) avoidance of unnecessary tape use (see Box 6-1). Additional protection of ecchymotic skin can be provided by applying transparent dressings, thin hydrocolloids, or low-adhesion foam dressings; keeping the arms and legs covered with roll gauze; or having the patient wear long sleeves and pants. However, when adhesive dressings are used on intact skin to prevent skin tears, the protocol should clearly indicate that the dressing is not changed routinely. It should be left undisturbed and allowed to fall off. As the edges of the dressing loosen, the loosened edges should be clipped rather than removing the entire dressing and applying a new dressing. More research is needed to explore the prevention of skin tears, such as the role of humectants, emollients, moisturizers, and skin cleansers (Mason, 1997).

The body of evidence concerning treatment of skin tears is sparse but growing. Transparent dressings, hydrocolloid dressings, SteriStrips, and foam have been used to stabilize the flap and cover the wound. However, Thomas, Blume, and Forman reported in a 1999 study that dressings with a high moisture vapor transmission rate (MVTR), such as those with a low-adhesive foam dressing, result in complete healing of 94% (16 of 17) category II and III skin tears within 21 days. This is in comparison with complete healing of only 65% (11 of 17) of skin tears when using a film dressing. The researchers suggest that film dressings keep the skin tear excessively moist and exacerbate the separation of the epidermis from the dermal papillae. These results underscore the importance of selecting dressings based on wound characteristics (see Chapter 19).

Appropriate tape application and removal techniques can also help prevent skin stripping. Proper tape application implies that the tape is applied without tension or "pinching" of the epidermis. Often, tape is applied appropriately after a surgical procedure, but as edema develops at the surgical site over the ensuing 24 hours, the tape begins to pull on the underlying skin. Blisters then develop under the tape. To alleviate the tension that develops as the skin becomes normally edematous after surgical manipulation, it may be advisable to remove and reapply dressings 24 hours after surgery.

Proper tape removal entails slowly peeling the tape away from the skin while stabilizing the skin. Solvents can be used to break the adhesive skin bond, although solvents have a drying effect on the skin. Plain tap water can often serve this purpose effectively. Some manufacturers recommend loosening the tape by pulling on one corner of the tape at an angle parallel with the skin. Solid-wafer skin barriers and thin hydrocolloids can also be applied to frame the wound; wound dressings are then secured by anchoring the tape to the surface of the barrier. One can easily apply and reapply the tape without traumatizing the epidermis. These skin barriers and hydrocolloid dressings can remain in place for several days.

Skin sealants may be applied to the skin before the tape is applied to provide protection from skin tears. Only alcohol-free skin sealants should be used when the skin is denuded or when contact with the wound edges is likely, because alcohol content can cause intense stinging. It is important to allow the skin sealant to dry completely before applying tape. Many central-line dressing kits are prepackaged with a skin sealant.

Unnecessary use of adhesives and tapes should be avoided, particularly on vulnerable, fragile skin. It is important to be creative when securing dressings without applying tape to the skin. For example, tubular stockinette gauze, roll gauze, or self-adhering tape can be used. In general, it is best to avoid applying adhesives in an area receiving radiation. A standardized care plan for patients at high risk for skin tears is provided in Box 6-3.

CHEMICAL FACTORS

The presence of irritating chemicals on the skin is a common source of skin damage. Solutions containing irritating chemicals include, but are not limited to, urine and fecal fluids from incontinence, povidone-iodine complex (Betadine), alkaline soaps, alcohol, skin cements, and drainage from percutaneous tubes. These substances alter one or more of the protective components of the stratum corneum such as the acid pH, or lipid and water-binding organic chemicals. Irritants extract water-binding chemicals and lipids from the stratum corneum, and the skin decompensates. Initially the skin becomes dry with erythema or an erythematous macular rash; fissures then develop (Habif, 2004) (Plate 8).

Dermatitis caused by chemical irritants is referred to as irritant contact dermatitis. Skin damage may be evident within only a few hours in the presence of a strong irritant (such as small bowel discharge). In fact, infants may develop an irritant contact dermatitis as soon as they pass a loose stool into the diaper. In other situations, repeat exposures over several days may be necessary such as when the irritant is weak, as with urine. Lesions are distributed in the areas that have been exposed to the offending agent. Chemically induced dermatitis is very uncomfortable for the patient since the chemicals often stimulate neurocutaneous pain receptors.

Chemical irritation can be prevented by (1) identification of patients at risk for chemical irritation, (2) preventing drainage around catheters or drains from contacting the skin, (3) avoiding the presence of harsh substances on the skin, (4) appropriate use of skin-care products (cleansers, barriers, adhesives, or solvents), and (5) use of containment devices.

Moisture-barrier ointments, gentle skin cleansing and creative uses of skin barriers, thin hydrocolloids, or low-adhesion foam dressings are the cornerstone to

BOX 6-3 Standardized Care Plan for Patients at High Risk for Skin Tears

1. Provide a safe environment:

a. Free room of obstacles that obstruct pathway around bed and bathroom.

b. Provide adequate lighting in resident's room.

c. Leave night-light on in bathroom with the door open.

d. Leave side rails down at night.

e. Make hourly rounds on resident.

f. Provide safe area for wandering.

g. Have resident wear anklet alarm.

h. Install bed alarm.

i. Provide well-fitting supportive shoes with skid-free soles.

j. Have family bring loose-fitting adaptive clothing with back closure.

k. Ensure that resident wears protective clothing for arms and legs (e.g., fleece-lined jogging suits, knee-length athletic socks, stockinette doubled).

l. Protect all areas of purpura.

m. Remove name tag when determined to be the cause of skin tears.

2. Maintain nutrition and hydration:

a. Obtain dietary consult.

b. Obtain physician's order for double portions or high protein snacks between meals.

c. Keep intake and output records.

d. Offer fluids between meals 2 times every shift.

e. Encourage fluids at every meal.

f. Use lotion on arms and legs twice daily.

g. Obtain order for ascorbic acid and zinc if resident is prone to skin tears with poor healing (vitamin C, 500 mg 4 times/day; zinc chelate, 50 mg 4 times/day).

h. Perform body checks twice daily, in morning and at bedtime.

3. Protect from self-inflicted injury or injury incurred during routine care:

a. Use wheelchair for transport only.

b. Pad wheelchair footrests.

c. Pad rough edges of tabletops and wheelchair trays.

d. Position resident with pillows and folded blankets to prevent head and arms from dangling over side of chair.

e. Use sling around chair legs to prevent resident's feet from falling off footrests.

f. Ensure smooth vinyl on wheelchair and recliner arms.

g. Pad wheelchair and recliner arms.

h. Use padding or cozy comforter to provide cushioning and protect skin while resident is up in recliner.

i. Use mechanical lift to transport resident.

j. Protect resident's arms and legs while in bed by padding side rails.

k. Get occupational or physical therapy consult if needed for positioning for safety.

l. Use lift sheet for positioning and moving resident.

m. Move resident by using palm of hands.

Reprinted with permission from White et al: Skin tears in frail elders: a practical approach to prevention, *Ger Nurs* 15(2):95-99, 1994.

the prevention of chemical irritation when patients are assessed to be at risk. For example, it should be anticipated that the patient with a low serum albumin level who is receiving antibiotics is at risk for developing diarrhea once enteral feedings are initiated. The nurse should initiate a care plan of gentle skin cleansing (no harsh soaps or rough cloths) and use of ointments to prevent chemical irritation (Habif, 2004). The infant with increased stooling frequency requires more frequent diaper changes, gentle cleansing, and appropriate use of ointments. Likewise, the adult may experience diarrhea for several reasons, such as gastrointestinal bleeding or antibiotic therapy. In most situations, diligent and appropriate use of moisture-barrier ointments can help prevent denudation or ulceration.

Containment devices may be indicated for both containment of contaminated stool for infection control purposes and/or when the frequency or volume of stool overwhelms moisture-barrier ointments and pastes. Rectal pouches are adhesive ostomy pouches specifically designed to fit the perianal contours and contain the incontinent stool. These products can be extremely cost-effective by protecting the skin from chemicals and moisture build-up, reducing linen changes, and freeing up nursing time for other types of care. Rectal pouches also preserve the patient's dignity by containing odor and feces. Step-by-step instructions to apply a rectal pouch are listed in Box 6-4.

Historically, rectal tubes designed for the purpose of enema and medication administration, as well as indwelling urinary catheters, have been attached to bedside bags for diverting and containing stool. This practice is not safe, since it has the potential to damage the anal sphincter and/or perforate the bowel. However, the FDA has approved two new indwelling bowel and fecal management systems that are designed to safely divert, collect, and contain potentially harmful and contaminated gastrointestinal waste without damaging the anal sphincter. The products are Zassi Bowel Management System (BMS) by Zassi Medical Evolutions in Fernandina Beach, Florida, and the Convetec Flexi-Seal FMS (Fecal Management System). It is important to review the manufacturer's instructions for each product to understand differences in features, indications and contraindications. Kim et al (2001) evaluated the Zazzi BMS on 21 patients in acute care. Researchers reported efficient evacuation with minimal leakage, improved perineal skin injury, and no anorectal mucosal injury. Echols et al (2004) evaluated 297 patients with the Zazzi BMS and 208 patients without the Zazzi BMS in a large burn center. Researchers noted that the patients using the Zazzi BMS system had decreased rates of urinary tract, soft tissue, skin, and blood stream infections. These studies highlight the potential these devices have beyond the scope of skin protection and into the realm of managing infection and cross-contamination.

Drainage around catheters and tubes should be managed in such a way that the drainage is either eliminated, when possible, or the skin is not directly exposed to the drainage. For example, when leakage occurs around a gastrostomy tube, the first step is to ascertain proper placement and stabilization of the tube. If drainage persists once this is accomplished, appropriate use of skin barriers (particularly moisture-barrier ointments, solid-wafer skin barriers, thin hydrocolloids, or foam dressings) is indicated. A solid-wafer skin barrier, hydrocolloid, or foam dressing can be trimmed to fit around a tube site and remain in place for several days, being changed only as it loosens at the tube site. When ointment is the selected treatment, it should be reapplied periodically throughout the day to ensure

---

BOX 6-4 Rectal Pouching Procedure

1. Assemble equipment: nonsterile gloves, pouch, skin-barrier paste, clip, cloth, bag for waste, razor.
2. Prepare pouch:
   a. Cut pouch opening to fit patient's anatomy as indicated.
   b. Remove paper backing from skin barrier and tape.
   c. Apply a thick bead of paste around the center opening; set aside.
3. Apply nonsterile gloves.
4. Remove and apply pouch:
   a. Loosen tape and gently push skin away from adhesive.
   b. Discard used pouch and save clip (if one is used).
   c. Remove any paste residue using a dry tissue.
   d. Wash skin with soft cloth and warm water; be sure to remove any greasy residue using a gentle soap and water. Rinse and dry thoroughly.
   e. Shave perianal hair, if present.
   f. To create a smooth adhesive surface, apply a bead of paste in the gluteal fold and between the anal opening and the scrotum or vagina.
   g. Before applying pouch, fold skin barrier surface of pouch vertically (lengthwise).
   h. Align pouch between scrotum or vagina and anal opening, and apply to skin.
   i. Slowly unfold pouch and adhesive to apply to skin in smooth fashion.
   j. Encourage seal by massaging the adhesive for 1 minute.
   k. Attach clip to open end of pouch or attach spout to straight drainage.
5. Change pouch only if it leaks.
6. Reposition patient carefully to avoid undue stress on pouch seal.

Note: Skin-barrier powders must be used to dry any denuded skin present before the pouch is applied.

adequate skin protection. However, ointments can never be used under an adhesive dressing. Regardless of the type of skin protection selected, gauze dressings are applied over the barrier to absorb drainage and are changed when damp.

The constant, prolonged presence of caustic substances against the skin can create chemical damage and jeopardize skin integrity. Damage to the skin around the wound can be prevented by (1) monitoring appropriate dressing technique so that gauze dressings contact only the wound bed and are not contacting surrounding intact skin and (2) bracketing the wound with skin barriers (ointments, solid wafers, skin sealants, or hydrocolloids).

Improper use of skin-care products such as skin cleansers, solvents, adhesives, and skin sealants can contribute to chemical irritation. Skin cleansers and solvents must be thoroughly rinsed from the skin to prevent build-up of harmful substances. Skin cleansers or soaps should be used sparingly to avoid disruption of the skin's normal acid pH. Skin sealants and adhesives, such as cements, must be allowed to dry adequately so that solvents evaporate before other products are applied.

VASCULAR DAMAGE

Ulcerations, particularly on the legs or feet, also occur as a result of venous hypertension, arterial insufficiency, or neuropathy, or a combination of these factors. Although these types of lesions commonly develop incidentally to benign trauma (i.e., by bumping against the leg of a chair), each ulcer has distinct distinguishing features, pathologic processes, and treatment regimen. Arterial ulcers, venous ulcers, and lymphedema wounds are discussed in detail in Chapter 15. Neuropathic ulcers, such as diabetic ulcers, are discussed in Chapter 16.

INFECTIOUS FACTORS

Many skin rashes or ulcers are indicative of an infectious process and can occur around wounds or be misinterpreted as a result of pressure, shear, or chemical irritation. Infections can be categorized according to infecting organism: fungus, bacteria, virus, or arthropod. The wound-care specialist may be the first person to observe some of these infections. In many cases, the wound care specialist will be responsible for identifying and managing the infections. A few key skin infections are summarized in this section.

Fungus

Candidiasis. Cutaneous candidiasis represents an epidermal infection with *Candida* spp., most commonly *C. albicans* (Plate 10). The primary lesion of candidiasis is a pustule or erythematous papules or plaques that may have associated scaling or crusting or a cheesy white exudate. Maceration is common. Lesions are typically beefy red, with satellite erythematous papules and pustules. When located in the skin folds (intertriginous areas), solid plaques of moist red lesions are commonly observed. Satellite lesions (outside the advancing edge of candidiasis) are an important diagnostic feature of candidiasis (Habif, 2004). Intact pustules are not always visible because opposing skin and clothing will unroof the pustule so that the lesion will appear to be a macule or papule. Pruritus is the key indicator of candidiasis and may be severe.

Predisposing factors include the presence of a moist environment, a hot and humid environment, tight underclothing, diabetes, and antibiotic therapy. Skin under damp surgical dressings, the perineum, the perineal area, and intertriginous areas (beneath pendulous breasts, overhanging abdominal folds, and inguinal skin folds) are typical moist areas and provide an excellent medium for yeast growth. Diabetes predisposes the patient to develop candidiasis because the associated increase in the amount of glucose in the saliva, sweat, and urine prevents bacteria from inhibiting yeast growth (Hooper and Goldman, 1999). Antibiotics predispose the patient to develop candidiasis by removing the competing organisms. An altered skin pH also increases susceptibility to yeast infection. Immunosuppressed patients and patients with irritant contact dermatitis are also vulnerable to candidiasis.

Folliculitis and contact dermatitis can be confused with candidiasis. Furthermore, candidiasis can be disguised by being superimposed on irritant contact dermatitis. The distribution and types of lesions is important to identifying the underlying problem. Folliculitis, the inflammation of a hair follicle, is characterized by the presence of pustules pierced in the center by a hair, whereas candidiasis causes nonfollicular pustules. Manifestations of contact dermatitis include erythema with papules, whereas pustules are unusual and warrant culture to rule out superimposed infection. Distribution can help distinguish contact dermatitis from candidiasis because a contact dermatitis is limited to the area in contact with the irritant.

Candidiasis is most often determined clinically by the signs, symptoms, and predisposing factors. Pruritus and burning at the site are common. The most relevant laboratory test to confirm candidiasis is a potassium hydroxide (KOH) preparation scraping. Scrapings from an intact pustule and the contents are needed to yield the best results. Budding spores and elongated pseudohyphae are observed. Because the skin can be colonized with *C. albicans* but not infected, swab cultures for *Candida* are not informative: such cultures cannot distinguish between infection and colonization (Habif, 2004).

Nonpharmacologic treatment includes reduction of predisposing factors, such as humidity, moisture, antibiotics, hyperglycemia, and tight-fitting clothes. Body powders (e.g., Zeasorb-AF) or wide-mesh gauze can be placed in intertriginous areas to absorb moisture. Prevention of moisture build-up is the most important intervention to prevent candidiasis. Box 6-5 lists strategies to prevent moisture build-up.

Burow's solution soaks followed by air-drying are soothing when maceration or severe pruritus are present. Topical antifungal creams may be applied twice daily for limited involvement, and antifungal powders may be used in less severe cases. When creams are used, they should be applied sparingly to reduce moisture entrapment. Because ointments can further trap moisture and therefore exacerbate the candidiasis, they are not preferred. Recalcitrant or severe fungal infections require orally administered therapy.

Bacterial

Folliculitis, impetigo, erysipelas, and staphylococcal scalded skin syndrome (SSSS), toxic shock syndrome, and necrotizing fasciitis are not necessarily frequently encountered in the typical practice of a wound care specialist. However, they pose significant complications and should be familiar to the wound care specialist. Many of the bacterial skin infections are caused by *Staphylococcus aureus*. Although *S. aureus* can be recovered from normal intact skin, especially in the nares, the axillae, and the groin, it is rarely a true member of resident bacterial flora (Leyden and Gately, 1995).

Folliculitis

Folliculitis is a bacterial infection that involves the hair follicle (Plate 9). *S. aureus* is the most common causative organism. The primary lesion is a pustule that is pierced by a hair, and secondary lesions are crusts and erythema. Folliculitis may be limited to the superficial area of the hair follicle or progress deeper into the follicle. Although most common on the scalp or the extremities, folliculitis may develop on any hairy body location, particularly under adhesive wound dressings.

Risk factors for developing folliculitis are diabetes mellitus, obesity, malnutrition, immunodeficiency, and chronic staphylococcal infections. Folliculitis may also develop as a secondary infection in the presence of excoriated skin (e.g., scabies, insect bites, and eczema).

Nonpharmacologic treatment includes the use of antibacterial soaps. Adhesives in the affected area should be avoided, and hair should be clipped rather than shaved. Oral antibiotics are required for deep folliculitis, which can lead to cellulitis or abscess formation.

Impetigo

Impetigo, most commonly seen in children, is a highly contagious superficial skin infection that is caused primarily by the gram-positive bacterium *S. aureus*, although *Streptococcus pyrogenes* may also be present. Impetigo may present clinically as bullous or nonbullous. The initial onset is a vesicle involving the superficial layer of the stratum corneum. The patient may experience itching and mild soreness, but systemic

---

BOX 6-5 **Strategies to Prevent Moisture Build-up**
....

- Dust intertriginous skin folds with absorbent skin barrier powders.
- Separate intertriginous skin folds with skin sealants (spray or wipes) and/or soft gauze.
- Use skin sealant, thin hydrocolloid, low-adhesion foam dressing, or solid-wafer skin barrier beneath dressings and around wounds.
- Change dressings before they become saturated.
- Use a support surface (if needed) with air-vent capabilities.

symptoms are very uncommon. Impetigo most often develops on seemingly intact skin, although it may also develop with minor breaks in the skin.

It is important to distinguish impetigo from herpes simplex. Herpes simplex can be distinguished from impetigo by culture and by early manifestations; herpes simplex begins with grouped, clear vesicles that are uniform in size, and it recurs at the same site.

Impetigo is often self-limited, resolving spontaneously, although it may also become chronic and/or recurrent. The treatment of choice for impetigo is topically administered 2% mupirocin cream (Bactroban). It has been shown to be as effective as oral erythromycin without the side affects (Habif, 2004). The cream should be applied 3 times daily until the lesions clear.

Bullous Impetigo.   Bullous impetigo develops when certain strains of *S. aureus* produce a specific epidermolytic toxin. While they may occur anywhere on the body, the most common location is the face. One or more vesicles enlarge, creating a superficial, fragile, clear fluid-filled bulla that gradually becomes filled with cloudy fluid. When the center of the bulla collapses, a rim of the bulla roof often remains, encircling the lesion. The center of the lesion then develops a thin, honey-colored crust. When this is removed, a red, inflamed, moist base is revealed that is exudative with serous fluid. Eventually the outer edges of the bulla become dry and flaky, and a crust forms. Bullous impetigo lesions have little if any surrounding erythema; they can range in size from 2 to 8 cm and remain for several months. Infants must be monitored for signs and symptoms of serious secondary infections such as septic arthritis and pneumonia.

Nonbullous Impetigo.   The lesions associated with nonbullous impetigo are asymptomatic, with minimal surrounding erythema present. Although lesions begin as small vesicles or pustules, they soon rupture, exposing a moist, red base that becomes crusted over. The most common sites affected are around the mouth, the nose, and the extremities. Generally the sequence of events is that the infectious agent is present on intact skin, and after minor trauma such as scratching, the skin is broken and an infection develops (Habif, 2004). During the early development of the lesions, group A beta-hemolytic streptococci may be isolated; however,

the lesions quickly become contaminated with staphylococci. Predisposing factors for streptococcal impetigo are warm, moist climates and poor hygiene.

Erysipelas

Erysipelas is an acute inflammatory form of cellulitis that occurs as a complication of a break in skin integrity such as with abrasions, or dry skin. Erysipelas differs from other types of cellulitis because it involves the cutaneous lymphatics, in the form of "streaking". This disease has a very high morbidity rate if left undiagnosed (up to 80% in infants and 75% in the elderly) (Hooper and Goldman, 1999).

Erysipelas most commonly occurs in infants, young children, and older adults. Additional risk factors include malnutrition, alcoholism, recent infections, stasis dermatitis, lymphedema, nephrotic syndrome, and diabetes mellitus. Small, seemingly insignificant breaks in the skin can serve as a portal of entry for the infection. The extremities and the face are the most common sites.

Erysipelas means "red skin," and the involved body part is characterized by well-demarcated erythema. (In contrast, cellulitis is less demarcated.) The classic primary lesion is a plaque, and the surrounding skin is erythematous, edematous, and painful. Secondary lesions are vesicles, bullae, and cutaneous hemorrhage. Associated lymphangitis is demonstrated by the presence of erythematous streaking over lymphatics draining the area of infection.

Erysipelas is usually diagnosed by clinical findings: sharply marginated erythema, edema, and/or streaking. Accompanying systemic complaints of fever, chills, malaise, and localized pain also raise suspicion for the presence of this condition. A culture (via needle aspiration) of any drainage from the advancing edge and skin biopsies are appropriate although often uninformative. When septicemia is suspected, a white blood cell count and blood cultures are warranted.

Nonpharmacologic interventions include bed rest, elevation of the affected extremity, and hot packs. Uncomplicated cases of erysipelas can be treated with oral antibiotics, whereas toxic, debilitated, and elderly patients or children with extensive facial involvement or any patient with rapid evolving erythema, pain, and swelling require intravenous antibiotics. Pain control measures are essential.

Staphylococcal Scalded Skin Syndrome

SSSS is a superficial blistering disease that results in superficial necrosis. SSSS is a cutaneous response to a circulating toxin released from a staphylococcal infection that may be distant from the affected area. The primary lesions are superficial bullae that may occur on the face, the neck, the axillae, and the groin. Secondarily, lesions develop superficial scales. Desquamation develops subsequent to the significant erythema. The skin may have a sandpaper feel. Significant pain is unusual for SSSS and, if present, suggests another diagnosis such as toxic epidermal necrolysis, a drug-induced necrosis of the epidermis.

Although it has been reported in adults, SSSS most commonly occurs in healthy children 6 years of age or younger (Habif, 2004). Mortality approaches 3% in adults with renal failure and in those who are immunocompromised.

Suspicious sites (nose, eyes, ears, throat, vagina) should be swabbed for microbial cultures to confirm the diagnosis. Bullae from the primary lesion usually yield cultures that are negative for bacteria. A frozen section of sloughing skin is needed to differentiate SSSS from a drug-induced skin reaction (toxic epidermal necrolysis). Full-thickness epidermal necrosis is inconsistent with SSSS and suggests a drug-induced process (Leyden and Gately, 1995).

Debridement and antibiotics are essential to manage the infection. Topical management of the desquamated skin should address exudate management, pain control, and maintenance of a moist environment. Foam dressings, superabsorbent dressings, sheet hydrogels, and alginates are preferred dressing options, and adhesives should be avoided. When massive tissue loss is apparent, the wound should be managed according to the principles for burn therapy as outlined in Chapter 18.

Toxic Shock Syndrome

Toxic shock syndrome is a bacterial infection with acute onset and widespread macular erythematous eruptions. The most common pathogen for this serious infection is *S. aureus*. Desquamation of the skin is highly characteristic of toxic shock syndrome and occurs 10 days to 3 weeks after onset. The primary body sites are the fingertips and plantar surface of the palms (Leyden and Gately, 1995). Treatment requires aggressive antibiotic therapy, and the mortality rate is approximately 7%. Local wound management is based on wound needs (e.g., exudate absorption), and topical dressings should be nonocclusive and nonadhesive.

Necrotizing Fasciitis

Necrotizing fasciitis is an uncommon but very serious subcutaneous tissue infection that spreads rapidly along the superficial fascial plane. The overall mortality rate from necrotizing fasciitis is quite variable: 20% in pediatric cases and anywhere from 6% to 73% in adults (Jallali, 2003). Necrotizing fasciitis is characterized by widespread necrosis of the fascia and deep subcutaneous tissue, with thrombosis of nutrient vessels and sloughing of overlying tissue. It usually occurs in the extremities after a minor operation or injury.

Initial signs of necrotizing fasciitis are pain, swelling at the site of the wound, chills, fever, toxemia, and rapidly spreading and painful cellulitis. The skin may initially appear normal over the cellulitis, but as the infectious process compromises blood supply the skin becomes erythematous, edematous, and reddish-purple to patchy blue gray. Bullae form within 3 to 5 days from onset and progress to necrosis of the skin, sloughing, and frank cutaneous gangrene. Pain is the main indicator of necrotizing fasciitis, and the pain is considered to be out of proportion for the extent of the skin damage (Jallali, 2005).

Necrotizing fasciitis can be detected by its dramatic clinical presentation and by probing the wound. When the affected area is probed with a hemostat through a limited incision, the instrument passes easily along a plane of superficial to deep fascia. This examination also helps to distinguish necrotizing fasciitis from cellulitis. This infection is most often polymicrobial; the most common monomicrobial infectious agent is group A streptococci (Habif, 2004).

Treatment is surgical intervention to debride all nonviable fascia and tissue. Surgical debridement must be prompt, extensive, and aggressive. Local wound care consists of close monitoring for further dissection, which indicates progression of the infection. Topical dressing recommendations are largely expert opinion-based or preference-based. Dressings should be used that meet the needs of the wound (e.g., fill dead space, absorb exudate), allow for frequent monitoring of the wound, and are nonadhesive and nonocclusive.

Viral

Viral infections, particularly herpes simplex virus (HSV) and varicella-zoster virus (VZV), are commonly triggered by stress and illness. It is important to recognize these highly contagious infections to facilitate prompt appropriate treatment and prevent spread to others.

Herpes Simplex

HSV infections of the epidermis are highly contagious and can be spread when a susceptible, noninfected person comes into direct contact (mucous membrane or broken skin) with a person shedding the virus. Viral shedding occurs even in the absence of symptoms. Most transmission of HSV occurs during periods of asymptomatic shedding (Whitley, Kimberlin, and Roizman, 1998). Consequently, HSV infection should be considered a chronic process rather than an intermittent process, and all HSV-infected people should be treated as potentially contagious. Furthermore, because the primary infection is often subclinical, a negative history of vesicles or blisters does not rule out previous HSV infection (Chandrasekar, 1999).

HSV has been divided into two types: HSV-1 (oral herpes) and HSV-2 (genital herpes). HSV-1 is associated with cold sores (fever blisters); genital and perianal herpes is caused by HSV-2. However, genital lesions from HSV-1 and oral lesions from HSV-2 are becoming more common, a trend that may be a consequence of sexual freedom and the ease of transmission. Ultimately, HSV lesions are not limited to the lips and genital area and may occur anywhere on the skin.

HSV infections have two phases: primary infection and secondary phase. During the primary infection, the virus becomes established in a nerve ganglion. HSV-1 most often occurs during childhood, whereas HSV-2 commonly occurs after sexual contact in sexually active individuals. Symptoms of the primary infection range from being undetectable to localized pain, headache, generalized aching, malaise, and tender regional adenopathy. Uniform, grouped vesicles develop on an erythematous base; the vesicles contain large numbers of infective viral particles. Vesicles soon become pustules that erode, drain, and crust (Plate 11). Primary lesions last for 2 to 6 weeks and heal without scarring. As the lesion heals, the virus enters the skin nerve endings and ascends through peripheral nerves to the dorsal root ganglia, where it remains in a latent stage.

Reactivation of the virus can occur in response to local trauma (abrasion, ultraviolet light) or systemic changes (such as stress, illness, fatigue, fever, and compromised immune system). The virus then travels back down the peripheral nerve to the site, or in the vicinity, of the initial infection to trigger a recurrence. Prodromal symptoms of burning at the site may precede the recurrence. The reactivated virus presents as vesicles on an erythematous base, or ulcers. Crusts cover the eruptions within 24 to 48 hours and are shed in approximately 12 days, exposing a reepithelialized surface (Hunter, Savin, and Dahl, 2002).

Clinical presentation of grouped vesicles on an erythematous base is a key indicator of HSV and can be confirmed with a Tzanck smear. However, the Tzanck smear is most reliable when the lesion sampled is a vesicle; the smear becomes less reliable with pustules, crusts, or ulcers.

Primary HSV-1 infections are generally asymptomatic. When symptoms are present, the lesions include painful vesicles or shallow ulcers on the lips or lower face or in the oral cavity, and they last for 2 to 3 weeks. Recurrent HSV-1 infections are foreshadowed by pain and tingling or a burning sensation 2 to 24 hours before the eruption of vesicles (Chandrasekar, 1999). Recurrent HSV-1 lasts about 2 days as vesicles, which then progress to pustules, ulcers, and eventually crusts. Complete healing occurs in 8 to 10 days.

Primary genital herpes (typically HSV-2 infection) lesions are initially macules and papules and are followed by vesicles, pustules, and ulcerations. Lesions may occur on the genitalia, the perineum, and the buttocks; are extremely painful; and persist for about 2 weeks. Spontaneous resolution of the primary infection is common. Recurrent genital herpes is less pronounced and lasts for 8 to 10 days. Ulcers are shallow and may or may not be painful.

Perianal ulcers are commonly misinterpreted as the result of pressure, chemical damage, or scabies (Plate 12). Therefore the differential diagnosis for ulcers located in the perianal area or on the buttocks must include HSV (Chandrasekar, 1999). Genital herpes can be distinguished from pressure sores in that the lesions are not limited to a bony prominence and are more typical over the fleshy part of the buttocks. Genital herpes in the perianal area can also be distinguished from chemical irritation (such as occurs with diarrhea) by the presence of several isolated ulcers rather than the confluence of superficial denudement or erythema that impinges on the anal opening.

In the clinical presentation, grouped vesicles on an erythematous base are highly suggestive of HSV regardless of body site. The most definitive method of confirming the infection is to unroof the intact vesicle so the vesicular fluid can be cultured. Rapid testing (within a few hours) can also be done with direct fluorescent antibody (DFA) examination. Commercially available kits also distinguish among HSV-1, HSV-2, and VZV.

Antiviral medications are effective in treating HSV infection and are available for topical, oral, and intravenous administration. Early initiation of oral acyclovir for genital herpes decreases healing time, viral shedding, and duration of pain.

Nursing care should be directed at keeping lesions dry, avoiding trauma, and providing comfort. Burow's solution (aluminum acetate) soaks and refrigerated hydrogel dressings can relieve the topical pain commonly associated with genital herpes lesions. When shedding HSV lesions are present, skin cleansing should be done cautiously so that spreading of the virus is avoided, particularly when the lesions are present on the buttocks.

Varicella-Zoster Virus

VZV causes varicella (chicken pox) and herpes zoster (shingles). VZV is highly contagious and is transmitted by direct contact with either vesicular fluid or airborne droplets from the infected host's respiratory tract. Airborne transmission as a mode for spreading VZV is very serious. Spread of varicella with no direct contact has been reported; the sole exposure was to air that flowed from the room of the infected individual to another room. Patients with herpes zoster are less contagious than patients with varicella (Cohen et al, 1999).

Herpes zoster is an infection within the epidermis that is characteristically unilateral and occurs along one or two adjacent dermatome distributions (Figure 6-2). Eruptions result from the reactivation of the VZV that entered the cutaneous nerves during a bout of chicken pox and has since remained dormant in the dorsal root ganglia. Reactivation can occur as a result of immunosuppression, fatigue, and emotional trauma and occurs in 15% of people (Cohen et al, 1999). The elderly may be predisposed to herpes zoster as a consequence of a potential decline in immunologic function. Individuals who are immunocompromised are at risk of developing VZV and experience more severe infections. These patients are more likely to develop disseminated disease with extensive skin lesions, pneumonia, hepatitis, or encephalitis (Cohen et al, 1999). Diagnosis is most often based on clinical appearance.

Herpes zoster has characteristic manifestations that begin with a burning pain, then erythema that evolves into a grouped unilateral vesicular rash along one or two dermatomes (Plate 13). Over the next few days, the clear vesicles become filled with purulent fluid (i.e., pustules form) that then rupture and crust over (Hunter et al, 2002). In some debilitated patients, the eruption may become more extensive and inflammatory, with necrosis or secondary infections developing. VZV in the immunocompromised patient may last from weeks to months, and the resulting ulcer may develop a black, adherent eschar. Pain that persists beyond 1 month after healing is called postherpetic neuralgia.

Treatment of herpes zoster is similar to that of HSV, with antiviral medications and Burow's solution to act as an astringent on the lesions. Like genital herpes, early initiation of systemic antiviral medications decreases healing time, viral shedding, and duration of pain. Lesions should not be occluded because this delays their healing (Chandrasekar, 1999). Analgesics may be necessary to control the pain associated with herpes zoster.

ARTHROPOD

Although most severe spider bites are attributed to the brown recluse spider, the bites that cause systemic poisoning are caused by one of five species of spiders within the genus *Loxosceles*; the brown recluse is one of these. It is impossible to know which species is responsible for the lesion without having actually seen the spider. A distinctive feature on the brown recluse spider

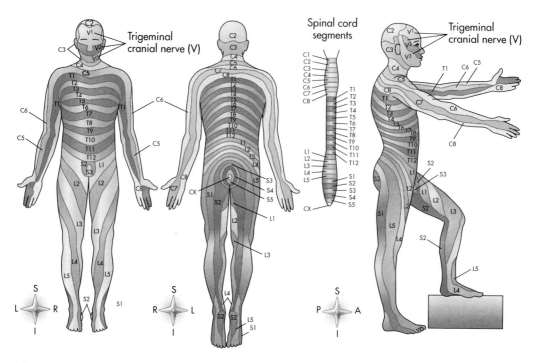

Fig. 6-2 Segmental dermatome distribution of spinal nerves to the front, back, and side of the body. Dermatomes are specific skin surface areas innervated by a single spinal nerve or group of spinal nerves. *C*, Cervical segments; *T*, thoracic segments; *L*, lumbar segments; *S*, sacral segments; *CX*, coccygeal segment. (From Thibodeau GA, Patton KT: *Anatomy and physiology*, ed 4, St Louis 1999, Mosby.)

is the fiddle-shaped mark. The brown recluse spider is usually shy and nocturnal; it tends to avoid humans and seek shelter in abandoned or infrequently-used buildings, attics, and basements. Bites generally occur when a person is disturbing a pile of wood or rocks, moving boxes that have been stored, or dressing in clothes that have been stored for a long period of time. The most common site for a *Loxosceles* spider bite is on the extremities, but they can also be found on the buttocks or the genitalia.

Manifestations of a brown recluse spider bite can range from small lesions with erythema to full-thickness necrotic wounds (known as necrotic arachnidism). Approximately 10% will develop severe a systemic reaction, known as loxoscelism and characterized by fever, nausea, hemolysis, and thrombocytopenia (Zeglin, 2005). Severity of the reaction depends upon the amount

of venom injected, the site of the bite, and host susceptibility. The very young, the elderly, and those individuals in poor physical condition are at highest risk for serious illness from a spider bite.

After a spider bite, the person may experience a mild burning sensation or no discomfort at all. Within 6 to 12 hours, itching, pain, and erythema develop around the bite. Because of the release of a necrolytic toxin, tissue necrosis can develop, indicated by a mottled, bluish discoloration that evolves into red bullae at the site of the bite. These severe lesions characteristically show a clinical presentation of a ring of blanching (due to vasoconstriction) and an outer ring of erythema that encircles the bite lesion (Zeglin, 2005).

The standard treatment of mild lesions is (1) thorough cleansing, (2) rest, (3) application of ice,

(4) compression, and (5) elevation. Oral antiinflammatory medications, an antihistamine, and tetanus vaccine may also be given. If cellulitis appears to be developing, antibiotics such as erythromycin are indicated (Zeglin, 2005). Topical dressings should provide a moist environment, absorb exudate, and be nonadhesive, so that the site can be easily monitored for signs of deterioration and cellulitis.

Treatment for severe necrotic lesions is controversial, but the following is indicated (Smith, Ickstadt, and Kucera, 1997): (1) application of an ice pack on the affected area (no heat), (2) administration of antibiotics to treat the secondary infection, (3) measures to control pain, (4) administration of tetanus toxoid, and (5) use of nonocclusive dressings to facilitate debridement and fill tissue loss. Patients with severe and rapidly progressing lesions may be given dapsone (Avlosulfon) therapy. However, it must be administered within hours of a bite to be effective. By inhibiting the spread of neutrophils, dapsone is believed to minimize tissue necrosis (Zeglin, 2005). Unfortunately, dapsone can have multiple moderate-to-severe, adverse effects. Alternative interventions include hyperbaric oxygenation, nitroglycerin patches, electric shock therapy, and heparin therapy, although there is no conclusive evidence for the effectiveness of these treatments. Systemic reactions and complications from the bite of a recluse spider include renal failure and coagulation disorders such as thrombocytopenia and disseminated intravascular coagulopathy (DIC) (Zeglin, 2005).

ALLERGIC FACTORS

Numerous allergic responses, both local and systemic, can be manifested on the skin. Because the wound care specialist is in a likely position to observe such a reaction, it is important to be able to describe the manifestations accurately and to report the assessment to the physician in a timely fashion. This section focuses on those allergic responses that are localized reactions to such things as adhesives, wound care products, or solutions. These types of skin damage are commonly referred to as allergic contact dermatitis.

Allergic contact dermatitis is an immunologic response to an allergen. Contact dermatitis occurs more readily in the presence of a preexisting skin disorder in which the cutaneous barrier is disrupted.

A true allergic dermatitis requires exposure to an allergen and has two phases:

1. The *sensitization phase* (the skin of a nonsensitized individual is exposed to a substance or chemical) transpires over a 7 to 10 day period. Small molecules from the allergen pass through the epidermis and attach to an epidermal protein found on the surface of the Langerhans' cell. From here these cells migrate through the dermis to the lymph nodes, where they present the allergen to T lymphocytes. Subsequently, effector and memory T lymphocytes proliferate in the lymph node, are released to circulate in the blood, and ultimately return to the skin. Here the body develops the ability to recognize the antigen when it reappears on the skin, and the T lymphocytes are now "primed" (Hunter, Savin, and Dahl, 2002).

2. When reexposed to the allergen, the *elicitation phase* occurs within 48 to 72 hours. Once the Langerhans' cell delivers the antigen to memory T cells in the skin, effector T cells begin to produce lymphokines. Inflammatory cells are summoned by the lymphokines, and allergic manifestations can be observed. Suppressor T cells are believed to end the inflammatory reaction.

An acute inflammatory response occurs within 48 hours of reexposure to an allergen. Clinical manifestations begin with erythema, followed by pruritus. Primary lesions are vesicles, bullae, papules, plaques, and wheals. Secondary lesions include moist desquamation, edema, fissure, excoriation, and crust (see Plates 6, 7, and 14). An acute reaction usually resolves in days to weeks, after the allergen has been removed.

The cause or source of the allergen may be obvious or obscured by other concurrent processes. A careful, detailed assessment and interview are imperative to identify the skin reaction as an allergic response. Common allergic sensitizers include poison ivy, nickel (used in jewelry), rosins, rubber compounds (used in elastic, gloves), benzocaine (used in antipruritic creams), paraphenylenediamine (a dye used to color hair), and preservatives. Topical preparations with one of the following ingredients are also common allergic offenders: aloe vera, fragrances, parabens, quarternium 15, diphenhydramine (Benedryl spray or Caladryl lotion), neomycin (Neosporin), and para-aminobenzoic acid (PABA) (Habif, 2004). Overuse of soaps, cleansers, moisturizers, and cosmetics can produce reactions. Many chemicals of similar structure cross-react; therefore a person who is sensitive to one product may be sensitive to several other products.

The location and distribution of the skin inflammation is an important clue in identification of the causative agent. Allergic contact dermatitis is localized to the skin where the product is applied, and involved areas typically have sharp margins. Therefore an allergic reaction to an adhesive, for example, will be the shape of the adhesive and will have well-defined borders. Allergic contact dermatitis can spread from the original site of application through inadvertent transfer of the allergen by the hands or, as the disease progresses, by the circulating T lymphocytes. However, the skin reaction begins and remains most severe in the area in which contact with the antigen occurred (Hunter, Savin, and Dahl, 2002).

Patch tests can be conducted to confirm the suspected agent that is causing the allergic reaction; however, these tests must be properly conducted and interpreted. Suspected allergens are applied to the skin and secured with tape. The patient's back is usually the preferred site for patch testing. After 48 hours, the patches are removed and the test site is assessed for skin damage, which is graded using a standard scale as described in Box 6-6. Although the patch test seems simple to apply and read, it is a complicated procedure that requires training and experience to obtain valid results (Rietschel and Fowler, 2001).

Simply avoiding contact with allergens can prevent allergic contact dermatitis. However, recognizing or identifying the potential allergen is the key to prevention and may not be an easy task.

When an allergic response is suspected, use of the offending product or chemical should be discontinued. Often a substitute can be used. Use of antiinflammatory medications may be warranted topically or systemically and is usually determined based on the severity of the allergic reaction.

INFLAMMATORY CONDITIONS LEADING TO ATYPICAL ULCERATIONS

Inflammatory conditions such as pyoderma granulosum and vasculitis-related ulcers precipitate atypical ulcerations that must be carefully assessed to avoid being misidentified as venous or arterial ulcers.

BOX 6-6 Scale for Interpretation of Patch Test Results

SCORE		SIGNIFIES
+	=	Weak (nonvesicular) positive reaction: erythema, infiltration, possibly papules
++	=	Strong (edematous or vesicular) positive reaction
+++	=	Extreme (spreading, bullous, ulcerative) positive reaction
−	=	Negative reaction
IR	=	Irritant reactions of different types
NT	=	Not tested
Macular erythema only is a doubtful reaction		

Adapted from Habif T: *Clinical dermatology: a color guide to diagnosis and therapy*, ed 4, St Louis, 2004, Mosby.

BOX 6-7 Systemic Diseases Associated with Pyoderma Granulosum

Ankylosing spondylitis
Rheumatoid arthritis
Sarcoidosis
Chronic active hepatitis
Inflammatory bowel disease
Monoclonal gammopathies
Myeloma

Pyoderma Granulosum

Pyoderma granulosum (PG) is a chronic neutrophilic inflammatory disease that can cause painful ulcerative lesions. Although associated with immune reaction and underlying systemic disorders (Box 6-7), 40% to 50% of cases are idiopathic (Goldstein and Goldstein, 1997; Margolis, 1993). When PG accompanies a systemic disease, it does not necessarily parallel the underlying disease. The pathophysiologic mechanism of PG is unknown. Histologically, the presence of numerous polymorphonuclear leukocytes creates a dense infiltrate of the dermis that can extend from the superficial dermis to the subcutaneous tissue (Hoffman, 1999).

PG has several different manifestations: ulcerative, pustular, bullous and vegetative (Powell, Su, and Perry, 1996). The most common presentation is the classical ulcerative form. This particular manifestation is commonly associated with inflammatory bowel disease, arthritis, or myeloproliferative disease. These extremely painful PG lesions begin with a nodule, pustules, or bullae that develop significant induration and erythema and progress to ulcers.

Common characteristics of the ulcerative PG lesion is that the wound edges are irregularly shaped, elevated, and violaceous (Plate 15). Ulcers are deep, exudative, and extremely tender. The wound base is often filled with yellow slough and/or islands of necrosis; wound edges are undermined. A band of erythema may extend from the wound edge, which defines the direction in which the ulcer will extend (Hoffman, 1999). Healing may be present along one edge of the ulcer while enlargement occurs along another edge. Ulcers heal slowly and leave an atrophic, irregular scar. The most common sites are the lower extremities (particularly the lower legs), although PG may also occur on the buttocks, the abdomen, the face, and the hands. A diagnostic characteristic of PG is a phenomenon known as pathergy, the abnormal and exaggerated inflammatory response to noxious stimuli. Patients often report the lesion developing after minor trauma, such as a bump against a piece of furniture.

PG is difficult to diagnose and is basically a disease of exclusion. It can be misdiagnosed as venous, arterial, neuropathic, vasculitic, or neoplastic wounds (Lorentzen and Gottrup, 1998). Diagnosis is based on clinical manifestations and a thorough examination in which other ulcerative skin disorders (e.g., vasculitis and infections) and psychosomatic illnesses have been excluded. A history and physical examination, skin biopsy for histology and microbiology, and an investigation for an associated illness constitute a thorough workup. The histopathologic findings are not specific for PG; however, they are supportive of the disease. Furthermore, the ulcer biopsy needs to be obtained from the erythematous margin of the wound to best demonstrate these histopathologic findings (Hoffman, 1999). This biopsy may trigger enlargement of the ulcer as a result of the pathergy response; however, biopsy is important to rule out vasculitic, vasoocclusive, and infectious causes (Hoffman, 1999). Laboratory tests

for antineutrophilic cytoplasmic antibodies (ANCA), antiphospholipid antibodies (anticardiolipin antibodies, lupus anticoagulant, rapid plasma reagin [RPR]) are important to obtain, again for the purpose of excluding other diseases that could account for these lesions. The diagnosis of pyoderma granulosum is reached only after this workup is complete.

The treatment of PG consists of a combination of systemic therapy and local wound care. Several treatments have been used to manage PG, and the most consistent, effective results have been obtained with corticosteroids. Large orally administered doses of prednisolone (60 to 120 mg) are given daily until the disease is under control as demonstrated by the reduction in pain and presence of granulation tissue. Although PG is not an infectious disease process, it can be complicated by infections (Hoffman, 1999). Dapsone has been useful in controlling the wound bioburden, particularly during the diagnostic workup.

Topical wound management should address wound needs, which include exudate management, protection from trauma, and a moist wound environment, and pain control. Typically, it will be necessary to manage the wound before its cause is known (Kelly, 2001). Because of the extreme pain that typifies PG, nonadhesive dressings are preferred. Debridement is achieved only through autolysis and regression of the disease process itself. Aggressive debridement is contraindicated, since it will lead to extension of the disease through the process of pathergy. In fact, local care should be delivered with great caution because of the tendency for pathergy to occur. Antibacterial topical dressings are often warranted to manage the wound bioburden and potential secondary bacterial infections (Coady, 2000).

Vasculitis

Vasculitis comprises a group of disorders that have in common the pathologic feature of inflammation of the blood vessels, endothelial swelling, and necrosis (Hunter, Savin, and Dahl, 2002). Vessels of any size can be affected, so any organ or system may be involved, resulting in a wide array of symptoms and clinical presentations (Jennette and Falk, 1997). Vasculitic ulcers that result in skin lesions are usually the sign of a complex process and may indicate a systemic disorder (Roenigk and Young, 1996). Most vasculitic syndromes are believed to have an immunologic etiology.

The size of the vessels involved (large, medium, or small) helps to characterize the skin manifestations. When a small vessel is affected, pinpoint areas of bleeding may develop, and small red or purple spots on the skin (petechiae) may appear, particularly on the leg. The inflammation of larger vessels causes the vessel to swell, producing a nodule that may be palpated. Blood flow will be impaired when the lumen of the blood vessel becomes narrowed or occluded from the edema; thus islands of ischemia or necrosis will develop on the skin, and tips of digits may become cold or ischemic.

Specific diseases that may have vasculitis as a prominent feature include rheumatoid arthritis, systemic lupus erythematosus, polyarteritis nodosa, hypersensitivity vasculitis, Wegener's granulomatosis, Sjögren's syndrome, cryoglobulinemia, scleroderma, and dermatomyositis (Roenigk and Young, 1996; Rubano and Kerstein, 1998).

The general signs and symptoms of vasculitis are fever, myalgias, arthralgias, and malaise. Patients sometimes describe a vague, flulike illness. Peripheral neuropathy may also be present. Other symptoms depend on the organ involved, which is determined by the specific disease. For example, cryoglobulinemic vasculitis is likely to involve renal and skin problems, Wegener's granulomatosis may lead to respiratory as well as renal involvement, and the vasculitis associated with Sjögren's syndrome attacks the brain, the lung, and the skin (Jennette and Falk, 1997).

Cutaneous features of vasculitis can vary depending on the disease, but there are certain common characteristics. The lesions can range from erythematous, nonblanching macules and/or nodules to hemorrhagic vesicles and palpable purpura, to necrotic lesions and ulceration. Skin biopsy is critical and is best taken from early lesions. Two or three sites might be needed to obtain the correct diagnosis (Roenigk and Young, 1996). Skin ulcers associated with vasculitis are frequently located on the lower extremities, making them difficult to distinguish from venous ulcers (Plate 16).

Treatment of vasculitic ulcers is aimed at control of the underlying disease process. Bed rest and administration of antihistamines, corticosteroids, and immunosuppressive agents are often necessary (Hunter, Savin, and Dahl, 2002). In cases associated with circulating immune complexes, plasmapheresis might be necessary.

Topical therapy includes debridement of necrotic tissue, prompt identification and treatment of infection, maintenance of a moist wound base, absorption of excess exudate, packing of any dead space, insulation, and protection from further trauma.

There are many similarities among the various vasculitic syndromes; however, there are some specific differences unique to some of the diseases. The unique features of rheumatoid arthritis, systemic lupus erythematosus, and polyarteritis nodosa are presented in Table 6-3.

Drug-Induced Vasculitis

In approximately 10% of patients with vasculitis, the cause is a drug reaction rather than a disease process. Drug-induced vasculitis is usually confined to the skin and will appear about 1 week after administration of the drug. The drugs bind to serum proteins, causing an immune-complex vasculitis (Jennette and Falk, 1997). The typical presentation is purpura and ulceration involving the lower extremities. Once systemic disease has been ruled out, treatment involves removal of the precipitating drug and symptomatic treatment. Antihistamines and nonsteroidal antiinflammatory drugs (NSAIDs) are most often prescribed. Corticosteroids may be added for more severe symptoms. Wound care is based on wound needs, and ulcers resolve spontaneously once the drug is removed.

INTRINSIC SKIN DISEASES ASSOCIATED WITH ULCERATION

Skin wounds may also develop as a manifestation of a disease process or as a complication associated with the treatment of a disease. In this section, four rare diseases that can trigger massive skin loss or skin necrosis and two blood dyscrasias are discussed.

Epidermolysis Bullosa

Epidermolysis bullosa (EB) is the name given to a group of similar diseases that have a tendency to develop blisters and erosions in the skin, and sometimes in mucous membranes, after mild mechanical trauma (Fine, Bauer, and Gedde-Dahl, 1999). EB is most often inherited, although there is a noninherited form (EB acquisita). There are many types of EB, and symptoms can range from mild, seasonal blistering to life-threatening

TABLE 6-3 Characteristics of Skin Lesions with Vasculitic Disorders

VASCULITIC DISORDER	DESCRIPTION	ULCER CHARACTERISTICS
Rheumatoid arthritis	• Not well understood • Associated with high levels of rheumatoid factor (RF) (Ikeda et al, 1998; Yamamoto, Ohkubo, Nishioka, 1995) • Evidence of venous insufficiency (McRorie, Ruckley, Nuki, 1998) • Limited ankle movement contributes to poor calf-muscle pump function and may place patient at risk for venous ulcer development	• Begin as palpable purpura and ecchymosis • May progress to ulceration • Shallow, well-demarcated, painful, and slow to heal • May require addition of compression therapy (McRorie, Ruckley, Nuki, 1998)
Systemic lupus erythematosus (SLE)	• Chronic immune disorder • Characterized by periods of exacerbation and remission • Affects multiple organs (skin, serosal surfaces, CNS, kidneys) and red blood cells • Circulating immune complexes and autoantibodies cause tissue damage and organ dysfunction • No single cause; influenced by environment, host immune responses and hormones • Common symptoms include fatigue, weight loss, fever, malaise • Butterfly rash (facial edema over cheeks and nose) is typical • Potential manifestations include seizures, hemiparesis, pericarditis, pleuritis, renal failure, nausea, vomiting, abdominal pain, and arthralgias	• Present as palpable purpura • Progress to ulceration • Occur on the malleolar area • Present as round lesions with erythematous borders • Wound may also have atrophy and loss of pigmentation (Rubano and Kerstein, 1998)
Polyarteritis nodosa (PAN)	• Medium and small vessel vasculitis • Necrotizing arteritis affecting small and medium-sized arteries of most organs • Involved organs commonly include kidney, liver, intestine, peripheral nerves, skin, and muscle • Characterized by fresh and healing lesions • Clinical manifestations include anorexia, weight loss, fever, and fatigue • Organ-specific manifestations include abdominal pain, myalgia, arthralgia, or paresthesia • Subcutaneous painful nodules of lower extremities may develop	• Skin involvement occurs in approximately 40% of patients • Lesions have a "punched out" appearance • Painful • Lesions may begin as purpura with urticaria before progressing to ulceration • May be a "starburst" pattern extending from the ulcer • Painful subcutaneous nodules present (Roenigk and Young, 1996; Rubano and Kerstein, 1998)

skin erosions (Schober-Flores, 2003). EB can affect every epithelial structure in the body, including the eyelids, conjunctivae, corneas, bowels, skin, and gums.

Inherited EB is rare, affecting 100,000 people, mostly children. (Fine, Bauer, and Gedde-Dahl, 1999). It is divided into three types: EB simplex (EBS), junctional EB (JEB), and dystrophic EB (DEB). At least 23 distinctive phenotypes of EB have been identified. Differences between the three types are based on ultrastructural levels of the skin within which the blisters develop. Immunofluorescence or electron microscopic studies of skin specimens are most reliable in establishing the diagnosis. Distinctive characteristics of EB are provided in Box 6-8.

Extracutaneous manifestations are common and may be gastrointestinal, ophthalmologic, or hematologic. The severity of these manifestations varies with the category of EB, as well as the subtype within that category. Gastrointestinal complications are a major source of symptoms and morbidity for all EB patients. The most severe problems are related to the oropharynx, esophagus, and proximal gut. The simple process of using

eating utensils and the passage of foods results in the formation of bullae that rupture, erode, and heal with scar formation. Strictures are inevitable, and nutritional problems develop.

Anemia is another major problem with EB and is multifactorial in origin. Poor nutrition resulting from painful oral blisters and esophageal strictures precipitates a deficiency in iron, trace metals, and protein, which contributes to anemia. Protein and blood are also lost through the chronic skin lesions typical of JEB and DEB.

The patient with EB is deprived of an epidermal barrier to bacterial invasion. *S. aureus* and other pathogens often colonize the chronic, nonhealing wound. Sepsis is a serious complication, especially in the infant. Judicious use of topical antibiotics is warranted to decrease bacterial flora and minimize the risk of soft tissue infection. Silver sulfadiazine cream is contraindicated in newborns under 8 weeks of age because of the increased risk of kernicterus (Caldwell-Brown et al, 1992). Topical antibiotics should not be used as a lubricating ointment because they are for

---

BOX 6-8 **Characteristics of Epidermolysis Bullosa (EB) by Category**

EB Simplex (EBS)
- Intraepidermal blisters
- Heals without scar formation
- Nails and teeth normal
- Occasional cutaneous blistering
- Autosomal dominant trait

Junctional EB (JEB)
- Autosomal recessive trait
- Blisters form at lamina lucida (between epidermis and basement membrane)
- Several subtypes with distinct clinical manifestations

Recessive Dystrophic EB (RDEB)
- Dystrophic scarring is distinctive feature that serves as clinical marker
- Separation at basement membrane zone deep to the basement membrane
- Recessive inheritance
- Blister formation results from even minimal mechanical trauma

- Blisters may be hemorrhagic
- Blisters eventually rupture to form slow-to-heal superficial ulcers that continue to be exposed to minimal mechanical trauma
- Healing always involves scarring so skin has atrophic and wrinkled appearance
- Elbows, knees, hands, and feet are sites of repeated trauma
- Predisposes patient to squamous cell cancer

Dominant Dystrophic EB (DDEB)
- Formation of blisters below the basement membrane
- Autosomal dominant inheritance
- Trauma-induced blisters form at birth or shortly thereafter
- Blisters heal with scar formation but are usually less extensive than the recessive form
- Predispose patient to squamous cell cancer

open lesions only. In the presence of cellulitis, systemic antibiotics are required (Marinkovich and Pham, 2005). Close monitoring of lesions and bacteriologic studies are imperative.

The primary objective in the care of patients with EB is to promote healing and prevent trauma (Schober-Flores, 2003). Nursing considerations include wound care, nutrition, education, and social support. Special precautions to minimize cutaneous trauma during select clinical procedures can be found in Table 6-4. Interventions such as the routine use of convoluted foam to pad rails, sheepskin, an air-fluidized support surface, and joint protectors are important. Low-adherence foam dressings or thin hydrocolloids may also be appropriate for protection of the hands or feet. However, if these are used, the dressing should be left in place and allowed to fall off rather than being removed and reapplied on a regular basis.

TABLE 6-4 Special Precautions to Minimize Cutaneous Trauma to Patients with DEB during Select Clinical Procedures

PROCEDURE	SUGGESTIONS
Blood pressure (BP) monitoring	Apply dressing under BP cuff.
Electrocardiogram monitoring	Use a nonadhesive plastic film such as Omiderm (which does not interfere with electrical conduction) as a barrier between the patient's skin and the adhesive of the electrode pads.
Urine collections (young children)	Wring out cloth diaper; do not apply urine bags containing adhesives.
Blood drawing	To cleanse skin, allow alcohol or Betadine swab to remain in place for 5 min without rubbing; place tourniquet over padding to protect skin; or apply direct pressure on vein using thumb in a parallel position to skin.
Parenteral therapy	Cut a piece of extra thin hydrocolloid dressing into a horseshoe shape and put dressing with adhesive backing side in contact with skin. Start the intravenous (IV) line between the legs of the horseshoe bandage, and tape the tubing onto the dressing. Secure IV with roller gauze, or place a snug-fitting piece of tube gauze such as Bandnet on extremity adjacent to IV and secure with tape to tube gauze.
Preoperative preparations: operating room, table, surgical drapes, and surgical scrub	Operating room table should be well-padded. Sheepskin covered by a table-sized burn pad such as Exudry, which has a double layer of meshed material to minimize friction, is advised. If positioning with pillows is necessary for patients with joint contractures, place Exudry pad between pillow and patient's skin. Sterile sheets of nonadherent mesh (Exudry Mesh or N-Interface) are placed under sterile drapes to protect exposed skin from friction. Fold mesh over edge of drape and secure with clamps as usual. Adhesive drapes are contraindicated. Apply antimicrobial solution to surgical site. Allow to remain on skin for 5 min, then irrigate to rinse. Repeat this process 3 times.
Mask-delivered anesthesia	Protect skin on face from possible shearing with a nonadherent foam or apply copious amount of petrolatum to face before applying mask.

Reprinted with permission from Caldwell-Brown D et al: Nursing aspects of EB: a comprehensive approach. In Lin AN, Carter DM, editors: *Epidermolysis bullosa: basic and clinical aspects,* New York, 1992, Springer-Verlag.

There is no single approach to wound care for managing EB lesions; rather, key principles should be followed to achieve desired objectives of containing exudate, avoiding trauma, preventing infection, and maintaining a moist environment (Schober-Flores, 2003). Nonadherent dressings are most appropriate and should be secured with roll gauze, tubular gauze, or a stockinette. Fenestrated, nonadherent dressings may be used so that wound moisture can pass through the fenestrations and be trapped by the cover dressing; ointments can also be applied over the fenestrated layer when trying to reduce wound bioburden. Creative dressing techniques are often necessary for difficult locations such as the digits or face. To avoid sensitization, the use of topical antibiotics is not recommended in the absence of very strong evidence that an infection exists. When infection is suspected—such as with the presence of increased drainage, odor, or wound pain—silver-impregnated dressings are appropriate. Temporary skin substitutes and bioengineered skin hold a great deal of promise for this dangerous disease. For further information about this disease, the Dystrophic Epidermolysis Bullosa Association of America (DEBRA) can be contacted at 141 Fifth Ave, New York, New York, 10010 (212-995-2220).

Calciphylaxis

Indurated, painful necrotic lesions with a violaceous discoloration characterize calciphylaxis, an extremely rare condition almost exclusively seen in patients with end-stage renal disease. Initially, patients develop painful, mottled skin lesions that progress to subcutaneous nodules and ulcerations that eventually become gangrenous. Subsequent infection and gangrene contribute to the high mortality rate associated with this disease (60%) (Budisavljevic, Cheek, and Ploth, 1996; Burkhart, Burkhart, and Mian, 1999). A distinctive finding with calciphylaxis is that peripheral pulses are intact because blood flow distal to the necrosis or deeper than the necrosis remains intact. This clinical assessment is critical in distinguishing the disease from other forms of peripheral vascular disease.

Histologically, microvascular calcification of the intima layer of the arteriole (and occasionally the media layer) is found. These calcifications precipitate a narrowing of the lumen, and arterial thrombosis is also occasionally observed. However, complete occlusion of the arteriole seldom develops. The primary cause for the accompanying ischemia is hyperplasia, another histologic change that occurs within the intima lining of the arteriole. The combination of microvascular calcification of the media layer and hyperplasia within the intima of arterioles with a diameter of approximately 0.04 to 0.1 mm is considered a histologic marker for calciphylaxis. These findings assist in differentiating this disease from peripheral arterial occlusion. Arteriole hyperplasia and microvascular calcification have also been reported in patients with normal renal function who have diabetes, multiple myeloma, breast cancer with hypercalcemia, or primary parathyroidism (Hafner et al, 1995; Khafif et al, 1990).

The etiology of calciphylaxis is as yet unknown. Hypercalcemia, hyperphosphatemia, and hyperparathyroidism are associated with the syndrome, although it also occurs in the absence of these abnormalities (Budisavljevic, Cheek, and Ploth, 1996; Ruggian, Maesaka, and Fishbane, 1996). Protein C functional deficiency that precipitates thrombosis in small blood vessels has been studied as a risk factor for calciphylaxis, although this deficiency is not consistently found (Hafner et al, 1995).

Treatment of calciphylaxis is neither universally standardized nor necessarily effective. Prompt recognition and treatment yield the best results. Systemically, normalization of abnormal calcium and phosphorus levels is warranted. Severe hyperparathyroidism may be managed pharmacologically or surgically. Antibiotics should be implemented to treat wound infection and to prevent sepsis. Most individuals who develop calciphylaxis require limb amputation and reconstructive surgery (Burkhart, Burkhart, and Mian, 1999).

Topical wound management should address specific wound needs: fill dead space, provide physiologic environment, and absorb exudate. Aggressive debridement is indicated to reduce the potential for wound infection. The severity of wound-related pain should be assessed regularly, and control measures for the pain should be implemented routinely and during wound procedures. Applications of split-thickness skin grafts have been successful (Snyder, Beylin, and Weiss, 2000).

Toxic Epidermal Necrolysis (TEN)

Toxic epidermal necrolysis (TEN) is a rare condition in which there is widespread loss of sheets of epidermis involving more than 10% of the body surface. TEN is seen in adults or children, usually as a drug reaction. Three main drug categories have been associated with TEN: antibiotics (sulfonamides, allopurinol, and ampicillin), anticonvulsants (phenytoin, carbamazepine, and phenobarbitol), and analgesics (acetaminophen and NSAIDs) (Clennett and Hosking, 2003). The mortality rate is high with TEN (30% to 40%), and death is usually the result of overwhelming sepsis.

Clinically, a generalized maculopapular rash develops, suddenly followed by widespread erythema. Within hours the skin becomes painful. With slight thumb pressure, the skin wrinkles, slides laterally, and separates from the dermis, a sign known as Nikolsky's sign (Habif, 2004). Large sheets of skin are sloughed. The entire epidermis is usually involved as well as mucous membranes (oral ulcers), the eyes (purulent conjunctivitis), and the respiratory tract (bronchopneumonia). A phase of fever and malaise resembling a viral illness will precede the clinical skin manifestations.

Diagnosis of TEN is by skin biopsy, and full-thickness epidermal damage is revealed. The differential diagnosis for TEN must include SSSS, which is distinguished by skin biopsy, and graft-versus-host disease (GVHD) of the skin, which is distinguished by history.

The patient with TEN should be managed as a burn patient because of temperature regulation problems, electrolyte disturbances, significant nutrition needs, and propensity to wound or skin infections. In fact, improved survival rates have been observed with the early recognition of TEN and referral to burn centers (Clennett and Hosking, 2003; Palmieri et al, 2002; Schulz et al, 2000). Box 6-9 lists a recommended treatment protocol. Temporary skin coverage is warranted; the use of systemic corticosteroids is not recommended. Intravenous administration of immunoglobulin G (IgG) appears to have beneficial results in patients with TEN (Viard et al, 1998).

Graft-versus-Host Disease (GVHD)

After allogeneic bone marrow transplantation (bone marrow from another individual), the transferred immune-competent cells have the potential to produce a severe reaction in the transplant patient. Clinically, acute GVHD occurs early after transplantation (less than 100 days). Chronic GVHD occurs after 100 days

BOX 6-9 Treatment Protocol for Toxic Epidermal Necrolysis

1. Patient is taken to the operating room on an urgent basis.
2. All loose skin and blisters are wiped vigorously with a rough washcloth moistened with normal saline solution. No detergents are used.
3. Porcine xenografts are applied to all raw surfaces and stapled in place.
4. The patient is transferred to a warmed, air-fluidized bed in the burn unit.
5. Initial fluid resuscitation is not required, but careful fluid and electrolyte monitoring is important.
6. The administration of oral corticosteroids is stopped unless medically necessary; they are tapered if possible.
7. Internal alimentation is established through a nasogastric feeding tube.
8. Systemic antibiotics are used only for specific infections.
9. Intense pulmonary toilet is established.
10. Physical therapy is begun on the day after operation.
11. Dislodged xenografts are replaced.
12. Pain is managed with a pain cocktail of methadone, hydroxyzine, and acetaminophen in cherry syrup. Intravenous narcotics are given as necessary. With the dermis covered, the wound becomes essentially pain-free.
13. Meticulous eye care is provided hourly. Each day the ophthalmologist removes conjunctival synechiae with a glass rod.
14. Central venous and bladder catheters are avoided.
15. The xenograft becomes brittle and desiccates as the wounds heal beneath it. These areas are trimmed each day.

Reprinted with permission from Habif TP: *Clinical dermatology: a color guide to diagnosis and therapy*, ed 4, St Louis, 2004, Mosby.

following transplantation. Risk factors that predispose the bone marrow transplantation patient to GVHD include recipient age (over 40 years), recipient history of blood transfusions, the conditioning regimen, the prophylaxis protocol, and the number of T cells infused (Alcoser and Burchett, 1999; Sullivan, 1999).

GVHD affects the skin, the gut, and the liver; it is a clinical diagnosis that cannot be confirmed by laboratory findings (Antin and Deeg, 2005). In the skin, cutaneous manifestations include a maculopapular rash that usually begins on the palms and then spreads to the face, the arms, the shoulders, and the ears. (Plate 17.) These may be asymptomatic, pruritic, or painful. In severe cases, generalized erythema, bullae, and desquamation may be present. GVHD may have the appearance of SSSS, a drug reaction, or toxic epidermal necrolysis. A skin biopsy is beneficial to differentiate among these three possibilities (Sullivan, 1999; Antin and Deeg, 2005).

TABLE 6-5   Characteristics of Skin Lesions with Blood Dyscrasias

BLOOD DYSCRASIA	PATHOLOGY	ULCER CHARACTERISTICS	TREATMENT
Sickle cell anemia	• Sickled blood cells are rigid • May clump together occluding the microcirculation • Damage to endothelium leads to thrombus formation (Eckman, 1996) • Altered vasomotor response, which can lead to a rise in capillary pressure and edema formation (Mohan et al, 1997)	• Exact etiology of the ulceration remains unclear • Located on lower leg near the malleolus • May be single or multiple • Can range significantly in size • Ulcers are well defined, vary in depth, and have raised borders (Eckman, 1996; Kerstein, 1996; Roenigk and Young, 1996) • Tend to be slow to heal • High rate of recurrence (Eckman, 1996)	• Control of edema (compression therapy and/or bed rest) • Systemic management of the underlying disease process (address anemia either pharmacologically or by transfusion) • Debridement • Prevention of infection • Protection from trauma • Pain management • Moist wound healing (such as with hydrocolloids [Cackovic, 1998; Chung, Cackovic, and Kerstein, 1996; Eckman, 1996])
Thalassemia	A microcytic anemia common in people of Mediterranean descent	Etiology related to a decreased hemoglobin and increased iron loading, making patients more susceptible to trauma	• Blood transfusions and iron-chelation therapy (Kerstein, 1996) • Topical care based on wound needs and moist wound-healing principles • Emphasis on insulating wound to prevent hypothermia • Protect wound from further trauma

Treatment of GVHD requires a combination of immunosuppressants and antiviral medications. To stimulate adequate neutrophil levels with these treatment regimens, growth-colony–stimulating factor is also given. Topical wound care requires attention to infection control, maintaining a physiologic wound environment, and pain management. Adhesive occlusive dressings are seldom desirable. Topical wound management should be determined collaboratively with input and discussion from the marrow transplantation team involved. For more detailed information concerning this disease, additional resources can be accessed (Ferrara, Cooke, and Deeg, 2005; Ringden, 2005; Thomas, 1999). Increasing use of autologous bone marrow stem cells for the treatment of cancer patients after lethal irradiation is greatly reducing the incidence of GVHD.

Blood Dyscrasias

Two types of blood dyscrasias may lead to chronic leg ulceration: sickle cell anemia and thalassemia. Their etiologies, ulcer characteristics, and treatments are summarized in Table 6-5.

SUMMARY

The intact skin provides the first line of defense against microbial invasion and trauma. Different factors can jeopardize the skin's integrity. It is important to be able to recognize the skin-related signs of these factors so that the factor can be eliminated or the intensity of the factor can be reduced substantially. Most of the time, the type of skin damage that the wound care specialist encounters is mechanical or vascular. Only with an in-depth skin assessment and history of the skin eruption can the etiology of the skin damage be identified and the negative sequelae arrested through appropriate prevention and treatment interventions.

Because the more rare inflammatory, infectious, or disease-related skin lesions often require prompt treatment to be effective, they should also be familiar to the wound care specialist. Although the underlying disease is the critical determinant for wound healing in these situations, the wound care specialist is an important partner and interdisciplinary team member because he or she can provide valuable recommendations for wound management that will best address the requirements of the wound and the needs of the patient.

SELF-ASSESSMENT EXERCISE

1. List seven factors known to damage the skin.
2. Which of the following is described as a lesion that is raised, solid, and less than 0.5 cm in diameter?
   a. Macule
   b. Papule
   c. Pustule
   d. Nodule
3. A blister that measures 1.5 cm in diameter may also be called which of the following?
   a. Bulla
   b. Pustule
   c. Vesicle
   d. Wheal
4. Distinguish between erosion and ulcer according to depth of tissue damage.
5. List at least four interventions to prevent skin stripping.
6. List three treatment options to prevent chemical skin irritation in a patient with diarrhea.
7. Which of the following accurately characterizes chemical skin irritation?
   a. Erythema with satellite lesions
   b. Erythema and erosion of skin
   c. Ulcerations with necrotic tissue in wound bed
   d. Ulcerations with pustules
8. Which of the following characterizes VZV?
   a. Requires prior exposure to genital herpes
   b. Is reactivated by mechanical trauma
   c. Consists of a bilateral vesicular rash
   d. Develops along one or two dermatomes
9. State the two phases of an allergic contact dermatitis.
10. Candidiasis can be described as which of the following?
   a. Macular rash with ulcerations
   b. Papular rash within the hair follicle
   c. Pustular erythematous rash
   d. Vesicular rash with plaque formation
11. Which of the following statements is true of herpes simplex virus?
   a. Initially develops as papules
   b. Secondary lesions consist of necrotic plaques
   c. Erythema signifies a secondary infection
   d. Vesicles are uniformly shaped and grouped
12. List three disease processes that can result in massive loss of epidermis.

REFERENCES

Alcoser PW, Burchett S: Bone marrow transplantation, *Am J Nurs* 99(6):26, 1999.

Antin JH, Deeg HJ: Clinical spectrum of acute graft-vs-host disease. In Ferrara JF, Cooke KR, Deeg HJ, editors: *Graft-vs-Host Disease,* ed 3, New York, 2005, Marcel Dekker.

Baranoski S: Skin tears, *Nurs Manage* 32(8):25, 2001.

Bettley FR: Some effects of soap on the skin, *Br Med J* 1:1675, 1960.

Bryant RA: Saving the skin from tape injuries, *Am J Nurs* 88(2):189, 1988.

Budisavljevic MN, Cheek D, Ploth DW: Calciphylaxis in chronic renal failure, *J Am Soc Nephrol* 7:978, 1996.

Burkhart CG, Burkhart CN, Mian A: Calciphylaxis: a case report and review of literature, *Wounds* 11(2):58, 1999.

Cackovic M et al: Leg ulceration in the sickle cell patient, *J Am Coll Surg* 187(3):30, 1998.

Caldwell-Brown D et al: Nursing aspects of EB; a comprehensive approach. In Lin AN, Carter DM, editors: *Epidermolysis bullosa: basic and clinical aspects,* New York, 1992, Springer-Verlag.

Chandrasekar PH: Identification and treatment of herpes lesions, *Adv Wound Care* 12(5):254, 1999.

Chung C, Cackovic M, Kerstein M: Leg ulcers in patients with sickle cell disease, *Adv Wound Care* 9(5):46, 1996.

Clennett S, Hosking G. Management of toxic epidermal necrolysis in a 15-year-old girl. *J Wound Care* 2003 Apr;12(4):151-154.

Coady K: The diagnosis and treatment of pyoderma gangraenosum, *J Wound Care* 9(6):282-285, 2000.

Cohen JI et al: Recent advances in varicella-zoster virus infection, *Ann Intern Med* 130:922, 1999.

Echols et al: Initial experience with a new system for the control and containment of fecal output for the protection of patients in a large burn center, *Chest* 126:862S-a, 2004.

Eckman J: Leg ulcers in sickle cell disease, *Hematol Oncol Clin North Am* 10(6):1333, 1996.

Ferrara JF, Cooke KR, Deeg HJ, editors: *Graft-vs-Host Disease,* ed 3, New York, 2005, Marcel Dekker.

Fine JD, Bauer EA, Gedde-Dahl T Jr: Inherited epidermolysis bullosa. Definition and historical overview. In: Fine JD et al, editors: *Epidermolysis bullosa. Clinical epidemiologic and laboratory advances and the findings of the National EB Registry,* Baltimore, Md., 1999, Johns Hopkins University Press.

Fontaine R, Risley S, Castellino R: A quantitative analysis of pressure and shear in the effectiveness of support surfaces, *J WOCN* 25:233, 1998.

Goldstein BG, Goldstein AD: *Practical dermatology,* ed 2, St Louis, 1997, Mosby.

Habif TP: *Clinical dermatology: a color guide to diagnosis and therapy,* ed 4, St Louis, 2004, Mosby.

Hafner J et al: Uremic small-artery disease with medial calcification and intimal hyperplasia (so-called calciphylaxis): a complication of chronic renal failure and benefit from parathyroidectomy, *J Am Acad Dermatol* 33:954, 1995.

Hoffman MD: Pyoderma gangrenosum, *Wounds* 11(Suppl B):2B, 1999.

Hooper BJ, Goldman MP: *Primary dermatologic care,* St Louis, 1999, Mosby.

Hunter JAA, Savin JA, Dahl MV: *Clinical Dermatology,* Oxford, 2002. Blackwell Science.

Ikeda E et al: Rheumatoid vasculitis in a patient with seronegative rheumatoid arthritis, *Eur J Dermatol* 8(4):268, 1998.

Jennette J, Falk R: Small-vessel vasculitis, *N Engl J Med* 337(21):1512, 1997.

Jallali N: Necrotising fasciitis: its etiology, diagnosis, and management, *J Wound Care* 12(8):297-300, 2003.

Kelly J: Pyoderma gangraenosum: exploring the treatment options, *J Wound Care* 10(4):125-128, 2001.

Kerstein M: The non-healing leg ulcer: peripheral vascular disease, chronic venous insufficiency, and ischemic vasculitis, *Ostomy Wound Manage* 42(Suppl 10A):19S, 1996.

Khafif RA et al: Calciphylaxis and systemic calcinosis: collective review, *Arch Intern Med* 150:956, 1990.

Kim J et al: Clinical application of continent anal plug in bedridden patients with intractable diarrhea, *Dis Colon Rectum* 44:1162-1167, 2001.

Leyden JJ, Gately LE III: Staphylococcal and streptococcal infections. In Sanders CV, Nesbitt LT: *The skin and infection,* Baltimore, Md., 1995, Williams and Wilkins.

Lin AN, Carter DM: Epidermolysis bullosa simples: a clinical overview. In Lin AN, Carter DM, editors: *Epidermolysis bullosa: basic and clinical aspects,* New York, 1992, Springer-Verlag.

Loeper JM et al: *Therapeutic positioning and skin care,* Minneapolis, 1986, Sister Kenny Institute.

Lorentzen H, Gottrup F: Misclassification errors of ulcerative pyoderma gangrenosum, *Wound Rep Reg* 6:A475, 1998.

Malone ML et al: The epidemiology of skin tears in the institutionalized elderly, *J Am Geriatr Soc* 39(6):591, 1991.

Margolis DJ: Dermatology of the lower extremity, *Ostomy Wound Manage* 39(5):36, 1993.

Marinkovich MP, Pham N: Epidermolysis bullosa available at http://www.emedicine.com/derm/topic/24.htm, Accessed March 30, 2005.

Mason SR: Type of soap and the incidence of skin tears among residents of a long-term care facility, *Ostomy Wound Manage* 43(8):26, 1997.

McGough-Csarny J, Kopac CA: Skin tears in institutionalized elderly: an epidemiological study, *Ostomy Wound Manage* 44(Suppl 3A):14S, 1998.

McRorie E, Ruckley C, Nuki G: The relevance of large-vessel vascular disease and restricted ankle movement to the aetiology of leg ulceration in rheumatoid arthritis, *Br J Rheumatol* 37(12):1295, 1998.

Mohan J et al: Postural vasoconstriction and leg ulceration in homozygous sickle cell disease, *Clin Science* 92:153, 1997.

Palmieri TL et al: A multicenter review of toxic epidermal necrolysis treated in the US burn centers at the end of the twentieth century, *J Burn Care Rehab* 23:87, 2002.

Payne RL, Martin ML: The epidemiology and management of skin tears in older adults, *Ostomy Wound Manage* 26:26, 1990.

Payne RL, Martin ML: Defining and classifying skin tears: need for a common language, *Ostomy Wound Manage* 39(5):16, 1993.

Powell FC, Su WPD, Perry HO: Pyoderma gangrenosum: classification and management, *J Am Acad Dermatol* 34:395, 1996.

Rietschel RL, Fowler JF Jr: *Fisher's contact dermatitis,* ed 5, Philadelphia, 2001, Lippincott, Williams & Wilkins.

Ringden O: Introduction to graft-versus-host disease, *Biol Blood Marrow Transplant* 11(2)(Suppl 2):17, 2005.

Roenigk H, Young J: Leg ulcers. In Young J, Olin J, Bartholomew J, editors: *Peripheral vascular diseases,* ed 2, St Louis, 1996, Mosby.

Rubano J, Kerstein M: Arterial insufficiency and vasculitides, *J WOCN* 25(3):147, 1998.

Ruggian JC, Maesaka JK, Fishbane S: Proximal calciphylaxis in four insulin-requiring diabetic hemodialysis patients, *Am J Kidney Dis* 28:409, 1996.

Schober-Flores C: Epidermolysis bullosa: the challenges of wound care, *Dermatol Nurse* 15(2):141, 2003.

Schulz JT et al: A 10-year experience with toxic epidermal necrolysis, *J Burn Care Rehab* 21:199, 2000.

Smith DB, Ickstadt J, Kucera J: Brown recluse spider bite, *J WOCN* 24(3):137, 1997.

Snyder RJ, Beylin M, Weiss SD: Calciphylaxis and its relation to end-stage renal disease: a literature review and case presentation, *Ostomy/Wound Management* 46(10):40, 2000.

Sullivan KM: Graft-versus-host disease. In Thomas ED, Blume KG, Forman SJ, editors: *Hematopoietic cell transplantation,* ed 2, Malden, Mass, 1999, Blackwell Science.

Thomas ED, Blume KG, Forman SJ, editors: *Hematopoietic cell transplantation*, ed 2, Malden, Mass, 1999, Blackwell Science.

Viard I et al: Inhibition of toxic epidermal necrolysis by blockade of CD95 with human intravenous immunoglobulin, *Science* 282:490, 1998.

White MW, Karam S, Cowell B: Skin tears in frail elders: a practical approach to prevention, *Geriatr Nurs* 15(2):95, 1994.

Whitley RJ, Kimberlin DW, Roizman B: Herpes simplex virus, *Clin Infect Dis* 26:541, 1998.

Yamamoto T, Ohkubo H, Nishioka K: Skin manifestations associated with rheumatoid arthritis, *J Dermatol* 22(5):324, 1995.

Zeglin D: Brown recluse spider bites, *AJN* 105(2):64-68, 2005.

CHAPTER

7 Patient Assessment and Evaluation of Healing

DENISE P. NIX

OBJECTIVES

1. Distinguish between assessment and evaluation of healing.
2. Describe the stages of pressure ulcers.
3. Distinguish between partial-thickness and full-thickness tissue loss.
4. List 10 indices of wound healing that should be assessed and recorded.
5. Identify clinical signs and symptoms of chronic wound infection.
6. Describe how to measure the length, width, depth, tunneling, and undermining of a wound.

Assessment provides the foundation for the plan of care and is critical for monitoring the effectiveness of the plan. Assessment is important for determining progress or deterioration. Documentation of assessment findings facilitates communication among caregivers. Because of the variety of etiologic, systemic, and local factors that are commonly involved in the pathogenesis of a wound, a comprehensive holistic assessment is essential to identify the factors that will have an impact on wound repair as well as the ability to maintain the integrity of the skin. Therefore, all patients with or without a wound require a comprehensive skin assessment. The patient with a wound requires additional assessment, which includes patient history and an analysis of probable underlying causes and cofactors.

The editors gratefully acknowledge Dr. Diane Cooper for her work on developing content for this chapter in the first and second editions of *Acute and Chronic Wounds Nursing Management*. Many of the comments and concepts she put forth in the previous editions are reflected in this chapter, and we are appreciative of her significant contribution.

SIGNIFICANCE

"What cannot be measured cannot be managed" (Woods et al, 1996). As with monitoring blood pressure, temperature, and pulse rate, those attending to wounds should never observe, care for, or make notations in a chart about a wound without objective criteria by which to reflect its present status.

The clinical value of measuring wounds for predicting healing has been established through a number of studies. However, researchers continue to debate which wound healing parameters accurately predict healing. Healing parameters include mean adjusted healing rate, 4-week healing rates, percentage change in area from baseline, and initial wound size. Tallman et al (1997), studied the mean adjusted healing rate of venous ulcers (i.e., measuring mean healing between all visits) and reported that a mean adjusted healing rate predicted complete healing as early as 3 weeks after initiating therapy ($p < 0.001$). Using percentage change in area from baseline to 4 weeks as the healing parameter, Kantor and Margolis (1998) reported that in venous ulcers the percentage change in area from baseline to 4 weeks predicted healing or nonhealing at 24 weeks ($p < 0.05$). Recently, initial wound size has been suggested to predict healing time. In a prospective study of 31 patients with neuropathic and neuro-ischemic ulcers, Zimny and colleagues (2002) demonstrated a linear relationship between wound radius and healing time, thus suggesting initial wound size may be used to predict healing time. In a prospective multicenter study with 203 patients with diabetic foot ulcers, 4-week healing rates were studied and found to be significantly correlated with healing at 12 weeks ($p < 0.01$) (Sheehan et al 2003).

The economics of health care impose additional motivation for conducting and documenting systematic

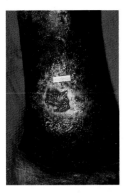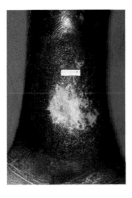

Plate 1 Partial-thickness venous ulcer healing by epithelialization. Resurfaced venous ulcer lacks normal dark pigmentation because of depth of damage (below basement membrane).

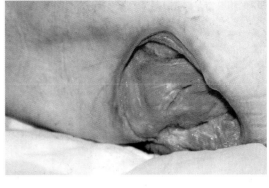

Plate 2 Stage IV pressure ulcer with exposed muscle.

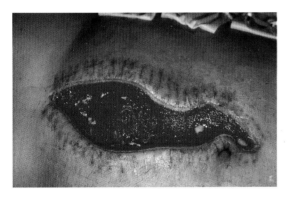

Plate 3 Full-thickness abdominal wound healing by secondary intention with healthy (red, cobblestone) granulation tissue and attached wound edges.

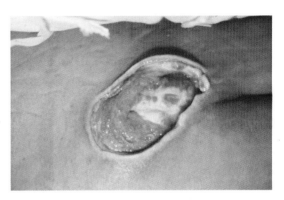

Plate 4 Stage IV sacral pressure ulcer wound edges are rolled (epibole) which is an impediment to wound healing.

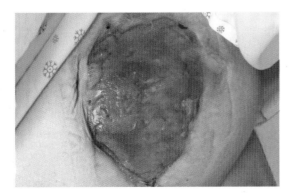

Plate 5a Wound clean, not granulating (note lack of red cobblestone appearance), suggesting heavy bacterial loads or other impediment to wound healing.

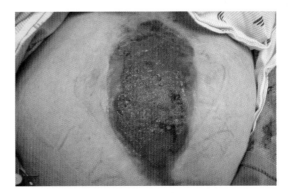

Plate 5b Same wound granulating after 1 week of topical antimicrobial use (note healthy red cobblestone appearance).

Plate 6 Primary Skin Lesions

Description	Examples		
A. Macule A flat, circumscribed area that is a change in the color of the skin; less than 1 cm in diameter	Freckles, flat moles (nevi), petechiae, measles, scarlet fever	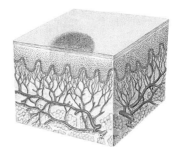	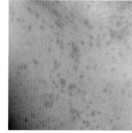 Measles. (From Habif, 1996.)
B. Papule An elevated, firm, circumscribed area; less than 1 cm in diameter	Wart (verruca), elevated moles, lichen planus	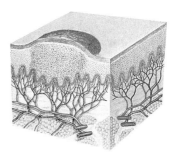	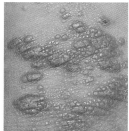 Lichen planus. (From Weston, Lane, Morelli, 1996.)
C. Patch A flat, nonpalpable, irregular-shaped macule greater than 1 cm in diameter	Vitiligo, port-wine stains, Mongolian spots, café au lait patch	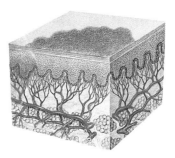	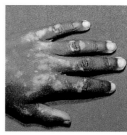 Vitiligo. (From Weston, Lane, Morelli, 1991.)
D. Plaque Elevated, firm, and rough lesion with flat top surface greater than 1 cm in diameter	Psoriasis, seborrheic and actinic keratoses	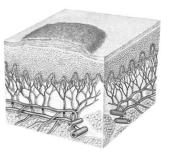	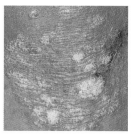 Plaque. (From Habif, 1996.)

Plate 6 Primary Skin Lesions—cont'd

Description	Examples

E. Wheal

Elevated, irregular-shaped area of cutaneous edema; solid, transient, variable diameter

Insect bites, urticaria, allergic reaction

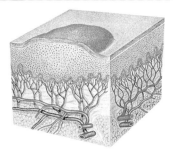

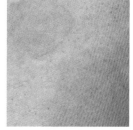

Wheal. (From Farrar et al, 1992.)

F. Nodule

Elevated, firm, circumscribed lesion; deeper in dermis than a papule; 1 to 2 cm in diameter

Erythema nodosum, lipomas

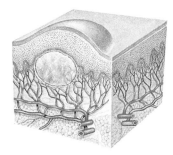

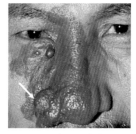

Hypertrophic nodule. (From Goldman, Fitzpatrick, 1994.)

G. Tumor

Elevated and solid lesion; may or may not be clearly demarcated; deeper in dermis; greater than 2 cm in diameter

Neoplasms, benign tumor, lipoma, hemangioma

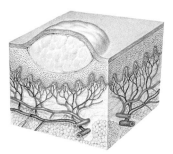

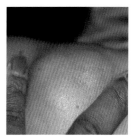

Lipoma. (From Lemmi, Lemmi, 2000.)

H. Vesicle

Elevated, circumscribed, superficial, not into dermis; filled with serous fluid; less than 1 cm in diameter

Varicella (chicken-pox), herpes zoster (shingles)

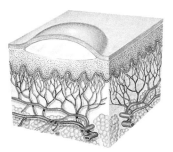

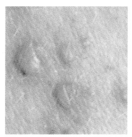

Vesicles caused by varicella. (From Farrar et al, 1992.)

Continued

Plate 6 Primary Skin Lesions—cont'd

Description	Examples

I. Bulla

Vesicle greater than 1 cm in diameter

Blister, pemphigus vulgaris

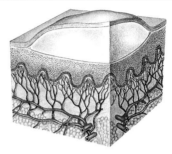

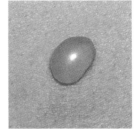

Blister. (From White, 1994.)

J. Pustule

Elevated, superficial lesion; similar to a vesicle but filled with purulent fluid

Impetigo, acne

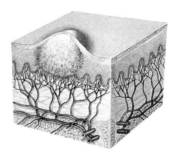

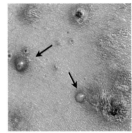

Acne. (From Weston, Lane, Morelli, 1996.)

K. Cyst

Elevated, circumscribed, encapsulated lesion; in dermis or subcutaneous layer; filled with liquid or semi-solid material

Sebaceous cyst, cystic acne

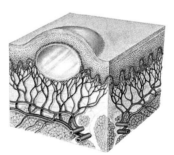

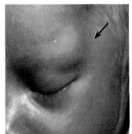

Sebaceous cyst. (From Weston, Lane, Morelli, 1996.)

L. Telangiectasia

Fine, irregular, red lines produced by capillary dilation

Telangiectasia in rosacea

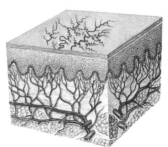

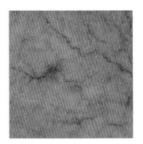

Telangiectasia. (From Lemmi, Lemmi, 2000.)

Plate 7 Secondary Skin Lesions

Description	Examples

A. Scale

Heaped-up, keratinized cells; flaky skin; irregular; thick or thin; dry or oily; variation in size

Flaking of skin with seborrheic dermatitis following scarlet fever, or flaking of skin following a drug reaction; dry skin

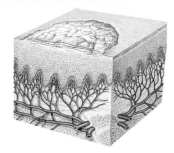

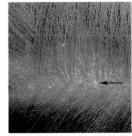

Fine Scaling. (From Baran, Dawher, Levene, 1991.)

B. Lichenification

Rough, thickened epidermis secondary to persistent rubbing, itching, or skin irritation; often involves flexor surface of extremity

Chronic dermatitis

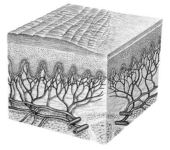

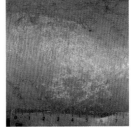

Lichenification. (From Lemmi, Lemmi, 2000.)

C. Keloid

Irregular-shaped, elevated, progressively enlarging scar; grows beyond the boundaries of the wound; caused by excessive collagen formation during healing

Keloid formation following surgery

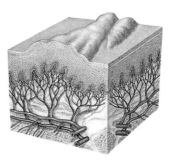

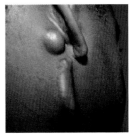

Keloid. (From Weston, Lane, Morelli, 1996.)

D. Scar

Thin to thick fibrous tissue that replaces normal skin following injury or laceration to the dermis

Healed wound or surgical incision

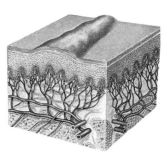

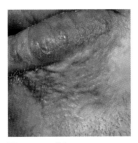

Hypertrophic scar. (From Goldman, Fitzpatrick, 1994.)

Continued

Plate 7 Secondary Skin Lesions

Description	Examples

E. Excoriation

Loss of the epidermis; linear hollowed-out, crusted area

Abrasion or scratch

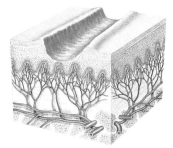

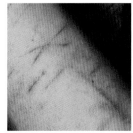

Excoriation from a tree branch. (From Lemmi, Lemmi, 2000.)

F. Fissure

Linear crack or break from the epidermis to the dermis; may be moist or dry

Athlete's foot, cracks at the corner of the mouth

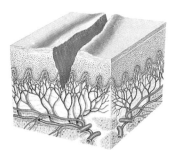

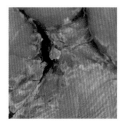

Scaling and fissures of tinea pedis. (From Lemmi, Lemmi, 2000.)

G. Erosion

Loss of part of the epidermis; depressed, moist, glistening; follows rupture of a vesicle or bulla

Varicella, variola after rupture

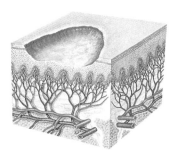

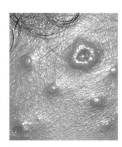

Erosion. (From Cohen, 1993.)

Plate 7 Secondary Skin Lesions—cont'd

Description	Examples

H. Ulcer

Loss of epidermis and dermis; concave; varies in size

Pressure ulcer

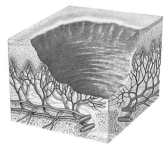

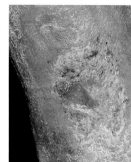

Venous insufficiency ulcer.
(From Habif, 1996.)

I. Crust

Dried serum, blood, or purulent exudates; slightly elevated; size varies; brown, red, black, tan, or straw-colored

Scab on abrasion, eczema

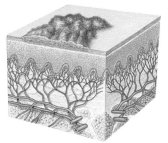

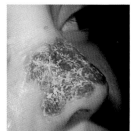

Scab.

J. Atrophy

Thinning of skin surface and loss of skin markings; skin translucent and paperlike

Striae; aged skin

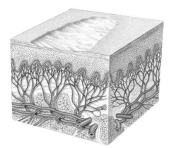

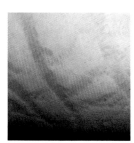

Striae.

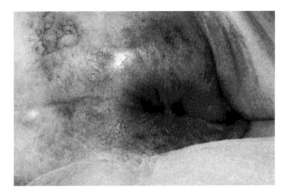

Plate 8 Irritant contact (chemical) dermatitis from fecal incontinence.

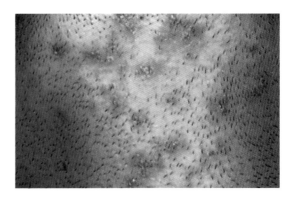

Plate 9 Folliculitis, infection of hair follicles resulting from inappropriate hair removal technique.

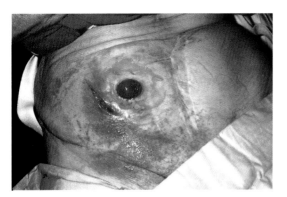

Plate 10 Patient with an ileostomy and incision placed to drain peristomal abscess. Chemical dermatitis present along inferior aspect of incision because of inadequate protection of skin from drainage. Candidiasis also present as indicated by satellite papular lesions and solid plaque-like rash advancing into groin and over suprapubic area.

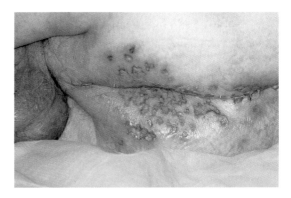

Plate 11 Herpes simplex on buttocks. Note cluster of vesicles on erythematous base.

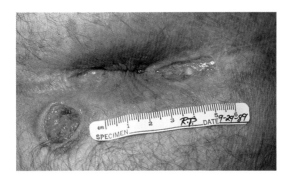

Plate 12 Perianal herpes simplex ulcers.

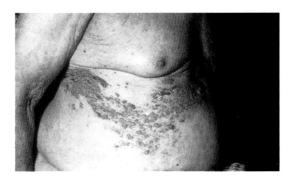

Plate 13 Herpes zoster involving simple thoracic dermatome. Vesicles are clustered and erythematous.

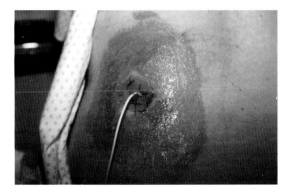

Plate 14 Moist desquamation after an allergic reaction in response to the second application of benzoin to a percutaneous nephrostomy site.

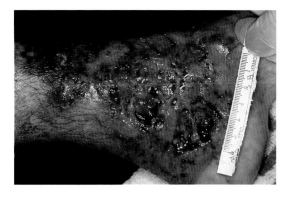

Plate 15 Classical ulceration form of pyoderma gangrenosum. Note violaceous (purple) color of skin surrounding ulcerations.

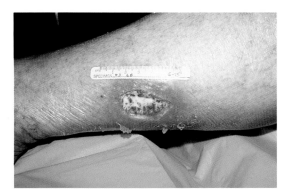

Plate 16 Vasculitic ulcer that developed in patient with rheumatoid arthritis. Wound bed has attached dry slough present, and surrounding skin is slightly erythematous.

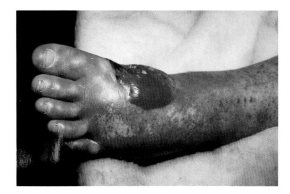

Plate 17 Graft-versus-host (GVHD) in patient after allogenic bone marrow transplantation. Edema, erythema, and bulla formation are present.

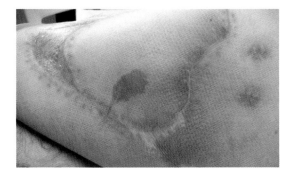

Plate 18 Right trochanter stage I pressure ulcer at surgical flap site.

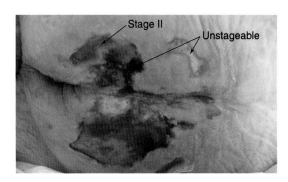

Plate 19 Sacral pressure ulcer, multiple stages of depth (note classic butterfly shape with additional chemical skin damage from incontinence).

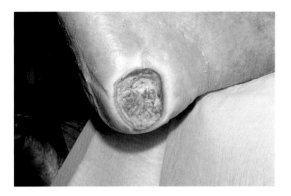

Plate 20 Right heel pressure ulcer with periwound maceration. Note this was previously a stage III ulcer that has recently developed a layer of slough in the wound bed.

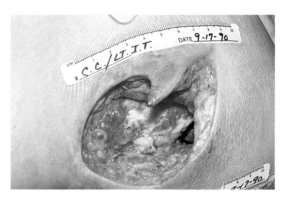

Plate 21 Left ischial tuberosity stage IV pressure ulcer.

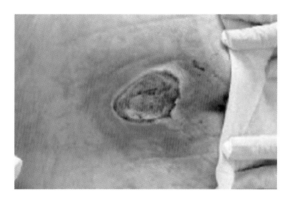

Plate 22 Sacral pressure ulcer with yellow nonadherent nonviable wound base. Periwound skin shows signs of deep tissue injury (DTI).

Wound Assessment: Anatomy of a Wound

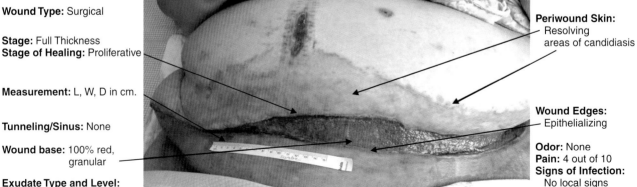

Wound Type: Surgical

Stage: Full Thickness
Stage of Healing: Proliferative

Measurement: L, W, D in cm.

Tunneling/Sinus: None

Wound base: 100% red, granular

Exudate Type and Level: Moderate, serosanguinous

Periwound Skin: Resolving areas of candidiasis

Wound Edges: Epithelializing

Odor: None
Pain: 4 out of 10
Signs of Infection: No local signs present

Plate 23 Anatomy of a wound.

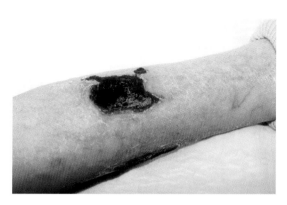

Plate 24 Arterial ulcer with dry, stable eschar covering. Note dry condition of leg.

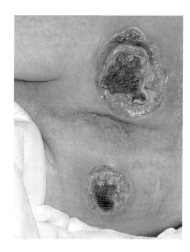

Plate 25 Bilateral ischial tuberosity pressure ulcers with eschar detaching from wound edges and softening in response to topical hydrogels. Cross hatching of eschar was initially performed and is visible in necrotic tissue.

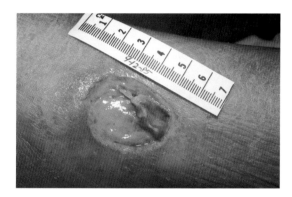

Plate 26 Arterial ulcer with loose and adherent yellow slough present in wound bed. Mild erythema present along left lateral edge.

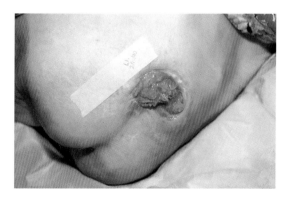

Plate 27 Healing stage III pressure ulcer with hypergranulation tissue present in wound bed.

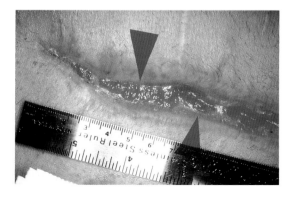

Plate 28 Surgical incision with epithelialization .

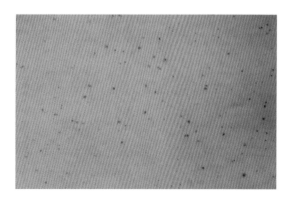

Plate 29 Petechiae on abdomen. Petechiae-red-purple nonblanchable discoloration less than 0.5 cm diameter. Cause: Intravascular defects, infection.

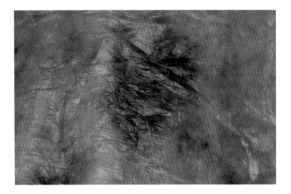

Plate 30 Senile purpura. Purpura—red. Purple nonblanchable discoloration greater than 0.5 cm diameter. [Cause: Intravascular defects, infection.]

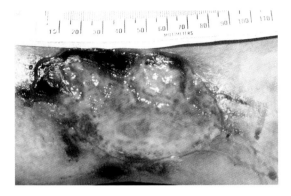

Plate 31a Highly exudative venous ulcer with slough present in wound bed and eschar present along superior aspect.

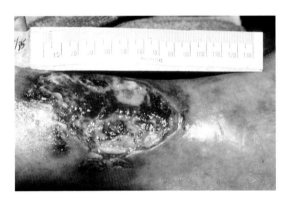

Plate 31b After 1 week of hydrocolloids and compression therapy, autolysis has occurred and venous ulcer has granulation tissue present. Amount of slough and eschar is reduced; remaining eschar is softened.

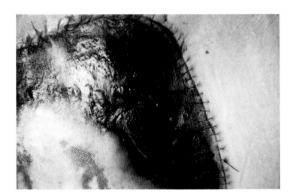

Plate 32 Approximated incision with intact sutures. This photograh illustrates the importance of documenting not only the condition of the incision but also the condition of the periwound skin.

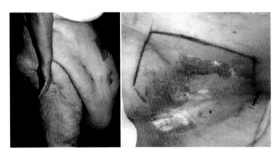

Plate 33 Abdomen of obese patient with skin breakdown under pannus due to pressure and moisture.

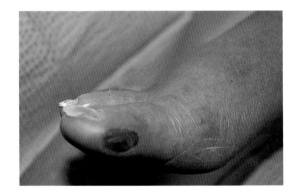

Plate 34 Arterial ulcer with necrotic base and halo of periwound erythema.

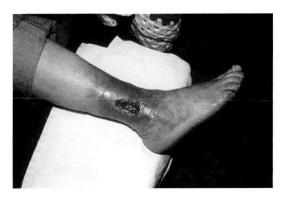

Plate 35 Typical appearance and location of venous ulcer. Surrounding skin has been moisturized to eliminate usual dry skin. Note hemosiderin staining of surrounding skin and ruddy red color of wound bed.

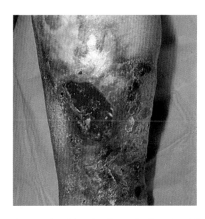

Plate 36 Atrophie blanche dermal sclerosis with dilated abnormal vasculature and ivory white plaques on the ankle or foot and hemosiderin borders.

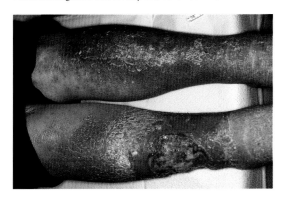

Plate 37 Venous dermatitis of lower leg. Note extensive hemosiderin staining and lipodermatosclerosis.

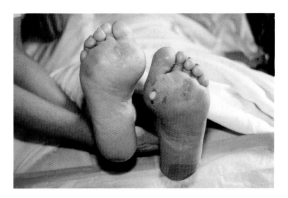

Plate 38 Neuropathic plantar ulcer on first metatarsal head after conservative debridement (packing is present in the ulcer). Note foot and toe deformities and callus formation in this patient with diabetes mellitus. Stage II pressure ulcers (blisters) are also present on both heels.

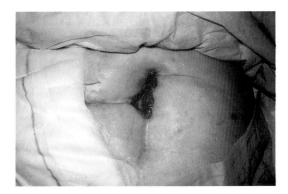

Plate 39 Patient with enterocutaneous fistula with irregular surrounding skin surfaces and depression along fistula-skin junction at inferior aspect and upper left aspect.

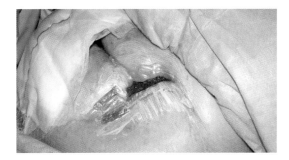

Plate 40 Tapered layers of solid-wafer skin barrier used to help level skin depression at inferior aspect. Skin-barrier paste has been applied to surrounding wound margins and in all three depressions (over skin-barrier wafer wedges) to level and protect the skin from effluent. Cement has been painted onto adhesive field (over paste and wedges) to increase adhesion.

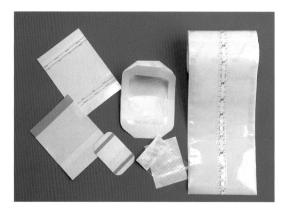

Plate 41 Variety of transparent film dressings.

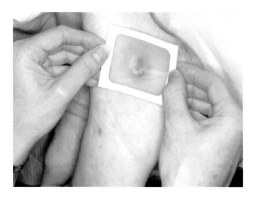

Plate 42 Application of a transparent dressing by a family member in the home setting.

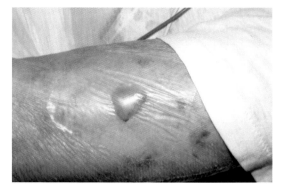

Plate 43 Transparent dressing prior to removal. Note collection of fluid under the dressing which is to be expected as autolysis occurs.

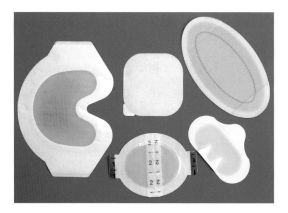

Plate 44 Variety of sizes and shapes of hydrocolloid dressings.

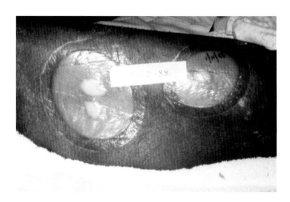

Plate 45 Hydrocolloid dressing prior to removal. Note the gel developing under the dressing which is expected as the wound exudate is absorbed by the hydrocolloid.

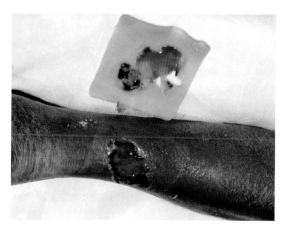

Plate 46 Hydrocolloid dressing after removal from a venous ulcer. Purulent appearing exudate is present on the dressing and the wound. This is expected with autolysis under a hydrocolloid dressing and should not be misinterpreted as evidence of an infection. Upon cleansing the wound bed is clean and granular.

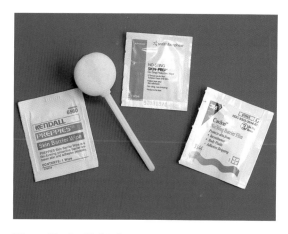

Plate 47 Liquid skin barrier (skin sealants).

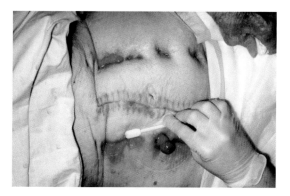

Plate 48 Application of liquid skin barrier to periwound skin of a granular full thickness abdominal wound resulting from retention sutures. The skin barrier is applied prior to dressing application to protect the periwound skin from adhesive and wound exudate.

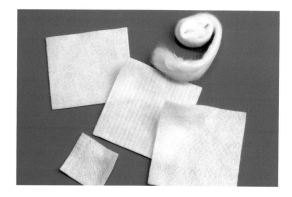

Plate 49 Variety of alginate dressings.

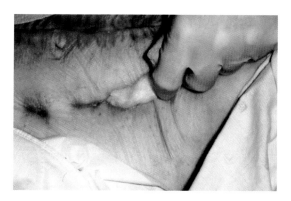

Plate 50 Alginate dressing applied to fill dead space and absorb exudate in a full thickness abdominal wound.

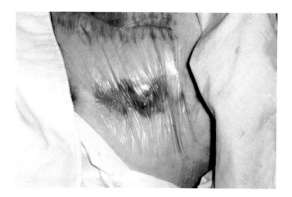

Plate 51 Alginate dressing (from Plate 50) has been secured with a secondary transparent dressing. Note two days later at the scheduled dressing change, the alginate formed an expected gel-like appearance as the wound fluid was absorbed. The periwound skin has been protected with liquid skin barrier.

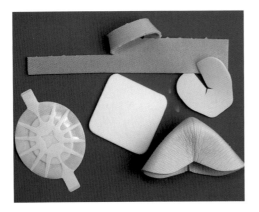

Plate 52 Variety of foam dressings.

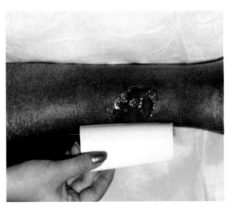

Plate 53 Application of foam dressing to venous ulcer by family member.

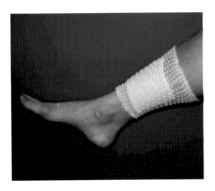

Plate 54 Foam dressing secured with stretch-net nonadherent secondary dressing.

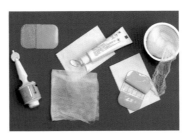

Plate 55 Variety of hydrogel dressings.

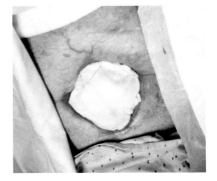

Plate 56 Hydrogel impregnated gauze is used to maintain a moist wound bed and fill dead space in this deep abdominal wound with undermining present.

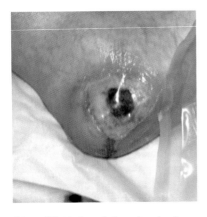

Plate 57 Hydrogel sheet dressing in place over a granular foot ulcer. This dressing overlaps onto intact periwound skin which is contraindicated with this particular brand of hydrogel dressing because of the risk of maceration of the periwound skin.

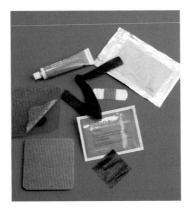

Plate 58 Antimicrobials are formulated into many different types of dressings.

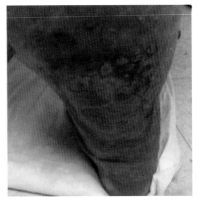

Plate 59 Silver staining. Epithelialized venous insufficiency ulcer on the posterior aspect of the lower leg. Note periwound staining secondary to the use of silver dressings.

See front matter for Plate Credits.

measurement of wound healing. Without objective criteria of the status or progress of repair, it is difficult for some treatments to be justified and for reimbursement to be appropriately assigned. Accurate and routine assessments are expected as the standard of care. Failure to assess the patient systematically also carries a great legal liability risk (Murphy, 1996). Without accurate, consistent, and retrievable documentation, it is very difficult to retrospectively create a clear picture of the patient's condition and of the care that was actually provided.

MONITORING, OBSERVATION, AND INSPECTION

Monitoring simply means keeping track or "watching." For instance, daily monitoring of a patient's skin may reveal a reddened area. This observation should then prompt an assessment by the appropriate staff so that additional information can be collected, interpreted and used for care plan development. When a patient has a wound, monitoring can occur independent of a dressing change. Specifically, a dressing intended to stay in place for several days need not be removed for monitoring purposes unless leakage, swelling, pain, or erythema around the dressing develops. If a dressing change is not indicated, the dressing and surrounding skin should be monitored and observations documented (van Rijswijk and Lyder, 2005); for example, "dressing dry and intact, surrounding skin within normal limits."

ASSESSMENT

Assessment includes the gathering of information and interpretation of that information. Assessment can be holistic, or limited to the skin or a wound.

Skin Assessment

All patients require a routine and systematic skin assessment, which includes daily evaluation of the integrity, temperature, texture and presence of lesions on the skin. Xerosis (pruritic, erythemic, dry, scaly, cracked, or fissured skin) is a problem for 59% to 85% of people older than 64 years yet is often ignored as a threat to the integrity of the skin. Xerosis is a result of the loss of natural moisturizing factors, barrier abilities, and epidermal water loss (Norman, 2003). It is uncomfortable and linked to pruritus, infection, skin tears and

pressure ulcers (AHCPR, 1994; Cole and Nesbitt, 2004; Guralnik et al 1988; Hunter et al, 2003; Klingman, 2000; White, Karam, and Cowell, 2000). The prevalence of xerosis and other potential and actual skin conditions that threaten the integrity of the skin underscores the importance of conducting and documenting daily, accurate skin assessment. Components of a skin assessment and examples of abnormalities (Bates, 1995) can be found in Table 7-1. Examples and descriptions of lesions are found in Chapter 6 (Table 6-1 and Plates 6 and 7). An example of a skin assessment documentation form can be found in Appendix C.

Holistic Assessment

Healing is a phenomenon made up of multiple processes (as described in Chapter 4), each of which must function properly for healing to result. Holistic assessment of a patient with a wound includes systemic, psychosocial, and local factors that affect wound healing. A certified wound specialist is specifically educated to conduct this type of holistic assessment in the patient with a wound. Holistic assessments are performed at least on admission and with any change of condition. Components of a holistic assessment are listed in Box 7-1. Diagnostic techniques used to assess some of the systemic factors that affect wound healing are presented in Table 7-2 and described in detail throughout Chapters 15 and 16.

Etiology/Type of Skin Damage. The initial holistic assessment must include the etiology of the wound. Etiology will drive intervention choices and strategies. For example, compression is a critical intervention for the successful management of the patient with a wound from venous hypertension, but compression is contraindicated for many patients with arterial disease (Chapter 15). Offloading is needed to heal a pressure ulcer (Chapter 13), whereas glucose must be managed to heal diabetic wounds (Chapter 16). Wound etiology will also give clues to the wound repair processes (Chapter 4). For example, venous wounds heal mostly by epithelialization and little depth is seen, whereas extensive pressure ulcer healing involves contraction, making wound depth an important aspect of assessment. Various types of skin damage are presented in Chapter 6 and throughout this text. Ability to understand and identify wound etiology is an important aspect of a holistic assessment and care plan development.

TABLE 7-1 Components/Techniques of a Skin Assessment and Examples of Abnormalities

COMPONENT	TECHNIQUE AND TIPS	EXAMPLE OF POSSIBLE ABNORMALITIES
Color	Visual inspection in good light Artificial light often distorts colors and masks jaundice Ask patients/family if they have noticed any skin color changes	Pallor with anemia, decreased blood flow, or arterial insufficiency Central cyanosis identified in lips, oral mucosa, or tongue may be seen in advanced lung disease, congestive heart failure, and when hemoglobin is abnormal or there is venous obstruction Yellow jaundice in sclera and skin with liver disease or excessive hemolysis of red blood cells Yellow on palms, soles, and face with high levels of carotene (carotenemia) Brown discoloration in lower extremities indicative of hemosiderin staining from venous insufficiency Redness may indicate erythema, an inflammatory response, or pressure ulcer
Moisture	Visual inspection in good light	Dry skin or xerosis with hypothyroidism
Temperature	Palpate using the back of fingers Normal skin is warm to the touch	Generalized increased warmth with fever or hyperthyroidism Local increased warmth with inflammation Coolness with hypothyroidism or poor vascularization
Olfaction	Note odor	Odor may indicate bacteria, metabolic acidosis, hygiene issues
Texture	Palpate using the back of fingers	Roughness in hypothyroidism
Mobility	Lift a fold of skin and note the ease with which it lifts up	Decreased mobility in edema
Turgor	Lift a fold of skin and note the speed with which it returns. Normally, skin returns quickly to baseline state	Decreased turgor in dehydration
Lesions	Observe any lesions of the skin, noting characteristics such as type, location, color, distribution, arrangement	See Plates 6 and 7
Skin injury	Skin should be intact If skin is open, assess for type of injury	See Chapter 6
Nails	Inspect and palpate fingernails and toenails	Clubbing of the fingers may be caused by lung problems
	Note color, shape, and presence of lesions	Onycholysis is the painless separation of the nails from the nail bed. It begins distally and can be caused by many things
Hair	Inspect and palpate Note quantity, distribution, and texture	*Alopecia* refers to hair loss; diffuse, patchy or total *Hirsutism* means excessive body hair

BOX 7-1   Assessment Parameters

Holistic Assessment

1. Etiology/type of skin damage
2. Duration of wound
3. Wound assessment (see below)
4. Factors that impede healing
   - Comorbid conditions (e.g., malignancy, diabetes, cardiac, respiratory, and renal issues)
   - Medications (corticosteroids, cancer medications, immunosuppressants)
   - Impaired access to appropriate resources
   - Host infection
   - Pressure ulcer risk factors
   - Decreased oxygenation and tissue perfusion
   - Alteration in nutrition and hydration
   - Psychosocial barriers (family support, financial resources, etc.)

Wound Assessment

1. Anatomic location of wound
2. Extent of tissue loss (i.e., stage)
3. Characteristics of wound base
4. Type of tissue
5. Percentage of wound containing each type of tissue observed
6. Dimensions of wound in cm (length, width, depth, tunneling, undermining)
7. Exudate (amount, type)
8. Odor
9. Wound edges
10. Periwound skin
11. Presence or absence of local signs of infection
12. Wound pain

TABLE 7-2   Physiologic Parameters that Determine Potential for Wound Healing

PARAMETER	MEASUREMENT APPROACH
Oxygen status	Transcutaneous oxygen
Bacterial status	Tissue biopsy
Vessel compliance	Ankle-brachial index
Neuropathy	Monofilament testing

Factors That Impede Healing. Identification of factors that impede healing is a critical component of a holistic assessment of a patient with a wound. Factors that impede healing are described in Chapter 4 and listed in Box 7-1.

Duration of Wound. The "age" of the wound deserves careful consideration; the 5-day-old surgical wound that shows no signs of a healing ridge may indicate pending dehiscence (Hunt and Van Winkle, 1997). A 4-week-old pressure ulcer that has not improved despite optimal care is suggestive of the presence of cofactors that have not been adequately addressed, such as unresolved pressure, malnutrition, or infection. Guidelines for pressure ulcers and arterial wounds recommend referral and biopsy consideration for wounds that are unresponsive to 2 to 4 weeks of appropriate therapies (WOCN Society 2002 and 2003). Given a clear understanding of healing, these wounds are out of synchronization and must be evaluated in light of what mechanisms might have altered the normal course of the healing trajectory.

Focused Wound Assessment

A focused wound assessment is more limited than a holistic assessment. Wound assessment refers to a collection of data that characterizes the status of the wound and the periwound skin (see Plate 23). Conducting a focused wound assessment is a skill and requires training, ideally by a certified wound specialist. Frequency of wound assessment is widely variable and will be discussed later in this chapter.

Anatomic Location. Assessment and documentation of the proper anatomic location of the wound is important to provide an accurate description of the wound to colleagues as well as clues about the etiology. Anatomic locations such as the sacrum and the coccyx must be clearly delineated. The location of a wound on the plantar surface of the foot can be further specified by terms such as metatarsal head. Anatomic location will also convey plan of care needs. For example, a wound on the ischial tuberosity should prompt caregivers to explore the patient's sitting surface. A typical venous ulcer commonly appears on the medial aspect of the lower leg and will require compression. A patient with diabetes and a plantar surface foot ulcer typically has neuropathy and will need adequate blood glucose control and off loading.

Extent of Tissue Involvement. Assessment of the wound to determine the extent of tissue involvement is an essential aspect of wound evaluation. The extent of tissue damage guides the selection of interventions appropriate to restore tissue integrity, and also provides some information about the length of time that the healing process may require. Prior to assessment, the wound must be cleansed of loose debris, particulate matter, or dressing residue. Extent of tissue involvement can be described as partial-thickness or full-thickness, or in terms of staging of tissue layers or classification systems.

Partial-thickness and full-thickness. A partial-thickness wound is confined to the skin layers; damage does not penetrate below the dermis and may be limited to the epidermal layers only. These wounds heal primarily by reepithelialization (Plate 1). A full-thickness wound indicates that the epidermis and dermis have been damaged into the subcutaneous tissue or beyond; tissue loss extends below the dermis (Plates 2-5). Wound repair will occur by neovascularization, fibroplasia, contraction, and then epithelial migration from the wound edges. Partial-thickness and full-thickness can be used to describe most wounds but are not precise terms for specific types of tissue loss and the depth of the wound. A full-thickness wound, for example, can expose subcutaneous tissue, or it may extend to bone.

Classification systems for non–pressure-related wounds. Classification systems for diabetic and vascular wounds describe "grades" of wounds according to levels of tissue involvement and additional factors such as history of previous ulceration, presence of bony deformity, presence and severity of ischemia, and presence and severity of infection (Armstrong, Lavery, and Harkless, 1996; Crawford and Fields-Varnado, 2004; Lavery, Armstrong, and Harkless, 1997). Several of these tools are presented in chapters 15 and 16. As described in Chapter 6, the Payne-Martin classification system for skin tears (Box 6-2) classifies skin tears according to amount of tissue loss. Methods to determine the extent of a burn injury are presented in Chapter 18. As with all classification systems, however, these systems only tell a small part of the story. Classification systems should be used as part of a comprehensive systematic assessment.

Pressure ulcer staging. Staging of tissue layers provides increased uniformity of language and a beginning basis for evaluation of protocols. Shea (1975) first described a method for classifying wounds according to tissue layers, which has subsequently undergone revision (Knighton et al, 1986; Lavery, Armstrong, and Harkless, 1997; NPUAP, 1998; NPUAP, 1999; Percoraro and Reiber, 1990; WOCN Society, 2003). Accurate staging requires knowledge of the anatomy of skin and deeper tissue layers, the ability to recognize these tissues, and the ability to differentiate between them. Careful evaluation of the wound bed facilitates accurate staging. Staging wounds is a complex skill that can take time to develop. The Wound, Ostomy Continence Nurses Society (WOCN Society, 2003) and the National Pressure Ulcer Advisory Panel (NPUAP, 1999) have advanced a 4-stage classification system as described in Box 7-2. This system was designed for use with pressure-induced ulcers only. Examples of Stage I-IV pressure ulcers are provide in Plates 18-21.

Darker skin tones. It is difficult to identify stage I pressure ulcers in darker skin tones. Redness and other color changes are not as detectable on darker skin tones. Therefore other observable, pressure-related alterations of intact skin as compared with the adjacent or opposite area on the body should be documented. Such indicators include changes in skin tissue consistency (firm or boggy feel), sensation (pain, itching), and temperature (Henderson et al, 1997; Sprigle et al, 2001).

Unable to stage. The staging system is based on the ability to assess the type of tissue in the wound bed. Therefore, a wound bed covered with necrotic tissue cannot be accurately staged. In such situations, "unable to stage" or "unstageable" should be documented. If the ulcer is covered with necrotic tissue, the wound is full-thickness and at least a stage III. But it is considered "unstageable" because accurately assessing the extent of tissue damage is not possible. In these instances however, regulating agencies may instruct assessors to designate the wound as stage IV for coding purposes (van Rijswijk and Lyder, 2005).

Reverse staging. The practice of reverse staging, where the wound is described as progressing from a stage III to a stage II to a stage I pressure ulcer

BOX 7-2 NPUAP Pressure Ulcer Staging*

Stage I
An observable, pressure-related alteration of intact skin whose indicators, as compared with the adjacent or opposite area on the body, may include changes in one of more of the following: skin temperature (warmth or coolness), tissue consistency (firm or boggy feel) and sensation (pain, itching). The ulcer appears as a defined area of persistent redness in lightly pigmented skin, whereas in darker skin tones the ulcer may appear with persistent red, blue, or purple hues.

Stage II
Partial-thickness skin loss involving epidermis, dermis, or both. The ulcer is superficial and presents clinically as an abrasion, blister, or shallow crater.

Stage III
Full-thickness skin loss involving damage or necrosis of subcutaneous tissue, which may extend down to but not through underlying fascia. The ulcer presents clinically as a deep crater with or without undermining of adjacent tissue.

Stage IV
Full-thickness skin loss with extensive destruction, tissue necrosis, or damage to muscle, bone, or supporting structures (such as tendon or joint capsule). Undermining and sinus tracts also may be associated with stage 4 pressure ulcers.

Reproduction of the National Pressure Ulcer Advisory Panel (NPUAP) materials in this document does not imply endorsement by the NPUAP of any products, organizations, companies, or any statements made by an organization or company.
*Note: If the wound involves necrotic tissue, staging cannot be confirmed until the wound base is viable. NPUAP, 2006.

is incorrect. Once layers of tissue and supporting structures are gone (such as with full-thickness wounds) they are not replaced. Instead, the wound is filled with granulation tissue. The staging system is to be used to describe the wound in its most severe state, and once accurately described, these descriptor levels endure, even in the presence of healing (NPUAP, 2005). Negative outcomes of reverse staging can lead to (1) denial of acute or skilled care after stage IV ulcers have

been restaged as stage II ulcers; (2) withdrawal of pressure-reducing support surfaces when ulcers "healed" from stage III or stage IV to stage II; and (3) lower fees paid to extended-care facilities for care of patients with healing stages III and stage IV ulcers that were reclassified as stage II or stage I pressure ulcers. Therefore a stage III pressure ulcer that appears to be granulating and resurfacing is described as a healing stage III pressure ulcer (Maklebust, 1997).

Deep tissue injury (DTI). Recently the concept of deep tissue injury (DTI) has been advanced as a classification. The proposed definition for (DTI) by the NPUAP is "a pressure-related injury to subcutaneous tissues under intact skin. Initially, these lesions have the appearance of a deep bruise. These lesions may herald the subsequent development of a stage III-IV pressure ulcer even with optimal treatment"(NPUAP, 2002). Described by clinicians as a purple pressure ulcer, a blister, or a bruise on a bony prominence, these lesions are expected to deteriorate (Ankrom et al, 2005). Plate 22 is an example of a wound with deep tissue injury.

Rapid deterioration of the DTI may be due to the effects of reperfusion, which can be more severe than the ischemia-induced injury itself (Black, 2003; Peirce, Skalak, and Rodeheaver, 2000). When there is a long duration of ischemia, the predominant mechanism for damage is hypoxia alone. With shorter periods of ischemia, the indirect or reperfusion-mediated damage becomes increasingly more important. In animal models, Parks and Granger (1988) reported that intestinal injury induced by 3 hours of ischemia with 1 hour of reperfusion is several times greater than the injury observed after 4 hours of ischemia alone.

Differential diagnosis. Ankrom et al (2005) describes several skin conditions that should be included in the differential diagnosis of deep tissue injury:
- *Bruise:* the extravasation of blood in the tissues as a result of blunt force impact to the body. Usually about 2 weeks is required for a bruise to heal under normal conditions. History of trauma is common.
- *Calciphylaxis:* vascular calcification and skin necrosis most common in patients with a long-standing history of chronic renal failure and

renal replacement therapy. Lesions may have a violaceous hue and be excruciatingly tender and extremely firm. Lesions are most commonly seen on the lower extremities, not bony prominences. The incidence of these lesions is very low in general patient populations.

- *Hematoma:* deep-seated purple nodule from clotted blood, usually associated with trauma.
- *Fournier's gangrene:* intensely painful necrotizing fasciitis of the perineum. May manifest initially as cellulitis.
- *Perirectal abscess:* first sign is commonly a dull, aching, or throbbing pain in the perianal area. The pain worsens when sitting and immediately before defecation; the pain abates after defecation. A tender, fluctuant mass may be palpated at the anal verge. These abscesses can open to reveal large cavities, which can be confused with deep pressure ulcers.
- *Stage I pressure ulcers:* the current definition of stage I pressure ulcers includes deep tissue injury in its earliest presentation, when it appears like a bruise. Labeling deep tissue injury as a stage I pressure ulcer can give an inaccurate impression that the skin damage is minor and will resolve with offloading. However, if enough tissue damage and reperfusion has already occurred, no amount of offloading will prevent sloughing of tissue to reveal the extent of damage. As patients move from one facility to another, this situation can lead to inappropriate care citations or medical malpractice claims for an injury that originated elsewhere.
- *Stage II pressure ulcers:* the definition of stage II pressure ulcers includes blisters. However, deep tissue injury may present as a serum blister or a blood blister. In addition, a large area of deep tissue injury can evolve without blister formation but with loss of the outermost cutaneous layers days after the initial injury. In these situations, the expected deterioration of these kinds of injury differentiates them from the typical, minor, stage II pressure ulcers, which should heal in a short period of time.

Percentage and Type of Tissue in Wound Base.
The type of tissue in the wound bed should be assessed and documented. Viable tissue (e.g., granulation,

epithelialization, muscle, or subcutaneous tissue) must be distinguished from nonviable tissue. Many wounds contain a combination of tissue types and should be described in percentages. For example "50% of the wound bed contains eschar and 50% contains granulation tissue." Type and amount is important because it indicates to what extent the wound is progressing toward healing. Healing wounds are characterized by increasing amounts of granulation tissue and decreasing amounts of necrotic tissue.

The supposition that all red wounds are healthy should be rejected: there are both healthy and unhealthy shades of red. Appropriate terms for wound bed description are important. Evaluating tissue type by a single variable, such as color alone, is limiting and trivializes the healing process. New epithelial tissue is light pink and dry (Plate 1). Healthy granulation tissue is characteristically described as beefy, red, moist, and cobblestone- or berry-like in appearance (Plate 3). In contrast, a wound base that is smooth and red but *lacks* the cobblestone- or berry-like appearance is considered "clean, nongranulating" (see Plate 5).

Deviations from an optimal state should be described carefully and correlated with conditions that may account for the abnormality such as those in the patient's fluid status, serum hemoglobin level, or nutrition, or colonization. Many of these factors affect collagen synthesis, new vessel formation, capillary stability, and hemoglobin formation and are therefore potentially reflected in tissue color and sheen (Rodeheaver, 1989).

Color, consistency, and adherence of the necrotic tissue to the wound bed should also be noted. The presence of nonviable tissue (or necrotic tissue) in the wound is often associated with altered tissue oxygenation, wound desiccation, or increased bacterial burden. As with viable tissue, color alone does not accurately describe nonviable tissue. Nonviable tissue can be yellow slough (Plate 26) or black eschar (Plate 24), but bone or tendon can also be yellow, and sutures can be black. Terms used to describe tissue and other descriptions used for wound assessment are presented in Table 7-3 and the Glossary.

Wound Size.
Measuring the size of the wound is a standard basic assessment parameter with numerous methods available for measurement of physical dimensions (Table 7-4). Measurement of wound

TABLE 7-3 Terms to Describe Types of Wound Base Tissue

Necrotic, nonviable, or devitalized	Tissue that has died and has therefore lost its physical properties and biologic activity
Eschar	Black or brown necrotic, devitalized tissue; tissue can be loose or firmly adherent; hard, soft, or boggy
Slough	Soft, moist, avascular (necrotic/devitalized) tissue; may be white, yellow, tan, or green; may be loose or firmly adherent
Granulation tissue	Pink/red moist tissue comprised of new blood vessels, connective tissue, fibroblasts, and inflammatory cells, fills an open wound when it starts to heal; typically appears deep pink or red; surface is granular, berry-like or cobblestone appearing
Clean, nongranulating	Absence of granulation wound surface appears smooth and red but not granular, and berry-like or cobblestone appearing
Epithelial	Regenerated epidermis across the wound surface; pink and dry in color

dimensions provides overall gross changes in size as an indicator of healing. Unfortunately, the measurement of wound size presents reliability problems as described by Bates-Jensen (1995):

1. Variations in the clinician's ability to define wound edge cannot be controlled.
2. Change in size occurs with debridement, yet the wound is better since necrotic tissue is removed.
3. Measuring the area is an imprecise method of determining depth.

Table 7-4 lists several two-dimensional (length and width) and three-dimensional (length, width, and depth) approaches to wound measurement. Each approach has its own advantages and disadvantages; some are more realistic in the laboratory setting than in the clinical setting (Berriss and Sangwine, 1997; Bohannon and Pfaller, 1983; Bulstrode, Goode, and

Scott, 1986; Ferrell, Artinian, and Sessing, 1995; Frantz and Johnson, 1992; Gilman, 1990; Gledhill and Waterfall, 1983; Harding, 1995; Hughes, 1983; Keast et al, 2004; Kundin,1985, 1989; Langemo et al, 1998; Liskay, Mion, and Davis, 1993; Plassman, Melhuish, and Harding, 1996; Resch et al, 1988; Thomas and Wysocki, 1990; Wood, Williams, and Hughes, 1977).

Accurate measurement of full-thickness wounds requires a three-dimensional approach. The most common form of measurement is the ruler-based linear method. Linear measurements provide an objective basis for evaluating the overall dimensions of a wound and provide greater objectivity than subjective appraisals of wound size. However, linear measurements can be problematic because the perimeter of open wounds is often irregular. As a result, it can be difficult to determine the best position on the wound surface from which to obtain the readings (Gorin et al, 1996). The rigor with which the measurement is obtained influences the results (Langemo et al, 1998). However, when repeated over time, linear measurements of wounds provide gross information regarding the trend of the wound-repair process.

The most common method for measuring wounds is done with a paper or plastic ruler. Measurements, recorded in centimeters or millimeters, should include length, width, and depth; and the extent and location of undermining and tunneling. To strengthen the measurement's value and accuracy, a consistent approach should be used, and the specific aspects of the wound used as landmarks stated in the policy and procedure manual or documented in the medical record. Wound area can be estimated by multiplying length by width by depth.

Measuring length, width, and depth. Length is measured by placing the ruler at the point of greatest length (or head-to-toe). Width is measured by placing the ruler at the point of greatest width (or side to side). (Doughty, 2004; Bates-Jensen, 1995; Bryant et al, 2001). (Figure 7-1). The most common method of obtaining wound depth is by inserting a cotton-tipped applicator into the wound bed and placing a mark on the applicator at the level of the skin (Figure 7-2). This mark is often simply the examiner's thumb and index finger, but it may also be an ink mark. The cotton-tipped applicator is then held against a metric ruler to determine the depth of the wound. Although this technique

TABLE 7-4 Methods of Physical Wound Measurement

METHOD	DESCRIPTION	ADVANTAGES	DISADVANTAGES
KUNDIN WOUND GAUGE	Three rulers placed at right angles Using a specific mathematic formula or formulas, one can ascertain the area of a surface lesion or the volume of wounds with depth	Measures irregular structures Three-dimensional approach	Problems with reliability when used by different clinicians Must be consistently placed over the same location of the open wound bed
PHOTOGRAPHY	Conventional camera, Polaroid, or digital camera	Facilitates both wound measurement and wound assessment Provides a template against which changes in wound status can be observed and compared	Two-dimensional approach Written consent required Storage of digital photos must be addressed Privacy with digital photos may be an issue Wound appearance can also be greatly modified as a consequence of the color-image processing, resolution, and calibration Camera and film can be expensive Skill required to operate the camera Serial photographs should be taken from the same distance, or even better from the same f-stop on the camera so that changes in the course of healing become apparent
PLANIMETRY	Wound surface area is calculated by multiplying length times width (L × W) Graph squares that are contained within a wound tracing or photograph on metric graph paper are counted and expressed in square centimeters (cm²)	Useful for large or irregularly-shaped wounds High reliability Computer-aided planimeters available	Inaccuracy may arise when estimating partial squares Time-consuming Two-dimensional approach Reliability decreases for smaller wounds

Continued

WOUND TRACINGS

External perimeter of the wound is traced using transparent paper or acetate and a marking pen

Inexpensive
Easy
Accessible with various dressing packages
Provides a pattern against which subsequent tracings can be compared

Two-dimensional approach
Some wounds may be difficult to trace because of their position on the body

STEREOPHOTOGRAMMETRY (SPG)

Combining video camera and software to videotape the wound and download onto a computer
Using a computer mouse, the length, width, and area of the wound is traced and software program calculates

Specific areas of interest such as the necrotic tissue can also be calculated by tracing the area
High reliability

Requires special training
Can be time consuming
Expensive
Two-dimensional approach

WOUND MOLDS

Alginate substance is placed into wounds
Substance thickens, is weighed
By calculating the weight over a series of molds, the status of the wound repair process can be assessed

Three-dimensional approach
Assesses volume
Properly stored molds provide some "permanence" of the reflection of the course of healing

Time-consuming
Difficult to perform
Infection-control and storage concerns
Impractical in most clinical settings

FOAM DRESSINGS

Similar to alginate molds
Various dressing materials (e.g., silicone elastomer, Silastic) are retained and reviewed serially

Similar advantages as wound molds
Measurement method can also provide local wound care

Similar disadvantages as wound molds

TABLE 7-4 Methods of Physical Wound Measurement—cont'd

METHOD	DESCRIPTION	ADVANTAGES	DISADVANTAGES
FLUID INSTILLATION	Solution (such as sterile water or saline) is instilled into the wound cavity, allowing it to fill to the perimeter Syringe or suction then extracts the fluid, and the amount is recorded	When carried out serially, with the patient in the same position each time that the measurement is taken, changes in the size of the wound cavity can be determined	Results are dependent on patient position Impractical
STRUCTURED LIGHT	The wound is illuminated with a set of parallel lights via a projector A camera connected to a computer then picks up the image Integrating the intersecting points, the computer produces a three-dimensional representation by triangulation	Three-dimensional approach More reliable results than either fluid instillation or wound molds with a standard deviation of 3% to 15%	Not applicable for undermined, very deep, and very large wounds Costly Not useful in the clinical setting
NEW TECHNOLOGY	Tracing grid, a depth indicator, and a battery operated digital tablet Measurements are recorded using a stylus. The system calculates percentage reduction in wound area from previous measurements	Three-dimensional approach Clinician can select additional factors to track such as undermining, epithelialization, or percentage of different tissue types	

is inherently imprecise (particularly with irregularly-shaped wound beds), serial measurements provide a trend in the dimensions indicating the presence or absence of healing.

Measuring tunneling and undermining. A tunnel is a channel that extends from any part of the wound through subcutaneous tissue or muscle (Figure 7-3). Undermining is tissue destruction that occurs under intact skin around the wound perimeter. Pressure ulcers that have been subjected to shear are often first seen with undermining. Undermining and tunneling can be documented by measuring depth and noting the location using the face of the clock as a guide. Using the clock method, the top of the wound (12 o'clock position) would point towards the patient's head, whereas the bottom of the wound (6 o'clock position) would point towards the feet. See examples in Figures 7-3 and 7-4.

Wound Exudate. Wound fluid contributes to the healing process when it contains the right mixture of growth factors and other components to stimulate tissue regeneration and cellular migration, debride necrotic tissue, and limit bacteria growth. The composition of fluid in the wound varies according to individual health and healing stages (Keast et al, 2004). The characteristics of wound exudate that should be assessed include amount, type, and odor. Amount can be assessed as none, light, moderate, or heavy (van Rijswijk and Lyder, 2005). Exudate quantity can vary with the type of wound (e.g., a venous ulcer may produce more exudate than an arterial ulcer). Wound containment systems can actually measure the amount of exudate. Exudate type can be described as clear, serosanguineous, sanguineous, purulent, yellow, tan, or green.

Odor. Odor can be described as absent, faint, moderate, or strong. Wound exudate characteristics will vary depending on wound moisture, organisms, and the amount of nonviable tissue. Extremely odorous, purulent exudate can be suggestive of an infection. However, it is important to note that most wounds have an odor. The type of dressing used can affect wound odor as well as hygiene and the presence of nonviable tissue (Keast et al, 2004).

Wound Edge. The edge, or rim, of the wound should be assessed as an integral part of wound evaluation.

Wound edges give information regarding epithelialization, chronicity, and even etiology. Ideally, the wound edges should be attached to the wound bed (Plate 3). Closed or rolled wound edges are usually an indication that the epithelial cells have migrated down and around the wound edges. This process is often referred to as epibole and is illustrated in Plate 4.

Periwound Area/Surrounding Skin. Assessment of the area around the wound should also be a part of routine wound assessment. Parameters of the periwound skin assessment include the following:

- color (erythema, white, blue)
- texture (moist, dry, indurated, boggy, macerated)
- skin temperature (warm, cool)
- integrity of the surrounding skin such as denudement, maceration, excoriation, stripping, erosion, papules, pustules, and lesions

Periwound assessment can give clues to the effectiveness of treatment choices or dressing application or removal technique. For example, maceration (Plate 20), dermatitis, or denudement of periwound skin occurs when exudate pools on intact skin for prolonged periods of time or when a moist dressing is inappropriately applied, left on too long, and/or overlaps onto intact skin. Periwound skin stripping may indicate inappropriate adhesive removal.

Venous/arterial insufficiency, infection, pressure damage, peripheral neuropathy, pyoderma gangrenosum, vasculitis, and calciphylaxis *may* present with distinct periwound features (Ferretti and Harkins, 2003). Table 7-5 list some pathologies that *may* be revealed through periwound skin inspection.

Bacterial Burden. Bacterial burden refers to more than just the total number of bacteria present; diversity, virulence, and interaction of organisms with each other and the body exert a cumulative and synergistic negative impact in the wound. The extent of bioburden is classified as contamination, colonization, critical colonization, and infection. Chapter 9 presents a thorough discussion of the assessment and management of bacterial burden and infection.

Contamination and colonization do not constitute infection. The skin is in constant contact with multiple microorganisms from various sources. The wound environment is not sterile; therefore a certain number of bacteria are inevitable in any wound. Given an intact

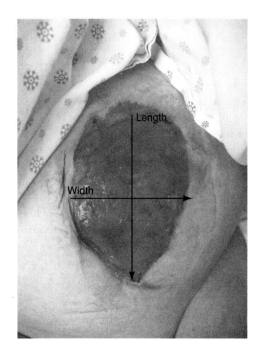

Fig. 7-1 Measuring wound length and width.

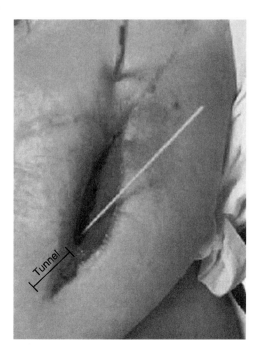

Fig. 7-3 Wound tunneling. Tunneling is present in this abdominal wound at the 7 o'clock position and measures 2 cm in length.

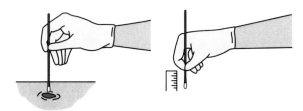

Fig. 7-2 Measuring wound depth.

immune system, the human body can usually phago-cytize bacteria present in a wound to balance host resistance and bacterial growth. Bacterial overload occurs when the balance of microorganisms present in the wound is upset by lowered host defense or increased bacteria quantity or strength. Infection is directly related to the number of organisms and to the virulence of the organisms, and is inversely related to host resistance as illustrated in Figure 9-1.

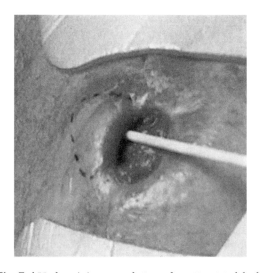

Fig. 7-4 Undermining extends 2 cm from 7 to 11 o'clock.

TABLE 7-5 Pathologies and Potential Periwound Features

PATHOLOGY	POTENTIAL PERIWOUND FEATURE
Venous insufficiency	Edema, brawny discoloration, hemosiderin-staining lipodermatosclerosis, dermatitis, scaling, weeping
Arterial	Pale, cool, dependent rubor, absent hair, xerosis
Infection	Erythema, pain, heat, swelling, induration
Pressure	Hyperemia, edema, induration, discoloration
Peripheral neuropathy	Insensate, edema, cellulitis, erythema, induration
Pyoderma gangrenosum	Ragged and boggy borders, elevated, dusky red, purple, edema halo
Vasculitis	Palpable, nonblanchable purpura in the skin may be associated with petechiae Nodules and vesicles may be present
Calciphylaxis	Dusky, purple, and palpable nodules progress to necrosis and ulceration Associated with renal disease May include mottled, reticulated patches and plaques with focal central necrosis
Candidiasis	Pustular erythematous satellite lesions

The presence or absence of local signs of infection should be documented as part of the assessment. Classic signs of infection include increased purulent exudate, induration, warmth, pain or tenderness, and erythema. Erythema alone does not indicate infection in the first 5 days of a surgical wound; in fact, it is expected as a normal inflammatory response. Patients who are immunosuppressed often mask many of the classic signs of infection, and new pain may be the only clue that something is off course.

Chronic wounds may also lack classic signs of infection, and they are prone to an excess number and variety of microorganisms. In chronic wounds, indicators of a subclinical infection or overwhelming bioburden include delayed healing despite optimal care, discolored or friable granulation tissue, pocketing or breakdown at the wound base, and/or foul odor. A "stagnant" wound despite optimal care may indicate critical colonization and will progress to infection without intervention (Gardner, 2001).

Unfortunately, wound cultures can be inconclusive. Techniques used to obtain wound culture greatly affect the accuracy of results. Infection takes place in viable tissue rather than necrotic tissue or exudate. Although a tissue biopsy of the wound is the gold standard for wound cultures, tissue biopsies are invasive and require a level of skill and resources that many settings lack. Therefore, quantitative swab cultures remain a reasonable alternative in clinical practice (Bill et al, 2001; WOCN Society, 2003).

BOX 7-3 Clinical Signs and Symptoms of Chronic Wound Infection

- New/increased slough
- Drainage excess, change in color/consistency
- Poor granulation tissue—friable, bright red, exuberant
- Redness, warmth around the wound
- Sudden high glucose in patient with diabetes
- Pain or tenderness
- Unusual odor
- Increased wound size/new areas of breakdown

Most infected wounds exhibit common "classic" signs and symptoms of infection (Box 7-3). However, some authors have noted subtle differences between wound types that may lead to early detection of critical colonization. Criteria for identifying these subtle changes in different wound types are being developed (Cutting and White, 2005). Managing bacteria is such an important factor in wound healing that this text has dedicated an entire chapter to wound infection diagnosis and management. Chapter 9 is a "must read" for any clinician assessing and treating wounds.

Wound Pain. As the fifth vital sign, pain has gained a much-deserved focus in today's health care environment. Yet wound pain is infrequently assessed and inadequately managed. Wound pain can indicate infection or deterioration as well as inappropriate or inadequate treatment choices. Pain can be directly related to patient satisfaction and has been shown to have a negative impact on wound-healing progress. Pain should be measured regularly and frequently with a validated pain assessment scale (Reddy et al, 2003). Chapter 25 provides a detailed discussion of the assessment and management of wound pain.

FREQUENCY OF WOUND ASSESSMENT

In general, the patient's overall condition wound severity, health care setting, type of dressings used, and goals determine the appropriate frequency of wound assessment. Since reassessment frequency is dependent on so many variables, it is common for the frequency interval to change over time and across care settings. A patient who is immunosuppressed and in acute care, for example, has a greater risk for developing a wound infection and may warrant more frequent monitoring. Once the patient is stable in long-term care, the "at-risk" patient's skin should be monitored daily but may only require a full wound assessment on admission and weekly. Once the patient is home, assessments are generally dependent on the frequency of home health worker or clinic visits. Family members should be instructed to make assessments between clinic visits and may be able and willing to monitor for trends.

The Wound Ostomy and Continence Nurses (WOCN) Society Guideline for Prevention and Management of Pressure Ulcers makes specific recommendations related to the frequency of monitoring, assessment, and evaluation of pressure ulcer healing. Patients at risk for skin breakdown should have a daily skin inspection (Bergstrom and Braden, 1992; WOCN Society, 2003). Pressure ulcers should be assessed and monitored at each dressing change, or sooner if the wound or the patient's condition deteriorates (van Rijswijk and Braden, 1999; WOCN Society, 2003). Evaluation of pressure ulcer healing should occur within 1 to 2 weeks, or sooner if the patient or wound condition deteriorates (van Rijswijk and Braden, 1999; van Rijswijk and Polansky, 1994; WOCN Society, 2003).

When selecting topical wound therapy, the frequency with which the wound should be assessed must be considered. A wound that has to be assessed daily, for example, should not be treated with a dressing that is designed to remain in place for several days. Conversely, some local wound care choices may warrant more frequent monitoring and/or assessments, at least initially,

to evaluate effectiveness (i.e., autolysis, absorptive capacity, etc.). Chapter 19 discusses the principles of wound management and the various features of local wound care options.

EVALUATION OF HEALING AND DOCUMENTATION TOOLS

Evaluation of healing involves wound assessment documented over time to reveal patterns and trends that indicate improvement or deterioration in the wound. In this way, assessment is linked to outcomes so that an evaluation of the plan of care can follow objective criteria.

Ideally, instruments to clinically measure the reparative process should be reliable and valid, clinically useful, theoretically-based, and provide a mechanism that systematically and objectively monitors the status of tissue healing. Valid and reliable instruments for use in the measurement of human healing have been identified, but in many cases come from a research rather than a clinical perspective. Although appropriate for clinical research, some may not be readily accessible or user-friendly for clinicians (Kantor and Margolis, 1998).

Clinicians should be familiar with the strengths and limitations of the several methods currently available to assess wound status. Staging and assessment tools are not designed to replace a comprehensive ongoing assessment. In addition, the clinician must develop an appreciation for the need to use a combination of evaluative modalities that allow one to assess wound status accurately and infer the quality of repair in relation to the normal healing trajectory (Cuddigan, 1997). Appendix C has examples of wound assessment documentation forms. Tools to evaluate healing are also located in Appendix C and presented next.

Asepsis Incision Assessment Tool

ASEPSIS is an acronym for seven wound assessment parameters. The ASEPSIS tool is reported to be the most frequently used assessment tool for surgical wound evaluation (Bruce et al, 2001). The tool was originally developed for patients undergoing cardiac surgery and later underwent validations studies with patients having general surgery (Byrne et al 1989; Wilson et al, 1986). When measures are repeated over time, a trend in the healing process is revealed. Chapter 11 presents the ASEPSIS tool and an in-depth discussion of the assessment and management of patients with acute wounds.

Wound Characteristics Instrument (WCI)

The WCI (Cooper, 1990, 1991), a criterion-referenced measurement, is a 17-item rating scale designed for use by clinicians evaluating the macroscopic (visible to the naked eye) characteristics of open, soft tissue, postsurgical wounds. Two sample items from the WCI are provided in Appendix C. In addition to encouraging the use of a common vocabulary among clinicians when open wounds are being discussed, this instrument directs the clinician to complete a wound assessment in a systematic manner. A systematic and consistent wound evaluation technique is essential to capture the subtle changes within a wound that can be otherwise easily overlooked.

The clinician using the WCI is directed to assess essential components or generic characteristics within the specific regions of the wound. For example, Plate 5 demonstrates the contrast in the presence of granulation. These observations are then ranked along a continuum from the optimal to the worst manifestations of that state. The WCI underwent reliability testing and both content and construct validity testing. Content validity scores by surgeon experts indicated a high level of agreement regarding the structural and generic characteristics of the open wound with an average congruency percentage at 90%. Construct validity and reliability testing by registered nurses indicated a range of difficulty scores among the items.

Pressure Sore Status Tool (PSST)

The PSST takes approximately 10 to 15 minutes to complete and addresses 15 macroscopic wound characteristics (Woodbury et al, 1999). Specific definitions are provided for each characteristic. Individual items are scored on a modified Likert scale (1, best for that characteristic; 5, worst). Individual items are summed, and the total provides a measure of overall wound status. The range of scores is from 13, which indicates tissue health, to 65, which indicates wound degeneration. Content validity of the PSST with a nine-member expert judge panel was 0.91. Interrater reliability coefficient was 0.915; intrarater reliability was 0.975 when used with wound care specialists in an acute care hospital. The interrater reliability of the PSST in long-term care with licensed practical nurses, registered nurses, and physical therapists who had no experience in wound care yielded a mean of 0.78; intrarater reliability for this group was 0.89, and agreement with an expert was 0.82. A benefit of the PSST is that it allows for tracking over time of each item or wound characteristic as well as of the total score. Thus each item can be monitored for improvement or deterioration. In this way, the PSST can be used to evaluate the effectiveness of specific interventions or achievement of short-term outcomes, such as to manage wound infection or to debride the wound (Bates-Jensen, 1995, 1997; Bates-Jensen, Vredevoe, and Brecht, 1992).

Pressure Ulcer Scale for Healing (PUSH)

The PUSH takes approximately 5 minutes to complete (Woodbury et al, 1999). The PUSH is a validated tool developed by the National Pressure Ulcer Advisory Panel (NPUAP) to monitor pressure ulcer healing over time. The PUSH tool is designed to monitor three parameters that are considered the most indicative of healing: size (length and width), exudate amount, and tissue type. Each parameter has at least four sublevels. The subscore for each parameter is totaled, and the overall total score is calculated ranging from 0 to 17 (0 = healed). A comparison of total scores measured over time provides an indication of wound improvement or deterioration (NPUAP, 1999; WOCN Society, 2003; Stotts et al, 2001; Stotts and Rodeheaver, 1997; Thomas et al, 1997).

Sussman Wound Healing Tool (SWHT)

The SWHT takes approximately 5 minutes to complete (Woodbury et al, 1999). The SWHT is an instrument developed to track physical therapy technologies used for wound healing. This device contains 10 variables that address wound attributes and 9 variables that address wound dimensions and extent of tissue damage. Attributes are assessed and determined by the tool to be good for healing or not good for healing. Necrosis, for example, is *not* good for healing and granulation is good for healing. Reliability and validity measures for the SWHT have not been reported (Sussman and Swanson, 1997).

Tool Selection

Several tools are available to enable the clinician to predict the development of wounds, classify existing wounds, measure existing wounds, and assess the status of a wound. Unfortunately, these methods have undergone varying degrees of testing and vary in reliability and validity. When selecting a tool, the clinician must first determine the parameters to be assessed. Once this determination is made, a decision can be made regarding which tool is most appropriate for the situation. When considering appropriateness, it is important to keep reliability and validity measures in mind. The clinician should select a tool in which the reliability and validity has been supported previously in a similar population and then assess its reliability for the specific application at hand, before assuming that the scores generated are valid (Strickland, 1995). The clinician must keep in mind that it is unrealistic to expect one instrument to be an adequate gauge of wound status. One tool will not capture all the information necessary to adequately describe and evaluate the dynamic nature of a wound. For example, wounds that are classified as stage III, or full-thickness, require additional descriptions of wound parameters (see Box 7-1).

SUMMARY

Few pathologic conditions are evaluated with a single instrument or parameter. The more intricate the process (e.g., congestive heart failure), the more clinicians rely on several measures (e.g., radiologic examination, physical examination, pulse characteristics, treadmill tests, hematocrit) to accurately capture a full description of the extent of the condition. Therefore, several parameters are required to best reflect the condition of the wound.

Recognizing the difference between simply measuring the dimensions of a wound and the more complex process of assessing the status of the wound's multiple components and healing status is essential to successful wound management and holistic patient care. It is clear that evaluating wounds as if they exist separately from the patient is not only inadequate, but also inconsistent with evidence-based practice.

SELF-ASSESSMENT EXERCISE

1. Distinguish between assessment and evaluation of healing.

2. Which of the following methods is an example of categorizing a wound by classification?
   a. Linear measurements
   b. Photographs
   c. Staging
   d. Wound molds
3. Blisters are an example of which stage of tissue loss?
   a. Stage I
   b. Stage II
   c. Stage III
   d. Stage IV
4. Distinguish between partial-thickness and full-thickness wounds.
5. List 10 indices of wound healing that should be assessed and recorded.
6. Describe necrotic, nonviable, or devitalized tissue.
7. Describe eschar.
8. Describe slough.

REFERENCES

Agency for Health Care Policy and Research (AHCPR): *Pressure ulcers in adults: prediction and prevention.* Clinical Practice Guideline No. 3, Rockville, Md, 1992, U.S. Department of Health and Human Services, Public Health Service, pub. No. 92-0047.

Ankrom M et al for the National Pressure Ulcer Advisory Panel (NPUAP): Pressure-related deep tissue injury under intact skin and the current pressure ulcer staging systems, *Adv Skin Wound Care* 18: 35-42, 2005.

Armstrong DG, Lavery LA, Harkless LB: Treatment-based classification system for assessment and care of diabetic feet, *Ostomy Wound Manage* 42(8):50, 1996.

Bates BA: The skin. In Bates BA, editor: *A guide to physical examination and history taking*, ed 6, Philadelphia, 1995, Lippincott.

Bates-Jensen BM: The pressure sore status tool: an outcome measure for pressure sores, *Top Geriatr Rehabil* 9(4):17, 1994.

Bates-Jensen BM: Indices to include in wound healing assessment, *Adv Wound Care* 8(4):28, 1995.

Bates-Jensen BM: The pressure sore status tool a few thousand assessments later, *Adv Wound Care* 10(5):65, 1997.

Bates-Jensen BM, Vredevoe DL, Brecht ML: Validity and reliability of the pressure sore status tool, *Decubitus* 5(6):20, 1992.

Bergstrom N, Braden B: A prospective study of pressure sore risk among institutionalized elderly, *J Am Geriatr Soc* Aug, 40(8):747 1992.

Berris WP, Sangwine SJ: Automatic quantitative analysis of healing skin wounds using colour digital image processing, Available on the Internet at www.smtl.co.uk/World-Wide-Wounds/1997/july/Berris/Berris.html, July, 1997.

Bill TJ et al: Quantitative swab culture versus tissue biopsy: a comparison in chronic wounds, *Ostomy Wound Manage* 47(1):34, 2001.

Black J: Deep tissue injury, *Wounds* 15(11): 380, 2003.

Bohannon RW, Pfaller BA: Documentation of wound surface area from tracings of wound perimeters, *Phys Ther* 63:1622, 1983.

Bruce J et al: The quality of measurement of surgical wound infection as the basis for monitoring: a systematic review, *J Hosp Infect* 49:99, 2001.

Bryant J et al: Reliability of wound measuring techniques in an outpatient wound center, *Ostomy Wound Manage* 2001:47: 44-51.

Bulstrode DJ, Goode AW, Scott PJ: Stereophotogrammetry for measuring rates of cutaneous healing: a comparison with conventional techniques, *Clin Sci* 71:437, 1986.

Byrne DJ et al: Postoperative wound scoring, *Biomed Pharm* 43:669, 1989.

Cole L, Nesbitt C: A three year multiphase pressure ulcer prevalence/incidence study in a regional referral hospital, *Ostomy Wound Management* 2004.

Cooper DM: Development and testing of an instrument to assess the visual characteristics of open, soft tissue wounds, doctoral dissertation, Philadelphia, 1990, University of Pennsylvania.

Cooper DM: Clinical assessment/measurement of healing: evolution and status, *Clin Materials* 8:263, 1991.

Crawford PE, Fields-Varnado M: *Guideline for management of wounds in patients with lower-extremity neuropathic disease.* WOCN Clinical Practice Guideline Series No. 3, Glenview, Ill, 2004, Wound, Ostomy and Continence Nurses Society.

Cuddigan J: Pressure ulcer classification: what do we have? What do we need? *Adv Wound Care* 10(5):13, 1997.

Cutting KF, White RJ: Criteria for identifying wound infection—revisited, *Ostomy Wound Manage* 51(1):28, 2005.

Doughty DB: Wound assessment: tips and techniques, *Adv Skin Wound Care* 17:369, 2004.

Ferrell BA, Artinian BM, Sessing D: The Sessing scale for assessment of pressure ulcer healing, *J Am Geriatr Soc* 43:37, 1995.

Ferretti DE, Harkins SM: Assessment of periwound skin. In Miline C, Corbett L, Dubuc D, editors: *Wound, ostomy, and continence nursing secrets,* Philadelphia, 2003, Hanley & Belfus.

Frantz RA, Johnson DA: Stereophotogrammetry and computerized image analysis: a 3-dimensional method of measuring wound healing, *Wounds* 4:58, 1992.

Gardner SE et al: A tool to assess clinical signs and symptoms of localized infection in chronic wounds: development and reliability, *Ostomy Wound Manage* 47(1):40, 2001.

Gilman TH: Parameter for measurement of wound closure, *Wounds* 2(3):95, 1990.

Gledhill T, Waterfall WE: Silastic foam: a new material for dressing wounds, *Can Med Assoc J* 128:685, 1983.

Gorin DR et al: The influence of wound geometry on the measurement of wound healing rates in clinical trials, *J Vasc Surg* 23(3):524, 1996.

Guralnik JM et al: Occurrence and predictors of pressure sores in the national health and nutrition examination follow-up, *J Am Geriatr Soc* 26(9):807, 1988.

Harding KG: Methods for assessing change in ulcer status, *Adv Wound Care* 8(4):37-42, 1995.

Henderson CT et al: Draft definition of stage I pressure ulcers: inclusion of persons with darkly pigmented skin. NPUAP Task Force on Stage I Definition and Darkly Pigmented Skin, *Adv Wound Care* 10(5):16-19, 1997.

Hughes LE: Wound measurement, *Can J Surg* 26:210, 1983.

Hunt, TK, Van Winkle W Jr: Normal repair. In Hunt TK, Dunphy JE, editors: *Fundamentals of wound management,* New York 1997, Appleton-Century-Crofts.

Hunter S et al: Clinical trial of a prevention and treatment protocol for skin breakdown in two nursing homes, *J WOCN* 30(5):250, 2003.

Kantor J, Margolis DJ: Efficacy and prognostic value of simple wound measurements, *Arch Dermatol* 134(12):1571, 1998.

Keast DH et al: Measure: a proposed assessment framework for developing best practice recommendations for wound assessment, *Wound Rep Regen* 5:S1, 2004.

Klingman A: Introduction. In Loden M, Maibach HI: *Dry skin and moisturizers chemistry and function,* Boca Raton, London, New York, Washington DC, 2000, CRC Press.

Knighton DR et al: Classification and treatment of chronic nonhealing wounds, *Ann Surg* 204:322, 1986.

Kundin JI: Designing and developing a new measuring instrument, *Periop Nurs Q* 1:40, 1985.

Kundin JI: A new way to size up a wound, *Am J Nurs* 89:206, 1989.

Langemo DK et al: Two-dimensional wound measurement: comparison of four techniques, *Adv Wound Care* 11:337, 1998.

Lavery LA, Armstrong DG, Harkless LB: Classification of diabetic foot wounds, *Ostomy Wound Manage* 43:44, 1997.

Levine ME: Holistic nursing, *Nurs Clin North Am* 6:253, 1971.

Liskay AM, Mion LC, Davis BR: Comparison of two devices for wound measurement, *Dermatol Nurs* 5:434, 1993.

Maklebust J: Policy implications of using reverse staging to monitor pressure ulcer status, *Adv Wound Care* 10(5):32-35. 1997.

Murphy RM: Legal and practical impact of clinical practice guidelines on nursing and medical practice, *Adv Wound Care* 9(5):31, 1996.

National Pressure Ulcer Advisory Panel (NPUAP): National Consensus Conference, Washington, DC, 1998.

National Pressure Ulcer Advisory Panel (NPUAP): Stage I assessment in darkly pigmented skin. Available on the Internet at www.npuap.org/positn4.htm. August, 1999.

National Pressure Ulcer Advisory Panel (NPUAP): Position statement on reverse staging: the facts about reverse staging in 2000. http:www.npuap.org, Accessed May 20, 2005.

National Pressure Ulcer Advisory Panel (NPUAP): NPUAP Staging Report Available on the Internet at http://www.npuap.org/positn6.html. Accessed February 06, 2006.

Norman RA: Geriatic dermatology in chronic care and rehabilitation, *Dermatol Ther* 16: 254, 2003.

Parks DS, Granger DN: Ischemia-reperfusion injury: a radical view, *Hepatology* 8(3):680, 1988.

Peirce SM, Skalak TC, Rodeheaver GT: Ischemia-reperfusion injury in chronic pressure ulcer formation: a skin model in the rat, *Wound Rep Regen* 8(1):68, 2000.

Percoraro RE, Reiber GE: Classification of wounds in diabetic amputees, *Wounds* 2:65, 1990.

Plassman P, Melhuish JM, Harding KG: Methods of measuring wound size: a comparative study, *Ostomy Wound Manage* 40(7):50, 1996.

Reddy M, Kohr R, Queen D, Keast D and Sibbald G: Practical treatment of wound pain and trauma: a patient centered approach. *Ostomy Wound Management* 49(4A Suppl):2-15, 2003.

Resch CS et al: Pressure sore volume measurement, *Am J Geriatr Soc* 36:444, 1988.

Rodeheaver G: Controversies in topical wound management, *Wounds* 1(1):19, 1989.

Shea JD: Pressure sores: classification and management, *Clin Orthop* 112:89, 1975.

Sheehan P et al: Percent change in wound area of diabetic foot ulcers over a 4 week period is a robust predictor of complete healing in a 12 week prospective trial, *Diabetes Care* 26:1879, 2003.

Sprigle S et al: Clinical skin temperature measurement to predict incipient pressure ulcers, *Adv Skin Wound Care* 14(3):133, 2001.

Stotts NA, Rodeheaver GT: Revision of the PUSH Tool using an expanded database, *Adv Wound Care* 10(5):107, 1997.

Stotts NA et al: An instrument to measure healing in pressure ulcers: development and validation of the pressure ulcer scale for healing (PUSH), *J Gerontol A Biol Sci Med Sci* 56(12):M795, 2001.

Strickland OL: Can reliability and validity be established? *J Nurs Manage* 3(2):91, 1995.

Sussman C, Swanson G: Utility of the Sussman Wound Healing Tool in predicting wound healing outcomes in physical therapy, *Adv Wound Care* 10(5):74, 1997.

Tallman P et al: Initial rate of healing predicts complete healing of venous ulcers, *Arch Dermatol* 133:1231, 1997.

Thomas AC, Wysocki AB: The healing wound: a comparison of three clinically useful methods of measurement, *Decubitus* 3:18, 1990.

Thomas DR et al: Pressure ulcer scale for healing: derivation and validation of the PUSH tool, *Adv Wound Care* 10(5):96, 1997.

van Rijswijk L, Braden BJ: Pressure ulcer patient and wound assessment: an AHCPR clinical practice guideline update, *Ostomy Wound Manage* 45(Suppl 1A):56S, 1999.

van Rijswijk L, Lyder C: Pressure ulcer prevention and care: implementing the revised guidance to surveyors for long-term care facilities, *Ostomy Wound Manage* 51(Suppl 4):7, 2005.

van Rijswijk L, Polansky M: Predictors of time to healing deep pressure ulcers, *Ostomy Wound Manage* 40(8):40, 1994.

White M, Karam S, Cowell B: Skin tears in frail elders: a practical approach to prevention, *Geriatric Nursing*, 12:116, 2000.

Wilson AP et al: A scoring method (ASEPSIS) for postoperative wound infections for use in clinical trials of antibiotic prophylaxis, *Lancet* 1(8476):311, 1986.

Wood RA, Williams RH, Hughes LE: Foam elastomer dressing in the management of open granulating wounds: experience with 250 patients, *Br J Surg* 64:554, 1977.

Woodbury MG et al: Pressure ulcer assessment instruments: a critical appraisal, *Ostomy Wound Manage* 45(5):42, 1999.

Woods FM et al: Current difficulties and the possible future directions in scar assessment, *Burns* 22(6):455, 1996.

Wound, Ostomy and Continence Nurses Society (WOCN Society) *Guideline for management of patients with lower extremity arterial disease*, WOCN clinical practice guideline series #1, Glenview IL, 2002, Author.

Wound, Ostomy and Continence Nurses Society (WOCN Society): *Guideline for management of pressure ulcers*, WOCN clinical practice guideline series #2, Glenview IL, 2003, Author.

Zimny S, Schatz S, Pfohl M: Determinants and estimation of healing times in diabetic foot ulcers, *J Diabetes Complications* 16:327, 2002.

8

Nutritional Assessment and Support

NANCY A. STOTTS

OBJECTIVES

1. Identify the effects of injury on metabolic needs.
2. Define malnutrition.
3. Compare and contrast the causes and signs of marasmus, kwashiorkor, and mixed marasmus-kwashiorkor.
4. Identify four reasons that obesity is a risk factor for impaired healing.
5. Identify two instruments to assess nutritional status.
6. Identify risk factors for malnutrition in a patient's history.
7. Describe the major physical findings of malnutrition.
8. Identify the laboratory test results that are consistent with malnutrition.
9. Identify the role of key nutrients needed for wound repair.
10. Compare and contrast at least 5 parameters that can be used to monitor nutritional status during nutritional support.

Nutrition is fundamental to normal cellular integrity and tissue repair. All phases of healing require nutrients. Lack of adequate nutrition is associated with increased morbidity and mortality in medical and surgical patients, a higher rate of hospital admission among older adults (Halsted, 2001-2004), decreased wound tensile strength, decreased T cell function, and decreased phagocytic activity (Williams and Barbul, 2003). Nursing has the primary responsibility for the initial nutritional assessment across settings (hospital, home care, and nursing home).

Early assessment is an effort to identify those individuals at-risk for and experiencing malnutrition; delay has been reported in nutritional assessment and treatment in this population (Brugler, DiPrinzio, and Bernstein, 1999). Timely intervention must be undertaken to mitigate the negative effects of inadequate nutrition and to support healing. It is important to recognize that both outpatients and inpatients are at risk for malnutrition; it follows that it is important for nutritional evaluation to be incorporated into all phases of care (Halsted, 2001-2004).

MALNUTRITION

Definition

Malnutrition is undernutrition or overnutrition that is caused by a deficit or excess of nutrients in the diet. Undernutrition occurs because intake is inadequate, the individual is unable to absorb nutrients, or lacks the capacity to metabolize substrates needed for normal function. Undernutrition is a major health problem in hospitalized patients and in those with acute and chronic illness. It is estimated that undernutrition is present in more than half of all hospitalized adults (Halsted, 2001-2004). Some patients are admitted to the hospital with undernutrition. Others develop undernutrition during hospitalization as a result of decreased intake, the hypermetabolic response that accompanies acute injury and inflammation, and an inability to metabolize nutrients (Halsted, 2001-2004). Certain populations have an increased incidence of known deficiencies. For example, older adults manifest low caloric intake, as well as insufficient intake of protein, zinc, and vitamin B_{12} (Seiler, 2001). Understanding who has a high incidence of various nutritional deficiencies should provide a focus for the nurse's nutritional assessment.

Undernutrition is generally divided into *protein-energy malnutrition* and *protein malnutrition*. Protein-energy malnutrition is sometimes called *marasmus*, and protein malnutrition is known as *kwashiorkor*. The terms marasmus and kwashiorkor come from Africa, where nutritional screening through the

World Health Organization revealed a high incidence of these problems (Jeliffe, 1966). Children were often first to develop malnutrition, marasmus, purely because the mother was unable to breast-feed and so the child received neither adequate calories nor protein. The etiology of kwashiorkor is different. Kwashiorkor is an African word meaning "first child–second child." It refers to the result of the protein-deficient diet given to the first child, as he or she is weaned to allow the second child to breast-feed. The first child (the weaned child) develops a predominantly protein malnutrition, characterized by thin arms and legs and an edematous abdomen. The breast-fed child does not experience malnutrition (Beers and Berkow, 1999-2004).

Protein-energy malnutrition is also known as protein-calorie malnutrition (PCM). It is more often seen in developed countries, and it is not limited to children. PCM often reflects the inadequate intake, absorption, or metabolism that occurs with illness in adults. PCM is seen in persons with chronic illnesses such as cancer and chronic heart failure. Severe weight loss, muscle wasting, and loss of adipose tissue characterize PCM (Collins, 2001a). The phenomenon of rapidly occurring protein-calorie malnutrition has been termed mixed protein-calorie malnutrition, or marasmus-kwashiorkor. It has an acute onset and is common in acutely ill persons and those who are hospitalized (Table 8-1). Understanding the processes that take place during malnutrition is important because it illustrates why specific assessment parameters are used and specific nutrients prescribed.

Pathophysiology

Starvation occurs when caloric intake is inadequate to meet metabolic needs. With inadequate intake, a series of compensatory processes is initiated to meet the glucose needs of essential tissues. Glycogen, stored in the liver, is mobilized for energy. Normally, the glycogen stores are exhausted in less than 24 hours, and then glucose needed for cellular activities is formed by the catabolism of muscle. There are no protein stores in the body, so when protein is used for gluconeogenesis, functional skeletal muscle and organs are destroyed (Bond and Heitkemper, 2003). Concomitantly, catecholamines are released and stimulate the breakdown of body fat and protein, and weight loss is rapid. The weight loss occurs from both the breakdown of protein and the osmotic diuresis that occurs as the byproducts of protein metabolism are excreted in the urine.

If intake still is less than the individual's metabolic needs after a few days, compensatory processes allow fat to become the primary energy source and for protein to be used at a much slower rate (Collins, 2001a). The brain adapts and uses ketones from fat metabolism for energy, the muscle releases less protein, and the kidney recycles the end products of protein metabolism for glucose (Bond and Heitkemper, 2003). Because fat has more than twice as many calories per gram of tissue than protein (9 calories/g compared with 4 calories), weight loss is slowed. Protein is converted to glucose for use by only a few tissues (e.g., red blood cells, fibroblasts, and renal medulla). During this time, changes in

TABLE 8-1 Malnutrition: Cause and Manifestations

TYPE OF MALNUTRITION	CAUSE	MANIFESTATIONS
Protein-calorie malnutrition (marasmus)	Inadequate protein and calories	Gradual weight loss Visceral protein levels are preserved Immune function is well preserved
Protein malnutrition (kwashiorkor)	Inadequate protein with adequate carbohydrate and fat	Rapid onset with loss of visceral protein Skeletal muscle mass is well preserved
Mixed protein-calorie malnutrition (marasmus-kwashiorkor)	Inadequate protein and calories	Acute onset Common in hospitalized patients Low visceral protein Presents with rapid weight loss and fat and muscle wasting

fat stores are gradual, as are declines in muscle stores. Weight loss is slowed during this period. Serum measurements reflecting protein status decline gradually (Beers and Berkow, 1999-2004).

When fat stores are depleted, protein again is the primary energy source. Rapid depletion occurs. Skeletal muscle size rapidly decreases, and serum protein levels fall. If treatment is not prompt, death will ensue (Table 8-2).

Stress and Starvation

With injury, there is an increased metabolic rate owing to the release of catecholamines at the time of tissue damage. The degree of hypermetabolism is directly related to the severity of injury. For example, severe burns cause greater increase in metabolic rate than uncomplicated surgery. The inflammatory response is elicited concomitantly. Cortisol released from the adrenal cortex enhances protein catabolism, amino

TABLE 8-2 Manifestations of Starvation

TYPE OF STARVATION	MANIFESTATIONS
Brief	Increased nitrogen in urine
	Increased urine output
	Rapid weight loss
	Decreased muscle mass
	Low normal glucose and insulin levels
Prolonged	Slow weight loss
	Slow loss of muscle mass
	Increased urinary ammonia
	Decreased urinary nitrogen
	Metabolic acidosis, usually compensated
Premorbid	Cachectic appearance
	Rapid weight loss
	Decreased midarm muscle circumference
	Increased creatinine/height index
	Increased urinary urea
	Decreased serum albumin
	Decreased transferrin
	Decreased lymphocyte count
	Anergy to recall antigens

acid mobilization, and hepatic glucose production (Bond and Heitkemper, 2003). The compensatory decreased metabolic rate is over-ridden and cytokines, including transforming growth factor α and interleukin-6 (Il-6), contribute to the stress response. During this period of hypermetabolism, caloric needs increase, and protein requirements increase disproportionately. The hypermetabolic demands decrease gradually, and if no additional insult occurs, the metabolic needs return to baseline within 10 to 14 days of the acute injury. This process is seen in the surgical patient who has an uncomplicated postoperative course.

In healthy persons who are wounded, inadequate intake for a brief period of up to 5 to 7 days is usually not a problem. During this time, there is a combination of hypermetabolism and starvation. The hypermetabolic response is a physiologic response to injury and results in increased energy needs. At the same time, these patients usually have inadequate intake, which makes it necessary for them to use their body substrate to meet their metabolic needs. They usually have a brief but rapid decrease in weight. When they return to their normal diet, they regain the lost weight (Williams and Barbul, 2003). Should the cause of the stress not be resolved or an additional stress occur, such as might be seen in infection following injury, the patient with a wound is set up for a downward spiral.

Excessive Intake as Malnutrition

On the other end of the continuum of malnutrition is overnutrition, seen as obesity. Obese patients may develop wound-healing problems such as delayed wound healing (Mathison, 2003), dehiscence, and infection (Gallagher, 2003). They often have concomitant medical problems that include diabetes, hypertension and poor oxygenation from pulmonary restrictive disease (Mathison, 2003). Because fat tissue is not as well perfused as muscular tissue, the obese patient is at increased risk for delayed healing and infection. Mobility may also be a problem, placing the obese patient at risk for pneumonia or deep venous thrombosis.

Caloric requirements are directly related to weight, so obese patients need more calories for maintenance than persons of normal weight. On the other hand, given equal health, the obese person's ability to tolerate prolonged starvation is better than the person of normal weight because of greater fat stores.

The excess weight of an obese patient does not necessarily reflect adequate nutritional health. Protein deficiency as well as low levels of vitamins and minerals may be present. Because weight is greater than normal, nutritional evaluation of obese persons is often incorrectly deferred (Gallagher, 2003). Obese patients with a wound needs exogenous nutrients to heal, so a weight-loss diet is generally not recommended. To support wound healing, the priority in care is to meet the caloric, protein, and nutritional needs of the obese patient (Collins, 2003).

Nutrient Needs for Healing

Normal healing requires adequate protein, fat, and carbohydrates, as well as vitamins and minerals. Deficiencies in any of the nutrients may result in impaired or delayed healing. The specific alteration may vary, in part, according to the defect (e.g., protein is needed for antibody formation). Normally, dietary intake provides the building blocks for repair and tissue replacement. Most diets are a combination of protein, carbohydrate, fat, vitamins, and minerals, so deficiencies of individual nutrients are uncommon. A balanced diet is ideal, as no single nutrient has been shown to accelerate healing (Langer et al, 2003). When nutrient intake is not adequate, a referral is made and the dietician performs an individual evaluation and makes a dietary recommendation.

With injury, more calories and substrates are needed for healing than in an uninjured state. Calories are needed purely for the energy needs of the body, that is, walking, breathing, and so on. About one half to three fifths of an individual's caloric needs are met through carbohydrates, 20% to 25% through fats, and the remainder derives from protein.

Carbohydrates are turned to glucose and are available immediately for ATP formation. They provide the energy for phagocytosis and the development of collagen. Glucose levels must be kept within normal limits to facilitate healing; excessive levels result in impaired healing. Glucose is important to prevent the use of protein as an energy source. Fats are important for development and stability of cell membranes (both intracellular and cell wall). Fats also participate actively in various aspects of the inflammatory response to injury and thus in healing. The type of fat ingested determines the type of prostaglandins produced.

Omega-3 fatty acids favor prostaglandins-E3 (PGE_3) and leukotrienes, and they participate in inflammation, vasoconstriction, and platelet aggregation. Omega-6 fatty acids generate a preponderance of PGE_1 and PGE_2, vasodilators, and antiinflammatory agents (Lewis, 2002).

Protein needs are disproportionally increased after injury, and a protein deficiency can prolong a person's healing time (MacKay and Miller, 2003). Proteins are made of amino acids and are necessary to generate acute phase proteins, including collagen and proteoglycans (Lewis, 2002). Arginine, a nonessential amino acid, is necessary for healing because it supports the immune response for collagen formation (Williams and Barbul, 2003). Arginine cannot be metabolized at an adequate rate in times of metabolic stress and therefore must be provided exogenously (Collins, 2004). Similarly, glutamine cannot be produced at an adequate rate during times of stress and, when provided exogenously, plays an important role in protein-sparing. Older adults are often protein-deficient since they have proportionally greater daily protein requirements than younger persons; at the same time, their intake of protein is often inadequate. During times of limited intake, the older adult is at risk for undernutrition (Zulkowski and Albrecht, 2003).

All of the vitamins are needed for tissue repair and regeneration because of their various functions in normal cellular metabolism (Table 8-3). Vitamins A and C are especially critical in healing. Vitamin A is fat-soluble and important in various steps in the deposition of collagen. Collagen is the most important component in scar formation and maintaining wound closure. In persons treated with corticosteroids, Vitamin A is an important antagonist; it reverses all the effects of corticosteroids except their impairment of contracture.

Vitamin C is a water-soluble vitamin. It is a cofactor in collagen formation and functions to enable complement to perform its functions. Vitamin C works synergistically with vitamin E to prevent oxidative cell damage. Lack of vitamin C can result in impaired collagen formation. Should vitamin C intake cease, it takes 2 to 3 months for stores to become depleted.

Among the minerals, zinc and iron have received the most attention in the context of wound healing. Zinc is important because of its role in enzyme systems, immunocompetence, and collagen formation (Lewis, 2002). Zinc supplementation enhances collagen formation in those with zinc deficiency. In persons with normal zinc levels, supplementation has not been shown to alter healing. Supplementation in those who are not in need may result in disruption of normal phagocytic activity, and it may cause copper deficiency. Copper deficiency may result in weaker scar tissue and decreased tensile strength.

Iron is important in hemoglobin for transport of oxygen. Persons with anemia who are not able to compensate for low oxygen with increased circulation rates may experience impaired collagen formation and ineffective phagocytic activity.

Water and balanced electrolytes are the sea in which these various nutrients function. Adequate hydration and electrolytes provide the physiologic space in which healing can occur.

NUTRITIONAL ASSESSMENT

Nutritional assessment is the basis for subsequent therapy. It identifies the presence of or risk for malnutrition and specific nutrient deficiencies. The data derived from a nutritional assessment provide the basis for developing a nutritional plan. Nutritional assessment can be performed using an instrument specifically designed for diagnosis of malnutrition or by combining the results of the history, physical examination, and laboratory work. The history and physical examination are the oldest and probably the most widely used evaluations of nutritional status. Initial nutritional assessment provides baseline data regarding a person's nutritional status and should be done at admission or as early as possible following admission (Shepherd, 2003). The Joint Commission for Accreditation of Health Care Organizations recommends nutritional assessment within 24 hours of admission (JCAHO, 2003). Reassessments reflect changes in status and effects of interventions. For those who are in acute care, stays of greater than a week necessitate nutritional reassessment. In the nursing home, weight loss or a change in status precipitate nutritional reassessment. In homecare, it is important to be vigilant to changes in patient status and incorporate nutritional parameters as the situation warrants.

The nurse often is the first person to perform the nutritional assessment. If the nurse fails to recognize nutritional risk or malnutrition, the patient may not be referred for a period and may experience deterioration

TABLE 8-3 The Role of Nutrients in Wound Healing

NUTRIENT	ROLE IN HEALING
Protein	Fibroplasia
	Angiogenesis
	Collagen formation and wound remodeling
	Immune function
	Precursor nitric oxide
Carbohydrates	Energy supply
	Protein sparing
	By-product of lactate
	Angiogenesis
Fat	Formation and stability of cell walls and intracellular organelles
	Inflammation
Vitamin A*	Epithelialization
	Wound closure
	Inflammatory response
	Angiogenesis
	Collagen formation
B vitamins	Cofactor in enzyme systems
	Immune response
	Synthesis of protein, fat, and carbohydrate
Vitamin C	Collagen synthesis
	Capillary wall integrity
	Fibroblast function
	Immunologic function
	Antioxidant
Vitamin D*	Calcium metabolism for building and maintaining bone
Vitamin E*	Unknown in relation to wound healing
	Antioxidant
Vitamin K*	Coagulation
Copper	Cross-linking of collagen
	Erythropoiesis
Iron	Collagen formation
	Leukocyte function
	Oxygen transport
Magnesium	Protein synthesis
Zinc	Collagen formation
	Protein synthesis
	Cell membrane stability
	Host defenses

*Fat-soluble vitamins.

during that period. Referral may be made to a dietician or a multidisciplinary nutritional support team (dieticians, nurses, pharmacists, physicians).

Nutritional Assessment Tools

When a specific nutritional tool is incorporated into assessment, it is important to select an approach that is easy to use, can be implemented by the members of the team, and has sufficient reliability and validity to accurately identify any problems. Samples of nutritional assessment tools will be provided in Appendix C and discussed in this section. The *Nutritional Screening Initiative* is one such tool. Developed for use with geriatric patients (deGroot et al, 1998), this tool includes a nutritional screening that can be performed during annual provider visits and at regular intervals. The screening instrument explores social and environmental factors such as whether the person eats alone, drinks alcohol, and has enough money to buy food. Identification of those individuals at risk triggers a more comprehensive assessment including a nutritional assessment, functional assessment, and evaluation for depression. The screening is easy to use on a regular basis and can be completed by the patient. The professional is able to take the data from the screening and perform more detailed assessment to quantify the nature of the nutritional problem. The assessment is the basis for problem identification and mobilizing the resources that are appropriate to meet the specific needs identified.

Another nutritional assessment tool is the *Mini Nutritional Assessment (MNA)*. The MNA is a reliable and valid 18-item tool consisting of anthropometric assessment, general assessment, dietary assessment, and subjective assessment. It is completed in a variety of health care settings and has been shown to detect malnutrition, especially in an elderly population (Guigoz, Lauque, and Vellas, 2002; Ruiz-Lopez et al, 2003).

Subjective Global Assessment (SGA) has been advocated as a strategy to assess nutritional status. It involves a focused history and physical examination where the parameters for assessment are delineated. At the end of the data collection, the examiner determines whether the person has (1) no malnutrition, (2) possible or mild malnutrition, or (3) significant malnutrition (Hoffer, 2001). Validity and reliability of this approach have been established, but the subjective nature of the analysis requires more sophisticated skills and more time than a staff nurse normally would have during admission. An advanced practice nurse, a physician, or the nutritional support team more frequently uses this assessment.

Patient History

Most information about a patient is derived from the history, and it gives focus to the physical examination and laboratory work. Many admission assessments structure how the history is taken and it is important to cluster significant dimensions to determine whether nutritional risk or deficit is present.

The *history* provides a chronologic picture of the person's nutritional health. Initially, the person's chief complaint and present illnesses are elicited. General health, major adult illnesses, and childhood illnesses are elicited. Prior surgery, functional limitations, and emotional status are all evaluated as related to nutrient intake. The social history is important, including personal history, home conditions, and environment. The history concludes with a review of systems (Seidel et al, 2002).

Conditions or diseases that have produced alterations in ingestion, digestion, absorption, and metabolism are elicited with the history. Box 8-1 lists common conditions that suggest malnutrition is present or may be a risk factor.

Issues related to obtaining and preparing food may also affect intake. These include limited income, environment at mealtime, social isolation, inability to purchase and prepare meals, and educational level. Specific information obtained by history includes usual weight, weight changes, change in the pattern

---

BOX 8-1 Risk Factors for Malnutrition

- Conditions that cause hypermetabolism
- Treatment with immunosuppressive drugs
- Weight loss
- Changes in appetite
- Food intolerances
- Dietary restrictions
- Lack of teeth, or poorly fitting dentures
- Inability to feed oneself
- Altered smell or taste
- Need to restrict intake for tests

or variety of food ingested, changes in appetite, and signs and symptoms of related problems (e.g., nausea, vomiting, anorexia, and diarrhea).

Physical Examination

Generally, the information gleamed from the patient's history will help to guide the type of assessments that are warranted during the physical examination. While no single physical finding is diagnostic of malnutrition, many different signs and symptoms are associated with specific nutritional alterations such as coarse hair or thin skin (Table 8-4). These are not specific, so the examiner must consider explanations other than nutritional alterations for the findings, such as disease process, medication side effects, metabolic alterations, age-related alterations, and the half-life of nutrients suspected as being deficient. Physical findings are often used to confirm suspicions raised with the history or the laboratory work. For those at risk of or with early malnutrition, the physical findings for malnutrition may be subtle or absent, because some signs do not appear until the malnutrition becomes advanced. With overt malnutrition, anthropometric changes often are key findings. Furthermore, obese patients are especially difficult to evaluate because their weight may mask the skeletal muscle wasting of malnutrition (Kyle et al, 2002).

Anthropometric measures are easy to perform and are pivotal in the evaluation of nutritional status. A person's hydration status is also taken into account, since total body water can affect anthropometric measures such as weight (Williams and Barbul, 2003; Thomas et al, 2000). Anthropometric parameters include weight, midarm muscle circumference, skin-fold measurements, and head circumference (Box 8-2).

Weight is the cornerstone in the diagnosis of malnutrition and can be used alone or in relation to height or frame size. Box 8-3 lists examples of weight-related indicators of malnutrition. Weight is often considered in relation to height. Recent tables for interpretation of these parameters are based on the National Research Council data on weight and height, the dietary guidelines, and the body mass index (BMI). The BMI is calculated by dividing weight in kilograms by height in meters squared and most often is used to determine whether people are underweight or overweight. BMI is a predictor of morbidity and mortality (Gallagher, 2003; Collins, 2001a). BMI is not always perfectly correlated with fat distribution; therefore it should be considered

---

BOX 8-2 Nutritional Assessment: Anthropometric Measures

Weight
Height
Body Mass Index (BMI)
Mid-upper arm circumference (measures muscle mass, bones and skin)
Midarm muscle circumference (measures lean body mass)
Skin fold (measures fat stores)
Head circumference (measures child's growth)

BOX 8-3 Weight-Related Indicators of Malnutrition

- A loss of 10% of usual weight in the last 3 months
- Body weight <90% of ideal body weight, *or*
- Body mass index (BMI) <18.5 kg/meter^2

From Halsted, 2001-2004.

TABLE 8-4 Physical Findings Associated with Nutritional Deficiencies

	SIGNS AND SYMPTOMS	RELATED NUTRITIONAL DEFICIENCY
SKIN MANIFESTATIONS	Dermatitis	Protein, calories, zinc, vitamin A
	Petechiae (Plate 29)	Vitamin C
MUSCLES	Weakness	Protein, calories
	Weight loss, wasting	Protein, calories
MOUTH	Glossitis	Riboflavin, niacin
	Bleeding	Vitamins A, C, and K

in conjunction with other assessment findings (Kyle et al, 2002). Also, the Centers for Disease Control and Prevention (CDC) advise that age and sex can affect the relationship between BMI and body fat in that women and older persons have a greater proportion of fat than do younger persons or men.

Arm muscle circumference and skin-fold measurement were initially employed in underdeveloped countries using only very basic instruments to evaluate the nutritional status of the population (Jeliffe, 1966). There are standards in the United States for specific age groups and for a limited number of minority populations (Frisancho, 1984; Gray and Gray, 1979; Marshall et al, 1999). Mid-upper arm circumference (MAC) is a measure of muscle mass, bones, and skin. It is used to calculate midarm muscle circumference (MAMC) as a measure of lean body mass (Stotts and Bergstrom, 2004). A decrease in arm muscle mass occurs with muscle disease and nutritional deficiencies.

Fat stores are measured with skin-fold measures. A skin-fold caliper is used to evaluate skin-fold thickness. Several sites are possible to use such as scapula, waist, and triceps; the triceps site is most frequently used. Fat stores do not change rapidly, thus skin-fold thickness is not a sensitive measure of malnutrition. It may be a useful measure in older adults, where body weight is stable or perhaps even increased, yet the lean mass is decreasing and fat content increasing (Bond and Heitkemper, 2003). Dieticians, advanced practice nurses, and the specialized nutritional support team may perform arm muscle circumference and skin-fold measurements, and low levels documented in the progress report indicate undernutrition.

Head circumference is used in children to evaluate their growth. Measurements are compared with tables of norms, allowing head size to be classified in percentiles. Chronic undernutrition results in a delay in the growth of the head, and its identification and treatment are important so that permanent damage does not occur (Mascarenhas, Zemel, and Stallings, 1998). Although performed primarily by dieticians, it is important to understand what the tests measure to appreciate the relevance of the findings.

Laboratory Data

Biochemical parameters reflect the end product of ingestion, digestion, absorption, and metabolism of nutrients.

Biochemical measurements offer a simple and minimally invasive strategy to evaluate nutritional status.

Serum proteins are biochemical indicators of malnutrition (Stotts and Bergstrom, 2004). They are synthesized by the liver and vary primarily in their rate of turnover. Table 8-5 lists the serum protein measures frequently used to evaluate protein status. Hydration status is important to the validity of all of them, with dehydration producing falsely elevated serum levels and overhydration producing false negative values. It should be noted that posture and circadian rhythm can also affect hydration and the accuracy of the values.

Serum albumin is probably the most frequently measured of these laboratory parameters. Albumin has a long half-life (18 to 20 days), is not sensitive to rapid changes in nutritional status, and in prolonged and premorbid starvation its levels fall only late (Bond and Heitkemper, 2003; Stotts and Bergstrom, 2004). Serum albumin is not an appropriate measurement to use for the diagnosis of either recent or mild-to-moderate malnutrition. Decreased albumin levels have long been associated with increased morbidity and mortality in medical and surgical patients (Seltzer et al, 1979) and intensive care patients (Seltzer et al, 1981).

It takes at least 2 to 3 weeks of nutritional treatment to raise albumin levels. Since albumin is formed in the liver, liver function should be considered when evaluating albumin levels. Liver disease causes the hepatocytes to lose their capacity to synthesize albumin (Collins, 2001b).

Transferrin, another component frequently measured to evaluate protein status, has a shorter half-life (8 to 10 days) and a smaller body pool. Its major function is to transport iron. Usually about one third of the body's transferrin is bound to iron. Transferrin level is affected by many factors other than protein-calorie malnutrition, so it is not sufficiently sensitive or specific

TABLE 8-5 Plasma Protein Levels: Normal and with Malnutrition

VISCERAL PROTEIN	NORMAL	MALNUTRITION
Serum albumin	3.5-5.5 g/dl	<3.5 g/dl
Transferrin	200-400 mg/dl	≤100 mg/dl
Prealbumin	16-35 mg/dl	<16 mg/dl

to be a meaningful measurement. For example, a deficiency of iron such as that frequently seen with protein-calorie malnutrition stimulates hepatic synthesis, so very high levels result. At the other extreme, inflammatory states, liver disease, and some anemias result in depressed transferrin levels (Stotts and Bergstrom, 2004).

Prealbumin is a plasma protein with a short half-life (2 days). It is also known as thyroxin-binding prealbumin and transthyretin (Stotts and Bergstrom, 2004). It is involved in thyroxine and vitamin A transport. Because of its short half-life, prealbumin decreases quickly when protein or calorie intake is decreased. In contrast, it responds quickly when exogenous nutrients are provided. Prealbumin is an excellent measure of nutritional status because it reflects not only what has been ingested but also what has been able to be absorbed, digested, and metabolized. On the other hand, prealbumin is sensitive to the inflammatory response and decreases rapidly with a decrease in protein synthesis.

Less commonly measured, retinol-binding protein is a plasma protein with a very short half-life (12 hours) and very low serum levels. It participates in the transport of vitamin A, and its response follows that of prealbumin. Although it has a theoretic advantage over other plasma proteins by virtue of its short half-life, its low normal values and the technical difficulties in its measurement have limited its usefulness compared to other measures of nutrient status (Stotts and Bergstrom, 2004).

Creatinine levels are another measure of protein status that has been used for more than 20 years in nutritional support settings to evaluate lean body mass. Since creatinine gives an indirect measure of skeletal muscle mass, it is considered to be a measure of long-term protein status (Bond and Heitkemper, 2003). Creatinine assessment is complex because it requires normal renal function and urinary output, the ability to accurately collect a 24-hour urine, adequate hydration, and that the patient not be on prolonged periods of bedrest and not have had a recent high-protein meal. Nutritional status is evaluated using a 24-hour urine creatinine excretion divided by normal creatinine for height, producing a creatinine height index (CHI). CHI of 40% to 60% reflects minimal protein depletion whereas a CHI of less than 40% indicates severe nutrition depletion (Lewis, 2002). Age-specific tables are used to interpret the findings.

Basic to the discussion of protein status is the concept of nitrogen balance. The concept is that nitrogen turnover is in balance (i.e., intake and loss from the body are carefully regulated and under normal nutritional circumstances closely approximate each other). Anabolism and repair require positive nitrogen balance. Negative nitrogen balance is a reflection of catabolism.

The immune system is very sensitive to protein status because protein is a major constituent of immune system components such as antibodies and lymphocytes. Consequently, gross tests of immune function, such as total lymphocyte count (TLC), also reflect protein status. Lymphocytes constitute a variable percentage of the circulating white blood cells and are reported in a white blood cell differential. The TLC is calculated by multiplying the percentage of lymphocytes by the white cell count. The normal level is 1500 to 3000 cells/mm^3. Below-normal levels may be a reflection of malnutrition; however, TLC may also be depressed by chemotherapy, autoimmune diseases, stress, and infection, including HIV (Lewis, 2002; Stotts and Bergstrom, 2004).

Evaluation of hydration status is an integral part of nutritional assessment. Table 8-6 lists laboratory measures of adequate and inadequate hydration.

TABLE 8-6 **Laboratory Measures of Adequate Hydration**

LAB TEST	NORMAL VALUES	DEHYDRATION
Serum sodium	135-150 mEq/L	>150 mEq/L
Osmolality	285 to 295 mOsm/kg H$_2$O	>295 mOsm/kg H$_2$O
Blood urea nitrogen (BUN)*	7 to 23 mg/dl	Elevated
BUN-Creatinine ratio	10:1	>25:1
Urine specific gravity	1.003 to 1.028	>1.028

*In the absence of renal insufficiency/failure.

NUTRITIONAL SUPPORT

Referral for Definitive Nutritional Support

The patient at risk for or with existing malnutrition needs to be brought to the attention of the health care team so that appropriate nutrients are provided. Depending on the individual institution's system, the appropriate action is to refer the patient to the dietician and notify the physician of the findings, or call the nutritional support team.

Nutritional Support for Persons with Wounds

Nutritional support therapy should provide a balanced intake of necessary nutrients based on the person's energy and protein requirements. Because a person's nutritional needs are dependent on many variables (such as age, sex, height, weight, presence of severe wasting or obesity, current disease state, severity of illness, and the presence and severity of a wound), it may be an oversimplification to give a range of calories and protein that a patient with wounds will require.

It is useful to remember that a healthy person requires approximately 0.8 g of protein per kilogram per 24 hours. Our best data about needs come from the pressure ulcer literature, where it is estimated that persons with pressure ulcers need more protein, about 1.0-1.5 g protein/kg of body weight/24 hr for total protein. Caloric needs must be individualized but are about 35 to 40 calories/kg of body weight/24 hr for total calories (AHCPR, 1994). In general, a patient with a wound needs adequate calories and increased amounts of protein (1.25 to 2.0 g/kg/24 hr). Daily vitamin and mineral needs also are increased to 1600 to 2000 retinol equivalents of vitamin A, 100 to 1000 mg of vitamin C, 15 to 30 mg of zinc, 200% of the recommended dietary allowance (RDA) of the B vitamins, and 20 to 30 mg of iron (Beers and Berkow, 1999-2004). There is some discussion in the literature about over-feeding patients. The issue arises from the fact that we don't know exactly what the needs of patients are. This is an especially important problem in acutely ill persons with unstable metabolic status, where excess calories may result in increased levels of carbon dioxide, acidosis, and impaired recovery (McClave, Snider, and Spain, 1999).

The preferred route of support is oral and, whenever possible, the gastrointestinal tract should be used for feeding. If the patient's intake is not adequate with oral feeding, then one of the various approaches to the gastrointestinal tract used for tube feedings is selected to supplement or supplant the oral feeding. When the gastrointestinal tract cannot be used, parenteral nutrition is the route of choice. Further information on management of persons using nutritional support is available in several textbooks (Halsted, 2001-2004; Beers and Berkow, 1999-2004).

SUMMARY

Nutritional assessment and support play an important role in wound healing. All patients with wounds should have their nutritional status evaluated. A thorough nutritional assessment should reveal the risk for or presence of malnutrition and provide the necessary information to develop an individualized nutritional plan of care. The nutritional status should be evaluated at baseline and at regular intervals to determine the effectiveness of the nutritional plan.

SELF-ASSESSMENT EXERCISE

1. Which of the following is a usual result of major penetrating traumatic injuries with associated wounds?
   a. Increased metabolic rate for 10 to 14 days after injury
   b. Decreased metabolic rate to help conserve energy for the first 2 to 5 days after injury
   c. Decreased metabolic rate for 48 hours, and then increased for the following 10 to 14 days
   d. Unknown metabolic consequences (cannot be determined without more information)

2. Which of the following permits definitive diagnosis of malnutrition?
   a. 10-pound weight loss in 1 year
   b. BMI ≤ 16
   c. Albumin 4.0 g/dl
   d. Petechiae

3. FD is a 65-year-old male who is retired and lives alone. He is healthy except for a venous ulcer on his high leg, and he needs a "water pill for his high blood pressure." He does not eat breakfast or lunch but goes to the local restaurant every evening for dinner. Over the past 3 months he has lost 15 pounds. Your initial suspicion is that he has which of the following?
   a. Protein-calorie malnutrition
   b. Protein malnutrition
   c. Depression
   d. Chronic dehydration

4. Which of the following explains why obesity is a risk factor for poor healing?
   a. Fat is more poorly perfused than lean tissue.
   b. Many obese people are dehydrated.
   c. Obese persons are often hypotensive.
   d. Skin is pulled tight by obesity.

5. Which of the following are symptoms of brief starvation with hypermetabolism?
   a. Slow weight loss and low albumin
   b. Slow weight loss and normal albumin
   c. Rapid weight loss and low albumin
   d. Rapid weight loss and normal albumin

6. Which of the following findings in the history indicate risk of malnutrition?
   a. Eating alone
   b Inability to prepare one's own food
   c. Low income
   d. All of the above

7. Vitamin C is essential to which of the following?
   a. WBC synthesis
   b. Collagen formation
   c. Angiogenesis
   d. Cell wall formation

8. Which of the following describes protein needs for repair after injury?
   a. They decrease because of reduced BMR.
   b. They decrease to conserve losses.
   c. They increase to provide energy for basal functions.
   d. They increase to support anabolism.

9. What is the ideal way to feed a person with a healing wound?
   a. Enterally with an NG tube because it is the least time consuming
   b. Parenterally because of the low infection rate and reduced risk of aspiration
   c. Orally because it maintains gut function and enhances independence
   d. It doesn't matter—there is no ideal in feeding a person with a wound.

10. Anabolism over the last 2 to 3 days of feeding with either enteral or parenteral nutrition is most accurately evaluated with which of the following?
   a. Weight change
   b. Serum albumin
   c. Blood urea nitrogen (BUN)-creatinine level
   d. Prealbumin

REFERENCES

Agency for Health Care Policy and Research (AHCPR): *Treatment of pressure ulcers in adults*, Rockville, MD, 1994, U. S. Department of Health and Human Services, AHCPR Publication No. 95-0652.

Beers MH, Berkow R, editors: *The Merck Manual*, ed 17, On-line, 1999-2004, http://www.merck.com/mrkshared/mmanual/home.jsp

Bond EF, Heitkemper MH: Protein-calorie malnutrition. In Carrieri-Kohlman V, Lindsey AM, West CM, editors: *Pathophysiological phenomena in nursing: human responses to illness*, St. Louis, 2003, Saunders.

Brugler L, DiPrinzio MJ, Bernstein L: The five-year evolution of a malnutrition treatment program in a community hospital, *Jt Comm J Qual Improv* 4:191, 1999.

Collins N: Assessment and treatment of involuntary weight loss and protein-calorie malnutrition, *Adv Skin Wound Care* 13(Suppl 1):4, 2001a.

Collins, N: The difference between albumin and prealbumin, *Adv Skin Wound Care* 14(5):235, 2001b.

Collins N: Obesity and wound healing, *Adv Skin Wound Care* 16(1):45, 2003.

Collins N: Arginine and wound healing, *Adv Skin Wound Care* 14(1):16, 2004.

deGroot LC et al: Evaluating DETERMINE Your Nutritional Health Checklist and the Mini Nutritional Assessment tool to identify nutritional problems in elderly Europeans, *Eur J Clin Nutr* 52(12):877, 1998.

Frisancho AR: New standards of weight and body composition by frame size and height for assessment of nutritional status of adults and the elderly, *Am J Clin Nutr* 40:808, 1984.

Gallagher S, Gates JL: Obesity, panniculitis, panniculectomy, and wound care: understanding the challenges, *J WOCN* 30(6):334, 2003.

Gray GE, Gray LK: Validity of anthropometric norms used in the assessment of hospitalized patients, *J Parenter Enteral Nutr* 3:366, 1979.

Guigoz Y, Laugue S, Vellas BJ: Identifying the elderly at risk for malnutrition: The Mini Nutritional Assessment, *Clin Geriatr Med* 18(4):737, 2002.

Halsted CH: Malnutrition and nutritional assessment. In Braunwald E et al, editors: *Harrison's Principles of Internal Medicine*, ed 15, On-line. 2001-2004. University of California San Francisco Web site: http://harrisons.accessmedicine.com/server-java/Arknoid/amed/harrison, Accessed July 10, 2004.

Hoffer LJ: Clinical nutrition: 1. Protein-energy malnutrition in the inpatient, *CMAJ* 165(19):1345, 2001.

Jeliffe DB: Direct nutritional assessment of human groups. In *The Assessment of Nutritional Status of the Community*, Geneva, Switzerland, World Health Organization Monograph, No. 53, 1966.

Joint Commission on Accreditation of Healthcare Organizations (JCAHO): Comprehensive accreditation manual for hospitals: the official handbook (CAMH), Chicago, 2003, Author.

Kyle UG et al: Body composition of 995 acutely ill or chronically ill patients at hospital admission: a controlled population study, *J Am Diet Assoc* 102(7):944, 2002.

Langer G et al: Nutritional interventions for preventing and treating pressure ulcers (Cochrane review). In: *The Cochrane Library*, Issue 2, Chichester, UK, 2003, John Wiley & Sons.

Lewis B: Nutrition and wound healing. In Kloth LC, McCulloch, JM, editors: *Wound healing: alternatives in management*, ed 3, Philadelphia, 2002, FA Davis.

MacKay D, Miller AL: Nutrition support for wound healing, *Altern Med Rev* 8(4):359, 2003.

Marshall JA et al: Indicators of nutritional risk in a rural elderly Hispanic and non-Hispanic white population: San Luis Valley Health and Aging Study, *J Am Diet Assoc* 99(3):315, 1999.

Mascarenhas MR, Zemel B, Stallings VA: Nutritional assessment in pediatrics, *Nutrition* 14(1):105, 1998.

Mathison CJ: Skin and wound care challenges in the hospitalized morbidly obese patient, *J WOCN* 30(2):78, 2003.

McClave SA, Snider HL, Spain DA: Preoperative issues in clinical nutrition, *Chest* 115:64S, 1999.

Ruiz-Lopez MD et al: Nutritional risk in institutionalized older women determined by the mini nutritional assessment test: what are the main factors? *Nutrition* 19(9):767, 2003.

Seidel HM et al, editors: *Mosby's guide to physical assessment*, Philadelphia, 2002, Mosby.

Seiler WO: Clinical pictures of malnutrition in ill elderly subjects, *Nutrition* 17(6):496, 2001.

Seltzer MH et al: Instant nutritional assessment, *J Parenter Enteral Nutr* 3(3):157, 1979.

Seltzer MH et al: Instant nutritional assessment in the intensive care unit, *JPEN J Parenter Enteral Nutr* 5(1):70, 1981.

Shepherd A: Nutrition for optimum wound healing, *Nurs Standard* 18(6):55, 2003.

Stotts NA, Bergstrom N: Measuring dietary intake and nutritional outcomes. In Frank-Stromborg M, Olsen SJ, editors: *Instruments for health-care research*, ed 3, Sudbury, Mass, 2004, Jones and Bartlett.

Thomas DR et al: Nutritional management in long-term care: development of a clinical guideline. Council for nutritional strategies in long-term care, *J Gerontol A Biol Sci Med Sci* 55(12):M725, 2000.

Williams JZ, Barbul A: Nutrition and wound healing, *Surg Clin North Am* 83(3):571, 2003.

Zulkowski K, Albrecht D: How nutrition and aging affect wound healing, *Nursing* 33(8):70, 2003.

9

Wound Infection: Diagnosis and Management

....

NANCY A. STOTTS

OBJECTIVES

1. Identify four reasons that wound infection is a significant problem.
2. Compare and contrast contamination, colonization, critical colonization, and wound infection.
3. Describe the pathophysiology of wound infection.
4. Describe the concept and relevance of wound bioburden.
5. Compare and contrast signs and symptoms of infection in acute and chronic wounds.
6. Identify risk factors for wound infection.
7. Propose how to obtain a wound culture by biopsy, aspiration, and swab.
8. Interpret laboratory data indicative of a wound infection.
9. Understand the interaction among the host defenses, the organism's defenses, and the environment in the development of wound infection.
10. Understand therapies frequently used to treat wound infection.

INFECTION AS A SIGNIFICANT PROBLEM

Wound infection is a serious problem. It results in increased admission to critical care, length of hospital stay, cost of care, and death (Fleischmann et al, 2003; Kirkland et al, 1999). Osteomyelitis may occur and increase the patient's risk of bacteremia, sepsis, and multisystem organ failure (Bonham, 2001).

Acute and chronic wounds are both at risk of infection. Acute wounds are those that have a rapid onset and normally heal as predicted (Lazarus et al, 1994). Surgical wounds are the predominant acute wound. More than 20 million surgeries are performed in the United States each year, and about 2.8% of those develop surgical site infection (Barie, 2002; Hall and Defrances, 2001). In fact, infection is the most frequent postsurgical complication, seen in about 38%

of those diagnosed with nosocomial infection. Most deaths caused by wound infection involve infections of organs or body cavities (Mangram et al, 1999).

One study conducted in a community hospital showed that surgical patients from all specialties with surgical site infection are admitted to an intensive care unit 60% more often than those without surgical site infection. Death was twice as frequent, and readmission to the hospital was 5 times more likely to occur in those with surgical site infection compared to patients without (Kirkland et al, 1999).

Chronic wounds do not heal in a timely manner for a return to full function and structural integrity (Lazarus et al, 1994). Major types of chronic wounds are pressure ulcers, vascular ulcers, diabetic ulcers, traumatic wounds, ischemic arterial ulcers, and nonhealing surgical wounds. Chronic wounds are a prevalent problem, as can be seen from the data on pressure ulcers, vascular ulcers, and diabetic ulcers. The prevalence of stage II or deeper pressure ulcers is 1.2% to 11.3% (Allman, 1997). In long-term care, about 10% of residents have one or more pressure ulcers on admission (Baumgarten et al, 2003).

Vascular disease results in alterations in blood flow, often to the lower extremities. About 70% to 80% of vascular ulcers are venous, 10% to 15% are arterial, and the rest are mixed. Trauma to ischemic lower extremities results in an ulcer. The underlying vascular pathology produces a relative hypoxia that contributes to delayed healing and infection (Falanga, 2004; Schultz et al, 2003; Stadelmann, Digenis, and Tobin, 1998).

Diabetic patients are at risk for foot ulcer infection because of hyperglycemia and neuropathy. The ulcer often occurs because of repeated trauma to an insensate foot, frequently without the awareness of the individual. Necrosis occurs deep in the foot architecture, and when the wound necrosis extends through to the skin, the wound becomes contaminated. The wound often is deep, warm, and full of necrotic material, an ideal environment to support organisms. Cultures often show multiple organisms, including gram-positive and gram-negative organisms, aerobes, and anaerobes (Steed, 2004). Amputation may be needed because of uncontrolled infection in the lower extremities of persons with diabetes. Chapter 16 provides more detail about infection in the patient with a neuropathic wound.

BIOBURDEN AS A CONCEPT

The presence of bacteria in the wound creates a burden on the wound healing process. This burden is due to the fact that bacteria compete for the limited supply of oxygen and nutrients in the wound. Bioburden refers to more than just the total number of bacteria present; diversity, virulence, and interaction of organisms with each other and the body are also integral to the negative impact of microorganisms in the wound. Achieving sterility in a wound is not possible, so the objective must be to achieve a host-manageable bioburden.

MICROBIAL STATES OF A WOUND (INFECTION CONTINUUM)

Initially the wound is contaminated by aerobic and anaerobic bacteria. Over a short period, the microbial environment increases and becomes more diverse (polymicrobial). See Figure 9-1.

Contamination

Contamination is the presence of nonreplicating microorganisms on the wound surface. Contaminating microorganisms arise from normal flora (e.g., skin, peri-wound), external environment (e.g., bed linen, devices), and endogenous sources (e.g., feces, urine). The contaminants themselves are not visible to care providers and do not elicit a response from the body.

Colonization

Colonization refers to the presence of replicating bacteria without a host reaction or clinical signs and symptoms of infection. It is important to note that the bacteria in this phase are not pathogenic and do not necessitate treatment with systemic or local antibiotics. Inappropriate use of antibiotics during this phase is

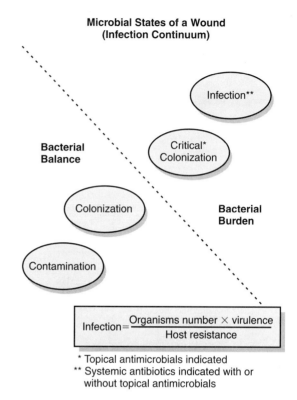

Microbial States of a Wound (Infection Continuum)

$$Infection = \frac{Organisms\ number \times virulence}{Host\ resistance}$$

* Topical antimicrobials indicated
** Systemic antibiotics indicated with or without topical antimicrobials

Fig. 9-1 Microbial states of a wound (infection continuum).

one of the many factors that have contributed to the prevalence of antibiotic-resistant organisms.

Critical Colonization

As the wound bioburden increases and further overwhelms the host, the wound reaches a period of critical colonization. Critical colonization is a term recently coined to describe a wound that is arrested in healing as a result of the bioburden (Bowler, Duerden and Armstrong, 2001; Edwards and Harding, 2004; Sibbald et al, 2001). During the critical colonization state, organisms remain on the surface of the wound and have not yet invaded the soft tissue. Therefore, systemic response to the microbial load (i.e., fever or leukocytosis) is not present. Visually, granulation tissue may not appear healthy. For example, the wound appear clean but not granular, lacking the red cobblestone appearance indicative of healthy granulation tissue (see Plate 5). Interestingly, the microorganisms that colonize wounds do not always match the microorganisms that actually cause wound infection (Bowler, Duerden, and Armstrong, 2001). Important indicators of this phase must be identified so that progression to infection can be prevented through appropriate use of topical antimicrobials.

Infection

Infection is present when microorganisms invade tissues and there is a systemic response to them (Edwards and Harding, 2004; Mangram et al, 1999; Robson, 1997). The clinical presentation of wound infection depends on whether the wound is acute or chronic as well as on the ability of the host to mount an inflammatory response.

Infected *acute* wounds usually demonstrate signs of local inflammation and pus formation or increased exudate. When cultured, infection in acute wounds is diagnosed by the presence of 10^5 microorganisms per gram of tissue or greater, or the presence of any level of β–hemolytic streptococcus (Falanga, 2004; Mangram et al, 1999; Robson, 1997).

Infection in *chronic* wounds is often subtle, as seen in change in the exudate, increased pain, and delayed healing (Bowler, Duerden, and Armstrong, 2001; Edwards and Harding, 2004; Gardner et al, 2001). Box 9-1 lists signs and symptoms of infection in chronic wounds. Chronic wounds are usually polymicrobial and characterized by high levels of resident bacteria. If the organisms are gram-negative as often is seen with chronic wounds, unusual odor occurs. Fever and leukocytosis may

be present. Occasionally with infection, hypothermia is seen, indicating a poor central nervous system response and poor potential for a positive outcome. Generally, it is agreed that culture results for chronic wound infections show more than 10^5 organisms per gram of tissue, or as few as 10^3 organisms/gram of tissue if a virulent organism such as β-hemolytic streptococcus is present (Edwards and Harding, 2004; Robson, 1997).

In older persons, infection in acute and chronic wounds may present merely as changes in cognitive level and a subtle decrease in activity level (Johnson, Lyons, and Covinsky, 2003). Further investigation is needed in older people to make the definitive diagnosis of wound infection.

FACTORS THAT EFFECT THE MICROBIAL STATE OF A CHRONIC WOUND

Host Defenses

Infection occurs when the homeostatic balance among the host, the organism, and the environment is disrupted. An intact dermal layer is the host's first line of defense. With wounds the protection offered by the skin is lost. Normal flora is present on the skin, and it may affect the response to the wound inoculum. The skin's normal flora varies by site; for example, the organisms expected in the groin are not the same as those seen on the face. Normal flora helps control invasion of the skin by other microorganisms. While normal skin flora sometimes invades a wound, infection often is due to contamination from body fluids (e.g., stool) or from cross-contamination (Bello et al, 2001; Bowler, Duerden, and Armstrong, 2001; Edwards and Harding, 2004).

The relationship between microorganisms and the host is kept in balance by an extensive set of host defense mechanisms (Bowler, Duerden, and Armstrong, 2001). When organisms invade tissues, the body's immune system is stimulated. The inflammatory response occurs and brings white blood cells (WBCs) and enzymes into the affected tissues. Lymphocytes are stimulated and release lymphokines that recruit neutrophils and monocytes to the area of injury. Once mobilized, the host's neutrophils phagocytose invading organisms. Exudate increases because of the enhanced capillary permeability and the increased number of cells recruited to the area. If this is the individual's first exposure to an organism, antibodies must be generated

---

BOX 9-1 Signs and Symptoms of Infection in Chronic Wounds

- New/increased slough[a]
- Drainage excess, change in color/consistency[ab]
- Poor granulation tissue—friable, bright red, exuberant[ab]
- Redness, warmth around the wound[b]
- Sudden high glucose in patient with diabetes[b]
- Pain or tenderness[bc]
- Unusual odor[bc]
- Increased wound size/new areas of breakdown[c]

[a]Cutting and Harding, 1994; [b]Stotts and Whitney, 1999; [c]Gardner, Frantz, Doebbeling, 2001.

to provide ongoing protection. For those with prior exposure, existing antibodies are activated to fight the bioburden. The interleukins mediate the acute phase response that is characterized by redness, warmth, swelling, pain, and impaired function (Falanga, 2004; Park and Barbul, 2004).

The host's response leads to resolution of the problem, a localization of the infection, or chronic inflammation. *Resolution* of the problem is seen in clearing of the infection. *Localization of the infection* is manifest as an abscess or pus. The *chronic inflammatory response* results in an increase in the number of monocytes and lymphocytes at the site. With chronic inflammation, monocytes are converted to tissue macrophages and become the long-term phagocytic cells in the wound. Fibroblast proliferation is supported during this phase, leading to increased fibrotic tissue in the area of chronic inflammation. Proinflammatory cytokines such as interleukin-1 (IL-1) and tumor necrosis factor alpha (TNFα) increase. Matrix metalloproteases (MMPs) are generated, and the quantity of tissue inhibitors of metalloproteases (TIMPs) is decreased. This interaction results in inhibition of growth factors and continuation of the cycle of impaired healing (Falanga, 2004; Tarnuzzer and Schultz 1996).

Microorganisms' Defenses

Microorganisms have several weapons to fight the body's defenses including toxins, adherence factors, evasive factors, and invasive factors (Bowler, Duerden, and Armstrong, 2001; Porth, 2002).

Toxins. Both endotoxins and exotoxins destroy or alter the normal function of the host's cells. *Endotoxins* are lipids and polysaccharides that are located in the cell wall of gram-negative organisms. When released, they activate the regulatory systems of the body (e.g., clotting, and inflammation). *Exotoxins* are proteins released from bacteria that enzymatically inactivate or modify cells, causing them to die or disrupting their normal cellular functioning (Edwards and Harding, 2004). Excessive activity in these systems may result in increased capillary permeability, leakage of fluid out of the vasculature, coagulopathies, and ultimately even shock.

Adherence of the Organism. Infection depends on the adherence of the organism to the host's body. Attachment requires that the organism bond with a receptor using a ligand. Some receptors are site-specific

(e.g., mucous membrane), others are cell-specific (e.g., T lymphocytes), and others are nonspecific (e.g., moist surface). Colonization and ultimately invasion of the tissue by microorganisms cannot occur without attachment (Bowler, Duerden, and Armstrong, 2001; Porth, 2002).

Some organisms can alter the environment in which they live so that the host's immune system cannot locate them and/or has difficulty destroying them. These *evasive factors* include capsules, slime, and mucous layers. Attention has been given to the role of biofilm in the defense of organisms. Biofilm is a polysaccharide matrix in which organisms live on the surface of wounds. The organisms produce the polysaccharide matrix in which they live and develop a relationship so they live in a harmonious community. The number of organisms is limited by nutrient availability. Bacteria within the biofilm respond to signals from other bacteria in the community to change their phenotype, increasing the difficulty of identifying an antibiotic that is effective in clearing the organisms from the tissue. The matrix protects the organism from invasion by other organisms, from phagocytic cells, and from antibiotics (Edwards and Harding, 2004). Recent data show that biofilm forms within hours of exposure to microorganisms. Future preventive measures and therapy will have to be initiated soon after contamination to prevent biofilm and treat its sequelae (Harrison-Balestra, et al, 2003).

Invasive Factors. Invasive factors are the fourth type of microorganism defense. They allow the microorganism to penetrate the host tissue. Most of these invasive factors are enzymes (e.g., proteases) that break down cells and allow the microorganism to enter the tissue (Porth, 2002). The host defenses and the microorganism's mechanisms compete. If the microorganism overwhelms the host's defenses, infection occurs (Bowler, Duerden, and Armstrong, 2001; Edwards and Harding, 2004; Gardner et al, 2001; Robson, 1997).

Environmental Factors

The local wound environment is important in the genesis of wound infection. Organisms proliferate in an environment rich in necrotic material and slough. The dead tissue provides a medium for the growth of the invading microorganisms. These stimulate the inflammatory mediators and cytokines and release enzymes that break down the protein. The enzymes degrade fibrin that is essential for fibroblast migration and maintenance of macrophage activity. The inflammatory response is augmented and prolonged. Exotoxins also are released from the organisms and inhibit migration of keratinocytes and fibroblasts (Schultz et al, 2003; Stadelmann, Digenis, and Tobin, 1998). The organisms use oxygen and contribute to the relative hypoxia seen in infected wounds (Falanga, 2004). Removal of necrotic material and slough is critical to reverse infection; debridement reduces the bacterial burden and decreases the factors that inhibit growth factors and migration of cells. In addition, if the environment is warm, moist, and slightly hypoxic, anaerobic organisms proliferate (Bowler, Duerden, and Armstrong, 2001; Edwards and Harding, 2004; Falanga, 2004; Steed, 2004).

ACUTE WOUND INFECTION

Chronic wounds are often more highly contaminated than acute wounds and become polymicrobial in a short period. This may be because they are open to the environment, often have necrotic material present, and have irregular surfaces that house microorganisms (Schultz et al, 2003; Edwards and Harding, 2004).

Surgical wound infection has been termed *surgical site infection* (SSI). It occurs within 30 days of surgery, or within 1 year if an implant has been inserted and the infection involves the site of the surgery. SSI is an incision infection or organ/space infection (Mangram et al, 1999). *Superficial incision infection* involves only skin and subcutaneous tissue at the incision. *Deep incision infection* involves the deep tissues, including the muscles and fascia. *Infection of the organ/spaces* involves organs or body cavities that were manipulated during surgery. Criteria for diagnosing various types of SSI are listed in Table 9-1. A stitch abscess, infection of an episiotomy or a newborn circumcision site, and an infected burn are not classified as SSIs (Mangram et al, 1999).

Understanding who is at risk for SSI provides an opportunity to increase surveillance so early detection can occur and timely intervention can be initiated. There are many definitions of SSI and much data available about how SSI is measured and monitored (Bruce et al, 2001). In the United States, the large database created by the National Surgical Surveillance Initiative (NSSI) and made available through the Centers for Disease Control and Prevention (CDC) is considered the most accurate data available (Bruce et al, 2001).

TABLE 9-1   Criteria for Incisional and Organ/Space Surgical Site Infection

SUPERFICIAL SSI	DEEP INCISIONAL SSI	ORGAN/SPACE SSI
Purulent drainage	Purulent drainage	Purulent drainage
Positive wound culture	Incision dehisces or is opened by physician when the patient had one of the following: fever, local pain, tenderness (unless the site is culture negative)	Positive wound culture
At least one of the following signs or symptoms of infection pain or tenderness, local swelling, redness, or heat	An abscess or other evidence of infection found on examination, x-ray study, or histopathology	Abscess or other evidence of infection found on examination, x-ray study, or histopathology
Superficial incision is deliberately opened by a surgeon unless incision culture is negative		
Diagnosis by a surgeon or attending physician	Diagnosis by a surgeon or attending physician	Diagnosis by a surgeon or attending physician

Modified from Guideline for prevention of surgical site infection, 1999. www.cdc.gov/ncidod/dhqp/pdf/guidelines/ssi.pdf accessed April, 20, 2006.

TABLE 9-2 Risk Factors for Surgical Site Infection

	Smith et al, 2004	Kompatscher et al, 2003	Malone et al, 2002	Barie, 2002	Mangram et al, 1999
Obesity	X			X	X
Intraoperative Hypotension	X				
Surgery Longer Than 2 hours		X			
Diabetes Mellitus			X	X	X
Malnutrition			X	X	X
Low Hematocrit			X	X	
Ascites			X	X	
Steroid use				X	X
Age Extremes				X	X
Remote Infection				X	X
Chronic Inflammation				X	
Hypercholesteremia				X	
Hypoxemia				X	
Peripheral Vascular Disease				X	
Prior Site Radiation				X	
Recent Operation				X	
Skin Carrier of *Staphylococcus*				X	
Skin Disease In Area				X	
Nicotine Use					X
Perioperative Blood Products					X

See chapter references for study citations.

BOX 9-2 Risk Factors for Wound Infection Elicited through History

- Lack of healing after 2 weeks in a clean wound
- Deficiencies of vitamins and minerals: vitamins A, B, C, D, or K; minerals zinc, copper, or magnesium
- Diseases: liver, kidney, or heart failure; diabetes
- Drugs: corticosteroids, nonsteroidal antiinflammatory drugs, chemotherapeutic agents
- Foreign debris: sutures
- Immunodeficiency
- Ischemia/hypoxia
- Hypothermia
- Necrotic material
- Remote infection
- Smoking/tobacco use

Table 9-2 shows that risk factors for SSI vary by study. Risk factors that occur in more than one of the studies cited include obesity, diabetes, malnutrition, low hematocrit, ascites, steroid use, age extremes, and remote infection. For surgical wounds where prophylactic antibiotics are used, administration within 30 minutes of surgery is recommended (Barie, 2002; Mangram, 1999). Chapters 11 and 21 provide a detailed discussion of acute surgical and traumatic wounds.

DIAGNOSIS OF INFECTION

The diagnosis of wound infection is made using a combination of history, physical examination, and laboratory work. This triad gives the provider a holistic view of the patient.

History

Risk factors for wound infection that should be elicited through history are listed in Box 9-2. The history is critical in the diagnostic process because the findings from it focus the physical examination and the laboratory work. The history is obtained from the patient and/or caregiver and available records. The initial focus is on when the wound occurred, how it occurred, the environment in which it occurred, the presence of a systemic infection, and the effects of prior treatments on healing and infection. The provider needs to understand whether the wound is chronic or acute, because this information will help direct the plan of treatment. Important data to elicit in the history pertain to the patient and systemic characteristics. Factors to include are age, cognitive ability, functional ability, level of mobility, caregiver ability, medications, nutritional status, and concurrent conditions such as diabetes, venous and arterial disease, and liver and kidney function (Stotts and Whitney, 1999).

Physical Examination

The physical examination is pivotal in the diagnosis of infection. Along with the classic signs of inflammation, one should also pay close attention to the characteristics of the drainage from the wound. The inflammation process is natural and expected; however, if inflammation persists for 5 days, infection should be suspected. Immunosuppressed patients, as well as those who are malnourished, diabetic, or receiving corticosteroids or chemotherapy, may have a slower or less pronounced inflammatory response.

Data from the physical examination for surgical patients must be categorized according to the Criteria for Diagnosis of Incision and Organ/Space SSI that were created by the CDC (see Table 9-1). Chronic wounds may present with more subtle symptoms. The caregiver should be alert to a change in the amount or character of exudate, redness, and warmth around the wound; poor-quality granulation tissue; pain and tenderness that did not previously exist; and a change in wound odor. A sudden high glucose level also is a heralding sign of infection. Table 9-1 and Box 9-1 list the signs of acute and chronic wound infection. Although most infected wounds exhibit common "classical" criteria for infection, authors have drawn attention to the subtle differences between wound types that may lead to early detection of critical colonization. Criteria for identifying infection in different wound types are currently being developed (Cutting and White 2005).

Laboratory Tests

Complete Blood Count (CBC). Laboratory tests also play an important role in the diagnosis of infection. A *complete blood count (CBC)* should be obtained when infection is suspected. It is a quick and relatively noninvasive test that with infection shows an increase in the number of WBCs. The differential may show an increase in bands or immature neutrophils. This is called a "shift to the left" and denotes increased production of leukocytes such that immature leukocytes are released into the blood stream; this shift indicates mobilization of the body to fight the invading organisms.

Wound Cultures

While there is controversy about the meaning of the number and types of organisms present in chronic wounds, cultures are indicated when signs of infection are present (see Box 9-1) or when a clean wound does not show any progress in healing in 2 weeks (AHCPR, 1994; Falanga, 2004; Cutting and Harding, 1994; Gardner et al, 2001; Stotts and Whitney, 1999).

A wound culture is performed to identify the number of organisms present, to diagnose infection, to identify the organism causing the infection, and to identify the antibiotic that will kill the organism. Clinical indications for culture are listed in Box 9-3. Wound culture is used to examine tissue for aerobic and anaerobic organisms. It also can be used to obtain a specimen for a Gram stain, a method recognized as a rapid diagnostic technique to identify infection (Duke, Robson, and Krizek, 1972; Levine et al, 1976). For a Gram stain, the tissue fluid is placed on a slide, treated with various stains, and viewed under a microscope. In wounds where swabs yielded fewer than 10^5 organisms, a Gram stain shows no bacteria and the

---

BOX 9-3 Clinical Indications for a Wound Culture

- Local signs of infection: pus, change in odor or character of exudates, redness, induration, change in wound odor
- Systemic signs of infection: fever, leukocytosis
- Suddenly elevated glucose
- Pain in neuropathic extremity
- Lack of healing after 2 weeks in a clean wound despite optimal care

culture is negative. Results from a Gram stain can be expected in 20 minutes, a preliminary culture report in 24 hours, and a final culture and sensitivity within 48 hours.

A wound culture must be taken from clean, healthy-appearing tissue (Stotts, 1995). Because infection involves the tissue, it is important to culture the tissue rather than pus, slough, eschar, or necrotic material. Although a laboratory report will be produced if pus, eschar, or necrotic tissue is cultured, the results will reflect the microflora of that site and will not provide an accurate profile of the microflora in the tissue. In fact, the results will be a false report—the only question is the type of error. It could be false-positive (organisms present in the area that is cultured but not present in the tissue), false-negative (organisms not present in the area that is cultured but present in the tissue), or a chance agreement (area that is cultured and tissue have the same result). A false-negative is problematic in that the patient has an infection and needs to have it treated. The patient's condition may deteriorate if the patient is not treated. A false-positive is problematic in that the patient is treated when there is not a need, increasing the risk of side effects of the antibiotic and the development of organism resistance. The probability that the number and type of organisms in the area that is cultured is the same as that in the tissue is small; data indicate that even within the same wound tissue, the number and types of organisms vary (Levine et al, 1976).

The three major types of wound cultures are *wound biopsy, needle aspiration culture*, and *swab culture*. The advantages and disadvantages to each technique is described below. It should be noted, that a culture may not accurately represent the microorganisms in the entire wound, because it gives only a sample of the organisms present in the particular section of the wound from which the culture was obtained (Steer et al, 1996). Box 9-4 lists tips for successful and accurate wound culture regardless of the culture method used.

Wound biopsy for culture is removal of a piece of tissue with a scalpel or punch biopsy. The wound may be anesthetized topically rather than by injection as the topical anesthetic does not affect the fluid balance in the tissue and so will not affect the culture results. The open wound is cleansed with a nonantiseptic sterile solution. A biopsy specimen is taken from the tissue with

---

BOX 9-4 Tips on Wound Culturing

- Obtain the culture before administering antibiotics.
- Obtain the culture from clean tissue.
- Collect the specimen using sterile technique.
- Do not contaminate the specimen when placing it in the container.
- Collect sufficient specimen for examination.
- If a Gram stain will be done, obtain enough specimen.
- Place the specimen in an appropriate container.
- Complete the laboratory slip to provide clinical data for the microbiologist.
- Transport quickly to the laboratory to keep the organisms viable.

---

a scalpel or punch biopsy, and bleeding is controlled. Once in the laboratory, the specimen is processed and plated (Robson and Heggers, 1969).

The tissue biopsy is considered the gold standard for wound culture (Mangram et al, 1999; Robson, 1967; Stotts and Whitney, 1999). A physician or wound care specialist with special training performs the biopsy. One of the limitations of the technique is that many facilities do not process tissue for culture and therefore the method cannot be used. In addition, obtaining a tissue culture requires disruption of the wound, so healing may be delayed, and it may cause the patient pain because it requires cutting living tissue.

Needle aspiration involves insertion of a needle in the tissue adjacent to the wound to aspirate tissue fluid. Negative pressure is applied, and the needle tip is inserted into the tissue in several directions in order to obtain wound exudate. Organisms present in the tissue are detected by the aspirated tissue fluid (Lee, Turnidge, and McDonald, 1985). Intact skin next to the wound is disinfected and allowed to dry. Fanning the area to speed drying is not recommended because it allows the organisms in the environment to settle on the biopsy site. Equipment needed is a 10-ml disposable syringe and a 22-gauge needle. About 0.5 ml of air is drawn into the syringe, and the needle is inserted through intact skin adjacent to the wound. Suction is applied by withdrawing the plunger to the 10-ml mark. The needle is moved backward and forward at different angles for 2 to 4 explorations. After the needle is withdrawn from the tissue, excess air is removed from the syringe and the syringe is capped. The aspirated fluid is plated in the laboratory. If tissue is extracted using this technique, it is processed as described for tissue biopsy.

With the aspiration technique, the operator needs to understand the structures being penetrated by the needle. The risk of inadvertent needle damage is the major threat of this technique. When compared to tissue biopsy, needle aspiration tends to underestimate the number of organisms (Rudensky et al, 1992).

The *swab technique* is the third type of culture and the most commonly performed. The method of Levine and colleagues (1976) is recommended for swab culture. The wound is cleansed with a nonantiseptic sterile solution. The swab or applicator is moistened with normal saline (without preservative), because the moistened swab provides more precise data than a dry swab (Georgiade et al, 1970). The end of a sterile alginate applicator is rotated in 1 cm^2 of clean tissue in the open wound. Pressure is applied to the swab to elicit tissue fluid. When the tip of the swab is saturated, it is inserted into the appropriate sterile container and transported to the laboratory. If a Gram stain is to be performed, a second swab is obtained from the same clean tissue site.

A common criticism to the swab technique is that it can reflect the presence of organisms on the ulcer surface rather than in the tissue where infection occurs (Pellizzer et al, 2001; Starr and MacLeod, 2003). This criticism can be addressed by utilizing the Levin technique appropriately and consistently.

The swab technique probably is the most frequently used, since it requires the fewest clinical skills and most laboratories are accustomed to performing the analysis. Synthesis of data by the Wound, Ostomy Continence Nurses (WOCN) Society has led to its recommendation that for pressure ulcer management, quantitative or semiquantitative swab cultures are a reasonable alternative to biopsy in the clinical setting (Bill et al, 2001; Herruzo-Cabrera et al, 1992; Ratliff and Rodeheaver, 2002; WOCN Society, 2003).

Newer Diagnostic Techniques

Newer techniques are available for the diagnosis of infection. One is a test for antigens identified with immunoassay or radioimmune assay. Another is detection of antibodies in host sera. The RNA or DNA of organisms may be identified with Northern, Southern, or Western blot techniques. Also, polymer chain reactions may be used to detect organism DNA (Singhal and Zammit, 2002). These sophisticated tests currently are used primarily in research. Some authors predict that these techniques will be increasingly used to determine the host's immune response and ability to fight infection (Costerton et al, 1999).

Osteomyelitis

Osteomyelitis, infection of the bone, is a special case of wound infection and not easily diagnosed. Osteomyelitis is suspected when the wound is healing poorly, with or without systemic manifestations of infection, such as fever, leukocytosis, and any signs of sepsis (Bonham, 2001). Bone biopsy is the gold standard for diagnosing ostomyelitis. It can be performed on hospitalized patients at the bedside or in an outpatient setting, although it most frequently is done intraoperatively as part of surgery. However, how often the bone biopsy is used in clinical setting is unknown (Bonham, 2001). More commonly, probing to bone is used in the clinical area to diagnose osteomyelitis in patients with diabetes (Grayson et al, 1995). Exposure of bone or the ability to probe to bone has a positive predictive validity of 89% and a negative predictive validity of 56%. There is no reason to believe that diagnosis of osteomyelitis is different for patients with diabetes than in others with chronic wounds.

Because of the invasive nature of bone biopsy, a number of noninvasive diagnostic tests for diagnosing osteomyelitis have been explored including magnetic resonance imaging (MRI), x-ray, bone scans (three-phase), Tc 99m-labeled antigranulocyte antibody scintillography, and In leukocytes scans. A series of small studies has shown MRI to be effective (Bonham, 2001). Another study reported that MRI demonstrated the presence of osteomyelitis with 98% sensitivity and 89% of specificity compared to the standard bone biopsy (Livesley and Chow, 2002). Although these diagnostic tests are useful and have predictive validity, they are expensive and not used routinely. As a result therefore, there is no consistent gold standard or community standard that is the reference standard for diagnosing osteomyelitis, making clinical diagnosis subjective and providing a challenge to people who are performing studies in this area.

TREATMENT OF WOUND INFECTION

Wounds do not heal until infection is eradicated. The goal of care during this phase of the healing trajectory is reduction of bioburden without damaging healthy tissue. Local treatment includes cleansing, debridement, and appropriate topical therapy. Systemic treatment includes antibiotics, oxygenation and nutrition.*

Local Treatment of Wound Infection

Cleansing. Local care of chronic wounds has largely been driven by pressure ulcer care, and cleansing of the wound at each dressing change is recommended (AHCPR, 1994; WOCN Society, 2003). Cleansing using water or normal saline is aimed at reducing surface contaminant and metabolic byproducts, rather than curing the infection. All wound cleansing should be done with a pressure between 4 and 15 psi (AHCPR, 1994). Nontoxic, commercial wound cleansers may be used, and contain surfactants that enhance their effectiveness. A dressing that absorbs exudate and keeps the wound moist is then applied. Analysis of data by the WOCN Society suggests that no specific dressing is superior to others (WOCN Society, 2003), although bacterial burden or infection was not a dependent variable in studies reviewed. Wound cleansing and dressing selection is discussed in more detail in Chapter 19.

Debridement. Debridement is the most important local treatment, because it removes dead tissue and foreign materials to improve or facilitate the wound healing process (Edwards and Harding, 2004; Singhal, Reis, and Kerstein, 2001; Steed, 2004). Debridement can be performed surgically, chemically, or through autolysis and is discussed in Chapter 10.

Topical Therapy. Appropriate topical therapy addresses the needs of each wound and is discussed in Chapter 19. Topical antimicrobials are sometimes indicated to reduce wound bioburden (Figure 9-2). The purpose of topical antimicrobials is to reduce the number of organisms on the surface of the wound so that they do not become adherent or contribute to the potential for infection. Topical animicrobials consist of antiseptics, antibiotics, and elemental antimicrobials.

Antiseptics. Antiseptics nonselectively kill or inhibit the growth of microorganisms on external surfaces of the body. Examples of antiseptics are listed in Box 9-5. Historically antiseptics were used for decontaminating infected wounds. Today, their use is generally discouraged, because their cellular toxicity exceeds their bactericidal activity (AHCPR, 1994; WOCN Society, 2001). Some clinicians report using topical antiseptics in clinical care (Edwards and Harding, 2004; Falanga, 2004; Schultz et al, 2004). However, use should be restricted to a limited time frame (1 to 2 weeks) and for very specific indications.

Topical antibiotics. Examples of topical antibiotics are listed in Box 9-6. Topical antibiotics are presumed to be effective if the invading organisms have not developed resistance. When topical agents are used, the agent should be carefully selected, based on the specific organism that has been identified (Stadelmann, Digenis, and Tobin, 1998). The effect of *triple antibiotic ointment* to prevent soft tissue infection has been studied in pilot work. Pilot work shows a lower rate of infection with triple antibiotic when compared to mupirocin, although not statistically less (Hood, Hood, Shermock, Emerman, 2004). Without a control group that receives a placebo, it is difficult to evaluate the value of these treatments.

Topical elemental antimicrobials. Examples of topical elemental antimicrobials are listed in Box 9-7. The formulation of the agent is important to its effectiveness. For example, elemental iodine kills a number of cells important to healing, but when formulated as *cadexomer iodine* gel, it contains microspheres that absorb bacteria while slowly releasing iodine (Stadelmann, Digenis, and Tobin, 1998; Zhou et al, 2002). An in vitro study examined the effect of varying concentrations of cadexomer iodine on the viability of human fibroblasts in culture. At concentrations of up to 0.45%, cadexomer iodine is nontoxic to fibroblasts and causes no structural damage to the cells. Biopsies of chronic wounds treated with cadexomer iodine show reepithelialization. Bacteria are found trapped within the cadexomer beads (Zhou et al, 2002).

Silver has been used widely as a topical agent because of its bacteriostatic properties. Silver is a noble metal

---

*The concept of wound bed preparation (debridement, bacterial balance, exudate management) is widely accepted (Schultz et al, 2003); however, it is designed for care of chronic wounds, and the treatment model presented in this chapter is more comprehensive.

Agent	Vehicle	*Staph. Aureus*	*Streptococcus*	*Pseudomonas*	Comments
f Cadexomer Iodine (Iodosorb)	Yellow-brown powder/paste/ointment	MRSA ✓	✓	✓	Releases iodine slowly, less toxic to granulating tissue; broad spectrum, including virus and fungus
Gentamicin sulphate cream/ointment	Alcohol cream base or petrolateum ointment	✓	✓	✓	Good broad spectrum vs gram negatives
f Metroidazole gel/cream	Wax-glycerin cream and carbogel 940/propylene glycol gel				Good choice for MRSA; excellent topical penetration
f Mupuricin 2% cream/ointment	Propylene glycol ointment	MRSA ✓	✓		Good choice for MRSA; excellent topical penetration
f Polymyxin B sulphate-Gramacidin	Cream	MRSA ✓	✓	✓	Broad spectrum; low cost; ointment contains bacitracin, a new sensitizer
Polymyxin B sulphate-Bacitracin zinc-neomycin*	Ointment	✓	✓	✓	Neomycin is a potent sensitizer and may cross-react, in 40% of cases, to aminoglycosides
f Silver sulfadiazine	Water-miscible cream	MRSA ✓	✓	✓	Do not use in self-sensitive individuals
f Silver (ionized)	Absorbent bilayered sheet, burn dressing, alginate, foam and other forms	MRSA ✓	✓	✓	Ionized silver is activated with sterile water. Saline will precipitate the silver chloride

Source: Fowler et al, 2003.
*Contains common sensitizer. *MRSA*=methicillin-resistant *Staphylococcus aureus*, f=preferred products.

Fig. 9-2 Topical antimicrobial indications.

that possesses an antimicrobial effect when it is oxidized to silver ions (Bowler, 2004). Silver has been used in wound care for its bacteriostatic properties. It comes in creams, pure silver, or a sustained release form incorporated into a dressing. Silver sulfadiazine (2% to 7%), for example, has been shown to reduce bacterial density, vascular margination, and migration of inflammatory cells (Fumal et al, 2002). Practitioners use dressings impregnated with silver since they demonstrate antimicrobial effects on broad-spectrum organisms (Bowler, 2004). Silver released in a moist environment enhances the rate of reepithelialization by 40% in a meshed skin graft as compared to treatment with antibiotic solution (Demling and DeSanti, 2002). Despite the current absence of negative systemic or local consequences, use of elemental antimicrobials should be judicious and limited to 2 to 4 weeks, similar to the approach used with

BOX 9-5 Examples of Topical Antiseptics

• •

- Acidic acid
- Alcohol
- Aluminum salt
- Betadine
- Boric acid
- Chlorhexidine
- Gentian violet
- Hexachloraphene
- Hydrogen peroxide
- Hypochlorite (Dakin's solution)

BOX 9-6 Examples of Topical Antibiotics

• •

Gram-Positive (+)

- Mupirocin
- Garamycin

Gram-Positive or Gram-Negative (+/−)

- Bacitracin
- Neomycin
- Mafenide acetate
- Nitrofurazone
- Sulfamylon

Anaerobic

- Mafenide acetate
- Metronidazole

BOX 9-7 Examples of Topical Elemental Antimicrobials

• •

- Silver sulfadiazine cream
- Silver-impregnated dressings
- Cadexomer iodine
- Copper
- Zinc
- Gold

antibiotics, and each wound should receive individualized consideration.

Additional Treatments. It is reported that negative pressure wound therapy (NPWT), electrical stimulation, and hyperbaric oxygen therapy (HBO) have a role in the treatment of infected wounds. Each of these interventions has its own set of indications, contraindications, advantages and disadvantages which are discussed in greater detail in Chapter 20.

Systemic Treatment of Wound Infection

Antibiotics. Antibiotics are appropriate when there is a systemic response to infection such as cellulitis, leukocytosis, or fever (Stadelmann, Digenis, and Tobin, 1998; Stotts and Whitney, 1999). Barie (2002) recommends the following principles be used to guide the selection of antibiotics: the agent should be safe, have a narrow but adequate spectrum of coverage, not be used frequently/routinely to avoid the resistance that is seen with overuse, and be prescribed for an effective but brief period. When antibiotics are used, it is critical that the blood level be maintained so the therapeutic effect can be achieved. This means that the timing of administration of antibiotics is critical.

Oxygen. Providing a physiologic environment for healing has long been a cornerstone of care of patients, especially those with wounds. Some data indicate an important link between wound infection and oxygenation. Early data from Knighton (1990) showed that an increased fraction of inspired oxygen (FiO_2) (45% compared with 12% and 21%) resulted in better clearing of bacteria in an animal model. More recently, a randomized clinical trial of intraoperative supplemental oxygen (30% versus 80%) showed that significantly fewer patients in the higher oxygen group developed SSI in the 30-day postoperative period (Grief et al, 2000). In contrast, a randomized clinical trial that compared FiO_2 levels of 35% and 80% showed that at 14 days after surgery, those who received higher levels of oxygen had greater SSI and more than twice the length of hospitalization (Pryor et al, 2004). This study has been criticized by a number of physicians for its design flaws (Hopf, Hunt, and Rosen, 2004). It is important to recognize that both groups in these large randomized clinical trials received supplemental oxygen, suggesting its value as a general principal. Whether supraoxygenation at an FiO_2 of 80% is beneficial remains to be resolved. Further work will be needed to resolve this controversy.

Other dimensions of providing for control of wound infection related to oxygenation and perfusion are *pain control, avoidance of smoking,* and *control of ambient temperature.* Pain control, at least in the acute wound setting, has been shown to be related to tissue oxygenation and infection (Akca et al, 1999). Smoking cessation has been shown to be important for prevention of wound infection in both ambulatory and inpatient surgery settings (Mylers et al, 2002; Sorensen, Karlsmark, and Gottrup, 2003). Cessation for 4 weeks is effective in reducing wound infection rates, although abstinence for less time has little benefit (Sorensen, Karlsmark, and Gottrup, 2003; Sorensen and Jorgensen, 2003). Providing for normothermia immediately after surgery is important in reducing the rate of wound infection (Sessler and Akca, 2002).

Nutrition and Fluid. In the nutrition literature, there is little information about the effect of feeding on infection. A meta-analysis (n = 837 patients) explored the effect of the preoperative practice of providing nothing by mouth in gastrointestinal (GI) surgery patients versus feeding patients orally or by tube into the small bowel (Lewis et al, 2001). Early feeding resulted in significantly lower overall infection rates, but not specifically surgical site infection. The trade-off in early feeding was significantly greater vomiting occurring among those fed earlier. The authors conclude that early feeding may be of value and should be considered, especially in the GI population, where risk of infection is great.

Of importance in examining the role of both oxygen and nutrition in infection is the recent study among surgical patients that explored administering varying volumes of fluid intraoperatively. Colon surgery patients were randomized to receive either the usual or additional fluids. Those who received additional fluids had higher tissue oxygen levels postoperatively (Arkilic et al, 2003). Preliminary work with nursing home patients with pressure ulcers showed that supplemental fluid given to those with low tissue oxygen resulted in improved tissue oxygen (Stotts and Hopf, 2003). Although neither study examined infection rate, these studies emphasize the importance of adequate fluid to deliver oxygen and nutrients to the site of injury and infection.

PSYCHOLOGICAL SUPPORT AND EDUCATION

There are only anecdotal data about patients' psychologic response to having a wound infection, the sociologic adaptations that take place, and the effect of the wound infection and its treatment on the family unit. Addressing psychosocial issues and inclusion of the family and/or involvement of social services in the plan of care may prove to be pivotal to patient outcomes. Effective recovery may require comprehensive assessment and mobilization of the needed resources to address the patient and the wound infection.

With the length of hospitalization decreasing, more care is provided in the home. Patients with wounds are at risk for infection, and it is not clear that they are able to identify infection when it is present (Seaman and Lammers, 1991). Further work is needed to help persons with wounds and their families understand and appreciate how to identify infection when it is present.

SELF-ASSESSMENT EXERCISE

1. Infection is when microorganisms do which of the following?
   a. Reside on the surface of the wound
   b. Invade the tissue
   c. Multiply on the wound
   d. Reside on the surface and multiply there
2. Which of the following statements accurately characterizes colonization of a wound?
   a. Colonization is associated with a fever and local inflammation of the wound.
   b. Colonization is manifested by delayed healing.
   c. Colonization is diagnosed with a culture result of 105 organisms/gram of tissue or more.
   d. Colonization is often present and is not indicative of an infection.
3. Mr. H is a 35-year-old man with an open wound of his foot caused when he was dragged by a tractor in a farm accident 3 days ago. He does not have insurance and so did not seek medical assistance at the time of the injury. He comes today because he has shaking chills. By history he is a healthy, active adult. On physical examination you find that he has abrasions over his legs, but x-ray examination shows no fracture. The wound involves the plantar surface of his foot, where a full thickness triangular flap is visible; but the wound is filled with eschar and its depth cannot be evaluated.

The entire foot is reddened, swollen, and hot. He is alert, oriented, and concerned. The major risk factor for infection in this man is which of the following?

a. Local wound environment because of the contamination

b. Malnutrition because he has not eaten well as a result of his fever

c. Ischemia resulting from trauma to the foot and leg

d. Immunosuppression resulting from the stress of the injury

4. All of the following define surgical site infection except which feature?

a. Less than 10^5 organisms/gram of tissue

b. Redness, induration, and local warmth surrounding a wound

c. Purulent drainage

d. Increased WBCs

5. Which of the following cause you to suspect infection in a 63-year-old man with diabetes who is seen with a neuropathic ulcer located on the left plantar surface of his foot?

a. Pain at the ulcer site

b. Sudden low glucose level

c. 10^3 organisms/gram of tissue or more

d. Delayed healing

6. You inadvertently contaminated a culture when you were obtaining it. How should the findings be interpreted?

a. False-positive. The laboratory work shows infection when it really is not present.

b. False-negative. The laboratory work shows no infection when in fact it is present.

c. False. You cannot know if the patient had infection because of the contamination.

d. Accurate. A little contamination is expected because the skin is always contaminated.

7. In a culture obtained by aspiration, what would you expect the number of organisms to be?

a. More than by swab culture

b. More than by tissue biopsy

c. The same as by swab culture

d. Fewer than on tissue biopsy

8. To get the most accurate culture, it is important that the specimen be taken from which of the following?

a. Pus

b. Necrotic tissue or slough

c. Exudate

d. Healthy wound tissue

9. Which of the following must be included in the comprehensive wound treatment of a 47-year-old patient with an open wound of the abdomen secondary to a retroperitoneal abscess?

a. Wet-to-dry dressings

b. Pain control

c. Debridement of granulation tissue

d. Treatment for depression

REFERENCES

Agency for Health Care Policy and Research (AHCPR): *Treatment of pressure ulcers in adults*, Rockville, MD, 1994, U. S. Department of Health and Human services, AHCPR Publication No. 95-0652.

Akca O et al: Postoperative pain and subcutaneous oxygen tension, *Lancet* 354(9172):41, 1999.

Allman RM: Pressure ulcer prevalence, incidence, risk factors, and impact, *Clin Geriatr Med* 13:421, 1997.

Alvarez OM et al: A prospective, randomized, comparative study of collagenase and papain/urea formulations, *Wounds* 14:293, 2002.

Arkilic CF et al: Supplemental perioperative fluid administration increases tissue oxygen pressure, *Surgery* 133(1):49, 2003.

Barie PS: Surgical site infections: epidemiology and prevention, *Surg Infect* 3:S9, 2002.

Baumgarten M et al: Pressure ulcers and the transition to long-term care, *Adv Skin Wound Care* 16(6):299, 2003.

Bello YM et al: Infection and wound healing, *Wounds* 13(4):127, 2001.

Bill TJ et al: Quantitative swab culture versus tissue biopsy: a comparison in chronic wounds, *Ostomy Wound Manage* 47(1):34, 2001.

Bonham P: A critical review of the literature. Part I: diagnosing osteomyelitis in patients with diabetes and foot ulcers, *J WOCN* 28(2):73, 2001.

Bowler PG, Duerden BI, Armstrong DG: Wound microbiology and associated approaches to wound management, *Clin Microbiol Rev* 14(2):244, 2001.

Bowler PG, Jones SA, Walker M, Parsons D: J Burn Care Rehabil. Microbicidal properties of a silver-containing hydrofiber dressing against a variety of burn wound pathogens. Mar-Apr;25(2):192-196, 2004.

Bruce J et al: The measurement and monitoring of surgical adverse events, *Health Technical Assess* 5(22):1, 2001.

Costerton JW, Stewart PS, Greenberg EP: Bacterial biofilms: a common cause of persistent infections, *Science* 284(5418):1318, 1999.

Cutting KF, Harding KGH: Criteria for identifying wound infection. *J Wound Care* 3:198, 1994.

Cutting KF, White RJ: Criteria for identifying wound infection-revisited, *Ostomy Wound Manage* 51(1):28, 2005.

Demling RH, DeSanti L: The rate of re-epithelialization across meshed skin grafts is increased with exposure to silver, *Burns* 28(3):264, 2002.

Duke WF, Robson MC, Krizek TJ: Civilian wounds, their bacterial flora and rate of infection, *Surg Forum* 23(0):518, 1972.

Edwards R, Harding KG: Bacteria and wound healing, *Curr Opin Infect Dis* 17(2):91, 2004.

Falanga V: The chronic wound: impaired healing and solutions in the context of wound bed preparation, *Blood Cells Mol Dis* 31:88, 2004.

Fleischmann KE et al: Association between cardiac and noncardiac complications in patients undergoing noncardiac surgery: outcomes and effects on length of stay, *Am J Med* 115(7):515, 2003.

Fowler EM et al: Wound care for persons with diabetes, *Home Healthcare Nurse* 21(8):531, 2003.

Fumal I et al: The beneficial toxicity paradox of antimicrobials in leg ulcer healing impaired by a polymicrobial flora: a proof-of-concept study, *Dermatology* 204(Suppl 1):70, 2002.

Gardner SE, Frantz RA, Doebbeling BN: The validity of the clinical signs and symptoms used to identify localized chronic wound infection, *Wound Repair Regen* 9(3):178, 2001.

Georgiade NG et al: A comparison of methods for the quantitation of bacteria in burn wounds, experimental evaluation, *Am J Clin Pathol* 53(1):35, 1970.

Grayson MI et al: Probing to bone in infected pedal ulcers. A clinical sign of underlying osteomyelitis in diabetic patients, *JAMA* 273:721, 1995.

Grief R et al: Supplemental perioperative oxygen to reduce the incidence of surgical-wound infection. Outcomes research group, *N Engl J Med* 342(3):161, 2000.

Hall MJ, DeFrances CJ: *2001 National hospital discharge survey.* Advanced Data from Vital and Health Statistics, No. 332, Hyattsville, MD, 2003, National Center for Health Statistics.

Harrison-Balestra C et al: A wound-isolated *Pseudomonas aeruginosa* grows a biofilm in vitro within 10 hours and is visualized by light microscopy, *Dermatol Surg* 29(6):631, 2003.

Herruzo-Cabrera R et al: Diagnosis of local infection of a burn by semi-quantitative culture of the eschar surface, *J Burn Care Rehabil* 13(6):639, 1992.

Hood R, Hood R, Shermock KM, Emerman C: A prospective, random-ized pilot evaluation of topical triple antibiotic versus mupirocin for the prevention of uncomplicated soft tissue wound infection, *Am J Emerg Med* 22(1):1, 2004.

Hopf HW, Hunt TK, Rosen N: Comment on: Supplemental oxygen and risk of surgical site infection, *JAMA* 291(16):1956, 2004.

Johnson CB, Lyons WL, Covinsky KE: Geriatric medicine. In Tierney LM Jr, McPhee SJ, Papadakis MA, editors: *Current medical diagnosis and treatment 2003,* New York, 2003, Lange Medical Books/McGraw-Hill.

Kirkland KB et al: The impact of surgical-site infection in the 1990's: attributable mortality, excess length of hospitalization, and extra costs, *Infect Control Hosp Epidemiol* 20(11):725, 1999.

Knighton DR et al: Oxygen as an antibiotic. The effect of inspired oxygen on bacterial clearance, *Arch Surg* 125(1):97, 1990.

Kompatscher P et al: Comparison of the incidence and predicted risk of surgical site infection after breast reconstruction, *Anesthetic Plast Surg* 27(4):308, 2003.

Lazarus GS et al: Definition and guidelines for assessment of wounds and evaluation of healing, *Arch Dermatol* 130:489, 1994.

Levine NS et al: The quantitative swab culture and smear: a quick, simple method for determining the number of viable aerobic bacteria on open wounds, *J Trauma* 16(2):89, 1976.

Lee P, Turnidge J, McDonald PJ: Fine-needle aspiration biopsy in diag-nosis of soft tissue infections, *J Clin Microbiol* 22(1):80, 1985.

Livesley NJ, Chow AW: Infected pressure ulcers in elderly individuals, *Clin Infect Dis* 35(11):1390, 2002. E-pub 2002 Nov 04.

Malone DL et al: Surgical site infections: reanalysis of risk factors, *J Surg Res* 103(1):89, 2002.

Mangram AJ et al: Guideline for prevention of surgical site infection, 1999. Centers for Disease Control and Prevention (CDC) Hospital Infection Control Practices Advisory Committee, *Am J Infect Control* 27(2):97, 1999.

Mylers PS et al: Risk of respiratory complications and wound infection in patients undergoing ambulatory surgery: smokers versus nonsmokers, *Anesthesiology* 97(4):842, 2002.

Park JE, Barbul A: Understanding the role of immune regulation in wound healing. *Am J Surg* 187(5A):11S, 2004.

Pellizzer G et al: Deep tissue biopsy vs. superficial swab culture monitor-ing in the microbiological assessment of limb-threatening diabetic foot infection, *Diabet Med* 18(10):822, 2001.

Porth CM: *Pathophysiology: concepts of altered health states,* ed 6, Philadelphia, 2002, Lippincott.

Pryor KO et al: Surgical site infection and the routine use of periopera-tive hyperoxia in a general surgical population: a randomized controlled trial, *JAMA* 291(1):79, 2004.

Ratliff CR, Rodeheaver GT: Correlation of semi-quantitative swab cultures to quantitative swab cultures from chronic wounds, *Wounds* 14:329, 2002.

Robson MC: Wound infection. A failure of wound healing caused by an imbalance of bacteria, *Surg Clin North Am* 77(3):637, 1997.

Robson MC, Heggers JP: Bacterial quantification of open wounds, *Mil Med* 134(1):19, 1969.

Rodeheaver GT: Pressure ulcer debridement and cleansing: a review of current literature, *Ostomy Wound Manage* 45(Suppl 1A):80S, 1999.

Rudensky R et al: Infected pressure sores: Comparison of methods for bacterial identification, *South Med J* 85(9):901, 1992.

Schultz GS et al: Wound bed preparation: a systematic approach to wound management, *Wound Rep Reg* 11:1, 2003.

Seaman M, Lammers R: Inability of patients to self-diagnose wound infections, *J Emerg Med* 9:215, 1991.

Sessler DL, Akca O: Nonpharmacological prevention of surgical wound infections, *Clin Infect Dis* 35(1):1397, 2002.

Sibbald RG et al: Screening evaluation of an ionized nanocrystalline silver dressing in chronic wound care, *Ostomy Wound Management* 47:38, 2001.

Singhal A, Reis ED, Kerstein MD: Options for nonsurgical debridement of necrotic wounds, *Adv Skin Wound Care* 14(2):96, 2001.

Singhal H, Zammit C: Wound infection, *E-medicine* July 23, 2002. http://emedicine.com/med/topic2422.htm. Accessed June 1, 2004.

Smith RL et al: Wound infection after elective colorectal resection, *Ann Surg* 239(5):599, 2004.

Sorensen LT, Jorgensen T: Short-term pre-operative smoking cessation intervention does not affect postoperative complications in colorectal surgery: a randomized clinical trial, *Colorectal Dis* 5(4):347, 2003.

Sorensen LT, Karlsmark T, Gottrup F: Abstinence from smoking reduces incisional wound infection: a randomized controlled trial, *Ann Surg* 238(1):1, 2003.

Stadelmann WJ, Digenis AG, Tobin GR: Impediments to wound healing, *Am J Surg* 176(Suppl 2A):39S, 1998.

Starr S, MacLeod T: Wound swabbing technique, *Nurs Times* 99(5):57, 2003.

Steed DL: Debridement, *Am J Surg* 187(Suppl May 2004):71S, 2004.

Steer JA et al: Quantitative microbiology in the management of burn patients. I. Correlation between quantitative and qualitative burn wound biopsy culture and surface alginate swab culture, *Burns* 22(3):173, 1996.

Stotts NA: Determination of bacterial burden in wounds, *Adv Wound Care* 8(4 Suppl):46, 1995.

Stotts NA, Hopf HW: The link between tissue oxygen and hydration in nursing home residents with pressure ulcers: preliminary data, *J WOCN* 30(4):184, 2003.

Stotts NA, Whitney JD: Identifying and evaluating wound infection, *Home Healthcare Nurse* 17(3):159, 1999.

Tarnuzzer RW, Schultz, GS: Biochemical analysis of acute and chronic wound environments, *Wound Rep Regen* 4:321, 1996.

Wound Ostomy and Continence Nurses (WOCN) Society: *Guideline for prevention and management of pressure ulcers* (series) Glenview, IL, 2003, Author.

Zhou LH et al: Slow release iodine preparation and wound healing: in vitro effects consistent with lack of in vivo toxicity in human chronic wounds, *Br J Dermatol* Mar;146(3):365, 2002.

10 *Wound Debridement*

JANET M. RAMUNDO

OBJECTIVES

1. Describe the role of debridement in the wound-healing process.
2. Distinguish between selective and nonselective debridement.
3. Compare and contrast four methods of debridement: autolysis, chemical, mechanical, and sharp.
4. Describe the appropriate technique for wet-to-dry dressings, conservative sharp debridement, and high-pressure wound irrigations.
5. List debridement options for infected wounds.
6. Describe at least five factors to consider when selecting a debridement approach.
7. For each method of debridement, list two advantages, disadvantages, and relevant precautions.

Debridement is the removal of nonviable tissue and foreign matter from a wound and is a naturally occurring event in the wound-repair process. During the inflammatory phase, neutrophils and macrophages digest and remove "used" platelets, cellular debris, and avascular injured tissue from the wound area. However, with the accumulation of significant amounts of damaged tissue, this natural process becomes overwhelmed and insufficient. Buildup of necrotic tissue then places considerable phagocytic demand on the wound and retards wound healing. Consequently, debridement of necrotic tissue is an essential objective of topical therapy and a critical component of optimal wound management (AHCPR, 1994; Goode and Thomas, 1997; Robson, 1997; Stotts and Hunt, 1997; WOCN Society, 2003). Debridement is an integral component of wound bed preparation, along with bacterial balance and moisture balance (Falanga, 2002; Sibbald et al, 2000).

With the limited research conducted thus far, debridement is believed to achieve several objectives:

1. Debridement reduces the bioburden of the wound. Because devitalized tissue supports the growth of bacteria, the presence of necrotic tissue places the patient at risk for wound infection and sepsis. Using external measures to remove the necrotic tissue and foreign matter reduces the volume of pathogenic microbes present in the wound.
2. Debridement controls and potentially prevents wound infections, particularly in the deteriorating wound.
3. Debridement facilitates visualization of the wound wall and base. In the presence of necrotic tissue, accurate and thorough assessment of the viable tissue is hampered (Rolstad and Harris, 1997).
4. At a molecular level, debridement interrupts the cycle of the chronic wound so that protease and cytokine levels more closely approximate those of the acute wound (Schultz, 1999).

Necrotic tissue can appear in various forms. Eschar has the firm, dry, leathery appearance of desiccated and compressed tissue layers (Plate 24). When the tissue is kept moist, the devitalized tissue, which is called slough, remains soft and may be brown, yellow, or gray in appearance (Plate 25). Slough may be adherent to the wound bed and edges, or loosely adherent and stringy (Plate 26). Components of slough include fibrin, bacteria, intact leukocytes, cell debris, serous exudate, and significant quantities of deoxyribonucleic acid (DNA) (Thomas, 1990b). Once the eschar is removed, slough is often visible covering the wound bed. Maintaining a moist wound environment is essential because continued exposure to air dehydrates slough, causing it to return to a hard, leathery state (Bale, 1997a).

Debridement is indicated for any wound, acute or chronic, when necrotic tissue (which may be slough or eschar) or foreign bodies are present. It is also indicated when the wound is infected. Once the wound bed is clean and viable tissue is present, debridement is no longer indicated.

Contraindications to debridement also exist. Dry, stable (i.e., noninfected, or nonfluctuant) ischemic wounds or those with dry gangrene should not be debrided until perfusion to the extremity has improved (Bale, 1997b; Bates-Jensen, 1998). Measurement of vascular status, including an ankle-brachial index (ABI), is an important component of the assessment process when considering debridement in a patient with lower leg ulceration. Debridement is also contraindicated for stable eschar covered heels (i.e., absence of edema, erythema, fluctuance or drainage). Treatment goals should be consistent with the goals and lifestyle of the individual (AHCPR, 1994).

METHODS OF DEBRIDEMENT

Several methods of debridement are available for removal of devitalized tissue from necrotic wounds. Debridement methods are classified as either selective (only necrotic tissue is removed) or nonselective (viable tissue is removed along with the nonviable tissue). More specifically, debridement is classified by the actual mechanism of action: autolysis, chemical, mechanical, or sharp (conservative or surgical). Although one method of debridement may be the primary approach selected to rid the wound of necrotic tissue, debridement typically involves a combination of methods.

Autolysis

Description. Autolysis is the lysis of necrotic tissue by the body's white blood cells and enzymes, which enter the wound site during the normal inflammatory process. Proteolytic, fibrinolytic, and collagenolytic enzymes are released to digest the devitalized tissue present in the wound (Rodeheaver et al, 1994). Autolysis is a selective method of debridement that leaves healthy tissue intact.

Autolysis, a naturally occurring physiologic process, occurs in a moist, vascular environment. The primary requirements for debridement via autolysis include a moist wound environment, adequate leukocyte function, and an adequate neutrophil count. Autolysis is enhanced or supported by applying a moisture-retentive dressing to the necrotic wound and allowing it to remain undisturbed for a reasonable length of time. By maintaining a moist wound environment, the cellular structures that are essential for phagocytosis (neutrophils and macrophages) remain intact and are not prematurely destroyed through desiccation. Since an important role of macrophages is to produce growth factors, the presence of healthy macrophages in the wound fluid supports the continued production of growth factors.

Wound dressings support autolysis if they add or maintain moisture at the wound surface. Semiocclusive dressings trap enzyme-rich wound exudate at the wound site and are very effective at detaching eschar from the surrounding skin and wound base.

Directions for Use. Dressing selection is based on the condition of the wound base, depth of the wound, presence of tunnels or undermining, volume of wound exudate, and the patient's condition. When the wound base is dry, a dressing that will add moisture, such as a hydrogel, should be used. If absorption is needed, a dressing should be selected that will absorb excess exudate without dehydrating the wound surface, such as an alginate dressing for a highly exudative wound or a hydrocolloid for the slightly exudative wound.

Autolysis can be used alone or in combination with other debridement techniques. Autolysis is automatically employed any time a moisture-retentive dressing is used. However autolysis as a sole method of debridement is only recommended for noninfected wounds with a limited volume of necrotic tissue. The moisture-retentive dressing selected to achieve autolysis is dependent upon the wound needs as described in Chapter 19. Many times it becomes necessary to combine dressings to meet the wound's needs and achieve debridement. For example, an alginate dressing and composite dressing may be best for an exudative wound that has tissue depth (Bryant and Rolstad, 1998). Promotion of autolysis is an important adjuvant to all debridement modalities so that cellular desiccation through air exposure and the resulting buildup of necrotic tissue is avoided. For example, after surgical sharp debridement of a pressure ulcer, the application of a hydrogel-impregnated gauze maintains a moist wound environment, thus preventing tissue desiccation and promoting continued softening and loosening of residual necrotic tissue.

Autolysis is considered by some practitioners to be a slower process than other debridement methods (Mosher et al, 1999). The time frame for autolysis to occur varies depending on the size of the wound and the amount and type of necrotic tissue. Generally, progress should be observed within 72 to 96 hours (Alvarez, 1988). Initially, the black eschar will loosen from the edges, become soft, change to brown or gray in color, and eventually transform into stringy yellow slough. It is critical to monitor the wound closely during the autolysis process, because as the wound debrides, the full wound bed and walls are exposed and the true extent of the wound is revealed.

Consequently, the wound will increase in length, width, and depth, necessitating a change in the therapy. Reassessment of the wound needs based on the changing wound dimensions is essential so that the most appropriate and effective dressing is used.

Precautions. It is important to use the most appropriate dressing for the wound when the objective is to debride by autolysis. Autolysis can be achieved with a variety of moisture-retentive dressings. The type of dressing used for autolysis must be selected based on the wound needs and the patient's status. Indications for each dressing as discussed in Chapter 19 must also be followed. For example, a transparent dressing is inappropriate for debridement of a wound that has depth and is heavily exudative. Instead, a dressing such as an alginate is warranted, because it will fill the wound depth and absorb the exudate. Likewise, a patient who is severely neutropenic (absolute neutrophil count of less than 500 mm^3) is at risk for severe infection or sepsis (Bodey et al, 1966). In these patients, it may be that debridement by autolysis is unrealistic and may be harmful, because the number of viable neutrophils available in the wound fluid may be diminished and could be overwhelmed by even the slightest increase in the number of bacteria present at the wound site. In the presence of neutropenia, alternatives to autolysis such as chemical debridement should be considered (see Figure 10-1).

Autolysis should not be the primary method of debridement in a wound with advancing cellulitis because of the length of time it takes to debride. In these situations the goal must be to debride the wound as quickly as possible. In addition, if the infection is due to anaerobic bacteria, any dressing that maintains a layer of fluid between the wound bed and dressing will provide some degree of occlusion, which may promote further growth of the anaerobic bacteria. However, if the infection is addressed and local symptoms have subsided (e.g., erythema, induration, and odorous exudate), autolysis may be used safely.

Debridement by autolysis compares favorably with other methods of debridement in terms of effectiveness (Colins, Kurning, and Yuon, 1996; Mulder et al, 1993). However, there are some precautions to note. Periwound maceration can develop when wound exudate has continued contact with intact skin. Logically, as nonviable tissue is liquefied, the volume of wound exudate will increase and the potential for maceration is increased. Liquid barrier film or skin barriers may be applied to the surrounding skin as prophylaxis. In addition, dressings should be selected and changed at appropriate time intervals so as to manage exudate levels and reduce the likelihood of maceration.

Fear and lack of familiarity with the process can also present problems. Clinicians, patients, and family members unfamiliar with the process of autolysis can misinterpret the collection of wound exudate and the accompanying odor as indicative of an infection. Consequently, they may want to change the dressing as soon as fluid appears, so reassurance and education is necessary. It is important to emphasize that the wound exudate contains phagocytic cells and growth factors that are essential to wound repair. The fear that moisture-retentive dressings promote an infection must be allayed. In fact, wounds treated with moisture-retentive dressings are less likely to become infected than wounds treated with conventional dressings because dressings are impermeable to exogenous bacteria, viable neutrophils, and other natural substances that inhibit bacterial growth, accumulate and are retained at the wound site, and the volume of necrotic tissue is reduced (Eaglstein, 1993; Hutchinson, 1989; Lawrence, 1994). Plate 31 shows the appearance of a wound before and after autolysis.

Chemical

Necrotic wound tissue can also be removed through a chemical process such as with enzymes, sodium hypochlorite (Dakin's solution), and maggots. Silver nitrate is also a method of chemical debridement; however, its use is generally limited to epibole (closed or rolled wound edges) and hypergranulation (see Chapters 4 and 7 and Plates 4 and 27).

Enzymes

Description. Topical application of exogenous enzymes is a selective method of debridement. Enzymes are derived from various sources (e.g., krill, crab, papaya, bovine extract, and bacteria) and are applied topically to the necrotic tissue. They are capable of inducing changes in the substrate against which they are effective and result in the breakdown of necrotic tissue. There are two commercially available enzymes: collagenase, and papain/urea combination. Table 10-1 provides a description of these commonly used enzymes.

Enzymes work in one of two ways: (1) by directly digesting the components of slough (e.g., fibrin, bacteria, leukocytes, cell debris, serous exudate, and DNA) or (2) by dissolving the collagen "anchors" that secure the avascular tissue to the underlying wound bed (Boxer et al, 1969). Ideally, the type of enzyme selected should correlate with the type of tissue found on the wound surface. Hebda and Lo (2001) conducted in vitro studies of collagenase and papain/urea on native and denatured collagenous substrates similar to what would be found in chronic wounds and burns. They reported that papain/urea was more effective on fibrin and collagenase was more effective on elastin. Unfortunately, there is little to guide the clinician in identifying the predominant substrate in a chronic wound. Both were more effective on denatured protein (such as seen in burns).

Directions for use. Enzymes require specific conditions, which vary from product to product, to be effective. Manufacturer's guidelines must be followed carefully to optimize the enzyme's effectiveness. Heavy metals, which can be found in many wound cleansers and other commonly used topical wound products, inactivate enzymes. Examples of heavy metals include silver and zinc. These products should be rinsed thoroughly from the wound before applying an enzyme.

Enzymes require a specific pH range, but testing for pH is not a common practice among clinicians. Because enzymes are not effective in a dry environment, eschar must be crosshatched to allow penetration of the enzyme, and the wound surface must be kept moist. Crosshatching the eschar is achieved by using a scalpel to make several slits the length and width of the eschar.

To avoid damaging the viable wound base beneath the necrotic tissue and causing pain, these slits are shallow and do not penetrate the depth of the necrotic tissue. Once the eschar begins to separate or demarcate from the surrounding skin, the enzyme can be applied to the wound edges along the line of demarcation to hasten separation. At this point, conservative sharp debridement can be used to remove softened necrotic tissue. Enzymes can then be continued, or another debridement technique such as autolysis can be instituted. Enzymes should be discontinued once viable tissue is revealed and necrotic tissue is removed.

The frequency of dressing changes ranges from daily to as often as 3 times daily depending on the type of enzyme used. The most appropriate type of cover dressing to use is not well researched. Manufacturer's guidelines suggest moist gauze dressings for papain/urea and dry gauze dressings for collagenase. However, these recommendations are based on safety and efficacy studies conducted before the advent of modern, moisture-retentive dressings (Boxer et al, 1969; Lee and Ambrus, 1975; Rao, Sane, and Georgier, 1975).

Although not researched, it appears that most dressings can be used safely with enzymes, including gauze, hydrogels, and transparent film dressings. The cover dressing that is selected should require the same frequency of application as the enzyme. Because enzymes are typically applied at least daily, dressings that are intended to remain in place for several days are not cost-effective in combination with enzyme preparations. Enzymatic debridement can be augmented further by using a moisture-retentive dressing. However, while this appears to facilitate more rapid debridement, the wound should be observed frequently and assessed carefully for infection. Collagenase has been safely combined with polymyxin B sulfate/bacitracin in the management of partial-thickness burns (Soroff and Sasvary, 1994).

Because these enzymes are selective, damage to viable tissue in the wound bed should not occur if the dressing is continued once debridement is completed and viable tissue is exposed. However, this practice is not advocated. More appropriate dressings are available at a fraction of the cost and should be implemented once the wound is debrided. Transient erythema and irritation, particularly when preparations containing papain come into contact with intact skin, have been,

TABLE 10-1 Enzyme Comparison

ENZYME	DESCRIPTION	SOURCE	MECHANISM OF ACTION	DOSAGE	APPLICATION GUIDELINES
Collagenase	Sterile enzyme debriding agent containing collagenase in white petrolatum (e.g., Santyl ointment)	Derived from *Clostridium* bacteria	• Digests native and denatured collagen, therefore effective on the "holding strands" and denatured collagen in the slough • Does not attack collagen in healthy tissue and newly forming granulation tissue	Administer once daily	• Optimal pH range: 6 to 8 • Activity adversely affected by detergents; hexachlorophene and heavy metal ions, such as mercury, zinc, and silver, will inactivate the enzyme; flush wound with saline before applying enzyme • Avoid soaks containing metal ions or acidic solutions such as Burrow's solution: metal ion and low pH will inactivate enzyme • Hydrogen peroxide and Dakin's solution compatible with enzyme • In wounds with depth, apply with tongue depressor; if wound is shallow, enzyme can be applied directly to gauze dressing • Crosshatch eschar with #10 blade to allow penetration
Papain/urea combination	• Combined papain and urea in a hydrophilic ointment base (e.g., Accuzyme, Panafil White) • Also available in combination with chlorophyllin copper complex sodium (e.g., Panafil, Gladase)	Derived from papaya	• Papain is a proteolytic enzyme that digests nonviable protein and is harmless to viable tissue • Papain is ineffective alone and requires activators (i.e., urea) to stimulate digestive potency • Urea is a denaturant of proteins and works as an activator to render the protein more susceptible to enzymatic attack by papain • Chlorophyllin copper complex sodium controls inflammation and reduces wound odor	Daily or twice-daily application	• Hydrogen peroxide may inactivate • Salts of heavy metals such as lead, silver, and mercury may inactivate • Active at pH range from 3 to 12

reported (Berger, 1993). Barrier ointments may be used to protect the periwound skin. Occasionally, patients report transient burning at the wound site with the application of enzymes.

Precautions. Enzymatic debridement has several disadvantages. Enzymes are a prescription item, so there are cost and reimbursement implications to their use. The frequent dressing changes dictate considerable commitment on the part of the caregiver (the patient, the family, or staff) that may not always be reasonable or acceptable. Enzymatic debridement is slow; the length of time required to achieve debridement may range from several days to weeks.

The major frustration about enzymatic debridement is the lack of research to guide clinical use and decision making. As previously mentioned, there is little research to guide the selection of the type of enzyme to use. Alvarez and colleagues (2000, 2002) reported increased effectiveness with papain/urea when compared with collagenase, but the study sample was small and there was little impact on healing rate. Another study showed favorable comparison between collagenase and surgical debridement on pediatric patients with partial-thickness burns (Ozcan et al, 2002). Although the enzyme's active ingredient is effective against specific types of necrotic tissue (e.g., denatured protein, denatured collagen, fibrin), it is unclear how this affects the enzyme's clinical effectiveness. It is very difficult to identify the specific type or predominant type of tissue present in the necrotic material. Currently, decisions about which product to use are based on availability, cost, ease, frequency of application, and familiarity with the product.

Few clinical trials comparing the effectiveness of enzymatic debridement with other enzymes and other debridement methods are available, and many of these studies were done with a product that is no longer commercially available (Hobson et al, 1998; Mekkes, Zeegelaar, and Westerhof, 1998). In a nonexperimental design using a complicated statistical technique employing decision analysis and computer modeling, Mosher and colleagues (1999) reported collagenase to have a greater likelihood of achieving a complete debridement of a full-thickness, noninfected pressure ulcer at 2 weeks than fibrinolysin, autolysis, or wet-to-dry dressings. This report, however, is difficult to apply clinically and requires clinical validation. Existing research uses several research designs and reports various endpoints, so consistency or consensus is lacking concerning effectiveness outcomes such as time required to debride (Glyantsev and Adamyan, 1997; Hobson et al, 1998; Mekkes, Zeegelaar, and Westerhof, 1998; Mosher et al, 1999).

Dakin's Solution. Dakin's solution (diluted sodium hypochlorite solution) has a long history of being used to cleanse and debride wounds and was originally used as a topical disinfectant for wounds sustained in war. The primary action of Dakin's solution is to exert antimicrobial effects and odor control. As a debriding agent, Dakin's solution is nonselective because of its cytotoxic properties.

Description. Dakin's solution denatures protein, therefore rendering it more easily removed from the wound. Loosening of the slough also facilitates debridement by other methods.

Directions for use. Dakin's solution is applied by saturating gauze with the solution, lightly packing it into the wound, and applying a gauze cover dressing. It is changed twice daily if the goal is debridement. Periwound skin protection should be provided with ointments, skin sealants, or solid-wafer skin barriers.

Dakin's solution is probably most appropriately used when there is a large amount of slough on the wound bed and the wound is infected or malodorous. Dakin's solution should be considered a short-term treatment (less than 10 days). Once infection and odor are under control, another debridement method should be selected to complete the process. Alternative dressing and debridement techniques should be implemented as the amount of slough decreases, exposing viable tissue.

The use of Dakin's solution for debridement is controversial (Monroe, 1992). Thomas (1990a, 1991) reports that hypochlorites are ineffective for the purpose of debridement based on findings that approximately 100 ml of 0.25% chlorine solution was needed to liquefy 1 g of slough, and that necrotic tissue remained unchanged after 24 hours of immersion in a chlorine solution.

Precautions. There is conflicting evidence linking the use of Dakin's solution and cytotoxicity, but some studies indicate that at a dilution of 0.025%, sodium hypochlorite can be an effective antimicrobial and still remain noncytotoxic (Heggers et al, 1991). Concentrations greater than 0.025% should be avoided, because higher concentrations may be toxic and pose a risk of damage to fibroblasts, resulting in an impaired wound-healing process (Rodeheaver, 1990).

Maggots. Originating from the battlefield, maggots are another method of chemical debridement. Physicians noted anecdotal reports from medics who observed the rapid removal of necrotic tissue when maggots were present on the wound bed. This technique has also been referred to as biologic debridement, or biosurgery. Because its mechanism of action is chemical in nature, this text discusses maggot therapy as a means of chemical debridement.

Description. Therapeutic maggot therapy involves sterilizing the eggs of *Lucilia sericata* (the greenbottle fly). Once they hatch (again, under sterile conditions) the sterile larvae are introduced into the wound bed. It is theorized that larvae secrete proteolytic enzymes, including collagenase, that break down the necrotic tissue. It is also believed that the larvae ingest microorganisms, which are then destroyed. Because of this reported action and the emergence of resistant organisms, there is renewed interest in maggot therapy in some centers, and more research is available to support this therapy (Sherman 2003, 2002; Thomas et al, 1996; Wallina et al, 2002; Wolff and Hanson, 2003).

Directions for use. Generally maggot therapy is considered for use in wounds that have not responded to conventional methods of debridement. The main benefit is the rapid debridement of necrotic tissue along with odor control. There may be some antimicrobial effects as well, although this claim is based on anecdotal reports. Some researchers are investigating the effects of maggots on fibroblasts and extracellular matrix (ECM) interaction and enhancement of healing beyond the debridement effects (Chambers et al, 2003; Horobin et al, 2003).

Precautions. Although there are no reported side effects, care should be taken to avoid having the larvae come in contact with healthy skin, since this could result in the proteolytic enzymes causing damage. The main disadvantage to maggot therapy is the sensation of crawling that some patients experience, but confinement of the larvae to the wound bed decreases this sensation. One dressing that has been devised for use with maggot therapy is comprised of hydrocolloid to protect the periwound skin, a mesh net over the wound to contain the larvae, and an absorbent pad to contain exudate (Sherman, 1997).

Mechanical

Mechanical modes of debridement include wet-to-dry gauze dressings, irrigation, and whirlpool. These techniques represent selective and nonselective modes of debridement.

Wet-to-Dry Debridement
Description. Wet-to-dry dressings have been the conventional treatment for debridement for decades (Mulder 1995; Turner, 1997). This method removes necrotic tissue and absorbs small amounts of exudate, but since it is a nonselective method of debridement, exposed healthy tissue in the wound is damaged.

Directions for use. Wet-to-dry mechanical debridement is most commonly used with heavily necrotic wounds. It is also used with infected wounds, thus allowing frequent visualization of the affected area. However, once the infection has resolved, a more selective method of debridement should be initiated.

Wet-to-dry debridement consists of applying saline-moistened gauze to the wound bed and allowing it to dry on the wound, trapping debris. Once dry, usually 4 to 6 hours after application, the dressing is pulled off the wound along with the trapped debris, the wound is cleansed, and the saline-moistened gauze reapplied. This process is continued until viable tissue is apparent, which takes several days to weeks.

Appropriate technique and dressing materials are critical for effective wet-to-dry debridement. Gauze should be moistened (not dripping wet) when applied to the wound, and although the gauze should contact the entire wound surface, it should not be packed tightly into the wound. Wet-to-dry gauze dressings must be allowed to dry out before removal, hence the need to avoid oversaturation of the gauze.

The most effective type of dressing material for wet-to-dry gauze dressings is an open-weave cotton fabric because it provides a combination of mildly abrasive qualities and adherent properties (Hall and Ponder, 1992; Mulder, 1995; Ponder and Krasner, 1993). Nonwoven gauze is generally ineffective because the fiber composition does not allow tissue adherence.

Precautions. Several disadvantages are associated with wet-to-dry debridement. To be effective, the procedure for preparing, applying, and removing the wet-to-dry dressing must be strictly followed. Unfortunately, the dressing change is rarely performed correctly. Gauze that is moistened immediately before removal minimizes the removal of debris (Goode and Thomas, 1997). The removal of the dressing can trigger acute noncyclic wound pain (see Chapter 25) for the patient and necessitate analgesia. Wet-to-dry dressings are a nonselective mode of debridement, so granulation tissue and epithelial tissue are also removed along with the necrotic tissue. Moistening the gauze before application with an excess amount of saline will also prevent the dressing from drying out as it should as well as increase the risk of periwound maceration (Rodeheaver et al, 1994). In addition, when the wound is exudative, wet-to-dry gauze dressings provide insufficient absorption, again macerating periwound skin. Wet-to-dry dressings are labor-intensive because they must be changed more than once per day. This technique is also complicated in that there are many steps involved that require a judgement call for correct execution. Finally, the steps involved in moistening the gauze provide ample opportunity to contaminate the gauze and break sterile technique or even clean technique, thus posing a risk of infection.

The use of wet-to-dry dressings is a controversial debridement method. Some wound care experts even consider gauze to be contraindicated as a wound contact dressing (Turner, 1997). However, wet-to-dry dressings remain a prevalent technique. This may be due to the ready availability of gauze, the perception that it is inexpensive, training, or simply force of habit. For most clinicians, until randomized clinical trials comparing wet-to-dry debridement with other methods of debridement are conducted, the appropriateness and effectiveness of wet-to-dry dressings will continue to be debated. Nonetheless, most experts in wound care agree that the use of wet-to-dry dressings should be restricted to heavily necrotic wounds and discontinued when viable tissue is present.

Irrigation. Another method of removing debris mechanically is through wound irrigation with pressurized fluids. There are two common methods of wound irrigation: high-pressure irrigation and pulsatile high-pressure lavage.

High-pressure irrigation

Description. Irrigation of the necrotic wound with fluid delivered at 8 to 12 pounds per square inch (psi), such as with a 35-ml syringe and a 19-gauge angiocatheter, is referred to as high-pressure irrigation. This procedure provides adequate force to remove debris without damaging healthy tissue or inoculating the underlying tissue with bacteria (Wheeler et al, 1976). Pressures below 4 psi, such as that provided by a bulb syringe, are not sufficient to remove eschar and slough from the wound base. These recommendations are also outlined in the AHCPR Pressure Ulcer Treatment Guideline (1994).

Directions for use. Normal saline is the most commonly recommended irrigant used with high-pressure irrigation. Occasionally, antimicrobial solutions such as Dakin's solution may be used for a short period when the wound is infected. Although these solutions precipitate cytotoxic effects on healthy wound cells, Rodeheaver (1990) suggests that unless an antiseptic is particularly toxic, brief contact with tissue will not impair wound healing. However, Lawrence (1997) states that "there is little evidence to suggest that irrigating with antiseptics significantly alters the bacteriological content of wounds". In a study conducted by Stringer, Lawrence, and Lilly (1983), no bacteriologic benefit was noted among "dirty wounds" irrigated with one of three popular antiseptics or physiologic saline.

High-pressure irrigation can be achieved with commercially available products that attach to saline bags so that a continuous flow of irrigation solution can be delivered to the wound at consistent, acceptable pressures. Prepackaged canisters of pressurized saline are also available and deliver the wound irrigant at an appropriate range of pressure.

Precautions. Delivering fluid under pressure to the wound bed can cause dissemination of wound bacteria over a wide area, exposing the patient and care provider to potential contamination. Consequently, personal protective equipment (i.e., mask, gloves, gown, and goggles) should be worn by the care provider during this procedure when "splash" is expected.

Pulsatile high-pressure lavage

Description. An alternative to high-pressure irrigation is pulsatile high-pressure lavage. These machines provide intermittent high-pressure irrigation combined with suction to remove the irrigant and debris. The apparatus allows adjustment of pressure to higher levels to remove debris. Pulsatile high-pressure lavage loosens necrotic tissue, facilitating removal by other methods of debridement, and may be used as an alternative to whirlpool. Pulsatile high-pressure lavage is an effective tool for removing larger amounts of debris, but efficacy studies are needed to determine its place in debridement and effects on wound healing. Morgan and Hoelscher (2000) reviewed the use of pulsatile high pressure lavage on 28 home care patients and noted favorable outcomes in a noncontrolled study.

Directions for use. The amount of solution needed depends on the size of the wound. Moist gauze is the most commonly used wound dressing; between pulsatile lavage due to the frequency of treatment. Pulsatile high-pressure lavage is best discontinued once the wound is clean.

Precautions. The main disadvantage to pulsatile high-pressure lavage is the cost. The hose and tip are designed for 1-time use, and necrotic wounds may require twice-daily treatments. Pressure settings should be maintained at 8 to 15 psi for debridement. Higher pressures are not appropriate because there may be inoculation of underlying tissue and damage to any granulation tissue (AHCPR, 1994). Caution should be used when irrigating with pulsatile high-pressure lavage to avoid blood vessels, graft sites, and exposed muscle, tendon, and bone. Patients on anticoagulant therapy should be observed carefully for any bleeding, and treatment should be immediately discontinued if bleeding occurs. As with high-pressure irrigation, personal protective equipment for the provider is necessary. Moreover, with pulsatile high-pressure lavage, treatment should be delivered in an enclosed area separate from any other patients to avoid contamination with mist (Loehne, 1998).

Whirlpool

Description. Whirlpool is commonly used to remove bacteria and debris from the surface of large wounds. Additional benefits include softening and loosening of adherent necrotic tissue and cleansing and removal of wound exudate. The vigorous action and hydration may contribute to the debridement effects; however, research to support this is minimal (Frantz, 1997).

Directions for use. Whirlpool is indicated for trunk or extremity wounds located on a body area that can be immersed in the tank. Wounds appropriate for whirlpool are usually large with a significant amount of necrotic material covering the wound surface. Water is the most common type of solution used, with an optimal temperature of 37° C (Sussman, 1998).

Questions have been raised about the efficacy of whirlpool alone in removing bacteria and debris from the wound surface (Frantz, 1997; Sussman, 1998). Although there is some reduction in bacterial load, this is actually thought to be the result of forceful rinsing after immersion rather than the action of the whirlpool alone (Neiderhuber, Stribley, and Koepke, 1975). Therefore it is probably the irrigation action rather than the whirlpool that decreases the surface bacteria. Burke and colleagues (1998) examined the effects of hydrotherapy on pressure ulcer healing and found significant improvement in the treatment group when compared with the control group. Sharp debridement was performed on all study patients before initiation of treatment; nutrition was not addressed.

Precautions. Vasodilatation, which leads to increased circulation to the affected area, naturally occurs with whirlpool therapy. However, vasodilatation is not always desirable. McCulloch and Boyd (1992) demonstrated an increase in lower leg edema in patients with venous ulcers after whirlpool therapy. This effect was attributed to a combination of the whirlpool action and the dependent position of the leg during the therapy.

Consequently, the pathophysiology of the wound must be considered before selecting whirlpool therapy. Increasing circulation in the extremity of patients with venous insufficiency contributes to venous congestion. In the presence of advanced arterial disease, the vessels in the leg are likely to be maximally dilated, so there is questionable benefit, and the added stress locally may increase metabolic demands. Also, whirlpool therapy must be used cautiously in the patient with diabetes who may not be able to detect temperature changes because of sensory or autonomic neuropathy.

Concerns also exist about cross-contamination between patients who use the whirlpool. According to Lawrence (1997), "Wound bacteria readily contaminate bath water." Although it is common practice to add antiseptic solution to the water, these additives may exert deleterious effects on the wound.

Sharp

Sharp debridement is also referred to as instrumental debridement and requires the use of surgical instruments. Sharp debridement can be done sequentially in a conservative fashion (conservative sharp wound debridement), or it can be done surgically (surgical sharp debridement).

Conservative Sharp Wound Debridement

Description. Conservative sharp wound debridement, also known as conservative instrumental debridement, is a selective debridement method for removal of loosely adherent, nonviable tissue using sterile instruments (e.g., forceps, or "pick-ups," scissors, and scalpel with #10 and #15 blades). Conservative sharp debridement is probably the most aggressive type of debridement performed by non–physician health care providers such as certified wound care specialists. When done correctly, the procedure is not aggressive enough to harm viable tissue and there is little likelihood of blood loss. Therefore the risks to the patient are minimal.

Professional and educational qualifications required to perform conservative sharp debridement have been proposed by numerous experts (Fowler, 1992; Gordon, 1996; Razor and Martin, 1991; Tomaselli, 1995). While some states consider conservative sharp debridement to be within the scope of practice for registered nurses, most states consider this a delegated medical function. A variety of other requirements may also have to be satisfied, depending on the nurse practice act specific to the state and the employer's requirements.

Directions for use. The basic principles of conservative sharp debridement include the following:
1. Decrease the likelihood of infection by using sterile instruments, using sterile technique, and preparing the site for debridement with an antiseptic (e.g., Betadine or a chlorhexidine solution such as Hibiclens).
2. Establish a plane of dissection by holding the necrotic tissue taut to clearly visualize the plane of dissection.
3. Avoid all vascular tissues and tissues that are not clearly identified.
4. Irrigate the wound following the procedure.

Conservative sharp debridement has several advantages. It removes the necrotic tissue more quickly than the previously discussed methods and can be accomplished in a serial manner. This method of debridement can be combined with other debridement techniques (autolysis or enzymatic) to shorten this phase of wound care. Theoretically, a more rapid approach to debridement decreases the body's expenditure of energy during a time of high resource use. Furthermore, because of the low risk involved, conservative sharp debridement can be performed in a variety of settings by non–physician clinicians who are skilled and credentialed in this technique. Therefore conservative sharp debridement of necrotic wounds is a viable option for patients residing in nonacute care settings and does not require transfer to a hospital.

It is impossible to make a "blanket statement" about the exact requirements that must be met for a nurse to be authorized to perform this procedure (Box 10-1). Wound care nurses and physical therapists interested in seeking approval to perform conservative sharp debridement should consult their particular state practice acts and individual facility requirements.

A sample policy and procedure on conservative sharp debridement is provided in Box 10-2. Before implementing these policies and procedures, they

---

BOX 10-1 Conservative Sharp Wound Debridement: Question/Qualifications to Consider

1. Is conservative sharp debridement covered under the clinician's state practice act?
2. Are specialty education, training, and credentials in conservative sharp debridement required by the state or employer?
3. Are formal knowledge and skill updates required on a periodic basis?
4. Has the individual's professional organization or employer delineated specific guidelines related to conservative sharp debridement?
5. Are policies, procedures, and protocols in place for conservative sharp debridement?
6. Is conservative sharp debridement considered part of the clinician's clinical privileges, or is a physician's order required for each incident of conservative sharp debridement?
7. What level of physician supervision, if any, is required for conservative sharp debridement?
8. Does the employer provide malpractice insurance coverage for conservative sharp debridement?
9. Does the clinician carry malpractice insurance to cover conservative sharp debridement?

BOX 10-2 Policy and Procedure: Conservative Sharp Wound Debridement

I. Purpose

The purpose of this policy and procedure is to outline the process by which an RN with certification in wound care may remove devitalized tissue by conservative sharp wound debridement.

II. Policy

- Any RN performing conservative sharp wound debridement will have additional didactic education in the skill.
- Any RN performing conservative sharp wound debridement will have additional laboratory education to develop the skill.
- Any RN performing conservative sharp wound debridement will participate in a clinical practicum involving patients with wounds.
- Documentation of the above will be filed with the individual's other credentialing information. (This is determined by practice setting.)

III. Authority and Responsibility

- The individual performing conservative sharp wound debridement will provide documentation of education and competency.
- An order from the attending physician will be obtained before the procedure, or physician practice protocols will be in effect permitting the procedure.
- Obtain consent from the patient or appropriate representative. (This is determined by practice setting.)

IV. Definitions

Conservative sharp wound debridement is the removal of loose, avascular tissue using surgical instruments (e.g., scissors, scalpel, forceps) without inflicting pain or precipitating bleeding.

V. Procedure

1. Explain procedure to patient
2. Obtain consent (this is determined by practice setting)
3. Assemble equipment:
   a. Forceps with teeth
   b. Scalpel handle with #15 blades
   c. Silver nitrate sticks
   d. Curved iris scissors
   e. Surgical gel foam or silver nitrate stick
   f. Gauze sponges
   g. Normal saline
   h. Clean gloves
4. Wash hands
5. Prepare work surface
6. Position patient for procedure
7. Ensure adequate lighting
8. Apply clean gloves
9. Remove old dressing and discard
10. Wash hands, apply clean gloves
11. Prep site with antiseptic (Betadine or Hibiclens if iodine allergy)
12. Grasp loosely adherent tissue with forceps; pull tautly, exposing a clear line of dissection
13. Cut or snip loose tissue
14. Irrigate wound with normal saline
15. For minor bleeding, apply silver nitrate, gel foam, or pressure
16. Apply appropriate dressing
17. Document procedure and patient's response to procedure

VI. References

- State-by-state nurse practice acts
- Tomaselli N: WOCN Society position statement: conservative sharp wound debridement for registered nurses, *J WOCN* 22(1):32A (www.wocn.org) 1995.

should be evaluated and approved by the organization in which the wound care specialist operates or is employed.

Precautions. A disadvantage of conservative sharp debridement is that, depending on the size of the ulcer and the amount of necrotic tissue involved, it could conceivably take weeks to remove all of the nonviable tissue. It may also be an uncomfortable procedure for the patient, so the need for analgesia either topically or systemically should be considered.

Although blood loss is not expected during conservative sharp debridement, it remains a possibility. As a result, the patient should be assessed for factors that place him or her at risk for clotting problems if a vessel is accidentally severed. Factors to consider include medications (e.g., heparin, warfarin, high-dose nonsteroidal antiinflammatory drugs [NSAIDs], and antibiotics) and pathologic conditions (e.g., thrombocytopenia, impaired liver function, vitamin K deficiency, and malnutrition). When any of these factors is present, the wound care specialist should confer with the physician before proceeding with conservative sharp debridement.

Infected wounds present unique considerations for conservative sharp debridement. In general, there is the potential for transient bacteremia after debridement of wounds, particularly when the wound is infected. Transient bacteremia in a patient who is nutritionally compromised, leukopenic, or otherwise immunocompromised can be devastating. Unfortunately, there is a lack of research concerning the relationship between sharp debridement and transient bacteremia. Therefore a cautious, conservative approach is warranted.

Theoretically, surgical sharp debridement is the preferred method of debriding most infected wounds. Realistically, this is not always an option because of either the patient's condition or the setting. In these situations, serial conservative sharp debridements can be conducted by the non–physician wound care provider, but only in conjunction with appropriate antibiotic coverage. Although systemic antibiotics may not penetrate the necrotic tissue to reduce the bacterial load in the wound, they should reduce the potential for systemic dissemination of the pathogens. Topical antiseptic solutions may also be instrumental in reducing the bioburden of the wound. The wound care specialist should be in compliance with policies of the facility or agency concerning the management of infected wounds.

Surgical Sharp Wound Debridement

Description. Surgical sharp wound debridement, also known as surgical debridement, is usually reserved for those cases requiring the removal of massive amounts of tissue or involving a life-threatening infectious process that dictates immediate removal of necrotic tissue to effectively treat the patient (Haury et al, 1978). Surgical debridement inherently implies aggressive removal of necrotic tissue. In most cases, it is a one-time procedure carried out by a surgeon in the operating room, although there are necrotic processes (e.g., necrotizing fasciitis) that require serial debridement. If the patient is unstable or unable to withstand the anesthesia required for such procedures, surgical debridement may be performed under a local or spinal anesthetic. When indicated, the surgeon may choose to perform a less aggressive sharp debridement at the bedside using a local anesthetic.

Directions for use. Surgical debridement is the fastest method for removing large amounts of necrotic tissue. It has also been demonstrated to stimulate wound repair in diabetic ulcers, theorized to be a result of correcting the imbalance of cytokines and proteases in chronic wound fluids, thus converting the detrimental molecular environment of a chronic wound into a pseudoacute wound molecular environment (Schultz, 1999; Steed et al, 1996). Two other studies report improved outcomes with neuropathic foot ulcers when sharp debridement was performed (Kumagi, 1998; Piaggesi, 1998).

Surgical debridement is beyond the scope of practice of most-nonphysician providers such as the wound care nurse and physical therapist.

Precautions. Disadvantages of surgical debridement include increased direct risks to the patient in terms of anesthesia risks, bleeding, and sepsis. As stated previously, it is common to see transient bacteremia after a wound is debrided. Most healthy individuals can withstand such events. Unfortunately, many infected wounds occur in people who are not in optimal health; therefore the transient bacteremia could progress to systemic infection and patient death. Due to the possibility of transient bacteremia, interventions should be employed to prevent or control it, such as using sterile technique and instruments and perioperative antibiotics. Because of its obvious aggressive nature, some viable tissue may be sacrificed during surgical debridement (Linder and Morris, 1990).

Another disadvantage of surgical debridement is that it may add tremendously to the overall costs of treating the patient. The condition of the patient, the aggressive nature of this procedure, and the higher level of care required after debridement often require hospitalization.

Laser Debridement

Description. Laser debridement, a form of surgical sharp debridement, uses focused beams of light to cauterize, vaporize, or slice through tissue. Several light sources for lasers are available: argon, CO_2, neodymium yttrium aluminum garnet (Nd:YAG), and tunable (Habif, 1996). Each type of laser emits light at a specific wavelength, and different body tissues absorb different wavelengths. The part of the tissue that absorbs the light is called the chromophore (e.g., water is the chromophore for the CO_2, laser, and hemoglobin is the chromophore for the argon laser). When the chromophore absorbs the light, it is quickly heated and vaporized. When the beam of light is tightly focused, it is capable of cutting through human tissue like a knife (Raz, 1995).

Directions for use. The choice of which laser to use is often dictated by the specifics of the problem at hand (e.g., the extent of the necrosis, location of the wound). Historically, continuous wave CO_2 lasers were often used to debride necrotic tissue. Advantages of laser debridement are that the wound bed is sterilized, and that most severed vessels are cauterized (Flemming, Frame, and Dhillion, 1986; Slutzki, Sharif, and Bornstein, 1977). Animal studies using a laser to debride partial-thickness burns have demonstrated improved healing (Lam et al, 2002) and similar results to sharp debridement, but with hemostasis and no disturbance of periwound skin (Graham, 2002).

Precautions. Disadvantages of laser debridement include risk of injury to adjacent healthy tissue and therefore delayed healing. More current work with pulsed laser beams rather than the continuous laser beams has decreased these negative effects (Glatter et al, 1998; Smith et al, 1997). Unfortunately, this method is not available in all settings.

SELECTION OF DEBRIDEMENT METHOD

The method of debridement selected is affected by individual patient situations and by clinician skill. Three general principles guide the selection of the most appropriate debridement process: (1) urgency of the need for debridement, 2) the skill level of the care provider, and 3) availability of products and supplies. Clinicians must assess the wound characteristics, wound-treatment goals, patient status or comorbidities, and the clinician's own clinical experience and competence.

Wound Characteristics

Type of Necrotic Tissue. The type of necrotic tissue in the wound guides the selection of debridement method. Eschar responds to autolysis, enzymes (with crosshatching), and either conservative or surgical sharp debridement. Slough is managed with autolysis, sharp debridement, wet-to-dry dressings, and high pressure lavage. When slough is unresponsive to these techniques, enzymes can be considered.

Presence of Wound Infection. The presence of an infected wound with necrotic tissue is another critical determinant of method. Infection dictates that rapid debridement is imperative.

Wound-Treatment Goals

The overall goals for the wound should also be considered. First it must be decided whether debridement is appropriate. When to pursue debridement is then prioritized according to the patient's condition and the wound treatment goal (whether the goal is to heal the wound or to prevent deterioration of the wound).

Occasionally, it may be necessary to forego debridement in light of other more urgent needs of the patient. Such a decision must include input from the patient, the patient's significant others, and the primary care provider. Even if the goal is not to heal the wound, debridement of necrotic tissue will also control unpleasant wound odors, making the environment more comfortable for the patient, family, and caregivers.

Wound debridement may be delayed in some circumstances. For example, when a necrotic but noninfected ulcer is found on a patient who is critically ill, unstable, or severely neutropenic, it may be prudent to delay the debridement until the patient's condition improves. Because necrotic tissue harbors microbes, transient bacteremia can still occur after sharp debridement of noninfected wounds and overwhelm the patient's immune system. Postponement of debridement can help to reduce this likelihood.

When eschar covers a stable, noninfected wound on an ischemic extremity, and when dry eschar covers a pressure ulcer located on the heel, debridement is not indicated (AHCPR, 1994). The presence of a wound infection (edema, erythema, fluctuance or drainage) dictates reevaluation of the plan of care and debridement is warranted.

Patient Status and Comorbidities

The patient's history and coexisting morbidities such as neutropenia and clotting disorders also affect the selection of debridement method. Autolysis should not be expected in the presence of severe neutropenia (absolute neutrophil count of less than 500 mm³) because there are an insufficient number of neutrophils available to respond to the wound demands. Generally, the wound will appear stagnant during this time. Debridement by autolysis should be postponed until the neutrophil count climbs over 1000 mm³. However, chemical debridement using enzymes is an effective option in the presence of neutropenia. Awareness of any clotting disorders or anticoagulant medication use is also critical when considering conservative sharp debridement.

Wound pain is another critical determinant of debridement method selection. Patients experiencing wound pain may benefit from the less painful debridement modalities such as autolysis or enzymatic debridement. Other types of debridement such as wet-to-dry, conservative sharp, and surgical sharp may trigger or exacerbate pain. The patient's pain status during dressing changes and while resting should be assessed; prophylactic analgesia should be administered topically or systemically.

Clinician Experience and Competence

Although debridement methods such as autolysis, wound irrigations, wet-to-dry dressings, and enzymes are ideally initiated under the direction of the physician or wound care specialist, they are procedures that can be performed by nurses, physical therapists, the patient, and caregivers. However, the more aggressive methods of debridement, specifically sharp debridement, require a level of skill and competence. Conservative sharp debridement should be performed only by a wound care specialist or physician with demonstrated and documented competence. The wound care specialist must also be in compliance with his or her scope of practice, state nurse practice act, and institutional policies. Surgical sharp debridement and laser debridement are only performed by physicians. Algorithms are available to guide the clinician in selecting the appropriate debridement method. Although they are based on expert opinion and have not been validated, these algorithms can serve as a useful starting point for decision making (Figure 10-1).

ASSESSMENT OF THE DEBRIDEMENT PROCESS

The methods of wound debridement typically employed by the non–physician wound care specialist do not immediately yield a completely clean wound; therefore the wound must be closely monitored for indicators of progression of the debridement process.

Deterioration of the wound requires reevaluation of the treatment selected. Assessment parameters include wound dimensions, volume of exudate, odor, type of tissue present, and condition of the periwound skin. Wound dimensions typically increase as the necrotic tissue is removed from the wound. Early in the debridement process, the wound is commonly exudative; this should decrease as the necrotic tissue is removed. As the underlying tissue is exposed, healthy viable tissue in the wound base should be present. When using autolysis, enzymes, or wet-to-dry dressings, a gradual transition in the type of necrotic tissue present in the wound base should be observed and documented. Hydrated eschar becomes gray and soft; firmly adherent slough becomes loose and stringy. When the wound is infected, a decrease in the periwound erythema and induration should be observed after debridement. If the patient was febrile or had leukocytosis before initiating debridement, a decrease should be observed as the necrotic tissue is removed and the bacterial load is reduced. However, these clinical changes may also be attributed to antibiotic therapy.

SUMMARY

Debridement is a critical component of topical therapy for necrotic wounds. The wound care specialist should be knowledgeable about the various methods available for debridement and should discuss the options with the patient's physician and the patient so the most appropriate wound-management choice can be made. Debridement methods are not used in isolation; rather, they are used in combination and modified as the wound conditions change. For example, an eschar-covered, noninfected wound may be crosshatched and covered with a hydrogel sheet. As the eschar softens, it may then be possible to use conservative sharp debridement to facilitate removal of the bulk of the residual eschar, and to then continue use of the hydrogel or select another moisture-retentive dressing, depending on the wound needs. Close supervision of the patient and accurate wound assessments during the debridement phase are essential to ensure an outcome consistent with the stated wound goals.

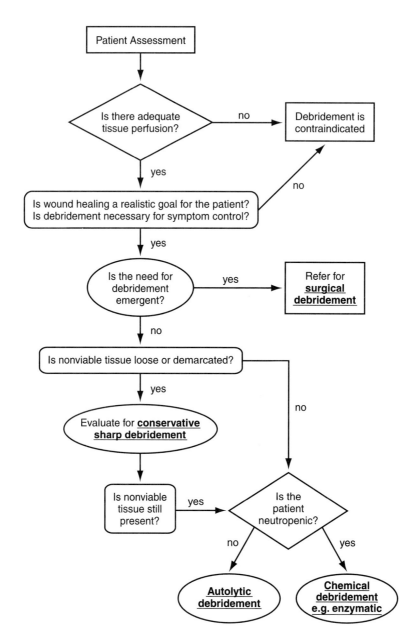

Fig. 10-1 Debridement algorithm.

SELF-ASSESSMENT EXERCISE

1. Which of the following methods of debridement is nonselective?
   a. Autolysis
   b. High-pressure irrigation
   c. Enzymes
   d. Surgical sharp
2. High-pressure wound irrigation requires which of the following?
   a. A bulb syringe
   b. Daily dressing changes
   c. Personal protective gear
   d. Expensive equipment
3. List three considerations in the use of enzymatic debridement.
4. Selection of debridement approach is guided by all of the following EXCEPT:
   a. Patient's age
   b. Presence of wound infection
   c. Extent and type of necrotic tissue
   d. Clinician experience
5. The risk of transient bacteremia is associated with which of the following debridement techniques?
   a. Autolysis
   b. Conservative sharp
   c. Enzymes
   d. Wet-to-dry dressings

REFERENCES

Agency for Health Care Policy and Research (AHCPR): *Treatment of pressure ulcers in adults*, Rockville, MD, 1994, U.S. Department of Health and Human Services, AHCPR Publication No. 95-0652.

Alvarez O: Moist environment for healing: matching the dressing to the wound, *Ostomy Wound Manage* 21:64, 1988.

Alvarez, O et al: Chemical debridement of pressure ulcers: a prospective, randomized comparative trial of collagenase and papain/urea formulations, *Wounds* 12(2):15, 2000.

Alvarez O et al: A prospective, randomized, comparative study of collagenase and papain-urea for pressure ulcer debridement, *Wounds* 14:293, 2002.

Bale S: A guide to wound debridement, *J Wound Care* 6(4):179, 1997a.

Bale S: Principles of wound intervention. In Bale S, Jones V, editors: *Wound care nursing: a patient-centred approach*, London, 1997b, Baillière Tindall.

Bates-Jensen B: Management of necrotic tissue. In Sussman C, Bates-Jensen B, editors: *Wound care*, Gaithersberg, Md, 1998, Aspen.

Berger M: Enzymatic debriding preparations, *Ostomy Wound Manage* 39(5):61, 1993.

Bodey GP et al: Quantitative relationship between circulating leukocytes and infection in patients with acute leukemia, *Ann Intern Med* 64(2):328, 1966.

Boxer A et al: Debridement of dermal ulcers and decubiti with collagenase, *Geriatrics* 24:75, 1969.

Bryant R, Rolstad BS: *Autolysis white paper*, St Paul, Minn, 1998, 3M Health Care.

Burke E et al: Effects of hydrotherapy on pressure ulcer healing, *Am J Phys Med Rehabil* 77(5):394,1998.

Chambers L et al: Degradation of extracellular matrix components by defined proteinases from the greenbottle larva *Lucilia sericata* used for the clinical debridement of non-healing wounds, *Br J Dermatol* 148:14, 2003.

Colins D, Kurning P, Yuon C: Managing sloughy pressure sores, *J Wound Care* 5(10):44, 1996.

Eaglstein WH: Occlusive dressings, *J Dermatol Surg Oncol* 19:715, 1993.

Falanga V: Wound bed preparation and the role of enzymes; a case for multiple actions of the therapeutic agents, *Wounds* 14:47, 2002.

Flemming A, Frame J, Dhillion R: Skin edge necrosis in irradiated tissue after carbon dioxide laser excision of tumor, *Lasers Med Sci* 1:263, 1986.

Fowler E: Instrumental/sharp debridement of non-viable tissue in wounds, *Ostomy Wound Manage* 38(8):26, 1992.

Frantz R: Adjunctive therapy for ulcer care, *Clin Geriatr Med* 13(3):553, 1997.

Glatter D et al: Carbon dioxide laser ablation with immediate autografting in a full-thickness porcine burn model, *Ann Surg* 228(2):257, 1998.

Glyantsev SP, Adamyan AA: Crab collagenase in wound debridement, *J Wound Care* 6(1):13, 1997.

Goode P, Thomas D: Pressure ulcers: local wound care, *Clin Geriatr Med* 13(3):543, 1997.

Gordon B: Conservative sharp wound debridement, *J WOCN* 23(3):137, 1996.

Graham JS et al: Efficacy of laser debridement with autologous split-thickness skin grafting in promoting improved healing of deep cutaneous sulfur mustard burns, *Burns* 28:719, 2002.

Habif TP, editor: *Clinical dermatology: a color guide to diagnosis and therapy*, ed 3, St Louis, 1996, Mosby.

Hall S, Ponder R: Non-woven wound care products, *Ostomy Wound Manage* 38(6):24, 1992.

Haury B et al: Debridement: an essential component of traumatic wound care, *Am J Surg* 135(2):126, 1978.

Hebda PA, Lo C: Biochemistry of wound healing: the effects of active ingredients of standard debriding agents—papain and collagenase—on digestion of native and denatured collagenous substrates, fibrin and elastin, *Wounds* 13:190, 2001.

Heggers JP et al: Bacteriocidal and wound healing properties of sodium hypochlorite solutions: the 1991 Lindberg Award, *J Burn Care Rehabil* 12:420, 1991.

Hobson D et al: Development and use of a quantitative method to evaluate the action of enzymatic wound debriding agents in vitro, *Wounds* 10(4):105, 1998.

Horobin AJ et al: Maggots and wound healing: an investigation of the effects of secretions from *Lucilia sericata* larvae upon interactions between human dermal fibroblasts and extracellular matrix components, *Br J Dermatol* 148:923, 2003.

Hutchinson JJ: Prevalence of wound infection under occlusive dressings: a collected survey of reported research, *Wounds* 1(2):123, 1989.

Kumagi SG et al: Treatment of diabetic (neuropathic) ulcers with two-stage debridement and closure, *Foot Ankle Internat* 19(9):649, 1998.

Lam DG, Rice P, Brown R: The treatment of Lewisite burns with laser debridement—lasablation, *Burns* 28(1):19, 2002.

Lawrence JC: Dressings and wound infection, *Am J Surg* 167(1A):215, 1994.

Lawrence JC: Wound irrigation: an update on irrigating fluids and their effect on wounds, *J Wound Care* 6(1):23, 1997.

Lee L, Ambrus J: Collagenase therapy for decubitus ulcers, *Geriatrics* 30:91, 1975.

Linder M, Morris D: The surgical management of pressure ulcers: a systematic approach based on staging, *Decubitus* 3(2):32, 1990.

Loehne HL: Pulsatile lavage with concurrent suction. In Sussman C, Bates-Jensen B, editors: *Wound care*, Gaithersburg, Md, 1998, Aspen.

McCulloch J, Boyd V: The effects of whirlpool and the dependent position on lower extremity, *J Orthop Sports Phys Ther* 16(4):169, 1992.

Mekkes J, Zeegelaar J, Westerhof W: Quantitative and objective evaluation of wound debriding properties of collagenase and fibrinolysin/deoxyribonuclease in a necrotic ulcer animal model, *Arch Dermatol Res* 290:152, 1998.

Monroe D: Hypochlorites: a review of the evidence, *J Wound Care* 1(4):44, 1992.

Morgan D, Hoelscher J: Pulsed lavage: promoting comfort and healing in home care, *Ostomy Wound Manage* 46(4):44, 2000.

Mosher BA et al: Outcomes of four methods of debridement using a decision analysis methodology, *Adv Wound Care* 12(2):81–88, 1999.

Mulder G: Evaluation of three non-woven sponges in the debridement of chronic wounds, *Ostomy Wound Manage* 41(3):62, 1995.

Mulder G et al: Controlled randomized study of a hypertonic gel for the debridement of a dry eschar in chronic wounds, *Wounds* 5(3):112, 1993.

Neiderhuber S, Stribley R, Koepke G: Reduction of skin bacterial load with use of the therapeutic whirlpool, *Phys Ther* 55(5):482, 1975.

Ozcan C, Ergun O, Celik A, Corduk N, Ozok G: Enzymatic debridement of burn wound with collagenase in children with partial thickness burns, *Burns* 28:791, 2002.

Piaggesi A et al: Conservative surgical approach versus non-surgical management for diabetic neuropathic foot ulcers: a randomized trial. *Diabet Med.* 15(5):412-7,1998.

Ponder R, Krasner D: Gauzes and related dressings, *Ostomy Wound Manage* 39(5):48, 1991.

Rao D, Sane P, Georgier E: Collagenase in the treatment of dermal and decubitus ulcers, *J Am Geriatr Soc* 23(1):22, 1975.

Raz K: Laser physics, *Clin Dermatol* 13:11, 1995.

Razor B, Martin L: Validating sharp wound debridement, *J ET Nurs* 18(3):105, 1991.

Robson M: Wound infection: a failure of wound healing caused by an imbalance of bacteria, *Surg Clin North Am* 77(3):637, 1997.

Rodeheaver GT: Influence of antiseptics on wound healing. In Wesley AJ, Thomson PD, Hutchinson JJ, editors: *International forum on wound microbiology*, Princeton, 1990, Excerpta Medica.

Rodeheaver GT et al: Wound healing and wound management: focus on debridement, *Adv Wound Care* 7(1):22, 1994.

Rolstad BS, Harris A: Management of deterioration in cutaneous wounds. In Krasner D, Kane D, editors: *Chronic wound care*, ed 2, Wayne, Penn, 1997, Health Management Publications.

Schultz G: Molecular regulation of the wound environment. In Bryant RA, editor: *Acute and chronic wounds: nursing management*, ed 2, St Louis, 1999, Mosby.

Sherman R: A new dressing design for use with maggot therapy, *Plast Reconstr Surg* 100(2):451, 1997.

Sherman R: Maggot vs conservative debridement therapy for the treatment of pressure ulcers, *Wound Rep Regen* 10(4):208, 2002.

Sherman R: Maggot therapy for treating diabetic foot ulcers unresponsive to conventional therapy, *Diabetes Care* 26(2):446, 2003.

Sibbald RG et al: Preparing the wound bed—debridement, bacterial balance and moisture balance, *Ostomy Wound Manage* 46(11):14, 2000.

Slutzki S, Sharif R, Bornstein L: Use of the carbon dioxide laser for large excisions with minimal blood loss, *Plast Reconstr Surg* 60:250, 1977.

Smith K et al: Depth of morphologic skin damage and viability after one, two, and three passes of a high-energy, short pulse CO_2 laser (Tru-Pulse) in pig skin, *J Am Acad Dermatol* 37(2):204, 1997.

Soroff HS, Sasvary DH: Collagenase ointment and polymyxin B sulfate/bacitracin spray vs. silver sulfadiazine cream in partial thickness burns: a pilot study, *J Burn Care Rehabil* 15:13, 1994.

Steed DL et al: Effect of extensive debridement and treatment on the healing of diabetic foot ulcer, *J Am Coll Surg* 183:61, 1996.

Stotts N, Hunt T: Managing bacterial colonization and infection, *Clin Geriatr Med* 13(3):65, 1997.

Stringer MD, Lawrence JC, Lilly HA: Antiseptics and the casualty wound, *J Hosp Infect* 4:410, 1983.

Sussman C: Whirlpool. In Sussman C, Bates-Jensen B, editors: *Wound care*, Gaithersberg, Md, 1998, Aspen.

Thomas S: Eusol revisited, *Dressing Times* 3:1, 1990a.

Thomas S: *Wound management and dressings*, London, 1990b, Pharmaceutical Press.

Thomas S: Evidence fails to justify use of hypochlorite, *J Tissue Viabil* 1:9, 1991.

Thomas S et al: Using larvae in modern wound management, *J Wound Care* 5(2):60, 1996.

Tomaselli N: WOCN position statement: conservative sharp wound debridement for registered nurses, *J WOCN* 22(1):32A, 1995.

Turner TD: The development of wound management products. In Krasner D, Kane D, editors: *Chronic wound care*, ed 2, Wayne, Penn, 1997, Health Management Publications.

Wheeler C et al: Side effects of high pressure irrigation, *Surg Gynecol Obstet* 143(5):775, 1976.

Wallina U et al: Biosurgery supports granulation and debridement in chronic wounds—clinical data and remittance spectroscopy measurement, *Internat J Dermatol* 41(10):635, 2002.

Wolff H, Hansson C: Larval therapy—an effective method of ulcer debridement, *Clin Exper Dermatol* 28(2):134, 2003.

Wound Ostomy Continence Nursing (WOCN) Society: *Guideline for prevention and management of pressure ulcers* (series), Glenview, IL, 2003, Author.

Acute Surgical and Traumatic Wounds

JOANNE D. WHITNEY

OBJECTIVES

1. Identify and describe two factors that impair acute wound–repair processes.
2. Describe the microcirculation of an acute surgical or traumatic wound environment.
3. Discuss the effects of an activated sympathetic nervous system on acute wound–repair processes.
4. Differentiate among the roles of wound tissue oxygen and arterial oxygen in wound repair.
5. Describe five interventions to increase tissue oxygen or improve healing in acute surgical and traumatic wounds.

The phenomenon of healing is an inescapable component of the human experience. The challenge of repairing bodily injury is complex. Tissue injury, whether accidental or planned, initiates a series of biochemical events directed toward reestablishing vascular and cellular integrity. During tissue repair, wound healing is vulnerable to disruption by a number of factors. Failure at any step of the sequence may impair wound healing and confer significant morbidity and cost. In acute wounds, there is a growing recognition that inadequate wound healing and complications such as surgical site infection likely have their origins early in the healing process, when tissue breaking strength is low and physiologic responses may not be optimal (Dubay and Franz, 2003).

The editors gratefully acknowledge Judith M. West and Michael L. Gimbel for their work on developing this chapter for the first and second editions of *Acute And Chronic Wounds, Nursing Management.* Many of the comments and concepts they put forth in the previous editions are reflected in this chapter, and we are appreciative of their significant contribution.

A great deal has been learned about tissue repair over the last decade, although much of the information that has been acquired has not become standard in everyday clinical practice. The literature is a guide to a new understanding of the importance of adequate blood flow to peripheral tissues to supply oxygen for optimal wound healing and resistance to infection. This chapter addresses factors that influence acute wound repair including autonomic nervous system (ANS) activation, fluids supplemental oxygen, hypothermia, warming, tobacco use, and glucose control. Interventions for modifying these factors to achieve better wound-tissue perfusion and healing responses are discussed.

FACTORS IN THE REPAIR OF THE ACUTE WOUND

Oxygen

Availability of oxygen (PO_2) to the local wound area is essential for the wound-healing processes. These processes include oxidative bacterial killing and resistance to infection (Babior, 1978; Hohn et al, 1976; Knighton, Halliday, and Hunt, 1984), collagen synthesis and fibroplasia (Niinikoski, 1969), angiogenesis (Knighton, Silver, and Hunt, 1981), and epithelialization (Pai and Hunt, 1972). Decreased local wound oxygen (tissue hypoxia) is a major contributor to wound complications (Goodson et al, 1987; Jönsson, Hunt, and Mathes, 1988; Knighton, Halliday, and Hunt, 1984). Additionally, oxygen-derived reactive oxygen species (ROS) are believed to participate in signaling and coordinating the repair process (Sen et al, 2002).

Peripheral tissues may become hypoxic from direct traumatic or surgical injury to vessels or from blood volume loss and vasoconstriction of regional vasculature. Wound-tissue oxygen delivery may be impaired unless conditions of diminished peripheral perfusion are anticipated and corrected. Correction of adrenergic vasoconstrictive stimuli, particularly cold, pain, and volume loss, elevates PO_2 (Akca et al, 1999; Hopf et al, 1997; West, 1994) and leads to fewer postoperative infections (Kurz et al, 1996). The degree of regional tissue perfusion regulates the supply of oxygen and is therefore the prime determinant of the competency of wound healing. Strategies to optimize perfusion by addressing specific sympathetic nervous system activators are described in Table 11-1.

Arterial oxygen levels are not necessarily reflective of tissue oxygen delivery. Although the PaO_2 of 90 mm Hg in a healthy volunteer breathing room air maintains a wound PO_2 of 50 mm Hg or greater, the postoperative patient experiencing pain, cold, fear, or periodic desaturation will exhibit predictably low oxygen levels within the wound. This observation led to an approach to adrenergic activation as an etiology for wound hypoxia (West, 1990).

Clinicians must demonstrate an awareness and understanding of the ways in which the injured may be at risk for wound complications given the patient's constellation of preinjury vulnerabilities. Wound-tissue hypoxia occurs to some extent at the time of injury in everyone, regardless of age or state of health (Silver, 1980). Early recognition and treatment of perfusion deficits translates to improved clinical outcome.

The type and extent of tissue loss can characterize human wounds. Whether the surgeon's scalpel or other trauma causes a wound, viability of tissue will determine the course and quality of healing. Incisions closed during elective surgery under the best of aseptic conditions appear to have the fewest reparative obstacles to healing. However, any tissue injury disrupts vascular supply. All wounds are relatively hypoxic at the center, in the range of 0 to 5 mm Hg (Silver, 1969). After oxygen leaves the red blood cells (RBCs) in the capillaries, it diffuses into the wound space. The driving force of diffusion is partial pressure. In wounds, damage to the microvasculature, vasoconstriction, and intravascular fluid overload markedly increase intercapillary distances (Goodson et al, 1979; Heughan, Niinikoski, and Hunt, 1972; Hunt and Hopf, 1997). In animal studies done in ear chamber wounds, the mean oxygen tensions were 0 to 3 mm Hg in the wound center dead space, 5 to 15 mm Hg in the growing edge, and 20 to 30 mm Hg in the newly vascularized area with early fibroblast proliferation. The steepest fall in oxygen occurred in the tissue within the first 25 microns of the wound edge (Niinikoski, Heughan, and Hunt, 1972; Silver, 1969).

Clinicians may assume that tissue hypoxia is present in all wounds. In most perioperative circumstances, oxygen supply to healing tissue can be enhanced (Chang et al, 1983; Hopf et al, 1997; Kurz et al, 1996; West, 1990). All surgical and traumatic wounds warrant concern

TABLE 11-1 **Strategies to Support Acute Wound Healing**

SYMPATHETIC NERVOUS SYSTEM ACTIVATORS	INTERVENTIONS TO OPTIMIZE PERFUSION
Cold	Provide active warming to maintain normothermia in the perioperative period.
	Increase warmth by covering feet with socks or slippers, applying blankets or sweaters, and facilitating postoperative warming with warm blankets.
	Prevent heat loss, and prevent shivering.
Pain	Medicate for comfort (adequate pain control).
	Seek additional measures for pain control such as repositioning and relaxation.
Fear	Provide patient teaching to reduce fear related to procedures or knowledge deficits.
	Administer medications as needed to reduce anxiety and fear.
Pharmacologic	Discontinue beta blockers, when possible.
Smoking	Refer patient to a tobacco cessation program.
	Advise patient to not smoke 2 to 4 weeks before surgery, and after surgery only when incision is completely healed.
	Encourage successful completion of entire program.
Hyperglycemia	Maintain glucose level between 80-180 mg/dl.

and effort. The acute surgical wound is often cited as an example of a healthy, potentially "uncomplicated" wound that will heal "uneventfully" if left unperturbed. However, most of the clinically relevant literature on healing addresses chronic or problematic wounds. At what points is the repair process stressed, compromised, or aborted? When and why does an acute wound, expected to have an uncomplicated and fairly predictable course, make the transition to a chronic and problematic wound? Hunt and Silver have focused attention on the study of events in the cellular microenvironment to discover how living tissue repairs itself when damaged (Hunt, Zederfeldt and Goldstick, 1969; Silver, 1969; Silver, 1980). Explanation of the nature of the healing (as opposed to the nonhealing) wound environments, and development of therapies designed to selectively modify the wound environment continue to be major foci of current wound-healing research (Gimbel and Hunt, 1999; Harding, Morris, and Patel, 2002).

Stress

Stress may be defined as the body's primitive protective response to injury or anticipated injury. Cannon (1970) revealed the mechanisms that activate the autonomic nervous system to respond to stress. He directly observed the constriction of blood vessels in peripheral tissues during stress in animals. The mediators of the sympathetic and adrenal response to stress, epinephrine and norepinephrine, induce profound vasoconstriction in subcutaneous and skin blood vessels supplying peripheral tissues (Rowell, 1986). Sympathetic activation in the postoperative period is a function of severing of afferent nerves, hypovolemia, fear, pain, and cold rather than anesthesia (Halter, Pflug, and Porte, 1977). Catecholamines may remain elevated for days after surgery (Derbyshire and Smith, 1984; Halter, Pflug, and Porte, 1977), and concentrations vary with length and severity of surgery (Chernow et al, 1987). This is illustrated by comparing the difference in norepinephrine levels observed following arthroscopy of the knee and total knee replacement in Figure 11-1 (Clark et al, unpublished data). Norepinephrine is increased threefold in the early postoperative hours (Derbyshire and Smith, 1984), peaking with the patient's first expression of pain (Niinikoski, Heughan, and Hunt, 1972).

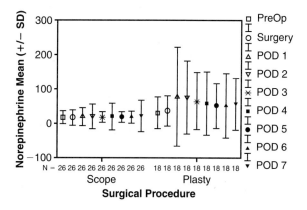

Fig. 11-1 Comparison of norepinephrine levels in patients having either arthroscopy or arthroplasty of the knee. (Clark et al, Unpublished data.)

The relationship of tissue oxygen and perfusion of various tissues is well established (Gosain et al, 1991; Gottrup et al, 1987; Jönsson et al, 1991). Evidence of how stress limits perfusion has been demonstrated by infusion of exogenous epinephrine in healthy subjects. In this study designed to mimic the body's response to stress, increasing levels of epinephrine decreased the level of subcutaneous tissue oxygen 45%, whereas heart rate and arterial P_{O_2} did not markedly change (Jensen et al, 1985).

In addition to the effects of stress-related ANS activity, changes in immune response mediated by psychologic stress are also believed to have a negative effect on healing (Kiecolt-Glaser et al, 2002). Preoperative stress has been shown to delay healing in oral surgery (Marucha, Kiecolt-Glaser, Favagehi, 1998). In patients undergoing inguinal hernia repair, higher levels of preoperative stress lowered the amounts of interleukin-1 and matrix metalloproteinase-9 found in wound fluid in the first 20 postoperative hours (Broadbent et al, 2003). These results suggest that increased stress before surgery reduces the early inflammatory response to injury and, potentially, subsequent postsurgical wound healing.

Hypothermia

The effects of temperature on the amount of vasomotor tone primarily determine cutaneous capillary blood flow. Cooling increases norepinephrine affinity to α-adrenergic receptors on vascular smooth muscle. This augments the response of cutaneous vessels to autonomic activation, which increases constrictive vessel tensions up to fivefold (Vanhoutte, Verbeuren, and Webb, 1981).

Hypothermia-induced vasoconstriction has decreased subcutaneous oxygen tension in anesthetized volunteers (FiO_2 of 0.6 mm Hg) to a mean of 50 mm Hg (Sheffield et al, 1992). Furthermore, a lower blood temperature also shifts the oxyhemoglobin curve to the left, thereby increasing the amount of oxygen carried in the blood but decreasing the amount of oxygen released (Severinghaus, 1958). This effect may exacerbate tissue hypoxia induced by peripheral vasoconstriction.

Virtually all anesthetic agents are vasodilators and may cause a rapid initial decrease in core temperature (1° C to 2° C) during the first hour after the induction of anesthesia. (Sessler, 1993). Internal redistribution of body heat from core to periphery is exacerbated by conductive and evaporative losses as a result of visceral exposure in a cold environment (Roe, 1971). Rapid initial body heat loss may be limited by heating the operating room and aggressive preoperative warming (Morris, 1971). Preinduction warming may nearly prevent rapid initial body heat loss (Hynson and Sessler, 1992).

Adverse consequences of perioperative body heat loss are significant and include prolonged hypothermia, postoperative warming time, and shivering. Shivering in the elderly, although rare, is dangerous because oxygen demand may increase by 400% to 500% (Bay, Nunn, and Prys-Roberts, 1968). This drastic increase in oxygen demand increases cardiac workload. Increased oxygen consumption has been shown to coincide with core decrements of 0.3° C to 1.2° C (Roe et al, 1966). Prolonged postoperative hypothermia is associated with increased mortality (Slotman, Jed, and Burchard, 1985) and myocardial ischemia (Frank et al, 1993). Animal studies demonstrate that the harmful effects of cooling are proportional to the duration of the cooling period. In a series of canine studies comparing incised wounds of cooled limbs with contralateral uncooled limbs similarly wounded, there was a higher incidence of infection after delayed primary closure of the cooled limbs (Large and Heinbecker, 1944). The cooled limb wounds had less tensile strength, and sections taken immediately after cooling showed no histologic evidence of response to injury (inflammation).

Hyperglycemia

Another important factor contributing to the potential for infection and failed healing is diabetes mellitus, which affects a large portion of the increasingly aging population undergoing surgical procedures. Diabetes is associated with increased hospital costs and length of hospital stay after cardiac surgery (Estrada et al, 2003). Elevated blood glucose levels are associated with significant reduction in the phagocytic ability of neutrophils and diminished wound strength (Goodson, 1979). Hyperglycemia, defined as whole-blood glucose above 200 mg/dl, in the 48 hours after surgery is associated with development of surgical site infection (SSI) in cardiothoracic surgery patients (Latham et al, 2001). This prospective study also demonstrated that patients previously undiagnosed with diabetes who were identified during the study based on hemoglobin A1c values above 7%, were at higher risk for SSI. Perhaps the single most advantageous action that can be taken to minimize this risk is to prevent postoperative hyperglycemia. Current recommendations for patients with cardiovascular disease advocate for protocol-based, aggressive glycemic control to achieve individualized target blood glucose levels, generally between 80 to 180 mg/dl (Trence, Kelly, and Hirsch, 2003). Careful monitoring and control of diabetes should extend well into the postoperative period to optimize the healing environment during the months of collagen remodeling.

Tobacco

Smoking is associated with poor wound outcomes through the catecholamine-mediated vasoconstrictive effects of nicotine and increases in carbon monoxide that reduce blood oxygen content (Gottrup, 2004). Vasoconstrictive effects resulting in significant decreases in tissue oxygen tension occur after smoking a single cigarette, and tissue oxygen requires an hour to return to baseline levels (Jensen et al, 1991). Reductions in tissue oxygen translate clinically into lower amounts of collagen production and reduced wound strength (Jorgensen et al, 1998). Recent studies document the significance of smoking as a factor that impairs healing. Smoking is the single most predictive factor of wound complications in patients having elective hip or knee replacements (Moller et al, 2003). Forty-seven percent of patients undergoing abdominoplasty who smoked had wound complications, compared to 14.7% of those who did not smoke (Manassa, Hertl and

Olbrisch, 2003). Because of the reductions in tissue oxygen supply when smoking and the substantial time needed for levels to recover, all patients with wounds should be advised to abstain from smoking. The optimal period for abstaining from smoking before surgery has not yet been determined. However, at least one study has shown that 2 weeks is inadequate to limit wound-related problems, and a longer period is likely to be needed (Sorensen and Jorgensen, 2003).

Obesity

Wound healing problems are more likely in patients who are overweight, and this is a growing national problem. In excess of 44 million Americans are considered obese (body mass index greater than or equal to 30); this represents an increase in population obesity rates of 74% since 1991 (CDC, 2001). Individuals with severe obesity often suffer from a number of related health problems. These include both serious and disabling conditions such as type II diabetes, hypertension, coronary artery disease, sleep apnea, venous stasis disease and lower extremity ulcers, osteoarthritis, urinary incontinence, gastro-esophageal reflux disease, fatty liver, cholelithiasis, and depression (Mun et al, 2001). Reduction of obesity is one of the objectives for the improvement of health in the United States designated in Healthy People 2010 (U.S. Department of Health and Human Services, 2000). For individuals with morbid obesity and for whom conventional weight loss treatments have proved unsuccessful, surgery is an effective treatment option (Colquitt et al, 2003). Recognition of this has led to increasing demand for and acceptance of this type of surgery in the treatment of obesity (Brolin, 2002). However, the incidence of postsurgical wound complications in patients with obesity compared to those of normal weight is high, with reported rates of 15% to 22% (Israelsson and Jönsson, 1997; Vastine, et al 1999; Winiarsky, Barth, and Lotke 1998). Fried and colleagues reported 15% of patients undergoing gastric resection for obesity experienced wound complications. Because of this increased vulnerability to wound complications, extra vigilance and measures to assure peripheral perfusion must be taken in surgical patients who are obese, including interventions for pain control and stress reduction, fluid repletion, warming, and nutrition. Obesity is addressed in greater detail in Chapter 14.

Nutrition

Presurgical morbidity is another critical variable, which may dramatically tip the balance against a favorable healing outcome. Poor nutrition before surgery correlates with decreased quality and quantity of collagen deposition (Goodson et al, 1987). Rapid preoperative replenishing of nutrients is effective in reducing postoperative wound complications (Hopf et al, 1997). Nutrition is addressed in greater detail in Chapter 8.

INTERVENTIONS THAT SUPPORT ACUTE WOUND HEALING

Warming

Aggressive intraoperative warming and rapid postoperative warming are effective modalities for minimizing the risks of prolonged hypothermia (Hynson and Sessler, 1992). Sympathetic vasoconstriction can be overcome by warmth to provide uncomplicated healing. In a large study combining intraoperative and postoperative warming, wound infection rates were reduced by 60% (Kurz et al, 1996).

Results of systemic warming studies suggest the importance of maintaining core temperature regulation in the perioperative and early postoperative periods. In addition, local wound temperature modification using controlled warming improves blood flow directly to sites of injury and may benefit healing. Heat applied in the form of a plastic-sealed moistened towel to small, experimental wounds in hospitalized patients produced threefold increases in perfusion and an average 39.5 torr increase in local oxygen tension (Rabkin and Hunt, 1987). Applying local controlled warming at 35° to 45° C increased tissue oxygen in a dose-dependent fashion in four healthy volunteers, with oxygen increases continuing for 30 minutes after warming (Ikeda et al, 1998). Further testing of local controlled warming applied over subcutaneous test wounds, using a 2-hour on/off cycle for 1 week in 10 volunteer subjects, increased tissue oxygen levels by 50% (West, Hopf, and Hunt, 1996). Though collagen deposition in warmed wounds was not increased compared to control in this small sample, these studies clearly demonstrate that local warming effectively increases blood flow and tissue oxygen.

Local warming has been evaluated in a small number of surgical wound studies. Plattner and colleagues (2000) applied local warming to abdominal incisions of 40 patients, showing significantly higher tissue oxygen in the immediate recovery period and on the first postoperative day. In a large, single-blind, randomized study (N = 421 patients having breast, varicose vein, or hernia repair surgeries), preoperative local warming was compared to systemic warming or no warming of any type (Melling et al, 2001). Patients received 30 minutes of systemic warming, local warming to the planned surgical site, or standard preoperative care (no warming). Infection rates of 4% with local warming, 6% with systemic warming and 14% with no warming were documented. In a pilot study of 54 patients at high risk for wound complications (gastric bypass and colectomy procedures) warming during postanesthesia recovery and the first postoperative day showed fewer complications with local warming (22%) compared to standard incision care (37%) (Whitney, Dellinger, and Wickline, 2004).

Supplemental Fluid and Oxygen

A growing number of researchers have suggested that inspiration of increased oxygen concentration (FiO_2) be routinely prescribed for postoperative patients during the first few days after surgery to increase oxygen delivery to the reparative site. Relatively low levels of supplemental oxygen (28%) in the first 24 to 36 postoperative hours have been shown to increase tissue oxygen tension in patients undergoing below-the-knee amputation and cervical laminectomy procedures (Butler et al, 1987; Whitney et al, 2001). This practice is especially emphasized in patients undergoing lengthy abdominal or pelvic procedures. However, it is important to recognize that correcting tissue hypoxia requires more than simply providing increased FiO_2 to increase the arterial saturation (SaO_2) and arterial PO_2. Wound PO_2 may remain unchanged even while the patient is breathing additional oxygen. In one study of patients who underwent general surgery, approximately 30% had reduced tissue oxygen tension levels despite adequate urine output and arterial oxygen levels (Chang et al, 1983). This finding results from the early postoperative compartmental fluid shifts, in which kidney perfusion is restored at the expense of peripheral vasculature vasoconstriction.

Jönsson and colleagues (1987) demonstrated that tissue oxygen levels could be corrected with infusion of fluids, and that a fluid bolus of 250 ml of normal saline was sufficient in most cases. In well-perfused patients, tissue oxygen pressure continues to rise as PaO_2 rises. Subsequent clinical studies where supplemental fluids were provided perioperatively continue to support this as an effective method of improving wound tissue PO_2. In patients having abdominal and colon surgeries, those receiving aggressive fluid repletion (defined as maintenance levels of 16 to 18 ml/kg/hour during surgery and one hour postoperatively) or for the first 24 postsurgery hours (an average 1.1 L increase above standard fluids) showed significantly higher wound PO_2 compared to patients receiving standard fluids (Arkilic et al, 2003; Hartmann, Jönssen, and Zederfeldt, 1992). Higher levels of collagen deposition were associated with the increased fluids and improved wound oxygen status (Hartmann, Jönssen, and Zederfeldt, 1992). Supporting the critical relationship between vascular volume and tissue oxygen, fluid repletion along with supplemental oxygen effectively raises wound PO_2. This was demonstrated in a randomized trial of 500 patients, half of whom received 80% oxygen during surgery, compared to 30% for the other half. Those in the higher oxygen group had significantly higher tissue oxygen levels and fewer wound infections (Greif et al, 2000).

The clinical findings of these studies justify in general the practices of assuring patients are well hydrated and the provision of oxygen to support wound healing. It is recommended that supplemental oxygen be given in the presence of good peripheral perfusion during surgery for infection control and for 3 days postoperatively to support collage synthesis (Chikungwa and Jönsson, 2002). Further clarity of the optimal dosage and duration of supplemental oxygen to achieve healing and avoid complications has yet to be determined. A recent study testing the use of 80% oxygen perioperatively in general surgery patients did not confirm the findings of Greif and colleagues (Pryor et al, 2004), and illustrates the need for additional studies to elucidate dosage and timing issues.

In a prospective randomized trial, aggressive postoperative warming and pain control increased the wound PO_2 to 70 mm Hg within 4 to 6 hours, a level nearly equal to that of normal volunteers (West, 1994). In addition, the actively rewarmed patients having undergone lengthy abdominal surgeries were given a 1-liter fluid bolus to replace fluids lost as urine during the diuresis, which commonly accompanies hypothermia and vasoconstriction. Trauma patients have demonstrated improved regional perfusion after warming and adequate fluid resuscitation (Knudson et al, 1997). Patients who are well perfused and oxygenated rarely develop wound infections (Hopf et al, 1997).

Hypovolemia is a powerful physiologic vasoconstrictor. Therefore volume replacement must coincide with postoperative warming to benefit peripheral perfusion. Core temperature is not a clinically useful indicator in this equation. Skin surface temperatures do correlate with fingertip blood flow; a forearm-minus-fingertip difference of 4° C defines a state of peripheral vasoconstriction. However, this method is not yet commonly used in practice (Rubinstein and Sessler, 1990).

ASSESSMENT OF HEALING IN THE ACUTE WOUND

One problem in making clinically useful decisions about wounds is that the wrong things may be measured at the wrong times. What is happening in the wound microenvironment may be discovered by sampling the wound itself (wound fluid, tissue, or oxygen tension). Infection, for example, is a function of bacteria *in* the tissue, not *on* the tissue. Just as myocardial dysfunction is confirmed by enzymes in the blood, and thyroid alterations may be detectable by blood analysis, wound oxygen has become a useful measure of perfusion. Wound oxygen is a clinically valid and reliable index that responds more rapidly to intravascular fluid shifts than do blood pressure and pulse. When adequate oxygen is available for wound fibroblasts, collagen formation and wound tensile strength can be achieved. Collagen maturation then continues for months after wounding.

Although low periwound oxygen is a feature of most wounds initially, continued and unexplained hypoxia is of particular importance. Wound healing is proportional to local oxygen tension. Transcutaneous oxygen tension ($tcPO_2$) is a useful, noninvasive way to assess the adequacy of tissue oxygenation near a wound or suture line in relationship to FiO_2 (Figure 11-2). Defining the contribution of hypoxia in the context of the recent history of the patient and time from wounding clarifies why wound PO_2 is low. Tests can be conducted to reveal the wound's responsiveness to factors such as local warming, vasodilating drugs, oxygen therapies, sympathetic blockade, positioning,

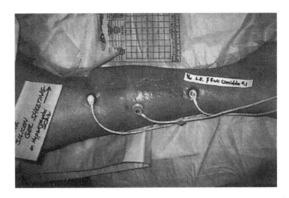

Fig. 11-2 Technique of obtaining $tcPO_2$ in lower leg wounds.

pain, and anxiety management (Figure 11-3). For example, during an oxygen challenge in the absence of vasoconstriction, there will be significant oxygen diffusion into the capillary-perfused wound edge. Simple, effective, and conservative corrective therapy can then be initiated. Since improved wound PO_2 is a real measure of wound healing progress, serial measurements of damaged tissue can be obtained during the course of healing.

Clinically, there is no single method of assessing healing of acute wounds. Deposition of collagen in the wound begins immediately in the inflammatory phase and peaks during the proliferative phase, approximately 4 to 21 days after wounding. When healing progresses normally, the clinician can detect the accumulation of new tissue synthesis by palpating what is referred to as the healing ridge in an approximated wound. The healing ridge presents as induration beneath the skin extending to about 1 cm on each side of the wound between 5 and 9 days after wounding. This is an expected positive sign. Lack of a ridge is cause for concern, and interventions to reduce mechanical strain on the wound must be instituted promptly. Hunt and Dunphy (1979) point out that "almost all dehiscences occur by the fifth to eighth postoperative day in patients who have not yet developed a cutaneous healing ridge and about half are associated with infection." Furthermore, they state that when a healing ridge is present, even retention sutures can be removed because the risk of separation has passed.

Acute wound complications can be evaluated on the basis of specific parameters using the ASEPSIS

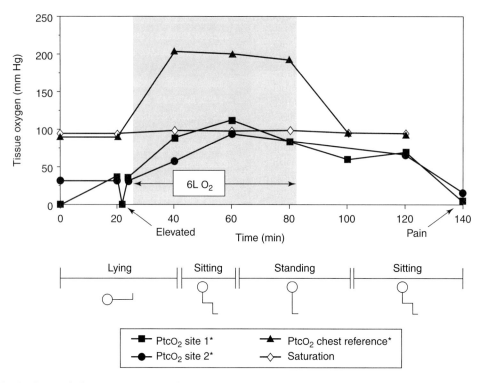

Fig. 11-3 Graph demonstrating wound responsiveness to position changes and oxygen challenge. Wound Po$_2$ measurement with the patient breathing Fio$_2$ 0.21 (room air), and then with a supplemental challenge at Fio$_2$ 0.50 or greater, allows one to see how the periwound microvasculature is able to respond. Notice that only the oxygen challenge, not the chest reference, is affected by position changes. The tcPo$_2$ for site 1 is lower than for site 2 and for the chest reference in both the lying and sitting positions. However, it does demonstrate a response to 6 liters of oxygen.

scoring tool ASEPSIS is an acronym for seven wound assessment parameters. The ASEPSIS tool is reported to be the most frequently used quantitative tool for surgical wound evaluation (Bruce et al, 2001). The ASEPSIS method was originally developed in cardiac surgery patients to evaluate characteristics of the surgical incision associated with infection (Wilson et al, 1986a). In a validation study, ASEPSIS was reported to be as sensitive and significantly more specific than other clinical indicators of wound problems or when compared to wound assessments made using standard definitions of wound infections (Wilson et al, 1990). Interrater reliability of 0.96 has been reported in patients having general surgery (Byrne et al, 1989). Similar reliability has been shown for sternal and leg wounds of patients

after cardiac surgery (Wilson et al, 1986b). Summed scores over wound assessments performed each day for the first 5 postoperative days indicate severity of infection or complication (see Box 11-1). Chapter 9 provides information related to surgical incision infection.

INCISIONAL CARE

Regardless of origin, wounds progress through the same phases of the reparative process: inflammation, angiogenesis, fibroplasia and matrix deposition, and epithelialization. Knowledgeable assessments of the patient's surgical incision site include evaluation of the primary dressing, epithelial resurfacing, wound closure, healing ridge, and local changes at the wound site that may signal infection.

BOX 11-1 ASEPSIS Scoring Tool for Evaluating Acute Wound Complications

CRITERION		POSSIBLE POINTS
A = Additional therapy	Antibiotics	10
	Debridement under general anesthesia	10
	Drainage of pus under general anesthesia	5
S = Serous exudate*		Daily 0-5
E = Erythema*		Daily 0-5
P = Purulent exudate*		Daily 0-10
S = Separation of deep tissue*		Daily 9-10
I = Isolation of bacteria		10
S = (hospital) Stay greater than 14 days.		5

*Given scores only on day 5 of first 7 postoperative days

Instructions for use

The proportion of the wound, as measured to the nearest 10% of its length for each characteristic, is assigned a numerical score.

Score Interpretation

0-10	=	Satisfactory healing
11-20	=	Disturbance of healing
21-30	=	Minor wound infection
31-40	=	Moderate wound infection
> 40	=	Severe wound infection

From Wilson APR et al: A scoring method (ASEPSIS) for postoperative wound infections for use in clinical trials of antibiotic prophylaxis, *Lancet* 1(8476):311, 1986.

Dressings serve the purposes of providing initial protection, exudate absorption, and thermal insulation for acute wounds. There is scant research to direct caregivers as to the preferred dressing for the surgical wound. One recent study of 737 patients having cardiac surgery reported no differences in wound infection or healing between dry absorbent, hydrocolloid, and hydroactive dressings for closed sternotomy wounds (Wynne et al, 2004). Comfort and cost analysis in the study showed dry absorbent dressings to be the least expensive and most comfortable. Interestingly, there are some data to suggest that dressings that provide some level of pressure or compression may actually impede local tissue perfusion (Plattner et al, 2000). This was based on the observation that wounds covered with dressings that provide some level of pressure had tissue oxygen levels 12 mm Hg lower than wounds with less constrictive covers. In the interest of supporting oxygen

delivery to acute wounds, avoiding extra pressure over the wound seems prudent unless required for hemostasis.

Surgical dressings are typically removed 48 to 72 hours following injury, which is consistent with Centers for Disease Control and Prevention (CDC) guidelines for the prevention of surgical site infections (Mangram et al, 1999). Resurfacing of the wound closed by primary intention occurs within 2 to 3 days after wounding because of the presence of intact epithelial appendages, such as hair follicles, and the relatively short distance that cells in the interrupted epithelial tissue must traverse. Although the incisional wound does not have the structural integrity (tensile strength) to withstand force at this time, by postoperative day 2 or 3, the incision is "sealed" and impenetrable to bacteria. Despite this fact, many patients prefer that the wound remain covered. As healing evolves, some incisions begin to itch as a result of wound contraction or simply dry skin. Desire to view the surgical scar is personal. The presence of a dressing allows patients to gradually incorporate changes in body image. Although an incisional dressing may no longer be necessary once epithelial cells have resurfaced the wound, a soft dressing placed over the suture line often limits local irritation and provides additional comfort and support, particularly as the patient begins to wear street clothes.

PATIENT EDUCATION

The knowledgeable nurse employs a theory-based assessment and coordinated therapeutic plan to optimize wound care within the context of a larger plan, including patient teaching and necessary follow-up. Patients in acute care settings require instruction in wound care, fluid replacement, avoidance of dehydration, use of tobacco, and practical ways to conserve body heat. Unfortunately, this instruction occurs frequently at a time when the patient is fatigued and somewhat overwhelmed by the entire surgical experience. Teaching, in this case, is best done succinctly and should be reinforced by providing the patient or family member with written guidelines. Follow-up of understanding and emphasis on healthy postoperative behaviors at clinic appointments reinforces initial teaching.

SUMMARY

All components of repair must be enhanced, step by step, to keep the wound "healing." Study results emphasize the need for perioperative intervention in order to support healing optimally and avoid acute wound complications. From the onset of injury, any interference with oxygen delivery to any degree will proportionately compromise reparative processes and increase susceptibility to infection (Hunt and Dunphy, 1979). Similarly, glycemic control in the perioperative period appears critical to normal repair. Maintaining tissue perfusion and glucose homeostasis must be incorporated among first-line interventions to assure rapid, uncomplicated repair of acute wounds.

SELF-ASSESSMENT EXERCISE

1. State two factors that are associated with reduced acute wound healing, and describe their mechanisms of limiting healing.

2. Define three observable characteristics of a healing acute surgical wound.
3. True or false: urine output 50 ml/hr correlates well with adequate wound P_{O_2}.
4. True or false: PaO_2 is a measure of tissue oxygen.
5. State four nursing interventions to optimize wound-tissue perfusion.
6. Describe the significance of the healing ridge in an acute surgical wound.
7. State five contributors to sympathetic nervous system activation.
8. To optimize the phagocytic ability of neutrophils, in what range should blood glucose levels be maintained?
   a. Between 40 and 80 mg/dl
   b. Between 80 and 180 mg/dl
   c. Below 150 mg/dl
   d. Below 200 mg/dl
9. Adequate oxygen is best provided to healing tissue by the following combined interventions:
   a. Oxygen to keep arterial saturation at 95% and pain control
   b. Supplemental fluids, pain control, and rapid rewarming
   c. Supplemental fluids, active warming, and oxygen
   d. Supplemental colloids, warm blankets, and pain control

REFERENCES

Akca O: Postoperative pain and subcutaneous oxygen tension, *Lancet* 354:41, 1999.

Arkilic CF et al: Supplemental perioperative fluid administration increases tissue oxygen pressure, *Surgery* 133:49, 2003.

Babior BM: Oxygen-dependent microbial killing by phagocytes, *N Engl J Med* 198:659, 1978.

Bay J, Nunn JF, Prys-Roberts C: Factors influencing arterial P_{O_2} during recovery from anaesthesia, *Br J Anaesthesia* 40:398, 1968.

Broadbent E et al: Psychological stress impairs early wound repair following surgery, *Psychosom Med* 65:865, 2003.

Brolin RE: Bariatric surgery and long-term control of morbid obesity, *JAMA* 288:2793, 2002.

Bruce J et al: The quality of measurement of surgical wound infection as the basis for monitoring: a systematic review, *J Hosp Infect* 49:99, 2001.

Butler CM et al: The effect of adjuvant oxygen therapy on transcutaneous P_{O_2} and healing in the below-knee amputees, *Prosthet Orth Int* 11:10, 1987.

Byrne D et al: Postoperative wound scoring, *Biomed Pharm* 43:669, 1989.

Cannon WB: *Bodily changes in pain, hunger, fear and rage: an account of recent researches into the function of emotional excitement,* College Park, Md, 1970, McGrath.

Center For Disease Control and Prevention (CDC): *1991-2001 Prevalence of obesity among U.S. adults, by characteristics,* http://www.cdc.gov/nccdphp/dnpa/obesity/trend/prev_char.htm. Accessed June 2004.

Chang N et al: Direct measurement of wound and tissue oxygen tension in postoperative patients, *Ann Surg* 197:470, 1983.

Chernow B et al: Hormonal responses to graded surgical stress, *Arch Intern Med* 147(7):1273, 1987.

Chikungwa MT, Jönsson K: The need for peri-operative supplemental oxygen, *Cent Afr J Med* 48:72, 2002.

Clark SJ et al: The effects of stress response on wound healing, Unpublished data.

Colquitt J et al: *Cochrane Database Syst Rev* 2: CD003641, 2003.

Derbyshire D, Smith G: Sympathoadrenal responses to anaesthesia and surgery, *Br J Anaesth* 56:725, 1984.

Dubay DA, Franz MG: Acute wound healing: the biology of acute wound failure, *Surg Clin North Am* 83:463, 2003.

Estrada CA et al: Outcomes and preoperative hyperglycemia in patients with or without diabetes mellitus undergoing coronary artery bypass grafting, *Ann Thorac Surg* 75;1392, 2003.

Frank SM et al: Unintentional hypothermia is associated with postoperative myocardial ischemia: the Perioperative Ischemia Randomized Anesthesia Trial Study Group, *Anesthesiology* 78:468, 1993.

Fried M et al: Bariatric surgery at the 1st Surgical Department in Prague: history and some technical aspects, *Obes Surg* 7:22, 1997.

Gimbel M, Hunt T: Wound healing and hyperbaric oxygen. In Kindwall E, Whelan H, editors: *Hyperbaric medicine practice*, Flagstaff, Az, 1999, Best Publishing.

Goodson W: Wound healing and the diabetic patient, *Surg Gynecol Obstet* 149:600, 1979.

Goodson W et al: Wound oxygen tension of large vs small wounds in man, *Surg Forum* 30:92, 1979.

Goodson W et al: The influence of a brief preoperative illness on postoperative healing, *Ann Surg* 205:250, 1987.

Gosain A et al: Tissue oxygen tension and other indicators of blood loss or organ perfusion during graded hemorrhage, *Surgery* 109:523, 1991.

Gottrup F et al: Directly measured tissue oxygen tension and arterial oxygen tension assess tissue perfusion, *Crit Care Med* 15:1030, 1987.

Gottrup F: Oxygen in wound healing and infection, *World J Surg* 28:312, 2004.

Greif R et al: Supplemental perioperative oxygen to reduce the incidence of surgical-wound infection, *N Engl J Med* 342:161, 2000.

Halter JB, Pflug AE, Porte D Jr: Mechanism of plasma catecholamine increases during surgical stress in man, *J Clin Endocrinol Metab* 45(5):936, 1977.

Harding KG, Morris HL, Patel GK: Science, medicine and the future. Healing chronic wounds, *BMJ* 324:160, 2002.

Hartmann M, Jönsson K, Zederfeldt B: Effect of tissue perfusion and oxygenation on accumulation of collage in healing wounds, *Eur J Surg* 158:521, 1992.

Heughan C, Niinikoski J, Hunt TK: Effect of excessive infusion of saline solution on tissue oxygen transport, *Surg Gynecol Obstet* 135:257, 1972.

Hohn DC et al: Effect of O_2 tension on microbicidal function of leukocytes in wounds and in vitro, *Surg Forum* 27:18, 1976.

Hopf HW et al: Wound tissue oxygen tension predicts the risk of wound infection in surgical patients, *Arch Surg* 132:997, 1997.

Hunt TK, Zederfeldt B, Goldstick TK: Oxygen and healing. *Am J Surg* 118(4):521-525, 1969.

Hunt TK, Dunphy JE: *Fundamentals of wound management*, New York, 1979, Appleton Century Crofts.

Hunt TK, Hopf H: Wound healing and wound infection: what surgeons and anesthesiologists can do, *Surg Clin North Am* 77:587, 1997.

Hynson JM, Sessler DI: Intraoperative warming therapies: a comparison of three devices, *J Clin Anesth* 4:194, 1992.

Israelsson LA, Jönsson T: Overweight and healing of midline incisions: the importance of suture technique, *Eur J Surg* 163:175, 1997.

Ikeda T et al: Local radiant heating increases subcutaneous oxygen tension, *Am J Surg* 175:33, 1998.

Jensen JA et al: Epinephrine lowers subcutaneous wound oxygen tension, *Curr Surg* 42(6):472, 1985.

Jensen JA et al: Cigarette smoking decreases tissue oxygen, *Arch Surg* 126:1131, 1991.

Jönsson K et al: Assessment of perfusion in postoperative patients using tissue oxygen measurements, *Br J Surg* 74:263, 1987.

Jönsson K et al: Tissue oxygenation, anemia, and perfusion in relation to wound healing in surgical patients, *Ann Surg* 214:605, 1991.

Jönsson K, Hunt TK, Mathes SJ: Oxygen as an isolated variable influences resistance to infection, *Ann Surg* 208:783, 1988.

Jorgensen et al: Less collagen production in smokers, *Surgery* 123:450, 1998.

Kiecolt-Glaser JK et al: Psychoneuroimmunology and psychosomatic medicine: back to the future, *Psychosom Med* 64:15, 2002.

Knighton DR, Halliday B, Hunt TK: Oxygen as an antibiotic: the effect of inspired oxygen on infection, *Arch Surg* 119:199, 1984.

Knighton DR, Silver IA, Hunt TK: Regulation of wound-healing angiogenesis—effect of oxygen gradients and inspired oxygen concentration, *Surgery* 90:262, 1981.

Knudson MM et al: Use of tissue oxygen tension measurements during resuscitation from hemorrhagic shock, *J Trauma* 42:608, 1997.

Kurz A et al: Perioperative normothermia to reduce the incidence of surgical-wound infection and shorten hospitalization, *N Engl J Med* 334:1209, 1996.

Large A, Heinbecker P: The effect of cooling on wound healing, *Ann Surg* 120:727, 1944.

Latham RL et al: The association of diabetes and glucose control with surgical-site infections among cardiothoracic surgery patients, *Infect Cont Hosp Epidemiol* 22:607, 2001.

Manassa, EH, Hertl CH, Olbrisch, RR: Wound healing problems in smokers and nonsmokers after 132 abdominoplasties *Plastic & Reconstructive Surgery*. 111(6):2082-2087, 2003.

Manassa EH, Hertl CH, Olbrisch RR: Wound healing problems in smokers and nonsmokers after 132 abdominoplasties, *Plast Recon Surg* 111:2082, 2003.

Mangram AJ et al: Guideline for prevention of surgical site infection, 1999, *Infect Control Hosp Epidemiol* 20:247, 1999.

Melling AC et al: Effects of preoperative warming on the incidence of wound infection after clean surgery: a randomized controlled trial, *Lancet* 358:876, 2001.

Moller AM et al: Effect of smoking on early complications after elective orthopaedic surgery, *J Cone Joint Surg* 85:178, 2003.

Morris RH: Influence of ambient temperature on patient temperature during intraabdominal surgery, *Ann Surg* 173:230, 1971.

Mun EC, Blackburn GL, Matthews JB: Current status of medical and surgical therapy for obesity, *Gastroenterology* 120:660, 2001.

Niinikoski J: Effect of oxygen supply on wound healing and formation of experimental granulation tissue, *Acta Physiol Scand* 1969:1, 1969.

Niinikoski J, Heughan C, Hunt TK: Oxygen tensions in human wounds, *J Surg Res* 12:77, 1972.

Pai MP, Hunt TK: Effect of varying oxygen tensions on healing of open wounds, *Surg Gynecol Obstet* 135:756, 1972.

Plattner O et al: The influence of two surgical bandage systems on wound tissue oxygen tension, *Arch Surg* 135:818, 2000.

Pryor KO et al: Surgical site infection and the routine use of perioperative hyperoxia in a general surgical population, *JAMA* 291:79, 2004.

Rabkin JM, Hunt TK: Local heat increases blood flow and oxygen tension in wounds, *Arch Surg* 122:221, 1987.

Roe CF: Effect of bowel exposure on body temperature during surgical operations, *Am J Surg* 122:13, 1971.

Roe CF et al: The influence of body temperature on early postoperative oxygen consumption, *Surgery* 60:85, 1966.

Rowell LB: *Human circulation: regulation during physical stress*, New York, 1986, Oxford University Press.

Rubinstein EH, Sessler DI: Skin-surface temperature gradients correlate with fingertip blood flow in humans, *Anesthesiology* 73:541, 1990.

Sen CK et al: Oxygen, oxidants, and antioxidants in wound healing. An emerging paradigm, *Ann NY Acad Sci* 957:239, 2002.

Sessler DI: Perianesthetic thermoregulation and heat balance in humans, *FASEB J* 7:638, 1993.

Severinghaus J: Oxyhaemoglobin dissociation curve correction for temperature and pH variation in human blood, *J Appl Physiol* 12:485, 1958.

Sheffield CW et al: Thermoregulatory vasoconstriction decreases subcutaneous oxygen tension in anesthetized volunteers, *Anesthesiology* 77:A96, 1992.

Silver IA: The measurement of oxygen tension in healing tissue, *Prog Resp Res* 3:124, 1969.

Silver IA: The physiology of wound healing. In Hunt T, editor: *Wound healing and wound infection: theory and surgical practice*, New York, 1980, Appleton-Century-Crofts.

Slotman GJ, Jed EH, Burchard KW: Adverse effects of hypothermia in postoperative patients, *Am J Surg* 49:495, 1985.

Sorensen LT, Jorgensen T: Short-term pre-operative smoking cessation intervention does not affect postoperative complications in colorectal surgery: a randomized clinical trial, *Colorectal Dis* 5:347, 2003.

Trence DL, Kelly JL, Hirsch IB: The rationale and management of hyperglycemia for in-patients with cardiovascular disease: time for change, *J Clin Endocrinol Metab* 88:2430, 2003.

U.S. Department of Health and Human Services: *Healthy People 2010* (Conference Edition), Washington DC, 2000, Government Printing Office.

Vanhoutte PM, Verbeuren TJ, Webb RC: Local modulation of adrenergic neuroeffector interaction in the blood vessel well, *Physiol Rev* 61:151, 1981.

Vastine VL et al: Wound complications of abdominoplasty in obese patients, *Ann Plas Surg* 42:34, 1999.

West JM: Wound healing in the surgical patient: influence of the perioperative stress response on perfusion, *AACN Clin Issues Crit Care Nurs* 1(3):595, 1990.

West JM: *The effect of postoperative forced-air rewarming on subcutaneous tissue oxygen tension and wound healing in hypothermic abdominal surgery patients*, San Francisco, 1994, University of California, San Francisco.

West JM, Hopf H, Hunt T: A radiant-heat bandage increases abdominal subcutaneous oxygen tension and temperature, *Wound Rep Regen* 4:A134, 1996.

Whitney JD et al: Tissue and wound healing effects of short duration postoperative oxygen therapy, *Bio Res Nurs* 2:206, 2001.

Whitney JD, Dellinger EP, Wickline M: Warming surgical wounds: effects on healing and wound complications, *Wound Rep Regen* 12:A8, 2004.

Wilson APR et al: A scoring method (ASEPSIS) for postoperative wound infections for use in clinical trials of antibiotic prophylaxis, *Lancet* 1(8476):311, 1986a.

Wilson APR et al: Repeatability of ASEPSIS wound scoring method, *Lancet* 849:1208, 1986b.

Wilson APR et al: The use of the wound scoring method "ASEPSIS" in postoperative wound surveillance, *J Hosp Infect* 16:297, 1990.

Winiarsky R, Barth P, Lotke P: Total knee arthroplasty in morbidly obese patients, *J Bone Joint Surg Am* 80:1770, 1998.

Wynne R, Botti M, Stedman H, Holsworth L, Harinos M, Flavell O, Manterfield C: Effect of three wound dressings on infection, healing comfort, and cost in patients with sternotomy wounds: a randomized trial. *Chest* 125(1):43-49, 2004.

12 Mechanical Forces: Pressure, Shear, and Friction

BARBARA PIEPER

OBJECTIVES

1. Describe the incidence and prevalence of pressure ulcers in various clinical settings and vulnerable patient populations.
2. Define pressure ulcer.
3. Identify the three most common locations for pressure ulcers to develop.
4. Describe the role of subcutaneous tissue and muscle in preventing pressure ulcers.
5. Describe the role of the causative factors for pressure ulcer formation.
6. Differentiate among the terms capillary pressure, capillary closing pressure, and tissue interface pressure.
7. Describe the phenomena of reactive hyperemia, blanching erythema, and nonblanching erythema.
8. Describe the pathophysiologic consequences of pressure damage, including the changes that occur at the cellular level and the cone-shaped pressure gradient.
9. List five variables that influence the extent of tissue damage as a consequence of pressure.
10. Describe the four components of a pressure ulcer prevention program.
11. Compare and contrast the Braden Scale and the Norton Scale for pressure ulcer risk assessment including reliability, validity, specificity, and sensitivity.
12. Distinguish between a pressure ulcer risk assessment and a skin assessment.
13. Discuss pain associated with a pressure ulcer.
14. Relate quality improvement and legal aspects of pressure ulcers.

Pressure ulcers present a significant health care threat to patients with restricted mobility or chronic disease and to older patients. Because of this threat, more documents are being published about pressure ulcers such as the National Pressure Ulcer Advisory Panel, *Pressure Ulcers in America: Prevalence, Incidence, and Implications for the Future* (NPUAP, 2001), the Wound Ostomy and Continence Nurses (WOCN) Society *Guideline for Prevention and Management of Pressure Ulcers* (WOCN Society, 2003), the Canadian Association of Wound Care guideline (Dolynchuk et al, 2000), and *Healthy People 2010* (U.S. Department of Health and Human Services, 2000). In addition, the development of an avoidable pressure ulcer in a person assessed at low risk in long-term care is considered a sentinel event (Ayello and Braden, 2002). At least 1.7 million people develop pressure ulcers annually, costing $2.2 to $3.6 billion (Beckrich and Aronovitch, 1998; Bergstrom et al, 1994). Besides monetary costs there is pain, disfigurement, suffering, and loss of productive time (Langemo et al, 2000).

Facility-associated pressure ulcers add to the patient's length of stay, delay the patient's recuperation, and increase the patient's risk for developing complications. In addition, pressure ulcers often necessitate hospitalization (in certain patient populations such as the elderly and patients with a spinal cord injury) because of sepsis or the need for debridement or surgical repair. At a time of increasingly scarce health care dollars, pressure ulcers consume intense resources in the form of dressing changes, nursing care, physical therapy, medications, nutritional support, and clinician services. Pressure ulcers have been examined in terms of their effects on mortality rates. Residents with a pressure ulcer in long-term care had a relative risk of dying of 2.37, but after adjusting for 16 other measures, the risk declined to 1.45 (Berlowitz et al, 1997). Pressure ulcers are not an independent predictor of mortality but a marker for underlying disease severity and other comorbidities (Allman, 1998; Berlowitz et al, 1997; Brown, 2003).

ECONOMIC EFFECTS

The financial cost of pressure ulcers to the U.S. health economy is a matter of conjecture. The literature reports a range of costs for pressure ulcer management. Kumar and colleagues (2004) studied four categories of skin ulcers and found pressure ulcers had the highest associated total costs per person (mean = $8,745) and for hospitalization and physician visits. Allman (1998) and Allman and colleagues (1999) calculated the mean cost per admission for patients who develop a pressure ulcer as $37,288 as opposed to $13,924 for patients who did not. After adjusting for admission characteristics, the mean cost for each patient who developed a pressure ulcer was $14,260 as opposed to $12,382 for those who did not (Allman, 1998; Allman et al, 1999). Patients who developed pressure ulcers compared to patients without them were more likely to develop nosocomial infections and other hospital complications (Allman et al, 1999). Xakellis and colleagues (2001) studied the cost of preventing and treating pressure ulcers in long-term care. They noted that the cost of pressure ulcer treatment per person decreased from $640 in 1994 to $140 in 1997; but the cost of prevention per person rose from $130 in 1995 to $158 in 1997.

Unfortunately, research about the costs that are incurred while a pressure ulcer is being managed must be viewed cautiously; the studies are not all comparable. Some studies account for all costs: room, nursing care, supplies, medications, physician fees, and so forth. Other studies examine only direct costs, such as the supplies or medications specifically indicated for that particular problem. There are many opinions in the literature about costs.

SCOPE OF THE PROBLEM

The scope of the pressure ulcer problem in the United States is examined in terms of the age and diagnosis of patient and the setting. Statistics about pressure ulcers vary because of how data were collected, variations in terminology about prevalence and incidence, concern about litigation, and political and social events that changed American healthcare in the 1990s (Baumgarten, 1998; Frantz, 1997; Lake, 1999).

The concepts of prevalence and incidence and methods for calculation are discussed in Chapter 1.

Prevalence

Pressure ulcer prevalence is defined by the WOCN Society (2004) as the number of patients with at least one pressure ulcer who exist in a given patient population at a given point of time.

In the United States, the Fifth National Pressure Ulcer Prevalence Study reported prevalence in acute care at 14.8%; this was a 4.6% increase over the Fourth National study (Amlung, Miller, and Bosley, 2001; Barczak et al, 1997). Prevalence of pressure ulcers in acute care settings ranges from 10.1% to 17%; 2.3% to 28% in long-term care; and 0% to 29% in home care (NPUAP, 2001). The discrepancies in prevalence can be attributed to the fact that some studies include intact pressure-damaged skin (stage 1), whereas other studies exclude such lesions. Prevalence is lower when intact pressure-damaged skin is *excluded* from the sample. In contrast, erroneous *inclusion* of patients with ordinary hyperemic responses such as intact pressure-damaged skin will *over*estimate prevalence. Pressure ulcers in dark-skinned persons may also be missed (Lyder et al, 1998; NPUAP, 2001). Some skin changes, such as candidiasis or herpetic lesions, may be misclassified as pressure ulcers (Pieper et al, 1997b). Data collectors must accurately distinguish between pressure ulcers and other causes of erythema and skin ulcerations.

Incidence

Incidence is defined by the WOCN Society (2004) as the number of patients who initially were ulcer-free who develop a pressure ulcer within a particular time in a defined population. Incidence measures new conditions (e.g., pressure ulcers) and is therefore considered more reflective of the quality of care within that setting. It is a measure used to evaluate the effects of preventive and therapeutic interventions. Determining the incidence of pressure ulcers is inherently difficult because such studies require longitudinal observations. As with prevalence, incidence will vary by setting. The incidence of pressure ulcers in acute care ranges from 0.4% to 38%; in long-term care, from 2.2% to 23.9%; and in home care, from 0% to 17% (NPUAP, 2001).

There are considerable methodologic issues that surround the calculation of incidence. For example, defining who is at risk (the number used in the denominator of the incidence formula) can have a significant influence on the resulting value, which may actually overestimate or underestimate the true frequency of the condition. Consequently, variation in reports of incidence may reflect a real difference in frequency of the condition or simply different data-collection techniques, definitions, and methods. Although differences in methodology make it difficult to compare incidence from one setting or report to that from another, it remains an important measure. Consistency in data collection technique within the health care setting is essential to generate data that can be compared over time (Gallagher, 1997). National standards for the definition of terms and the process for conducting prevalence and incidence studies will also increase the comparability of this kind of data (WOCN Society, 2004).

Vulnerable Patient Populations

The group that experiences pressure ulcers most frequently is over 65 years of age; this may be the result of conditions that result in immobility and physiologic changes to the skin (NPUAP, 2001). The elderly account for 50% of all hospital admissions in the United States, and up to 75% of the elderly experience a decrease in functional abilities from hospital admission to discharge (Zulkowski and Kindsfater, 2000). For persons admitted to long-term care, 10.3% to 18.4% have one or more pressure ulcers on admission (Baumgarten et al, 2003; Siem et al, 2003).

Pressure ulcer prevalence for persons with spinal cord injuries ranges from 10.2% to 30% (NPUAP, 2001). Eighty-five percent of them will develop a pressure ulcer at some point in life (Niazi et al, 1997). The incidence of pressure ulcers in patients with a spinal cord injury is 20% to 31% (NPUAP, 2001).

Children may also develop pressure ulcers, primarily in the occipital region in infants and toddlers and on the sacrum in the young child (Quigley and Curley, 1996). The prevalence of pressure ulcers in pediatric intensive care units has been reported as high as 27% and 20% in neonatal intensive care units. Most ulcers develop within two days of admission. Among noncritical hospitalized children, a prevalence of 0.47%-13%

and an incidence of 0.29%-6% has been cited (Waterlow, 1997; Baldwin, 2002; Curley, 2003; Groeneveld et al, 2004, NPUAP, 2005).

The incidence of pressure ulcers in surgical patients ranges from 4% to 45% (NPUAP, 2001). The etiology of pressure ulcers in the surgical patient is unclear; preoperative variables frequently examined include patient's age, nutritional status and comorbidities such as diabetes. Intraoperative variables under investigation include time on the operating room table, hypotensive episodes, and type of procedure (Aronovitch, 1998; Price et al, 2005). Unfortunately, tissue damage may become apparent within hours or delayed for up to 3 days. Initial manifestations may be skin discoloration (e.g., bruising) that evolves into blister formation or necrosis. Because this process transpires over several days (i.e., 2-6), isolating the time of the original injury is complicated (Price et al, 2005). Since the length of surgery and other variables for the surgical patient cannot be changed, the surgical team must aim to decrease pressure and shear during the procedure (Schoonhoven et al, 2002).

TERMINOLOGY

Over the years, several terms have been used to describe pressure ulcers: *bedsore, decubitus ulcer, decubiti,* and *pressure sore. Pressure ulcer* is the accepted term because it is more accurate and descriptive.

The origin of the term *bedsore* is not known, but it predates the term *decubitus. Decubitus,* a Latin word referring to the reclining position (Fox and Bradley, 1803), dates from 1747 when the French used it to mean "bedsore" (Arnold, 1983). However, this term is inaccurate, because it does not convey the tissue destruction associated with these lesions, and because these lesions result from positions other than the lying position (such as sitting). Furthermore, although *decubiti* is used as the plural form of *decubitus,* it also is incorrect. *Decubitus* is a fourth-declension Latin noun, and "fourth declension nouns form their plural with the ending –us" (Arnold, 1983). Therefore the plural of *decubitus* is *decubitus*; the English plural *decubitus ulcers* is better.

A pressure ulcer is defined as localized areas of tissue necrosis that tends to develop when soft tissue is compressed between a bony prominence and an external surface for a prolonged period (Panel for the

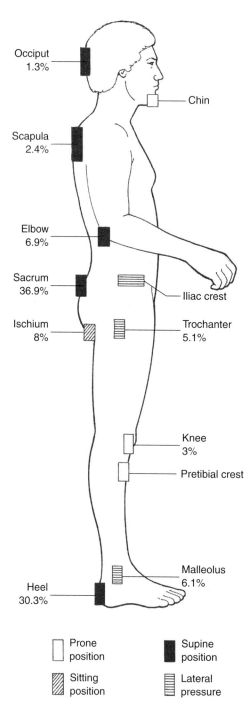

Fig. 12-1 Sites for pressure ulcers and frequency of ulceration per site. Note: This illustration does not include sites for device related pressure ulcers which may not involve bony prominences.

Prediction and Prevention of Pressure Ulcers in Adults, 1992; WOCN Society, 2003). The NPUAP defined a pressure ulcer as any lesion caused by unrelieved pressure resulting in damage of underlying tissue (NPUAP, 2001). These are usually located over bony prominences and are staged according to the extent of observable tissue damage (NPUAP, 2001).

Pressure ulcers occur most commonly over a bony prominence such as the sacrum, the ischial tuberosity, the trochanter, and the calcaneus; however, they may develop anywhere on the body (e.g., underneath a cast, splint, or cervical collar). Figure 12-1 shows common sites for pressure ulcers and frequency of ulceration per site. The majority of pressure ulcers occur in the pelvis. However, the most common locations are the sacrum and the heels.

Bony locations are the areas most prone to pressure ulcer formation because a person's body weight is concentrated on these areas when resting on an unyielding surface. Those who have atrophy of the subcutaneous and muscle tissue layers are at even greater risk for the "mechanical load" of pressure and thus increased soft tissue and capillary compression. The coccyx, the sacrum, and the heel are particularly vulnerable because less soft tissue is present between the bone and skin.

CAUSATIVE FACTORS

Pressure is the major causative factor in pressure ulcer formation. However, several factors play a role in determining whether pressure is sufficient to create an ulcer. The pathologic effect of excessive pressure on soft tissue can be attributed to (1) intensity of pressure, (2) duration of pressure, and (3) tissue tolerance (the ability of both the skin and its supporting structures to endure pressure without adverse sequelae). Braden and Bergstrom (1987) presented a model of the factors that contribute to the intensity and duration of pressure ulcers (Figure 12-2), in combination with intrinsic and extrinsic factors that affect tissue tolerance.

INTENSITY OF PRESSURE

To understand the importance of intensity of pressure, it is important to review the terms capillary pressure and capillary closing pressure. *Capillary pressure* tends to move fluid outward through the capillary membrane (Boulpaep, 2003). Exact capillary pressure is not

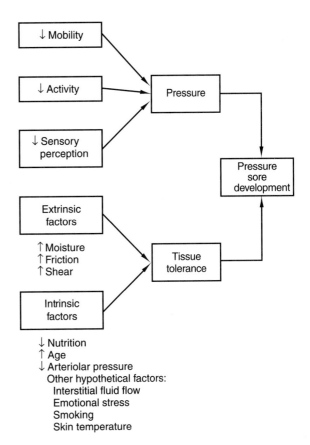

Fig. 12-2 Factors contributing to the development of pressure ulcers. (From Rehablilitation Nursing 12(1), 9. Adapted with permission of Association of Rehabilitation Nurses, 4700 W. Lake Avenue, Glenview, IL 60025. Copyright © 2004 Association of Rehabilitation Nurses.)

known because of the difficulty of obtaining the measurement. Various methods have been used to estimate capillary pressure.

One method used to measure capillary pressure was by direct cannulation of the capillary with a microscopic glass pipette. A manometer is then attached to the pipette, and a pressure reading is obtained. Capillary pressures have been obtained in animals and in the fingernails of humans using this method. Using such techniques, capillary pressures have been reported as follows: 32 mm Hg in the arteriolar limb, 12 mm Hg in the venous limb, and 20 mm Hg in the midcapillary (Landis, 1930) (Figure 12-3). Capillary pressures are reported as 35 mm Hg at the arterial end, 15 mm Hg at the venous end, and about 25 mm Hg in the middle

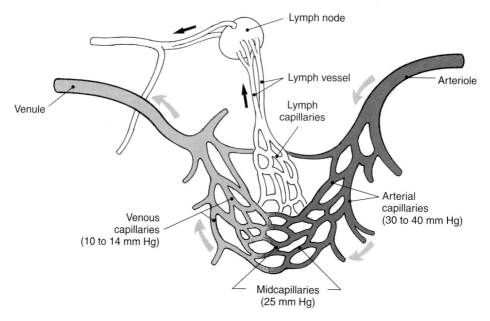

Fig. 12-3 Capillary pressure within the capillary bed.

of the capillary (Boulpaep, 2003). Two indirect methods to measure capillary pressure have been reported and result in a pressure termed the *functional capillary pressure*, or the pressure (17 mm Hg) believed necessary to keep the capillary system open and functional (Guyton and Hall, 1996).

The term *capillary closing pressure*, or *critical closing pressure*, describes the minimal amount of pressure required to collapse a capillary (Burton and Yamada, 1951). Tissue anoxia develops when externally applied pressure causes vessels to collapse. It is believed that the amount of pressure required to collapse capillaries must exceed capillary pressure. It is common to use capillary pressures of 12 to 32 mm Hg as the numerical "standard" for capillary closing pressure.

To quantify the intensity of pressure being applied externally to the skin, one measures the interface pressures. Numerous studies have been conducted to measure interface pressures (Kosiak, 1961; Kosiak et al, 1958; Lindan, 1961). These studies have shown that the interface pressures attained while one is in the sitting or supine position commonly exceed capillary pressures (Bennett et al, 1984).

In 1961, Lindan used an experimental "bed" to calculate the pressure distribution over the skin of a healthy adult male in the supine, prone, side lying, and sitting positions. The range of interface pressures was from 10 to 100 mm Hg. Interface readings as high as 300 mm Hg have been obtained over the ischial tuberosity of healthy, able-bodied male subjects when sitting in an unpadded chair (Kosiak, 1961).

Fortunately, interface pressures in excess of capillary pressure will not routinely result in ischemia. Healthy people with normal sensation regularly shift their weight in response to the discomfort associated with capillary closure and tissue hypoxia. Unfortunately, pathologic processes such as spinal cord injury or sedation impair a person's ability to recognize or respond to this discomfort. Tissue hypoxia can then develop and progress to tissue anoxia and cellular death.

DURATION OF PRESSURE

Duration of pressure is an important factor that influences the detrimental effects of pressure and must be considered in tandem with intensity of pressure. An inverse relationship exists between duration and intensity of pressure in creating tissue ischemia (Brooks and Duncan, 1940; Kosiak, 1961; Trumble, 1930). Specifically, low-intensity pressures over a long period can create tissue damage, just as high-intensity pressure can over a short period (Figure 12-4).

Husain (1953) underscored the significance of the relationship between duration and intensity of pressure. Husain found that a 100 mm Hg pressure applied to rat muscle for 2 hours was sufficient to produce only microscopic changes in the muscle. The same pressure applied for 6 hours, however, was sufficient to produce complete muscle degeneration.

TISSUE TOLERANCE

Tissue tolerance is the third factor that determines the pathologic effect of excessive pressure and describes the condition or integrity of the skin and supporting structures that influence the skin's ability to redistribute the applied pressure. Compression of tissue against skeletal structures and the resulting tissue ischemia can be avoided by effective redistribution of pressure.

The concept of tissue tolerance was first discussed in the literature in 1930 by Trumble, who recognized the need to identify how much pressure skin could "tolerate."

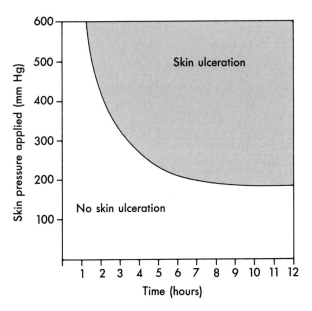

Fig. 12-4 Graph demonstrating relationship between intensity and duration of pressure. (From Kosiak M: Etiology of decubitus ulcers, *Arch Phys Med Rehabil* 42:191, 1961.)

Later, Husain (1953) introduced the concept of sensitizing the tissue to pressure and consequently to ischemia. Rat muscle was sensitized with a pressure of 100 mm Hg applied for 2 hours. Seventy-two hours later, a mere 50 mm Hg pressure applied to the same tissue caused muscle degeneration in only 1 hour. This muscle destruction resulted during the second application of pressure, even though the intensity and duration of pressure were lower than the initial intensity and duration. This finding has significant implications for the patient population at risk for pressure ulcers. It indicates that episodes of deep tissue ischemia can occur without cutaneous manifestations, and that such episodes can sensitize the patient's skin. Small increments of pressure, even if only slightly above normal capillary pressure ranges, may then result in breakdown.

Tissue tolerance is influenced by the ability of the skin and underlying structures (e.g., blood vessels, interstitial fluid, collagen) to "work together as a set of parallel springs that transmit load from the surface of the tissue to the skeleton inside" (Krouskop, 1983). Several factors can alter the ability of the soft tissue to perform this task.

Extrinsic Factors that Affect Tissue Tolerance

Shear. Shear was first described in 1958 as a contributing element in pressure ulcers (Reichel, 1958). Shear is caused by the interplay of gravity and friction. It exerts force parallel to the skin and is the result of both gravity pushing down on the body and resistance (friction) between the patient and a surface, such as the bed or chair. For example, when the head of the bed is elevated, the effect of gravity on the body is to pull the body down toward the foot of the bed. In contrast, the resistance generated by the bed surface tends to hold the body in place. However, what is actually held in place is the skin, whereas the weight of the skeleton continues to pull the body downward.

Because the skin does not move freely, the primary effect of shear occurs at the deeper fascial level of the tissues overlying the bony prominence. Blood vessels, which are anchored at the point of exit through the fascia, are stretched and angulated when exposed to shear. This force also dissects the tissues "in the plane of greater concentration which is observed clinically as a large area of undermining which extends circumferentially" (Reichel, 1958).

Shear causes much of the damage often observed with pressure ulcers. In fact, some lesions that may result solely from shear are misinterpreted to be pressure ulcers. According to Bennett and Lee (1988), as many as 40% of injuries that might actually be shear injuries are reported as pressure ulcers. Vascular occlusion is enhanced if shear and pressure occur together (Kanj, Wilking, and Phillips, 1998). For example, when the head of the bed is elevated more than 30 degrees, shear force occurs in the sacrococcygeal region. The sliding of the body transmits pressure to the sacrum and the deep fascia; the outer skin is fixed because of friction with the bed. The vessels in the deep superficial fascia angulate, leading to thrombosis and undermining of the dermis (see Chapter 6, Figure 6-3).

Friction. Friction is a significant factor in pressure ulcer development because it acts in concert with gravity to cause shear. Alone, its ability to cause skin damage is confined to the epidermal and upper dermal layers. In its mildest form, friction abrades the epidermis and dermis similarly to a mild burn, and such skin damage is often reported as a "sheet burn." This type of damage most frequently develops in patients who are restless. To avoid friction when moving up in bed, a patient who can lift independently should do so with a lift device or with use of the hands and arms. A patient who is dependent in care may need two caregivers to assist with moving up in bed while using a lift sheet to prevent the body from dragging.

However, when friction acts with gravity the effect of the two factors is synergistic, and the outcome is shear. It is not possible to have shear without friction. However, it is possible to have friction without significant shear (such as from moving the palm of the hand repeatedly against a bed sheet).

Moisture. Moisture, specifically incontinence, is frequently cited in the literature as a predisposing factor to pressure ulcer development (Braden and Bergstrom, 1987). The mechanism may be that moisture alters the resiliency of the epidermis to external forces. According to Adams and Hunter (1969) both shear and friction are increased in the presence of mild to moderate moisture. However, it appears that shear and friction actually decrease in the presence of profuse moisture. Studies have shown that the high-moisture environment created by urinary incontinence is not a major factor in the production of pressure ulcers (Allman et al, 1986; Shannon and Skorga, 1989). In a small study with healthy women, sustained skin wetness increased the vulnerability to pressure-induced blood flow reduction (Mayrovitz and Sims, 2001). More research about the role of moisture is needed.

Intrinsic Factors that Affect Tissue Tolerance

Nutritional Debilitation. Approximately 3% to 50% of hospitalized patients suffer from malnutrition; in the general population, 25% of older Americans are malnourished (Wellman, 1997). A nutritional assessment helps to identify the presence of malnutrition, assess its severity, and determine baseline data to evaluate nutritional interventions. Guenter and colleagues (2000) examined nutritional status of newly hospitalized patients with stages III and IV pressure ulcers and noted that a majority of them were below usual body weight, had low prealbumin levels, and were not taking enough nutrition to meet their needs. As age increased, the percentage of nutritional intake decreased (Guenter et al, 2000). The nutritional assessment should include anthropometric data (weight and body mass index), biochemical data (serum albumin, serum transferrin, total lymphocyte count, nitrogen balance, serum prealbumin, and serum retinol-binding protein), clinical data, and dietary history (Flanigan, 1997; Strauss and Margolis, 1996). Serum albumin and body weight are valuable gauges of nutrition (Fife et al, 2001), yet decreases in either may indicate poor health rather than poor nutritional intake (Evans-Stoner, 1997; Wellman, 1997; Zulkowski and Kindsfater, 2000). Nutritional assessment tools (Appendix C and Chapter 8) and dietary consultation are helpful in documenting nutritional status.

Although good nutrition is necessary for wound healing, the role of significant nutritional debilitation in producing pressure ulcers is often less appreciated. In hospitals and long-term care facilities, impaired nutritional intake, lower dietary protein intake, impaired ability to self-feed, and recent weight loss have been identified as independent predictors of pressure ulcer development (Allman et al, 1995; Bergstrom and Braden, 1992; Brandeis et al, 1990; Berlowitz and Wilking, 1989; Chernoff, 1996). Even though 52% of patients in one study were assessed with poor nutritional status, 65% of them did not receive orders for nutritional supplements or nutritional consultation (Zulkowski and Kindsfater, 2000). A Cochrane evaluation of enteral and parenteral nutrition on pressure ulcer prevention and treatment was not able to draw conclusions about their effect because of the small number of studies and methodologic issues with the studies (Langer et al, 2004). Research is needed to determine if improving dietary intake reduces the incidence of pressure ulcers.

Severe protein deficiency renders soft tissue more susceptible to breakdown when exposed to local pressure, because hypoproteinemia alters oncotic pressure and causes edema formation. Oxygen diffusion and transport of nutrients in ischemic and edematous tissue are compromised. In addition, there is a decreased resistance to infection with low protein levels because of the effect on the immune system (Thomas, 1997c).

Malnutrition has also been associated with altered tissue regeneration and inflammatory reaction; increased postoperative complications; increased risk of infection, sepsis, and death; and increased length of stay (Strauss and Margolis, 1996; Thomas, 1997c).

Certain vitamin deficiencies, particularly of vitamins A, C, and E, may also contribute to pressure ulcer development. Vitamin A has a role in epithelial integrity, collagen synthesis, and humoral and cell-mediated protective mechanisms against infection (Flanigan, 1997; Thomas, 1997b). Vitamin A deficiency delays reepithelialization, collagen synthesis, and cellular cohesion. Vitamin C plays a part in collagen synthesis, wound repair, and immune function (Collins, 2004). Vitamin C deficiency compromises collagen production and immune system function and results in capillary fragility. Vitamin E deficiency may decrease cell-mediated immunity and may also increase tissue damage from toxic free radicals. All nutrients have a positive role. Still, there are questions regarding how much supplementation of nutrients will positively affect outcomes (Thomas, 1996). Using creative methods, nutrition should be maintained or enhanced as long as possible.

Advanced Age. Several changes occur in the skin and its supporting structures with aging. A flattening of the dermoepidermal junction occurs; there is less nutrient exchange and less resistance to shear force.

With aging there is a gradual atrophy and greater heterogeneity of blood and lymph vessels of human skin (Ryan, 2004). Intraepidermal nerve fibers decrease (Chang, Lin, and Hsieh, 2004). Skin tears occur more commonly. There is a loss of dermal thickness; the skin appears paper-thin and nearly transparent. Aging skin experiences decreased epidermal turnover, decreased surface barrier function, decreased sensory perception, decreased delayed and immediate hypersensitivity reaction, increased vascular fragility, loss of subcutaneous fat, and clustering of melanocytes (Kanj and Phillips, 2001). With these changes, the ability of the soft tissue to distribute the mechanical load without compromising blood flow is impaired.

These changes combine with many other age-related changes that occur in other body systems to make the skin more vulnerable to pressure, shear, and friction (Jones and Millman, 1990). For example, studies have shown that the blood flow in the area of the ischial tuberosity while one is sitting on an unpadded surface is lower in paraplegic and geriatric populations than in normal patients.

Low Blood Pressure. When Trumble (1930) identified the need to study tissue tolerance, he looked at the amount of external pressure needed to create skin "pain" in relationship to the patient's blood pressure instead of capillary pressure. He postulated that "skin pressure tolerance varies slightly with blood pressure."

In fact, systolic blood pressures below 100 mm Hg and diastolic pressures below 60 mm Hg have been associated with pressure ulcer development (Bergstrom, 1997; Gosnell, 1973; Moolten, 1972). Mayrovitz and colleagues (2003), in a study about heels, noted that persons with lower blood pressure need lower levels of pressure to the heels. When interface pressures are near diastolic pressure, little if any functional pressure redistribution is realized. Hypotension may shunt blood flow away from the skin to more vital organs, thus decreasing the skin tolerance for pressure by allowing capillaries to close at lower levels of interface pressure.

Stress. Psychosocial issues such as emotional stress have been associated with pressure ulcer formation (Rintala, 1995). Hospitalization can be a stressor. Up to 75% of elderly experience a decrease in functional ability from hospital admission to discharge

(Zulkowski and Kindsfater, 2000). Cortisol may be the trigger for lowered tissue tolerance when a person is under stress. One stress for older adults is relocation to a long-term care facility. Cortisol is the primary gluco-corticoid secreted when a person is exposed to a stressor and lacks appropriate coping mechanisms to mediate the stress-related hormonal response (Braden, 1990; Krouskop, 1983).

There are two mechanisms by which cortisol might decrease the ability of the skin to absorb mechanical load:

1. Cortisol may alter the mechanical properties of the skin by disproportionately increasing the rate of collagen degradation over collagen synthesis (Cohen, Diegelmann, and Johnson, 1977; Rodriquez et al, 1989). Loss of skin collagen has been associated with the development of pressure ulcers among patients with spinal cord injury.

2. Glucocorticoids may trigger structural changes in connective tissue and may affect cellular metabolism by interfering with the diffusion of water, salt, and nutrients between the capillary bed and the cells.

Some research has reported that a causal relationship between cortisol and pressure ulcers cannot be inferred (Braden, 1998). Many factors affect cortisol such as advanced age, immobility, body fat, recent surgery, stroke, and malnutrition.

Smoking. Smoking may be a predictor of pressure ulcer formation (Salzberg et al, 1998). Cigarette smoking has been reported to correlate positively with the presence of pressure ulcers in a group of patients with spinal cord injury (Lamid and El Ghatit, 1983). The incidence and extent of existing ulcers was greater in those patients with higher pack-per-year histories. In addition, patients who smoke have been reported to have higher recurrence rates of pressure ulcers.

Elevated Body Temperature. Elevated body temperature has been associated with pressure ulcer development (Allman et al, 1986; Braden and Bergstrom, 1987; Gosnell, 1973). Although the mechanism of this association between elevated body temperature and pressure ulcer development is not proven, it may be related to increased oxygen demand in already anoxic tissue.

Miscellaneous Factors. Other conditions, such as those that create sluggish blood flow, anemia, blood dyscrasias, or poor oxygen perfusion, may also be significant intrinsic factors jeopardizing tissue tolerance (Kanj, Wilking, and Phillips, 1998; Niazi et al, 1997; Schmid-Schönbein, Rieger, and Fischer, 1980). For example, greater tissue damage has been associated with increased blood viscosity and high hematocrit level. This may explain why dehydration is sometimes mentioned as a contributing factor in pressure ulcer development. The elderly may experience low subcutaneous oxygen; fluid administration may increase tissue oxygen (Stotts and Hopf, 2003). The morbidly obese are at risk for pressure ulcers owing to the inability to turn themselves, underlying diseases, improper equipment and lack of adequate pressure redistribution, inadequate staff numbers, or staff not trained in how to turn and move the patient (Knudson and Gallagher, 2003; Mathison, 2003). The Minimum Data Set Plus has been examined for items associated with pressure ulcer prevalence in newly institutionalized elderly patients (Zulkowski, 1998). Strongly associated factors were serum albumin, dependence for transfer, bowel incontinence, history of resolved or healed pressure ulcer, and absence of Alzheimer's disease or non-Alzheimer's dementia. Elderly in home care and at risk for pressure ulcers by the Outcome and Assessment Information Set (OASIS) were those limited in activity to bed, dependent in dressing, incontinent of urine, needing assistance with transferring, using oxygen, and having a current fracture (Bergquist, 2003).

PATHOPHYSIOLOGIC CHANGES

Clinical Presentation

The pathophysiologic tissue changes that occur with pressure ulcer formation are a predictable series of events (Parish, Witkowski, and Crissey, 1983). Clinical presentation can vary from nonblanching erythema to ecchymosis and then to frank necrosis. Assessment and classification of pressure ulcers is discussed in Chapter 7.

Obstruction of capillary blood flow by externally applied pressure creates tissue ischemia (hypoxia). If the pressure is removed in a short period, blood flow returns and the skin can be seen to flush. This phenomenon, known as *reactive hyperemia*, is a compensatory mechanism whereby blood vessels in the pressure area dilate in an attempt to overcome the ischemic episode. Reactive hyperemia by definition is transient and may also be described as blanching erythema. Blanching erythema is an area of erythema that becomes white (blanches) when compressed with a finger. The erythema promptly returns when the compression is removed. The site may be painful for the patient with intact sensation. Blanching erythema is an early indication of pressure and will usually resolve without tissue loss if pressure is reduced or eliminated.

When the hyperemia persists, deeper tissue damage should be suspected. Nonblanching erythema is a more serious sign of impaired blood supply and suggests that tissue destruction is imminent or has already occurred; it results from damage to blood vessels and extravasation of blood into the tissues. The color of the skin can be an intense bright red to dark red or purple. Many people misdiagnose pressure-induced nonblanching erythema as a hematoma or ecchymosis. When deep tissue damage is also present, the area is often either indurated or boggy when palpated. Nonblanching erythema attributable to ischemia is seldom reversible.

Cellular Response

When pressure occludes capillaries, a complex series of events is set into motion. Surrounding tissues become deprived of oxygen, and nutrients and metabolic wastes begin to accumulate in the tissue. Damaged capillaries become more permeable and leak fluid into the interstitial space to cause edema. Because perfusion through edematous tissue is slowed, tissue hypoxia worsens. Cellular death ensues, and more metabolic wastes are released into the surrounding tissue. Tissue inflammation is exacerbated, and more cellular death occurs (Figure 12-5).

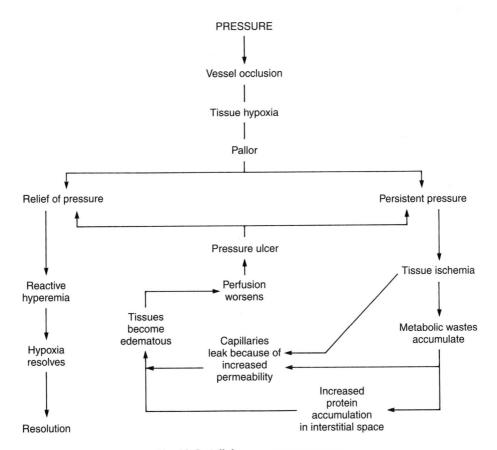

Fig. 12-5 Cellular response to pressure.

Muscle Response

Muscle damage may occur with pressure ulcers and is more significant than the cutaneous damage. Pressure is highest at the point of contact between the soft tissue (such as muscle or fascia) and the bony prominence (Kosiak, 1961). This cone-shaped pressure gradient indicates that deep pressure ulcers initially form at the bone–soft tissue interface, not the skin surface, and extend outward to the skin (Figure 12-6) (Shea, 1975). Thus deep tissue damage may occur with relatively little initial superficial evidence of damage to alert caregivers of its extensiveness. The skin damage seen in pressure ulcers is often referred to as the "tip of the iceberg" because a larger area of necrosis and ischemia is assumed to be present at the tissue-bone interface.

It has been further suggested that muscle damage is more extensive than skin damage because the muscle is more sensitive to the effects of ischemia (Cherry et al, 1980). In addition, atrophied, scarred, or secondarily infected tissue has an increased susceptibility to pressure (Yarkony, 1994). An understanding of the structure of the vascular system allows one to form a rationale for this enhanced muscle damage.

The vascular circulation can be divided into three sections: segmental, perforator, and cutaneous (Daniel and Kerrigan, 1979). The segmental system is composed of the main arterial vessels arising from the aorta. The perforator system supplies the muscles but also serves as an interchange supply to the skin. The cutaneous system consists of arteries, capillary beds, and veins draining at different levels of the skin and serves

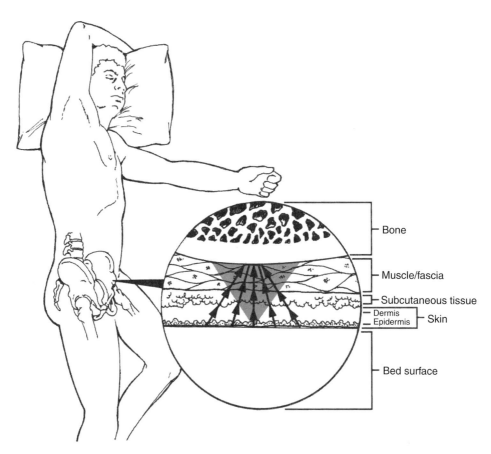

Fig. 12-6 Diagram of extent of tissue damage at muscle and skin levels.

to provide thermoregulation and limited nutritional support. This indicates that occlusion of the perforator system may initiate muscle damage and may also create some of the cutaneous ischemia. The significance of the perforator blood flow to skin damage has been demonstrated when musculocutaneous flaps have been elevated surgically.

"Interruption of the blood supply to the muscle can lead to skin necrosis, emphasizing the importance of the relationship of the physiological blood supply to the skin from underlying muscle. It is reasonable to suspect that the same type of tissue breakdown or necrosis could result from pressure-induced muscle ischemia in bedridden patients, and that in some cases the cutaneous lesions are secondary to the impaired muscle circulation" (Daniel and Kerrigan, 1979).

Because the skin receives its blood supply from both the perforator and the cutaneous systems, the skin actually receives more blood than necessary to meet metabolic needs (Parish, Witkowski, and Crissey, 1983). It is possible that the occlusion of "perforators" may be of more significance than the occlusion of the cutaneous system and may produce more extensive tissue damage.

Variables Influencing Extent of Tissue Damage

If pressure is not relieved, ischemic changes occur as a consequence of decreased perfusion; however, the occlusion also triggers a cascade of events that further intensifies the extent of tissue ischemia. Hence the tissue damage typically seen with pressure is precipitated by pressure but then worsened by events such as venous thrombus formation, endothelial cell damage, redistribution of blood supply in ischemic tissue, alteration in lymphatic flow, and alterations in interstitial fluid composition.

Externally applied high pressures, even when applied for a short duration, damage the blood vessels directly, which in turn causes tissue ischemia. In 1961, Kosiak described the changes in larger vessels and the formation of venous thrombi, which impair the normal reactive hyperemia that should occur once pressure is removed. Tissue remains ischemic even after the pressure has been alleviated.

Compression of the capillary wall also damages the endothelium (Cherry, Ryan, and Ellis, 1974). Once pressure is removed and reperfusion begins, the damaged

endothelial cells are shed into the bloodstream and proceed to occlude the blood vessel. As the endothelium is shed, platelets are activated by the underlying collagen and clot formation is triggered. Furthermore, damaged endothelial cells lose their usual anticoagulant characteristics and release thrombogenic substances that exacerbate vessel occlusion and ultimately cause increased tissue ischemia.

The redistribution of the blood supply that occurs in ischemic skin further aggravates pressure-induced tissue hypoxia. Because of the externally applied pressure, blood flow to surface capillaries is reduced, and such reduction renders them more vulnerable and more permeable than before. The extent of ischemia created can be further worsened when neutrophils are present in the tissue, because their resting oxygen demands are 30 times greater than those of resting epithelial cells (Ryan, 1980).

Alteration in the lymphatic flow and the composition of the interstitial fluid also affects pressure-induced ischemia (Reuler and Cooney, 1981). Lymphatic flow in pressure-damaged skin ceases. Likewise, the normal movement of interstitial fluid is inhibited by both the pressure and the ischemia. Consequently, protein is retained in the interstitial tissues, causing increased interstitial oncotic pressure, edema formation, dehydration of the cells, and tissue irritation.

In summary, extensive or extended pressure occludes blood flow, lymphatic flow, and interstitial fluid movement. Tissues are deprived of oxygen and nutrients, and toxic metabolic products accumulate. Interstitial fluids retain proteins that dehydrate cells and irritate tissues. The ensuing tissue acidosis, capillary permeability, and edema contribute to cellular death.

To reduce the incidence of pressure ulcers, it is essential to understand the risk factors for pressure ulcer development. With an in-depth review of the etiology of pressure ulcer formation and the pathophysiologic process involved, factors that must be addressed in a pressure ulcer prevention program become apparent.

PRESSURE ULCER PREVENTION PROGRAM

In 1992, a research-based practice guideline for the prediction and prevention of pressure ulcers was released by a panel of private sector and multidisciplinary health care members convened by the Agency for

Healthcare Research and Quality (AHRQ) (Bergstrom et al, 1994; Panel for the Prediction and Prevention of Pressure Ulcers in Adults, 1992). Subsequently, other organizations worldwide have written pressure ulcer prevention and treatment guidelines. A formal, comprehensive pressure ulcer prevention program developed from evidenced-based research is essential to effectively prevent pressure ulcers. Components of a pressure ulcer prevention program include (1) risk assessment, (2) systematic skin assessment, (3) reducing risk factors, (4) patient, family and staff education, and (5) evaluation. Such a program is best developed and implemented with a multidisciplinary team who can provide a holistic approach. Typically, members of this team should consist of representatives from nursing, medicine, physical therapy, occupational therapy, and nutritional support. An algorithm for pressure ulcer prediction and prevention is presented in Figure 12-7. Research has documented that pressure ulcer incidence

decreases after prevention programs (Robinson et al, 2003), but is difficult for staff and may require an examination of barriers and a management focus to sustain them (Bryant and Rolstad, 2001; Xakellis et al, 2001).

Risk Assessment

Pressure ulcer prevention programs establish guidelines that allocate resources and describe activities aimed at decreasing the probability that a patient will develop a pressure ulcer. When allocating resources for pressure ulcer prevention, three options exist:

1. Assume that all patients are at risk and use preventive resources on all patients.
2. Depend on clinical judgment and intuitive sense to identify those patients at risk.
3. Use a risk assessment tool to identify patients who are at risk.

The assumption that all patients are at risk and that preventive measures should be universally applied is

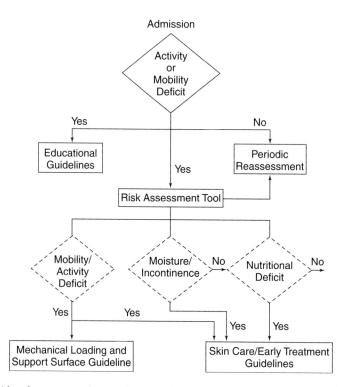

Fig. 12-7 Algorithm for pressure ulcer prediction and prevention (Agency for Healthcare Research and Quality, or AHRQ).

difficult to defend in most settings and likely represents an extremely inefficient use of resources. To treat all patients in such settings as being at risk is a tremendously wasteful approach to care. However, such an approach is probably acceptable practice in neurologic centers, especially spinal cord rehabilitation, where the degree of immobility is so profound that all patients should be considered at risk.

The accuracy of clinical judgment and intuitive sense in identifying those at risk has not been studied extensively, but Bergstrom, Demuth, and Braden (1987) found that using a risk-assessment tool led to more accurate identification of those patients who would develop a pressure ulcer than the nurse's "best guess." Furthermore, clinical judgment is likely to be much less reliable (consistent) than risk scales because it will be based on highly variable individual experience and knowledge. Risk scales should be both more reliable and more accurate than clinical judgment, and they may also enhance the judgment of the novice nurse and focus the attention of the expert nurse.

The most cost-efficient method of implementing a pressure ulcer prevention program is to use a risk-assessment scale so that those patients who are most in need of preventive care can be targeted. Risk assessment scales have become an essential ingredient in a pressure ulcer prevention program. Risk assessment facilitates prevention primarily by distinguishing those who are at risk for developing a pressure ulcer from those who are not, thus allowing for judicious allocation of resources. The second function of this type of assessment is to identify the extent to which a person exhibits a specific risk factor, thus prompting the implementation of appropriate risk reduction interventions. With consistency in risk assessment and interpretation of this risk, system wide policies concerning risk reduction interventions can be established.

Risk Assessment Tools. Screening tests vary in terms of cost, invasiveness, use (ease of use, time required), reliability, and predictive validity. Although the cost-benefit ratio of a screening tool can be a particularly difficult determination, it should be considered. How high a cost can be tolerated for detection on a per-case basis? What kind of costs are either incurred or avoided based on the outcome of the test? How often would a test have to be repeated to effectively identify those at highest risk? The selection of screening tests

entails practical and ethical considerations. For example, interface pressure measurement might be an excellent predictor of pressure ulcer risk yet is impractical for routine screening.

The rating scale is the most common screening tool used to identify patients at risk for pressure ulcer development. Commonly used risk assessment tools can be found in Appendix C. Although rating scales have the advantage of being low-cost and noninvasive, a critical evaluation of their performance is necessary. Specifically, information concerning reliability and validity is crucial. Does the tool accurately predict the development of a pressure ulcer (validity)? When rating the same patient simultaneously, do different raters consistently assign the same rating (reliability)? In addition, several related questions should be considered. Does the educational background (registered nurse [RN], licensed practical nurse [LPN], nurse aide [NA]) of the rater, or the shift during which the rater worked, affect reliability? Is the scale consistent in predicting pressure ulcer development regardless of age? Does patient population (such as nursing home, acute care, or critical care) affect the predictive ability of the scale? Does the timing of the assessment influence the predictive validity?

Common measures of predictive validity are sensitivity, specificity, predictive power of positive results, and predictive power of negative results (Table 12-1) (Baumgarten, 1998; Frantz, 1997). Sensitivity and specificity are the two measures that best reflect predictive validity; these measures are less likely to be influenced by the pressure ulcer prevalence of different patient populations (Baumgarten, 1998; Eager, 1997; Frantz, 1997). Sensitivity addresses the following question: What percentage of patients who developed pressure ulcers was identified by the screening tool as being at risk (true-positives)? Specificity addresses the following question: Of the patients who did not develop a pressure ulcer, what percentage was identified by the screening tool as being at no risk (true-negatives)?

Rating scales can also create false-positive and false-negative results. Patients who were predicted to develop a pressure ulcer but do not are referred to as false-positives, whereas patients who are predicted to remain pressure ulcer–free and do not are referred to as false-negatives. Both sensitivity and the predictive value of negative results are influenced by the number

TABLE 12-1   **Definitions of Measures of Validity for Screening Tools to Predict Development of Pressure Sores (PS+/PS–)**

	PS+	PS–	
Positive test	TP (true positive)	FP (false positive)	PVP
Negative test	FN (false negative)	TN (true negative)	PVN
	$Sensitivity = \dfrac{TP}{TP+FN}$	$Specificity = \dfrac{TN}{TN+FP}$	

Sensitivity: Answers the question: How well does the tool predict disease? Interpreted as: Of those who become PS+, the precentage who had a positive test.
Specificity: Answers the question: How accurately does the tool rule out people who will not develop disease. Interpreted as: Of those who remained PS–, the percentage who had a negative test.
Predictive value of positive results (PVP): Answers the question: How well does the tool predict who will develop the disease? Interpreted as: Of those who had a positive test, the percentage who became PS+. (AKA *PPV:* Positive predictive value).
Predictive value of negative results (PVN): Answers the question: How well does the tool predict who will not develop the disease? Interpreted as: Of those who had a negative test, the percentage who remained PS–. (AKA *NPV:* Negative predictive value).

of false-negatives; the number of false-positives influences specificity and the predictive value of positive results.

The ideal screening test would be 100% sensitive and 100% specific, but this is rarely achieved, even by tests intended for diagnosis rather than screening. This ideal is still less likely to be achieved when one is attempting to predict a condition that is preventable. Nevertheless, these measures of predictive validity are invaluable when one compares the results of various instruments for screening. Table 12-2 shows reliability and validity data on selected risk assessment tools.

Several instruments designed to predict the risk of pressure ulcers have been reported in the literature. These instruments use summative rating scales based on contributing factors and specify critical scores for identifying patients are risk. Two commonly used scales are the Norton Scale and the Braden Scale. A preoperative risk assessment tool is under development (Price et al, 2006).

Norton scale. Doreen Norton developed the first pressure ulcer risk assessment scale (Norton, 1996). The Norton scale has been studied extensively (Goldstone and Goldstone, 1982; Goldstone and Roberts, 1980; Haalboom, den Boer, and Buskens, 1999; Lincoln et al, 1986, Roberts and Goldstone, 1979) and consists of five parameters: physical condition, mental state, activity, mobility, and incontinence. Each parameter is rated on a scale of 1 to 4, with one- or two-word

descriptors for each rating. The sum of the ratings for all five parameters yields a score that can range from 5 to 20, with lower scores indicating increased risk.

Norton found an almost linear relationship between the scores of the elderly patients and the incidence of pressure ulcers, with a score of 14 indicating the "onset of risk" (although subsequent publications would place risk at 15 or 16 [Norton, 1996]) and a score of 12 or below indicating a high risk for pressure ulcer formation (WOCN Society, 2003). Sensitivity ranges from 81% to 92% for the Norton scale which indicates the ability of the tool to predict risk when risk is present. Specificity, the extent to which the tool predicts risk when no risk is present, ranges from 36% to 59% (Goldstone and Goldstone, 1982; Lincoln et al, 1986; Pang and Wong, 1998; Roberts and Goldstone, 1979). When tested with other scales, the Norton scale was able to predict the development of pressure ulcers (Haalboom, den Boer, and Buskens, 1999).

Braden scale. The Braden scale (Bergstrom, Demuth, and Braden, 1987; Bergstrom et al, 1987; Braden and Bergstrom, 1989) is composed of six subscales that conceptually reflect degrees of sensory perception, skin moisture, physical activity, nutritional intake, friction and shear, and ability to change and control body position. All subscales are rated from 1 to 4, except for the friction and shear subscale, which is rated from 1 to 3. Each rating is accompanied by a brief description of criteria for assigning the rating.

Potential scores range from 4 to 23. Interpretation of Braden scale scores has evolved with research. Initially, a hospitalized adult patient with a score of 16 or below was considered at risk (Bergstrom et al, 1987). Further research in three types of settings identified the critical cutoff score as 18 (Bergstrom et al, 1998). A score of 18 results in higher overprediction but decreases the number of false-negatives (Bergstrom et al, 1998). Braden scale scores are also examined by categories based on the percentage of patients who can be expected to develop pressure ulcers: 15-18 at risk; 13-14 moderate risk; 10-12 high risk; and 9 and lower very high risk (Ayello and Braden, 2002). In a small study, Lyder and colleagues (1998) concluded that the Braden scale did not predict pressure ulcer risk in African American and Hispanic elders and identified a need for further research. Some investigators examine subscales of the Braden scale score as a way to look at risk (Fisher, Wells, and Harrison, 2004).

The Braden scale has undergone testing in many clinical settings, and validity has been established by expert opinion. Raters have been RNs, LPNs, and NAs. Data demonstrate that the Braden scale is highly reliable when used by RNs. Sensitivity ranges from 29% to 100% and specificity from 34% to 100% (Aronovitch, 1998; Bergstrom et al, 1998; Bergstrom, Demuth, and Braden, 1987; Bergstrom et al, 1987; Braden and Bergstrom, 1989; Capobianco and McDonald, 1996; Pang and Wong, 1998; Ramundo, 1995). Quigley and Curley (1996) adapted the Braden scale for use with acutely ill children, naming it the Braden Q. The Braden Q has face and content validity and test-retest reliability (NPUAP, 2001). The Braden scale continues to be translated into many languages and is used worldwide. The instrument continues to be tested in different cultures and countries.

Implementing Risk Assessment. When implementing the risk-assessment component of a pressure ulcer prevention program, one must make several decisions. It must first be determined what caregiver can perform the assessment. Since only RNs have been found to reliably use any of these scales, it seems wise to specify that assessments be performed by RNs whenever possible. Personnel who were untrained in use of the tool were found to be at an unacceptably low percentage of agreement in the interrater reliability test in which raters were LPNs and NAs. Therefore in

settings where LPNs or NAs are the predominant bedside caregivers, the RN must train these personnel in the correct use of the tool. Furthermore, the assessment of the RN should be validated until there is consistently no more than 1 point difference in the total score assigned to any patient.

Another decision involves the timing of risk assessment. Admission assessment is important because it allows the nurse to identify those at highest risk; however, the nurse is rarely able to learn enough during the admission assessment to accurately identify lesser degrees of risk. For this reason, patients must be reassessed. The timing of risk reassessment is affected by the clinical setting. In long-term care, most patients who develop a pressure ulcer do so within the first 2 weeks of admission (Bergstrom and Braden, 1992; Vyhlidal, 1997). Kemp and colleagues (1993) reported that 61% of the individuals who developed a pressure ulcer did so within 10 days of admission. This was substantiated by Fife and colleagues (2001), who reported that 68% of all ulcers developed within 7 days for patients admitted to a neurologic unit. These reports substantiate the importance of reassessment at properly timed intervals.

In acute care, risk assessment is done upon admission and every 48 hours, or whenever the patient's condition changes (Ayello and Braden, 2002; WOCN Society, 2003). Persons in long-term care are evaluated upon admission, reassessed weekly for the first 4 weeks, and monthly and quarterly after that or when the person's condition changes. In home care, the person is assessed at the first visit, or "on admission," and reassessed each visit. None of these tools requires more than 30 seconds to complete when the nurse is familiar with the patient, so frequent assessment should not be burdensome.

The use of risk assessment scales should be increased in all health care settings (Siem et al, 2003). However, risk assessment involves more than simply determining the patient's score on an assessment tool. It involves synthesizing risk factors identified through use of a risk-assessment tool with knowledge of additional contributing factors and nursing judgment based on experience. While a pressure ulcer risk score is important data, knowledge of the score without recognition of the specific deficits contributing to that score is insufficient for determining a program of prevention.

TABLE 12-2-A Reliability and Validity Data on Selected Risk Assessment Tools: Braden Scale

AUTHOR	STATISTICS	RATERS	SETTING	N	AGE RANGE	AGE MEAN	AGE SD	% SENSITIVITY	% SPECIFICITY
Schoonhaven et al (2002)	Area under the curve 0.56 PPV 7.1% NPV 94.5%	Research nurse	Netherlands, 2 hospitals (surgical, internal medicine, neurologic and geriatric units) Risk score <16	1,229	>18 yr	60.1 yr	16.7 yr	46.2%	60.4%
VanMarum et al (2000)		Nurses	Netherlands, nursing home Risk cutoff score = 15	220	>64 yr	79 yr	3 yrs	Extrapolated from graph: 55%	Extrapolated from graph: 72%
Lyder et al (1999)	Blacks ≥75 yr: PPV 100%; NPV 60% Blacks ≤74 yr: PPV 77%; NPV 50% Latino/Hispanics ≤74 yr: 60%; NPV 50%	3 research nurses, each having a specific role and blinded throughout the study	United States, urban teaching tertiary-care hospital Blacks (n = 52) and Latino Hispanics (n = 22) Risk cut-off score = 18	74	60-99 yr	72 yr	8.3 yr	Blacks ≥75 yr: 81% Blacks ≤74 yr: 77% Latino/Hispanics ≤74 yr: 90%	Blacks ≥75 yr: 100% Blacks ≤74 yr: 50% Latino/Hispanics ≤74 yr: 14%
Halfens, Van Achterberg, and Bal (2000)	Interrater reliability of total scale .86. Interrater reliability of individual risk factors .71-.86 Internal consistency (Cronbach's alpha) 0.78 Stability of scale 0.52	Nurses	Netherlands, 3 hospitals; 11 wards Risk cut-off score = 20	320		60.9 yr	18.3 yr	73.1%	73.7%

TABLE 12-2-A Reliability and Validity Data on Selected Risk Assessment Tools: Braden Scale

AUTHOR	STATISTICS	RATERS	SETTING	N	AGE RANGE	AGE MEAN	AGE SD	% SENSITIVITY	% SPECIFICITY
Bergquist and Frantz (2001)	PPV 11% NPV: given by week	Written records; retrospective Collected by PI	Home health; non-hospice patients Risk cut-off score = 19	1,711; Braden available on 1,696	60-101	(PU+) = 78.78 yr (PU–) = 76.28 yr	(PU+) = 8.38 yr (PU–) = 8.56 yr	61%	68%
Fife et al (2001)	For risk cut-off score = 16: —FN 0% —FP 81.9% —Accuracy 44.1% For risk cut-off score = 13: —PPV 27.3% —FN 1.8% —Accuracy 68.9%	10 trained nurses	Neurologic ICU; neurologic intermediate care Risk cut-off scores = 16 and ≤13	186	14-95			91.4% for risk cut-off score: ≤13	
Bergstrom and Braden (2002)	Black patients: —Accuracy 76% —PPV 17%; —NPV 97% —Area under the curve 0.82 White patients: —Accuracy 75% —PPV 41% —NPV 92% —Area under the curve 0.75		6 settings: 2 VAMC; 2 tertiary-care hospitals; 2 SNFs Comparison of Braden scale among black and white patients Risk cut-off score = 18	843 (white: 666; black: 159; other: 18)	White 19-97 Black 19-99	White 58.09 Black 63.12	White 16.65 Black 15.92	White 70% Black 75%	White 77% Black 76%

Continued

TABLE 12-2, B Reliability and Validity Data on Selected Risk Assessment Tools: Norton Scale

AUTHOR	STATISTICS	RATERS	SETTING	N	AGE RANGE	AGE MEAN	AGE SD	% SENSITIVITY	% SPECIFICITY
Schoonhoven et al (2002)	PPV 8.1% NPV 94.9% Area under the curve 0.55	Research nurse	Netherlands, 2 hospitals (surgical, internal medicine, neurologic, and geriatric units) Risk score: <16	1,229	>18 yr	60.1 yr	16.7 yr	43.5%	67.8%
Curley et al (2003) Braden Q Scale—Pediatrics	90% agreement PPV 15% NPV 98% Area under the curve 0.83	Site investigators and research assistants	3 pediatric ICUs Cut-off score = 16	322	21 days-8 yr	36 months	29 months	88%	58%
Seongsook, Ihnsook, and Younghee (2004)	Overall validity and area under the curve 0.707. PV 37% NPV 95%	3 research nurses	Korea (3 ICUs) Cut-off score = 16	125 with 112 for final analysis	≥21 yr	62 yr		97%	26%

PPV, Positive predictive value; NPV, negative predictive value; PU+, pressure ulcer–positive; PU–, pressure ulcer–negative; ICU, intensive care unit. FN, false negative (rate); FP, false positive (rate); VAMC, Veteran's Administration Medical Center; SNF, skilled nursing facility; PI, principle investigator.

Systematic Skin Assessment

Systematic skin assessments should also be conducted (and documented) at least once per day on persons at risk. Skin inspection may be done when bathing, dressing, or assisting a patient. The WOCN Society (2003) recommends removing special garments, shoes, heel and elbow protectors, orthotic devices, restraints, and protective wear during skin inspection. Special attention should be directed to specific, vulnerable pressure points for bed- or chair-bound individuals; supine position (occiput, sacrum, and heels), sitting position (ischial tuberosities and coccyx), and side-lying position (trochanters). Components of a skin assessment can be found in Chapter 7. An example of a skin assessment documentation form can be found in Appendix C.

Reducing Risk Factors

Identification of factors (intrinsic and extrinsic) that place the patient at risk for developing a pressure ulcer is, in itself, insufficient to prevent pressure ulcers. Risk assessment must serve as a basis to identify measures that will alleviate, reduce, or minimize the negative effects of identified risk factors.

To reduce risk factors, it is imperative to ascertain which risk factors are present for an individual patient. The individual activity, mobility, nutrition and sensory perception subscale score on the Braden scale risk-assessment tool can also be used to provide an indication of specific risk so that risk-reduction strategies can be better tailored to meet that individual's needs (Vyhlidal et al, 1997). For example, when the nutrition subscale is rated poor or probably inadequate, efforts are needed to improve the patient's nutritional status. Protein, calories, vitamins, and minerals are essential to support the wound-repair process and prevent extension of the ulcer (Dolynchuk et al, 2000; WOCN Society, 2003). Nutritional support may be in the form of snacks, oral supplements, adjunctive tube feedings, or parenteral nutrition. The method selected is guided by the extent of the patient's nutritional needs, patient/family desires, and the goals of care. For patients with pressure ulcers, 35 to 40 kcalories/kg of body weight/day and 1 to 1.5 grams protein/kg of body weight may be recommended (WOCN Society, 2003). The use of vitamin C and zinc supplements and other dietary supplements requires further research (WOCN Society, 2003). A Cochrane review was not able to draw conclusions on the use of parental or enteral nutrition on pressure ulcer treatment (Langer et al, 2004).

Because pressure is the causative factor of pressure ulcers, reduction or elimination of the interface pressure is essential. Pressure redistribution can be achieved with repositioning and support surfaces. Positions that may result in pressure ulcer formation, such as supine, sitting, or an operative position, must be determined. Therefore the patient who spends much of their time sitting in a chair is prone to pressure ulcer formation over the ischial tuberosities and requires pressure redistribution in the chair rather than the bed.

Coexisting factors predisposing to pressure ulcer formation must also be assessed. Reduction of pressure alone is not sufficient if the patient is subjected to shear, friction, or fungal infection, for example. Interventions appropriate for prevention of these types of skin damage are discussed in detail in Chapter 6. Interventions to prevent skin breakdown based on Braden Score and pressure ulcer risk are located in Appendix B.

Positioning. For many years, frequent repositioning of the patient has been recommended to prevent capillary occlusion, tissue ischemia, and pressure ulceration (Kosiak, 1958; Scales, 1976; Trumble, 1930). In 1961, Kosiak recommended the frequency of repositioning to be hourly to every 2 hours, based on the interface pressure readings from healthy, able-bodied subjects. Although repositioning does not reduce intensity of pressure, it does reduce the duration, which is the more critical element of pressure ulcer formation. Turning frequency lacks strength of research evidence to draw scientific conclusions and should be challenged with research (Salcido, 2004). More frequent turning may be indicated by the patient's assessment. An every-2-hour turning schedule for a hemodynamically unstable patient may not be appropriate. In such instances, minor shifts of the shoulders and hips can be implemented for pressure redistribution. The WOCN Society (2003) recommends a regular and frequent turning and repositioning schedule for bed- and chair-bound patients; at least every 2 to 4 hours on a group 2 or 3 mattress or at least every 2 hours on a group 1 mattress. Turning is necessary even when pressure-redistribution support surfaces are used (Bergstrom, 1997; Patterson and Bennett, 1995). The effectiveness of small shifts in body weight, such as those accomplished by placing a small folded towel under different parts, remains to be demonstrated (Bergstrom, 1997; WOCN Society, 2003).

Unfortunately, because capillary closing pressures vary among persons and pressure points, the frequency of repositioning required to prevent ischemia is variable and unknown. Furthermore, there are many other factors that impinge on the frequency of repositioning such as pain, hemodynamic instability, and staffing. Therefore frequent repositioning alone may not be sufficient to prevent tissue ischemia.

When repositioning it is essential to avoid the 90-degree side-lying position (Bergstrom, 1997; Schmid-Schönbein, Rieger, and Fischer, 1980), because this position exerts such intense pressure directly over the trochanter. Instead, the 30-degree lateral position as described by Seiler and Stahelin (1985) should be used alternately with the supine position (Figure 12-8) (Panel for the Prediction and Prevention of Pressure Ulcers in Adults, 1992). The head of the bed should be lowered 1 hour after meals or tube feedings (WOCN Society, 2003). Keeping the head of the bed at an angle of 30 degrees or less, consistent with the patient's medical condition, prevents shear. If lower elevation levels of the head of bed cannot be maintained, the sacral region must be frequently monitored for effects of pressure.

Because heels have a small surface area and a large underlying bony surface, they are prime sites for pressure ulcer development. Although the hyperemic response seen during pressure redistribution tends to compensate for flow deficits, persons with diabetes mellitus may have diminished hyperemic response to pressure redistribution of the heels (Mayrovitz and Sims, 2004). Kerstein (2002) reported that of 53 diabetic patients with hospital-acquired heel ulcers, 38% had amputation of the ipsilateral leg. Persons with diabetes need extra diligence in preventing heel pressure ulcers. Pressure relief to the heels should be provided by pillow elevation or pressure redistribution can be provided with commercial products (WOCN Society, 2003). Wong and Stotts (2003) reviewed the research related to the prevention of heel pressure ulcers. Heel interface pressure is lower on a pressure redistribution surface than a conventional hospital mattress. Because support surfaces vary in their ability to reduce interface pressure under the heels, heel protection may be indicated in combination with the support surface. A variety of heel pressure redistribution devices are commercially available, but which product is best has not yet been identified. Heel elevation with a bed pillow has been shown in some studies to be more effective than commercial

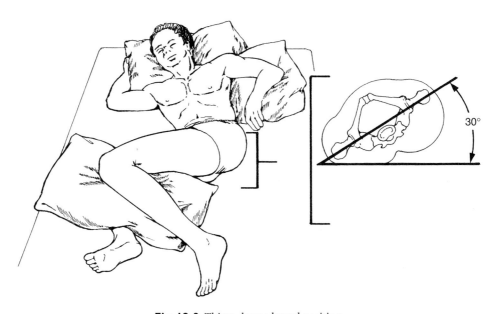

Fig. 12-8 Thirty-degree lateral position.

products (Wong and Stotts, 2003). Commercial products must be carefully evaluated for proper fit, patient activity level, and leg movement (Tymec, Pieper, and Vollman, 1997; Wong and Stotts, 2003).

A posted turning schedule is a reminder to a nurse or caregiver of the time to turn a patient and the position to use. (See Figure 12-9.) A patient's bony prominences should not touch; thus additional pillows to place between the legs and/or a positioning wedge may be needed. Unfortunately, positioning products and a turning schedule have been found to be lacking for patients at risk for pressure ulcers (Pieper et al, 1997a, 1998).

Patients who sit in a chair must also change position. A person who is dependent in care should have his or her position changed in a chair at least every hour (Panel for the Prediction and Prevention of Pressure Ulcers in Adults, 1992; WOCN Society, 2003). Those who are capable should shift their weight every 15 minutes. A change in position may include, for example, standing and reseating in a chair or elevating the legs. A patient should be properly positioned in a chair for postural alignment, distribution of weight, and balance and stability (Panel for the Prediction and Prevention of Pressure Ulcers in Adults, 1992). A pressure-reducing chair cushion should be used. Geyer and colleagues

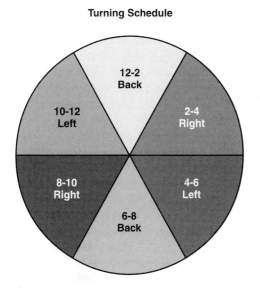

Turning Schedule

Fig. 12-9 Example of a turning schedule.

(2001) reported that pressure-reducing cushions were more effective in preventing ischial pressure ulcers; higher interface pressures were associated with a higher incidence of pressure ulcers. Unfortunately, a Cochrane review noted that seat cushions have not been adequately evaluated with research (Cullum et al, 2004).

Incontinence and Moisture Control. Patients who are incontinent should be cleaned as soon as possible after soiling and at intervals. Soap is a powerful degreaser that emulsifies fats and removes lipids, thus causing dryness. Soap also alters the skin's acid mantle, an effective antimicrobial. Specialized incontinence skin cleaners or soaps that are neutral in pH and contain a moisturizer are a better choice. Some are no-rinse and thus are convenient and save time for the care provider. The care provider should avoid excessive friction and scrubbing, which can further traumatize the skin (WOCN Society, 2003). Barrier ointments help to protect the skin from incontinence episodes. Underpads, diapers, and briefs that are absorbent and wick moisture away from the skin, a pouching device for urine or stool, a Food and Drug Administration–approved fecal containment or management device, or short-term use of an indwelling urinary catheter may have to be considered. Incontinence may increase the risk of perineal candidiasis or fungal infections. The skin exposed to urine or stool as a result of incontinence should be assessed daily so that proper treatment can be determined. See Chapter 6 for more detail.

Outdated Interventions. Many devices used to prevent pressure in the past are now known to be deleterious. For example, foam or rubber rings (i.e., donuts) are never indicated to relieve pressure because they concentrate the intensity of the pressure to the surrounding tissue (Agris and Spira, 1979; WOCN Society, 2003). Although it may provide comfort, sheepskin has no effect on pressure and so is inappropriate for pressure prevention. Likewise, the practice of vigorous massaging of pressure points, which for many years was believed to stimulate circulation to areas injured by pressure, should be critically evaluated. Furthermore, extended massage may further injure ischemic, fragile capillaries. Massage cannot be recommended in preventing pressure ulcers (WOCN Society, 2003).

Support Surfaces. A cornerstone in the reduction or elimination of interface pressures is the use of support surfaces. These products reduce tissue interface pressures over the bony prominence by maximizing contact and redistributing weight over a large area (Bergstrom, 1997; Tallon, 1996; Whittemore, 1998). Support surfaces are available in a variety of sizes and shapes that are appropriate for beds, chairs, examining tables, and operating room tables. To select and use support surfaces efficiently and effectively, the wound care specialist must be knowledgeable of their indications, contraindications, advantages, and disadvantages. Chapter 13 presents detailed information about support surfaces.

Education

The final component of a pressure ulcer prevention program is education. Pressure ulcer care and prevention is not a passive process for the patient or caregivers. Education of the patient, staff, caregivers, and family members is the key to effective prevention of pressure ulcers and to successful management of existing pressure ulcers (Xakellis et al, 1998). Teaching provides information and enhances skill development. Optimally the patient and primary caregivers have an understanding of the cause of pressure ulcer formation, the significance of factors contributing to pressure injury, preventive measures, the significance of nutrition in wound repair, skin inspection, skin assessment and the indicators of wound healing (WOCN Society, 2003). All health care personnel providing care to the patient must appreciate the role that they play in pressure ulcer prevention.

Formal patient education programs are common for patients with a spinal cord injury in rehabilitation centers. These could serve as a model for similar educational programs for patients with any chronic disease that limits mobility as the disease progresses and increases risk for pressure injury (e.g., multiple sclerosis, terminal cancer). Teaching materials about pressure ulcer prevention and treatment should be left with the patient. Examples of patient education handouts can be found in Appendix D. Educational materials for patients must be at an appropriate reading level, be evaluated for design features such as organization, writing style, appeal, and appearance, and include family members (Wilson and Williams, 2003; WOCN Society, 2003). It may be helpful to request that caregivers come to the hospital to work with a nurse to learn techniques of care before a patient's discharge.

Likewise, high-risk patients should be routinely assessed, specifically for indications of pressure damage.

Evaluation

Once a plan for reducing or eliminating pressure is developed and the plan is implemented, the effectiveness of the intervention (turning, support surface, etc.) should be evaluated at regular intervals. Daily skin inspection should provide the information needed to determine if the pressure redistribution plan is sufficient or requires modification. As a general rule, resolution of the intensity of erythema, if present, should become apparent within 24 hours of placement upon a support surface. A patient's risk for pressure ulcer formation will vary as their overall condition changes; therefore routine and regular reassessment and modification of the plan of care is warranted.

Evaluation of the overall pressure ulcer prevention program can be accomplished with pressure ulcer incidence studies. An effective pressure ulcer prevention program should yield a low incidence of pressure ulcers. Additional measures of the impact of a pressure ulcer prevention program may include staff knowledge, trends in support surface utilization (volume and type of surface), frequency of risk and skin assessment and reassessment and correlation of risk score with appropriate level of intervention.

MANAGEMENT OF PRESSURE ULCERS

Pressure ulcers must be managed by utilizing three principles of wound management, which are discussed in Chapter 19. Control and elimination of causative factors is the first principle of wound management. Continued use of preventive measures even when the patient has a pressure ulcer is critical to the successful management of pressure ulcers (WOCN Society, 2003). The second principle of wound management involves supporting the host (i.e., optimize nutrition and control blood glucose levels). Finally, the third principle is to provide a physiologic wound environment. Historically, pressure ulcers have been managed with a variety of poorly researched or scientifically unsubstantiated treatment modalities. The heat lamp, antacids, and insulin are just a few therapies that should be put to rest.

Evidence based guidelines should be the basis of all pressure ulcer prevention and treatment programs.

The AHRQ clinical practice guidelines, *Treatment of Pressure Ulcers* (Bergstrom et al, 1994), the WOCN Society (2003), and the Canadian Association for Wound Care (Dolynchuk et al, 2000) address assessment, managing tissue loads, ulcer care, managing bacterial colonization and infection, operative repair, education, and quality improvement.

PRESSURE ULCER HEALING

Measuring healing of pressure ulcers requires accurate measurement with tools that are consistent, reliable, and easily used by staff (Thomas, 1997a; Xakellis and Frantz, 1997). Measurement may include photography, wound dimensions, exudate characteristics, and predominant tissue in the ulcer (Eager, 1997; Ovington, 1997; Xakellis and Frantz, 1996). Some instruments include scored wound descriptors, such as the Pressure Sore Status Tool (PSST), the Sussman Wound Healing Tool, the Sessing Scale, the Wound Healing Scale, and the Pressure Ulcer Scale for Healing (PUSH) (Bates-Jensen, 1997; Ferrell, 1997b; Krasner, 1997; PUSH Task Force, 1997; Sussman and Swanson, 1997; Thomas, 1997a). A sample of these instruments is located in Appendix C and are discussed in Ch. 7.

Pressure ulcer staging should not be used to indicate pressure ulcer healing, and the pressure ulcer should never be "down-staged" or reverse-staged. According to NPUAP (2001) the statement about reverse staging, pressure ulcer healing does not replace lost muscle, subcutaneous fat, or dermis but instead the wound is filled with scar tissue. Therefore, reverse staging does not accurately characterize the physiologic changes of the pressure ulcer. Pressure ulcer healing is complicated by many comorbid conditions, and outcomes may be unpredictable. Some intermediate outcomes of healing may also be included, such as resolution of infection, decreased pain, enhanced quality of life, treatment costs, or change in caregiver burden (Allman and Fowler, 1995).

The time to heal a pressure ulcer is variable. Stage II pressure ulcers have a mean or median time to heal ranging from 8.7 to 38 days (van Rijswijk, 1995). The median time to heal a stage III or stage IV pressure ulcer has been reported as 69 days with the percentage reduction in ulcer area after 2 weeks of treatment as an independent predictor of time to heal (van Rijswijk, 1995). Healing rates are lower for stage III and stage IV ulcers than for stage 2 ulcers in all health care settings (Allman, 1995). Complete wound closure may not be a practical way to assess healing because of prolonged healing time, patient's loss to follow-up, and changing care goals (Ferrell, 1997a). In a study in long-term care, pressure ulcer healing was associated with higher body weight, lower body temperature, and lower ulcer stage (Kramer and Kearney, 2000).

QUALITY OF LIFE AND PSYCHOSOCIAL NEEDS

Pressure ulcers may affect psychosocial needs and quality of life in terms of occurrence, recurrence, ulcer characteristics, and ulcer demands. Pressure ulcers may cause social isolation and add burden and frustration for the patient, the family and care providers (Dolynchuk et al, 2000). Most quality-of-life research is about persons with spinal cord injury (Rintala, 1995). Quality-of-life research studies are small, and additional research is needed (Rintala, 1995). It is important to assess the patient's social networks, the patient's living space and environment, and the patient's mental status, learning needs, and personal goals (Dolynchuk et al, 2000). Functional and financial status should also be considered along with psychosocial needs and quality of life (see Chapter 26). Pain associated with pressure ulcers must be assessed. Pain assessment and management is discussed in detail in Chapter 25.

QUALITY IMPROVEMENT

Continuous quality improvement looks for problems that exist in care delivery and attempts to correct them. Pressure ulcers are often viewed as a quality of care marker in health care settings. There is a need for health care agencies to improve pressure ulcer prevention (Bates-Jensen et al, 2003; Lyder et al, 2001; Siem et al, 2003). Quality of care may be examined by reviewing medical records to determine if the care delivered was acceptable or appropriate as well as the use of standards and guidelines. The method to collect quality data must be reliable and valid. The use and recording of prevention methods or risk assessment may be found to be lacking (Lyder et al, 2001; Pieper et al, 1997b). Educational programs and decision charts may assist health care workers to enhance quality of care (Kiernan, 1997; Letourneau and Jensen,

1998; Moore and Wise, 1997; Suntken et al, 1996; Xakellis and Frantz, 1997). Education about pressure ulcers should be integrated into medical and nursing school curricula. The pressure ulcer knowledge of geriatric fellows was reported to require improvement, with most knowledge obtained from bedside rounds, nurses, lectures, and textbooks (Odierna and Zeleznik, 2003). The health professional's knowledge about pressure ulcers has to be updated (Pieper and Mattern, 1997; Pieper and Mott, 1995). Unfortunately, none of the approaches—blame, monetary compensation, measures of pressure ulcer neglect—has resulted in a sustainable improvement in the incidence rates or management of pressure ulcers (Meehan, 2000). The team approach, as described in Chapter 2, is necessary to accommodate the increasing complexity of patients as well the ever changing amount of literature and level of evidence.

Research is needed about the prevention and treatment of pressure ulcers. Pressure ulcers comprise 0.06% of indexed publications with descriptive studies being published most frequently (Halfens and Haalboom, 2001). Scientific evidence articles on which to base care remain limited. The current investment in research is small compared to treatment expenditures. Research funds represent 0.5% of the $3.6 billion annual cost of pressure ulcers (Zanca et al, 2003). Professional organizations continue to set priorities for pressure ulcer research.

LEGAL CONCERNS

An issue in medical malpractice is whether the practitioner met the standard of care, namely that exercised by other practitioners in the same line of practice under the same or similar circumstances (Murphy, 1996). Pressure ulcers may be viewed as an indicator of neglect. Documentation is critical and should be done in detail. Concerns are raised when there are numerous and varying descriptions of the pressure ulcer, lack of evidence of ordered care, and a failure to match or monitor a treatment protocol. Photographs document many aspects of wound assessment and may be used during litigation. Health professionals must constantly ask if prevention and/or treatment follow evidence-based practice and if they are effective. If not, what are criteria for changing care? It is important to document whenever interventions are performed, patient instructions are given, or a patient refuses care. The medical record is a central component in litigation because it presents decisions, rationale, treatments, and outcomes (Knowlton, 2003). Documentation must be thorough; what is missing may be more significant than what is present (Knowlton, 2003).

SUMMARY

Pressure ulcers are a global health concern because, for the most part, they are a costly preventable complication. As a consequence of unrelieved pressure, capillaries are occluded and tissue damage ensues; the extent of tissue damage being influenced by numerous variables. Pressure ulcer prevention requires a comprehensive multidisciplinary plan that includes (1) risk assessment, (2) regular and routine skin assessment, (3) reducing risk factors, (4) patient, family and staff education, and (5) evaluation. When familiar with the pathologic process of tissue destruction caused by unrelieved pressure, appropriate interventions can be implemented.

SELF-ASSESSMENT EXERCISE

1. Why are the data describing the prevalence of pressure ulcer formation in hospitals, nursing homes, and high-risk populations so varied?
2. Define pressure ulcer.
3. What is the role of muscle in preventing pressure ulcers?
   a. Muscle redistributes pressure load.
   b. Muscle provides the blood supply to the skin.
   c. Muscle enables blood vessels to resist shear injury.
   d. Muscle concentrates pressure over the bony prominence.
4. State the three factors that play a role in determining the negative effects of pressure.
5. What is the common range of capillary closing pressure?
   a. 5 to 15 mm Hg
   b. 12 to 32 mm Hg
   c. 10 to 20 mm Hg
   d. 15 to 45 mm Hg
6. Which of the following defines capillary closing pressure?
   a. Pressure required to maintain a patent capillary
   b. Difference in pressures between the arteriolar end of the capillary and the venous end
   c. Pressure needed to occlude the capillary blood flow
   d. Mean capillary pressure

7. Explain why it is difficult to accurately assign a numerical value to capillary closing pressure.

8. Tissue interface pressure is believed to be an indirect measure of which of the following?
   a. Capillary closing pressure
   b. Mean capillary pressure
   c. Pressure being exerted on a capillary
   d. Pressure required to maintain a patent capillary

9. Explain the relationship between tissue interface pressure and capillary closing pressure.

10. Describe how intensity of pressure and duration of pressure affect tissue ischemia.

11. Which of the following are major factors that contribute to pressure ulcer development?
    a. Shear, smoking, and friction
    b. Age, smoking, and blood pressure
    c. Nutrition and stress
    d. Shear, friction, and nutritional debilitation

12. Which of the following statements about blanching erythema is false?
    a. It resolves once pressure is removed.
    b. It indicates deep tissue damage.
    c. It is an area of erythema that turns white when compressed.
    d. It implies that pressure is not adequately relieved or reduced.

13. State four variables that influence the extent of tissue damage associated with pressure.

14. State at least two variables that contribute to cellular death in a pressure-damaged area.

15. The undermining that is commonly observed with pressure ulcers may be the result of which process?
    a. Shear
    b. Friction
    c. Maceration
    d. Advanced age

REFERENCES

Adams T, Hunter WS: Modification of skin mechanical properties by eccrine sweat gland activity, *J Appl Physiol* 26:417, 1969.

Agris J, Spira M: Pressure ulcers: prevalence and treatment, *Clin Symp* 31(5):21, 1979.

Allman RM: The impact of pressure ulcers on health care costs and mortality, *Adv Wound Care* 11(3 Suppl):2, 1998.

Allman RM, Fowler E: Expected outcomes for the treatment of pressure ulcers, *Adv Wound Care* 8(4):28, 1995.

Allman RM et al: Pressure sores among hospitalized patients, *Ann Intern Med* 105:3371, 1986.

Allman RM et al: Pressure ulcer risk factors among hospitalized patients with activity limitations, *JAMA* 273:865, 1995.

Allman RM et al: Pressure ulcers, hospital complications, and disease severity: impact on hospital costs and length of stay, *Adv Wound Care* 12(1):22, 1999.

Amlung SR, Miller WL, Bosley LM: The 1999 national pressure ulcer prevalence survey: a benchmarking approach, *Adv Skin Wound Care* 14:297, 2001.

Arnold HL: Decubitus: the word. In Parish LC, Witkowski JA, Crissey JT: *The decubitus ulcer*, New York, 1983, Masson.

Aronovitch SA: Intraoperative acquired pressure ulcer prevalence: a national study, *Adv Wound Care* 11(3 Suppl):8, 1998.

Ayello EA, Braden B: How and why to do pressure ulcer risk assessment, *Adv Skin Wound Care* 15:125, 2002.

Baldwin KM: Incidence and prevalence of pressure ulcers in children, *Adv Skin Wound Care* 15:121, 2002.

Barczak CA et al: Fourth national pressure ulcer prevalence survey, *Adv Wound Care* 10(4):18, 1997.

Bates-Jensen BM: The pressure sore status tool a few thousand assessments later, *Adv Wound Care* 10(5):65, 1997.

Bates-Jensen BM et al: The minimum data set pressure ulcer indicator: does it reflect differences in care processes related to pressure ulcer prevention and treatment in nursing homes? *J Am Geriatr Soc* 51(9):1203, 2003.

Baumgarten M: Designing prevalence and incidence studies, *Adv Wound Care* 11(6):287, 1998.

Baumgarten M et al: Pressure ulcers and the transition to long-term care, *Adv Skin Wound Care* 16:299, 2003.

Beckrich K, Aronovitch SA: Hospital-acquired pressure ulcers: a comparison of costs in medical versus surgical patients, *Adv Wound Care* 11(3 Suppl):2, 1998.

Bennett LM et al: Skin stress and blood flow in sitting paraplegic patients, *Arch Phys Med Rehabil* 65:1861, 1984.

Bennett LM, Lee BY: Vertical shear existence in animal pressure threshold experiments, *Decubitus* 1:18, 1988.

Bergquist S: Pressure ulcer prediction in older adults receiving home health care: implications for use with the OASIS, *Adv Skin Wound Care* 16:132, 2003.

Bergquist S, Frantz R: Braden scale: validity in community-based older adults receiving home health care, *Appl Nurs Res* 14:36, 2001.

Bergstrom NI: Strategies for preventing pressure ulcers, *Clin Geriatr Med* 13(3):437, 1997.

Bergstrom NI, Braden B: A prospective study of pressure sore risk among institutionalized elderly, *J Am Geriatr Soc* 40:747, 1992.

Bergstrom N, Braden BJ: Predictive validity of the Braden scale among black and white subjects, *Nurs Res* 51:398, 2002.

Bergstrom NI, Demuth PJ, Braden B: A clinical trial of the Braden scale for predicting pressure sore risk, *Nurs Clin North Am* 22(2):4171, 1987.

Bergstrom NI et al: The Braden scale for predicting pressure sore risk, *Nurs Res* 36(4):2051, 1987.

Bergstrom NI et al: *Treatment of pressure ulcers*, Clinical Practice Guideline #15, Rockville, Md, 1994, USDHHS, PHS, AHCPR, Pub. No. 95-0652.

Bergstrom NI et al: Predicting pressure ulcer risk: a multisite study of the predictive validity of the Braden scale, *Nurs Res* 47(5):261, 1998.

Berlowitz DR et al: Effect of pressure ulcers on the survival of long-term care residents, *J Gerontol* 52A(2):M106, 1997.

Berlowitz DR, Wilking SVB: Risk factors for pressure sore: a comparison on cross-sectional and cohort-derived data, *J Am Geriatr Soc* 37:1043, 1989.

Boulpaep EL: The microcirculation. In Boron WF, Boulpaep EL, editors: *Medical Physiology*, Philadelphia, 2003, WB Saunders.

Braden BJ: *Emotional stress and pressure sore formation among the elderly recently relocated to a nursing home: key aspects of recovery: improving mobility, rest, and nutrition*, New York, 1990, Springer.

Braden BJ: The relationship between stress and pressure sore formation, *Ostomy Wound Manage* 44(3A):26S, 1998.

Braden BJ, Bergstrom N: A conceptual schema for the study of the etiology of pressure sores, *Rehabil Nurs* 12(1):81, 1987.

Braden BJ, Bergstrom N: Clinical utility of the Braden scale for predicting pressure sore risk, *Decubitus* 2(3):441, 1989.

Brandeis GH et al: The epidemiology and natural history of pressure ulcers in elderly nursing home residents, *JAMA* 264(22):2905, 1990.

Brooks B, Duncan W: Effects of pressure on tissues, *Arch Surg* 40:696, 1940.

Brown G: Long-term outcomes of full-thickness pressure ulcers: healing and mortality, *Ostomy Wound Manage* 49(10):42, 2003.

Bryant RA, Rolstad BS: Utilizing a systems approach to implement pressure ulcer prediction and prevention, *Ostomy Wound Manage* 47(9):26, 2001.

Burton AC, Yamada S: Relation between blood pressure and flow in the human forearm, *J Appl Physiol* 4:3291, 1951.

Capobianco ML, McDonald DD: Factors affecting the predictive validity of the Braden scale, *Adv Wound Care* 9(6):32, 1996.

Chang YC, Lin WM, Hsieh ST: Effects of aging on human skin innervation, *Neuroreport* 15(1):149, 2004.

Chernoff R: Policy: nutrition standards for treatment of pressure ulcers, *Nutr Rev* 54(1):S43, 1996.

Cherry GW et al: Functional microcirculatory changes after flap elevation: possible factor in flap failure, *Plast Surg Forum* 3:2061, 1980.

Cherry GW, Ryan TJ, Ellis J: Decreased fibrinolysis in reperfused ischemic tissue, *Thromb Diathesis Haemorrhag* 32:659, 1974.

Cohen IK, Diegelmann RF, Johnson MJ: Effect of corticosteroids on collagen synthesis, *Surgery* 82(1):151, 1977.

Collins N: Adding vitamin C to the wound management mix, *Adv Skin Wound Care* 17:109, 2004.

Cullum N et al: Beds, mattresses and cushions for pressure sore prevention and treatment, *Cochrane Database Syst Rev* 2, 2004.

Curley MAQ et al: Predicting pressure ulcer risk in pediatric patients: The Braden Q scale, *Nurs Res* 52:22, 2003.

Dallam L et al: Pressure ulcer pain: assessment and quantification, *J WOCN* 22:211, 1995.

Daniel RK, Kerrigan CL: Skin flaps: an anatomical and hemodynamic approach, *Clin Plast Surg* 6:181, 1979.

Dolynchuk K et al: Best practices for the prevention and treatment of pressure ulcers, *Ostomy Wound Manage* 46(11):38, 2000.

Eager CA: Monitoring wound healing in the home health arena, *Adv Wound Care* 10(5):54, 1997.

Evans-Stoner N: Nutritional assessment: a practical approach, *Nurs Clin North Am* 32:637, 1997.

Ferrell BA: Assessment of healing, *Clin Geriatr Med* 13(3):575, 1997a.

Ferrell BA: The Sessing scale for measurement of pressure ulcer healing, *Adv Wound Care* 10(4):78, 1997b.

Fife C et al: Incidence of pressure ulcers in a neurologic intensive care unit, *Crit Care Med* 29:283, 2001.

Fisher AR, Wells G, Harrison MB: Factors associated with pressure ulcers in adults in acute care hospitals, *Adv Skin Wound Care* 17:80, 2004.

Flanigan KH: Nutritional aspects of wound healing, *Adv Wound Care* 10(3):48, 1997.

Fletcher J: Pressure-relieving equipment: criteria and selection, *Br J Nurs* 6(6):323, 1997.

Fox J, Bradley R: *A new medical dictionary*, London, 1803, Darton & Harvey.

Frantz RA: Measuring prevalence and incidence of pressure ulcers, *Adv Wound Care* 10(1):21, 1997.

Gallagher SM: Outcomes in clinical practice: pressure ulcer prevalence and incidence studies, *Ostomy Wound Manage* 43(1):28, 1997.

Geyer MJ et al: A randomized control trial to evaluate pressure-reducing seat cushions for elderly wheelchair users, *Adv Skin Wound Care* 14:120, 2001.

Goldstone LA, Goldstone J: The Norton score: an early warning of pressure sores? *J Adv Nurs* 1:4191, 1982.

Goldstone LA, Roberts BV: A preliminary discriminant function analysis of elderly orthopaedic patients who will or will not contract a pressure sore, *Int J Nurs Stud* 17(5):171, 1980.

Gosnell DJ: An assessment tool to identify pressure sores, *Nurs Res* 22(1):551, 1973.

Groeneveld A et al: The prevalence of pressure ulcers in a tertiary care pediatric and adult hospital, *J WOCN* 31:108-120, 2004.

Guenter P et al: Survey of nutritional status in newly hospitalized patients with stage III or stage IV pressure ulcers, *Adv Skin Wound Care* 13:164, 2000.

Guyton AC, Hall JE: *Textbook of medical physiology*, Philadelphia, 1996, WB Saunders.

Haalboom JR, den Boer J, Buskens E: Risk-assessment tools in the prevention of pressure ulcers, *Ostomy Wound Manage* 45(2):20, 1999.

Halfens RJD, Haalboom JRE: A historical overview of pressure ulcer literature of the past 35 years, *Ostomy Wound Manage* 47(11):36, 2001.

Halfens RJD, Van Achterberg T, Bal RM: Validity and reliability of the Braden scale and the influence of other risk factors: a multi-centre prospective study, *Int J Nurs Stud* 37:313, 2000.

Husain T: An experimental study of some pressure effects on tissues, with reference to the bedsore problem, *J Pathol Bacteriol* 66:3471, 1953.

Jones PL, Millman A: Wound healing and the aged patient, *Nurs Clin North Am* 25:2631, 1990.

Kanj LF, Phillips TJ: Skin problems in the elderly, *Wounds* 13(3):93, 2001.

Kanj LF, Wilking SVB, Phillips TJ: Pressure ulcers, *J Am Acad Dermatol* 38(4):517, 1998.

Kemp MG et al: The role of support surfaces and patient attributes in preventing pressure ulcers in elderly patients, *Res Nurs Health* 16:89, 1993.

Kerstein MD: Heel ulcerations in the diabetic patient, *Wounds* 14(6):212, 2002.

Kiernan M: Pressure sores: adopting the principles of risk management, *Br J Nurs* 6(6):329, 1997.

Knowlton SP: The medical record: treatment tool or litigation device? *Adv Skin Wound Care* 16:97, 2003.

Knudsen AM, Gallagher S: Care of the obese patient with pressure ulcers, *J WOCN* 30(2):111, 2003.

Kosiak M: Etiology of decubitus ulcers, *Arch Phys Med Rehabil* 42:191, 1961.

Kosiak M et al: Evaluation of pressure as a factor in the production of ischial ulcers, *Arch Phys Med Rehabil* 39:623, 1958.

Kramer JD, Kearney M: Patient, wound, and treatment characteristics associated with healing in pressure ulcers, *Adv Skin Wound Care* 13:17, 2000.

Krasner D: Using a gentler hand: reflections on patients with pressure ulcers who experience pain, *Ostomy Wound Manage* 42:20, 1996.

Krasner D: Wound healing scale, version 1.0: a proposal, *Adv Wound Care* 10(5):82, 1997.

Krouskop TA: A synthesis of the factors that contribute to pressure sore formation, *Med Hypotheses* 11(2):2551, 1983.

Kumar RN et al: Direct health care costs of four common skin ulcers in New Mexico Medicaid fee-for-service patients, *Adv Skin Wound Care* 17:143, 2004.

Lake NO: Measuring incidence and prevalence of pressure ulcers for intergroup comparison, *Adv Wound Care* 12:31, 1999.

Lamid S, El Ghatit AZ: Smoking, spasticity and pressure sores in spinal cord injured patients, *Am J Phys Med* 62(6):300, 1983.

Landis EM: Micro-injection studies of capillary blood pressure in human skin, *Heart* 15:209, 1930.

Langemo DK et al: The lived experience of having a pressure ulcer: a qualitative analysis, *Adv Skin Wound Care* 13:225, 2000.

Langer G et al: Nutritional interventions for preventing and treating pressure ulcers, *Cochrane Database of Systematic Reviews* 2, 2004.

Letourneau S, Jensen L: Impact of a decision tree on chronic wound care, *J WOCN* 25(5):240, 1998.

Lincoln R et al: Use of the Norton pressure sore risk assessment scoring system with elderly patients in acute care, *J Enterostom Ther* 13:171, 1986.

Lindan O: Etiology of decubitus ulcers: an experimental study, *Arch Phys Med Rehabil* 42:774, 1961.

Lyder CH et al: Validating the Braden scale for the prediction of pressure ulcer risk in blacks and Latino/Hispanic elders: a pilot study, *Ostomy Wound Manage* 44(3A):42, 1998.

Lyder CH et al: The Braden Scale for pressure ulcer risk: evaluating the predictive validity in Black and Latino/Hispanic elders, *Appl Nurs Res* 12:60, 1999.

Lyder CH et al: Quality of care for hospitalized medicare patients at risk for pressure ulcers, *Arch Intern Med* 161:1549, 2001.

Mathison CJ: Skin and wound care challenges in the hospitalized morbidly obese patient, *J WOCN* 30:78, 2003.

Mayrovitz HN, Sims N: Biophysical effects of water and synthetic urine on skin, *Adv Skin Wound Care* 14:302, 2001.

Mayrovitz HN, Sims N: Effects of support surface relief pressures on heel skin blood flow in persons with and without diabetes mellitus, *Adv Skin Wound Care* 17:197, 2004.

Mayrovitz HN et al: Effects of support surface relief pressures on heel skin blood perfusion, *Adv Skin Wound Care* 16:141, 2003.

Meehan M: Beyond the pressure ulcer blame game: reflections for the future, *Ostomy Wound Manage* 46(5):46, 2000.

Moolten SE: Bedsores in the chronically ill patient, *Arch Phys Med Rehabil* 53:4301, 1972.

Moore SM, Wise L: Reducing nosocomial pressure ulcers, *J Nurs Adm* 27(10):28, 1997.

Murphy RN: Legal and practical impact of clinical practice guidelines on nursing and medical practices, *Adv Wound Care* 9:31, 1996.

National Pressure Ulcer Advisory Panel (NPUAP), Cuddigan J, Ayello EA, Sussman C, editors: *Pressure ulcers in America: prevalence, incidence, and implications for the future*, Reston, Va, 2001, Author.

National Pressure Ulcer Advisory Panel (NPUAP): *Pressure ulcers in neonates and children*, Reston, Va, 2005, Author.

Niazi ZBM et al: Recurrence of initial pressure ulcer in persons with spinal cord injuries, *Adv Wound Care* 10(3):38, 1997.

Norton D: Calculating the risk: reflections on the Norton scale, *Adv Wound Care* 9(6):38, 1996.

Odierna E, Zeleznik J: Pressure ulcer education: a pilot study of the knowledge and clinical confidence of geriatric fellows, *Adv Skin Wound Care* 16(1):26, 2003.

Ovington LG: What is needed to monitor healing in the outpatient clinic setting? *Adv Wound Care* 10(5):58, 1997.

Panel for the Prediction and Prevention of Pressure Ulcers in Adults: *Pressure ulcers in adults: prediction and prevention*. Clinical Practice Guideline, 1992, AHCPR Pub. No. 92-0047.

Pang SM, Wong TK: Predicting pressure sore risk with the Norton, Braden, and Waterlow scales in a Hong Kong rehabilitation hospital, *Nurs Res* 47(3):147, 1998.

Parish LC, Witkowski JA, Crissey JT: *The decubitus ulcer*, New York, 1983, Masson.

Patterson JA, Bennett RG: Prevention and treatment of pressure sores, *J Am Geriat Soc* 43:919, 1995.

Pieper B, Mattern J: Critical care nurses' knowledge of pressure ulcer prevention, *Ostomy Wound Manage* 43(3):22, 1997.

Pieper B, Mott M: Nurses' knowledge of pressure ulcer prevention, staging and description, *Adv Wound Care* 8(3):34, 1995.

Pieper B et al: Presence of pressure ulcer prevention methods used among patients considered at risk versus those considered not at risk, *J WOCN* 24:191, 1997a.

Pieper B et al: The occurrence of skin lesions in ill persons, *Dermatol Nurs* 9(2):91, 1997b.

Pieper B et al: Risk factors, prevention methods, and wound care for patients with pressure ulcers, *Clin Nurse Spec* 12:7, 1998.

Price MC et al: Development of a risk assessment tool for intraoperative pressure ulcers, *J WOCN* 32:19, 2005.

PUSH Task Force: Pressure ulcer scale for healing: derivation and validation of the PUSH Tool, *Adv Wound Care* 10(5):96, 1997.

Quigley SM, Curley MAQ: Skin integrity in the pediatric population: preventing and managing pressure ulcers, *J Soc Pediatr Nurs* 1(1):7, 1996.

Quirino J et al: Pain in pressure ulcers, *Wounds* 15(12):381, 2003.

Ramundo JM: Reliability and validity of the Braden scale in the home care setting, *J WOCN* 22(3):128, 1995.

Reichel SM: Shearing force as a factor in decubitus ulcers in paraplegics, *JAMA* 166:762, 1958.

Reuler JB, Cooney TG: The pressure sore: pathophysiology and principles of management, *Ann Intern Med* 94(5):6611, 1981.

Rintala DH: Quality of life considerations, *Adv Wound Care* 8(4):28, 1995.

Roberts BV, Goldstone LA: A survey of pressure sores in the over sixties on two orthopaedic wards, *Int J Nurs Stud* 16:3551, 1979.

Robinson C et al: Determining the efficacy of a pressure ulcer prevention program by collecting prevalence and incidence data: a unit-based effort, *Ostomy Wound Manage* 49(5):44, 2003.

Rodriquez G et al: Collagen metabolite excretion as a predictor of bone and skin-related complications in spinal cord injury, *Arch Phys Med Rehabil* 70(6):4421, 1989.

Ryan T: The ageing of the blood supply and the lymphatic drainage of the skin, *Micron* 35(3):161, 2004.

Ryan TJ: Microvascularization in psoriasis, blood vessels, lymphatics and tissue fluid, *Pharmacol Ther* 10:27, 1980.

Salzberg CA et al: Predicting and preventing pressure ulcers in adults with paralysis, *Adv Wound Care* 11(5):237, 1998.

Salcido R: Patient turning schedules: why and how often? *Adv Skin Wound Care* 17:156, 2004.

Scales JT: Pressure on the patient. In Kenedi RM, Cowden JM, editors: *Bedsore biomechanics*, London, 1976, University Park Press.

Schmid-Schönbein H, Rieger H, Fischer T: Blood fluidity as a consequence of red cell fluidity: flow properties of blood and flow behavior of blood in vascular diseases, *Angiology* 31:3011, 1980.

Schoonhoven L et al: Risk indicators for pressure ulcers during surgery, *Appl Nurs Res* 15(3):163, 2002.

Schoonhoven L et al, for the pre PURSE study group: Prospective cohort study of routine use of risk assessment scales for prediction of pressure ulcers, *BMJ* 325:797, 2002.

Seiler WO, Stahelin HB: Decubitus ulcers: preventive techniques for the elderly patient, *Geriatrics* 40(7):531, 1985.

Seongsook J, Ihnsook J, Younghee L: Validity of pressure ulcer risk assessment scales; Cubbin and Jackson, Braden, and Douglas scale, *Int J Nurs Stud* 41:199, 2004.

Shannon ML, Skorga P: Pressure ulcer prevalence in two general hospitals, *Decubitus* 2:38, 1989.

Shea JD: Pressure sores: classification and management, *Clin Orthop* (112):891, 1975.

Siem CA et al: Skin assessment and pressure ulcer care in hospital-based skilled nursing facilities, *Ostomy Wound Manage* 49(6):42, 2003.

Stotts NA, Hopf HW: The link between tissue oxygen and hydration in nursing home residents with pressure ulcers: preliminary data, *J WOCN* 30:184, 2003.

Strauss EA, Margolis DJ: Malnutrition in patients with pressure ulcers: morbidity, mortality, and clinically practical assessment, *Adv Wound Care* 9:37, 1996.

Suntken G et al: Implementation of a comprehensive skin care program across care settings using the AHCPR pressure ulcer prevention and treatment guidelines, *Ostomy Wound Manage* 42(2):20, 1996.

Sussman C, Swanson G: Utility of the Sussman Wound Healing Tool in predicting wound healing outcomes in physical therapy, *Adv Wound Care* 10(5):74, 1997.

Tallon RW: Support surfaces: therapeutic and performance insights, *Nurs Manage* 27(9):57, 1996.

Thomas DR: Nutritional factors affecting wound healing, *Ostomy Wound Manage* 42:40, 1996.

Thomas DR: Existing tools: are they meeting the challenges of pressure ulcer healing? *Adv Wound Care* 10(5):86, 1997a.

Thomas DR: Specific nutritional factors in wound healing, *Adv Wound Care* 10(4):40, 1997b.

Thomas DR: The role of nutrition in prevention and healing of pressure ulcers, *Clin Geriatr Med* 13(3):497, 1997c.

Thomson CW et al: Fluidized-bead bed in the intensive-therapy unit, *Lancet* 1:568, 1980.

Trumble HC: The skin tolerance for pressure and pressure sores, *Med J Aust* 2:7241, 1930.

Tymec AC, Pieper B, Vollman K: A comparison of two pressure-relieving devices on the prevention of heel pressure ulcers, *Adv Wound Care* 10:39, 1997.

U.S. Department of Health and Human Services: *Healthy People 2010*, Washington, D.C., 2000, Author.

Van Marum RJ et al: The Dutch pressure sore assessment score or the Norton scale for identifying at-risk nursing home patients? *Age Ageing* 29:63, 2000.

van Rijswijk L: Frequency of reassessment of pressure ulcers, *Adv Wound Care* 8:28, 1995.

Vyhlidal S et al: Mattress replacement or foam overlay? A prospective study on the incidence of pressure ulcers, *Appl Nurs Res* 10(3):111, 1997.

Waterlow JA. Pressure sore risk assessment in children, *Paediatr Nurs* 9(6):21, 1997.

Wellman NS: A case manager's guide to nutrition screening and intervention, *J Case Manage* 3:12, 1997.

Whittemore R: Pressure-reduction support surfaces: a review of the literature, *J WOCN* 25:6, 1998.

Wilson FL, Williams BN: Assessing the readability of skin care and pressure ulcer patient education materials, *J WOCN* 30:224, 2003.

Wong VK, Stotts NA: Physiology and prevention of heel ulcers: the state of science, *J WOCN* 30:191, 2003.

Wound, Ostomy and Continence Nurses (WOCN) Society: *Guideline for prevention and management of pressure ulcers*, Glenview, Il, 2003, Author.

Wound, Ostomy and Continence Nurses (WOCN) Society: *Prevalence and incidence: a toolkit for clinicians*, Glenview, Il, 2004, Author.

Xakellis GC et al: Cost-effectiveness of an intensive pressure ulcer prevention protocol in long-term care, *Adv Wound Care* 11(1):22, 1998.

Xakellis GC et al: Translating pressure ulcer guidelines into practice: it's harder than it sounds, *Adv Skin Wound Care* 14:249, 2001.

Yarkony GM: Pressure ulcers: a review, *Arch Phys Med Rehabil* 75:908, 1994.

Zanca JM et al: For the National Pressure Ulcer Advisory Panel (NPUAP): Pressure ulcer research funding in America: creation and analysis of an on-line database, *Adv Skin Wound Care* 16:190, 2003.

Zulkowski K: MDS RAP items associated with pressure ulcer prevalence in newly institutionalized elderly: Study 1, *Ostomy Wound Manage* 44(11):40, 1998.

Zulkowski K, Kindsfater D: Examination of care-planning needs for elderly newly admitted to an acute care setting, *Ostomy Wound Manage* 46(1):32, 2000.

13 *Support Surfaces*

DENISE P. NIX

OBJECTIVES

1. List three limitations to the reliance of capillary closing values for support surface evaluation.
2. List four factors to consider when interpreting the significance of interface tissue pressure readings.
3. List four functions of a support surface.
4. Identify four types of support surfaces.
5. Compare advantages and disadvantages of four support surface mediums.

A support surface is a device that redistributes pressure. Depending on the composition of the support surface and its mechanism of action, the support surface may also reduce shear, friction, and moisture. Support surfaces are available in differing sizes and shapes and are made for chairs as well as horizontal surfaces such as beds, examining tables, and operating room (OR) tables.

Though many claims are made as to effectiveness, few clinical trials are available to support those claims; limitations are common in the numbers of patients and statistical validation (Rithalia and Kenney, 2001). The WOCN Society (2003) reports insufficient evidence to specify any particular brand of support surface for pressure ulcer prevention. Experts agree that the following measures be taken:

1. At-risk individuals should be placed on a pressure-redistribution support surface rather than a standard hospital mattress.
2. Pressure redistribution should be used in the operating room for the at-risk individual.

3. The individual with a stage III or stage IV pressure ulcer or who has multiple ulcers over several turning surfaces needs a therapeutic support surface.
4. The chair-bound individual with a pressure ulcer located on a sitting surface should limit sitting time and use cushions (gel or air) that provide pressure redistribution.
5. The support surface should serve as an adjunct to and not a replacement for turning and positioning.

It is essential that health care practitioners responsible for support surface selection be knowledgeable about product functions, indications, contraindications, advantages, and disadvantages. Selecting an appropriate support surface for the patient requires the critical analysis of several factors: (1) the condition of the wound (wound assessment), (2) the presence of risk factors for pressure ulcer development, (3) the patient's rehabilitation needs, (4) discharge plans, (5) staffing, and (6) product maintenance.

When a support surface intervention is warranted, the patient's documented plan of care must include the following:

1. Education of the patient and caregiver on pressure ulcer prevention and management
2. Regular skin assessment
3. Routine pressure ulcer risk assessment
4. Appropriate turning and repositioning
5. Appropriate wound care including ongoing assessments and evaluation of healing
6. Management of moisture and incontinence
7. Nutritional support (assessment and intervention) that is consistent with the patient's overall goals

SUPPORT SURFACE FEATURES

Pressure Redistribution

Support surfaces are designed to prevent pressure ulcers or promote the healing of wounds by reducing or eliminating tissue interface pressure. Most of these devices reduce interface pressure by conforming to the contours of the body so that pressure is redistributed over a larger surface area rather than concentrated on a more circumscribed location. Pressure redistribution is accomplished through *immersion* and *envelopment*. *Immersion* allows the pressure to be spread out over the surrounding area rather than directly over a bony prominence. Immersion is dependent on factors such as the stiffness and thickness of the support surface and flexibility of the cover. *Envelopment* refers to the ability of the support surface to conform to irregularities (i.e., clothing, bedding, bony prominences) without causing a substantial increase in pressure (Brienza and Geyer, 2005).

Capillary Closing Pressure. Historically, the terms *pressure reduction* and *pressure relief* were used to describe support surface function.* By measuring an applied load (the patient's weight) over a small area, tissue interface pressure was obtained; this measure was used to determine the effectiveness of the support surface (Rithalia and Kenney, 2001). When the skin-resting surface interface pressure decreased to near capillary closing pressures, the support surface was interpreted as being less likely to interrupt or occlude capillary blood flow. Therefore, the surface was categorized as pressure-relieving (therapeutic) when the skin-resting surface interface pressure was consistently below 32 mm Hg, and pressure-reducing (preventive) when the skin-resting surface interface pressure remained above 32 mm Hg, but less than a standard hospital mattress.

In fact, as it turns out, there has been an excessive degree of reliance on capillary pressure values as an absolute indication of support surface effectiveness. Le et al (1984) points out the following limitations to the reliance on capillary closing values:

- Capillary closing values are based on measurements of the fingertips of young healthy males.
- Lower capillary pressures have been reported in older patients.

- Tissue interface pressures do not ensure that blood flow through the capillaries is unimpeded.
- Pressure is 3 to 5 times greater at the bone than at the surface of the skin.

Interface Pressure Measurement. Interface tissue pressure is the force per unit area that acts perpendicularly between the body and the support surface. Several factors affect interface tissue pressure: (1) the stiffness of the support surface, (2) the composition of the body tissue, and (3) the geometry of the body being supported (WOCN Society, 2003).

In a Cochrane review conducted by Cullum and colleagues (2004), 29 randomized controlled trials (RCTs) were evaluated and it was concluded "that interface pressure measurements have not been demonstrated to reliably predict the clinical performance of support surfaces." However because tissue interface pressure is the method currently being used to evaluate support surfaces and their ability to reduce pressure, it is important to understand how that interface pressure is calculated. Interface pressure is a measurement obtained by placement of a sensor between the skin and the resting surface (Figure 13-1). Thus, when interpreting the significance of reported pressure readings, it is important to consider several factors (Reger et al, 1988):

- The range of pressure readings obtained per site and the number of readings conducted per site should be reported, instead of one single pressure reading per site.

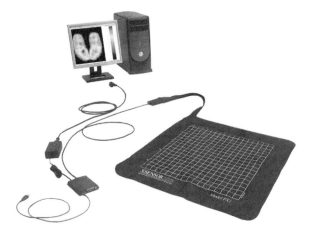

Fig. 13-1 Pressure mapping device. (Xsensor® Pressure Mapping System. Courtesy The ROHO Group, Belleville, IL.)

---

*The terms pressure reduction and pressure relief are outdated and have been replaced by pressure redistribution.

- The procedure used to acquire the pressure reading should be described.
- The population tested should be described (i.e., healthy subjects as opposed to patients with comorbid conditions).
- Researchers should state how often equipment was recalibrated, because sensors are fragile and may malfunction.
- Factors known to affect the results of interface pressure measurements should be disclosed (transducer size and shape, the load shape and its interaction with the support material, the method of equilibrium detection, and the uniformity of the measurement technique).
- Uniformity of the measurement technique is necessary, because the skill of the person taking the readings may also make a difference.

The importance of the shape of the load is exemplified by the fact that a healthy person with normal muscle mass will support and distribute weight more effectively than a debilitated person. As a result, the healthy subject will usually demonstrate lower pressure readings than the debilitated subject.

Skin tissue perfusion, assessed by using heated transcutaneous oxygen ($tcPO_2$) and carbon dioxide ($tcPCO_2$) sensors has also been investigated. Both blood gas use and tissue interface pressure measurement remain limited in their value, and therefore carefully constructed clinical trials are still needed in this area (Rithalia and Kenney, 2001).

Control of Temperature, Moisture, Friction, and Shear

In addition to reducing tissue interface pressure, support surfaces can reduce shear, friction, and moisture; factors that collectively contribute greatly to skin breakdown.

An increase in temperature can be uncomfortable as well as contribute to skin breakdown. The support surface should not make the patient perspire yet should be designed to help maintain normal skin temperature (Brienza and Geyer, 2005). Surfaces with porous cover material through which air can flow will help reduce moisture between the body and support surface (Fleck, 2001). Support surface features that affect moisture and temperature are generally related to the type of medium used and are described later in this chapter.

The support surface cover should allow for low-friction positioning without too much sliding. Many mattress covers are manufactured with a slick surface, such as Gortex, that aid in the reduction of friction and shear. Regardless of support surface, caregivers must provide essential interventions to prevent pressure, friction, and shear such as lifting the patient during repositioning (rather than dragging the patient) and limiting the degree and length of time to which the head of bed is elevated. Additional interventions to reduce these mechanical factors are discussed in Chapters 6 and 12.

CATEGORIES OF SUPPORT SURFACES

Support surfaces are categorized by (1) extent of pressure redistribution, (2) form of the device, (3) power source, (4) redistribution medium, and (5) Medicare reimbursement group (See Box 13-1 and Table 13-1).

Degree of Pressure Redistribution

The extent to which a support surface reduces the tissue interface pressure can be categorized as preventive (pressure is reduced but not consistently below 32 mm Hg) or therapeutic (pressure is consistently reduced to below 32 mm Hg). *Preventive* intervention support surfaces are used for patients at risk for skin breakdown or as part of a treatment plan for a partial thickness ulcer. *Therapeutic* support surfaces are generally intended for patients with advanced wounds such as stages III and IV pressure ulcers (Mackey, 2005).

Form of Device

Numerous forms of support surface devices are available for the patient in the supine position as well as the sitting position. The device may be a supplement to the existing sleep surface, replace the sleep surface, or completely replace the bed frame in addition to the sleep surface.

Chair Cushions. The patient's risk for pressure ulcer development is not limited to the time spent in bed. Pressure also exists (particularly on the ischial tuberosity and calcaneous) while the patient is sitting in a chair. Historically, many devices have been used in the chair in an attempt to reduce pressure and are now known to be deleterious. For example, rings or donut devices are never indicated to reduce pressure, because

BOX 13-1 Categories of Support Surfaces

1. Extent of Pressure Redistribution
- Preventive intervention
- Therapeutic intervention

2. Form of the Device
- Chair Cushions
- Overlay
- Mattress replacement
- Specialty Bed Systems
- Operating Room Pads

3. Power Source
- Powered or dynamic (i.e., low air–loss, alternating pressure)
- Nonpowered or static (i.e., foam mattress and overlays)

4. Redistribution Medium
- Foam
- Water
- Gel
- Air
  Nonpowered (static)
  Cyclical (i.e., alternating pressure)
  Powered Continuous Flow (i.e., Low air–loss)
  Air Fluidized

5. Reimbursement Group
- Group 1
- Group 2
- Group 3

they concentrate the intensity of the pressure to the surrounding tissue (WOCN Society, 2003). Although this chapter predominantly discusses horizontal support surfaces, several of the technologies described in this chapter are available in the form of a chair cushion. Seating surfaces can be customized to allow for pressure reduction as well as sitting stabilization, which will decrease friction and shear forces resulting from involuntary movement in the chair.

Mattress Overlays. Mattress overlays are a category of support surfaces that are placed on top of an existing mattress. Because overlays are applied over an existing mattress, they increase the height of the bed and may complicate patient transfers and alter the fit of linen. Gel, water, and some air-filled overlays are intended for multiple-patient use. By contrast, others are for single-patient use only and present environmental concerns relative to disposal of the product. Storage of the standard hospital bed while a specialty bed is in use may be difficult; an overlay requires less storage space than an entire mattress or bed.

Replacement Mattresses. Replacement mattresses are complete hospital mattresses that are placed on the bed frame in place of the standard mattress. Many facilities have realized improved skin and wound outcomes by purchasing pressure-reducing mattresses to replace standard mattresses for the prevention of pressure ulcers (Cullum et al, 2004; Gray, Cooper and Stringfellow, 2001). Replacement mattresses vary in design as well as function and can be rented or purchased. The types of replacement mattresses available range from prevention products intended for "at-risk" patients to therapeutic dynamic products intended for patients with an existing pressure ulcer.

Specialty Bed Systems. Specialty bed systems are entire bed units that integrate the therapy surface into the bed frame unit and are used in place of a hospital bed. These can be rented or purchased. With the specialty bed system, the features of the frame will have to be evaluated along with the features of the mattress. Frames come in different widths and lengths and will support a specified amount of weight. Some frames have the ability to fold for storage or when transporting a patient. Most frames today are electric, but some alternatives are available. When selecting a frame, consideration should be given to the population served by the product, as well as the setting in which it will be used. Many options are available with frames such as built-in scales and call lights. Frame selection should be based on the needs of the patient population and setting.

Power Source

Support surfaces vary in the power source used to deliver pressure reduction: they are *powered* or *nonpowered,* or static. The nonpowered support surface has the advantage of requiring no electricity and less maintenance time and cost. The support surface that requires power is attached to a simple control panel or a more complicated computer, both of which require a

TABLE 13-1 Medicare B Reimbursement Criteria for Support Surfaces

GROUP	REIMBURSEMENT CRITERIA	PRODUCT EXAMPLES
1 (Preventive Intervention)	Patient meets either of the following two scenarios: Scenario 1 Completely immobile; i.e., patient cannot make changes in body position without assistance OR Scenario 2 Limited mobility or any stage ulcer on the trunk or pelvis and one of the following: • Impaired nutritional status • Fecal or urinary incontinence • Altered sensory perception • Compromised circulatory status	Foam dry overlay or mattress Air overlay or mattress Alternating pressure pad with pump Gel overlay or mattress Water mattress or overlay
2 (Therapeutic Intervention)	Patient meets either of the following 3 scenarios: Scenario 1 Multiple stage II pressure ulcers on the trunk or pelvis and: • A comprehensive ulcer treatment program for at least the past month, which has included the use of an appropriate group 1 support surface. • The ulcers have worsened or remained the same over the past month. Scenario 2 Large or multiple stage III or IV pressure ulcer(s) on the trunk or pelvis. Scenario 3 Recent myocutaneous flap or skin graft for a pressure ulcer on the trunk or pelvis (surgery within the past 60 days). The patient has been on a Group 2 or 3 support surface immediately prior to a recent discharge from a hospital or nursing facility.	Nonpowered advanced air or fluid overlay Powered overlay and mattress Powered alternating pressure mattress Low–air loss mattress
3 (Air-fluidized beds)	Patient meets all of the following criteria: • Stage III or stage IV pressure ulcer • Bedridden or chair-bound as a result of severely limited mobility • In the absence of the air-fluidized bed, the patient would require institutionalization • The air-fluidized bed is ordered in writing by the patient's attending physician based upon a comprehensive assessment and evaluation • A comprehensive ulcer treatment program, including the use of an appropriate group 2 surface, has been in place for at least 1 month with no improvement of the ulcer • A physician directs the treatment regimen on a monthly basis • All other alternative equipment has been considered and ruled out • Moist dressings are protected with an impervious cover • Structure support is adequate for support the weight of the bed • Electrical system is sufficient for the anticipated increase in consumption • Absence of coexisting pulmonary disease • Caregiver is willing and able to provide the type of care required on an air-fluidized bed.	Clinitron fluid air

*Examples are included for reference only and are not intended to be inclusive. Each product must meet specific requirements for reimbursement.
Source: http://www.wocn.org/publications/facts/pdf/medicare_part_b.pdf Accessed August 24, 2005.

motor to operate. Unlike the static support surface, the motor generates some degree of sound. However, powered systems have the advantage of offering additional features such as low air–loss, alternating pressure, and lateral rotation.

Redistribution Medium

Different types of medium are used to reduce or redistribute the tissue interface pressure: foam, water, gel, and air. These mediums can be used alone to create the support surface or in combination with other mediums. The various mediums, along with their unique features, advantages, and disadvantages, are summarized and described here. All support surfaces, regardless of medium, function best with less linen between the patient and the surface.

Foam. Foam support surfaces are lightweight and designed to conform to bony prominences to enhance pressure redistribution and reduce shearing forces. Foam is available (mattresses, cushions, and overlays). Foam can be the sole medium or it can be used in combination with air or gel. One foam product, for example, has sections that can be removed so a gel pad can be inserted. Many foam overlays and cushions are indicated for single-patient use, whereas most foam mattress replacements are intended for multiple-patient use over a limited period specified by warranty (e.g., 2 to 5 years).

The effectiveness of foam products varies greatly according to features such as height, density, indentation deflection, open cells, or closed cells. Base height refers to the height of the foam from the base to where the convolutions begin (Figure 13-2). Density is the weight of the foam per cubic foot. The indentation load deflection (ILD), a measurement of the firmness of the foam, is determined by the number of pounds needed to indent a foam piece to a depth of 25% of the thickness of the foam. This measures compressibility and conformability and indicates the ability of the

foam to distribute mechanical load. Therefore a low ILD about 30 pounds, is preferred. Manufacturer guidelines will state the amount of body weight that the foam product will support and its duration of use.

High-specification foam has been effective in decreasing the incidence of pressure ulcers in fairly high-risk patients including the elderly and patients with fractures of the neck and femur (Cullum et al, 2000). Viscoelastic foam is open-celled and temperature-sensitive. If the temperature of the foam gets close to the same as a person's body, it tends to conform in a manner similar to a gel.

The disadvantage to foam products is their tendency to increase skin temperature as air becomes trapped in the foam cells (Nicholson et al, 1999). The life span is limited because over time and with extended use, foam degrades and loses resilience. When used for long-term pressure reduction, staff or family must examine the product at intervals and replace the foam when it's effectiveness appears reduced. Disposal of foam raises environmental concerns. If the product is not effectively covered, infection control problems can occur as fluids from wounds, incontinence, and perspiration are absorbed into the foam. Additionally, the fire-retardant capability of foam products may be altered if it becomes wet; a key reason why many facilities no longer use foam overlays.

If a foam overlay is used, the following features are recommended for pressure reduction (Krouskop and Garber, 1987; Whittemore, 1998):

- Base height of 3 to 4 inches
- Density of 1.3 to 1.6 pounds per cubic foot
- ILD of about 30 pounds
- Ratio of 60% ILD to 25% ILD of 2.5 or greater

Water. Water-filled overlays and waterbeds have long been used to reduce interface pressure (Siegel, Vistness, and Laub, 1973). Several studies have demonstrated that the waterbed provides significantly lower interface pressure than a hospital mattress (Sloan, Brown, and Larson, 1977; Wells and Geden, 1984). According to Berecek (1975), pressure points are eliminated because the function of the waterbed is based on Pascal's law: "The weight of a body floating on a fluid system is evenly distributed over the entire supporting system."

Waterbeds require electricity for a heater to control the temperature. They are heavy and must be drained

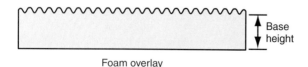

Foam overlay

Fig. 13-2 Measuring the depth of foam overlay.

to move. Water support surfaces have the potential to leak if damaged. Water can become unevenly distributed during head or foot of bed elevation. Procedures such as repositioning, CPR, and transferring can be difficult on a water support surface. Although water-filled devices are popular for the home, their many disadvantages (i.e., leaks, weight, maintenance) make them inappropriate for acute care or long-term care settings.

Gel. Gel products are constructed of Silastic (silicone elastomer), silicone, or polyvinyl chloride (Berecek, 1975) and are available alone or in combination with foam. Gel surfaces are nonpowered, and because they are available in several device forms (cushions and pads, overlays, and mattress replacements), gel products can be used in the bed, chair, exam table, and operating table. Most gel support systems are intended for multiple-patient use. Gel surfaces exhibit a low surface tension and allow for pressure redistribution by conforming to the body, allowing maximum surface contact and equalization of pressure. Because of the consistency of the medium, gels have been found to be effective in the prevention of shear (Fleck, 1997). Gel surfaces are easy to clean and require no electricity. Disadvantages of gel support surfaces are that they tend to be heavy and difficult to repair. They also lack airflow for moisture control and have been reported to increase skin temperature after periods of unrelieved sitting (Brienza and Geyer, 2005).

Air. When air is used as the redistribution medium, it can be nonpowered (such as with an air mattress), powered (e.g., low air–loss mattress), cyclical (such as with an alternating air mattress), or fluidized (such as with a high air–loss bed system).

Nonpowered (Static). Nonpowered (i.e., static) air support surfaces consist of interconnected, single-bladder, longitudinal, or latitudinal cells (Figure 13-3). The static air support surface is available in several forms: cushion or pad, mattress, and overlay. Static air may be the sole redistribution medium or be combined with other mediums; these may be rented or purchased. Most static air support surfaces (not all) are easy to clean and can be reused. Pressure redistribution with an air product requires adequate immersion of the body into the product.

A literature review conducted by Whittemore (1998) reported that numerous investigators have

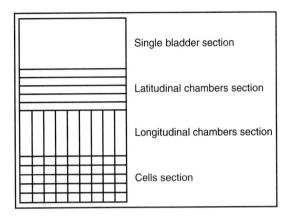

Fig. 13-3 Interconnected, single bladder, longitudinal or latitudinal cells

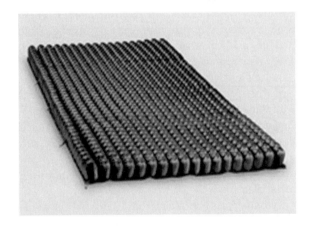

Fig. 13-4 Nonpowered static air support surface; consists of hundreds of individual air cells. (Courtesy the ROHO Group, Belleville, IL.)

examined static air overlays and documented significant lower mean tissue interface pressures as compared with a standard hospital mattress. Static air-filled overlays may be used with moderate- and high-risk patients as long as the product is maintained (WOCN Society, 2003).

One type of nonpowered air overlay consists of hundreds of individual air cells (Figure 13-4). Unlike other static air overlays, this product is appropriate (and reimbursed) as a therapeutic support surface. This surface is adjustable and can be customized to conform to any shape to minimize bottoming out.

Much like gel support surfaces, the consistency of the medium allows for maximum surface contact, equalization of pressure, and low friction and shear. This individual air cell technology is also available in chair cushions and table pads and can be custom-built for a variety of uses (Fleck, 1997). Air-filled overlays may not be effective in preventing pressure ulcers if they are overinflated, underinflated, or punctured. Inflation must be checked daily.

Cyclical (Alternating). *Alternating pressure* (AP) surfaces are powered and available in the form of overlays and mattress replacements. Rather than increasing the surface area through immersion and envelopment, pressure is redistributed by shifting the body weight. Alternating air surfaces have chambers or cylinders arranged in various patterns. Air or fluid is then pumped through the chambers at periodic intervals to inflate or deflate the chambers in opposite phases. These products constantly change pressure points and create pressure gradients that enhance blood flow (McLeod, 1997; Whittemore, 1998).

Alternating pressure mattresses have been associated with lower incidence of pressure ulcers compared with standard mattresses. Products that alternate pressure are believed to improve blood flow to contacted tissues (Hickerson et al, 2000). Moisture control and temperature control with AP products will depend on the characteristics of the cover and supporting material.

Pulsating pressure differs from AP in that the duration of peak inflation is shorter and the cycling time is more frequent. Pulsating pressure appears to help increase lymphatic flow (Gunther and Brofeldt, 1996). Alternating pressure and pulsating pressure can be found in combination with foam and low air–loss products.

Continuous lateral rotation therapy (CLRT) rotates the patient in a regular pattern around a longitudinal (i.e., head to foot) axis of 40 degrees or less to each side. Kinetic therapy is defined as the side-to-side rotation of 40 degrees or more to each side. These therapies have been used for the past 30 years for the prevention and treatment of selected cardiorespiratory conditions. More recently, CLRT has been incorporated into some of the low air–loss support surfaces and hospital replacement mattresses, as well as an air/foam combination mattress, so the patient requiring lateral rotation can also have pressure reduction. Despite the number of published studies on CLRT and its effects on cardiorespiratory conditions, drawing firm conclusions regarding effectiveness with cardiorespiratory is difficult owing to the variety of uncontrolled variables involved. Knowledge of CLRT for pressure-related skin damage is limited. One descriptive study with 30 patients, on CLRT incorporated into a foam mattress replacement, noted no new pressure ulcer development, while trunk and pelvis wounds improved (Anderson and Rappl, 2004). Regardless of bed type, CLRT does not eliminate the need for routine manual repositioning.

Low–air loss. Powered continuous flow support surfaces are low air–loss products, which are available in the form of overlays, mattresses bed systems, and even chair cushions. A low air–loss surface consists of a series of connected air-filled pillows that run across the support surface. The amount of pressure in each pillow is controlled and can be calibrated to the needs of the individual patient, based on height of the person and his or her weight and its distribution. A pump provides airflow in a continuous pattern, since the covering of the mattress is porous, allowing for the leaking of air (Figure 13-5). The pressure reduction is achieved as the patient settles down into the mattress, distributing weight more evenly. There may be an additional surface placed at the base of the product, such as foam or air pillows, when "bottoming out" is problematic.

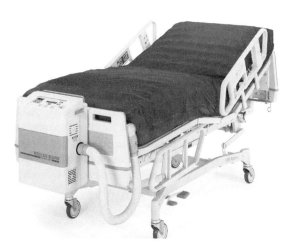

Fig. 13-5 Low air–loss support surface. Flexicair Eclipse Low Airloss Therapy Unit. (Courtesy Hill-Rom Services, Inc.)

The smooth covers for low air–loss surfaces are generally made of nylon or polytetrafluoroethylene fabric and have a low coefficient of friction. The covers are waterproof, impermeable to bacteria, and easy to clean. In order to receive the benefits of low air–loss, only air-permeable pads should be used under the patient so the high-moisture vapor-permeable cover can allow movement of air through the pores of the cover along the surface of the skin. This feature may either prevent maceration or desiccate the wound bed, depending on the amount of moisture and the size, configuration, and number of pores in the cover (Weaver and Jester, 1994). Low air–loss support surfaces have a feature that instantly inflates the cushions to make positioning much easier. In the event that CPR is required, low air–loss support surfaces have a special control that instantly flattens the surface.

Low air–loss beds have been reported as effective treatments and may improve healing rates (Allman et al, 1987; Cullum et al, 2000; Ferrell, Osterweil and Christianson, 1993; Jackson et al, 1988; WOCN Society, 2003). However, these surfaces can be costly, and they require electricity and special pads that cost more than the standard pad. This type of support surface is contraindicated for patients with an unstable spine. Patients on low air–loss surfaces have an increased risk of bed entrapment, especially if the device is not properly adjusted. It is imperative that clinicians and involved staff are familiar with the manufacturer's recommended instructions for use. Once the proper weight setting is established, it would be prudent to record the setting to assure continuity of product use.

Some low air–loss surfaces include pulsation therapy, lateral rotation, and air-fluidized technology. Bennett and colleagues (1998) examined use of a low air–loss hydrotherapy bed with incontinent hospitalized patients. Some patients experienced hypothermia, and staff, patients, and family members expressed some degree of dissatisfaction. Unfortunately, an insufficient number of patients with pressure ulcers were followed long enough to assess the effect on pressure ulcer healing.

Air-fluidized. Air fluidized, or high air–loss beds (Figure 13-6), initially developed to treat persons with burns, consist of a bed frame containing silicone-coated beads and incorporating both air and fluid support (Tallon, 1996). Fluidization of the beads occurs when

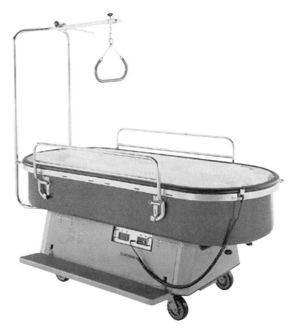

Fig. 13-6 High air–loss support surface. (Courtesy Hill-Rom Services, Inc.)

air is pumped through the beads, making them behave like a liquid. The person "floats" on a sheet with one third of the body above the surface and the rest of the body immersed in the warm, dry, fluidized beads (Holzapfel, 1993). High air–loss beds allow body fluids to flow freely through the sheet. This must be pressurized at all times to prevent contamination (Peltier, Poppe, and Twomey, 1987). When the air-fluidized bed is turned off, it quickly becomes firm enough for cardiopulmonary resuscitation or for repositioning the patient for dressing changes.

Air-fluidized beds are recommended for patients with burns, myocutaneous skin flaps and multiple stage III or stage IV pressure ulcers. They may be used to rewarm a person with hypothermia, since they can quickly narrow the gap between the core and peripheral temperatures, thus reducing vasoconstriction and improving peripheral circulation. This may reduce shivering and the subsequently increased oxygen demand. Patients with severe, debilitating pain are often more comfortable on this bed because of its "cocooning" effect. Furthermore, appetite is reported to improve with air-fluidized therapy, which may correlate with the pain control provided by the bed (Jackson et al, 1988).

Although evidence indicates that air-fluidized beds enhance pressure ulcer healing rates, occipital and calcaneous tissue interface pressures may remain sufficient to occlude capillary perfusion. Occipital and calcaneous ulcers have been reported to develop in patients while on the air-fluidized bed surface (Parish and Witkowski, 1980). Ochs and colleagues (2005), using a subset of retrospectively collected National Pressure Ulcer Long-Term Care Study data, compared pressure ulcer outcomes of 664 residents placed on several types of support surfaces including air fluidized, low air–loss, powered and nonpowered overlays, and hospital replacement mattresses. Results indicated that residents placed on air-fluidized support surfaces had larger and deeper pressure ulcers and higher illness severity scores than residents placed on the other support surfaces. However, residents using air-fluidized surfaces had better healing rates, fewer emergency visits, and fewer hospital admissions. Findings, although significant, warrant more research to control variables such as initial wound size, use of dressing, debridement, nutritional status and presence of infection and incontinence.

In the institutional environment, these products are not ideally suited to facility ownership because of the complexity and the high costs of maintenance. Air-fluidized products are generally the most expensive rental product in the specialty bed category. Because air-fluidized beds are heavy, they may not be safe for use in older homes. Air-fluidized beds are not recommended for ambulatory patients, or the patient with pulmonary disease or unstable spine. Negative factors associated with use of air-fluidized therapy include calcium loss from long bones owing to the weightless environment, disorientation of the individual on the surface, as well as similar drying issues noted in the low air–loss surfaces. Air-fluidized products have a warming feature for the pressurized air, which can be comforting or harmful depending on the overall condition of the patient.

Air-fluidized therapy in the lower half of the bed has been combined with low air-loss in the upper portion of the surface to create the bed that is adjustable for the patient who needs to be more upright. This bed is similar in size to a hospital bed, the head is readily adjustable, and it is lighter than a total air-fluidized system.

PRODUCT SELECTION

Selecting specialty surfaces for an institution or agency presents many challenges. Generally, one product alone is not sufficient for any institution, and a range of products is required. Table 13-2 lists several factors that should guide the development of a formulary of support surfaces for the institution or agency. However, once a decision is made, attention must turn to educating the staff as to appropriate use of the products.

Guidelines for selecting a support surface for a specific patient are also necessary to facilitate appropriate staff decision making and proper product use (Jay, 1997; Tallon, 1996; Whittemore, 1998). Unfortunately there is a paucity of research to guide decision making or to compare product effectiveness. Therefore, product selection will depend on desired functions, the product's indications, contraindications, advantages and disadvantages, and the payer source. Ultimately, the patient's clinical condition must be analyzed; the particular product selected should meet the patient's needs (Dukich and O'Connor, 2001). Table 13-3 lists several factors to consider when selecting a support surface for an individual patient.

Bariatric Options

Offloading for the obese patient is critical to provide, yet extremely difficult to achieve in a manner that is safe for the patient as well as the staff. Furthermore, the size of the routine hospital bed precludes the ability of the obese patient to effectively reposition for any period of time. Unfortunately, once a pressure ulcer develops in this type of patient, healing is even more complicated because of the location of the wound, the presence of skin folds, and the decreased vascularity of adipose tissue. As a result, pressure prevention in this patient population has received a surge of attention. Bariatric support surfaces are available in foam, air, gel and water with features such as low-friction covers and moisture dissipation and others discussed in this chapter. Care of the obese patient as well as specific benefits related to bariatric beds are presented in Chapter 14 and Table 14-1.

Reimbursement

Finally, payers reimburse support surfaces according to specific criteria. Table 13-1 provides the Medicare

TABLE 13-2 Factors Guiding Support Surface Selection for an Institution or Agency

	FACTORS	EXAMPLES
1.	Typical needs of patient population	A rehabilitation setting will require a support surface that allows the patient to gradually decrease dependence on others and utilize a variety of transfer methods.
2.	Continuum of support surfaces	A variety of surfaces should be accessible to assure the patient can be moved from one type of product to another as their condition and needs changes.
3.	Procedures performed within the institution	Settings where many grafts or flaps are performed will need access to specialty beds and appropriate "stepdown" support surfaces. Duration and type of surgical procedures are becoming increasingly recognized as factors contributing to pressure ulcer formation and require support surfaces for the OR and exam rooms.
4.	Cost of the support surface	Some devices are available on a rental basis, whereas others have a one-time fee. The cost of the device should be considered with the length of time the product will be used, goals for use, and length of product efficacy.
5.	Indirect costs	Time commitment of the staff to use the product must be considered as well as labor required for set up, maintenance and cleaning. The ease with which the product can be used and maintained is important to minimize staff time required to not only use the device but to learn how to use the device.
6.	Electrical costs	The number of units in service can increase utility costs and should be considered.
7.	Company performance and service	Services such as setup, maintenance, storage, and disposal may be provided. The company's shipping and delivery policy and guarantee should be reviewed. Some companies provide in-service programs for the staff. A trial of the product may be possible and practical.
8.	Regulatory issues	The company should provide documentation of essential regulatory approvals such as UL Listing and ISO 9001 conformity by manufacturer.

TABLE 13-3 Factors Guiding Support Surface Selection for an Individual Patient

FACTORS	EXAMPLES
Wound extent and location	Therapeutic support surface is indicated for the patient with stages III or IV pressure ulcers or ulcers that involve multiple turning surfaces.
Mobility/activity	Repositioning by the patient or staff is feasible. Independent functioning by the patient remains possible
Comfort	Powered surfaces produce noise, which may be intolerable for some patients Patient must be comfortable and able to sleep on the support surface Product may produce heat and make patient too warm
Body size	Patient's weight does not exceed maximum weight for the support surface The obese patient requires a bariatric support surface On select surfaces, the patient with a thin body build may have higher tissue interface pressures

Part B reimbursement criteria for support surfaces. Reimbursement criteria change as technology and knowledge about support surfaces and wounds evolve. It is important to contact insurance companies, health maintenance organizations (HMOs), Medicaid, and Medicare for the most up-to-date information. Payer sources can change as the patient moves through the continuum of care, and it is critical that the clinician work with the appropriate liaisons and provide documentation stating the rationale for product selections.

SAFETY

Use of adult specialty beds in the rotation mode is ineffective for small children because their small bodies are confined to one section or pillow of the surface. (McCord et al, 2004). Low air–loss beds are designed for adults and do not provide options to accommodate the height and weight of small children. Children and infants can sink into and between cushions (McLane et al, 2004).

Product service requirements should be detailed in the manual along with life expectancy and what to do if problems arise. Staff education is critical to ensure safety and correct use (setup and maintenance) so the device's effectiveness is not jeopardized. Staff education should be provided to housekeeping, safety, maintenance, infection control, code team, staff nurses, and the wound care staff.

Most products have a correct and incorrect method for setup that will greatly affect their pressure redistribution capabilities. For example, some support surface products have different materials under the head and the foot sections; therefore the surface must be placed in the correct position on the bed frame. Other support surface devices must be adjusted according to the patient's size and weight.

Many devices, such as the low air–loss surfaces, are equipped with a feature to rapidly deflate the bed for CPR. Any surface that raises the patient higher in the bed or creates more distance between the resting surface and the bed frame and side rails increases the risk for entrapment and falls. When the support surface increases the risk of entrapment or falls, additional monitoring will be necessary. When possible, the support surface that minimizes height and gaps should be selected.

The surface must not ignite easily or promote bacterial growth. Mattress covers should be flame-resistant, impermeable to bacteria, and durable enough to prevent any damage that will allow bacteria to enter inside. It is essential to consult the manufacturer's instructions for proper cleaning and maintenance and other instructions for use. Some support surfaces will not maintain infection control standards if used with more than one patient. Others have removable components within the mattress for individualized pressure redistribution that may be beneficial to one patient but harmful to another if not replaced or placed properly. In addition, if the components are not handled correctly, bacteria can be transferred as the components are moved around.

RENTING VERSUS OWNING

For many facilities, renting support surfaces is the best option. Renting enables access to the most current technology free of any concerns about the need to update equipment. Renting support surfaces places the responsibility of maintenance and much of the liability for malfunctioning equipment with the rental company. Companies that rent equipment generally provide inservices to educate the staff on safety issues and proper use of the equipment.

Costs may be as variable as the technology, ranging from as little as a few dollars to roughly $150.00 per day in rental costs. Some health care companies negotiate individual contracts with manufacturers, based on volume of product used. However, with the introduction of PPS (Prospective Payment System) some businesses have decided to look at the efficacy of owning surfaces, rather than continuing to pay rental fees.

When purchasing a product, it is important to note the warranty, the manufacturer's guidelines for weight limits, and instructions for use, maintenance, and cleaning. Some warranties allow for full mattress replacement as indicated over a specified time frame. Others are prorated and allow for the full replacement cost initially; however, as the product ages over time, the amount of this reimbursement decreases. Maintenance of support surfaces varies with the type of design, composition, and technology. For example, some support surfaces have heel zones or head zones and must be placed on the bed frame in a specific direction. Others have to be turned (or flipped) regularly to maintain efficacy, and checked for wear, proper inflation, and resilience. Other important features include a water-repellent, antimicrobial top cover, a flame-retardant feature, and a waterproof, antibacterial bottom cover.

All purchased items should be marked with the month and year of delivery, preferably with indelible ink and in a consistent location. The designated department should keep a corresponding list so maintenance work and warranty claims can be handled efficiently. Unfortunately, this is an area that has been greatly ignored, with many facilities unaware of the age and condition of their frames and surfaces.

If a complete bed system or frame is purchased, it is important to note that some frames are not designed to accommodate the mattress manufactured by a competing company. Clearly this will restrict the options for that facility's support surface formulary.

EVALUATION OF EFFECTIVENESS

Once a product is selected, its effectiveness for any given patient must be reevaluated at regular intervals. The same factors that guide support surface selection for an individual should also guide the decision to discontinue or change a support surface. For example, when a support surface is initiated because of the presence of erythema over a bony prominence, the site should be monitored to ensure that the extent or intensity of the erythema is not increasing and, ideally, is decreasing.

An evaluation of the effectiveness of the facility's support surface formulary should include a review of the advantages and disadvantages for the patient population served as well as the needs of the staff. Ideally, the advantages should far outweigh the disadvantages. Factors that should be addressed during an evaluation of a support surface are listed in Box 13-2.

SUMMARY

Well-designed clinical research on the effectiveness of various support surface devices is needed. Ideally, clinical trials should measure the effects of the particular support surface on outcomes such as incidence, comfort, cost, and satisfaction. Small sample sizes may increase the risk of "false-positives" (i.e., lead to the conclusion that a product makes a significant difference when it does not). In addition, the sample size

---

BOX 13-2 Queries for Evaluating Support Surface Effectiveness

Patient Factors

- Has there been a decrease in factors that place a patient at risk for pressure ulcers?
- Has mobility become impaired because of the support surface?
- Is the patient comfortable?
- Can the patient sleep?
- Does the patient bottom out after the bed is properly adjusted?
- Is the wound improving?

Facility Factors

- Do accessible, standardized, or contracted support surfaces include enough variety of methods to meet the changing needs of all patients?
- Do the support surfaces meet the needs of the facility in the most cost-effective way possible after all costs (direct and indirect) are calculated?
- Is the staff competent with set up, maintenance, and cleaning?
- Do patients express overall satisfaction with the products?
- Does staff express overall satisfaction with the products?
- Is there an increase in entrapment, back injuries, or falls?
- Does product live up to claims?
- Does company live up to promises for support and value added services?
- Do the products conform with essential regulations?

---

should be the appropriate size to allow for the most relevant and meaningful type of statistical analysis.

It is the responsibility of care providers involved in product selection to maintain up-to-date knowledge regarding factors relevant to support surface selection. The prudent wound care practitioner must be familiar with the operation, indications, and contraindications of the specialty support surface products in the facility, the agency, or patient's home.

SELF-ASSESSMENT EXERCISE

1. List the forms of support surfaces devices.
2. List four functions of a support surface.
3. All nonpowered support surfaces for the bed are for prevention only: true or false?
4. Describe three limitations to using capillary closing values to evaluate the effectiveness of a support surface.
5. Discuss four factors that guide the interpretation of the significance of interface tissue pressure readings.
6. Once a patient is placed on a support surface, he or she should remain on that surface until the wound has closed: true or false?

REFERENCES

Allman RM et al: Air-fluidized beds or conventional therapy for pressure sores, *Ann Intern Med* 107:641, 1987.

Anderson C, Rappl L: Lateral rotation mattresses for wound healing, *Ostomy Wound Manage* 50(4): 50–62, 2004.

Bennett RG et al: Low airloss hydrotherapy versus standard care for incontinent hospitalized patients, *J Am Geriatr Soc* 45:569, 1998.

Berecek KH: Treatment of decubitus ulcers, *Nurs Clin North Am* 10(1):171-210, 1975.

Brienza DM, Geyer MJ: Using support surfaces to manage tissue integrity, *Adv Skin Wound Care* 18(3):151-157, 2005.

Cullum N et al: Systematic reviews of wound care management: (5) beds; (6) compression; (7) laser therapy, therapeutic ultrasound, electrotherapy and electromagnetic therapy, *Health Technology Assessment* 5(9):1-237, 2000.

Cullum N et al: *Beds, mattresses and cushions for pressure sore prevention and treatment* (Cochrane Review), The Cochrane Library, No. 2, Chichester, UK, 2004, John Wiley and Sons.

Dukich J, O'Connor D: Impact of practice guidelines on support surface selection, incidence of pressure ulcers and fiscal dollars, *Ostomy Wound Management* 47(3):44-53, 2001.

Ferrell BA, Osterweil D, Christenson P: A randomized trial of low-air-loss beds for treatment of pressure ulcers, *JAMA*, 269(4):494, 1993.

Fleck CA: Support Surfaces: criteria and selection. In Krasner DL, Rodeheaver GT, editors: *Chronic Wound Care*, ed 2, Wayne, Penn, 1997, Health Management Publications 116-21, 1996.

Gray D, Cooper PJ, Stringfellow, S: Evaluating pressure-reducing foam mattresses and electric bed frames, *Br J Nurs* 10(Suppl 22):s23, 2001.

Gunther R, Brofeldt B. Increased lymphatic flow: effect of a pulsating air suspension bed system. *Wounds*, 8:134–40, 1996.

Hickerson WL et al: Comparison of total body tissue interface pressure of specialized pressure relieving mattresses, *Wound Rep Regen* 8(4):325, 2000.

Holzapfel SK: Support surfaces and their use in the prevention and treatment of pressure ulcers, *J ET Nurs* 20(6):251, 1993.

Jackson BS et al: The effects of a therapeutic bed on pressure ulcers: an experimental study, *J Enterostom Ther* 15:220, 1988.

Jay R: Other considerations in selecting a support surface, *Adv Wound Care* 10(7):37, 1997.

Krouskop TA, Garber SL: The role of technology in the prevention of pressure sores, *Ostomy Wound Manage* 16:45, 1987.

Le KM et al: An in-depth look at pressure sores using monolithic silicon pressure sensors, *Plast Reconstr Surg* 74(6):745, 1984.

Mackey D: Support surfaces: beds, mattresses, overlays-oh my! *Nurs Clin North Am*, 40(2):251-265, 2005.

McCord S, McElvain V, Sachdeva R, Schwartz P, Jefferson LS. Risk factors associated with pressure ulcers in the pediatric intensive care unit. *J Wound Ostomy Continence Nurs.* Jul-Aug;31(4):179-183, 2004.

McLane KM, Bookout K, McCord S, McCain J, Jefferson LS. The 2003 national pediatric pressure ulcer and skin breakdown prevalence survey: a multisite study. *J Wound Ostomy Continence Nurs.* Jul-Aug;31(4):168-178, 2004.

McLeod R: Other considerations in selecting a good support surface, *Adv Wound Care* 10(7):37, 1997.

Nicholson GP et al: A method for determining the heat transfer and water vapour permeability of patient support systems, *Med Eng Phys* 21(10):701, 1999.

Ochs RF et al: Comparison of air-fluidized therapy with other support surfaces used to treat pressure ulcers in nursing home residents, *Ostomy Wound Manage* 51(2):38, 2005.

Parish LC, Witkowski JA: Clinitron therapy and the decubitus ulcer: preliminary dermatologic studies, *Dermatology* 19:517, 1980.

Peltier GL, Poppe SR, Twomey JA: Controlled air suspension: an advantage in burn care, *J Burn Care Rehabil* 8(6):558, 1987.

Reger, SI et al: Correlation of transducer systems for monitoring tissue interface pressures, *J Clin Engineer* 13(5):365, 1988.

Rithalia S, Kenney L: The art and science of evaluating patient support surfaces, http://www.worldwidewounds.com/2001/september, Accessed on August 20, 2005.

Siegel RJ, Vistness LM, Laub DR: Use of waterbed for prevention of pressure sores, *Plast Reconstr Surg* 51:81, 1973.

Sloan DR, Brown RD, Larson DL: Evaluation of a simplified water mattress in the prevention and treatment of pressure sores, *Plast Reconstr Surg* 60(4):5961, 1977.

Tallon RW: Support surfaces: therapeutic and performance insights, *Nurs Manage* 27(9):57, 1996.

Wells P, Geden E: Paraplegic body-support pressure on convoluted foam, waterbed, and standard mattresses, *Res Nurs Health* 7:127, 1984.

Weaver V, Jester J: A clinical tool: updated readings on tissue interface pressures, *Ostomy Wound Manage* 40(5):34, 38, 1994.

Whittemore R: Pressure-reduction support surfaces: a review of the literature, *J WOCN* 25:6, 1998.

WOCN Society: *Guideline for management of pressure ulcers*, WOCN Clinical Practice Guideline Series #2, Glenview, Ill, 2003, Author.

14 *Skin Care Needs of the Obese Patient*

SUSAN GALLAGHER CAMDEN

OBJECTIVES

1. Define obesity.
2. Describe necessary accommodations in the physical environment for the obese patient.
3. Identify risk factors for three common skin complications in the obese patient population.
4. Discuss two common pulmonary complications in the obese patient population.

Health care problems associated with obesity include diabetes, hypertension, soft tissue infection, some cancers, impaired circulation, and others, each of which interferes with the patient's level of health, in general, and skin care, specifically. These comorbidities affect the morbidly obese patient disproportionately, and at younger age. Many authors contend that from the onset, the obese patient is at a disadvantage because diagnosis is difficult and procedures are technically more complicated (Kral, Strauss, and Wise, 2000). Many hospitals report concerns because of inadequate equipment and personnel to accommodate the needs of larger patients (Kramer and Gallagher, 2004). However, recent advances in information, intervention, equipment, and education have helped reduce some of these risks (Gallagher et al, 2004a).

The skin, which is the largest organ of the body, is at particular risk for injury in the health care setting, especially in the presence of obesity. The changing demographics of obesity and factors that place the patient at risk are presented in this chapter. Prevention of common and predictable skin breakdown is discussed. Early assessment and intervention of skin injury is reviewed, along with the value of an interdisciplinary approach. Preplanning activities including a bariatric task force, criteria-based protocol, basic competency

development, and outcomes are discussed. Barriers to change are reviewed.

DEFINING OBESITY

Obesity is defined as a body mass index (BMI) of 30 or greater; morbid obesity is defined as a body mass index greater than 40. (See Box 14-1.)

Bariatrics is a term derived from the Greek word *baros* and refers to the practice of health care relating to the treatment of obesity and associated conditions (Gallagher, 2004b). The American Society for Bariatric Surgery (2001) defines obesity as a lifelong, progressive, life-threatening, genetically related, multifactorial disease of excess fat storage with multiple comorbidities. Others describe obesity as simply the excessive accumulation of body fat, which manifests as slow, steady, progressive increase in body weight. In one sense the cause of obesity is straightforward—the state of expending less energy that the amount consumed. But in another sense, the etiologies of obesity are intangible, involving the complex individual regulation of body weight—specifically, body fat. This individual regulation is the unknown factor in weight management (Knudsen and Gallagher, 2003). Regardless, according to the National Institutes of Health, obesity is simply a diagnostic category that represents a complex and multifactorial disease (Kuczmarski et al, 1994).

BOX 14-1 Body Mass Index Categories

Underweight = less than 18.5
Normal weight = 18.5 to 24.9
Overweight = 25 to 29.9
Obesity = 30 or more

Source: National Heart, Lung, and Blood Institute, Bethesda, MD.

CHANGING DEMOGRAPHICS

Sixty-seven percent of Americans are overweight, 10% to 25% are considered obese, and 3% to 10% are morbidly obese (Gallagher, 2003). Morbid obesity, once a very rare occurrence in America, has quadrupled since the 1980s to 6 million. Studies suggest a substantial increase in obesity among all age, ethnic, racial, and socioeconomic groups (Lanz et al, 1998). In the early 1960s, only a quarter of Americans were overweight, today over two thirds of this country's adults are overweight, as are 25% of its children.

Obesity has an economic, physical, and emotional impact on our patients. Americans spend close to $117 billion on obesity-related health problems, and $33 billion are spent annually in attempts to control or lose weight. Despite efforts at weight loss, Americans continue to gain weight, with obesity reaching epidemic proportions. Obesity is a factor in 5 of the 10 leading causes of death (Knudsen and Gallagher, 2003), and is considered the second most common cause of preventable death in the United States (Fox, 1995). In addition to the physiologic costs, some authors argue that obesity is associated with emotional conditions such as situational depression, altered self-esteem, and social isolation (Charles, 1987). On the other hand, others argue that it is society's response to the obese person that leads to these emotional conditions, which includes prejudice and discrimination (Gallagher et al, 2004b).

STEREOTYPES ABOUT OBESITY

Obese Americans chose neither to be overweight nor to experience widespread prejudice and discrimination (Gustafson, 1997). Failure to provide just, fair intervention is often based on inadequate policies and procedures that are, in turn, justified by blaming the patient for conditions that are simply the result of his or her body weight. This attitude creates a barrier to change. Health care clinicians need to ensure a safe haven from obesity-related prejudice and discrimination, which often stems from misunderstanding as to the etiologies of obesity (Gallagher, 1997). Although related, the terms prejudice and discrimination hold very different meanings. Prejudice is described as a prejudgment, and most health care providers carry some form of prejudgment toward a particular category of patient. On the other hand, discrimination refers to action based on this prejudgment (Gallagher, 2004e). Overweight Americans

experience both. Prejudice against obese people is observed at a very young age. For example, children as young as 6 years old describe silhouettes of obese children as lazy, stupid, and ugly. According to this study, prejudice toward the obese child is observed regardless of race or socioeconomic status (Staffieri, 1967). Children are not the only ones who hold a prejudice against the overweight person; health care clinicians are also often biased against the larger patient (Thone, 1997). It is even observed among obese persons themselves (Maiman et al, 1992). In a culture that worships thinness, obese patients experience discrimination in schools, the workplace, and health care settings (Faulcbaum and Choban, 1998).

The problem is that from a historic perspective, obesity has been perceived as a problem of self-discipline. However, recent discoveries suggest that this is far from the truth. There is no debate that weight gain occurs when intake, meaning food intake, exceeds output, meaning activity—but the real mystery behind balancing body weight depends on a number of other factors. Genetics, gender, physiology, biochemistry, neuroscience, as well as cultural, environmental, and psychosocial factors influence weight and its regulation (Torpey, 2003). Health care clinicians best serve their patients when they recognize obesity as the chronic, multifactorial condition that it is.

The problem with prejudice and discrimination is that they pose barriers to care regardless of practice setting or professional discipline. The overwhelming misunderstanding of obesity is likely to interfere with preplanning efforts, access to services, and resource allocation. Although this misunderstanding is not universal, it is pervasive enough to pose obstacles, and clinicians interested in making changes will need to recognize these barriers.

COMMON SKIN COMPLICATIONS IN THE OBESE POPULATION

Pressure Ulcers

Pressure ulcers are the result of pressure, friction, and shear. Other contributing factors include moisture, dehydration, and malnutrition; however, immobility is at the heart of pressure ulcer formation. Pressure ulcers typically occur over a bony prominence and develop because of the inability to adequately reposition the patient—this is particularly true among very heavy patients. In addition, obese patients can be at risk for atypical or unusual pressure ulcers, which can result from pressure within skin folds, from tubes or catheters, or from an ill-fitting chair or wheelchair.

Pressure within skin folds can be sufficient to cause skin breakdown (Plate 33). Tubes and catheters burrow into skin folds, which can further erode the skin surface. Pressure from side rails and armrests not designed to accommodate a larger person can cause pressure ulcers on the patient's hips. One way this atypical skin breakdown can be minimized is by using properly sized equipment. In addition, the patient needs to be repositioned at least every 2 hours, as do tubes and catheters. Tubes should be placed so that the patient does not rest on them. Tube and catheter holders may be helpful in this step. In the event that the patient has a large abdominal panniculus, it too must be repositioned to prevent pressure injury beneath the panniculus. Patients who are alert are able to physically lift the pannus off of the suprapubic area. If clinically appropriate, the dependent, weak, or unconscious patient can be placed in the side-lying position, and the pannus lifted away from the underlying skin surface, allowing air flow to the regions and pressure redistribution.

Bariatric beds with pressure redistribution mattresses reduce the risk of pressure ulcers, promote patient independence, improve clinical outcomes, decrease staff workload and help control unnecessary costs (Mathison, 2003). Much like other support surfaces, bariatric support surfaces are available in foam, air, gel and water features such as low-friction covers and moisture dissipation which are discussed in detail in Chapter 13. Specific benefits related to bariatric bed features for the patient, staff and facility are presented in Table 14-1 (Kramer and Gallagher, 2004). Use of a support surface with lateral rotation therapy is often regarded as the standard of care for certain pulmonary situations; however, it can also serve to ensure sufficient repositioning for a very large patient, whose need for frequent turning may otherwise pose a realistic challenge. Despite the value of rotation therapy in prevention and treatment of skin injury among obese patients, it is still necessary to take precautions to prevent friction and shear. Correct pressure settings, fitting the patient to the appropriately sized surface, and assessment for skin changes can meet these precautions (Gallagher, 2002).

Candidiasis

The increased prevalence of diabetes mellitus among obese patients places them at risk for candidiasis, since diabetes is a major risk factor. *Candida albicans* is a yeast-like fungus that thrives in a dark, moist environment, such as within skin folds. These organisms are principally found among mammals, and are inhabitants of the mouth, gastrointestinal tract, and vagina. There are over 80 species of *Candida*. Most human infections are from *C. albicans* or *C. tropicalis*. In fact, *C. albicans* is one of the most, if not the most, common perpetrator of human disease. In addition to diabetes mellitus, factors that contribute to candidiasis include immunocompromised states, infection, chronic steroid and antibiotic use, hyperhidrosis, and obesity. Many obese patients report chronic candidal involvement. Yeast generally affects an intertriginous area, which are areas where skin contacts skin. When an individual is hospitalized, moisture from urine, perspiration, or wound drainage exacerbates this chronic but otherwise mild condition. Clinically, candidiasis is characterized by scaling erythema and small pustules that appear as macules when unroofed. Patients often complain of itching or burning. If the condition progresses without intervention, it can lead to fissuring and maceration. In the face of associated pruritus, patients may scratch the skin surface, further compromising skin integrity. This can lead to a secondary bacterial invasion.

Candidiasis is manageable in a number of ways. The first is to eliminate excessive moisture to the skin surface. Locally, an antifungal powder can be applied after the skin is cleaned and dried. For a dry, flaking surface, an antifungal cream can be helpful. See Chapter 6 for more information related to candidiasis.

Chemical Dermatitis due to Incontinence

Moisture and chemical irritants are risk factors for skin breakdown; therefore incontinence can threaten skin integrity. Predisposing factors for urinary incontinence include gender, genetics, race, culture, neurology, anatomy, and collagen status. Urinary incontinence is greater in women for all age groups. Increased BMI has been presented as a risk factor for developing incontinence and as an explanation for failed therapy. For example, studies independent of age suggest a direct correlation between increased BMI and urinary

TABLE 14-1 The Benefits of Bariatric Beds Features for Patient, Care Staff, and Facility

FEATURE	PATIENT BENEFIT	STAFF BENEFIT	COST BENEFIT/RISK REDUCTION
600- to 1000-lb capacity	• Safely supports weight • Eliminates fear of the bed breaking	Reduced risk of injury during cares	• Reduces risk of patient injury (and possible litigation) if bed breaks • Reduces risk of workman's compensation injury
Integrated scale	• Safer, more dignified and less time consuming than loading docks • More accurate than portable under mattress scales	• Saves time • More accurate	Reduces risk of inappropriate treatment resulting from inaccurate weights
Expandable surface width	Enhances patient participation by allowing room for proper repositioning to prevent skin breakdown	Bed width is a safe distance to prevent back injuries from over reaching	• Reduces risk of workman's compensation injury • Reduces risk for nosocomial pressure ulcer development • Reduces risk for litigation and citations from regulating agencies for nosocomial pressure ulcers
Trendelenburg/ Reverse Trendelenburg	Decreases friction on back when "boosting"	Helps with gravity-assisted "boosting" for fewer lifting injuries	Reduces risk of workman's compensation injury
Cardiochair	Increases mobility decreases cardiac and pulmonary decompostion, leading to faster recovery	Helps patient mobility, decreases staff lifting, and transfers	• Reduces risk of workman's compensation injury • Reduces length of stay by decreasing the effects of immobility • Reduces risk of workman's compensation injury
Trapeze	Increases mobility and independence, decreases friction on skin	Decreases staff lifting, decreasing staff injury	• Reduces length of stay by decreasing the effects of immobility • Reduces risk for nosocomial pressure ulcer development • Reduces risk for litigation and citations from regulating agencies for nosocomial pressure ulcers
Supportive mattress	Prevents skin breakdown from pressure, friction, and moisture	Eases transfers and turning of patients	• Reduces risk of workman's compensation injury • Reduces length of stay by decreasing the effects of immobility • Reduces risk for nosocomial pressure ulcer development • Reduces risk for litigation and citations from regulating agencies for nosocomial pressure ulcers • Immobility

Modified from Kramer K, Gallagher S: WOC nurses as advocates for patients who are morbidly obese: A case study promoting use of bariatric beds, *JWOCN* 31(1):276, 2004.

incontinence (Engel, Burgio, and Matthews, 1991). Sleep apnea, a condition associated with obesity, can lead to decreases in oxygen tension and to relative central nervous system hypoxia. Both of these clinical conditions cause increased excitability of autonomic neurons. Urgency, urge incontinence, and enuresis can be improved with continuous positive pressure ventilation (Steers and Suratt, 1997).

Many otherwise continent persons develop short-term incontinence when physically dependent in health care settings. This may occur because of medication, delays in locating a caregiver to place the patient on the bedpan, or simply because the patient can't reach a commode in time to prevent an incontinent episode. Also, patients are frequently reluctant to ask for assistance with hygiene. Patients need to be reminded that the goal of health care providers is to serve their needs. Maintaining clean, dry skin is the objective, and if the patient needs assistance in this effort, caregivers are available to help.

After each incontinent episode, clean the entire affected area with an incontinence cleanser, and then rinse and dry it. Patients report that drying the buttocks, perineal area, and between folds with an institutionally-approved blow dryer on the cool setting is more comfortable than towel drying. This technique may be less traumatic to the outermost layer of skin. Failure to provide clinicians with properly fitting gloves could serve as a barrier to adequate cleansing. Most organizations have access to elbow length gloves—a product specialist can locate this resource.

If skin breakdown occurs despite preventive efforts, an aggressive plan of care is indicated. A moisture barrier ointment can serve as a protective barrier to chemicals in urine or stool. Few moisture barrier ointments adhere to weeping or moist areas of superficial breakdown. A light coat of protective (i.e., skin barrier) powder applied to the moist areas may increase adherence of the moisture barrier ointment, thus more completely protecting the skin surface from the irritating chemicals found in stool and urine. If these are ineffective, a skin barrier paste should be considered. Food and Drug Administration–approved fecal containment devices may also be considered and are discussed in Chapter 6.

Foot Pain

Because the feet carry a person's entire weight, heavier individuals are prone to wear-and-tear injuries, since some activities can create loads on the feet as large as 4 times the body's weight. Patients should be reminded that foot pain could signal other serious medical conditions such as arthritis, nerve and circulatory disorders, and diabetes.

Foot care, especially among the obese population, can require special attention. Persons receiving outpatient wound care may find issues as simple as transportation challenging, and once the patient arrives in the outpatient setting, the physical environment may serve as a deterrent to care. Consider accommodations in the physical environment that promote patient safety and comfort. (See Box 14-2.)

A podiatry consultation can be essential to the care of the obese patient with foot pain. When the joints of the feet are involved, medication, physical therapy, exercise, orthotics, braces, specially designed shoes, and surgery are among the tools used to relieve pain and restore feet to as near normal function as possible (Medical Network, 2004).

THE SURGICAL EXPERIENCE

The surgical experience predisposes the patient to skin injury, since surgery may increase the patient's length of stay and dependency or immobility because of pain, sedation, or the fear of falling. Although the patient

---

BOX 14-2 Accommodations in the Physical Environment for the Obese Patient

Large blood pressure cuff
Long needles
Larger tracheostomy ties
Longer abdominal binders
Large gowns/drapes
Elbow-length gloves for incontinence clean-up
Beds wide enough for effective repositioning
Support surfaces
Overhead trapeze to facilitate repositioning
Bariatric lifts for moving the patient safely
Bedside commode (appropriate size)
Wide wheelchair with pressure-reducing cushion
Walker with proper support
Size-friendly art and magazines
Larger clinic exam tables anchored to the floor with adequate step
Sturdy, armless chairs for clinic waiting rooms

may be awake and alert shortly after surgery, extra personnel and supportive equipment are required to transfer the patient, taking care not to create shearing injury or place undue stress on incisions (Gallagher, 2004d). Patients can experience complications, such as pressure ulcers or respiratory complications, because of immobility and physical dependence (Gallagher, 1998). Early activity is encouraged because this decreases the chances of immobility-related complications (Gallagher, 2005). Some patients will fail to progress postoperatively, either because of surgical complications or a critical condition. Unless the patient can be mobilized in critical care, deconditioning can occur very rapidly, thus increasing the risk for skin and wound-related complications. A physical therapy consultation within 24 hours of an intensive care unit admission may be valuable to (1) evaluate for and demonstrate immobility-related equipment, and (2) offer passive and active exercises aimed at reducing problems associated with deconditioning.

Larger patients require closer observation because of comorbid conditions, and sometimes because of failed postoperative extubation or intraoperative complications, and could require intensive care. Like all patients, this population requires routine monitoring of vital signs and documentation of physiologic progress including blood pressure, pulse, quality and number of respirations per minute, temperature, coughing, and deep breathing. However, when caring for the obese patient it is especially important to assess the skin (Davidson and Callery, 2001). Documentation is critical, since the patient's condition can rapidly change and having a baseline will be important.

After surgery, patients seem to breathe more easily when the bed is at 30 degrees, since this reduces the weight of the abdominal adipose tissue, which can otherwise press against the diaphragm (Lasater-Erhard, 1995). The challenge in terms of skin care is that patients who fear shortness of breath may refuse repositioning from this 30-degree, semi-Fowler's position, thus placing them at risk for sacral pressure injury. Introducing pressure redistribution early in the admission may reduce some of this risk, along with patient and clinical education designed to improve awareness about it. Care plans require modification to address or prevent skin breakdown.

Incisions and Sutured Wounds

Incised and sutured wounds are expected to create a water-tight seal within 48 hours; however, wound healing can be delayed in some obese patients. Blood supply to fatty tissue may be insufficient to provide an adequate amount of oxygen and nutrients (Gallagher and Gates, 2003): which may interfere with wound healing and increase the risk of wound dehiscence. Wound healing may also be delayed if the patient has a diet that lacks essential vitamins and nutrients. Wound healing can be delayed if the wound is within a skin fold, where excess moisture and bacteria can accumulate. Ostomies may be more difficult to manage because of abdominal irregularities; a well-placed and constructed stoma will be critical to avoid some of the challenges that can occur in caring for the patient with an ostomy (Gallagher and Gates, 2004). Excess abdominal fat also increases the tension at the wound edges (Gallagher, 2002). To reduce the occurrence of abdominal wound separation, some clinicians use a surgical binder to support the area; however, safety considerations need to be addressed when using binders. The binder should rest no higher than 4 cm below the xiphoid process. Additionally, in order promote adequate ventilation, it is important that the binder is not too constrictive. To ensure the binder is not too tight, 2.5 cm of space should exist between the skin and the binder. Binders are especially important when the patient ambulates. Some patients find the binders so comfortable that they ask to leave the binder on at all times. Careful assessment under the binder will reveal any signs of early pressure-related breakdown where the edges of the binder meet the skin (Gallagher, 2004c).

Hypoventilation Syndrome and Sleep Apnea

Morbidly obese patients tend to have pulmonary problems, two in particular: obesity hypoventilation syndrome (OHS) and sleep apnea (OSA). OHS is an acute respiratory condition wherein the weight of fatty tissue on the rib cage and chest prevents the chest wall from expanding fully. Because patients are unable to breathe in and out fully, ventilatory insufficiency can occur (Gallagher, 1998).

Sleep apnea usually occurs when the patient is asleep in the supine position. The weight of the excess fatty tissue in the neck causes the throat to narrow, severely restricting or even cutting off breathing for seconds or even minutes at a time. Breathing can be made easier by keeping the patient in the semi-Fowler's position, which takes some of the pressure off the diaphragm for the reasons described earlier. Mobilizing the patient as early as possible will also help. At home, many patients manage the problems of nighttime sleep apnea with the use of a continuous positive airway pressure (CPAP) machine (Shinohara et al, 1997). However, in the health care setting, some patients use bilevel positive airway pressure (BiPAP) for a short time after extubation.

Tracheostomy Care

If long-term ventilator support becomes necessary, performing a tracheostomy can be especially challenging if the trachea is buried deep within fatty tissue. A large wound may be needed in order to locate the trachea. This larger wound can lead to complications such as bleeding, infection, or damage to the surrounding tissue. Postoperative tracheostomy care, therefore, must include steps to protect the peristomal skin, manage the tracheostomy, and contain wound drainage. Locally, a nonadhesive moisture-absorbing dressing is helpful in achieving this goal. To compound this dilemma, standard-sized "trach" tubes may be inadequate for use with patients with larger necks. In addition, narrow cloth "trach" ties can burrow deep within the folds of neck, further damaging the skin; to prevent this sort of damage, clinicians have used thicker or wider ties.

QUALITY IMPROVEMENT

Even with good education, clinical skills, and motivation, it can still prove impossible for the wound care clinician to deliver safe, effective skin and wound care. Clinicians across the country are looking with an element of frustration for creative strategies to achieve this goal. Policies and procedures typically assist in providing care for complex, costly patient groups by employing a standardized criteria-based method of delivering care. In managing the skin care needs of the obese patient, preplanning for equipment is an essential first step (Box 14-2) however, it simply is not sufficient to adequately prevent the costly, predictable complications that occur in caring for obese patients

and their skin. A comprehensive, interdisciplinary patient care approach is necessary to provide safe patient care in a timely, cost-effective manner, and prevent caregiver injury. This approach should include (1) a bariatric task force, (2) a criteria-based protocol, which includes preplanning equipment, (3) competencies/skill set, and (4) outcome measurement efforts.

Bariatric Task Force

The bariatric task force is an interdisciplinary quality improvement effort designed to address ongoing issues and ideas. The value of an interdisciplinary approach cannot be overlooked. Pharmacists, physical/ occupational and respiratory therapists, physicians, clinical nurse specialists, the wound, ostomy continence/ enterostomal therapy (WOC/ET) nurse, and others can be essential in planning care. Each member of the team brings a unique and important perspective (Gallagher et al, 2004). The entire health care team must be diligent in caring for the morbidly obese patient.

Criteria-Based Protocol

Health care facilities should have a plan in place for the special skin care needs of the morbidly obese patient. This could include resources such as equipment or clinical experts. A criteria-based protocol is simply preplanning based on specifically designated criteria. The patient's weight, BMI, body width, and clinical condition serve as such criteria (Gallagher, 1999). Actual weight is particularly useful, because if the weight limit of equipment is exceeded, then breakage, failure to function properly, or patient or caregiver injury can occur. Body width is described as the patient's body at his or her widest point, which could be at the hips, the shoulders or across the belly when side-lying. Further, any clinical condition that interferes with mobility such as pain, sedation, fear, or resistance to participating in care places the patient at risk. Criteria-based protocols should be designed to meet the needs of the patient by ensuring access to resources, such as specialty equipment and clinical experts, in a timely, cost-effective manner (Gallagher et al, 2004b).

Communication and timing is critical to prevent the costly, predictable, and often preventable complications associated with caring for very complex patients.

Although sometimes difficult to arrange, a face-to-face interdisciplinary conference, which is planned within 24 hours of admission may prevent costly intervention later (DeRuiter, Meitteunen, and Sauder, 2001). Consider including the patient's significant other, as this person may offer insight into the patient's special needs. Documentation of meetings, individual goals, and corresponding intervention may protect the institution from legal action. This level of accountability also outlines more fully each clinician's responsibilities, and when the timing is right smoothes the transition from one practice setting to another.

Competency Skill Sets

It is easy to minimize the challenges that basic care of the obese patient can present. Typically simple tasks such as repositioning and urinal placement can require several staff members and skills to accomplish these tasks safely and effectively. Education to ensure basic skills or competencies is imperative. Consider conducting a survey to determine the actual learning needs of clinicians. Members of the bariatric task force serve as a pool of experts to develop lesson plans and education addressing identified clinical needs. For example, when clinicians are seeking information pertaining to caregiver safety, a physical/occupational therapist, nurse expert, risk manager, and patient member of the task force could develop a 1-hour module to teach these skills.

Outcomes Measurement

In order to ensure success of a comprehensive bariatric program, it is essential to monitor and collect relevant and appropriate outcomes. Patient and staff satisfaction, safety, and complications are among the issues that should be monitored.

SUMMARY

With obesity on the rise, wound care clinicians are increasingly responsible for managing the needs of this complex patient population. Although equipment is a helpful adjunct to care, it is never a substitute for care. Numerous resources are available to clinicians across practice settings, and use of resources in a timely and appropriate manner is thought to improve measurable therapeutic, satisfaction, and cost outcomes; coordinating these resources in the form of a comprehensive

bariatric care plan may ensure the most favorable outcome. The obese patient poses many care challenges, and it is in the interest of health care organizations to meet these skin and wound care challenges in a clinically, ethically, and legally sound manner.

SELF-ASSESSMENT EXERCISE

1. Morbid obesity is defined as a body mass index of which of the following?
   a. Greater than 40
   b. Greater than between 30-35
   c. Between 35 and 40
   d. Between 30 and 35
2. Literature suggests a direct correlation between increased BMI and urinary incontinence: true or false?
3. Discuss two factors that delay wound healing in obese patients.
4. Which of the following interventions will reduce the risk of abdominal wound dehiscence in the obese patient?
   a. Montgomery straps
   b. Transparent dressing
   c. Abdominal binder
   d. SteriStrips
5. Describe obesity hypoventilation syndrome (OHS).

REFERENCES

American Society of Bariatric Surgeons: Rationale for the surgical treatment of morbid obesity, 2001, www.asbs.org; Accessed February 12, 2005.

Charles S: Psychological evaluation of morbidly obese patients, *Gastroenterol Clinics of North Am* 16(3):41-47, 1987.

Davidson J, Callery C: Care of the obesity surgery patient requiring immediate-level care or intensive care, *Obesity Surg* 11:93-97, 2001.

DeRuiter H-P, Meitteunen E, Sauder K: Improving safety for caregivers through collaborative practice, *J Heathcare Safety Compliance Infection Control* 5(2):61, 2001.

Engel BT, Burgio KL, and Matthews KA: Prevalence incidence and correlates of urinary incontinence in healthy middle aged women, *J Urol* 46(5):1255, 1991.

Faulcbaum L, Choban P: Surgical implications of obesity, *Ann Rev Med* 49:215, 1998.

Fox HR: Discrimination: alive and well in the United States, *Obesity Surg* 5:352, 1995.

Gallagher S: Morbid obesity: a chronic disease with an impact on wounds and related problems, *Ostomy Wound Manage* 43(5):18, 1997.

Gallagher S: Caring for obese patients, *Nursing* 98(3):32HN1, 1998.

Gallagher S: Restructuring the therapeutic environment to promote care and safety for the obese patient, *J WOCN* 26:292, 1999.

Gallagher S: Obesity and the skin care in the critical care area, *Crit Care Nurs Q* 25(1):69, 2002.

Gallagher S: Panniculectomy, documentation, reimbursement and the WOCN, *J WOCN* 30(2):72, 2003.

Gallagher S: Bariatrics: considering mobility, patient safety, and caregiver injury. In: Charney W, Hudson A, editor: *Back injury among healthcare workers*, Baton Rouge, 2004a, Lewis Publishers.

Gallagher S: Nursing management of the patient having panniculectomy surgery, *Nursing* 34(12):52-62, 2004c.

Gallagher S: Shedding weight with bariatric surgery, *Nursing* 34(3):58, 2004d.

Gallagher S: Understanding compassion, sensitivity, and the obese patient, *Bariatric Times* 1(1):1, 2004e.

Gallagher S: Issues of caregiver injury: addressing the needs of a changing population, *Bariatric Times* 2(1):1, 2005.

Gallagher S, Gates J: Obesity, panniculitis, panniculectomy, and wound care: understanding the challenges, *J WOCN* 30:334, 2003.

Gallagher S, Gates J: Challenges of ostomy care and obesity, *Ostomy Wound Management* 50(9):38, 2004.

Gallagher S et al: Criteria-based protocols and the obese patient: planning care for a high-risk population, *Ostomy Wound Management* 50(5):32, 2004a.

Gallagher S et al: Preplanning protocols for skin and wound care in obese patients, *Adv Skin Wound Care* 17(8):436, 2004b.

Gustafson NJ: *Managing obesity and eating disorders*, South Easton, Mass, 1997, Western Schools Press.

Knudsen AM, Gallagher S: Care of the obese patient with pressure ulcers, *J WOCN* 30:111, 2003.

Kral JG, Strauss RJ, Wise L: Perioperative risk management in obese patients. In Deitel M: *Surgery for the morbidly obese patient*, North York, Canada, 2000, FD-Communications.

Kramer K, Gallagher S: WOC nurses as advocates for patients who are morbidly obese: A case study promoting use of bariatric beds, *J WOCN* 31(1):276, 2004.

Kuczmarski RJ et al: Increasing prevalence of overweight among US adults. The National Health and Nutrition Examination surveys, 1960 to 1991, *JAMA* 272:205, 1994.

Lanz P et al: Socioeconomic factors, health behavior and mortality, *JAMA* 279(2):1703, 1998.

Lasater-Erhard M: The effect of patient position of arterial oxygen saturation, *Crit Care Nurs Q*, 15:31, 1995.

Maiman LA et al: Attitudes toward obesity and the obese among professionals, *J Am Diet Assoc*, 74:331, 1992.

Mathison CJ: Skin and wound care challenges in the hospitalized morbidly obese patient, *J Wound Ostomy Continence Nurs*, 30(2):78-83, 2003.

Medical Network: Foot problems: foot problems as symptoms and warning signs, 1999-2001; http://alegent.iqhealth.com//atoz/foot/symptoms.htm; Accessed April 1, 2004.

Shinohara E et al: Visceral fat accumulation as an important risk factor for obstructive sleep apnea syndrome in obese subjects, *J Intern Med* 241:11, 1997.

Staffieri JR: A study of social stereotype of body image in children, *J Pers Soc Psychol* 7:101, 1967.

Steers WD, Suratt PM: Sleep apnea as a cause of daytime and nocturnal enuresis, *Lancet* 349(9069):1604, 1997.

Thone RR: *Fat: a fate worse than death*, New York, 1997, Harrington Park Press.

Torpey J: Obesity, *JAMA* 289(14):1880, 2003.

15

Lower-Extremity Ulcers of Vascular Etiology

DOROTHY B. DOUGHTY & RHONDA HOLBROOK

OBJECTIVES

1. Identify the key elements of assessment for the patient with a lower-extremity ulcer of vascular etiology.
2. Describe the indications, procedure, and interpretation for ankle-brachial index and toe-brachial index.
3. Compare and contrast venous and arterial ulcers in terms of etiologic factors, risk factors, pathophysiology, typical presentation, and principles of management.
4. Outline a patient teaching plan for the individual with ischemic disease of the lower extremity, to include lifestyle changes to maximize perfusion and measures to prevent trauma.
5. Define the term *critical limb ischemia,* including assessment parameters and implications for management.
6. Identify indications and options for surgical revascularization and for surgical correction of venous insufficiency.
7. Describe pharmacologic options for management of arterial and venous ulcers.
8. Describe the principles underlying effective compression therapy for the individual with chronic venous insufficiency, including indications and contraindications for use.
9. Explain the mechanism of action and indications for use of the following: short stretch bandages, long stretch bandages, compression stockings, and intermittent pneumatic compression devices.
10. Explain how lymphedema differs from venous edema in terms of pathology, presentation, and management.
11. Identify adjunctive therapies that may be of benefit to the patient with an arterial or venous ulcer.

Leg ulcers affect approximately 2.5 million people in the United States (WOCN Society, 2002). Approximately 70% of these ulcers are caused primarily by chronic venous insufficiency (CVI), with 20% to 25% being attributed to arterial or mixed disease (Nelson and Bradley, 2003). It is difficult to accurately determine the prevalence and incidence of these ulcers since they represent a complication of an underlying systemic disease process and may not be reported separately. In addition, these ulcers may be "underreported" to health care providers; one study suggests that many patients care for their own wounds without consulting a physician or alternate care provider (Nelzen, Bergqvist, and Lindhagen, 1996).

While the exact prevalence of leg ulcers may be unclear, the impact of these ulcers on the health care system and the patient is becoming increasingly evident. The cost of treatment for venous ulcers alone is estimated to be $1 billion per year in the United States (WOCN Society, 2005a; Valencia et al, 2001). In addition to the fiscal impact, there is the impact on the individual and family, specifically significant pain, disability, and interference with activities of daily living (Franks and Moffatt, 1998; Liew et al, 2000; Phillips et al, 1994). The importance of an accurate diagnosis and lifelong management for these patients cannot be overstated. Patient education is a major component of any successful wound management program and will be discussed with examples throughout this chapter. (See Appendix D for patient teaching tools.)

To manage the patient with a lower-extremity ulcer effectively, the wound care provider must be knowledgeable regarding the various pathologies involved and must be skilled in assessment and management strategies (Choucair and Fivenson, 2001). Diagnosis and management of these patients is complicated by the fact that many patients present with "mixed" disease. For example, a patient with an ulcer caused by lower-extremity venous disease (LEVD) may have coexisting arterial disease that precludes standard compression therapy and that further compromises the patient's ability to heal. Similarly, the patient with an ulcer caused by lower-extremity arterial disease (LEAD) may have coexisting edema that must be effectively managed if the ulcer is to heal.

Wound care specialists must be alert to the possibility that a lower-extremity wound may result from vasculitis, pressure, neuropathy, pyoderma gangrenosum, calciphylaxis, arthropod bites, or malignant processes (Chapters 6, 16, and 22). This chapter will address the general assessment of the lower limb and the unique pathology, presentation, and management of ulcers caused by LEVD, LEAD, and lymphedema. It is important to remember that the ulcer is secondary to the underlying etiology and that other cofactors affect healing such as nutrition and infection.

TERMINOLOGY

There are a wide variety of terms that are used to describe lower-extremity venous and arterial disease. Lower-extremity venous disease (LEVD) is also referred to as chronic venous insufficiency (CVI) and venous stasis. Lower-extremity arterial disease (LEAD) is also referred to as peripheral arterial disease (PAD), peripheral vascular disease (PVD), or peripheral arterial occlusive disease (PAOD).

ASSESSMENT OF THE LOWER EXTREMITY

Effective management of a lower extremity ulcer is always dependent on accurate determination of the underlying etiologic factors; thus the clinician must be knowledgeable regarding clinical presentation and skilled in differential assessment. Critical assessment parameters include the general appearance of the limb, perfusion, sensory function, range of motion, pain, and ankle-brachial index.

General Appearance of the Limb

Limb appearance should be compared with that of the contralateral limb to identify or rule out trophic changes. For example, thinning of the epidermis, loss of hair growth, and thickened nails are often associated with, but are not diagnostic of, arterial disease. Conversely, edema, varicosities (dilated, swollen, tortuous), hemosiderin staining, and dermatitis may be indicative of venous insufficiency. These findings will be discussed in greater detail later in the chapter.

Edema. Edema is a localized or generalized abnormal accumulation of fluid in the tissues (WOCN Society, 2005a). Edema causes swelling that may obscure the appearance of normal anatomy. To determine the presence of edema in the lower extremities, compare the appearance of one extremity with the other, noting the relative size and prominence of veins, tendons, and bones. Presence of edema is a significant finding and should be investigated.

The extent of edema is assessed by pressing firmly but gently with the index finger for several seconds on the dorsum of each foot, behind each medial malleolus, and over the shins. Edema is "pitting" when there is a visible depression that does not rapidly refill and resume its original contour (Figure 15-1). Box 15-1 is a 1- to 4-point scale that describes the severity of the edema (Seidel et al, 2003). Because there are a variety of 3- and 4-point scales used in clinical practice, it is important to document the type of scale used (e.g., 3+ pitting edema on a 1 to 4 point scale). Ideally, the categories should be defined on the documentation form where the assessment is recorded so terminology is used consistently.

Patterns associated with edema should be noted. For example, dependent edema describes the accumulation of fluid in the lowest body parts such as the feet

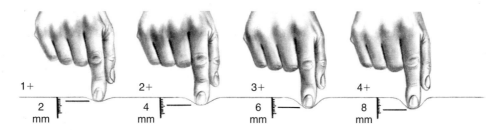

Fig. 15-1 Assessing for pitting edema. (From Cannobio MM: *Cardiovascular disorders,* St Louis, 1990, Mosby.)

BOX 15-1 Grading Scale for the Severity of Edema
....

1+ Slight pitting, no visible distortion, disappears rapidly

2+ A somewhat deeper pit than in 1+; but again, no readily detectable distortion, and it disappears in 10-15 seconds

3+ The pit is noticeably deep and may last more than a minute; the dependent extremity looks fuller and swollen

4+ The pit is very deep and lasts as long as 2-5 minutes, and the dependent extremity is grossly distorted

From Seidel HM et al, editors: Blood vessels. In *Mosby's guide to physical examination*, ed 6, St Louis, 2006, Mosby, Elsevier Science.

BOX 15-2 Assessment of Elevational Pallor
....

1. Raise leg to a 60-degree angle for 15 to 60 seconds
2. Observe the amount of time it takes for pallor to appear:
   • Pallor within 25 seconds indicates severe occlusive disease
   • Pallor within 25-40 seconds indicates moderate occlusive disease
   • Pallor within 40-60 seconds indicates mild occlusive disease

From Seidel HM et al, editors: Blood vessels. In *Mosby's guide to physical examination*, ed 6, St Louis, 2006, Mosby, Elsevier Science.

and legs (WOCN Society, 2005a). With lower-extremity venous disease, dependent edema generally develops gradually, worsens with prolonged standing, and diminishes when the patient rests in a recumbent position with the legs elevated. However, the pattern of edema associated with lymphedema does not resolve with leg elevation. Types of edema are distinguished in Table 15-1 and described later in the chapter.

Color Changes. Color changes in one or both legs provide additional information; specifically, they reflect the adequacy of arterial perfusion.

Elevational pallor. With the leg raised to a 60-degree angle for 15 to 60 seconds, the examiner observes for a visible color change. Normally, color should not change. When perfusion is impaired, pallor is observed in fair-skinned individuals and gray (ashen) hues are observed in dark-skinned individuals. Box 15-2 correlates the severity of occlusion with the amount of time it takes for the color change (pallor or gray tones) to be observed (Cantwell-Gab, 1996; Lesho, Manngold, and Gey, 2004; Rockson and Cooke, 1998).

Dependent rubor. The examiner observes for the development of rubor by placing the leg in a dependent position. Rubor is a purple-red discoloration of the lower limb that develops as a result of the retention of deoxygenated blood in the dilated skin capillaries. The normal leg will remain a healthy color when dependent.

Perfusion

Skin temperature, color, quality of pulses, venous filling time, and ankle-brachial index (ABI) are additional parameters used to assess perfusion (Seidel et al, 2003).

Venous Filling Time. Venous filling time (also known as venous refill time) is a visual assessment measuring the time it takes for foot veins to fill while the leg is in a dependent position. Normally the veins on the dorsum of the foot will fill in 15 to 20 seconds when the leg is placed in a dependent position from a horizontal position. A filling time of more than 20 seconds usually indicates occlusive disease (WOCN Society, 2002).

Capillary Refill. Box 15-3 explains how and why capillary refill time is assessed (Seidel et al, 2003). The capillary bed joins the arterial and the venous systems. The time it takes for the capillary bed to fill after it is occluded by pressure (capillary refill time) gives some indication of the health of the system. Delayed capillary refill (greater than 3 seconds) may indicate LEAD (WOCN Society, 2002). However, the patient with arterial disease may have normal capillary refill, because the emptied vessels may refill in a retrograde manner from surrounding veins even if arterial inflow is markedly impaired or absent. Environmental factors such as temperature may also influence the results of capillary refill time; therefore the assessment is vulnerable to considerable subjective interpretation and should be used only to confirm a clinical judgment.

TABLE 15-1   **Venous Edema, Lymphedema, and Lipedema**

	VENOUS EDEMA	LYMPHEDEMA	LIPEDEMA
DISTRIBUTION	• Ankle to knee • May have limited foot involvement • Usually unilateral	• Toes to groin • Usually unilateral	• Ankle to groin • Bilateral and symmetrical
CHARACTERISTICS	• Pitting edema of variable severity • In long-standing disease, nonpitting edema may result from tissue fibrosis	• Brawny, nonpitting edema • Skin and soft tissue changes common, i.e., papilloma formation and hyperkeratosis • Positive Stemmer sign an early indicator (not possible to pinch fold of skin over dorsum of second toe) *Advanced disease-* Elephantiasis: loss of normal architecture/massive enlargement of limb	• Soft, rubbery tissue • Pain on palpation common • Painful bruising common • Negative Stemmer sign • Abnormal fat distribution extends to involve hips
MANAGEMENT	• Elevation and compression (toes to knees) primary approaches • Intermittent pneumatic compression typically beneficial • Surgery sometimes beneficial	• Elevation and standard compression beneficial only in early stages • Manual lymphatic drainage and inelastic compression key elements of management • Intermittent pneumatic compression frequently contraindicated	• No effective treatment available • Management focus: treatment of any comorbidities; patient education, and support
RISK FACTORS	• Deep vein thrombosis or thrombophlebitis • Thrombophilia • Obesity or multiple pregnancies • Sedentary lifestyle • Calf muscle pump failure	• Filariasis (third-world countries) • Radical cancer surgery plus radiation • Long-standing venous disease • Vein harvesting/reconstruction	• Heredity

BOX 15-3 Assessment of Capillary Refill

- Blanch the toenail bed with a sustained pressure of several seconds
- Release the pressure
- Observe the time elapsed before the nail regains full color
- In the presence of arterial occlusion, refill time will take longer than 2-3 seconds
  Caution: decreased temperature can prolong capillary refill time.

Data from Seidel HM et al, editors: Blood vessels. In *Mosby's guide to physical examination,* ed 6, St Louis, 2006, Mosby, Elsevier Science.

Skin Temperature. Skin temperature of the leg is assessed by palpating lightly with the palmar surface of the fingers and hands, moving from proximal to distal and comparing the right leg with the left leg and the right foot with the left foot. Findings of unilateral coolness and a sudden marked change from proximal to distal, are possible indicators of lower-extremity arterial disease (Wipke-Tevis and Sae-Sia, 2004). In contrast, patients with LEVD have been shown to have higher skin temperatures at the ankle (WOCN Society, 2005a; Kelechi et al, 2003).

Auscultation for Bruits. The arteries of the lower limb may be auscultated for bruits, which are heard as blowing or rushing sounds through the bell of a stethoscope. Presence of a bruit is indicative of arterial narrowing (Dillavou and Kahn, 2003; Lesho, Manngold, and Gey, 2004).

Assessment of Pulses. Pulses should be compared with the contralateral pulse and should be assessed in a proximal-to-distal approach. Normally pedal pulses can be palpated at both the dorsalis pedis and the posterior tibialis location (Figure 15-2).

The best way to document pulses is to use descriptive terms such as present or absent followed by clarifying terms such as weak or bounding. Box 15-4 presents a 0 to 4 point scale that describes the amplitude of the pulse (Seidel et al, 2003). As previously stated, since there are a variety of 3 and 4 point scales used in clinical practice, it is important that the type of scale is communicated (e.g., 3+ pedal pulses on a 0 to 4 point scale).

Presence or absence of *palpable* pulses is not diagnostic of lower-extremity arterial disease (LEAD). If pulses are palpable, the patient may still have LEAD. If pulses are not palpable, a Doppler probe must be used to determine the presence or absence of pulses. Absence of both pulses is indicative of LEAD (WOCN Society, 2002).

Ankle-Brachial Index (ABI). The ankle-brachial index (ABI), also known as the ankle-arm index, is a simple bedside comparison of perfusion pressures in the lower leg with those in the upper arm using a blood pressure cuff and a Doppler probe (Figure 15-3). The Doppler probe that generates the correct frequency (in megahertz, or MHz) for assessment of skin level vessels is a 5- to 7-MHz probe (Aronow, 2004; Schainfeld, 2001). This noninvasive test is used to screen patients for evidence of significant arterial insufficiency and to identify patients who require further workup. The procedure for conducting an ABI is outlined in Box 15-5. Table 15-2, pg. 265 provides guidelines for interpretation of ABI ankle, and toe pressure measurements. ABI mea-surements provide only an indirect measure of peripheral perfusion and cannot be considered accurate in patients with noncompressible vessels (e.g., the patient with diabetes and vessel calcification). Therefore, patients with diabetes who have clinical evidence of ischemia but normal or elevated ABI measurements should be referred for more definitive testing such as transcutaneous oxygen pressure ($tcPO_2$) (WOCN Society, 2002; Gibbons, 2003; WOCN Society, 2005b).

Toe-Brachial Index (TBI). An alternative to the ABI is the toe-brachial index (TBI), also known as the toe-arm index. Toe pressures are generally more accurate in the presence of vessel calcification because these vessels are much less likely to be calcified. This procedure is performed in exactly the same manner as the ABI test, except a toe cuff is placed around the great toe or the second toe and the Doppler probe is placed against the distal toe surface to monitor the pulse signal. A normal TBI value is greater than 0.6 (Bonham, 2003; WOCN Society, 2002).

Sensory Function

A focused sensory exam is an essential component of any lower-extremity assessment. Sensory assessment (the ability to feel pain, pressure, temperature changes, and friction in the lower extremities and feet) is

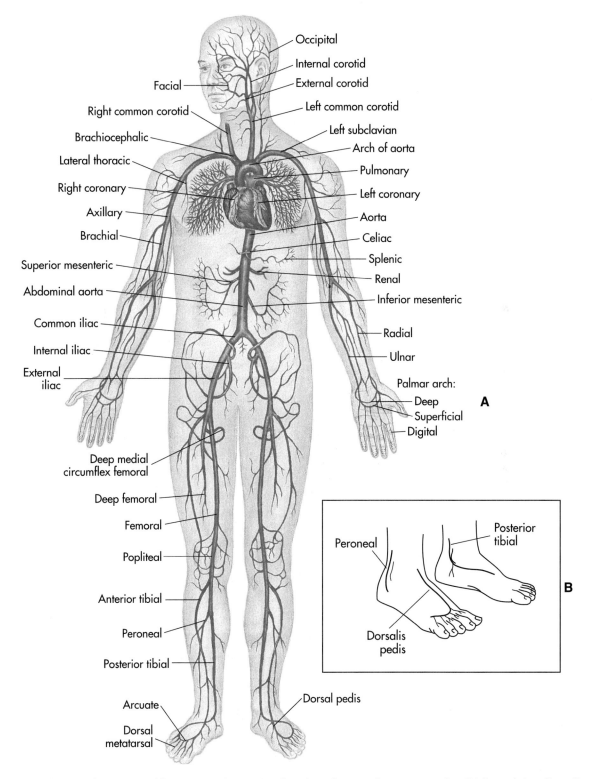

Fig. 15-2 Arterial structure of lower extremity. **A,** Note location of peroneal artery, posterior tibialis, and dorsalis pedis. **B,** Note location of peroneal artery, posterior tibialis, and dorsalis pedis. (**A,** From Seidel HM et al, editors: Blood vessels. In *Mosby's guide to physical examination,* ed 5, St Louis, 2006, Mosby, Elsevier Science.)

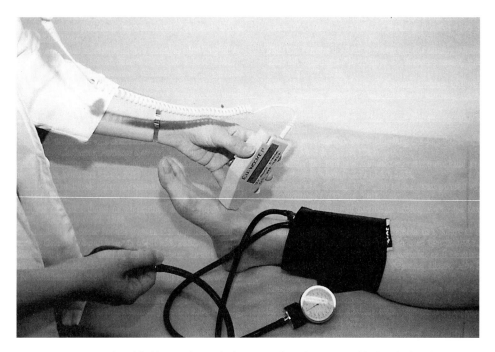

Fig. 15-3 A hand-held Doppler probe being used to obtain an ankle-brachial index.

BOX 15-5 Procedure for Performing an Ankle-Brachial Index (ABI)

....

1. Place patient in a supine position for at least 10 minutes before the test.
2. Obtain the brachial pressure in each arm using Doppler probe. Record the highest brachial pressure.
3. Place an appropriately-sized cuff around the lower leg 2.5 cm above the malleolus.
4. Apply acoustic gel over the dorsalis pedis pulse location.
5. Hold the Doppler probe over the pedal pulse according to manufacturer guidelines (e.g., "pen-style" Dopplers should be held at a 45-degree angle). Be careful not to occlude the artery with excessive pressure; hold the probe lightly!
6. Inflate the cuff to a level 20 to 30 mm Hg above the point that the pulse is no longer audible.
7. Slowly deflate the cuff while monitoring for the return of the pulse signal. The point at which the arterial signal returns is recorded as the dorsalis pedis pressure.
8. Apply acoustic gel over the posterior tibial pulse location and repeat this procedure. The higher of the two values is used to determine the ABI.
9. Calculate the ABI by dividing the higher of the two ankle pressures by the higher of the two brachial pressures.

TABLE 15-2 Interpretation of Ankle-Brachial Index (ABI), Ankle Pressures (AP), and Toe Pressures (TP) Results

ABI VALUE	INTERPRETATION/CLINICAL SIGNIFICANCE
ABI ≥ 1.0 to 1.3	"Normal" range
ABI ≤ 0.6 to 0.8	Borderline perfusion
ABI ≤ 0.5	Severe ischemia; wound healing unlikely unless revascularization can be accomplished.
ABI ≤ 0.4	Critical limb ischemia
AP < 40	Limb threatened
TP < 30	
> 1.3	Abnormally high range, typically because of calcification of the vessel wall in the patient with diabetes
	Renders ABI test invalid as a measure of peripheral perfusion

WOCN Society, 2002.

particularly relevant to the patient with a lower-extremity wound. Failure to detect touch indicates loss of protective sensation, and warrants caution if applying compression wraps (because the patient may not sense ischemic changes in a timely manner) (Bonham, 2003; Phillips, 2001). Sensorimotor assessment is discussed in greater detail in Chapter 16.

Range of Motion of the Ankle Joint

The calf muscle pump is a critical contributor to normal venous return. Normal function of the calf muscle pump is dependent on a normally moving ankle joint. A "normal" walking motion requires flexion of the ankle joint past the 90-degree position. Therefore, routine assessment of ankle range of motion should be incorporated into the physical assessment of a patient with known or suspected venous disease (Orsted, Radke, and Gorst, 2001).

Pain

The wound care provider must assess verbal and nonverbal indicators of pain. Pain in the lower extremity is typically the first indication of LEAD. The patient should therefore be questioned regarding when the pain occurs, as well as the location, duration, intensity, and relieving factors, all of which provide clues to etiology (Table 15-3). In patients with arterial disease, pain location and characteristics suggest the level and severity of the occlusion. In general, pain occurs one joint distal to the occlusion as outlined in Table 15-4.

The three categories of ischemic pain are described in Box 15-6. Intermittent claudication is typically described as "cramping," whereas rest pain is usually perceived as a "constant deep aching pain." Some patients interpret claudication as the "leg giving out" or "leg fatigue" rather than pain; therefore it is important to ask questions concerning activity tolerance. Exacerbating and relieving factors help to verify the etiology of the pain and also the severity of the occlusion. For example, nocturnal pain that is relieved by dependency is characteristic of ischemic pain involving marked vessel occlusion. In contrast, leg pain that is relieved by elevation is more consistent with a venous etiology, and the patient with diabetes who complains of leg pain relieved by walking is probably experiencing neuropathic pain (Gibbons, 2003; Lewis, 2001; Newman, 2000; Wipke-Tevis and Sae-Sia, 2004). See Chapter 24 for more detail of assessment and management of wound pain.

DIAGNOSTIC TESTS FOR THE LOWER EXTREMITY

For the vast majority of patients, a thorough history and physical is sufficient to identify the ulcer as either venous or arterial in origin and to identify any additional factors that should be considered in providing therapy (de Araujo et al, 2003). When the diagnosis is unclear, or when surgical intervention is contemplated, additional diagnostic studies may be indicated to delineate the specific anatomic and functional abnormalities. Specific vascular studies can identify the components of the vascular system involved in the disease process, the specific pathologic process, the anatomic level of the lesions or dysfunction, and the severity of the dysfunction. The most commonly used noninvasive diagnostic tests for venous insufficiency include simple "tourniquet" tests, plethysmography studies, and duplex imaging or ultrasonography; the

TABLE 15-3 **Pain Assessment for Patient with Lower Leg Ulcer**

FACTORS TO BE ASSESSED	TYPICAL FINDINGS		
	VENOUS	ARTERIAL	NEUROPATHIC
CHARACTERISTICS	Dull Aching	Intermittent claudication Nocturnal pain Rest pain (see Box 15-6)	Burning/tingling "Pins and needles" "Shooting"
SEVERITY	Variable Typically moderate to severe	Variable Frequently severe	Variable Commonly severe
EXACERBATING FACTORS	Dependency Increased edema Infection	Elevation Activity Infection	Variable Inactivity sometimes a precipitating factor

RELIEVING FACTORS	Elevation
	Edema control
	Reduction of
	  bacterial burden
		Dependency
		Rest
		Reduction of bacterial
		  burden
			Activity such as
			  walking

TABLE 15-4 **Correlation between Site of Occlusion and Location of Pain**

SITE OF OCCLUSION	LOCATION OF PAIN
Ileofemoral arteries	Thighs and buttocks; calves
Superficial femoral artery	Calf
Infrapopliteal	Foot

From Cimminiello, C: PAD: Epidemiology and pathophysiology, *Thrombosis Res* 106(6):V295, 2002.

BOX 15-6 **Categories of Ischemic Pain**

- *Intermittent claudication* is pain that occurs only with moderate to heavy activity and is relieved by approximately 10 minutes of rest. This type of pain typically occurs when the involved vessel is approximately 50% occluded.
- *Nocturnal pain* develops as the occlusion worsens. This type of pain occurs when the patient is in bed and is caused by the combination of leg elevation and reduced cardiac output.
- *Rest pain* refers to pain that occurs in the absence of activity and with the legs in a dependent position; rest pain signals advanced occlusive disease (typically >90% occlusion).

WOCN Society, 2002.

most common diagnostic tests of the arterial system include pulse volume recordings, segmental pressure analysis, transcutaneous oxygen measurements, and magnetic resonance angiography (MRA) (WOCN Society, 2002).

Invasive vascular studies such as venography or arteriography may be warranted to further assess anatomy of the venous or arterial system, especially for patients in whom surgical intervention is being contemplated.

Noninvasive Testing for Venous Disease

Tourniquet Testing. There are various types of tourniquet tests that can be done; Perthes' test is one of the simplest. In this test, a tourniquet is applied above the knee with the patient standing; the patient is then instructed to ambulate, and the clinician assesses for increased distention of superficial varicosities. Positive findings suggest incompetence in the deep venous system (Paquette and Falanga, 2002).

Plethysmography Studies. These studies use noninvasive techniques to determine the amount of blood in the extremity in different positions and during various maneuvers, and specifically to determine the amount of time required for the veins to refill after being emptied. Photoplethysmography uses light reflection as an indicator of blood volume, whereas air plethysmography uses air-filled cuffs to determine changes in venous volume. For example, with photo-plethysmography, the light sensor is placed 10 cm above the medial malleolus and the patient is instructed to sit with legs bent and feet on the floor and to perform a series of dorsiflexions. In the absence of venous insufficiency and reflux, venous refill time following these maneuvers is greater than 20 seconds; refill times of less than 20 seconds indicate that the veins are refilling rapidly because of reflux, and are considered diagnostic of venous insufficiency (Wipke-Tevis and Sae-Sia, 2004). However, plethysmography does not provide visualization of the venous system and therefore has limited value when compared to other studies now available, specifically color duplex ultrasonography (Min, Khilnani, and Golia, 2003).

Duplex Imaging. Duplex ultrasound imaging with or without color has become the preferred study for assessing venous disease; it is now considered the "gold standard" because it is noninvasive and has a high degree of sensitivity. Duplex imaging produces images of blood flow through the vessels, pinpointing the anatomic site of reflux, obstruction such as deep vein thrombus, or abnormal vein walls (de Araujo, et al, 2003; Jansen, Lawall, and Diehm, 2003; WOCN Society, 2005; Kalra and Gloviczki, 2003; Min, Khilnani, and Golia, 2003; Weingarten, 2001).

Noninvasive Testing for Arterial Disease

Pulse Volume Recordings and Doppler Waveform Studies. A pulse volume recording provides a reflection of actual perfusion volume. This test is typically performed using a machine with pneumatic cuffs. The cuff is inflated to a preset level, and the machine provides a tracing that reflects the change in blood volume occurring within that limb segment over the course of the cardiac cycle. A similar tracing of flow within a single vessel may be obtained using a Doppler probe; this tracing is commonly referred to as a Doppler waveform study. Pulse volume recordings and Doppler waveform studies of normal vessels are described as triphasic (Figure 15-4, *A*). They clearly demonstrate a systolic peak, a dicrotic notch representing blood flow reversal during early diastole, and a diastolic wave. With mild atherosclerotic disease, the waveform becomes biphasic, and with advanced disease the waveform becomes monophasic (Figure 15-4, *B*) or severely blunted (Figure 15-4, *C*) (Aronow, 2004).

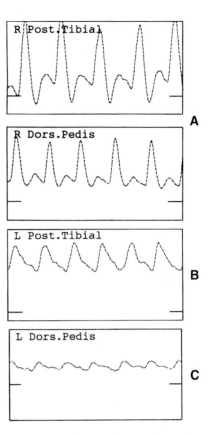

Fig. 15-4 A, Normal Doppler waveforms from normal vessels (right posterior tibialis and right dorsalis pedis). Signal is triphasic, showing systolic peak, dicrotic notch representing blood flow reversal during early diastole, and a diastolic wave. **B,** Doppler waveform study of vessel with moderately severe occlusive disease as evidenced by a monophasic waveform. **C,** Doppler waveform study of vessel with advanced occlusive disease. Note that waveform is severely blunted.

Segmental Pressure Recordings. These recordings are used to determine the level of occlusion. Cuffs are placed at thigh level, below the knee, and just above the ankle. A Doppler probe is used to localize the most distal pulses (dorsalis pedis and posterior tibialis), and the ankle cuff is inflated until the arterial signal is obliterated. The cuff is then deflated until the arterial signal is again audible. The pressure at which the signal is heard is recorded as the ankle systolic pressure. The procedure is then repeated with inflation of the "below-the-knee" cuff and then with the thigh cuff. Each pressure is then compared with the adjacent pressure. Differences of more than 20 mm Hg indicate an occlusive lesion located between the two involved cuffs (Gahtan, 1998).

Transcutaneous Oxygen Pressure Measurements. Transcutaneous oxygen pressure measurements ($TcPO_2$) provide information about the adequacy of oxygen delivery to the skin and underlying tissues. Values above 40 mm Hg generally indicate sufficient oxygen to support wound repair, values between 20 and 40 mm Hg are considered equivocal in terms of wound healing, and values below 20 mm Hg generally indicate marked ischemia and the inability to heal (WOCN Society, 2002; Moon, 1998).

Magnetic Resonance Angiography (MRA). Advances in magnetic resonance imaging provide improved visualization of the arterial lumen and atherosclerotic plaques. The major advantages of the MRA are increased safety; it is noninvasive and does not require the use of contrast (Lewis, 2001).

Invasive Testing

Venography. Venography, an invasive study that requires injection of a radiopaque dye into the lower-extremity veins, details the venous system in the leg. Venography studies were commonly used until the late 1980s to identify the severity of deep vein incompetence. However, this is an invasive study with significant potential for complications and limited diagnostic value, and it has largely been replaced by duplex ultrasound imaging (Min, Khilnani, and Golia, 2003).

Arteriography. Arteriography has been the gold standard in assessment of LEAD; however, the arteriogram is an invasive procedure that provides anatomic data only and is therefore restricted to patients in whom surgical intervention is planned (Aly et al, 1998). Digital subtraction angiography (DSA) is a specialized arteriography that uses computerized fluoroscopy to enhance visualization. The image before contrast injection is electronically subtracted from the post-contrast images, leaving only the opacified vessels on the final image. Advantages of DSA include increased visualization of smaller vessels, and increased safety (because injecting the contrast via

vein reduces the risk of hemorrhage and thrombosis) (Lewis, 2001).

ARTERIAL ULCERS

Arterial ulcers occur as a result of severe tissue ischemia and are therefore extremely painful. In addition, an ischemic ulcer represents potential limb loss. These lesions are generally refractory to healing unless tissue perfusion can be improved, and are prone to progress to invasive infection and/or gangrene, which may necessitate amputation (WOCN Society, 2002). The treatment plan for these patients must be multifaceted, including measures to maximize perfusion and minimize the risk of infection, ongoing assessment for deterioration in wound or tissue status, and interventions to reduce pain. Since effective management of the ischemic limb frequently requires significant lifestyle modifications, patient education regarding care options and needed lifestyle changes is an essential element of the management plan.

Epidemiology

LEAD increases with age and is higher among men. It is very difficult to accurately determine the prevalence of LEAD. Rates vary widely depending on the particular study and the inclusion criteria. When the inclusion criteria define LEAD as the presence of intermittent claudication, prevalence ranges from a low of 2% to 6% (in individuals under 50 years of age) to a high of 20% or more in individuals over the age of 80 (Aronow, 2004; Boulton, 2001; Cimminiello, 2002). When the inclusion criteria are based on noninvasive testing, such as ankle-brachial index (ABI) measurements, the prevalence of significant disease (defined as ABI of less than 0.9), is considerably higher (Newman, 2000; Schainfeld, 2001).

In fact, many "asymptomatic" patients diagnosed with LEAD by noninvasive testing actually do experience symptoms. They frequently report impaired mobility, leg weakness, and reduced activity levels, which are incorrectly attributed to aging or other conditions. Ischemic changes in the muscle and the resulting limitations in activity may serve to "mask" the presence of intermittent claudication.

There is a significant "overlap" between individuals with LEAD and individuals with CAD (coronary artery disease). As a result, screening for asymptomatic LEAD is effective in identifying individuals with asymptomatic CAD who will benefit from treatment (Cimminiello, 2002; Newman, 2000; Schainfeld, 2001).

Of individuals with intermittent claudication, 15% to 20% progress to the point of critical limb ischemia (Box 15-7). This high-risk group of patients comprises about 1% of the general population over age 50 and represents the individuals who are at risk for limb loss and who may require aggressive revascularization (Cimminiello, 2002).

Etiology

The most common cause of LEAD and arterial ulceration among older adults is atherosclerosis involving the peripheral circulation. In the young adult population, LEAD is typically due to premature atherosclerotic disease or thromboangiitis obliterans (Buerger's disease, or arteriosclerosis obliterans). Both of these processes are uncommon and occur almost exclusively in heavy smokers (Mills, 2003). Arterial ulcers may also occur as a result of uncommon etiologic factors such as arterial trauma, entrapment syndromes, or acute embolic syndromes (Rockson and Cooke, 1998).

Atherosclerosis. Atherosclerotic disease can occur in any vessel in the body. In the peripheral circulation the aortic, iliac, femoral, and popliteal arteries are the vessels most commonly affected (Dillavou and Kahn, 2003). The pathology of atherosclerotic disease is not yet completely understood but is known to involve two primary processes in addition to other, related ones: plaque formation and enlargement, which causes narrowing of the vessel lumen; and endothelial injury, which triggers an inflammatory process that

ultimately results in fibrosis and hardening of the vessel wall (Lewis, 2001).

Plaque formation begins with the lesion known as a "fatty streak," which is a gray or pearly white lesion that adheres to the intima (inner layer of the arterial wall). This lesion consists of a lipid core and a connective tissue covering. As further lipid accumulation occurs, the plaque enlarges, which results in progressive narrowing of the vessel lumen. Over time the plaques become hardened, as a result of the deposition of calcium salts and cholesterol crystals; this causes loss of vessel elasticity and further compromises blood flow (Lewis, 2001).

The second process contributing to vessel narrowing and hardening is triggered by damage to the vessel lining. Endothelial damage results in areas where the intimal lining is denuded; platelets aggregate over these denuded areas, causing clot formation and the subsequent release of growth factors. The growth factors stimulate mitosis of the vascular smooth muscle cells and also promote synthesis of connective tissue proteins such as collagen. The end result is the thickening and fibrosis of the vessel wall, which further contributes to narrowing and hardening of the involved arteries (Lewis, 2001). Clinically these changes result in a chronic reduction in blood flow to the tissues and a loss of the ability to respond with increased blood flow when metabolic demands are increased (Lewis, 2001; Reininger, Graf, and Reininger, 1996). In addition, acute vessel occlusion may occur as a result of sudden plaque enlargement or plaque rupture (Rockson and Cooke, 1998).

Thromboangiitis Obliterans (Buerger's Disease). Thromboangiitis obliterans, also known as Buerger's disease and arteriosclerosis obliterans, is a rare condition almost exclusively limited to young adults (under 50 years of age) who are heavy smokers (Mills, 2003). The disease typically involves the distal veins and arteries in both the upper and lower extremities. The lesions cause significant pain (claudication), and there is a high incidence of digit or limb amputation but no increase in mortality. The cause of the disease is not known but does not involve plaque formation or hypercoagulability. Instead the lesions appear to be inflammatory in origin, which suggests an autoimmune process (Mills, 2003; Olin, 2000).

BOX 15-7 Indicators of Critical Limb Ischemia

- Nonpalpable pulses
- ABI ≤ 0.4
- $TcPO_2 < 20$ mm Hg
- Rest pain
- Ulceration or gangrene

Patients may first be seen with complaints of cold sensitivity, rest pain, pedal claudication, digital ulceration, or gangrene. Ulceration may occur spontaneously but more commonly is precipitated by minor trauma. The disease process is always bilateral and frequently involves all four limbs. The most effective management is elimination of tobacco, which provides consistent interruption of the disease process; other reported treatment options include sympathectomy and vascular endothelial growth factor gene therapy (Olin, 2000).

Risk Factors for Lower Extremity Arterial Disease (LEAD)

Risk factors for LEAD are the same as those for coronary artery disease and include both reversible and irreversible factors as summarized in Box 15-8 (Cimminiello, 2002; Dieter, 2002). Tobacco use is the factor most predictive of LEAD; 80% of individuals with symptomatic LEAD report a history of tobacco use. The by-products of tobacco include nicotine, carbon monoxide, and hydrogen cyanide. As both a vasoconstrictor and a promoter of platelet aggregation and clot formation, nicotine is a significant contributor to peripheral arterial disease (Newman, 2000).

Diabetes mellitus is another major risk factor and an important prognostic variable for the progression to severe ischemia. Specific pathologic features associated with diabetes that contribute to LEAD include increased plaque formation, increased red blood cell (RBC) rigidity, increased blood viscosity and coagulability, hypertrophy of the vascular smooth muscle, and increased vascular resistance (Gibbons, 2003). Insulin resistance and hyperinsulinemia may be one causative factor for hypertrophy of vascular smooth muscle, even in the early stages of the disease (insulin is known to be a vascular growth factor). Elevated insulin levels may also help to explain the development of LEAD among nondiabetic patients (Cimminiello, 2002; Schainfeld, 2001). Patients with diabetes and LEAD typically exhibit much more severe and advanced disease at earlier ages. In addition, their risk of ischemic ulceration, gangrene, and amputation is significantly increased (Boulton, 2001; Gibbons, 2003; Lewis, 2001). The differences in the presentation and progression among patients with diabetes as compared with nondiabetics are highlighted in Box 15-9 (Gibbons, 2003; Lewis, 2001). The patient with diabetes and LEAD is at particular risk for ischemia and gangrene of the toes as a result of one or more of the following:

- advanced atherosclerosis with thrombosis
- formation of microthrombi as a result of infection
- reduced blood flow secondary to vasopressor medications
- cholesterol emboli resulting in "blue toe syndrome" or in painful petechiae and livedo reticularis

Homocystinemia is a rare autosomal dominant disease that is known to contribute to endothelial injury, platelet aggregation, and early onset of severe atherosclerotic disease. The abnormal metabolism of homocysteine (a thiol-containing amino acid) can be easily normalized through administration of vitamin B_6,

---

BOX 15-8 Lower-Extremity Arterial Disease: Reversible vs Irreversible Factors
••

Reversible
- Hypertension (controlled)
- Diabetes (controlled)
- Cigarette smoking
- Hypercholesterolemia (controlled)
- Obesity
- Sedentary lifestyle

Irreversible factors
- Male gender
- Strong family history

BOX 15-9 Lower-Extremity Arterial Disease in the Diabetic Population vs the Nondiabetic Population
••

- Onset at earlier age
- Faster progression to critical ischemia/increased risk of limb loss
- Most commonly involved vessels are infrapopliteal (i.e., tibial and peroneal)
- Multisegmental occlusions and multivessel disease common
- Disease usually bilateral as opposed to unilateral
- May require vascular reconstruction

vitamin B12, and/or folic acid (de Jong, 2001; Taylor, 2003), a fact that underscores the importance of early detection and patient education.

The link between hypertension and LEAD is currently thought to be the vessel wall changes associated with hypertension, though data are conflicting and inconclusive (Cimminiello, 2002; Lesho, Manngold, and Gey, 2004; Lewis, 2001). While treatment with antihypertensive medication has not been shown to improve LEAD outcomes, it is an essential element of care owing to its impact on morbidity from cardiovascular and cerebrovascular disease (Lesho, Manngold, and Gey, 2004).

Elevated cholesterol levels, especially elevated low-density lipoproteins (LDLs), play an important pathogenic role in endothelial injury and the development of atherosclerosis and are therefore an important risk factor for the development of atherosclerosis and LEAD (Lewis, 2001; Schainfeld, 2001).

Pathology of Arterial Ulceration

The exact pathologic mechanisms producing ulceration in the ischemic limb have not been clearly defined. Ulceration is believed to result from (1) progressive occlusion leading to cellular ischemia and necrosis; (2) minor trauma, which results in a nonhealing wound owing to the damaged vessels' inability to meet the increased demands for oxygen associated with tissue injury and the healing process; and/or (3) external occlusive pressures such as heel pressure in a patient who is bed-bound (Lewis, 2001).

Assessment Findings Unique to the Patient with LEAD

The components of assessment for any patient who is seen with signs or symptoms of LEAD include the patient history, physical examination, and simple, noninvasive vascular studies. Select patients may require more complex or invasive vascular studies.

Patient History. The patient interview should include queries regarding any past illnesses or surgical procedures. Specific questions should be posed regarding any cardiovascular symptoms or "problems with circulation." Patient history includes general state of health, medication use (prescription and over-the-counter), and risk factors for LEAD as previously discussed and summarized in Box 15-10.

BOX 15-10 Lower-Extremity Arterial Disease and Arterial Ulcers: Components of a Focused Patient History
....

1. **Risk factors for arterial insufficiency**
   - Past and present tobacco use (to include type and amount)
   - Diabetes mellitus (include type, onset, past and present management)
   - History of hypertension or treatment with medications
   - History of high cholesterol levels and management
   - History of elevated homocysteine levels and treatment
   - History of angina, myocardial infarction, or cerebrovascular accident

2. **Pain**
   - Location
   - Characteristics of the pain (cramping versus constant deep aching pain)
   - Exacerbating and relieving factors

3. **Ulcer history**
   - Onset
   - Precipitating factors (e.g., minor trauma, bed rest)
   - Past and present management
   - Progress or regression in healing

Lower Extremity Characteristics. Trophic changes alone are not diagnostic of arterial insufficiency and should be interpreted cautiously. Ischemic skin changes that may be indicative of LEAD include thinning of the epidermis; alopecia; dry, taut, shiny skin; and dystrophic nails. Color changes include elevational pallor (See Box 15-2) or greyish hue for darkly pigmented skin, dependent rubor, and purpura. There may be a delayed capillary refill and prolonged venous filling time. Extremities may be cool unilaterally or have a sudden marked change from proximal to distal. Pulses **may** be diminished or absent. The ankle pressure will be lower than 50 mm Hg, toe pressures lower than 30 mm Hg, and the ABI will be 0.9 or less.

Ischemic pain. Pain is typically the first indication of LEAD. The patient should therefore be questioned regarding the presence of pain and its location and characteristics. Pain location and characteristics suggest the level and severity of the occlusion. In general, pain occurs one joint distal to the occlusion as outlined in Table 15-4.

The three categories of ischemic pain are described in Box 15-6. The earlier section on "Pain" provides further details about the categories of ischemic pain. (Gibbons, 2003; Lewis, 2001; Newman, 2000; Wipke-Tevis and Sae-Sia, 2004).

Ulcer characteristics. The physical examination must include a comprehensive assessment of any ulcers (assessment is discussed in Chapter 7). Classic arterial ulcer characteristics are listed in Table 15-5 (see Plate 34). Arterial ulcers tend to be small and deep, dry or minimally exudative, and pale or necrotic with well-defined borders at distal body locations (e.g., toes) (WOCN Society, 2002; Wipke-Tevis and Sae-Sia, 2004).

Management of the Patient with Arterial Ulceration

Management of the patient with an arterial ulcer translates into measures to improve perfusion. The prognosis for wound healing is directly correlated with the patient's ability to deliver sufficient volumes of oxygen and nutrients to support the repair process. Perfusion and tissue oxygenation can be improved via surgical options, pharmacologic agents, lifestyle changes, and adjunctive therapies such as hyperbaric oxygen therapy and arterial flow augmentation using intermittent pneumatic compression devices. The specific interventions selected for the individual patient are determined by the severity of the ischemia, the patient's overall medical status and prognosis for healing, and the patient's preferences and priorities.

TABLE 15-5 Characteristics of Ischemic vs. Venous vs. Neuropathic Ulcers

	ARTERIAL	VENOUS	NEUROPATHIC
LOCATION	Tips of toes (spontaneous necrosis) Pressure points (e.g., heel or lateral foot) Areas of trauma (nonhealing wounds)	Between ankles and knees; "classic" location is medial malleolus	Plantar surface over metatarsal heads Areas of foot exposed to repetitive trauma (toes and sides of feet)
WOUND BED	Pale or necrotic	Dark red, "ruddy" May be covered with fibrinous slough	Typically red (if no coexisting ischemia)
EXUDATE	Minimal	Moderate to large amounts	Moderate to large amounts
WOUND EDGES	Well-defined	Poorly defined; irregular	Well-defined; frequently associated with callous formation
OTHER	Infection common but sign and symptoms muted Typically painful Typically associated with other indicators: ischemia; diminished/absent pulses; elevational pallor and dependent rubor; thin fragile skin	Edema common Hyperpigmentation surrounding skin common Feet typically warm with good pulses (if no coexisting arterial disease)	Infection common but signs and symptoms may be muted May or may not have coexisting ischemia

Surgical Options. Indications for lower-extremity angioplasty and bypass surgery include the following:

- Presence of an arterial ulcer and an ABI of less than 0.5 in a patient who is very unlikely to heal without surgical revascularization
- An ABI of greater than 0.5 in a patient who is a surgical candidate and who fails to respond to pharmacologic and behavioral therapy
- Presence of incapacitating claudication that interferes with the patient's work or lifestyle
- Presence of limb-threatening ischemia as manifested by rest pain, infection, and/or gangrene

Surgical intervention is generally an option as long as preoperative imaging studies demonstrate patent distal vessels. Options include bypass grafting, angioplasty, and placement of stents.

Bypass grafts. Bypass grafts are most commonly constructed using the patient's saphenous vein (Figure 15-5). If the saphenous veins are damaged, an upper extremity vein may be harvested or a synthetic graft may be used (Lewis, 2001; Wipke-Tevis and Sae-Sia, 2004). Bypass procedures involving vessels below the knee have better patency rates when veins are used for the graft, as opposed to synthetic grafts (Lewis, 2001).

Angioplasty. Angioplasty has frequently been advocated as a simpler and less invasive approach to revascularization than bypass grafting. However, angioplasty is generally not a good option for extensive occlusive disease or for lesions more than 10 cm in length. In addition, angioplasty may not be feasible in smaller vessels. Approximately one third of patients with severe ischemic disease of the lower leg are candidates for angioplasty, and initial results are generally good. Long-term patency rates have been disappointing but can be improved by long-term administration of anticoagulants or antiplatelet agents or by placement of impregnated vascular stents into the stenotic area immediately after angioplasty (Aronow, 2004; Ellozy and Carroccio, 2003; Wipke-Tevis and Sae-Sia, 2004).

Amputation. Amputation is reserved as the "treatment of last resort" and is indicated primarily for patients with irreversible ischemia (i.e., tissue necrosis) and invasive infection (Aronow, 2004; Palmer-Kazen and Wahlberg, 2003).

Pharmacologic Options. The mainstay of pharmacologic therapy for patients with LEAD include medications to reduce the risk of thrombotic events (anticoagulants and antiplatelet agents), antilipemics, and analgesics.

Antiplatelets. Antiplatelet agents work primarily by reducing platelet aggregation. The most commonly used antiplatelet agent is low- to medium-dose aspirin (75 to 325 mg/day): this is not thought to affect LEAD but does reduce cerebrovascular and cardiovascular complications (stroke and myocardial infarction) (WOCN Society, 2002).

Specific antiplatelet drugs include dipyridamole, cilostazol, and clopidrogel, which inhibit platelet activation by antagonizing specific receptors (Aronow, 2004; WOCN Society, 2002; Dillavou and Kahn, 2003; Lesho, Manngold, and Gey, 2004; Schainfeld, 2001). Cilostazol, which has both antiplatelet and vasodilatory effects, is currently the most commonly recommended drug for symptomatic LEAD. Benefits include increased distance the patient is able to walk (walking distance), reduced intermittent claudication, improved ABI, and favorable modification of plasma lipoprotein levels. Studies indicate that the addition of cilostazol may increase walking distance 100% over exercise alone. Contraindications include new onset of congestive heart failure (WOCN Society, 2002; Dillavou and Kahn, 2003; Lewis, 2001).

Vasodilators. Systemic vasodilators are generally contraindicated for patients with LEAD because the resulting vasodilatation may divert blood from the affected area (Lewis, 2001). However, l-arginine has been shown in controlled trials to be an effective local vasodilator and to improve walking distance in patients with LEAD; the recommended dosage is 6.6 g/day for 2 weeks (WOCN Society, 2002). A commonly used over-the-counter herbal supplement derived from *Gingko biloba* has also been shown to increase walking distance for individuals with intermittent claudication (Wipke-Tevis and Sae-Sia, 2004).

Hemorrheologics. Specific effects of hemorrheologic agents include reduced concentrations of fibrinogen, which reduces blood viscosity, and reduced rigidity and aggregation of red blood cells, which improves their deformability and ability to pass through narrow vessels. Pentoxifylline (Trental) is the agent currently approved by the Food and Drug Administration for LEAD. Unfortunately, studies demonstrate only minimal to moderate beneficial effects in clinical practice,

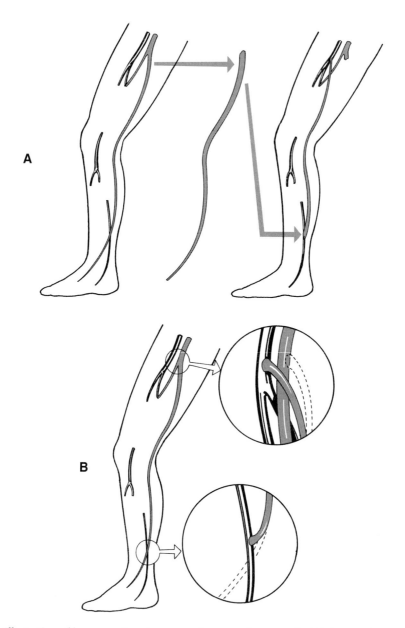

Fig. 15-5 Illustration of bypass grafts using an autologous saphenous vein (**A**) (reversed saphenous vein procedure) and in-situ procedure (**B**).

complicated by a fairly high incidence of gastro-intestinal side effects. If this agent is used for the treatment of LEAD, it should be given for 8 to 12 weeks at a dosage of 400 mg 3 times daily (with meals), at which point the patient should be evaluated for objective and subjective evidence of improvement. Failure to

demonstrate improvement should result in discontinuation (Aronow, 2004; Lesho, Manngold, and Gey, 2004; Lewis, 2001).

Antilipemics. Treatment of systemic atherosclerosis with lipid-lowering drugs helps to slow disease progression and reduces the severity of claudication.

Colestipol-niacin, simvastatin, and cholestyramine are currently considered the drugs of choice (Aronow, 2004; Lesho, Manngold, and Gey, 2004; Newman, 2000; Schainfeld, 2001).

Analgesics. Opioid analgesics may be required for patients with advanced ischemia to relieve the chronic pain and thus improve quality of life. Pain control will also address vasoconstriction caused by sympathetic stimulation (Wipke-Tevis and Sae-Sia, 2004).

Investigational agents. The pharmacologic agents discussed previously have limited ability to improve perfusion and no ability to induce new vessel growth. Therefore they are of limited benefit to patients with advanced ischemic disease and ulceration. Fortunately, there are several investigational agents and procedures that may prove beneficial in halting and/or reversing the atherosclerotic process, inducing selective vasodilatation, improving oxygen use by ischemic tissues, or promoting growth of new vessels; these include levacarnitine, prostaglandins, and angiogenic growth factors. It is hoped that continued research will identify new drugs that provide definitive clinical benefits, for example, reduction in rest pain and promotion of ulcer healing (Lewis, 2001; Schainfeld, 2001).

Lifestyle Changes. Currently, the ability to improve tissue perfusion and to promote wound healing depends in large part on the patient's ability to make appropriate lifestyle changes. Specifically, the patient must be counseled regarding strategies to modify correctable risk factors (Boxes 15-11 and 15-12), improve tissue perfusion (Box 15-13), and protect the compromised limb (Box 15-14). Lifestyle changes may be more difficult for the patient than either a surgical procedure or drug therapy; therefore effective introduction of such changes requires in-depth education and supportive, goal-directed patient counseling (Aronow, 2004; WOCN Society, 2002; Lesho, Manngold, and Gey, 2004; Lewis, 2001; Schainfeld, 2001).

The patient should be informed of the benefits of a *therapeutic walking program* (Box 15-15) and given a specific "walking prescription." The guidelines for therapeutic walking in the patient with LEAD usually address frequency, duration, and rate. A typical walking program involves 30-minute sessions at least 3 times per week; the patient is instructed to walk until near-maximal pain is reached in each session, and the program should last at least 6 months. If the patient

BOX 15-11 Goals and Strategies for Management of Lower-Extremity Arterial Disease

Goals
- Normalize blood pressure
- Normalize blood glucose levels
- Normalize serum cholesterol levels
- Eliminate tobacco use

Strategies
- Intensify patient education
- Monitor blood pressure, blood glucose levels, and serum cholesterol levels on a routine basis
- Aggressively modify the treatment plan to achieve and maintain as "near normal" a state as possible
- Initiate appropriate referrals

BOX 15-12 Interventions to Promote Cessation of Tobacco Use

1. General education concerning the negative effects of tobacco use on health status
2. Specific and consistent advice from health care team to eliminate tobacco use
3. Establishment of patient-provider contracts in which the patient commits to a date on which he or she will eliminate tobacco use
4. Anticipatory guidance (e.g., counseling to help the patient identify triggers for tobacco use and specific strategies for managing triggering events and situations)
5. General stress management and support
6. Appropriate use of adequate doses of nicotine replacement agents (nicotine replacement therapy) and/or medications for nicotine addiction
7. Frequent follow-up during the critical weeks after initial termination of tobacco use (either by phone or by office visit)
8. Appropriate counseling after any relapse on recognition that most individuals who successfully stop smoking have one to four relapses

with rest pain and an ischemic ulcer is not able to tolerate walking, a walking program may have to be delayed until the ulcer is healed and metabolic demands are reduced (Aronow, 2004; WOCN Society, 2002; Lesho, Manngold, and Gey, 2004; Lewis, 2001).

Hyperbaric Oxygen Therapy. Hyperbaric oxygen therapy increases the amount of oxygen dissolved in the plasma, which results in the delivery of "oxygen-enriched" blood to the tissues. It can be of particular benefit to the patient with an arterial ulcer since oxygen delivery is no longer dependent upon the ability of the red blood cell to traverse the narrowed vessels. Hyperbaric oxygen therapy is discussed in greater detail in Chapter 20.

Arterial flow augmentation using intermittent pneumatic compression devices. Augmentation of arterial

---

BOX 15-13 Measures to Improve Tissue Perfusion
....

- Maintenance of hydration (to reduce blood viscosity)
- Avoidance of cold, caffeine, and constrictive garments (to reduce vasoconstriction)
- Weight control (to reduce the workload of the ischemic limb)
- Planned graduated walking program (to improve tissue perfusion and oxygen use)
- Pain management (to prevent vasoconstriction)

BOX 15-15 Benefits of a Planned Graduated Walking Program
....

Physiologic benefits
- Adaptive changes within ischemic tissues, resulting in improved oxygen use at the cellular level (increased cellular levels of oxidative enzymes and leva-carnitine)
- Enhanced workload tolerance
- Reduced blood viscosity
- Promotion of weight loss
- Reduction of blood pressure
- General stress reduction
- Improved gait efficiency

Clinical benefits
- Improved exercise tolerance
- Reduced pain

BOX 15-14 Limb Preservation Strategies
....

Routine skin care
- Application of emollients after bathing to prevent cracking and fissures
- Careful drying between toes to prevent maceration
- Use of lamb's wool or foam toe "sleeves" to prevent interdigital friction and pressure

Measures to prevent mechanical trauma
- Avoidance of barefoot walking, even indoors, including consistent use of protective footwear (e.g., closed-toe shoes) to prevent inadvertent cuts or puncture wounds
- Inspection of shoes before wearing
- Careful fitting of shoes to prevent pressure, friction, or shear injuries
- If indicated, use of protective shin guards when working around house or yard

- Professional foot and nail care (or self-care of nails limited to conservative trimming and filing); no "bathroom surgery"

Measures to prevent thermal trauma
- Warm socks to be worn during cold weather to prevent vasoconstriction
- No use of hot water bottles, heating pads, or other thermal devices
- Hand or elbow checks of water temperature before bathing

Measures to prevent chemical trauma
- No use of antiseptic or chemical agents such as corn removers

General measures
- Daily inspection of feet and legs
- Prompt reporting of any minor injuries

flow using intermittent pneumatic compression devices appears promising for patients who are not candidates for revascularization or percutaneous angioplasty (WOCN Society, 2002; Labropoulos, 2002). Intermittent compression devices are discussed further in the section on venous ulcer management.

Topical Therapy. Topical therapy for arterial ulcers is based on the principles outlined in Chapter 19. Because of the potential for limb loss, of particular importance in the topical therapy of patients with ischemic wounds is the management of a dry, non-infected necrotic wound and the identification and management of infection.

Management of a dry, noninfected necrotic wound. Although necrotic tissue is clearly a potential medium for bacterial growth, a dry, intact eschar can also serve as a bacterial barrier. A closed wound surface is advantageous when managing a very poorly perfused wound in which any bacterial invasion is likely to result in clinical infection and limb loss. Current evidence supports maintenance of a closed wound when (1) the involved limb is clearly ischemic with limited or no potential for healing, (2) there are no indications of infection, and (3) the wound surface is dry and necrotic. The maintenance of a dry wound with frequent monitoring for any deterioration in wound status (i.e., any signs of infection) is the current standard (WOCN Society, 2002; Kunimoto, 2001b). A sample topical therapy protocol for this type of ulcer is outlined in Box 15-16.

Identification and management of infection. Prompt identification and aggressive treatment of any infection is critical when managing an ischemic wound. Because the ischemic wound is much less able to mount an inflammatory response, these patients are at risk for overlooked infections that can become severe (e.g., cellulitis and osteomyelitis). Therefore the wound care provider must be alert to subtle indicators of infection (as listed in Box 15-17) and must intervene promptly and aggressively, if limb loss is to be avoided (Wipke-Tevis and Sae-Sia, 2004). Management of the infected ischemic ulcer is dependent on aggressive and early debridement of all necrotic tissue, wicking of dead space to evacuate all wound fluid, and culture-based antibiotic therapy. The critically ischemic limb (i.e., the limb with no palpable pulses and an ABI lower than 0.4 to 0.5) should be revascularized if at all possible, once the necrotic tissue has been debrided

BOX 15-16 Topical Therapy for Dry, Necrotic, Uninfected Ischemic Wound

1. Inspect for subtle indicators of infection. If any signs or symptoms of infection develop, immediate referral for debridement and initiation of antibiotic therapy are critical.
2. Paint with antiseptic solution (e.g., povidone-iodine 10% solution); allow to dry.
3. Apply dry gauze dressing and secure with wrap gauze.

BOX 15-17 Indicators of Wound Infection in Ischemic Limbs

- Increased pain or edema or both
- Increased necrosis
- Fluctuance of the periwound tissues
- Faint halo of erythema surrounding the wound

and antibiotic therapy has been initiated. For the patient with critical ischemia in whom revascularization is not possible, amputation may be required if meticulous wound care coupled with antibiotic therapy is ineffective (WOCN Society, 2002; Schainfeld, 2001).

VENOUS ULCERS

Whereas arterial ulcers develop as a result of inadequate blood flow to the tissues (LEAD), venous ulcers occur as a result of impaired return of venous blood from the tissues to the heart, or chronic venous insufficiency (CVI). Venous ulcers are much more common, accounting for 70% to 90% of all leg ulcers (WOCN Society, 2005a; Valencia et al, 2001). These lesions develop as a result of skin and tissue changes caused by CVI and the associated ambulatory venous hypertension.

Management of patients with venous ulcers must include measures to optimize wound healing through reduction of edema, prevention of complications, and appropriate topical therapy to promote healing (de Araujo et al, 2003; Kunimoto, 2001b; Weingarten, 2001). Once the ulcer is healed, the emphasis shifts to long-term disease management to prevent recurrence.

Epidemiology

The exact prevalence of venous ulcers is not known, although prevalence estimates in developed countries range from less than 1% to more than 3% of the population (Kerstein, 2003; Phillips, 2001). Venous disease and venous ulcers occur in individuals as young as 20. "Peak" incidence is between the ages of 60 and 80 (de Araujo et al, 2003; Paquette and Falanga, 2002; Phillips, 2001; Weingarten, 2001). Although there seems to be no racial predilection, most studies report female gender as a risk factor (de Araujo et al, 2003; Kalra and Gloviczki, 2003; Paquette and Falanga, 2002).

LEVD affects approximately 6 to 7 million individuals in the United States, and about 1 million of these will develop ulcerations (WOCN Society, 2005; Valencia et al, 2001). The impact of venous disease is tremendous as it relates to the individual and costs to the health care system and society. Individuals with venous disease report pain, itching, anxiety, social isolation, and reduced ability to carry out usual activities as their areas of greatest concern (de Araujo et al, 2003; Ryan, Eager, and Sibbald, 2003; Weingarten, 2001). In contrast, nurses caring for these patients rated pain control as a less important aspect of care than wound healing and limb preservation, which indicates the need for increased awareness and focus on quality of life issues on the part of health care providers (Ryan, Eager, and Sibbald, 2003). Venous insufficiency and venous ulcers also have a major economic impact. The average lifetime cost of care for an individual with LEVD can exceed $40,000. The total cost for the care of LEVD in the United States is estimated to be more than 1 billion dollars per year (WOCN Society, 2005a; Simka and Majewski, 2003; Valencia et al, 2001; Weingarten, 2001).

The negative impact of venous ulcers is compounded by recurrence rates as high as 57% to 97%, which reflects the chronicity of the underlying condition. Frequent recurrence is also attributed to a failure to adequately address the primary problems of venous insufficiency and venous hypertension (WOCN Society, 2005a; Paquette and Falanga, 2002).

Etiology

Venous ulceration is a direct result of ambulatory venous hypertension from CVI. A clear understanding of the anatomy and physiology of the lower-extremity venous system provides the framework for an understanding of the pathology of LEVD, ambulatory venous hypertension, and venous ulceration. The venous system of the lower extremity includes three major components: deep veins, superficial veins, and perforator veins. The deep veins include the posterior and anterior tibial and the peroneal veins; these veins are located in the deep tissue adjacent to the calf muscle. The superficial venous system is also known as the saphenous system because the two major vessels are the greater saphenous vein (GSV) and lesser saphenous vein (LSV). These two vessels are located just below the superficial fascia, with multiple tributaries located in the superficial tissues (Figure 15-6) (Kalra and Gloviczki, 2003). The perforator veins "connect" the two systems, transporting blood from the superficial system into the deep system, from which point the blood is propelled back to the heart (Anwar et al, 2003).

All veins are equipped with one-way valves that support a unidirectional flow of blood toward the heart. Because these valves prevent reflux of blood from the high-pressure deep venous system to the low-pressure superficial venous system, they play an essential role in normal venous function. Further protection is provided by the fact that the perforator veins follow an oblique course through the fascia and muscle layers, which provides additional support for these connecting veins and their valves. The closed valves in the perforator veins prevent transmission of the high resting pressures back into the superficial system, so long as the valves remain competent (Anwar et al, 2003; Kalra and Gloviczki, 2003; Reichardt, 1999).

Returning blood from the feet and legs to the heart is a major physiologic challenge, since the blood must flow "uphill" against the forces of gravity. When an individual is standing upright, the gravitational force creates a column of hydrostatic pressure that equals about 90 mm Hg at the ankle. The primary mechanisms by which venous blood is returned to the heart are the smooth muscle tone within the venous walls, contraction of the calf muscles (gastrocnemius and soleus muscles), and the negative intrathoracic pressure created during inspiration. Of these three mechanisms, contraction of the calf muscle pump is by far the most critical (Anwar et al, 2003; Kalra and Gloviczki, 2003).

The calf muscle pump and one-way valves normally work together to propel venous blood back toward

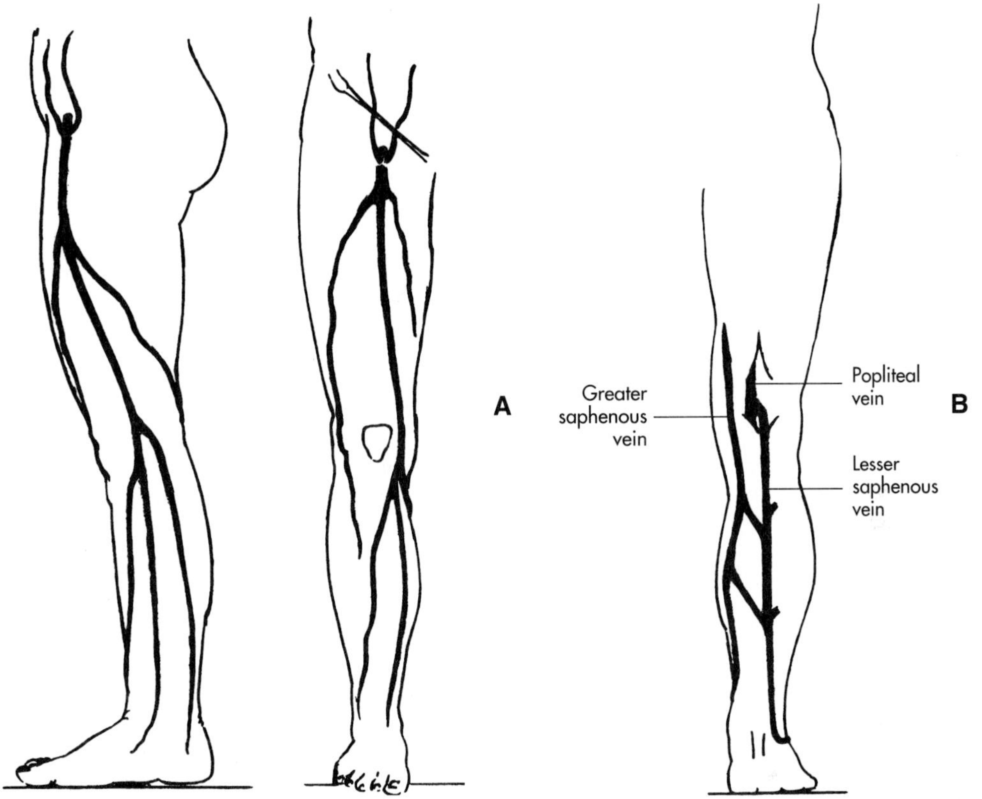

Fig. 15-6 A, Anatomy of greater saphenous vein with anterior and posterior branches. **B,** Anatomy of lesser saphenous vein and its communication with greater saphenous vein and the popliteal vein. (From Young JR, Olin JW, Bartholomew JR: *Peripheral vascular diseases*, ed 2, St Louis, 1996, Mosby.)

the heart. Calf muscle contraction forces the blood out of the deep veins and into the central circulation. While blood is being pumped from the deep veins, the one-way valves in the perforator system are closed to prevent backflow of blood into the superficial veins. As the calf muscle relaxes, the valves in the perforator veins open to permit the blood in the superficial system to flow into the deep veins. At the onset of calf muscle contraction, the pressures within the deep venous system peak at about 120 to 300 mm Hg. These pressures then fall rapidly as the veins empty and the calf muscle relaxes (Figure 15-7). Thus high resting (filling) pressures, but low walking (emptying) pressures, characterize normal venous function (Figure 15-8).

Pathology of LEVD. The two elements most critical to normal venous function are competent valves and a normally functioning calf muscle pump; normal venous tone also contributes to venous return. Loss of valvular competence permits reflux of blood from the deep veins and perforator veins into the superficial venous system. This condition is known as CVI or LEVD. Conditions that cause or contribute to valvular incompetence include those that cause direct damage to the valve leaflets and those that cause venous distention. Distention contributes to valve dysfunction by causing mechanical stretch that results in loss of coaptation of the valve leaflets. Incompetent valves subsequently contribute to venous hypertension.

Valve failure changes the normal unidirectional flow of blood into a "bidirectional" flow. As a result, blood can now reflux back into the superficial system, causing distention and congestion of the superficial veins and capillaries. This will manifest clinically as edema. At the same time, valvular dysfunction permits transmission

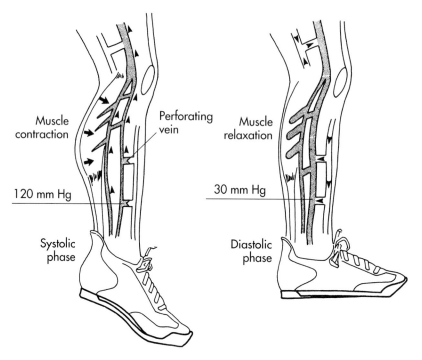

Fig. 15-7 Anatomy of the perforating (communicating) veins. During the systolic phase of calf muscle contraction, the one-way valves of the perforating veins are closed, which prevents deep to superficial blood flow. During the diastolic phase the valves of the perforating veins are open, allowing superficial-to-deep blood flow to refill the deep veins. (From O'Donnell TF Jr, Shepard AD: Chronic venous insufficiency. In Jarrett F, Hirsch SA, editors: *Vascular surgery of the lower extremities,* St Louis, 1996, Mosby.)

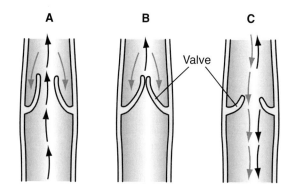

Fig. 15-8 Venous valves. **A,** Open valves allow forward blood flow. **B,** Closed valves prevent back flow. **C,** Incompetent valves unable to fully close, causing blood to flow backward and producing venous in sufficiency.

of the high pressures in the deep system to the superficial veins and tissues, resulting in varicosities and damage to the skin and soft tissues.

Ambulatory venous hypertension can result either from valvular incompetence or from failure of the calf muscle pump, or from some combination of the two factors. Incompetent valves are a factor in most cases. Any degree of calf muscle failure can cause or compound this scenario. When the calf muscle fails to contract effectively, the deep veins are incompletely emptied. This causes increased pressures within the deep system, which creates resistance to blood draining from the superficial veins. Resistance to flow creates congestion and distention of the superficial and perforator veins, which causes loss of valve coaptation. The incompetent valves then permit backward transmission of the high pressures in the deep system (Anwar et al, 2003; Kalra and Gloviczki, 2003).

Many patients have multisystem valvular incompetence (i.e., incompetent valves in at least two of the three venous systems). Perforator valve incompetence is particularly common and clinically significant. At least two thirds of patients with venous hypertension and venous ulcers have incompetent perforator valves, which can result in supramalleolar pressures well above 100 mm Hg and a "reflux rate" of more than 60 ml/min. When multiple valves become incompetent, the effect is magnified and clinically evident disease becomes much more likely (Anwar et al, 2003; Kalra and Gloviczki, 2003). Further study is needed to accurately quantify the impact of calf muscle failure.

Ultimately, the end result of prolonged venous hypertension is damage to the skin and soft tissues that renders these structures vulnerable to minor trauma and susceptible to spontaneous ulceration (Paquette and Falanga, 2002).

Classification of LEVD

CEAP is an acronym for a classification system for chronic venous insufficiency and stands for *c*linical indicators, *e*tiologic factors, *a*natomical location of the dysfunctional venous structures, and the specific *p*athophysiologic processes. This system is presented in Table 15-6 (Anwar et al, 2003; WOCN Society, 2005a; Weingarten, 2001).

Risk Factors for LEVD

Risk factors for LEVD include factors that lead to valvular or calf muscle dysfunction (Table 15-7).

Valvular Dysfunction. Numerous risk factors for valvular dysfunction have been identified and include the following (Bradbury et al, 2002; de Araujo et al, 2003; WOCN Society, 2005a; Kunimoto, 2001a; Paquette and Falanga, 2002; Phillips, 2001; Wipke-Tevis and Sae-Sia, 2004):

- obesity, which creates resistance to venous return owing to pressure on pelvic veins
- pregnancy, especially multiple pregnancies or pregnancies that are close together, because of increased pressure against pelvic veins and compromised venous return
- thrombophlebitis (e.g., deep venous thrombosis [DVT] or pulmonary embolism [PE]) which triggers an inflammatory response that may cause direct damage to the valve leaflets or may cause chronic partial deep vein obstruction due to incomplete recanalization of the vein, which in turn causes venous distention and valvular compromise
- leg trauma (e.g., fracture), which suggests undiagnosed damage to the vessel walls and valves
- thrombophilic conditions (e.g., protein S deficiency, protein C deficiency, and factor V [Leiden mutation]) which increase the coagulability of

TABLE 15-6 CEAP Classification for Lower-Extremity Venous Disease

CLINICAL INDICATORS	ETIOLOGIC FACTORS	ANATOMICAL DEFECTS (LOCATIONS)	PATHOPHYSIOLOGY
0 = No visible or palpable indicators of venous disease	Congenital Primary Secondary	Superficial system Deep system Perforator system Combination defects	Reflux Obstruction Combination of reflux and obstruction
1 = Telangiectases			
2 = Varicosities			
3 = Edema			
4 = Venous skin changes (hemosiderosis, dermatitis, lipodermatosclerosis)			
5 = Venous skin changes *plus* healed ulceration			
6 = Venous skin changes *plus* active ulceration			

TABLE 15-7 Key Elements of History for Patients with Lower-Extremity Ulcers

RISK FACTORS FOR LEG ULCERATION	FACTORS AFFECTING HEALING/ TREATMENT	HISTORY OF ULCER/ PRIOR TREATMENT	PATIENT CONCERNS
Venous	*Healing*	*History*	*Concerns*
Deep vein thrombosis (known or suspected) or leg trauma	Diabetes mellitus	Onset and duration of any precipitating event[‡]	Pain
Thrombophlebitis	Tobacco use	Previous ulcers	Itching
Venous disease (family history of venous disease)	Malnutrition (e.g., unplanned weight loss)		Anxiety
Thrombophilia	Medications*	*Treatment*	Impact on activities of daily living
Pregnancies		Treatments used to date and response:	Cost issues
Obesity	*Treatment*	surgical treatment	
Varicose veins	Cardiac disease/ heart failure[†]	pharmacologic treatment	Treatment goals and priorities
Intravenous drug use involving affected extremity	Activity level	compression therapy (type, duration, response, tolerance)[§]	Anticipated problems with treatment plan (e.g., ability to come to clinic, elevate legs, utilize compression stockings, etc.)
Arthritis or other conditions affecting calf muscle function			
Sedentary lifestyle or prolonged standing			
Ischemic			
Cardiovascular disease			
Hyperlipidemia			
Tobacco use			
Diabetes mellitus			
Hypertension			
Neuropathic			
Diabetes mellitus			
Spinal cord injury			

*Corticosteroids particularly deleterious to repair (at doses greater than 30 mg/day).
[†]Clinically significant heart failure is contraindication to compression therapy.
[‡]Duration longer than 6 months is negative predictor for wound healing.
[§]Venous ulcers that consistently fail to respond to compression therapy should be reevaluated to rule out malignant disease or missed diagnosis.

venous blood, thus increasing the risk of DVT and of microvascular thrombosis. Thrombophilic conditions have been identified in as many as 50% of patients with venous ulcers.

Calf Muscle Dysfunction. LEVD and ambulatory venous hypertension may also be caused or exacerbated by calf muscle dysfunction (Orsted, Radke, and Gorst, 2001). Compromise of the calf muscle pump results in incomplete emptying of the deep veins, and in turn causes venous distention, valvular compromise, and increased pressures within the venous system (ambulatory venous hypertension). Risk factors for compromised calf muscle function include the following:

- sedentary lifestyle
- occupations that require prolonged standing
- musculoskeletal conditions that compromise calf muscle function (e.g., paralysis, arthritis)
- advanced age, which is associated with decreased elasticity of the calf muscle tendon

- reduced mobility
- altered, "shuffling" gait that fails to induce calf muscle contraction

Note reduced mobility and gait do not relate to calf muscle dysfunction.

Pathology of Venous Ulceration

While the pathology of edema formation is fairly clear, the reason for its accompanying venous dermatitis, lipodermatosclerosis, and venous ulceration is not well understood. There are numerous conditions that result in edema formation (e.g., heart failure, hypoalbuminemia), yet these conditions do not lead to skin ulceration (Weingarten, 2001). This mystery is compounded by the fact that only a minority of patients with chronic venous disease actually progress to ulceration. There are currently three theories regarding the pathogenesis of venous ulcerations.

Fibrin Cuff Theory. Browse and Burnand (1982) initially postulated that capillary bed distention permitted leakage of large molecules such as fibrinogen into the dermal tissue, and that the fibrinogen then polymerized to form fibrin cuffs around the dermal capillaries. Subsequent studies confirmed the presence of fibrin cuffs in patients with venous ulcerations. Investigators also demonstrated reduced fibrinolytic activity, which helps to explain the persistence of these "cuffs." Initially these cuffs were thought to act as a physical barrier to the diffusion of oxygen and nutrients into the tissues. However, later studies demonstrated that transcutaneous oxygen levels are unchanged and venous ulcers can heal in the presence of fibrin cuffs (Roszinski and Schmeller, 1995). More recently, these cuffs have been thought to possibly act as a "trap" for growth factors and other substances that are necessary for the maintenance of normal tissue and the healing of wounded tissue (WOCN Society, 2005a).

The White Blood Cell Activation Theory. Venous hypertension is known to reduce the velocity of blood flow through the capillary bed. When the blood flow becomes sluggish, leukocytes begin to adhere to each other (leukocyte aggregation) and/or to the capillary walls (leukocyte margination) (Smith, 1996). Each of these processes can contribute to tissue damage. Leukocyte aggregation causes "plugging" of the capillaries, which results in tissue ischemia. Leukocyte margination causes migration of activated leukocytes into the surrounding tissues, where they release proteolytic enzymes and other inflammatory mediators that cause additional tissue damage (WOCN Society, 2005a; Van de Scheur and Falanga, 1997).

Trap Hypothesis. The trap hypothesis suggests that fibrin and other macromolecules leak out of the permeable capillary beds into the dermis. Consequently, they trap growth factors and matrix proteins, rendering them unavailable for maintenance of healthy tissue and wound repair (WOCN Society, 2005a; Van de Scheur and Falanga, 1997).

Combination Theory. Kalra and Gloviczki (2003) suggest that venous ulceration is actually caused by some combination of processes. The initiating event in venous ulceration and related skin changes is the extravasation of red blood cells (RBCs) and protein molecules (e.g., fibrinogen) into the soft tissues. As the RBCs and protein molecules break down, they release substances that are powerful chemoattractants for white blood cells (WBCs). It is the migration and activation of the WBCs that is the most significant pathologic event. These activated WBCs release inflammatory mediators and growth factors that cause tissue inflammation and dermal fibrosis. The inflammatory and fibrotic changes in the tissues render them very susceptible to ulceration, which can occur spontaneously or as a result of minor trauma.

Assessment Findings Unique to the Patient with LEVD

Patient History. Risk factors for LEVD should be identified through a complete patient history. Of particular importance would be risk factors that differentiate venous insufficiency from arterial disease and other pathologies that may cause ulceration in the lower extremity (see Table 15-7).

Lower Extremity Characteristics. Examination from the knee down to the medial malleolus of a patient with LEVD may reveal edema, hemosiderosis, dermatitis, atrophie blanche, varicose veins, ankle flaring, scarring from previous ulcers, or tinea pedis (WOCN Society, 2005a). Many of these findings are unique to the patient with LEVD and are described below.

Edema. Edema is a classic indicator of venous disease, because of the combination of capillary bed distention and elevated intracapillary pressures. The severity of the edema is variable, both from patient to patient and from time to time throughout the day. The classic pattern is pitting edema (Box 15-1 and Figure 15-1) that worsens with dependency and improves with elevation (Phillips, 2001). With prolonged disease and gradual fibrosis of the soft tissues, the edema may become "brawny," that is, nonpitting; thus the characteristics of the edema is one clue as to the duration of the underlying disease process. The distribution of the edema is also significant; venous edema primarily involves the lower leg, that is, between the ankle and the knee; whereas lymphedema and lipedema involve the entire extremity. See Table 15-1 for a comparison of the edema associated with these three conditions.

Hemosiderin staining (Hemosiderosis). Another "classic" indicator of venous disease is hemosiderosis, the discoloration of the soft tissue that results when the extravasated RBCs break down and release the pigment hemosiderin. The result is a gray-brown pigmentation of the skin known also as "hyperpigmentation" or "tissue staining" (de Araujo, et al, 2003; Lopez and Phillips, 1998; Reichardt, 1999) (Plate 35).

Varicosities. Varicose veins and telangiectasias are another prevalent finding in venous insufficiency. These are swollen and twisted veins that appear blue and close to the skin's surface. They may bulge, throb, and cause the legs to swell and feel heavy. They are most often seen in the back of the calf or the inside of the leg. Varicosities are caused by the combination of venous reflux and venous hypertension, which combine to produce the dilated and tortuous superficial veins known as "varicose veins." Varicosities are a clear indicator of LEVD and a predictor of venous ulceration. Patients with varicosities should manage their weight, exercise, and avoid crossing their legs and wearing constrictive garments (WOCN Society, 2005a).

Malleolar flare (ankle flare). Another common finding is a sunburst pattern of visible capillaries from distention of small veins inferior and distal to the medial malleolus known as ankle flare (Rudolph, 1998).

Atrophie blanche lesions. Atrophie blanche lesions (Plate 36) can be found in as many as one third of patients with LEVD. These lesions present as smooth white plaques of thin, atrophic tissue "speckled" with tortuous vessels on the ankle or foot with hemosiderin-pigmented borders. Sometimes mistaken for scars of healed ulcers, this clinical finding actually represents

spontaneously developing lesions. Prompt recognition is important because these areas are high risk for ulceration (owing to the thin, atrophic epidermis?) (de Araujo et al, 2003; WOCN Society, 2005a; Kunimoto, 2001a; Ryan, Eager, and Sibbald, 2003).

Lipodermatosclerosis. Lipodermatosclerosis (Plate 35), a term used to denote fibrosis, or "hardening," of the soft tissue in the lower leg, is indicative of long-standing venous disease. The fibrotic changes are typically confined to the gaiter, or "sock," area of the leg, which results in an inverted "champagne bottle" or "apple core" appearance of the affected lower leg (the fibrosis causes abnormal narrowing of the affected area, which contrasts sharply with the normal tissue in the proximal limb). These fibrotic changes are thought to result from a combination of fibrin deposits, compromised fibrinolysis, and the deposition of collagen in response to growth factors produced by activated WBCs (de Araujo et al, 2003; Kunimoto, 2001a; Paquette and Falanga, 2002). Lipodermatosclerosis is also referred to as hypodermitis sclerodermiformis (WOCN Society, 2005a).

Venous dermatitis. Dermatitis, or inflammation of the epidermis and dermis, in the gaiter area of the leg is a common and distressing feature of LEVD (Plate 25). Scaling, crusting, weeping, erosions, and intense itching and tremendous discomfort characterize this condition. These symptoms are often confused with those of cellulitis. Factors to distinguish between dermatitis and cellulitis are presented in Table 15-8 (WOCN Society, 2005a).

Venous dermatitis appears to be triggered by the presence of the inflammatory mediators (released by activated white blood cells) within the subcutaneous tissue and dermis. It is unclear why venous dermatitis is common among some patients and rare among others (WOCN Society, 2005a; Kunimoto, 2001a; Paquette and Falanga, 2002; Ryan, Eager, and Sibbald, 2003). Patients with venous insufficiency and venous ulcers are also more likely to develop irritant dermatitis in response to pooling of drainage onto the periwound skin. Allergic contact dermatitis may also develop in response to topical agents. These are issues that must be considered when selecting products for topical therapy (de Araujo et al, 2003; Kunimoto, 2001a).

Ulcer Characteristics. The classic venous ulcer is located around the medial malleolus, probably because

TABLE 15-8 **Comparing Dermatitis and Cellulitis**

	ECZEMA/DERMATITIS	CELLULITIS
SYMPTOMS	Afebrile Itching Varicose veins/DVT	May have fever Painful No relevant history
SIGNS	Normal temperature Erythema, inflammation May be tender Vesicles Crusting Lesions on other parts of the body, such as other leg and arms May be unilateral or bilateral	Elevated temperature Erythema, inflammation Tenderness One or a few bullae No crusting No lesions elsewhere Unilateral
PORTALS OF ENTRY	Not applicable	Usually unknown, but breaks in skin, ulcers, trauma, tinea pedis, and intertrigo are implicated
LABORATORY	Normal WBC count Negative blood cultures Skin swabs, *Staphylococcus aureus* common	High WBC count Usually negative blood cultures Skin swabs usually negative except for necrotic tissue

DVT, Deep vein thrombosis; *WBC,* white blood cell.
Note: It is acceptable to use compression therapy with LEVD even in the presence of acute dermatitis and cellulitis.
Source: WOCN Society, 2005.

this area is the point of greatest hydrostatic pressure (See Table 15-5). Typically, these ulcers are shallow and exudative, with a dark red wound base or a thin layer of yellow slough. Venous ulcers usually have irregular edges and periwound maceration, crusting, scaling and/or hemosiderin staining (Kunimoto, 2001a; Paquette and Falanga, 2002; Phillips, 2001; Wipke-Tevis and Sae-Sia, 2004) (Plate 35).

Ankle blowout syndrome. Ankle blowout syndrome refers to the rupture of small vessels around the medial malleolus and presents as a cluster of small and acutely painful ulcers. These patients typically obtain significant relief with the application of compression therapy, which helps to reverse the underlying venous hypertension (Kunimoto, 2001a).

Mixed venous and arterial ulcers. Concomitant arterial disease occurs in as many as 25% of patients with venous ulcers; these ulcers are referred to as "mixed etiology" (de Araujo et al, 2003; Kunimoto, 2001a; Nelzen, Bergqvist, and Lindhagen, 1997; Ryan, Eager, and Sibbald, 2003). Patients can also have a combination of arterial and diabetic ulcers and/or

venous ulcers and diabetic ulcers, but these are rarely referred to as "mixed etiology." The mixed venous-arterial ulcer is typically a venous ulcer that also has to some extent a component of arterial insufficiency. In fact, wounds that began specifically as a venous ulcer can, over time, develop an arterial insufficiency component and therefore evolve into a mixed venous-arterial ulcer.

Management

Primary strategies for correction of venous insufficiency and hypertension include compression therapy, limb elevation, and surgical procedures; adjunct measures include physical therapy and exercise to improve calf muscle function, pharmacologic agents, and routine leg elevation.

Compression therapy. Compression therapy is the application of externally applied pressure or static support to the lower extremity as a means of facilitating normal venous flow. Compression therapy was used as early as the seventeenth century (in the form of rigid lace-up stockings). In the twenty-first century, compression therapy remains the cornerstone of venous ulcer management (Cullum et al, 2003; Kantor and Margolis, 2003). It is acceptable to use compression therapy with LEVD even in the presence of acute dermatitis and cellulitis (WOCN Society, 2005a).

Although there are multiple compression therapy products and options, all have advantages and disadvantages, and patients report multiple problems with their use. In addition, compression therapy merely controls the underlying venous insufficiency; so most patients require long-term therapy to prevent recurrent ulceration (Wipke-Tevis and Sae-Sia, 2004). The clinician is therefore challenged to design the most clinically effective and "patient-friendly" system for each individual, based on knowledge of the currently available products as well as patient assessment data.

Mechanisms of action. All compression therapy products are designed to provide graduated pressure from the ankle to the knee and to support the calf muscle pump during ambulation and dorsiflexion; thus these products serve to "augment" venous return. In addition, most products compress the superficial tissues, thus increasing interstitial tissue pressure and partially collapsing the superficial veins. The increased interstitial tissue pressure serves to oppose leakage of fluid into the tissues and to return interstitial fluid to the blood stream, thus eliminating edema. Compression of the superficial veins promotes coaptation and normal function of the valves, and also increases the velocity of blood flow, which reduces the aggregation and extravasation of white blood cells (Choucair and Phillips, 1998; Kunimoto, 2001b; Spence and Cahall, 1996; Weingarten, 2001).

Level of compression. An important factor in compression therapy is the *level of compression*, that is, the amount of pressure exerted against the underlying tissue. The level of compression provided by currently available devices ranges from less than 20 mm Hg to more than 60 mm Hg at the ankle.

High levels. The amount of compression considered "therapeutic" for venous ulcer management is 30 to 40 mm Hg at the ankle. This level of compression has been demonstrated to be effective in controlling venous hypertension and preventing edema formation in most patients with venous disease (de Araujo et al, 2003; Kunimoto, 2001b; Paquette and Falanga, 2002; Phillips, 2001). Some clinicians recommend even higher levels of compression for patients with severe venous insufficiency, that is, 40 to 50 mm Hg (Phillips, 2001; Weingarten, 2001).

Lower (modified) levels. Despite the fact that optimal compression is represented by at least 30 mm Hg compressive force, some studies suggest that lower levels of compression are better than no compression at all. This is a significant consideration when caring for patients who are unable to tolerate optimal levels of compression or who have coexisting arterial disease that precludes high levels of sustained compression (WOCN Society, 2002; Cullum et al, 2004; WOCN Society, 2005a). Table 15-9 correlates ABI values with acceptable levels of compression for patients with LEVD and mixed venous/arterial etiology.

Compression options. Table 15-10 provides an overview of compression therapy options.

Compression devices can be categorized as (1) sustained or static (e.g., compression wraps, stockings, and orthoses) and (2) intermittent or dynamic (e.g., pneumatic pump devices). Sustained compression devices can be further classified according to their mechanism of action, that is, inelastic as opposed to elastic.

A critical issue in the use of compression products is correct application of wraps and proper fitting of stockings. Compression wraps are a particular challenge;

TABLE 15-9 Level of Compression Guide for Patients with Lower-Extremity Venous Disease and Mixed Venous/Arterial Etiology

THERAPEUTIC LEVEL UP TO 30 mm Hg AT ANKLE	MODIFIED (LOW LEVEL) UP TO 23 mm Hg AT ANKLE	NO STATIC COMPRESSION
ABI greater than 0.8 No evidence of acute heart failure	ABI greater than 0.5 to less than 0.8* No evidence of acute heart failure	ABI less than 0.5* Clinical evidence of acute heart failure

*Intermittent pneumatic compression may be considered in the absence of acute heart failure.

TABLE 15-10 Overview of Compression Therapy Devices

CLASSIFICATION	INDICATIONS OR CONTRAINDICATIONS	COMMENTS/ CONSIDERATIONS	EXAMPLES
Sustained (static)	• Contraindicated in patient with symptomatic heart failure • Contraindicated in patient with clinical evidence of peripheral arterial disease	• Must modify compression level if ABI greater than 0.5 to less than 0.8	
Elastic • Layered compression wraps	• Good choice for early treatment (to reduce edema and control exudate) because it is changed 1-2 times/week and is absorptive • Appropriate for both actively ambulating and sedentary patients	• Must be applied by professional • Need to lubricate intact skin to prevent excessive drying	• Profore and ProGuide by Smith and Nephew • Dynapress by Johnson and Johnson
• Reusable single-layer elastic wraps ("long stretch")	• Can be used for initial treatment or maintenance therapy	• May be applied by caregiver who has been trained (some have visual indicators to facilitate correct application) • Can be reused multiple times, so may be more cost-effective	• SurePress by ConvaTec
• Therapeutic compression stockings	Good option for later treatment and maintenance therapy (need to delay use until edema is reduced and exudate controlled)	• Must be correctly fitted • Must ensure patient is able to correctly don stockings • Must teach patient proper care and importance of replacement every 3-4 months • Medicare reimbursement available for patient with venous ulcer (need to obtain stocking before complete healing)	• Jobst, Juzo, Sig-Varis, Medi-Strumpf, Therapress Duo
Inelastic • Unna's boot	• Good choice for early treatment, i.e., until edema is reduced and exudate controlled • Good choice for patient who is actively ambulating; generally less effective with sedentary patient	• Must be applied by a professional • Need to cover with outer wrap, typically self-adherent compression wrap (e.g., Coban)	• ViscoPaste by Smith and Nephew

Continued

TABLE 15-10 Overview of Compression Therapy Devices—cont'd

CLASSIFICATION	INDICATIONS OR CONTRAINDICATIONS	COMMENTS/ CONSIDERATIONS	EXAMPLES
Inelastic—cont'd	• May be used in patient with borderline ABI, i.e., greater than 0.5 to less than 0.8		
• Short-stretch wrap	• Can be used for initial treatment or for maintenance therapy • Good choice for patient who is actively ambulating; generally less effective in sedentary patient • May be used in patient with borderline ABI, i.e., greater than 0.5 to less than 0.8	• May be applied by caregiver who has been trained • Can be reused multiple times, so may be more cost-effective • Lack of elasticity makes wrap more likely to slip out of place; may cover with self-adherent outer wrap	• Comprilan by Beiersdorf Jobst
• Orthosis	Good option for later treatment and maintenance therapy (need to delay use until edema is reduced)	• Must be correctly fitted • Easy to remove and apply because of Velcro closure mechanism • Bulky	• CircAcid by Coloplast
Intermittent (dynamic) pneumatic compression	• Can be used for patient with mixed disease (arterial and venous) • Contraindicated in patient with symptomatic heart failure	• Reimbursed by Medicare only if patient has failed 6-month trial of static compression therapy	• Huntleigh

High compression options	**Modified, reduced compression options**
• Layered compression wraps • Reusable single-layer elastic wraps ("long stretch") • Therapeutic compression stockings	• Therapeutic compression stockings (less than 30 mm Hg) • Modified layered compression wraps (e.g., Profore "light") • Unna's boot • Short-stretch wrap • Orthosis

studies indicate that nurses frequently apply the wrap with insufficient tension to produce therapeutic level pressures, even when they are "experienced" in compression bandaging. Training has been shown to significantly improve accuracy, but further studies are needed to quantify the interval at which this training should be repeated (Feben, 2003).

Sustained (static) compression. Compression wraps are one of the most commonly used compression products, especially during early therapy when limb volumes are changing rapidly as a result of edema reduction. Most wraps are applied by professionals and are left in place for 3 to 7 days; some also provide for significant absorption of exudate.

All compression wraps are designed based on LaPlace's law of physics, which is illustrated in Figure 15-9. LaPlace's law states that sub-bandage pressure is directly proportional to the tension and number of bandage layers and inversely proportional to leg circumference and bandage width. In other words, sub-bandage pressure is equal to the stretch (tension) applied to the wrap, multiplied by the number of layers, divided by the circumference of the leg multiplied by

the width of the bandage (Kunimoto, 2001b; Moffatt and O'Hare, 1995). LaPlace's law explains why application of a wrap with constant tension will create graduated pressure: because bandage tension is held constant while the circumference of the leg increases steadily from ankle to knee, the sub-bandage pressure will be highest at the ankle and lowest at the knee (Kunimoto, 2001b).

The most commonly used wraps are the nonelastic paste wrap (i.e., "Unna's boot"), the layered elastic wraps, and single layer short stretch bandages. There are no conclusive data indicating superiority of one type of

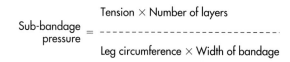

$$\text{Sub-bandage pressure} = \frac{\text{Tension} \times \text{Number of layers}}{\text{Leg circumference} \times \text{Width of bandage}}$$

Fig. 15-9 LaPlace's law of physics as it applies to compression bandaging. LaPlace's law demonstrates how compression therapy is a function of tension, number of layers, leg circumference, and bandage width. Increases in tension and/or layering increase sub-bandage pressure, whereas increases in leg circumference and/or bandage width decrease sub-bandage pressure.

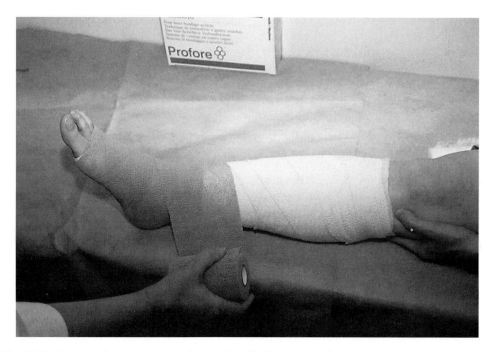

Fig. 15-10 Compression wraps: Unna's boot with self-adherent stretch cover-wrap. Note foot at 90° angle to leg.

wrap over another. The "wrap of choice" appears to differ according to geographic location; for example, Unna's boot is most commonly used in the United States, the layered wraps are most common in the United Kingdom, and the short stretch bandages are most common in Europe and Australia (Cullum et al, 2003).

Nonelastic compression. Nonelastic devices are designed to augment the function of the calf muscle pump; they provide limited compression at rest but effectively compress the calf during ambulation. Nonelastic devices are therefore indicated primarily for patients who are actively ambulating, and are safer for patients with coexisting arterial disease (de Araujo et al, 2003; Phillips, 2001). Examples of nonelastic compression methods include (1) the nonelastic paste bandage and (2) orthotic devices.

Nonelastic paste bandage. Dr. Paul Unna was the first to introduce use of a zinc paste bandage to create a conformable but inelastic "boot" around the leg; thus paste-type compression wraps are commonly referred to as *Unna's boot* (Weingarten, 2001). Today there are a number of gauze wraps that are used to provide an inelastic compression dressing; most are impregnated with zinc oxide, glycerine, and gelatine, though some also contain additional ingredients such as calamine (Wipke-Tevis and Sae-Sia, 2004). The bandage should be applied without tension beginning at the base of the toes and extending to the tibial tuberosity below the knee; the patient must be reminded to maintain the foot in a dorsiflexed position while the paste wrap is applied (Figure 15-10). Clinicians use a variety of techniques to ensure a smooth conformable "fit" to the inelastic bandage; for example, pleating, reverse folding, and cutting and restarting are all common and appropriate techniques (Wipke-Tevis and Sae-Sia, 2004). If the paste layer is left open to air, it dries to a "semicast" consistency. However, most commonly the paste layer is covered with an elastic bandage or a self-adherent wrap (e.g., Coban, 3M Company, Minneapolis, MN). This provides an "active compression" layer and also prevents soiling of clothing with the zinc paste bandage. (See Box 15-18 for a suggested procedure for paste bandage application.)

As noted earlier, nonelastic devices such as Unna's boot are most appropriate for actively ambulating patients because they work primarily by supporting the calf muscle pump. The Unna's boot should be changed when the patient detects a loosening of the boot or anytime the wrap becomes saturated with drainage (typically every 3 to 7 days).

Orthotic devices. The Circ-Aid Thera-Boot (Coloplast Corporation, Marietta, GA) is an orthotic device that works by augmenting calf pump function, in addition to providing a level of continuous compression (Figure 15-11). It consists of multiple Velcro straps that can be adjusted by the patient or caregiver for optimal fit and comfort. Although the device is bulky, the ability to adjust the product and the ease of removal and application may improve compliance among motivated individuals who are unable to tolerate other forms of compression therapy (Phillips, 2001). In addition, the ability to remove and reapply the device permits more frequent bathing and wound care.

ELASTIC COMPRESSION. Products with elasticity adapt to changes in limb volume and are therefore able to provide compression both at rest and during ambulation. These devices are better choices for patients who

---

BOX 15-18 **Procedure for Paste Bandage Application**

1. Apply gloves.
2. Gently wash extremity and dry.
3. Place patient in supine position with affected leg elevated. Foot and leg should be at a 90-degree angle.
4. Open all paste bandage wrappers and cover wrap. Estimate amount for at least two layers of paste bandaging on the leg.
5. Holding paste bandage roll in nondominant hand. Begin to apply bandage at base of toes.
6. Wrap twice around toes without using tension.
7. Continue wrapping bandage around foot, ankle, and heel, using a circular technique, with each strip overlapping the previous strip approximately 50% to 80%.
8. Smooth paste bandage while applying, and remove any wrinkles and folds (may pleat, reverse fold, or cut to assure smooth bandage).
9. Wrap up to knee and finish smoothing.
10. Remove gloves.
11. Apply cover wrap using recommended amount of tension (e.g., 50% stretch with Coban wrap).
12. Remove twice weekly, weekly, or every other week as indicated by leakage, hygiene, or anticipated decrease in edema.

are relatively sedentary or who have a "shuffling" gait that fails to engage the calf muscle (de Araujo et al, 2003; Phillips, 2001).

Layered bandage systems. Layered bandage systems combine nonelastic and elastic layers to provide

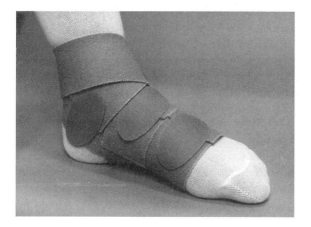

Fig. 15-11 Orthotic compression device: the Circ-Aid. (Courtesy Coloplast Corp., Marietta, Ga.)

sustained compression at rest and during activity. These systems are available as two-layer, three-layer, and four-layer systems; all provide one or two inner layers that afford padding of bony prominences and absorption of exudate, and one or two elastic layers that afford sustained compression. In many settings, these devices have become the "product of choice" for early intervention, owing to their ability to absorb exudate, adapt to changes in limb size, and provide sustained compression both at rest and with activity. In applying layered bandage systems, clinicians must follow manufacturers' guidelines in order to ensure therapeutic and safe levels of compression (Figure 15-12). For example, some wraps are designed to be applied with a spiral technique, whereas others require a figure-eight application to achieve optimal results. The most critical element of effective application is the correct degree of tension; insufficient tension compromises therapeutic outcomes whereas excessive tension places the patient at risk for tissue damage. Again, clinicians must base their application technique on manufacturers' guidelines and must continually monitor their clinical outcomes to

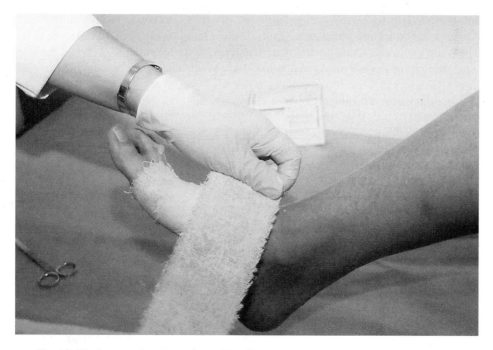

Fig. 15-12 Compression wraps: layered bandage system. (Profore J. Smith and Nephew, Ltd.).

assure that their technique is correct. Some products incorporate a visual indicator that helps to ensure the correct level of tension (Kunimoto, 2001b; Phillips, 2001; Wipke-Tevis and Sae-Sia, 2004).

Single-layer reusable compression wraps. Single-layer reusable compression wraps are available as nonelastic short-stretch wraps (e.g., Comprilan by Jobst) and as elastic long-stretch compression wraps (such as Surepress [Convatec]). The nonelastic short-stretch wraps provide high-level support for the calf muscle pump and excellent outcomes for the actively ambulating patient, but are ineffective with sedentary patients (Kunimoto, 2001b). In contrast, because elastic long-stretch compression wraps provide sustained compression, they can be used for both sedentary and actively ambulating patients.

A major advantage of single-layer reusable wraps is their "wash and reuse" feature; if there is a caregiver who can be taught to apply the wrap correctly, this feature permits more frequent removal for bathing and dressing changes and also contributes to cost-effective care. Many of these wraps incorporate a visual indicator of correct tension, which is advantageous when teaching a caregiver how to apply the wrap (Phillips, 2001; Wipke-Tevis and Sae-Sia, 2004).

A disadvantage of single layer reusable compression wraps is their limited conformability, which means they are more likely to slip out of place; this is particularly true of the short-stretch bandages. One approach to this problem is to add a self-adherent elastic wrap such as Coban (Phillips, 2001). While this technique holds the wrap in place, it adds cost, especially if the wrap is being changed frequently. Another potential problem with the short-stretch bandages is the possibility of pressure injury over bony prominences, especially in patients with small limbs; padding over bony prominences is beneficial in this situation.

Support stockings. Therapeutic support stockings are most commonly used for patients with stable venous insufficiency to prevent ulceration (either initial or recurrent). They may also be used for patients with an existing ulcer once the edema has been controlled and the limb circumference has stabilized. Stockings are generally not a good choice for compression during the initiation of therapy, owing to the rapid changes in limb circumference associated with edema reduction. Another relative contraindication for stocking use is severe lipodermatosclerosis, because the "inverted champagne bottle" configuration of the leg in this condition makes it difficult to obtain a good fit. Stockings are appropriate for sedentary as well as actively ambulating patients, because the elasticity of support stockings provides support both at rest and with activity.

Stockings are available in various levels of compression (Table 15-11), and in a variety of sizes, colors, and styles (e.g., open-toe as opposed to closed-toe and knee-high as opposed to thigh-high). Most patients

TABLE 15-11 **Compression Stockings: Levels of Compression**

	U.S. DEFINITION	U.K. DEFINITION	INDICATIONS
CLASS 1	20-30 mm Hg (light support)	14-17 mm Hg (light support)	Treatment of varicose veins
CLASS 2	30-40 mm Hg (medium support)	18-24 mm Hg (medium support)	U.S.: Venous ulcer treatment and prevention U.K.: Treatment of severe venous insufficiency and prevention venous ulcers
CLASS 3	40-50 mm Hg (strong support)	25-35 mm Hg (strong support)	U.S.: Treatment of refractory venous ulcers and lymphedema U.K.: Treatment and prevention of venous ulcers
CLASS 4	50-60 mm Hg (very strong support)	N/A	U.S.: Lymphedema U.K.: N/A

U.S., United States; *U.K.*, United Kingdom.

with venous ulceration are effectively managed with knee-high stockings, which are generally better tolerated; however, the stocking must be sized correctly, and the clinician must ensure the patient's ability to correctly don the stocking (Phillips, 2001; Weingarten, 2001). Patients should be instructed to purchase two pairs of stockings at a time, so that they have a pair to wear while the other pair is being laundered. Tips for stocking donning and key points to be covered in patient education are outlined in Box 15-19; Figure 15-13 illustrates devices to facilitate stocking application (Phillips, 2001; Wipke-Tevis and Sae-Sia, 2001).

Stockings are the "mainstay" of long-term compression. Unfortunately patients report multiple problems with their use, such as difficulty with application, comfort issues, and cost issues (there is very limited reimbursement for compression stockings, and they are costly) (Wipke-Tevis and Sae-Sia, 2004). It is therefore critical for the wound care clinician to educate the patient regarding the importance of compression, to discuss the various options, to *hear* the patient's concerns, and to *involve* the patient in decision making regarding both short-term and long-term management (Furlong, 2001).

Elastic stockinette type of sleeve. An alternative that provides consistent low-level compression is known as Elastocrepe or Tubigrip (WOCN Society, 2005a). According to the manufacturers, these products are elasticized stockinette sleeves that provide 18 to 20 mm Hg pressure when applied as a double layer.

Contraindications to sustained compression. Although most patients tolerate sustained compression well and respond favorably, the clinician must be aware of two contraindications to high-level sustained compression: uncompensated heart failure and coexisting peripheral arterial disease. Uncompensated (unstable) heart failure is a contraindication because mobilization of edema fluid into the systemic circulation

---

BOX 15-19 Patient Education Tips Regarding Compression Stockings

Tips for getting stockings on:
- Don stockings immediately upon arising
- Use rubber gloves to don stockings—they significantly improve grip!
- Consider use of a commercial device designed to facilitate stocking application:
    stocking "butler" (Jobst); easy-slide toe sleeves for open-toe stockings (Jobst, Juzo, Sig-Varis, Medi-Strumpf)
- Use a silky stocking "liner"
- Use a "layered" approach: either two-piece stockings (Therapress Duo) or two layers of lower-compression stockings (e.g., two layers of a stocking, each of which provides 15-mm Hg compression)

Care and management
- Purchase two pairs of stockings at a time to permit laundering
- Launder with mild detergent; line dry (follow manufacturer's guidelines)
- Replace stockings every 3 to 4 months to maintain therapeutic efficacy

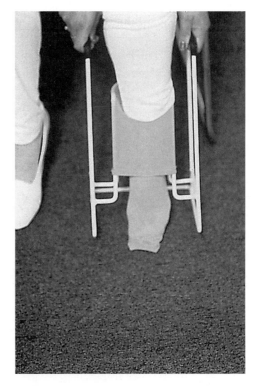

Fig. 15-13 Application of a therapeutic support stocking with a "stocking donner".

could increase preload volume and precipitate pulmonary edema (de Araujo et al, 2003; Weingarten, 2001). An ABI of 0.5 or less is a contraindication because the high levels of sustained tissue pressure exerted by compression devices could further compromise tissue perfusion and potentially cause ischemic tissue death (de Araujo et al, 2003; Weingarten, 2001). These contraindications to sustained compression reinforce the importance of thorough pretreatment evaluation to include cardiac history, any indicators of heart failure, and ABI measurements.

Patients without evidence of acute heart failure and an ABI of greater than 0.8 are candidates for *high-level compression therapy*. Patients with an ABI of greater than 0.5 to less than 0.8, or borderline cardiac status, are best managed with *low-level compression* (20- to 23-mm Hg compression at the ankle). Finally, patients with an ABI of 0.5 or less or acute heart failure are best managed with leg elevation but *no compression* (WOCN Society, 2002; Kunimoto, 2001b) (See Table 15-9).

Antiembolism hose/support (ace) bandages. Support bandages, most commonly known as Ace bandages, provide low levels of compression and are not considered therapeutic for patients with LEVD and venous ulceration. Ace-type bandages tend to stretch when the calf expands, and thus fail to provide calf muscle support during ambulation. In addition, they are very user-dependent and are frequently applied incorrectly. Antiembolism hose or stockings (15 to 17 mm Hg) are not designed for therapeutic compression (WOCN Society, 2005a).

Intermittent (dynamic) pneumatic compression (IPC). Dynamic compression therapy, commonly known as "intermittent pneumatic compression (IPC)," may be used for patients who are immobile or who need higher levels of compression than can be provided with stockings or wraps (LEVD). IPC involves use of an air pump to intermittently inflate a sleeve applied to the lower extremity (Figure 15-14). Intermittent compression can be used as adjunct therapy to sustained compression therapy, or as an alternative for patients who are unable to tolerate sustained compression (Kunimoto, 2001b). Typically, patients are instructed to apply the therapy once or twice daily for 1 to 2 hours each time. Intermittent compression devices vary in terms of the inflation-deflation cycle, amount of pressure

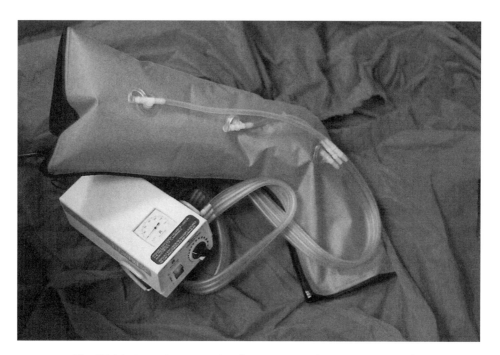

Fig. 15-14 Dynamic compression device: sequential compression therapy.

exerted against the leg, and the number of compartments in the sleeve. Single-compartment sleeves simply inflate and deflate on a cyclic basis, while multicompartment sleeves provide for sequential compression (i.e., a distal to proximal "milking" compression wave); computer-simulated models suggest that the sequential compression devices have the greatest impact on venous return (Chen et al, 2001).

There are a number of documented benefits of IPC therapy: mobilization of interstitial (edema) fluid back into the circulation, enhanced venous return, and increased arterial inflow (owing to the increased pressure gradient created by improved venous emptying). IPC is thought to exert antithrombotic and vasodilatory effects, possibly as a result of the marked increase in the velocity of blood flow and the resultant "shear stress" at the level of the endothelial cells (Chen et al, 2001).

IPC therapy may contribute to healing of long-standing venous ulcers that have "failed" standard compression therapy (Berliner, Ozbilgin, and Zarin, 2003; Mani, Vowden, and Nelson, 2004). In addition, these studies reported higher levels of patient satisfaction and adherence to therapy. In the United States, these devices are covered by Centers for Medicare and Medicaid Services only for patients with refractory edema and ulceration who have "failed" a 6-month trial of sustained compression therapy (Berliner, Ozbilgin, and Zarin, 2003).

IPC therapy is generally considered contraindicated for patients with uncompensated heart failure because of the potential for rapid fluid shifts causing further cardiac decompensation (de Araujo et al, 2003). However, it is an appropriate therapy for most patients with mixed arterial and venous disease, and may be beneficial for patients with pure arterial disease (Chen et al, 2001). It is generally not used for patients with an active thrombus because of the potential for embolism.

Limb Elevation. Limb elevation is a simple but effective strategy for improving venous return by the use of gravitational forces. This is an important component of management for any patient with venous insufficiency, but it is an *essential* element of therapy for patients who are unable to adhere to a compression therapy regimen. Patients should be taught to lie down and elevate the affected leg above the level of the heart for at least 1 to 2 hours twice daily, as well as during sleep. In addition, these patients should be taught to strictly avoid prolonged standing or prolonged sitting with the legs dependent. Periods of standing or sitting must be interspersed with walking. Asking the patient to keep a "legs-up" chart can reinforce the importance of leg elevation. This chart should then be reviewed at each visit (Kunimoto, 2001b; Wipke-Tevis and Sae-Sia, 2004).

Surgical Management. Surgical intervention is primarily indicated for the patient with significant lipodermatosclerosis or persistent or recurrent ulceration whose underlying pathology involves valvular incompetence; surgical intervention is of less benefit when there is significant outflow obstruction, as occurs with postthrombotic syndrome (Anwar et al, 2003).

The most commonly performed surgical procedures are *ligation* and *stripping of the superficial (saphenous) veins,* and *open* or *endoscopic ligation of incompetent perforator veins.* The procedure of choice depends on the components of the venous system that are incompetent (Anwar et al, 2003; Kalra and Gloviczki, 2003). For example, ligation and stripping of the saphenous veins is most effective when the valvular incompetence is limited to the superficial system. This procedure may also be of some benefit when there is concomitant involvement of the perforator system, but is of no benefit when the pathology involves the deep system (Kalra and Gloviczki, 2003). The procedure of choice for patients with significant perforator and/or deep vein incompetence is ligation of the incompetent perforator veins, which acts to prevent transmission of the elevated pressures within the deep system to the vulnerable superficial veins and tissues. This procedure may be combined with superficial vein stripping for patients who also have significant saphenous vein incompetence. In the past, ligation of perforator veins was performed as an open procedure (the Linton procedure). However, the current trend is to perform the procedure endoscopically, that is, the subfascial endoscopic perforator surgery (SEPS) procedure, when possible.

Better outcomes have been observed with the endoscopic approach as compared both to open surgical procedures and to conservative therapy alone, although there are no large randomized controlled trials to clearly define the role of this procedure in venous ulcer management. Current consensus is that the procedure should be reserved for patients with significant symptomatic venous insufficiency unresponsive to conservative medical management (Anwar et al, 2003; Kalra and Gloviczki, 2003; Lee et al, 2003; Russell and Logsdon, 2002; Tenbrook et al, 2004; Weingarten, 2001).

Patients with deep venous insufficiency who fail both conservative management and ligation of superficial and perforator veins should be considered for deep vein reconstruction (Kalra and Gloviczki, 2003). Patients who are considering surgical intervention should have a thorough diagnostic workup to clearly define the incompetent veins and to determine the presence and severity of outflow obstruction. In addition, patients must understand that surgical intervention does not guarantee long-term "cure" and that compression stockings will still be needed, at least short-term (Anwar et al, 2003).

Physical Therapy and Exercise. As explained earlier, normal function of the calf muscle pump is critical to venous return, and effective contraction of the calf muscle requires a mobile ankle and routine dorsiflexion beyond 90 degrees. Therefore a patient with reduced ankle mobility or a "shuffling" gait should have a physical therapy evaluation to determine if he or she could benefit from gait retraining and routine exercises to increase ankle strength and range of motion. A home-based exercise program including isotonic exercise can improve poor calf muscle and calf muscle pump function (WOCN Society, 2005). All patients with venous insufficiency should be encouraged to perform ankle pumps routinely when standing or sitting and to intersperse standing and sitting with walking (Kunimoto, 2001b; Orsted, Radke, and Gorst, 2001; Wipke-Tevis and Sae-Sia, 2004).

Weight Control. Obesity is one of the factors known to interfere with venous return and to increase the risk for LEVD. In fact morbid obesity can actually *cause* insufficiency in the deep venous system. In addition, significant obesity makes it very difficult for the patient to adhere to compression therapy and to avoid prolonged sitting. It is therefore important to educate patients regarding the relationship between weight and venous disease, and to strongly encourage patients to reduce their weight to a healthy level. Patients who are morbidly obese should be referred to a bariatric treatment center for evaluation and management (Phillips, 2001; Wipke-Tevis and Sae-Sia, 2004).

Pharmacologic therapy. Venous outflow obstruction, valvular failure, and CVI are structural and functional abnormalities that cannot be "corrected" pharmacologically. However, there are several pharmacologic agents that have demonstrated benefit in the management of venous disease, primarily as a result of their ability to interfere with the pathologic events that lead to skin and soft tissue changes, that is, leukocyte activation and migration. The three agents with documented efficacy in the management of venous disease are pentoxifylline (Trental), sulodexide and mesoglycan, micronized purified flavonoid fraction (Daflon), and horse chestnut seed extract (HCSE).

Pentoxifylline. In the United States, pentoxifylline (Trental) is the drug most commonly prescribed for venous disease and appears to be an effective adjunct to compression therapy. Its mechanism of action appears to be reduced aggregation of platelets and white blood cells, which reduces capillary plugging, and enhanced blood flow in the microcirculation, which reduces tissue ischemia (Jull, Waters, and Arroll, 2004; Kunimoto, 2001b; Phillips, 2001). Dosages of 400 mg orally 3 times daily can accelerate healing of venous ulcers and should be considered in slow-healing venous ulcers (WOCN Society, 2005a).

Pentoxifylline may also promote healing even in the absence of compression. However, the beneficial effects of pentoxifylline must be balanced against its potential adverse effects (e.g., diarrhea and nausea) and its cost. Therefore, pentoxifylline is generally reserved for patients who fail to respond to standard therapy as opposed to being used for routine care (Jull, Waters, and Arroll, 2004; Kunimoto, 2001b; Phillips, 2001).

Sulodexide and mesoglycan. Nelson and Bradley (2003) found that compression plus sulodexide (a glycosaminoglycan) or mesoglycan (a sulphated polysaccharide) increased the proportion of ulcers healed compared with compression alone.

Micronized purified flavonoid fraction (MPFF). Although not available in the United States, Europe and other countries have approved a phlebotropic drug known as micronized purified flavonoid fraction (Daflon) to improve outcomes for patients with LEVD. The specific mechanisms of action include that it (1) enhances venous tone, which promotes venous return; (2) reduces capillary permeability, which reduces edema formation; and (3) reduces expression of endothelial adhesion molecules, which reduces margination, activation, and migration of leukocytes.

These mechanisms reduce the release of inflammatory mediators, which is thought to be the primary pathologic event resulting in dermatitis, lipodermatosclerosis, and ulceration (Coleridge-Smith, 2003; Lyseng-Williamson and Perry, 2003; Simka and Majewski, 2003).

The combination of MPFF with standard therapy (compression plus topical therapy) resulted in a statistically significant improvement in healing rates when compared to standard therapy alone or to placebo in a double-blind trial, with a side effect profile comparable to placebo. In addition, cost analysis studies have shown a significant reduction in cost to healing when compared to conventional therapy. Finally, studies indicate a significant improvement in quality of life scores for patients with LEVD treated with MMPF (Coleridge-Smith, 2003; Lyseng-Williamson and Perry, 2003; Simka and Majewski, 2003).

Horse chestnut seed extract (HCSE). Another agent currently thought to be of benefit in the management of LEVD is the herbal agent horse chestnut seed extract (HCSE). Several placebo-controlled trials suggest that treatment with HCSE results in decreased pain and a significant reduction in edema as evidenced by leg volume measurement. Interestingly, one study reported comparable outcomes between HCSE and compression therapy. However, more study is needed to clearly identify the role of HCSE in treatment of patients with venous insufficiency and venous ulceration. The suggested dose is 250 mg 2 to 3 times daily (WOCN Society, 2005a; Pittler and Ernst, 2003).

Treat Dermatitis. As noted, dermatitis is a common issue in the management of patients with venous ulcers and leads to pruritus, weeping, and tenderness. Because venous dermatitis is often treated unsuccessfully as cellulitis, wound care specialists must recognize the difference between venous dermatitis and cellulitis (Table 15-8) of the leg (WOCN Society, 2005a). Inflammatory mediators released by activated leukocytes probably cause venous dermatitis, so the skin that is affected by the dermatitis is more vulnerable to irritants and allergens. Therefore ingredients in products should be reviewed for possible irritants. To avoid creating a "vicious cycle" in which one form of dermatitis leads to another, it should be treated promptly to control symptoms and break the inflammatory cycle. Low-dose, short-term (2 weeks) topical corticosteroids are usually sufficient. Patients with severe or nonresponsive dermatitis should be referred to dermatology for management (Bonham, 2003; Kunimoto, 2001b; Ryan, Eager, and Sibbald, 2003).

Topical Therapy. The initial focus in topical therapy is elimination of any necrotic tissue and identification and control of critical colonization or invasive infection, since necrosis and infection prolong the inflammatory phase and prevent healing. Necrotic tissue is easily identified; it typically presents as moist adherent slough and can be removed via enzymatic, instrumental, or autolytic debridement. (See Chapter 10 for additional guidance on debridement options.) Invasive infection, that is, cellulitis, is also easy to identify; indicators include erythema, induration, tenderness of the periwound tissue, and possibly systemic manifestations (e.g., fever, leukocytosis, and malaise). There is widespread agreement that cellulitis requires treatment with a broad-spectrum antibiotic; topical antimicrobials are insufficient because the infection involves the surrounding tissue (WOCN Society, 2005a; Kunimoto, 2001b; Ryan, Eager, and Sibbald, 2003).

A more challenging infectious complication is the condition sometimes known as "critical colonization"; a term used to denote a bacterial burden sufficient to interfere with the wound healing process, but insufficient to mount an invasive infection. Critical colonization must be recognized and treated if healing is to occur; thus the wound care clinician must be alert to the indicators (e.g., sudden deterioration in quality or quantity of granulation tissue; recurrent formation of thin layer of slough; increased wound pain; friable wound bed; and high-volume exudate). Since critical colonization represents a *surface* infection, topical agents such as sustained-release iodine and sustained-release silver are frequently used as "first intervention"; oral antibiotics may be required if there is inadequate response to topical agents (WOCN Society, 2005a; Kunimoto, 2001b; Ryan, Eager, and Sibbald, 2003). Critical colonization and bacterial burden are discussed in detail in Chapter 9.

Once a clean wound bed is established, the focus of topical therapy becomes exudate management and maintenance of a moist and protected wound surface. Patients with venous ulcers are at increased risk for both irritant contact dermatitis and allergic contact dermatitis. Therefore the wound care clinician must select products that effectively control exudate while minimizing the risk of a sensitivity reaction, and must incorporate periulcer skin protection into the management plan. An appropriate rule of thumb is to select dressings that will effectively manage the exudate and to minimize use of products with potential allergens. It is also beneficial to protect the peri-wound skin either with a petrolatum product or a skin sealant. Products that effectively control exudate include absorptive dressings such as alginates, hydrofibers, and foams. Products that are more likely to cause a sensitivity reaction include compounds with adhesives, neomycin, fragrance, lanolin, and preservatives (Bonham, 2003: Kunimoto, 2001b; Ryan, Eager, and Sibbald, 2003).

Interactive wound therapies. Unfortunately a significant number of venous ulcers fail to heal with "standard" management (compression therapy and optimal local wound care) (Paquette and Falanga, 2002). Factors associated with failure to heal include increased ulcer size (larger than 5 cm^2) and longer duration (longer than 6 months), as well as failure to show significant progress toward healing during the first 3 to 4 weeks of compression therapy. Coexisting arterial disease, persistence of fibrin throughout the wound bed, reduced mobility, and a history of vein ligation or knee or hip replacement are also negative prognostic indicators (Paquette and Falanga, 2002; Phillips, 2001).

When confronted with a wound that fails to progress, the clinician must carefully reevaluate the entire treatment plan to assure appropriateness, and should also consider biopsy to rule out malignancy. If the biopsy is negative and the management plan is appropriate, the most likely reason for failure to heal is the negative cellular environment of a chronic wound. In this case, the clinician should consider implementation of an interactive wound therapy, that is, a product or therapy designed to convert the chronic wound environment into an environment that supports repair. Specific therapies that have shown varying degrees of success in management of refractory venous ulcers include skin grafts, bioengineered human skin equivalents, negative-pressure wound therapy, ultrasound, and selected growth factors (Choucair, Faria, and Fivenson, 1998; de Araujo et al, 2003; Demling et al, 2004; Dolynchuk et al, 1999; Flemming and Cullum, 2003; Johnson, 2003; Omar et al, 2004; Paquette and Falanga, 2002;

Phillips, 2001). These therapies are discussed in greater detail in Chapters 5, 18 and 20.

Prevent Recurrence. With recurrence rates during the first 12 months following ulcer healing ranging between 26% and 69%, the emphasis in management must shift to prevention of recurrence once the ulcer is healed (Nelson, Bell-Syer, and Cullum, 2004). Conventional clinical wisdom supports lifelong use of compression therapy to control the underlying venous insufficiency and thereby prevent recurrent ulceration; it is an approach that makes biologic sense. However, relatively few studies are available that address the issues related to recurrent ulceration. There is a paucity of research that identifies the patients who are at greatest risk for recurrence, objectively defines the efficacy of continued compression, or establishes the appropriate level of compression needed to prevent recurrence.

Many patients fail to utilize compression consistently, for a variety of reasons (Furlong, 2001; Jull et al, 2004; Nelson et al, 2004). In one study, the two factors that were most predictive of patients' continued use of compression therapy were their perception of the value of compression, and the level of comfort/discomfort associated with the stockings (Jull et al, 2004). These findings clearly speak to the importance of effectively communicating to the patient the reasons for and the importance of continued use of compression, and the value of working *with* the patient to ensure that the stockings chosen are comfortable to wear. For example, this may mean placing the patient in a lower level of compression so they are able to apply the garment. While there is evidence suggesting that high-level compression may be more effective in preventing recurrence, there is also evidence that compliance rates are significantly higher with medium-level compression (Furlong, 2001; Jull et al, 2004; Nelson et al, 2004).

LYMPHEDEMA

Although edema formation is a consequence of venous disease, the extent, severity, and etiology of edema associated with lymphedema is much different. Similarly, the management of lymphedema differs in significant ways from the management of venous edema and venous ulcers. The wound care clinician must be knowledgeable of the pathology, differential assessment, and management of lymphedema so that a distinction between this disease and venous insufficiency can be made in a timely manner. Appropriate management of the weeping and inflamed skin, maceration, and ulcerations that commonly complicate lymphedema can then be provided (Macdonald, Sims, and Mayrovitz, 2003).

Epidemiology

The lymphatic system is the third component of the vascular system but the one that receives the least attention; similarly, lymphedema and related pathologies have received much less attention than the pathologies associated with venous and arterial ulcers. Worldwide, the most common cause of lymphedema is filariasis, a parasitic infection of the lymph nodes found in certain developing countries. In the Western world, there are two primary types of lymphedema: primary lymphedema and secondary lymphedema. Primary lymphedema is a rare condition caused by a congenital defect in the lymphatic system, whereas secondary lymphedema is a much more common condition that occurs as a result of damage to the lymphatics.

Etiology

Specific conditions associated with the development of lymphedema include chronic venous insufficiency and venous hypertension, trauma, cancer therapy (lymphadenectomy and radiation), vascular reconstruction, joint replacement, and harvesting of veins for coronary artery bypass procedures (Macdonald, Sims, and Mayrovitz, 2003; Sarvis, 2003; Tiwari et al, 2003). The incidence of lymphedema is expected to increase as a result of the increasing numbers of joint replacements, vascular procedures, and venous disease.

Normal Lymphatic Function. To understand lymphedema and its management, it is essential to have a basic understanding of normal lymphatic function. The lymphatic system consists of open-ended lymphatic capillaries, lymphatic vessels (lymph collectors), regional lymph nodes, and lymphatic ducts (Figure 15-15). There are several similarities between the venous system and the lymphatic system. The larger lymphatic vessels (the collectors) contain valves to promote one-way flow of lymph, and there is both a superficial and a deep lymphatic system. As is true of venous flow, lymph flow proceeds from the superficial to the deep system and from distal to proximal, facilitated by the respiratory cycle and by skeletal muscle contraction (Macdonald, Sims, and Mayrovitz, 2003).

A major function of the lymphatic system is the maintenance of normal plasma volume. Specifically, the lymphatic vessels absorb 2 to 4 liters of protein-rich fluid retained in the interstitial space daily, the product of the imbalance between diffusion of fluid out of the capillary bed (on the arterial side) and return of fluid to the capillary bed (on the venous side). This fluid is picked up by the lymphatic capillaries and eventually returned to the blood stream, thus maintaining normal plasma volume and preventing interstitial edema (Macdonald, Sims, and Mayrovitz, 2003; Villavicencio and Pikoulis, 1997). Further protection against edema is provided by the inherent reserve capacity of the lymphatic system; the capacity for lymph transport is considerably greater than the amount of lymph normally produced. The lymphatic system also has important secondary functions that include the removal of toxic substances and damaged cells from the tissues, protection against infection, and defense against the spread of malignancy. Lymph nodes, which are located at various points along the larger lymphatic channels, contain large numbers of lymphocytes. These lymphocytes "clear" the lymph of toxins, pathogens, and malignant cells (Terry, O'Brien, and Kerstein, 1998; Villavicencio and Pikoulis, 1997).

Pathology

Lymphedema occurs as a result of one of two pathologic processes: (1) a significant increase in lymph production that overwhelms the adaptive capacity of the lymphatic system, (a less common cause), or (2) a significant reduction in the capacity for lymph transport owing to lymphatic damage (the "usual" cause). Lymph node excision, radiation fibrosis, and long-standing venous disease are known to damage the lymphatic transport system. Chronic venous insufficiency and venous hypertension cause leakage of red blood cells and blood proteins into the tissues, which results in progressive dermal fibrosis. These fibrotic changes in the soft tissues result in progressive obstruction to lymphatic flow resulting from distortion or obliteration of the lymphatic channels (Macdonald, Sims, and Mayrovitz, 2003; Sarvis, 2003; Tiwari et al, 2003).

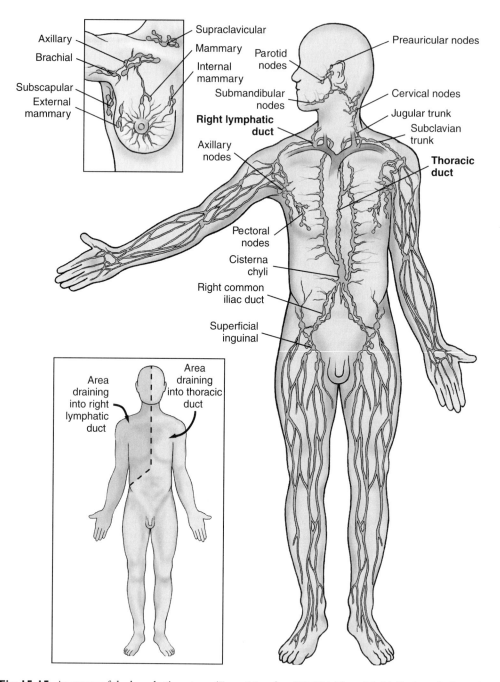

Fig. 15-15 Anatomy of the lymphatic system. (From Monahan FD, Neighbors M: *Medical surgical nursing: foundations for clinical practice*, ed 2, Philadelphia, 1998, Saunders.)

Regardless of the specific cause, the end result of compromised lymphatic return is the progressive accumulation of protein-rich fluid in the interstitial space, causing further fibrosis in the soft tissues and even greater lymphatic obstruction (Macdonald, Sims, and Mayrovitz, 2003).

Lymphedema is clinically staged as described in Table 15-12 (Macdonald, 2003). Severity is also classified according to the amount of edema in the limb: less than 20% larger than the unaffected limb is considered indicative of mild edema, while more than 40% larger than the unaffected limb signals severe edema (Macdonald, Sims, and Mayrovitz, 2003; Sarvis, 2003).

Patients with lymphedema are at high risk for recurrent infections, cellulitis, and lymphangitis because of the compromised function of the lymphatic system and the high protein content of the lymphatic fluid. Constant surveillance for signs of infection and prompt treatment are indicated since inflammation causes further fibrosis, which results in even greater obstruction to lymphatic drainage (Sarvis, 2003; Tiwari et al, 2003).

TABLE 15-12 **Stages of Lymphedema**

	MANIFESTATIONS
STAGE 1	Reversible pitting edema that begins distally (at the foot)
	Negative or borderline Stemmer sign
	No palpable fibrosis
STAGE 2	Minimally pitting or nonpitting (brawny) edema that is not reduced by simple measures such as elevation
	Positive Stemmer sign
	Pronounced fibrosis
	Hyperkeratosis (thickening of the skin)
	Papillomatosis (skin has a rough cobblestone appearance and texture)
STAGE 3	Lymphostatic elephantiasis (massive enlargement and distortion of the limb caused by breakdown of the skin's elastic components)
	Progressive fibrosis, hyperkeratosis, and papillomatosis
	Ulceration

Assessment Parameters

Initial diagnosis is made based on patient history and clinical presentation.

Patient History. Lymphedema should be suspected in the patient who has had an inguinal node dissection with or without radiation therapy. Gynecologic, prostate, or kidney cancer and melanoma are examples of diseases that are treated with node dissection. Lymphedema can occur immediately after surgery, within a few months, within a couple of years, or as long as 20 years after cancer therapy. The patient history with regard to joint surgery or coronary artery bypass should also be obtained. The presence of these factors in addition to the physical assessment findings should be sufficient to distinguish lymphedema from venous insufficiency.

Physical Assessment. The earliest clinical indicator is painless pitting edema, which progresses to brawny (nonpitting) edema and fibrotic changes in the skin and soft tissues (hyperkeratosis and papillomatosis). Eventually elephantiasis (loss of the elastic components of the skin resulting in massive distortion and enlargement of the limb) may develop. One clinical sign that is considered pathognomonic for lymphedema is a positive Stemmer sign, that is, when it is not possible to pinch a fold of skin at the base of the second toe, dorsal aspect (Macdonald, Sims, and Mayrovitz, 2003; Sarvis, 2003; Tiwari et al, 2003).

One condition that is sometimes mistaken for lymphedema is lipedema, a congenital disorder of lipid metabolism that occurs almost exclusively in women and typically manifests during puberty. Lipedema is characterized by abnormal distribution of fat and hyperplasia of fat cells, primarily in the lower extremities. The patient with lipedema is seen with symmetrically heavy hips and thighs, tissue that feels soft and rubbery, pain on palpation, swelling that ends at the ankles, a negative Stemmer sign, and reports of frequent bruising. Dieting has little effect on this condition, and there is no definitive treatment; management is focused on patient education and support, and treatment of any comorbidities. Lymphedema can occur as a complication of lipedema; in this case, management follows the principles outlined in a later section (Macdonald, Sims, and Mayrovitz, 2003; Tiwari et al, 2003).

Diagnostic Tests. Specific diagnostic studies are indicated when the diagnosis of lymphedema is unclear. Scans are often required to exclude other diagnoses

TABLE 15-13 Lymphedema: Treatment Components

INTERVENTION	DESIRED EFFECT	ACTION	CAUTIONS
Complex decongestive physiotherapy	Mobilization of retained lymph	Therapeutic massage to mobilize lymphatic fluid in channels adjacent and proximal to involved site, followed by massage of affected area Compression bandages applied immediately after treatment	Performed only by therapists trained in the technique Usually requires one to two treatments daily for 1 to 3 weeks
Sequential compression therapy	Mobilization of retained lymph	Dynamic compression pumps with limb sleeves compress lymphatics and mobilize lymph	Risk of displacing fluid to proximal leg or genitalia Risk of further damage to lymphatics
Limb elevation	Edema reduction	Counters the effect of gravity on lymph flow	Effective only in early phase of disease
Compression bandaging	Critical component of maintenance therapy Nonelastic or short-stretch bandages and custom-fitted sleeves or stockings most effective	Applies pressure to tissues to facilitate compression of lymph channels and movement of lymph from interstitial space into channels	Should provide 40- to 60-mm Hg sub-bandage pressure Replace regularly to prevent loss of therapeutic effectiveness
Exercises	Maintenance of lymph reduction	Stimulates the intact lymphatics to increase rate of lymph transport	Encourage to exercise involved limb with compression bandage or garment in place
Skin and nail care	Infection control during restorative and maintenance phases	Keeps skin supple and prevents breaks in skin to reduce risk of infection	May have standing prescription for antibiotics to be filled if signs of infection develop

that may account for edema formation such as tumor or deep vein thrombosis. When the diagnosis remains unclear, imaging studies such as lymphoscintigraphy may be performed to elucidate the structure and function of the lymphatic system (Macdonald, Sims, and Mayrovitz, 2003).

Management

Lymphedema is a chronic condition with no known cure. Positive clinical outcomes depend on prompt recognition of lymphedema and initiation of treatment designed to interrupt the "vicious cycle" of fluid retention, lymphatic obstruction, and soft-tissue fibrosis. Effective management of the patient with lymphedema requires a comprehensive lifelong program of exercise, massage, and compression garments and is most effectively carried out in a lymphedema center. The goals of lymphedema management include (1) mobilization of the "trapped" lymph from the interstitial space, (2) elimination of edema, (3) restoration of normal limb contours, (4) maintenance of the "restored" limb state, and (5) prevention of infection. Therapy can be divided into two main phases: restorative, or "volumetric reduction," and maintenance. The components of treatment are highlighted in Table 15-13, with key points highlighted in the following material (Macdonald, Sims, and Mayrovitz, 2003; Sarvis, 2003; Tiwari et al, 2003).

Manual Lymph Drainage (MLD). MLD is a key element of therapy for patients with moderate to severe lymphedema. MLD involves daily sessions with a highly trained therapist using specialized massage techniques to (1) activate the lymphatic channels proximal to the affected limb, (2) mobilize lymph in the proximal tissues, and (3) mobilize lymph in the distal tissues. MLD is accompanied by range of motion exercises, short-stretch compression bandages (worn between treatments), and meticulous skin care.

High-Level Compression Garments. High-level compression wraps and stockings are an essential component of therapy for all patients with lymphedema. These garments must be worn between treatment sessions during the restorative phase, and throughout the day and night thereafter. Intermittent pneumatic compression devices are frequently contraindicated in the management of lymphedema. When the distal tissues are compressed before the trapped lymph in the proximal tissues has been mobilized with MLD, adverse effects such as additional lymphatic damage and genital edema can develop.

Meticulous Skin Care. Meticulous skin care is essential to the prevention of infection. This includes daily monitoring for any evidence of infection, prompt treatment when infection does occur, and routine use of fragrance-free, lanolin-free emollients to prevent cracking of the skin.

Education. With proper education and care, lymphedema can be avoided, or if it develops, kept under control. Initially, these patients will require much encouragement to continue using appropriate compression therapy. In addition, compression must remain in place during the night, so there is very little "break" from compression therapy for the individual with lymphedema. Box 15-20 provides a list of special instructions to help the patient with lymphedema protect the affected limb from trauma.

BOX 15-20 Teaching Points for the Patient with Lymphedema

Avoid the sauna or hot tub.

Do not use a chemical hair remover.

Use an electric razor to avoid cuts or nicks in the skin.

Blood pressure, blood draws, etc., should all be taken from the unaffected limb.

When washing dishes or clothes, cleaning, or gardening, wear glove to protect the limb from heat and potential trauma.

Protect the lymphedema extremity from the sun at all times.

Protect the lymphedema extremity and foot from all types of trauma.

Apply sunscreen and bug spray on the lymphedema extremity when outside.

Only wear closed toe shoes (if the leg is the affected extremity).

Avoid heavy lifting with the affected limb (arm); do not carry handbag or bags on the shoulder of the affected side.

Do not restrict fluid intake or protein intake in an attempt to prevent fluid buildup.

Ongoing Research. Experimental research is exploring other treatment approaches such as heat therapy and drug therapy with benzopyrones. Surgical intervention (to establish venolymphatic anastomoses or to "debulk" the affected extremity) is associated with high complication rates and is limited to patients who fail medical therapy (Macdonald, Sims, and Mayrovitz, 2003; Tiwari et al, 2003).

SUMMARY

Lower-extremity ulcers are an increasingly common problem and may be caused by compromised function in any component of the circulatory system; that is, arterial, venous, or lymphatic. In addition, there are multiple other causes for lower-extremity ulcers; for example, vasculitic processes, autoimmune disorders, neuropathy, and metabolic derangements. To further complicate the picture, many patients have ulcers of mixed etiology or comorbidities that affect management and the potential for healing. Effective management of the patient with lower-extremity ulceration is therefore dependent on thorough and accurate assessment followed by an individualized treatment plan that addresses all etiologic factors as well as any comorbidities. The treatment plan must also focus heavily on patient education, since lower-extremity ulcers are typically a complication of a chronic disease process that persists even after the ulcer is healed.

SELF-ASSESSMENT EXERCISE

1. Rest pain is indicative of which of the following?
   a. Mild occlusive disease, such as with 25% occlusion
   b. Moderate occlusive disease, such as with 50% occlusion
   c. Advanced occlusive disease, such as with 90% occlusion
   d. Need for amputation
2. Risk factors for LEAD include which of the following?
   a. Alcoholism
   b. Hypertension
   c. Elevated HDL levels
   d. Diabetes insipidus
3. What type of pain is claudication?
   a. Pain that exists without precipitating activity
   b. Pain that develops when the patient elevates the legs
   c. Pain that is triggered by moderate to heavy activity
   d. Pain that worsens with rest
4. Which of the following ABI values is indicative of calcification of vessel wall in a person with diabetes?
   a. 0.95-1.3
   b. 0.5-0.95
   c. 0.5
   d. >1.3
5. List the classic characteristics of an arterial ulcer.
6. Which of the following describes when maintenance of an eschar-covered arterial ulcer is preferred?
   a. The involved limb can be revascularized.
   b. The wound surface is exudative.
   c. The wound is infected.
   d. Indications of infection are absent and there is limited potential for healing.
7. Describe how a competent venous system and the calf muscle pump work together to prevent venous hypertension.
8. Therapeutic level compression therapy is characterized by which of the following?
   a. 25 mm Hg compression at the ankle
   b. At least 20 mm Hg compression at the ankle but no more than 10 mm Hg at the knee (to ensure distal-to-proximal flow)
   c. At least 30 mm Hg compression at the ankle
   d. At least 40 mm Hg compression at the ankle
9. How should management be modified for the patient with a venous ulcer complicated by arterial disease, as evidenced by an ABI of 0.7?
   a. Use elevation to control edema; do not compress
   b. Use pneumatic compression or modify sustained compression to provide pressures in the 20 to 25 mm Hg range
   c. Recommend Trental (pentoxifylline) as an alternative to compression
   d. Delay any treatment until patient undergoes revascularization
10. Distinguish between elastic and nonelastic static compression products, and explain which is best for the sedentary patient.
11. Explain why the patient with long-standing venous disease is at risk for development of lymphedema.

REFERENCES

Aly S et al: Comparison of duplex imaging and arteriography in the evaluation of lower limb arteries, *Br J Surg* 85:1099, 1998.

Anwar S et al: Subfascial endoscopic perforator surgery: a review. *Hosp Med* 64(8):479, 2003.

Aronow, Wilbert: Management of peripheral arterial disease of the lower extremities in the elderly patients, *Caring for Vascular Leg Ulcers*, 59(2): 248-249, 2004.

Berliner E, Ozbilgin B, Zarin D: A systematic review of pneumatic compression for treatment of chronic venous insufficiency and venous ulcers, *J Vasc Surg* 37(3):539, 2003.

Bonham P: Assessment and management of patients with venous, arterial, and diabetic/neuropathic lower extremity wounds, *AACN Clin Issues Adv Pract Acute Crit Care* 14(4):442, 2003.

Boulton A: Peripheral arterial disease in diabetic and nondiabetic patients, *Diabetes Care* 24(8):1433, 2001.

Bradbury A et al: Thrombophilia and chronic venous ulceration, *Eur J Vasc Endovasc Surg* 24:97, 2002.

Browse N, Burnand K: The cause of venous ulceration, *Lancet* 28(292):243, 1982.

Cantwell-Gab K: Identifying chronic peripheral arterial disease, *Am J Nurs* 96(7):40, 1996.

Chen A et al: Intermittent pneumatic compression devices-physiological mechanisms of action, *Eur J Vasc Endovasc Surg* 21:383, 2001.

Choucair M, Phillips T: Compression therapy, *Dermatol Surg* 24:141, 1998.

Choucair M, Faria D, Fivenson D: Use of human skin equivalent in the successful treatment of chronic venous leg ulcers, *Wounds* 10(3):97, 1998.

Choucair M, Fivenson D: Leg ulcer diagnosis and management, *Dermatol Clin* 19(4):659, viii, 2001.

Cimminiello, C: PAD: Epidemiology and pathophysiology, *Thrombosis Res* 106(6): V295, 2002.

Coleridge-Smith P: From skin disorders to venous leg ulcers: pathophysiology and efficacy of Daflon 500 mg in ulcer healing, *Angiology* 54(Suppl 1):S45, 2003.

Cullum N et al: Compression for venous leg ulcers, Cochrane Library, The Cochrane Collaboration, *Cochrane Database Syst Rev* 2, 2003.

de Araujo T et al: Managing the patient with venous ulcers, *Ann Intern Med* 138(4):326, 2003.

de Jong S: Hyperhomocysteinaemia in patients with peripheral arterial occlusive disease, *Clin Chem Labor Med* 39(8):714, 2001.

Demling R et al: Small intestinal submucosa wound matrix and full-thickness venous ulcers: preliminary results, *Wounds* 16(1):18, 2004.

Dieter RS et al: The significance of lower extremity peripheral arterial disease, *Clin Cardiol* 25(1):3, 2002.

Dillavou E, Kahn M: Diagnosing and treating the 3 most common peripheral vasculopathies, *Geriatrics* 58(2): 37-42, 2003.

Dolynchuk K et al: The role of Apligraf in the treatment of venous leg ulcers, *Ostomy Wound Manage* 45(1):3, 1999.

Ellozy S, Carroccio A: Drug-eluting stents in peripheral vascular disease: eliminating restenosis, *Mount Sinai J Med* 70(6):417, 2003.

Feben K: How effective is training in compression bandaging techniques? *Br J Community Nurs* 8(2):80, 2003.

Flemming K, Cullum N: Therapeutic ultrasound for venous leg ulcers, Cochrane Library, Cochrane Collaboration, *Cochrane Database Syst Rev* 1:20, 2003.

Franks PJ, Moffatt CJ: Quality of life issues in patients with chronic wounds, *Wounds* 10(suppl E):1E, 1998.

Furlong W: Venous disease treatment and compliance: the nursing role, *Br J Nurs* 10(11Suppl):S18, 2001.

Gahtan V: The noninvasive vascular laboratory, *Surg Clin North Am* 78(4):507, 1998.

Gibbons G: Lower extremity bypass in patients with diabetic foot ulcers, *Surg Clin North Am* 83:659, 2003.

Jansen T, Lawall H, Diehm C: Diagnosis of arterial vascular diseases with duplex sonography, *NMW Fortschritte der Medizin* 145(37):45, 2003.

Johnson S: Low-frequency ultrasound to manage chronic venous leg ulcers, *Br J Nurs* 12(19 Suppl):S14, 2003.

Jull A, Waters J, Arroll B: Pentoxifylline for treating venous leg ulcers, *Lancet*, 359(9317):1550-1554, 2004.

Jull A et al: Factors influencing concordance with compression stockings after venous leg ulcer healing, *J Wound Care* 13(3):90, 2004.

Kalra M, Gloviczki P: Surgical treatment of venous ulcers: role of subfascial endoscopic perforator vein ligation, *Surg Clin North Am* 83:671, 2003.

Kantor J Margolis D: Management of leg ulcers, *Semin Cutaneous Med Surg* 22(3):212, 2003.

Kelechi TJ et al: Skin temperature and chronic venous insufficiency, *J WOCN* 30(1):17, 2003.

Kerstein M: Economics of quality ulcer care, *Dermatol Nurs* 15(1):59, 2003.

Kunimoto B: Assessment of venous leg ulcers: an indepth discussion of a literature-guided approach, *Ostomy Wound Manage* 47(5):38, 2001a.

Kunimoto B: Management and prevention of venous leg ulcers: a literature-guided approach, *Ostomy Wound Manage* 47(6):36, 2001b.

Labropoulos N: Intermittent pneumatic compression for the treatment of lower extremity arterial disease: a systematic review, *Vasc Med* 7(2):141, 2002.

Lee D et al: Subfascial endoscopic perforator surgery for venous ulcers, *Hong Kong Med J* 9(4):279, 2003.

Lesho E, Manngold J, Gey D: Management of peripheral arterial disease, *Am Fam Phys* 69(3):525, 2004.

Lewis C: Peripheral arterial disease of the lower extremity, *J Cardiovasc Nurs* 15(4):45, 2001.

Liew IH, Law KA, Sinha SN: Do leg ulcer clinics improve patients quality of life? *J Wound Care* 9(9):423, 2000.

Lopez A, Phillips T: Venous ulcers, *Wounds* 10(5):149, 1998.

Lyseng-Williamson K, Perry C: Micronised purified flavonoid fraction, *Drugs* 64(1):71, 2003.

Macdonald J, Sims N, Mayrovitz H: Lymphedema, lipedema, and the open wound: the role of compression therapy, *Surg Clin North Am* 83:639, 2003.

Mani R, Vowden K, Nelson E: Intermittent pneumatic compression for treating venous leg ulcers, The Cochrane Library, The Cochrane Collaboration, *Cochrane Database Syst Rev* 2004.

Mills JL Sr: Buerger's disease in the 21st century: diagnosis, clinical features, and therapy, *Semin Vasc Surg* 16(3):179, 2003.

Min R, Khilnani N, Golia P: Duplex ultrasound evaluation of lower extremity venous insufficiency, *J Vasc Intervent Radiol* 14(10):1233, 2003.

Moffatt C, O'Hare L: Venous leg ulcerations: treatment by high compression bandaging, *Ostomy Wound Manage* 41(4):16, 1995.

Moon R: Use of hyperbaric oxygen in the management of selected wounds, *Adv Wound Care* 11(7):332, 1998.

Nelson E, Bell-Syer S, Cullum N: Compression for preventing recurrence of venous ulcers, The Cochrane Library, The Cochrane Collaboration, *Cochrane Database Syst Rev*:1, 2004.

Nelson E, Bradley M: Dressings and topical agents for arterial leg ulcers. The Cochrane Library, The Cochrane Collaboration, *Cochrane Database Syst Rev* 2003.

Nelzen O, Bergqvist D, Lindhagen A: The prevalence of chronic lower limb ulceration has been underestimated: results of a validated population questionnaire, *Br J Surg* 83(2):255, 1996.

Nelzen O, Bergqvist D, Lindhagen A: Long-term prognosis for patients with chronic leg ulcers: a prospective cohort study. *Eur J Vasc Endovasc Surg* 1997 May;13(5):500-508, 1997.

Newman A: Peripheral arterial disease: insights from population studies of older adults, *J Am Geriatr Soc* 48(9):1157, 2000.

Olin, J: Thromboangiitis obliterans (Buerger's disease), *New Engl J Med* 343(12):864, 2000.

Omar A et al: Treatment of venous leg ulcers with dermagraft, *Eur J Vasc Endovasc Surg* 27(6):666, 2004.

Orsted H, Radke L, Gorst R: The impact of musculoskeletal changes on the dynamics of the calf muscle pump, *Ostomy Wound Manage* 47(10):18, 2001.

Palmer-Kazen Wahlberg E: Arteriogenesis in peripheral arterial disease, *Endothelium* 10(4):225, 2003.

Paquette D, Falanga V: Leg ulcers, *Geriatr Dermatol* 18(1):77, 2002.

Phillips T: Current approaches to venous ulcers and compression, *Dermatol Surg* 27:611, 2001.

Phillips T et al: A study of the impact of leg ulcers on quality of life: financial, social and psychological implications, *J Am Acad Dermatol* 31(1):49, 1994.

Pittler M, Ernst E: Horse chestnut seed extract for chronic venous insufficiency, *Cochrane Database Syst Rev* 1: CD003230, 2003.

Reichardt L: Venous ulceration: compression as the mainstay of therapy, *J WOCN* 26(1):39, 1999.

Reininger C, Graf J, Reininger A: Increased platelet and coagulatory activity indicate ongoing thrombogenesis in peripheral arterial disease, *Thrombosis Res* 82(6):523, 1996.

Rockson S, Cooke J: Peripheral arterial insufficiency: mechanisms, natural history, and therapeutic options, *Adv Intern Med* 43:253, 1998.

Roszinski J, Schmeller W: Differences between intracutaneous and transcutaneous skin oxygen tension in chronic venous insufficiency, *J Cardiovasc Surg* 36:407, 1995.

Rudolph D: Pathophysiology and management of venous ulcers, *J WOCN* 5(5):248, 1998.

Russell T, Logsdon A: Subfascial endoscopic perforator surgery: a surgical approach to halting venous ulceration, *J WOCN* 29(1):33, 2002.

Ryan S, Eager C, Sibbald G: Venous leg ulcer pain, *Ostomy Wound Manage* 49(4A Suppl):16, 2003.

Sarvis C: When lymphedema takes hold, *RN* 66(9):32, 2003.

Schainfeld R: Management of peripheral arterial disease and intermittent claudication, *JABFP* 14(6):443, 2001.

Seidel HM et al, editors: Blood Vessels. In *Mosby's guide to physical examination,* ed 5, St Louis, 2003, Mosby, Elsevier Science.

Simka M, Majewski E: The social and economic burden of venous leg ulcers: focus on the role of micronized purified flavonoid fraction adjuvant therapy, *Am J Clin Dermatol* 4(8):573, 2003.

Smith P: The microcirculation in venous hypertension, *Cardiovasc Res* 32:789, 1996.

Spence R, Cahall E: Inelastic versus elastic leg compression in chronic venous insufficiency: a comparison of limb size and venous hemodynamics, *J Vasc Surg* 24:783, 1996.

Taylor LM Jr: Elevated plasma homocysteine as risk factor for peripheral arterial disease—what is the evidence? *Semin Vasc Surg* 16(3):215, 2003.

Tenbrook J et al: Systematic review of outcomes after surgical management of venous disease incorporating subfascial endoscopic perforator surgery, *J Vasc Surg* 39(3):583, 2004.

Terry M, O'Brien S, Kerstein M: Lower-extremity edema: evaluation and diagnosis, *Wounds* 10(4):118, 1998.

Tiwari A et al: Differential diagnosis, investigation, and current treatment of lower limb lymphedema, *Arch Surg* 138(2):152, 2003.

Valencia I et al: Chronic venous insufficiency and venous leg ulceration, *J Am Acad Dermatol* 44:401, 2001.

Van de Scheur M, Falanga V: Pericapillary fibrin cuffs in venous disease, *Dermatol Surg* 23:955, 1997.

Villavicencio J, Pikoulis E: Lymphedema. In Raju S, Villavicencio J, editors: *Surgical management of venous disease*, Baltimore, Md, 1997, Williams & Wilkins.

Weingarten M: State-of-the-art treatment of chronic venous disease, *Clin Infect Dis* 32:949, 2001.

Wipke-Tevis D, Sae-Sia W: Caring for vascular leg ulcers, *Home Healthcare Nurse* 22(4):237, 2004.

Wound, Ostomy and Continence Nurses Society (WOCN Society): *Guideline for management of patients with lower extremity arterial disease*, WOCN clinical practice guideline series #1, Glenview IL, 2002, Author.

Wound, Ostomy, and Continence Nurses Society (WOCN Society): *Guideline for management of patients with lower extremity venous disease*, WOCN clinical practice guideline series #1, Glenview IL, 2005a, Author.

Wound, Ostomy, and Continence Nurses Society (WOCN Society): Ankle Brachial Index: Best Practice for Clinicians, Mt Laurel, NJ, 2005b, Author.

16 Neuropathic Wounds: The Diabetic Wound

VICKIE R. DRIVER, MARY ANNE LANDOWSKI, & J. L. MADSEN

OBJECTIVES

1. Describe the correlation of protective sensation with risk for diabetic foot ulcer.
2. Distinguish between the musculoskeletal foot deformities that lead to focal areas of high pressure in the patient with peripheral neuropathy.
3. Describe three types of neuropathy that may occur in the patient with diabetes.
4. Identify critical factors to be included in the history and physical examination of the patient with lower-extremity neuropathic disease.
5. Identify key components of a patient education program for the patient with lower-extremity neuropathic disease.

Lower-extremity neuropathic disease (LEND) develops as a result of damage to nerve structures. In the case of diabetic foot ulcers (DFU) the lower-extremity metabolic changes and peripheral arterial disease (PAD) exacerbate neuropathy. Diabetic foot ulcers are sometimes referred to as neurotrophic, trophic, perforating, or malperforans ulcers (Plate 38). Due to impaired perfusion, susceptibility to infection, neuropathy, biochemical abnormalities, repeated or continuous trauma or a combination of these factors ulcer healing is particularly challenging for the patients with diabetes who has LEND (Frykberg, 2003; Levin, 2001). This chapter presents the assessment, prevention and treatment for the management of the diabetic foot ulcer.

EPIDEMIOLOGY

The prevalence of diabetes in the United States is 6.3% of the population or 18.2 million people (2002 estimate) and increasing; of this, 5.2 million are undiagnosed. Type 2 diabetes is steadily increasing in the U.S. In the twelve years from 1990 to 2002, the prevalence of diagnosed diabetes doubled (CDCP, 2004b). The increasing prevalence of diabetes is due to a wide variety of causes; the obesity epidemic and an aging population head the list.

Using the national survey database, Behavioral Risk Factor Surveillance System (BRFSS), the Center for Disease Control and Prevention (2003), estimated a 12.7% prevalence of patients with diabetes who had a history of foot ulcers. In the BRFSS, foot ulcers are defined as "any sores or irritations on the feet that took greater than 4 weeks to heal." Reiber and colleagues (1995) estimate a slightly higher prevalence of DFU's during the lifetime of a patient with diabetes at 15%-20%. Within a given year, the incidence of patients with diabetes that develop foot ulcers ranges from 1.9%–2.6% (Abbott et al, 2002; Ramsey et al, 1999; Muller et al, 2002).

Foot ulcers precede lower extremity amputations (LEA) 85% of the time (Pecoraro et al, 1990; Larsson et al, 1998). The leading non-traumatic cause of lower extremity amputations in the United States is attributed to diabetes. Of all the non-traumatic amputations in the United States, 50%-75% are caused by DFU's (CDCP, 2001). The national average annual incidence of patients with diabetes having a lower extremity amputation (LEA) was approximately 5.5 per 1000 (age-adjusted) for the year 2001 (CDCP, 2004b). Thus, approximately 25% of diabetic foot ulcers result in a LEA.

In addition, the percentage of amputations in the diabetic population compared to total amputations appears to be increasing. Department of Veterans Affairs data shows in 1986, 59% of all amputations were because of diabetes. In 1998, 66% of all amputations were because of diabetes (Mayfield et al, 2000). In 1997 the total number of lower extremity amputations (LEAs) for patients with diabetes in the U.S.

peaked at 84,000 (excluding military healthcare facilities) and the total figure has remained above 80,000 annually since then (CDCP, 2004a). The rate of LEA for patients with diabetes is **28 times** greater than those individuals without diabetes. Furthermore, amputation of the contralateral limb within 2-3 years is 50-84% and 3 years after a patient with diabetes has a LEA, the mortality rate is 20-50% (Reiber et al, 1995).

ECONOMIC BURDEN

The economic burden of diabetes in the U.S. is enormous and growing. Direct medical and indirect expenditures due to diabetes in 2002 were estimated to be $132 billion (ADA, 2003a). LEAs in the patient with diabetes and their consequences represent a significant portion of these costs (not to mention the cost in quality of life). Ramsey et al (1999) estimated the two-year medical costs for a middle-aged male with a DFU to be $27,900, using 1992-1995 data from a private health maintenance organization. Harrington et al (2000), using Medicare data from 1995-1996, found a 20-week healing rate for DFUs to be only 31% and estimated the annual cost for lower extremity ulcer treatment in patients with diabetes to be $15,300, with 74% of the costs from inpatient charges.

The cost of care increases significantly when a DFU proceeds to amputation. The total event cost ranges from $23,700 for a toe amputation to $51,300 for above-the-knee amputation, using 2001 costs (Gordois et al, 2003). An earlier, comprehensive study of amputation costs from Sweden that includes all inpatient, outpatient, and home care costs over a 3-year period estimated a cost of $43,100 for a minor amputation and $63,100 for a major amputation (Apelqvist et al, 1995).

PATHOGENESIS

The origin and development of a DFU has several components. An in-depth causal pathway study, with two patient cohorts from different parts of the world, identified 32 unique causal pathways for developing foot ulcers. The study found three components present in the majority (63%) of the identified pathways: peripheral neuropathy, structural foot problems, and minor trauma (Reiber et al, 1999). In another study, peripheral neuropathy (PN) was the major contributing factor leading to the development of 90% of all foot ulcers (Boulton, 1994). Other, less prevalent causes were edema, callus, and peripheral ischemia resulting from PAD. Although infection is a very common factor (59%) associated with LEAs in the patient with diabetes, it is not a common cause leading to DFUs (Pecoraro and Reiber, 1990).

Neuropathy

PN is involved in 78% of DFUs (Reiber et al, 1999). The incidence of neuropathy in patients with diabetes appears to be linked to the duration of diabetes and, to some extent, to glycemic control. Prospective studies comparing patients with standard versus those with tighter control of blood glucose have shown patients with better glucose control to have better nerve conduction velocity as well as reductions in retinopathy and nephropathy (Diabetes Control and Complications Research Group, 1993). The exact etiology of peripheral neuropathy is unknown, but it is likely the result of metabolic events including the accrual of glucose, sorbitol, and fructose, a reduction in myo-inositol (needed for nerve conduction), and nerve ischemia due to reduction of the vessels in the vasa nervosum (Levin, 2002; Page and Chen, 1997; Veves and Sarnow, 1995). The predominant structural mechanism that is affected by the various metabolic components may be the microvascular component. Under normal conditions the arteriole-venule (AV) shunts in the sole of the foot are closed, and blood flow is through the nutrient capillaries (capillary dermal papillae loops). With diabetic neuropathy a decrease in the sympathetic innervation of the highly innervated AV shunts results in a greater dilation in the arterioles and leads to a shunting away of blood from the capillary dermal papillae loops. This results in lower skin temperature and a decrease in transcutaneous oxygen tension at the skin. Theoretically the metabolic components may be reversible, but structural component changes (shunting) apparently cannot be undone once changed (Pfeifer and Schumer, 1995; Tanneberg et al, 2001). A more detailed explanation of the many etiologic pathways that lead to diabetic neuropathy is beyond the scope of this chapter.

Neuropathy can be either focal or diffuse. *Focal* neuropathy can be divided into ischemic and entrapment types. Focal ischemic neuropathies are caused by an acute event to the nerves. Examples include cranial and femoral neuropathies. This type of neuropathy is characterized by a sudden onset and is asymmetric in distribution. Focal entrapment neuropathies occur when a nerve is compressed in a specific area of the body. These tend to be more progressive in development and are also often asymmetrically located. Examples of these are carpal tunnel and tarsal tunnel syndromes.

Diffuse neuropathy includes distal symmetric polyneuropathy and autonomic neuropathy. Diffuse neuropathies are due to abnormal structural, vascular, and metabolic conditions. These have a symmetric distribution and are progressive in nature. These are the neuropathies encountered frequently in patients with diabetes. Diffuse neuropathies are divided into distal symmetric polyneuropathy—which includes motor and sensory neuropathies—and autonomic neuropathy (Tanneberg et al, 2001).

As mentioned, neuropathy is a frequent risk factor for DFUs and can include (1) sensory nerves (controlling sensation), (2) motor nerves (controlling musculature), and (3) autonomic nerves (controlling functions such as sweating, vascular flow, and heart rate) (Sumpio, 2000; Tanneberg et al, 2001). Sensory, motor, and autonomic neuropathies represent the most common complication affecting the lower extremities of patients with diabetes (Armstrong and Lavery, 1998; Mulder, Armstrong, and Seaman, 2003). Although diabetes is the most common cause of lower-extremity neuropathy, other well-defined causes include uremia, acquired immunodeficiency syndrome (AIDs), nutritional deficiencies, nerve compression, trauma, fractures, prolonged use of crutches, tumors, radiation and cold exposure, certain medicines, systemic lupus erythematosus, and rheumatoid arthritis, among others (NINDS, 2003).

Sensory and Motor Neuropathy. Sensory and motor neuropathies are grouped under the frequently cited category of "peripheral neuropathy" (PN) rather than the distal symmetric polyneuropathy category. The vast peripheral nervous system connects the nerves running from the brain and spinal cord (the central nervous system) and transmits information to the rest of the body, that is, the arms, the legs, the hands, and the feet. This distal and dying-back progression is often referred to as a "stocking and glove" pattern.

In *sensory neuropathy* the loss of protective sensation leads to a lack of awareness of pain and temperature change, resulting in increased susceptibility to injury. However, the eventual lack of pain awareness is generally preceded by 8 to 10 years of painful neuropathy. Persons with this condition will have worse pain at night, and relief will come from movement rather than rest (Tanneberg et al, 2001). Once the painful phase ends, minor trauma caused by poor-fitting shoes or an acute injury can precipitate a chronic ulcer. Patients may not realize they have a foot wound for some time because of lack of sensation in their feet. The loss of pain sensation can reach to the knees.

Motor neuropathy affects the muscles required for normal foot movement and can result in muscle atrophy. The distal motor nerves are the most commonly affected and cause atrophy of the small intrinsic muscles of the foot. Often the wasting of the lumbrical and interosseous muscles of the foot will result in collapse of the arch (Sumpio, 2000). Cocked-up or claw toes, hammer toes (Figure 16-1), and weight redistribution from the toes to the metatarsal heads leads to increased pressures and subsequent ulceration (Grunfeld, 1991; Levin, 2002). Generally, patients with diabetes develop both kinds of distal symmetric polyneuropathy (Sumpio, 2000).

Autonomic Neuropathy. Autonomic neuropathy (AN)—a disease of the involuntary nervous system— can affect a wide range of organ systems throughout the body. Diabetic AN frequently coexists with other peripheral neuropathies and other diabetic complications (Vinik et al, 2003). AN results in decreased sweating, loss of skin temperature regulation, and abnormal blood flow in the soles of the feet. The resulting xerosis can precipitate fissures, cracks, callus, and finally ulceration (Mulder, Armstrong, and Seaman, 2003; Tanneberg et al, 2001).

Musculoskeletal Abnormalities

Foot deformities (see Figure 16-1) are very common in patients with diabetes and peripheral neuropathy and lead to focal areas of high pressure. Table 16-3 later in this chapter provides a brief description of selected foot malformations. These deformities are also associated with thinning of the fat pad under the metatarsal heads. DFUs are generally developed from repetitive stress on "hot spots" that develop from bone

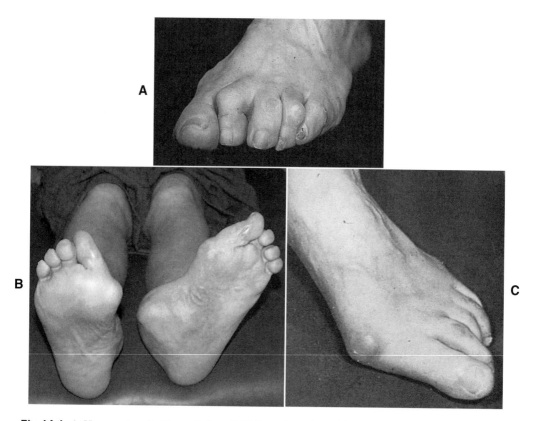

Fig. 16-1 **A,** Hammertoes. **B,** Charcot's foot. **C,** Hallux valgus (lateral deviation of the hallux) and bunions.
A, C From Seidel HM et al, editors: Blood vessels. In *Mosby's guide to physical examination*, ed 6, St Louis, 2006, Mosby, Elsevier Science. Courtesy Charles W. Bradley, DPM, MPA, and Caroline Harvey, DPM, California College of Podiatric Medicine; *B* From Bowker JH, Pfeifer MA: *Levin and O'Neal's The diabetic foot*, ed 6, St Louis, 2001, Mosby.

deformities and/or callus build-up (Levin, 2002). The areas at the top of the toes, the tips of the toes, and under the metatarsal heads are vulnerable to ulceration and infection. Atrophied or dislocated fat pads beneath the metatarsal heads increase the pressure under them. This can lead to skin loss or callus development and increases the risk of ulceration (Sumpio, 2000).

Associated callus can increase foot pressure by as much as 30% (Young et al, 1992). In the absence of neuropathy, the patient can feel the presence of a fissure, blister, or a bony prominence and will take corrective action. However, with neuropathy the protective response is diminished or even nonexistent.

Thus foot ulcers can get progressively worse before any action is taken (Bowering, 2001). Individuals with diabetic neuropathy have been known to walk around for days in shoes containing shoehorns. Abnormalities in foot biomechanics from the previously described deformities and possible ulceration often cause a dysfunctional gait. This leads to further damage to the structure of the foot.

Ankle Joint Equinus. Ankle joint equinus, defined as less than 0 degrees of ankle joint dorsiflexion, occurs in some patients with peripheral neuropathy. With ankle joint equinus the range of motion of the foot joint becomes limited, which increases pressure on the sole of the foot (Caselli et al, 2002; Daniels, 1998). Of all patients with diabetes, 10.3% develop ankle joint equinus; this risk increases with duration of disease (Lavery, Armstrong, and Boulton, 2002). High plantar pressures from ankle equinus can increase incidence of ulceration in patients with diabetes (Caselli et al, 2002).

Charcot's Foot. Charcot's foot or Charcot's neuroarthropathy (or arthropathy) is a classic, although relatively uncommon, diabetic foot deformity (Reiber, Boyko, and Smith, 1995). Lavery and colleagues (2003) found the incidence of Charcot's arthropathy for non-Hispanic whites with diabetes to be 11.7 per 1000 per year. A long duration of diabetes is an important factor in the development of Charcot's neuroarthropathy; over 80% of patients with Charcot's foot have diabetes for more than 10 years (Cofield, Morison, and Beabout, 1983).

The precise neural mechanism causing Charcot's foot is unknown, and a number of different theories have been proposed to explain the underlying etiology (Yu and Hudson, 2002). Despite conventional thinking that many diabetic lower extremities are ischemic, there is overwhelming evidence that many patients with diabetic neuropathy have increased blood and pooling in their feet. This condition has been directly correlated with decreased bone density in Charcot's foot, possibly as a result of autonomic neuropathy (Edmonds, Roberts, and Watkins, 1982; Young et al, 1995). Charcot's foot may well be due to a combination of neurotraumatic and neurovascular mechanisms (Yu and Hudson, 2002).

Eichenholz (1966) divided Charcot's disease progression into three radiographically different stages: *development, coalescence,* and *reconstruction.* Development represents the acute, destructive phase characterized by joint effusions, edema, subluxation, formation of bone and cartilage debris, intraarticular fractures, and bone fragmentation. This period is often initiated by minor trauma and aggravated by persistent ambulation. The stage of coalescence is marked by a reduction in edema, absorption of fine debris, and healing of fractures. The final phase of bone healing is reconstruction, in which further repair and remodeling of bones takes place along with fusion and rounding of large bone fragments and decreased joint mobility. Early diagnosis and treatment (i.e., offloading) in the

development stage is critical in treating this disease (Sanders and Frykberg, 2001).

The Charcot's foot is prone to increased pressures because of its deformity and possible bone or joint collapse. Thus the patient with Charcot's neuroarthropathy is 4 times more likely to develop a foot ulcer (Jeffcoate, 2003; Larsen, Fabrin, and Holstein, 2001; Yu and Hudson, 2002).

Peripheral Arterial Disease (PAD)

PAD is a major risk factor for lower-extremity amputation, particularly with patients who have diabetes, because the accompanying inadequate oxygenation and perfusion of tissues significantly impairs wound healing (Mulder, Armstrong, and Seaman, 2003). In a comparison between patients with diabetes and patients without diabetes and PAD, patients with diabetes were 5 times more likely to have an amputation (Jude et al, 2001).

The incidence of ischemic diabetic foot ulcers is relatively low. However, since over half of the people with PAD are asymptomatic, it is difficult to determine the true prevalence in patients with diabetes. Oyibo et al (2001) found that only 1% of new DFUs were ischemic—26% were neuroischemic, and 67% were neuropathic—whereas Reiber et al (1999) reported that ischemia was present in 35% of the DFUs. In contrast, in a recent study from England, only 16% of the new DFUs were ischemic, with 24% classed as neuroischemic.

Although ischemic or neuroischemic foot ulcers are relatively less common than neuropathic DFUs, they are more serious and lead to higher rates of amputation in patients with diabetes (Moulik, Mtonga, and Gill, 2003). Amputations of lower extremities in patients with diabetes are almost always due to multiple causes, including ischemia, infection, and neuropathy (Pecoraro and Reiber, 1990).

Relatively little is known about the biology of PAD in patients with diabetes; however, it is thought to be similar to other manifestations of atherosclerotic diseases such as coronary and carotid artery disease (ADA, 2003b). PAD typically results from gradual diameter reduction of the lower-extremity arteries and from the progression of atherosclerotic changes in arterial circulation in the lower extremities. Endothelial injury and resulting endothelial dysfunction occur in the earliest stages of the disease. The endothelial surface can be injured by various means including hyperlipidemia or diabetes (Levy, 2002). The atherosclerotic plaque that develops in the patient with diabetes and PAD is no different than that which develops in the patient without diabetes (Levin, 2002). The pattern of PAD in patients with diabetes is such that medium sized arteries, mainly at the popliteal trifurcation, are affected. However, there is sparing of the distal pedal vessels. Patients with advanced PAD also develop structural changes in skeletal muscle, including loss of type 2 fibers and muscle fiber denervation (Regensteiner et al, 1993).

Microvascular tissue perfusion, in contrast to macrocirculation, may also present problems for patients with diabetes. While PAD in persons with diabetes normally spares the small pedal arteries, microcirculation abnormalities are common in the foot as a result of neuropathy. Diabetic neuropathy impairs the nerve axon reflex and causes local vasodilation in response to a painful stimulus. The impaired vasodilation in diabetic neuropathic lower extremities can create a functional ischemia. The characteristics of the patient with LEAD in the presence of diabetes compared to the patient with LEAD in the absence of diabetes are listed in Chapter 15, Box 15-9.

ASSESSMENT

The components of assessment for any patient who is seen with signs or symptoms of LEND include the patient history and risk factors, physical examination, and simple noninvasive tests. Select patients may require more complex studies. Figure 16-2 is an example of an assessment form for patients with LEND.

Patient History

Patient history includes general state of health, a record of diabetic complications and treatments, walking difficulties, shoe problems, pain in the extremity, medications (prescribed and over-the-counter), glycosylated hemoglobin level, and risk factors for LEND and DFUs. Because DFUs can occur as a consequence of neuropathy and lower-extremity arterial disease (LEAD), specific questions should be posed regarding any LEAD risk factors (Chapter 15, Table 15-7).

Risk Factors

A number of studies have quantified the relative significance of various risk factors associated with the presence of foot ulceration. Lavery et al (1998) found that the risk of ulceration increases dramatically based on the number and type of risk factor associated with a patient with diabetes. They found the relative risk is increased by the following factors:
- 1.7 in persons with PN
- 12.1 in those with PN and foot deformity
- 36.4 in those with PN, foot deformity, and a history of previous amputation

In a large multicenter study that lasted 30 months, Pham et al (2000) analyzed the incidence of new foot ulceration in patients with diabetes with various measurable risk factors. Of the enrolled patients in their study, 29% developed one or more foot ulcers over the 30-month period (a very high incidence rate). Nearly all (99%) of these patients had a high neuropathy disability score (NDS) and/or a poor score on the Semmes-Weinstein monofilament examination (SWME) for sensation. Additional factors that yielded a statistically significant odds ratio for foot ulceration during the study include the following:
- gender (male)
- race (Native American)
- duration of diabetes (long)
- palpable pulses
- history of foot ulceration
- high vibration threshold score
- high foot pressures

It is apparent that foot ulcers often have a multifactorial etiology. Although the above studies list the most commonly associated risk factors, there are many others that the clinician must recognize in order to comprehensively assess a patient. Box 16-1 contains a list of the most commonly recognized risk factors for ulceration (Abbott et al, 2002; Armstrong and Lavery, 1998; Lavery et al, 1998). As with the presence of infection, vascular insufficiency has a much more important role in delaying wound healing and subsequent amputation than as a risk factor contributing to ulceration (Lavery et al, 1998).

Classification of Risk. Many specialized foot treatment clinics use a foot risk classification system for patients with diabetes to allocate resources such as

Foot Screening Examination

Name_____ID#_____

Age_____ Date_____/_____/_____

Past Medical History

DM Type I ☐ or Type II on Insulin ☐, Oral Agents ☐, Diet ☐, Hypertension ☐, CHF ☐, h/o MI ☐, h/o Heart Bypass ☐
PVD ☐, h/o LE Bypass ☐, Intermittent Claudication ☐, RA ☐, Retinopathy ☐, Nephropathy ☐, h/o Peripheral
Neuropathy ☐, h/o Foot Surgery ☐, h/o Foot Ulcer ☐, h/o Amputation ☐
HbA1c (and date):_____, Smoking HX ☐
Other Dx:

_____

Social History

Employed ☐, Retired ☐, Homemaker ☐, Indep Amb ☐, Walk w/ Assist ☐, Wheelchair ☐, Ambulation Distance
Unlimited ☐, Limited Community ☐, Homebound ☐, Non-ambulatory ☐, Exercise ☐; Walk ☐, Run ☐,
Weight Training ☐, #____days/wk

Other

	R			L		
	ROM	Strength	Pain	ROM	Strength	Pain
Ankle Dorsiflexion						
Ankle Plantarflexion						
Hallux Extension						
Hallux Flexion						

Fig. 16-2 Example of an assessment form for the patient with LEND.

Continued

Sensation-Vibration Sense

	R		L
Ankle	Y☐ N☐_____		Y☐ N☐_____
Great Toe	Y☐ N☐_____		Y☐ N☐_____

Semmes Weinstein (10g)

RIGHT   LEFT

Skin (location)

Dryness ☐_____ Redness ☐_____

Maceration ☐_____ Callus ☐_____

Pre-Ulcer ☐_____, Ulcer ☐_____

Vascular

	R		L
Dorsal Pedal Pulse	Y☐ N☐_____		Y☐ N☐_____
Posterior Tibial Pulse	Y☐ N☐_____		Y☐ N☐_____
Shiny, hairless, atrophic skin	Y☐ N☐_____		Y☐ N☐_____
Capillary refill <3 sec	Y☐ N☐_____		Y☐ N☐_____
Edema	Y☐ N☐_____		Y☐ N☐_____

Deformities

	R		L
Hammer/Claw Toes	Y☐ N☐_____		Y☐ N☐_____
Bunion/Tailor's Bunion	Y☐ N☐_____		Y☐ N☐_____
Planus/Cavus	Y☐ N☐_____		Y☐ N☐_____
Hallux Limitus	Y☐ N☐_____		Y☐ N☐_____
Bony Prominence	Y☐ N☐_____		Y☐ N☐_____
	Loc:_____		Loc:_____
Equinus/Calcaneus	Y☐ N☐_____		Y☐ N☐_____
Drop Foot	Y☐ N☐_____		Y☐ N☐_____
Charcot Fracture	Y☐ N☐_____		Y☐ N☐_____
Partial Foot Amputation	Y☐ N☐_____		Y☐ N☐_____

	R		L
Mobility/Vision	Y☐ N☐_____		Y☐ N☐_____
Able to SEE/IDENTIFY a Foot Mark	Y☐ N☐_____		Y☐ N☐_____
Able to REACH foot	Y☐ N☐_____		Y☐ N☐_____

Fig. 16-2, cont'd Example of an assessment form for the patient with LEND.

Footwear

Standard Y☐ N☐
Prescription Y☐ N☐

Describe:

Appropriate Y☐ N☐
Worn Y☐ N☐

ASSESSMENT

☐ **Low Risk**
Intact sensation + vascular flow, no bony prominence or deformity

☐ **Moderate Risk**
Intact sensation + vascular flow, bony prominence or deformity

☐ **High Risk**
Absent sensation +/or absent vascular flow, may have bony prominence, deformity, or prior h/o ulcer/amputation

Does patient realize their level of 'Risk' Y☐ N☐

PLAN/GOALS

☐ Consult to Limb Preservation Service_____

☐ Consult to Vascular Surgery_____

☐ Consult to Diabetes Clinic_____

☐ Consult for Orthotics_____

☐ Consult for Diabetic Shoes_____

TREATMENT PLAN

Routine Foot Screening Follow-Up: 6 mos ☐, 12 mos ☐
Palliative Care Follow-Up: 2 mos ☐, 3 mos ☐

Surgical Candidate ☐

Other:

_____

_____   _____
                        Signature   **Date**

Fig. 16-2, cont'd Example of an assessment form for the patient with LEND.

BOX 16-1 Diabetic Foot Ulcer Risk Factors

- Absence of protective sensation due to peripheral neuropathy
- Vascular insufficiency
- Structural deformities and callus formation
- Autonomic neuropathy causing decreased sweating, and dry feet
- Limited joint mobility
- Long duration of diabetes
- Long history of smoking
- Poor glucose control
- Obesity
- Impaired vision
- Past history of ulcer or amputation
- Male gender
- Increased age
- Ethnic background with high incidence of diabetes (i.e., Native American)
- Poor footwear inadequately protecting skin from high pressures

TABLE 16-1a Foot Risk Classification System

LOW RISK	MODERATE RISK	HIGH RISK
Diabetes	Diabetes	Diabetes
Intact sensation (neurologic)	Intact sensation (neurologic)	Absence of sensation (neurologic) AND/OR
Intact pulses (vascular)	Intact pulses (vascular)	Absence of pulses (vascular)
Absence of foot deformities	Presence of foot deformities	Presence or absence of foot deformities

From Driver et al, 2005.

TABLE 16-1b Generalized Management Considerations for Foot Risk Classifications

RISK CATEGORY	MANAGEMENT PLAN TO REDUCE RISK OF ULCERATION
Low	Education emphasizing disease control, proper shoe fit/design, daily self-inspection, and early reporting of foot injuries or breaks in skin
	Proper fitting/design footwear with orthotics as needed
	Annual follow-up for foot screening
	Follow as needed for skin/callus/nail care or orthosis
Moderate	Above, plus the following:
	Proper fitting/design footwear with orthotics as needed
	Routine follow-up every 6 months for foot examination
	Depth-inlay footwear, molded/modified orthosis may be required. If deformity causing pressure point and conservative measures fail, then make referral to foot and ankle care specialist
High	Above plus the following:
	May require modified or custom footwear
	Routine follow-up every 1 to 12 weeks for foot ulcer evaluation and callus/nail care
	Referral to foot and ankle care specialist

therapeutic shoes, education, and frequency of clinical visits (Peters and Lavery, 2001). *The International Working Group on the Diabetic Foot* (Apelqvist et al, 1999) recommends the following "international" system:

- Group 0 patients have diabetes but no other risk factors
- Group 1 includes those with diabetes and neuropathy
- Group 2 includes those with diabetes, neuropathy, vascular disease, and/or foot deformities
- Group 3 includes those with a history of foot ulcers or previous amputation and is further specified as:
  - Group 3A for those with history of foot ulcers
  - Group 3B for those with a previous amputation

Risk classification systems such as this one have been shown to be very effective in prediction of future DFUs (Lavery et al, 1998; Peters and Lavery, 2001; Rith-Najarian, Stolusky, and Gohdes, 1992). Additional risk classification systems are provided in Tables 16-1 and 16-2, and Chapter 17, Table 17-2.

Lower Extremity and Foot Physical Examination

Chapter 15 describes how to conduct a comprehensive lower extremity assessment and should be

TABLE 16-2 Lower-Extremity Amputation Prevention Program (LEAP) and Management Categories for the Foot

RISK CATEGORIES	MANAGEMENT CATEGORIES
"0" No loss of protective sensation of the feet	Education emphasizing disease control, proper shoe fit/design Follow up yearly for foot screen Follow as needed for skin, callus, nail care or orthosis
"1" Loss of protective sensation of the feet	Education emphasizing disease control, proper shoe fit/design, daily inspection, skin/nail care, early reporting of foot injuries Proper fitting/design footwear with soft inserts/soles Routine follow up every 3 to 6 months for foot/shoe examination and nail care
"2" Loss of protective sensation of the feet with either high pressure deformity or poor circulation	Education emphasizing disease control, proper shoe fit/design, daily inspection, skin/nail care, early reporting of foot injuries Depth-inlay footwear, molded/modified orthoses; modified shoes as needed; footwear with soft inserts/soles Routine follow-up every 1 to 3 months for foot/activity/footwear evaluation and callus/nail care
"3" History of plantar ulcer or neuropathic fracture	Education emphasizing disease control, proper fitting footwear, daily inspection, skin/nail/callus care, early reporting of foot injuries Depth-inlay footwear, molded/modified orthoses; modified/custom footwear, ankle footwear orthoses as needed Routine follow-up every 1 to 12 weeks for foot/activity/footwear evaluation and callus/nail care

Note: "Loss of protective sensation" is assessed with a Semmes-Weinstein monofilament examination using a 5.07 monofilament at 9 locations on each foot. Foot clinic visit frequency may vary based on individual patient needs.
From WOCN Society: *Guideline for management of wounds in patients with lower-extremity neuropathic disease,* WOCN Clinical Practice Guideline Series #3, Glenview IL, 2004, Author.

carefully reviewed. The following section will discuss the aspects of the lower extremity exam that is unique to the patient with LEND.

Protective Sensation. Screening for neuropathy can be done rapidly and reliably with a 5.07 (10-gram) SWME or the vibration tuning fork test by the on-off method (ADA, 1999; Perkins et al, 2001). The monofilament line used for the SWME test is normally mounted on a rigid paper holder. The line has been standardized to deliver a 10-gram force when pushed against an area of the foot. The patient should be placed in a room that is quiet and relaxed. Box 16-2 provides a procedure for conducting this exam, and it is illustrated in (Figure 16-3 *A, B*).

Pain. A detailed presentation for pain assessment and management can be found in Chapter 25. A description of neuropathic pain is an important assessment parameter and may be specific to the disease state. For example, impaired glucose tolerance can trigger a pain described as burning (Poncelet, 1998). In general, neuropathic pain varies in severity and is described as "burning," "tingling," "shooting," or "pins and needles." Activity can alleviate or exacerbate neuropathic pain. Because of the potential for LEAD, the patient should be assessed for ischemic pain (Chapter 15, Box 15-6).

Musculoskeletal Abnormalities. Loss of motor nerve function affects the intrinsic foot muscles. When imbalances due to weakening of the intrinsic muscles occur, it can cause changes in foot structure and gait and muscle wasting. Plantar fat pads also become displaced, and the metatarsal heads become prominent. These changes may predispose the patient to ulceration.

Each foot has 26 bones, 29 joints, and 42 muscles; thus there are numerous potential locations for problems (Levin, 2001). A few structural foot deformities are briefly described in Table 16-3 and include the

BOX 16-2 Procedure: Semmes-Weinstein 5.07 (10 gram) Monofilament Examination (SWME)

1. Explain procedure to the patient.
2. Position patient in a sitting position, resting patient's lower leg on the examiner's lap.
3. Demonstrate the monofilament on the patient's hand so that the patient will know what to anticipate.
4. Explain to the patient that when he/she feels the filament touching the skin, to respond with a "yes."
5. Have the patient close his or her eyes. The sites to be tested should be shown on the examination form.
6. Apply the monofilament perpendicular to the skin's surface. Apply sufficient force to cause the filament to buckle or bend, using a smooth, not a jabbing, motion.
7. The total duration of the approach, skin contact, and departure of the filament at each site should be approximately 1 to 2 seconds.
8. Apply the filament along the margin of the callus, ulcer, scar, and/or necrotic tissue; do NOT apply filament over these lesions.
9. Record and, if appropriate, map the results on the examination form.

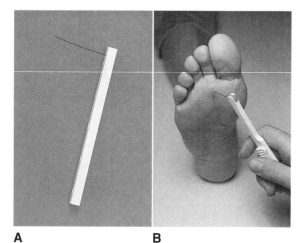

A   **B**

Fig. 16-3 A, Monofilament. **B,** Press the monofilament against the skin hard enough to allow it to bend. From Seidel HM et al, editors: Blood vessels. In *Mosby's guide to physical examination,* ed 5, St. Louis, 2003, Mosby, Elsevier Science.

following: pes cavus (high arch), hammer toes, mallet toes, claw toes, hallux valgus (lateral deviation of the hallux), prominent metatarsal heads, bunions, and Charcot's foot. Figure 16-1 provides illustrations of selected structural foot deformities.

Claw, hammer, and mallet toes are a sign of distal muscle atrophy and foot neuropathy. When muscles weaken, other muscles can overpower them, leading to contractures. *Hammer toe* is a contracture of the proximal joint, which is further from the front (or top) of the toe. *Mallet toe* refers to the distal joint, closer to the end of the toe, and is almost identical to hammer toe. When both joints are contracted, the condition is called a *claw toe.* Prominent metatarsal heads occur if one of the metatarsal bones is longer or lower than its neighboring bones. This may lead to uneven weight distribution between the heads and subsequent pain, callus, and ulceration. Bunions are caused by an enlarged head of the first metatarsal bone just below the first toe joint (ADA, 2004a).

When changes in the gait or foot structure are observed, the patient should be referred for more testing. Patients with Charcot's foot are normally seen with a rocker-bottom foot that is hot, erythematous, and edematous with bounding pedal pulses and prominent veins (Figure 16-1). Pain is normally, but not always, minimal in the early stages. The foot may be 10° F to 12° F warmer than the rest of the skin (Yu and Hudson, 2002). A history including an absence of trauma, the absence of a portal of entry for infection, and the absence of other signs of infection are suggestive of an acute Charcot's foot (Levin, 2002).

Vascular Status. The coexisting calcification of arteries that occurs with diabetes and PAD leaves the blood vessels difficult to compress and therefore difficult to assess (Levin, 2002; Sumpio, 2000). When unable to palpate pulses, a Doppler probe may be used and will allow the skilled examiner to denote whether pulses are triphasic, biphasic, or monophasic.

In the absence of pedal pulses, additional noninvasive vascular tests may be conducted to obtain a better indication of the condition: (1) segmental pressures (i.e., taken at the thigh, calf, and ankle); (2) toe pressures; or (3) transcutaneous oxygen readings (Bowering, 2001). Transcutaneous oximetry, or $tcPo_2$, is an assessment of the microcirculatory system, which can be impaired in persons with diabetes and peripheral neuropathy.

TABLE 16-3 Brief Descriptions for Selected Foot Malformations

MALFORMATION	CHARACTERISTICS
Plantar fasciitis	Heel pain caused by inflammation of the long band of connective tissue running from the calcaneous to the ball of the foot
Heel spurs	Bony growths on the underside, forepart of the calcaneous bone that may lead to plantar fasciitis
Bunions (hallux valgus)	The first joint of the large metatarsal slants outward with the tip angling toward the other toes; may lead to edema and tenderness
Hammer (claw) toes	Toes appear bent into a claw-like position; often seen in the second metatarsal when a bunion slants the large metatarsal toward and under it
Neuromas	Enlarged, benign growths of nerves, most commonly between the third and fourth toes caused by bones or other tissue rubbing against and irritating the nerves
Charcot's arthropathy	Disruption or disintegration of some of the foot and ankle joints frequently associated with diabetes resulting in erythema, edema and deformity
Pes cavus	High arch or instep
Pes covus	Flat foot

Zimny and colleagues (2001) found that patients with diabetes and neuropathy had significantly higher sitting to supine tcPO$_2$ differences than patients with diabetes only, indicating microcirculatory impairment.

The absence of pedal pulses despite the presence of popliteal pulses is a classic finding for patients with diabetes who also have PAD (ADA, 1999). If pedal pulses are not detectable with a Doppler device, an immediate referral to a vascular specialist is warranted. Refer to Chapter 15 for further information on vascular disease.

Skin temperature should be assessed in both feet. A difference in skin temperature may be an indication of trauma or fracture and/or infection. The temperature should be assessed with the back of the examiner's hand or by using an infrared temperature scanner. Research by Armstrong and colleagues (2003a) has shown that skin temperature is a poor indicator of vascular status or neuropathy, or as a predictor of future foot complications in diabetes patients. The only significant association found in this study was skin higher temperatures in those with Charcot's arthropathy.

As previously mentioned, the impaired vasodilation in diabetic, neuropathic lower extremities can create a functional ischemia. Symptoms of impaired microcirculation can include edema; altered skin characteristics (hair, nails, moisture); weak or absent pulses; skin discolorations; skin temperature changes; altered sensations; diminished arterial pulsations; skin color becoming pale on elevation; color not returning on lowering the leg; slow healing of lesions; cold extremities; and blue or purple skin color in dependent limb (Ackley, 2004).

Skin and Nail Condition. Skin and nail condition is an important component of assessment for the patient with LEND. Descriptions of foot lesions and nail disorders can be found in Chapter 17, Figures 17-4, 17-5 and Plate 7f. Loss of sweating may cause cracking of the skin and fissures that can become infected. The presence of eczema, dermatitis, and/or psoriasis should be noted. The web spaces (between the toes) should be examined for moisture and/or fungal problems. Document the patient's skin condition, including the presence of any corn, callus or preulcerative lesion (i.e., blister or hematoma) or open ulcers; these should be measured and drawn on the exam form. If there is coexisting vascular disease, additional skin changes may be apparent. Chapter 15, Table 15–5 lists characteristics of lower extremities and wounds with LEAD, LEND, and LEVD.

Callus formation is a natural protective response to repetitive stress. It is characterized by thickened hyperkeratotic skin. The problem with this buildup is that accumulation of callus can also increase pressure

25% to 30%, resulting in an ulcer below the callused area that is not visible to the examiner or palpable. Hemorrhage into a callus is a principle indicator of ulceration (WOCN Society, 2004). Although usually painless, in some cases a callus can cause pain because nerve endings close to the surface layers are irritated. Callus buildup is a result of a biomechanical problem. Unless the underlying cause is eliminated, callus will continue to occur. Based on the duration and the amount of pressure applied, the skin may eventually break down and an ulcer will develop.

Thickened nails are common. In addition, any abnormalities under the nail and any sign of nail infections should be noted. Nails bear the brunt of daily activities: running, walking, participating in sports, and just wearing shoes. When feet are abused and/or injured, a portion or all of the nail plate can be damaged. Repeated trauma, improper trimming, and minor injuries can result in nail problems. If the toe box is pressing down on the nails, bleeding may occur under the nail. Some nail disorders can also be hereditary. Ingrown toenails (onychocryptosis) may have a convex deformity. As pressure is exerted on the tissues, callus builds up. Nails that are red, brown, or black may indicate trauma (acute or chronic). Any discharge noted from around the nail or under the nail may indicate an infection process. Fungal infections are very common. A nail that curves inward in the corners is called a paronychia. If present, remove nail polish to better view the nails.

Footwear

Evaluation of the patient's shoes is as important as taking a good history and/or examining the patient's feet. As mentioned, the majority of injuries to the foot are not recognized by the person with diabetes because of neuropathy. Most skin injuries on the foot of the person with diabetes are on either the dorsal or plantar surfaces (Edmonds et al, 1986). Many ulcers on the dorsum are at sites of high pressure, where the patient's footwear creates a lesion that implies a biomechanical etiology (Apelqvist, Larsson, and Agardh, 1990). The following items should be investigated while evaluating the patient's shoes:

- Bulges on the outside of the shoes
- Wear patterns on the soles of the shoes
- Wearing down on the heels
- Worn lining inside the shoes
- Shoe cushioning
- Foreign objects in the shoes

Foot Imprints (Harris Mat). Although a number of commercial devices exist for barefoot or in-shoe plantar pressure measurement (Cavanagh, Hewitt, and Perry, 1992), an inexpensive method that can be used to identify areas of increased pressure and unequal weight distribution of the patients' feet is the Harris mat (Tanneberg et al, 2001). The mat (foot imprint system) has two compartments. One side of the mat is inked. Paper is then placed facing the inked surface. Two sheets are required; one for each foot. The inked side is closed, and the mat is reversed. The patient is asked to remove his or her shoes, leaving socks and/or hose on. The patient is asked to take a normal step down on the side that doesn't have ink. By stepping on the mat, an impression of the foot is left on the paper indicating areas of high pressure and uneven weight distribution (Figure 16-4). The use of the mat identifies high-risk areas and is a good motivator in getting patients to wear their orthotics, since they can see where problem areas exist.

Forefoot Test. The forefoot test illustrates to patients how well their shoes fit their feet. First, have the patient remove his or her socks and/or hose. Instruct the patient to stand on a piece of paper with both feet. Trace the outline of both feet on the paper Next, take the patient's shoes and just place the edge of the shoe over the traced outline. If any of the lines are visible, the shoes are too tight (Figure 16-5). Again, this is a very visual cue for the patient that helps them realize the importance of wearing shoes that fit their feet.

DFU Evaluation

The initial description of the foot ulcer is critical for the mapping of its development during treatment (Frykberg et al, 2000). Wound assessment and evaluation of healing are described in Chapter 7.

Characteristics of DFUs. Common locations and causes for DFUs are listed in Table 16-4. Ulcers with a LEND etiology may resemble a laceration, puncture, or blister with a rounded or oblong shape. The wound base may be necrotic, pink, or pale, with well-defined, smooth edges and small-to-moderate amounts of

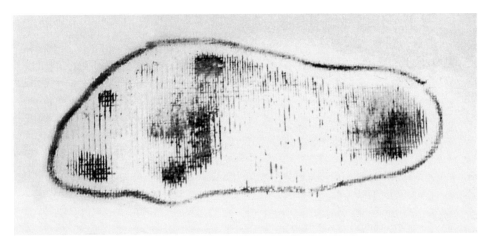

Fig. 16-4 Example of a Harris ink mat impression. (Courtesy David M. Osterman.)

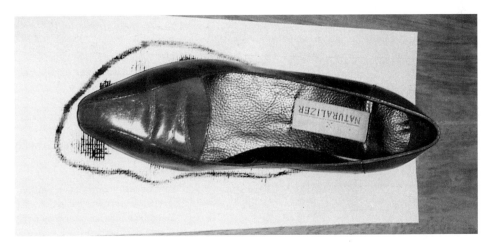

Fig. 16-5 Patient's shoes laid over traced image of feet. (Courtesy David M. Osterman.)

serous or clear exudate. The periwound skin often presents with callus.

DFU with LEAD. Although ischemic or neuro-ischemic foot ulcers are relatively less common than neuropathic DFUs, they are more serious and lead to higher rates of amputation in patients with diabetes (Moulik, Mtonga, and Gill, 2003). Amputations of lower extremities in patients with diabetes are almost always due to multiple causes, including ischemia, infection, and neuropathy (Pecoraro and Reiber, 1990).

A comparison of the characteristics of neuropathic, arterial, and venous wounds is listed in Chapter 15, Table 15-5. Trophic changes for arterial disease alone are not diagnostic of arterial insufficiency and should be interpreted cautiously. Characteristics of ischemic foot ulcers include pain, the absence of bleeding, and the presence of an underlying deformity or history of a trauma (Sumpio, 2000). Ischemic ulcers are uncommon on the dorsum, because perfusion is usually better and pressures are reduced (Sumpio, 2000).

TABLE 16-4 Common LEND Wound Sites and Causative Factors

Toe interphalangeal joints	Limited interphalangeal joint flexibility
Metatarsal head	High pressure, limited joint flexibility
Interdigital	Increased moisture, footwear too narrow, toe crowding, deformity
Bunion sites	Footwear too narrow, foot deformity
Dorsal toes	Hammer or claw toe deformity, footwear too shallow in toe box
Distal toes	Poor arterial perfusion, external force (heat), footwear too short
Midfoot (dorsal or plantar surface)	Charcot's fracture, external trauma
Heels	Unrelieved pressure

From WOCN Society: *Guideline for management of wounds in patients with lower-extremity neuropathic disease,* WOCN Clinical Practice Guideline Series #3, Glenview IL, 2004, Author.

TABLE 16-5a Wagner Ulcer Classification System

GRADE	DESCRIPTION
0	Preulcer No open lesions May have deformities, callus, or cellulitis
1	Superficial diabetic ulcer (partial or full thickness)
2	Full-thickness ulcer Penetrates through fat to tendon, joint capsule, or deep fascia without abscess or osteomyelitis
3	Deep ulcer with abscess, osteomyelitis, or joint sepsis
4	Gangrene localized to a portion of foot such as toes, forefoot, or heel
5	Extensive gangrene or necrosis to the point that the foot is beyond salvage

From Wagner FW: The dysvascular foot: a system for diagnosis and treatment, *Foot Ankle* 2:64, 1981.

Common symptoms include intermittent claudication, cold feet, thinning, shiny atrophic skin, hair loss (alopecia) on the feet and legs, and dystrophic nails.

Color changes include elevation pallor (Chapter 15, Box 15-2) or greyish hue for darkly pigmented skin, dependent rubor, and purpura. There may be a delayed capillary refill and prolonged venous filling time. Extremities may be cool unilaterally or have a sudden marked change from proximal to distal. Pulses may be diminished or absent. The ankle pressure will be less than 50 mm Hg, and the ankle-brachial index

TABLE 16-5b Wagner Ulcer Classification System (Modified)*

GRADE	DESCRIPTION
0	At-risk foot Preulcer No open lesions; skin intact May have deformities, erythematous areas of pressure or callus formation
1	Superficial ulcer Disruption of skin without extending into the subcutaneous fat layer Superficial infection with or without cellulitis may be present
2	Full-thickness ulcer Penetrates through fat to tendon or joint capsule, without abscess or osteomyelitis
3	Deep ulcer that may or may not probe to the bone, with abscess, osteomyelitis, or joint sepsis Includes deep plantar space infections or abscesses, necrotizing fasciitis, or tendon sheath infections.
4	Gangrene of a geographical portion of foot such as toes, forefoot, or heel The remainder of the foot is salvageable, though it may be infected
5	Gangrene of the whole foot beyond salvage Required limb- or life-sparing amputation

*A modification was added to the Wagner scale to identify ischemia and infection.
From WOCN Society: *Guideline for management of wounds in patients with lower-extremity neuropathic disease,* WOCN Clinical Practice Guideline Series #3, Glenview IL, 2004, Author.

(ABI) will be 0.9 or less (although unreliable in patients with diabetes). In the presence of diabetes, toe pressures should be measured; toe pressures lower than 30 mm Hg are indicative of LEAD.

DFU Classification. Numerous diabetic ulcer classification systems exist in the literature (Frykberg, 1991; Gibbons and Elipoulos, 1984; Lavery, Armstrong, and Harkless, 1996, Pecoraro and Reiber, 1990; Sims, Cavanaugh, and Ulbrecht, 1988; Van Acker et al; 2002; Wagner, 1981). These systems are useful for guiding future treatment regimes, communication between care providers, and prediction of future outcomes, and in conducting clinical trials. The various systems often include location, depth, necrotic characteristics, and presence of infection, ischemia, and/or neuropathy.

The widely used Wagner foot wound classification system (Table 16-5a) divides foot ulcers into six grades based on depth of the lesion and the presence of osteomyelitis or gangrene (Wagner, 1981). The Wagner system does not include presence of infection, ischemia, or neuropathy. The WOCN Society (2004) modified the Wagner system to identify ischemia and infection (Table 16-5b).

Another popular diabetic foot ulcer classification system—the University of Texas (UT) system (Table 16-6)—utilizes a matrix structure with four grades of wound depth and four associated stages to specify ischemia, infection, both ischemia and infection, or neither (Lavery, Armstrong, and Harkless, 1996). The UT system has been judged superior to the original Wagner system as a better predictor of patient outcomes (Oyibo et al, 2001). Another system is the size (Area and Depth) (SAD) classification system, which grades the wound according to area, depth, sepsis, quality of pulses, and accuracy of sensation (Table 16-7) (Macfarlane and Jeffcoate, 1999).

Infection. Infection rarely causes diabetic foot ulcers. Rather, ulcers provide a portal for the entry of pathogens. These microbes often thrive because of the impaired host response of the person with diabetes (ADA, 1999). As cited earlier, infection is a causal component in 59% of diabetic limb amputations

TABLE 16-6 **University of Texas at San Antonio Diabetic Wound Classification System**

STAGE	GRADE			
	0	*I*	*II*	*III*
A	Preulcerative or postulcerative lesion completely healed	Superficial wound not involving tendon, capsule, or bone	Wound penetrating to tendon or capsule	Wound penetrating to bone or joint
B	Preulcerative or postulcerative lesion completely epithelialized with infection	Superficial wound not involving tendon, capsule, or bone with infection	Wound penetrating to tendon or capsule with infection	Wound penetrating to bone or joint with infection
C	Preulcerative or postulcerative lesion completely epithelialized with ischemia	Superficial wound not involving tendon, capsule, or bone with ischemia	Wound penetrating to tendon or capsule with ischemia	Wound penetrating to bone or joint with ischemia
D	Preulcerative or postulcerative lesion completely epithelialized with infection and ischemia	Superficial wound not involving tendon, capsule, or bone with infection and ischemia	Wound penetrating to tendon or capsule with infection and ischemia	Wound penetrating to bone or joint with infection and ischemia

From Lavery LA, Armstrong DG, Harkless, LB: Classification of diabetic foot wounds, *J Foot Ankle Surg* 35:528, 1996.

TABLE 16-7 Size (Area and Depth) (SAD) Classification

GRADE	AREA	DEPTH	SEPSIS	ARTERIOPATHY	DENERVATION
0	Skin intact	Skin intact	No infection	Pedal pulses palpable	Pinprick sensation >VPT normal
1	<10 mm^2	Skin and subcutaneous tissue	Superficial slough or exudate	Diminution of both pulses or absence of one	Reduced or absent pinprick sensation VPT raised
2	10-30 mm^2	Tendon, joint, capsule, periosteum	Cellulitis	Absence of both pedal pulses	Neuropathy dominant: Palpable pedal pulses
3	>30 mm^2	Bone and/or joint spaces	Osteomyelitis	Gangrene	Charcot's foot

VPT = Vibration Perception Threshold.
From Macfarlane R, Jeffcoate W: Classification of diabetic foot ulcers: the size (area and depth) (SAD) system, *Diabetic Foot* 2(4):123, 1999.

(Pecoraro and Reiber, 1990). In a Swedish study, Eneroth, Apelqvist, and Stenstrom (1997) found that 42% of patients with diabetes with deep foot infections required LEAs, and 86% required surgery.

The person with diabetes is more prone to infection than the person without diabetes (Shah and Hux, 2003). However, infected diabetic foot wounds are often less symptomatic than nondiabetic wounds, exhibiting only subtle or even a complete absence of signs (Frykberg, 2003; Sibbald et al, 2000). In fact, recalcitrant hyperglycemia may be the only clinical finding indicating a severe infection of a DFU (Frykberg, 2002). The presence of probable infection needs to be noted during the initial examination, although culturing is best done after surgical debridement.

Curettage or sampling technique is important in obtaining useful culture results (to ensure confusing surface colonies are not included) (Dow, Browne, and Sibbald, 1999). Wound cultures should be taken by obtaining tissue from the debrided wound base or by aspirating pus. If swabs are the only option, ensure they are taken from the wound base (Lipsky, 2004). The "gold standard" for infection assessment is the quantitative biopsy (Frykberg, 2003; Sibbald et al, 2000). Evaluation does not end after initial culturing. Wounds must be continually monitored for bacterial colonization. Ulcers that do not show signs of infection need not be cultured (ADA, 1999).

TABLE 16-8 Signs of Limb-Threatening and Non–Limb-Threatening Diabetic Foot Infections

NON–LIMB-THREATENING	LIMB-THREATENING
Less than 2 cm of surrounding cellulitis	More than 2 cm of surrounding cellulitis
No systemic toxicity signs	Deep abscesses
No deep abscesses, osteomyelitis, or gangrene	osteomyelitis or gangrene

Like diabetic foot ulcers in general, classifying diabetic foot infections can be a useful process to determine appropriate treatment. Caputo and colleagues (1994) proposed three categories: non–limb-threatening, limb-threatening, and life-threatening. More recently, however, diabetic foot infections are subdivided into either non–limb-threatening and limb-threatening categories, with the understanding that the later classification can become life-threatening (ADA, 1999). Table 16-8 summarizes the characteristics of these two categories.

One of the most important assessments at this stage is wound depth and, more importantly, presence of osteomyelitis. Osteomyelitis is surprisingly common and is found in approximately 60% of moderate to severe diabetic foot ulcers (Eneroth, Apelqvist, and Stenstrom, 1997; Lipsky 1997). Thus, after initial

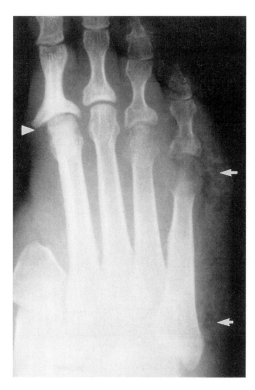

Fig. 16-6 MRI image of osteomyelitis in first metatarsal bone (lateral view). From Bowker JH, Pfeifer MA: *Levin and O'Neal's The diabetic foot*, ed 6, St Louis, 2001, Mosby.

descriptions are made, an examination of the ulcer is normally made with a blunt sterile probe. Either direct exposure of bone or a positive "probe to bone" test is used to determine presence of osteomyelitis (Grayson et al, 1995; Newman et al, 1991). Probing can also detect sinus tract formations and undermining along the ulcer margins (Frykberg, 2002). A number of methods are used for osteomyelitis verification including plain film x-rays, magnetic resonance imaging (MRI), and leucocyte scans with indium In 111 oxyquinoline (see Figures 16-6 and 16-7 for an x-ray image and an MRI of the same first metatarsal bone [lateral view] with osteomyelitis). Serial x-ray studies are indicated for all but the least severe chronic DFUs to evaluate for osteomyelitis. Early diagnosis of this complication is critical, but it is often undetected by physicians (Newman et al, 1991). In addition, previously unknown fractures were found in 22% of patients with neuropathic foot ulcers through radiography

(Cavanagh et al, 1994). If osteomyelitis is suspected, a referral to a foot and ankle specialist should be made immediately.

MANAGEMENT

The level of expertise and knowledge required to manage LEND and DFUs is constantly increasing. Because of the complex nature of DFUs and the numerous comorbidities that can occur in patients with diabetes, a multidisciplinary team approach to management is recommended (ADA, 1999; Frykberg, 2002; Driver et al, 2005). An ideal foot care team should include the following: (1) podiatric/orthopedic surgeon; (2) vascular surgeon; (3) infectious disease specialist; (4) endocrinologist or family practice or internal medicine physician; (5) orthopedic/podiatric technician; (6) certified wound care nurse; (7) orthotist; and (8) a certified diabetes educator (CDE). Numerous references from the United States and Europe literature document improvements in patient outcomes, including reduction of lower-extremity amputation rates, as a result of implementing a multidisciplinary approach to diabetic foot care (Bild et al, 1989; Edmonds et al, 1986; Meltzer et al, 2002; Muller et al, 2002; Van Houtum et al, 2003). However, health care providers frequently work in situations without this level and variety of expertise; thus, patients with diabetes who develop a foot problem will often need to be referred to consultants. In fact, the standards of medical care in diabetes recommend the referral of high-risk patients to foot specialists for surveillance and preventative care (ADA, 2004b).

As described earlier, diabetic neuropathy is associated with a reduced blood supply to the nerves, a microcirculatory network called the *vasa nervosum*. Currently, there is no prescription therapy in the United States approved to treat the underlying process of microvascular damage that leads to diabetic peripheral neuropathy. Recent research has demonstrated that capillary vascular perfusion is inversely correlated with the degree of peripheral neuropathy (Nabuurs-Franssen et al, 2002). This nerve ischemia leads to poor nerve function. Based on earlier research in Europe, in which certain prostacyclins (vasodilators) or their analogues have gained approval for critical limb ischemia treatment, Remodulin (United Therapeutics Corp.) is being tested for patients with diabetes and

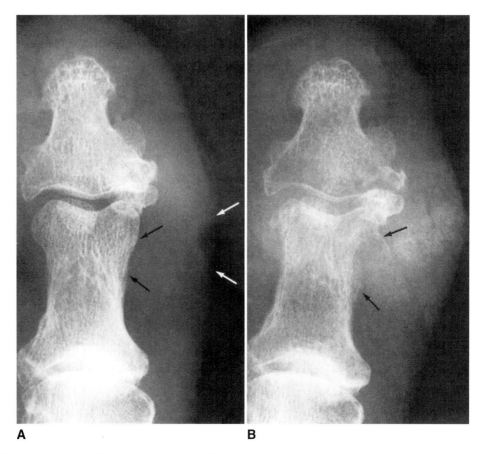

A **B**

Fig. 16-7 Osteomyelitis shown on X-ray of first metatarsal bone. From Bowker JH, Pfeifer MA: *Levin and O'Neal's The diabetic foot,* ed 6, St. Louis, 2001, Mosby.

neuropathic ulcers. Preliminary results demonstrated the treatment significantly increased lower limb blood flow in these patients (Mohler et al, 2000). Another new area of investigation for neuropathy treatment of the patient with diabetes involves the enzyme protein kinase C beta, or "PKC beta." Current hypotheses concerning the pathogenesis of diabetic neuropathy suggest that PKC beta (which is stimulated by hyperglycemia) may help explain the process that leads to microvascular dysfunction, impairment of endoneural blood flow, and damage of nerves (Vinik, 2003). The PKC beta inhibitor LY333531 (Ely Lily) is currently being tested and has shown encouraging results in improving diabetic peripheral neuropathy (Litchy et al, 2002).

Early Interventions (Prevention)

Careful and frequent inspection of the diabetic foot is the most effective and least expensive method for preventing DFUs and possible LEAs. Abnormalities, whether age-related, structural, or pathologic, can be assessed and documented. The American Diabetic Association (2004b) recommends patients with diabetes have a comprehensive **annual** foot examination.

At least 50% of all amputations due to diabetic neuropathy are preventable with early intervention (Reiber, Boyko, and Smith, 1995). Given the life-altering and life-threatening risks associated with the development of a DFU, it is incumbent upon the health care professional to identify patients with lower-extremity peripheral neuropathy as early as possible so that

BOX 16-3 Instructions for Care of Diabetic Feet

Inspection

- Inspect feet and toes daily for blisters, cuts, swelling, redness, or any other discolored area. If you are unable to see the bottom of your feet, use a mirror.
- Look for dry areas and cracks in the skin. Apply a thin coat of lubricating oil after bathing.
- If your vision is impaired, have a family member inspect your feet daily, and also trim nails and buff calluses when required.

Bathing

- Wash your feet daily. Dry them carefully, including between the toes. Test the water with hands or elbow to ensure it will not burn your feet.
- Do not soak your feet. Soaking actually dries the skin by removing natural oil and can cause maceration (wrinkled appearance).
- Apply moisturizing cream to feet (but not between the toes) after bathing.

Toenail care

- Cut toenails after bathing, when they are soft and easier to trim.
- Never cut nails too short. Leave $1/16$ to $1/8$ inch of the nail. Nails should be cut straight across the top or shaped to follow the contour of the toe. Sharp edges should be filed smooth with an emery board to avoid cutting adjacent toes.
- Ingrown nails or other problematic nails should be cared for by a foot care provider.
- Avoid using sharp objects to clean under the toenail.

Corns and calluses

- Do not use chemical corn or callus removers or corn pads. They can damage or burn the skin.
- When feet are dry, file away calluses with a pumice stone.
- Corns and calluses are a response to pressure from poorly fitting shoes. Change footwear to reduce these pressure "hot spots."
- Never use a razorblade yourself to reduce corns or calluses.

Shoes

- Do not walk barefoot, even in your home. Wear slippers with a rubber sole. Wear shoes and socks outside at all times.
- Ideally, shoes should have thick, flexible rubber soles, closed toes, and closed heels. Shoes should be sufficiently wide for your feet. Always avoid pointed-toe shoes or boots. Running or walking shoes are the best ones to buy. Do not depend on breaking in shoes. Buy them later in the day when feet are their largest.
- Inspect shoes for objects inside before you put them on.
- Wear new shoes for short periods each day, from 1 to 2 hours. Watch for signs of poor fit.
- Do not wear sandals with thongs between your toes.
- In winter, take special precautions to avoid foot damage from the cold.

Socks

- Wear clean socks every day. Avoid nylon socks as much as possible.
- Socks need to fit well, with no tight elastic at the top or seams.

Circulation

- Do not smoke; or if you do, stop!
- Exercise regularly.
- If your feet are cold, wear warm socks.
- Do not use a heating pad or a hot water bottle.

---

preventive interventions can be implemented. Preventive interventions for the patient with LEND must become a routine that the patient incorporates into everyday life. Specific instructions concerning inspection of the foot, bathing, nail care, care of corns and calluses, shoes, socks, and circulation should be enforced in writing and verbally as outlined in Box 16-3. Clearly, one of the most important components of the clinician's role is to provide patient education.

Using the patient's foot risk classification, a management plan (i.e., education, diagnostic studies, footwear recommendations, referrals, and follow-up visits) can be developed in order to minimize the odds of developing a foot ulcer (Driver, 2004). Tables 16-1, 16-2, and 17-2 are examples of programs that correlate specific preventive interventions with each level of risk. By implementing these early interventions and adhering to preventive interventions such as moisturizing the foot and inspecting the shoe before putting it on, the first two principles of wound management (i.e., control or eliminate causative factors, and provide systemic support to reduce existing and potential cofactors) are addressed.

Glycemic Control

As was discussed in the introduction, the prevalence of undiagnosed diabetes is approximately 30% of the total number of people in the United States with diabetes (CDCP, 2004a). A similar percentage of people admitted to the hospital for treatment will also have undiagnosed diabetes. A recent study by Umpierrez and colleagues (2002) documented that 31% of persons—with diabetes—admitted to an urban hospital had no known history of diabetes and were diagnosed during their stay.

Inadequate glycemic control is a key in the development of neuropathy in the extremity of the person with diabetes (Bowering, 2001). Hyperglycemia results in leukocyte dysfunction and suppression of lymphocytes, high blood pressure, and impaired endothelial function, among other dangers. Because of the impaired immune response, persons with hyperglycemia will respond poorly to a severe foot infection. Armstrong and colleagues (1996) found that 56% of persons being admitted for diabetic foot infections had normal white blood cell counts. Improved blood glucose levels will increase the immune defenses of patients and thus needs to be a component of clinical care of infected diabetic foot ulcers (Bagdade et al, 1978). If infected, elevated hemoglobin A (HbA_1c) may be the only sign from a patient with diabetes to alert the provider of the problem (Frykberg, 2003). Thus patients with diabetes must be managed with a high index of suspicion for soft tissue infection, deep space infection, and osteomyelitis.

Offloading

As mentioned in the examination section, pressure reduction is a basic principle involved in the prevention of foot ulcers and lower-extremity amputations as well as with the healing of existing DFUs. Numerous books, references, and websites discuss the various offloading modalities used for patients with DFUs or at risk for developing foot ulcers. Orthotists and pedorthists are frequently consulted for assistance in managing foot problems. Orthotists and pedorthists are trained specifically to make and fit orthopedic footwear (and other appliances) that can accommodate the patient with diabetes. Chapter 17, Table 17-3 shows methods and considerations for offloading the foot. The following section will discuss total contact cast (TCC), removable cast walkers (RCWs), and Achilles tendon lengthening (ATL).

Patients with DFUs require pressure relief during the healing phase. The total contact cast (TCC) has been shown to be very effective at pressure relief and healing of DFUs. The cast (Figure 16-8) is designed to equalize pressure loading of the plantar surface by equal "total contact "of the plantar skin with the cast material (Coleman, Brand, and Birke, 1984). While the patient ambulates, repetitive injury to the wound site is reduced (Lavery et al, 1997; Sinacore, 1996). A test of the effectiveness of the TCC, removable cast walkers (RCWs), and half-shoes to heal neuropathic DFUs demonstrated that patients with the TCC had significantly better healing rates at 12 weeks than those treated with the other two offloading modalities. Interestingly, patients with the TCCs were significantly less active than those with the half-shoes. There was no activity difference between patients with the TCC or the RCW (Armstrong et al, 2001). Armstrong and colleagues (2003b) devised an activity test of patients with DFUs wearing RCWs. Total daily activity was recorded per patient. In addition, unbeknownst to patients the daily activity of the RCW was also recorded. Results showed that patients only wore the RCW 28% of the time. A study involving 50 patients with neuropathic foot ulcerations compared healing rates of wounds offloaded with RCW to wounds offloaded with RCW wrapped with a cohesive bandage. Results showed that the wounds offloaded with the RCW wrapped with a cohesive bandage healed significantly sooner (p = 0.02) than the RCW that could be removed more easily (Armstrong et al, 2005). These studies suggest that protective footwear that is less easily removed may increase the odds of healing DFUs.

Options for offloading in addition to TCCs, RCWs, and half-shoes include bed rest, wheelchairs and,

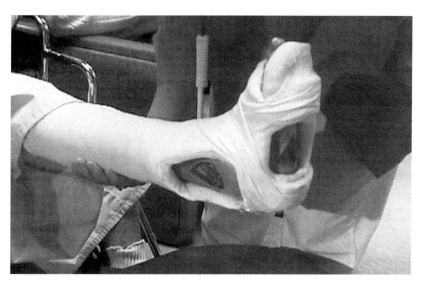

Fig. 16-8 Modified total contact cast applied to offload pressure from neuropathic plantar ulcer that developed after prolonged use of a multipodus boot (L'nard splint). By creating a window in the cast over the pressure ulcer located near the medial malleolus and a window over the plantar neuropathic ulcer, topical dressings can be reapplied without removing the cast. The cut-out portion or window of the cast can then be reapplied over the dressing and secured with self-adhering tape (Coban [3M]) to restore the integrity of the cast. (Courtesy Ted Tomter, RN, CWOCN, St. Joseph's Candler Health System, Savannah, Ga.)

if crutches are also employed, surgical shoes, custom sandals, healing shoes, cast shoes, and foam dressings (ADA, 1999). TCCs are absolutely contraindicated for patients with acute deep infection, sepsis, or gangrene. Relative contraindications include ulcers with depth greater than width, fragile skin, or excessive edema, noncompliant patients, or those who would be unstable with a cast (Sinacore and Mueller, 2001).

An additional topic that can be included under the heading of offloading is the prophylactic surgical procedure of Achilles tendon lengthening, sometimes referred to as tendo-Achilles lengthening or TAL. Patients who may be considered for this treatment include those with peripheral neuropathy and equinus contracture. Equinus causes high forefoot pressure that contributes to plantar surface ulceration (LaBorde, 2003). A randomized clinical trial testing patients with plantar DFUs compared the treatments (1) TCC with TAL and (2) TCC without TAL. The study showed that all ulcers in the TAL plus TCC group healed with the risk of recurrence 75% fewer at 7 months, and 52% fewer at 2 years than the TCC-only treatment (Mueller

et al, 2003). However, a follow-up study to this found that patients with the TAL plus TCC procedure had, surprisingly, decreased physical functioning compared to the TCC-alone patients after 8 months (Mueller et al, 2004).

Structural Foot Deformities. The traditional treatment for Charcot's arthropathy (without ulceration) is cast immobilization. Few patients require surgery for this condition. Before immobilization, compression bandages are applied at weekly intervals until all edema has subsided. This can last 2 to 3 weeks. A short non–weight-bearing cast is generally required for 12 to 16 weeks. The cast can be changed once or more times during this period. Gradual weight-bearing is started when the surface of the skin has returned to near-normal temperature (Yu and Hudson, 2002). Noninvasive bone stimulation such as electrostimulation can be a valuable adjunctive treatment for Charcot's arthropathy (Grady et al, 2000). If edema and inflammation persist, administration of pamidronate is recommended to prevent further deterioration (Guis et al, 1999). Table 16-9 shows the healing phases of Charcot's foot.

TABLE 16-9 The Healing Phases of Charcot's Foot

CLINICAL PRESENTATION	DISSOLUTION PHASE	COALESCENCE PHASE	REMODELING PHASE
Edema	May be profound	Decreased	Decreased
Erythema	May be severe	Generally absent	Generally absent
Temperature compared to contralateral foot	May be 3° C to 7° C increased	Generally more than 2° C increased	Generally less than 2° C increased
X-ray image	May demonstrate fractures, dislocations, and subluxations May not show abnormality during the earliest acute phase of injury	May demonstrate early consolidation, formation of bone callus	Demonstrates consolidation stability

From WOCN Society: *Guideline for management of wounds in patients with lower-extremity neuropathic disease,* WOCN Clinical Practice Guideline Series #3, Glenview IL, 2004, Author.

Pain Control

A variety of pharmacological interventions are available for the treatment of neuropathic pain and are presented in Chapter 25, Table 25-5. In some cases, it may be necessary to refer to pain clinic and neurologists for pain management (WOCN Society, 2004).

Wound Management

Chapter 19 describes the principles of wound management and goals of topical therapy. Specifically for treating diabetic foot wounds, Jeffcoate (2003) listed the priorities as follows: (1) aggressively treat infections; (2) establish whether ischemia is present and revascularization is required; (3) relieve pressure to the wound; and (4) improve the wound condition by debridement, dressings, and advanced care treatments where appropriate. In general, the principal goal in the treatment of diabetic foot ulcers is wound closure (Frykberg et al, 2000).

Debridement Level. Wound and callus debridement is an integral process in the management of diabetic foot wounds. Key benefits of debridement in the diabetic wound include removal of free-living bacteria (Robson, Stenberg, and Heggars, 1990); removal of bacteria "biofilms" (Serralta, 2001); stimulation of growth factors (Mulder and Vande Berg, 2002); removal of senescent cells (Vande Berg et al, 1998); and

removal of hyperproliferative nonmigratory tissue, that is, "callus" (Bowering, 2001; Steed et al, 1996).

Methods of debridement may change over time or be done in combination as conditions change. Surgical debridement is repeated as often as needed, depending on formation of new necrotic tissue. Weekly debridement is common and is commonly referred to as maintenance debridement (Frykberg et al, 2000).

When selecting a specific method of debridement of DFUs, many factors concerning the DFU must be considered: pain, arterial insufficiency, antiembolic medications, patient setting, resources, and characteristics of the wound, as well as the type of debridement. Methods of debridement and factors to consider for selection are discussed in detail in Chapter 10.

Considerations specific to patients with LEND and DFUs are highlighted by the ADA and the WOCN Society:

- Revascularization and surgical removal of necrotic tissue from an infected wound on an ischemic leg or foot is the treatment of choice for limb salvage.
- All ulcers with extensive cellulitis and/or osteomyelitis should be debrided and referred for pharmacologic (intravenous) intervention.

- Evidence is insufficient to support use of whirlpool or pulsatile jet irrigation in neuropathic ulcers.
- Caution must be exercised to prevent immersion burns from whirlpool because of reduced sensitivity in the neuropathic leg.
- Maintain dry, stable eschar on noninfected, ischemic, neuropathic wounds.

Infection. The assessment and treatment of infection is described in Chapter 9. The classification of the infection, allergies, the medical condition of the patient, and culture results (often not available initially) usually guide antibiotic therapy (Frykberg et al, 2000; Lipsky, 2000). The American Diabetes Association (1999) cites categories of infection for the patient with diabetes: limb-threatening infections, non–limb-threatening infections, and osteomyelitis.

For the patient with an ulcer that is not clinically uninfected, no antibiotics are recommended. It should be remembered that the patient with diabetes often does not show common symptoms of infection and thus must be monitored closely. Limb-threatening infections (Table 16-9) require immediate hospitalization. Additional conditions of limb-threatening infections may include necrotizing fasciitis, ischemia, hyperglycemia, and leukocytosis (American Diabetes Association, 1999; Eneroth, Apelqvist, and Stenstrom, 1997; Frykberg, 2003).

Patients with non–limb-threatening infections require immediate antibiotic therapy, generally the same day as the diagnosis. For mild and most moderate infections, therapy can be an oral agent, although certain patients may need parenteral therapy. Commonly used oral agents include cephalexin, clindamycin, levofloxacin, and amoxicillin/clavulanate. Trovafloxacin is appropriate for polymicrobial infections. Patients may be treated on an outpatient basis but only if certain criteria are met. Those who require surgical procedures, multiple diagnostic tests, or consultations or who are immunocompromised may be better treated and evaluated in a brief hospitalization.

Those with limb-threatening infections need to be hospitalized and treated parenterally with antibiotics. Empirical therapy for these infections should be broad in spectrum, including aerobic, gram-positive and gram-negative organisms, as well as resistant organisms. Examples of these antibiotic therapies include imipenem/cilastatin or vancomycin plus aztreonam plus metronidazole. Antibiotics should be reassessed when culture results are available.

Healing osteomyelitis with antibiotics alone is difficult but possible. Treatment usually lasts 6 weeks or more, usually with 1 to 2 weeks of parenteral therapy. Infected bones that can be easily resected should be removed to speed recovery and reduce the need for antibiotic therapy. Additional regimens for treating diabetic foot infections can be found in the new international consensus guidelines for diagnosing and treating infected diabetic feet (Frykberg, 2003; Lipsky, 2004).

Methicillin-resistant *Staphylococcus aureus* (MRSA) and other resistant bacteria are a major new challenge for treating DFU infections (Frykberg, 2003). Pfaller and colleagues (2001) using data from a multihospital study in the United States, reported that the percentage of MRSA of all *S. aureus* isolates increased from 22% to 34% from 1997 to 2000. In addition, vancomycin-resistant *S. aureus* (VRSA) has recently been found (Tenover et al, 2004). Vancomycin (Vancocin HCl, Eli Lilly) or linezolid (Zyvox, Pfizer) are frequently prescribed for control of MRSA.

Topical Wound Care. Evidence does not support the use of one dressing over the other for the treatment of DFUs (WOCN Society, 2004). Topical therapy for DFUs is based on the principles outlined in Chapter 19 and a formulary of multiple dressing options will be necessary to meet the needs of the wound as it changes characteristics such as size, depth, and exudate.

The increase in bacterial resistance to antibiotics has changed how some clinicians view the use of topical antimicrobials. There is a lack of consensus on the use of topical antimicrobial therapy for infected or ischemic neuropathic ulcers (WOCN Society, 2004). A short course of a topical antimicrobial may be considered if the ulcer has a high level of bacteria (WOCN Society, 2003). However, it should be noted that wounds treated with topical antimicrobials can develop resistant organisms overtime. Topical creams, ointments, and gels containing antimicrobials may also cause sensitivity reactions.

Advanced care has been described as "the use of drugs, devices, or treatment regimens that may be experimental, newly approved, or above and beyond treatment modalities routinely used in the general community for a specific medical problem. Advanced care may sometimes be the only means of rapidly and effectively attaining wound closure" (Mulder, Armstrong, and Seaman, 2003). Diabetic foot ulcers that are limb-threatening, based on ADA criteria, and require hospitalization, antibiotics, and debridement may not progress to this level (or any further) if early advanced care interventions are made. Early, advanced or "appropriate" care practices may in fact be more cost-effective than standard care practices for decreasing the incidence of LEAs (Apelqvist et al, 1995; Boulton, Meneses, and Ennis, 1999).

When confronted with a wound that fails to progress, the clinician must carefully reevaluate the entire treatment plan to assure appropriateness and should also consider biopsy to rule out malignancy. If the biopsy is negative and the management plan is appropriate, the most likely reason for failure to heal is the negative cellular environment of a chronic wound. In this case, the clinician should consider implementation of an interactive wound therapy, that is, a product or therapy designed to convert the chronic wound environment into an environment that supports repair (Driver, 2004). Specific therapies that have shown varying degrees of success in management of DFU include regenerative tissue matrix, negative-pressure wound therapy, hyperbaric oxygen therapy, angiogenic stimulators, and protease inhibitors (Armstrong et al, 2004; Boykin, 2000; Boykin, Crossland, and Cole, 1997; Brigido, Boc, and Lopez, 2004; Cianci, 1992; Cianci and Hunt, 1997; Cullen et al, 2004; DeFranzo et al, 2001; Eginton et al, 2003; Faglia et al, 1996; Holloway et al, 1993; Li and Li, 2003; Li, Tsakayannis, and Li, 2003; Margolis et al 2001; Mulder and Vande Berg, 2002; Ovington, 2004; Sihl, 1998; Steed et al, 1996; Trengrove et al, 1999). These therapies are discussed in greater detail in Chapters 5 and 20.

EDUCATION

Basic knowledge assessment in patients with diabetes, regardless of the length of time since diagnosis, often reveals a lack of understanding about the principles of diabetes self-management (Brown, 1999). Education must be relevant, simple, complete, and ongoing in order to assist the patient to achieve and maintain the highest possible level of functioning. However, education does not equal knowledge. It often takes the

presentation of material multiple times in different formats and by different health care team members to achieve understanding.

Major components of the patient's education plan require behavior change on the part of the patient, which can leave the patient feeling overwhelmed. However, education combined with behavioral therapies can be very effective for teaching coping strategies (Roter et al, 1998). Another study reported that focus groups rated the combined use of video vignettes and patient discussions highly, because the stories stimulated important discussion and patients were able to relate to the situations presented (Anderson and Funnell, 1999). The inability of the patient to follow through with a treatment plan should be carefully scrutinized and explored rather than assumed to be intentional or the patient erroneously being labeled as "noncompliant." There are many factors that contribute to an individual's ability to succeed or fail in the treatment plan. Key among these factors is expecting the patient to implement a therapy that he or she is physically unable to perform or that conflicts with another activity in his or her life. Probably the best advice to health care professionals was provided by Heisler and colleagues (2002), who stated that to facilitate patients' self-management, there is a need for a paradigm shift in the relations between provider and patients from directive to a more collaborative interactive style in which problems, treatment goals, and management stratagems are defined together. Strategies for achieving a sustainable plan are further discussed in Chapter 26.

Numerous studies have documented the success of diabetes and foot-care education in reducing the incidence of diabetic foot ulcers (Dargis et al, 1999; Litzelman et al, 1993; Malone et al, 1989; Ollendorf et al, 1998). Unfortunately, many of the studies documenting success of educational efforts at reducing diabetic foot problems compare comprehensive programs that may not exist in more operational settings. In other words, in real-world situations, both patients and providers face significant challenges in the areas of diabetes and diabetic foot care education. A study in south Texas showed those contextual factors such as time constraints, practice economics, and low reimbursement rather than physician knowledge and attitude affected caregivers' performance in delivering diabetes care education. The study also found that patients with a lower income had a decreased awareness of diabetic care principles (Larme and Pugh, 2001).

Appropriate measures should be implemented for patients who have limited mobility, cognitive problems, and visual difficulties. Other members of the family and/or friends can be employed to assist with visual assessments. Many patients diagnosed with diabetes participate in general diabetes self-management education (DSME) programs through their primary health care provider (ADA, 2004a). Some clinics include a preexamination and a postexamination test on diabetes and foot care knowledge. The test is scored at the time of the visit, and the patient is told that the test will be repeated at the end of the visit. Testing both before and after the exam provides an opportunity for the clinician to build on the patient's knowledge base.

It is imperative that patients understand the importance of daily foot exams, the implication of losing protective sensation, their risk for ulceration and amputation, and how to minimize or eliminate factors that place them at risk for ulceration and amputation. Printed educational materials can be helpful in "getting the message" across to them. Included in Box 16-3 and appendix D is an example of general foot care instructions that can be given to patients (Bowering, 2001; Wiersma-Bryant and Kraemer, 2000).

Teaching appropriate footwear selection (Chapter 17, Box 17-6) is a critical intervention. All patients need to pay special attention to the fit and the style of their shoes. They need to avoid tight-fitting, pointed-toe or open-toe shoes, thongs, or high heels. Shoes need to fit the foot. Also, shoes need to be able to breathe. Plastic shoes are inelastic and do not breathe. Finally, shoes should be adjustable with Velcro, laces, and/or buckles. Shoes with soft insoles to cushion feet may do well at reducing plantar pressure, but if the upper part of the shoes does not fit with the insole inserted, then injury to the dorsum may result (Cavanagh, Ulbrecht, and Caputo, 2001).

SUMMARY

Peripheral neuropathy, structural foot problems, and minor trauma are the primary causative factors for a DFU in the patient with LEND, and 25% of the patients with a DFU require LEA. The ultimate goals in the care of the patient with LEND and a DFU are to reduce the incidence of LEAs and to increase the frequency of minor or partial foot amputations as a percentage of all LEAs. A team approach is required for adequate management of the patient with LEND to adequately address the complex needs of this patient population: prevention of injury or trauma, frequent inspection, diligent daily foot care, education and support, and appropriate offloading (i.e., use of shoes and orthotics).

SELF-ASSESSMENT EXERCISE

1. Identify the types of neuropathy and the effects of each on skin integrity.
2. Which of the following is the primary cause of diabetic foot ulcers?
   a. Peripheral neuropathy
   b. Infection
   c. Edema
   d. Peripheral arterial disease
3. Which of the following findings are suggestive of osteomyelitis in the patient with a diabetic foot ulcer?
   a. Abnormal bone scan
   b. Nonhealing ulcer
   c. Abnormal x-ray study findings
   d. All of the above
4. Identify factors other than topical therapy that must be addressed in the management plan of a patient with a diabetic foot ulcer.
5. Identify routine precautions that one should include in the teaching of the patient with lower-extremity neuropathic disease.

REFERENCES

Abbott CA et al: The North-West Diabetes Foot Care Study: Incidence of, and risk factors for, new diabetic-foot ulceration in a community-based patient cohort, *Diabet Med* 19(5):377, 2002.
Ackley B: Nursing diagnosis: ineffective tissue perfusion: cerebral, renal, cardiopulmonary, GI, peripheral, Nursing Diagnosis Handbook; http://www1.us.elsevierhealth.com/MERLIN/Ackley/NDH/Constructor/index.cfm?plan=50; Accessed on July 13, 2004.
American Diabetes Association (ADA): Consensus Development Conference on Diabetic Foot Wound Care, 7-8 April 1999, Boston, Mass, *Diabetes Care* 22(8):1354, 1999.
American Diabetes Association (ADA): Economic costs of diabetes in the U.S. in 2002, *Diabetes Care* 26(3):917, 2003a.
American Diabetes Association (ADA): Peripheral arterial disease in people with diabetes, *Diabetes Care* 26(12):3333, 2003b.
American Diabetes Association (ADA): Preventative foot care in diabetes, *Diabetes Care* 27:S63, 2004a.
American Diabetes Association (ADA): Standards of medical care in diabetes, *Diabetes Care* 27(Suppl 1):S15, 2004b.

Anderson RM, Funnell MM: Theory is the cart, vision is the horse: reflections on research in diabetes patient education, *Diabetes Educ* 25:43, 1999.

Apelqvist J, Larsson J, Agardh CD: The influence of external precipitating factors and peripheral neuropathy on the development and outcome of diabetic foot ulcers, *J Diabetes Complications* 4:21, 1990.

Apelqvist J et al: Long-term costs for foot ulcers in diabetic patients in a multidisciplinary setting, *Foot Ankle Internat* 16:388, 1995.

Apelqvist J et al: International consensus on the diabetic foot. In: *The international working group on the diabetic foot*, Amsterdam, The Netherlands, 1999, John Wiley & Sons.

Armstrong DG et al: Off-loading the diabetic foot wound: a randomized clinical trial, *Diabetes Care* 24(6):1019, 2001.

Armstrong DG et al: Skin temperatures as a one time screening tool do not predict future diabetic foot complications, *J Am Pod Med Assn* 93(6):443, 2003a.

Armstrong DG et al: Activity patterns with diabetic foot ulceration: patients with active ulceration may not adhere to a standard pressure off-loading regimen, *Diabetes Care* 26(9):2595, 2003b.

Armstrong DG et al: Guidelines regarding negative pressure wound therapy (NPWT) in the diabetic foot, *Ostomy Wound Manage* 50(4 Suppl B):3S-21S, 2004.

Armstrong DG, Lavery LA: Diabetic foot ulcers: prevention, diagnosis, and classification, *Am Fam Physician* March: 15;57(6):1325-1332, 1337-8, 1998. Armstrong DG et al: Value of white blood cell count with differential in the acute diabetic foot infection, *J Am Pod Med Assoc* 86(5):224, 1996.

Armstrong DG, Lavery LA, Wu S, Boulton AJ. Evaluation of removable and irremovable cast walkers in the healing of diabetic foot wounds: a randomized controlled trial. Diabetes Care. Mar;28(3):551-554, 2005.

Bagdade JD, Stewart M, Walters E: Impaired granulocyte adherence: a reversible defect in patients with poorly controlled diabetes, *Diabetes* 27:677, 1978.

Bild DE et al: Lower-extremity amputation in people with diabetes. Epidemiology and prevention, *Diabetes Care* 12:24, 1989.

Boulton AJM: The diabetic foot: of neuropathic aetiology? *Diabetes Care* 17:557, 1994.

Boulton AJ, Meneses P, Ennis WJ: Diabetic foot ulcers: a framework for prevention and care, *Wound Repair Regen* 7(1):7, 1999.

Boykin JV Jr: The nitric oxide connection: hyperbaric oxygen therapy, becaplermin, and diabetic ulcer management, *Adv Skin Wound Care* 13(4):169, 2000.

Boykin JV Jr, Crossland MC, Cole LM: Wound healing management: enhancing patient outcomes and reducing costs, *J Healthc Resour Manag* 15:22, 1997.

Bowering CK: Diabetic foot ulcers, pathophysiology, assessment and therapy, *Can Fam Physician* 47:1007, 2001.

Brigido SA, Boc SF, Lopez RC: Effective management of major lower extremity wounds using an acellular regenerative tissue matrix: a pilot study, *Orthopedics* 27(1 Suppl):s145, 2004.

Brown, SA: Interventions to promote diabetes self-management: state of the science, *Diabetes Educ* 25:52, 1999.

Caselli A et al: The forefoot-to-rearfoot plantar pressure ratio is increased in severe diabetic neuropathy and can predict foot ulceration, *Diabetes Care* 25:1006, 2002.

Cavanagh PR, Hewitt FG, Perry JE: In-shoe plantar pressure measurement: a review, *Foot* 2:185, 1992.

Cavanagh PR et al: Radiographic abnormalities in the feet of patients with diabetic neuropathy, *Diabetes Care* 17:201, 1994.

Cavanagh PR, Ulbrecht JS, Caputo: The biomechanics of the foot in diabetes mellitus. In: Bowker JH, Pfeiffer MA, editors: *Levin and O'Neal's The diabetic foot*, ed 6, St Louis, 2001, Mosby.

Centers for Disease Control and Prevention (CDCP): National Health Interview Survey, Washington, DC: National Center for Health Statistics, 2001.

Centers for Disease Control and Prevention (CDCP): History of foot ulcer among persons with diabetes—United States, 2000-2002, *MMWR* 52 (45):1098, 2003.

Center for Disease Control and Prevention (CDCP): Data and trends, diabetes surveillance system. Nontraumatic lower extremity amputation with diabetes, http://www.cdc.gov/diabetes/statistics/lea/fig1.htm; Accessed April 23, 2004a.

Center for Disease Control and Prevention (CDCP): National Center for Chronic Disease Prevention and Health Promotion. Data and trends, diabetes surveillance system, Prevalence of diabetes, http://www.cdc.gov/diabetes/statistics/prev/national/figpersons.htm; Accessed May 16, 2004b.

Cianci PE: Adjunctive hyperbaric oxygen therapy in the treatment of the diabetic foot, *Wounds* 4:158, 1992.

Cianci PE, Hunt TK: Long term results of aggressive management of diabetic foot ulcers suggest significant cost effectiveness, *Wound Repair Regen* 5:141, 1997.

Cofield RH, Morison MJ, Beabout JW: Diabetic neuroarthropathy in the foot: patient characteristics and patterns of radiographic change, *Foot Ankle* 4:15, 1983.

Coleman WC, Brand PW, Birke JA: The total contact cast: a therapy for plantar ulceration on insensitive feet, *J Am Pod Med Assn* 74:548, 1984.

Cullen B et al: Mechanism of action of PROMOGRAN, a protease modulating matrix, for the treatment of diabetic foot ulcers, *Wound Repair Regen* 10(1):16, 2002.

Caputo GM et al: Assessment and management of foot disease in patients with diabetes, *N Engl J Med.* 331:854, 1994.

Daniels TR: Diabetic foot ulcerations: an overview, *Ostomy Wound Manage* 44(9):76, 1998.

Dargis V et al: Benefits of a multidisciplinary approach in the management of recurrent diabetic foot ulceration in Lithuania: a prospective study, *Diabetes Care* 22:1428, 1999.

DeFranzo AJ et al: The use of vacuum-assisted closure therapy for the treatment of lower-extremity wounds with exposed bone, *Plast Reconstr Surg* 108(5):1184, 2001.

Diabetes Control and Complications Research Group: The effect of intensive treatment of diabetes on the development and progression of long-term complications in insulin-dependent diabetes mellitus, *N Engl J Med* 329:977, 1993.

Dow G, Browne A, Sibbald RG: Infection in chronic wounds: controversies in diagnosis and treatment, *Ostomy Wound Manage* 45(8):23, 1999.

Driver VR, Madsen J, Goodman RA: Reducing amputation rates in patients with diabetes at a military medical center: the limb preservation service model, *Diabetes Care* 28(2): p. 248-253, 2005.

Driver VR: Treating the macro and micro wound environment of the diabetic patient::managing the whole patient, not the hole in the patient. *Foot and Ankle Quarterly-* 16(2): p. 47-56, 2004.

Edmonds ME, Roberts VC, Watkins PJ: Blood flow in the diabetic neuropathic foot, *Diabetologia* 22:9, 1982.

Edmonds ME et al: Improved survival of the diabetic foot: the role of a specialized foot clinic, *QJ Med* 60(232):763, 1986.

Eginton MT et al: A prospective, randomized evaluation of negative pressure dressings for diabetic foot wounds, *Ann Vasc Surg* 17(6):645, 2003.

Eichenholz SN: *Charcot joints*, Springfield, Ill, 1966, Charles C. Thomas.

Eneroth M, Apelqvist J, Stenstrom A: Clinical characteristics and outcome in 223 diabetic patients with deep foot infections, *Foot Ankle Int* 18(11):716, 1997.

Faglia E et al: Adjunctive systemic hyperbaric oxygen therapy in treatment of severe prevalently ischemic diabetic foot ulcers. A randomized study, *Diabetes Care* 19(12):1338, 1996.

Frykberg RG: Diabetic foot ulcerations. In: Frykberg RG, editor: *The high risk foot in diabetes*, New York, 1991, Churchill Livingstone.

Frykberg RG: Diabetic foot ulcers: pathogenesis and management, *Am Fam Physician* 66:1655, 2002.

Frykberg RG: An evidence-based approach to diabetic foot infections, *Am J Surg* 186/5A:44S, 2003.

Frykberg RG et al: *Diabetic foot disorders – a clinical practice guideline*, Brooklandville, Md, 2000, Data Trace Publishing.

Gibbons G, Eliopoulos G: Infection in the diabetic foot. In Kozak GP et al, editors: *Management of diabetic foot problems*, Philadelphia, 1984, WB Saunders.

Gordois A et al: The health care costs of diabetic peripheral neuropathy in the U.S., *Diabetes Care* 26:1790, 2003.

Grady JF et al: Use of electrostimulation in the treatment of diabetic neuropathy, *J Am Pod Med Assn* 90:287, 2000.

Grayson ML et al: Probing to bone in infected pedal ulcers. A clinical sign of underlying osteomyelitis in diabetic patients, *JAMA* 273(9):721, 1995.

Grunfeld C: Diabetic foot ulcers: etiology, treatment, and prevention, *Adv Intern Med* 37:103, 1991.

Guis S et al: Healing of Charcot's joint by pamidronate infusion, *J Rheumatol* 26:1843, 1999.

Harrington C et al: A cost analysis of diabetic lower-extremity ulcers, *Diabetes Care* 23:1333, 2000.

Heisler M et al: The relative importance of physician communication, participatory decision-making, and patient understanding in diabetes self-management, *J Gen Intern Med* 17:243, 2002.

Holloway GA et al: A randomized, controlled dose response trial of activated platelet supermatant, topical CT-102 in chronic, nonhealing, diabetic wounds, *Wounds* 5:160, 1993.

Jeffcoate WJ, Harding KG: Diabetic foot ulcers, *Lancet* (361):1545, 2003.

Jude EB et al: Peripheral arterial disease in diabetic and nondiabetic patients: a comparison of severity and outcome, *Diabetes Care* 24:1433, 2001.

Laborde, JM: Treatment of forefoot ulcers with tendon lengthenings, *J South Orthop Assn* 12(2):60, 2003.

Larme AC, Pugh JA: Evidence-based guidelines meet the real world, *Diabetes Care* 24:1728, 2001.

Larsen K, Fabrin J, Holstein PE: Incidence and management of ulcers in diabetic Charcot feet, *J Wound Care* 10(8):323, 2001.

Larsson J et al: Long term prognosis after healed amputations in patients with diabetes, *Clin Orthop* 350:149, 1998.

Lavery LA, Armstrong DG, Boulton AJM: Ankle equinus deformity and its relationship to high plantar pressure in a large population with diabetes mellitus, *J Am Pod Med Assn* 92(9):479, 2002.

Lavery LA, Armstrong DG, Harkless LB: Classification of diabetic foot wounds, *J Foot Ankle Surg* 35:528, 1996.

Lavery LA et al: Reducing plantar pressure in the neuropathic foot. A comparison of footwear, *Diabetes Care* 20:1706, 1997.

Lavery LA et al: Practical criteria for screening patients at high risk for diabetic foot ulceration, *Arch Intern Med* 158(2):157, 1998.

Lavery LA et al: Diabetic foot syndrome: evaluating the prevalence and incidence of foot pathology in Mexican Americans and non-Hispanic whites from a diabetes disease management cohort, *Diabetes Care*, 26(5):1435, 2003.

Levin ME: Pathogenesis and general management of foot lesions. In Bowker JH, Pfeiffer MA, editors: *Levin and O'Neal's The diabetic foot*, ed 6, St. Louis, 2001, Mosby.

Levin ME: Management of the diabetic foot: preventing amputation, *South Med J* 95(1):10, 2002.

Levy PJ: Epidemiology and pathophysiology of peripheral arterial disease, *Clin Cornerstone* 4(5):1, 2002.

Li WW, Li VW: Therapeutic angiogenesis for wound healing, *Wounds* 15(9 Suppl):2S, 2003.

Li WW, Tsakayannis D, Li VW: Angiogenesis: a control point for normal and delayed wound healing, *Contemp Surg* Nov(Suppl):5, 2003.

Lipsky BA: Osteomyelitis of the foot in diabetic patients, *Clin Infect Dis* 25:1318, 1997.

Lipsky BA: Antibiotic therapy of diabetic foot infections, *Wounds* 12 (suppl B):55B, 2000.

Lipsky BA: A report from the international consensus on diagnosing and treating the infected diabetic foot, *Diabetes Metab Res Rev* 20(Suppl 1):S68, 2004.

Litchy W et al: Diabetic peripheral neuropathy (DPN) assessed by neurological examination (NE) and composite scores (CS) is improved with LY 333531 treatment. Program and abstracts of the 62nd Scientific Sessions of the American Diabetes Association; June 14-18, San Francisco, California, 2002, Abstract 321-OR.

Litzelman DK et al: Reduction of lower-extremity clinical abnormalities with non-insulin dependent diabetes mellitus, *Ann Intern Med* 119:36, 1993.

Macfarlane R, Jeffcoate W: Classification of diabetic foot ulcers: the size (area and depth) (SAD) system, *Diabetic Foot* 2(4):123, 1999.

Malone JM et al: Prevention of amputation by diabetic education, *Am J Surg* 158(6):520, 1989.

Margolis DJ et al: Effectiveness of platelet releasate for the treatment of diabetic neuropathic foot ulcers, *Diabetes Care* 24:483, 2001.

Mayfield JA et al: Trends in lower limb amputation in the Veterans Health Administration, 1989-1998, *J Rehabil Res Dev* 37:23, 2000.

Meltzer DD et al: Decreasing amputation rates in patients with diabetes mellitus. An outcome study, *JAPMA* 92(8):425, 2002.

Mohler ER 3rd et al: Trial of a novel prostacyclin analog, UT-15, in patients with severe intermittent claudication, *Vasc Med* 5:231, 2000.

Moulik PK, Mtonga R, Gill GV: Amputation and mortality in new-onset foot ulcers stratified by etiology, *Diabetes Care* 26:491, 2003.

Mueller MJ et al: Effect of Achilles tendon lengthening on neuropathic plantar ulcers. A randomized clinical trial, *J Bone Joint Surg (Am)* 85:1436, 2003.

Mueller MJ et al: Impact of Achilles tendon lengthening on functional limitations and perceived disability in people with a neuropathic plantar ulcer, *Diabetes Care* 27(7):1559, 2004.

Mulder GD, Vande Berg JS: Cellular senescence and matrix metalloproteinase activity in chronic wounds, *J Am Podiatr Med Assoc* 92(1):34, 2002.

Mulder G, Armstrong DG, Seaman S: Standard, appropriate, and advanced care and medical-legal considerations. Part one—diabetic foot ulcerations, *Wounds* 15(4):92, 2003.

Muller IS et al: Foot ulceration and lower limb amputation in type 2 diabetic patients in Dutch primary health care, *Diabetes Care* 25:570, 2002.

Nabuurs-Franssen MH et al: The effect of polyneuropathy on foot microcirculation in Type II diabetes, *Diabetologia* 45(8):1164, 2002.

National Institute of Neurological Disorders and Stroke: National Institutes of Health. NINDS Peripheral Neuropathy Information Page, http://www.ninds.nih.gov/health_and_medical/disorders/peripheralneuropathy_doc.htm; Accessed December 1, 2003.

Newman LG et al: Unsuspected osteomyelitis in diabetic foot ulcers. Diagnosis and monitoring by leukocyte scanning with indium in 111 oxyquinoline, *JAMA* 266:1246, 1991.

Ollendorf DA et al: Potential economic benefits of lower-extremity amputation prevention strategies in diabetes, *Diabetes Care* 21(8):1240, 1998.

Ovington, L: Part 1. Overview of matrix metalloprotease modulation and growth factor protection in wound healing, http://www.woundsresearch.com/wnds/matrix/pt1.cfm, Accessed July 7, 2004.

Oyibo SO et al: A comparison of two diabetic foot ulcer classification systems: the Wagner and the University of Texas wound classification systems, *Diabetes Care* 24:84, 2001.

Page J, Chen E: Management of painful diabetic neuropathy—a treatment algorithm, *J Am Podiatr Med Assn* 87:370, 1997.

Pecoraro RE, Reiber GE: Classification of wounds in diabetic amputees, *Wounds* 2:65, 1990.

Pecoraro RE, Reiber GE, Burgess EM: Pathways to diabetic limb amputation. Basis for prevention, *Diabetes Care* 13:513, 1990.

Perkins BA et al: Simple screening tests for peripheral neuropathy in the diabetes clinic, *Diabetes Care* 24:250, 2001.

Peters EJG, Lavery L: Effectiveness of the diabetic foot risk classification system of the International Working Group on the Diabetic Foot, *Diabetes Care* 24:1442, 2001.

Pfaller MA et al: Trends in antimicrobial susceptibility of bacterial pathogens isolated from patients with bloodstream infections (BSI) in North America (NA): SENTRY Program, 1997-2000. Program and abstracts of the 41st Interscience Conference on Antimicrobial Agents and Chemotherapy, Chicago, Ill, Dec. 16-19, 2001.

Pfeifer MA, Schumer MP: Clinical trials of diabetic neuropathy: past, present and future, *Diabetes* 44:1335, 1995.

Pham H et al: Screening techniques to identify people at high risk for diabetic foot ulceration: a prospective multicenter trial, *Diabetes Care* 23(5):606, 2000.

Poncelet AN: An algorithm for the evaluation of peripheral neuropathy, *Am Fam Physician* 57:755, 1998.

Ramsey SD et al: Incidence, outcomes, and cost of foot ulcers in patients with diabetes, *Diabetes Care* 22:382, 1999.

Regensteiner JG et al: Chronic changes in skeletal muscle histology and function in peripheral arterial disease, *Circulation* 87:413, 1993.

Reiber GE, Boyko EJ, Smith DG: Lower extremity foot ulcers and amputations in diabetes. In *Diabetes in America*, ed 2, Bethesda, MD, 1995, National Institutes of Health.

Reiber GE et al: Causal pathways for incident lower-extremity ulcers in patients with diabetes from two settings, *Diabetes Care* 22(1):157, 1999.

Rith-Najarian SJ, Stolusky T, Gohdes DM: Identifying diabetic patients at high risk for lower-extremity amputation in a primary health care setting. A prospective evaluation of simple screening criteria, *Diabetes Care* 15:1386, 1992.

Robson MC, Stenberg BD, Heggars JP: Wound healing alterations caused by infection, *Clin Plast Surg* 17:485, 1990.

Roter DL et al: Effectiveness of interventions to improve patient compliance: a meta-analysis, *Med Care* 36:1138, 1998.

Sanders LJ, Frykberg RG: Charcot neuropathy of the foot. In Bowker JH, Pfeiffer MA, editors: *Levin and O'Neal's The diabetic foot*, ed 6, St Louis, 2001, Mosby.

Seidel HM et al, editors: Blood vessels. In *Mosby's guide to physical examination*, ed 5, St Louis, 2003, Mosby.

Serralta VW et al: Lifestyles of bacteria in wounds: presence of biofilms? *Wounds* 13(1):29, 2001.

Sibbald RG et al: Preparing the wound bed—debridement, bacterial balance, and moisture balance, *Ostomy Wound Manage* 46(11):14, 2000.

Shah BR, Hux JE: Quantifying the risk of infectious diseases for people with diabetes, *Diabetes Care* 26:510, 2003.

Sihl N: Diabetes and wound healing, *J Wound Care* 7:47, 1998.

Sims DS, Cavanaugh PR, Ulbrecht JS: Risk factors in the diabetic foot: recognition and management, *Phys Ther* 68:1887, 1988.

Sinacore DR: Total contact casting for diabetic neuropathic ulcers, *Phys Ther* 76:296, 1996.

Sinacore DR, Mueller MJ: Total-contact casting in the treatment of neuropathic ulcers. In: Bowker JH, Pfeiffer MA, editors: *Levin and O'Neal's The diabetic foot*, ed 6, St Louis, 2001, Mosby.

Steed DL et al: Effect of extensive debridement and treatment on the healing of diabetic foot ulcers. Diabetic Ulcer Study Group, *J Am Coll Surg* 183:61, 1996.

Sumpio B: Primary care: foot ulcers, *New Eng J Med* 343(1):787, 2000.

Tanneberg RJ et al: Neuropathic problems of the lower extremities in diabetic patients. In: Bowker JH, Pfeiffer MA, editors: *Levin and O'Neal's The diabetic foot*, ed 6, St Louis, 2001, Mosby.

Tenover FC et al: Vancomycin-resistant *Staphylococcus aureus* isolate from a patient in Pennsylvania, *Antimicrob Agents Chemother* 48(1):275, 2004.

Trengrove NI et al: Analysis of the acute and chronic wound environments: the role of proteases and their inhibitors, *Wound Repair Regen* 7(6):442, 1999.

Umpierrez GE et al: Hyperglycemia: an independent marker of in-hospital mortality in patients with undiagnosed diabetes, *J Clin Endocrinol Metab* 87:978, 2002.

Van Acker K et al: The choice of diabetic foot ulcer classification in relation to the final outcome, *Wounds* 14(1):16, 2002.

Vande Berg JS, Rudolph R, Hollan C, Haywood-Reid PL: Fibroblast senescence in pressure ulcers, *Wound Repair Regen* 6(1):38, 1998.

Van Houtum WH et al: *Reduction in diabetes lower extremity amputations in the Netherlands: 1991-2000*, 18th Internat. Diabetes Fed. Congress, Paris, Aug. 24-29, 2003.

Veves A, Sarnow M: Diagnosis, classification, and treatment of diabetic peripheral neuropathy, *Clin Podiatr Med Surg* 12:19, 1995.

Vinik AI et al: Diabetic autonomic neuropathy, *Diabetes Care* 26:1553, 2003.

Wagner FW: The dysvascular foot: a system for diagnosis and treatment, *Foot Ankle* 2:64, 1981.

Wiersma-Bryant LA, Kraemer BA: Vascular and neuropathic wounds: the diabetic wound. In Bryant RA, editor: *Acute and chronic wounds—nursing management*, ed 2, St Louis, 2000, Mosby.

WOCN Society: *Guideline for management of wounds in patients with lower-extremity neuropathic disease*, WOCN Clinical Practice Guideline Series #3, Glenview IL, 2004, Author.

Young MJ et al: The effect of callus removal on dynamic plantar foot pressures in diabetic patients, *Diabetic Med* 9:55, 1992.

Young MJ et al: Osteopenia, neurological dysfunction, and the development of Charcot neuroarthropathy, *Diabetes Care* 18:34, 1995.

Yu GV, Hudson JR: Evaluation and treatment of stage 0 Charcot's neuroarthropathy of the foot and ankle, *J Am Pod Med Assn* 92(4):210, 2002.

Zimny S et al: Early detection of microcirculatory impairment in diabetic patients with foot at risk, *Diabetes Care* 24:1810, 2001.

Foot and Nail Care

·····································

TARA L. BEUSCHER

OBJECTIVES

1. Correlate patient history information with the potential for foot problems.
2. Describe the structure and function of the foot and nails.
3. Identify the key features of manifestations and management of foot malformations (e.g., bunions, hammer toes).
4. Describe common foot lesions including etiology, symptoms, manifestations, treatment, and prevention.
5. Distinguish between two toenail disorders and their treatments.
6. Develop an appropriate plan for routine care of the foot.

Foot problems occur in the lives of at least 75% of Americans (Menz, Pod, and Lord, 2001). Most people mistakenly believe that discomfort and pain are normal or should be expected. Foot ailments may stem from the cumulative impact of a lifetime of abuse and neglect, or they may be hereditary, or they may be symptomatic of an underlying disease process. A number of systemic diseases precipitate foot pathology.

Health care providers frequently overlook foot screening for a number of reasons such as lack of interest, reimbursement, knowledge, or time (Cameron, 2002). Although it is often overlooked, foot screening and education should be done in conjunction with routine skin assessment (Pelican, Barbieri, and Blair, 1990; Williams, 2001). This includes (1) routine screening and early detection, (2) education regarding prevention and treatment measures, (3) collaborative goal setting, and (4) routine follow up through monitoring and case management (Cameron, 2002).

This chapter will describe anatomy, common pathology, prevention, assessment, and interventions associated with foot and nails. Specific problems related

to the patient with lower-extremity neuropathic disease (LEND) are addressed in Chapter 16.

QUALITY OF LIFE

Foot diseases and their treatments have a tremendous impact on the quality of life (Brod, 1998; Katsambas et al, 2005). In fact, patients with diabetes who have foot ulcers report a poorer quality of life than patients with diabetes who have amputations (Price and Harding, 2000).

The number of patients whose quality of life is affected by their foot disease varies considerably from country to country (Katsambas et al, 2005). This may be a consequence of attributes and perceptions of health and illness by various cultures as well as the possibility that foot conditions may be managed more effectively in some countries (Drake et al, 1999).

Overall, foot disease has a significantly greater effect on the quality of life of women than of men with regards to the experience of pain, discomfort in walking, and embarrassment (Katsambas et al, 2005; Leveille et al, 1998). One explanation could be that many types of shoes typically worn by women are tighter-fitting, thus increasing the risk of developing toenail onychomycosis, which is associated with pain and discomfort in walking (Drake et al, 1999).

The Achilles Project, a large-scale survey of foot diseases conducted in 17 countries (15 European countries, Israel, and South Africa) assessed the quality of life of 45,593 patients with foot disease. Study participants were surveyed to assess the extent of pain and discomfort in walking, and to what extent their condition contributed to embarrassment or limitations in their activities of daily living (ADLs). The results revealed that 40.3% experienced discomfort in walking, 30.7% had pain, 27.3% had embarrassment, and 19.6% experienced limitations in their ADLs. All four quality of life measures were present in 7% of the patients (Benvenuti et al, 1995; Katsambas, 2005)

STRUCTURE AND FUNCTION

The human foot contains a quarter of all the bones in the body (specifically, 26 bones), 33 joints, and a network of more than 100 tendons, muscles, and ligaments, blood vessels, nerves, and nails. An average day of walking brings a force equal to several hundred tons to bear on the feet; feet are more subject to injury than any other part of the body.

The rear, mid-, and forefoot comprise the three main functional units of the foot. All units must work together to provide both flexibility and rigidity. Of the 26 bones in each foot there are 14 phalanges (toe bones), 5 metatarsals (instep bones), and 7 tarsals (anklebones) (Figure 17-1).

The plantar arch runs the length of the foot, touches the ground only at the ball of the foot and at the heel bone (calcaneous), and is thickly padded at both ends. A thick pad of fat also underlies the calcaneous. The metatarsal arch runs crosswise under the instep. The lateral arch runs lengthwise along the outside of the foot. In the ankle, the talus contacts the lower tibia and fibula.

Nails are made of epidermal cells converted to hard plates of keratin (Figure 17-2). The highly vascular nail bed lies beneath the plate, giving the nail its pink color. The stratum corneum layer of the skin covering the nail root is the eponychium (cuticle), which forms a seal between the nail and toe preventing foreign matter from entering. The paronychium is the soft tissue surrounding the nail border (Scher et al, 2003; Seidel et al, 2003). Nails on the foot can take 1 year or more to grow out completely.

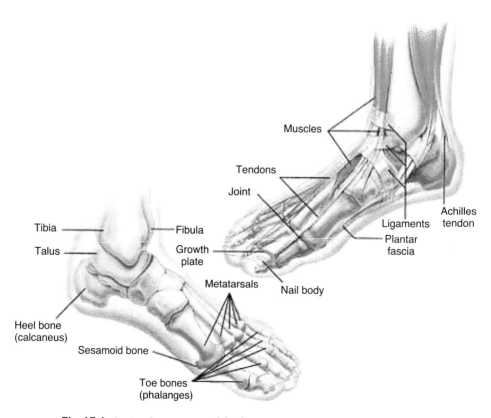

Fig. 17-1 Anatomic structures of the foot. (From Fort Worth Orthopaedics, 2003.)

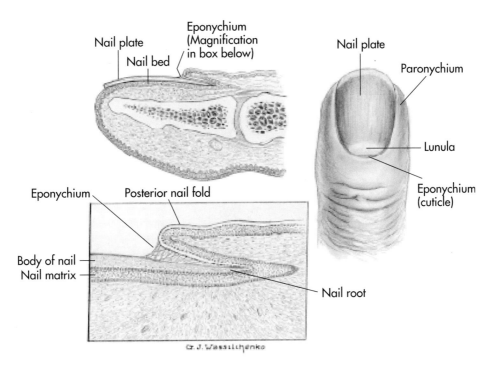

Fig. 17-2 Anatomic structures of the nail. (From Thompson JM et al: *Mosby's Clinical Nursing*, ed 5, St Louis, Mosby, 2002.)

PATHOLOGY

Many conditions or circumstances such as obesity, anemia, renal insufficiency, gout, warfarin therapy, Raynaud's disease, immunosuppression, and recurrent cellulitis can greatly affect the integrity and function of the foot (Leveille et al, 1998). The 33 joints in each foot must accommodate an extraordinary weight load, making the feet particularly susceptible to arthritic inflammation and swelling of the cartilage and lining of the joints. Individuals over 50 years of age are at greatest risk for arthritis. Osteoarthritis is the most common form of arthritis and is associated with aging, injury, or overuse. In contrast, rheumatoid arthritis is an autoimmune disorder. The foot is one of the first places for osteoporosis to appear. A stress fracture of the foot is often its first sign.

Repetitive stress of the foot leads to a variety of normal age-associated changes (Bryant and Beinlich, 1999; George, 1993; Resnick 1997; Turner and Quine, 1996). With age, the foot becomes wider, longer, and flatter. The fat pad on the bottom of the calcaneous thins out, whereas the foot and ankle lose some range

of motion, become stiff, and contribute to some loss of balance with ambulation (Mathias, Nayak, and Isaacs, 1986; Podsiadlo and Richardson, 1991).

Impaired Circulation and Sensation

Any impairment in circulation or sensation contributes to problems with the foot. Lower-extremity arterial disease (LEAD), lower-extremity venous disease (LEVD), and lower-extremity neuropathic disease (LEND) are underlying pathologies such as neuropathy and edema of the legs and feet. These pathologies are discussed in great detail in chapters 15 and 16. Decreased foot sensation also occurs with syphilis, leprosy, myelomeningocele, syringomyelia, hereditary neuropathies, and traumatic nerve injury. Any sensory impairment and loss of protective pain sensation places the patient at increased risk of ulceration, infection, and amputation (Adler et al, 1999; Younes, Albsoul, and Awad, 2004).

Foot Malformations

Brief descriptions and examples of foot malformations are presented in Chapter 16 Table 16-3, Figure 16-1.

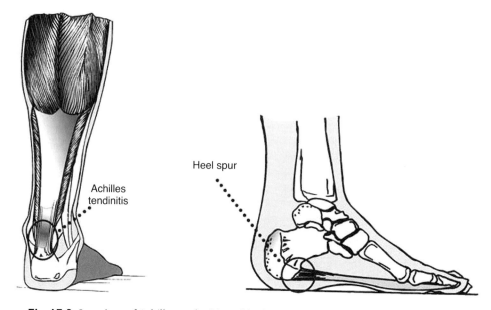

Fig. 17-3 Locations of Achilles tendonitis and heel spurs. (From *Am Physical Therapy Assoc*, 1996.)

Plantar Fasciitis and Heel Spurs. Plantar fasciitis is heel pain caused by inflammation of the long band of connective tissue running from the calcaneous to the ball of the foot (Lemont, Ammirati, and Usen, 2003). Plantar fasciitis can be painful and is usually caused by faulty biomechanics that place too much stress on the calcaneus bone, ligaments, or nerves in the area (Jolly, Zgonis, and Hendrix, 2005; La Porta and La Fata, 2005). Plantar fasciitis can cause or be caused by heel spurs (the bony growths on the underside, foremost part of the calcaneous bone, as seen in Figure 17-3) (Aldridge, 2004; Lemont et al, 2003). Stress on the calcaneous bone can result from poorly made footwear and walking or jumping on hard surfaces. Arthritis, gout, ankylosing spondylitis, Reiter's syndrome, tarsal tunnel syndrome, radiculopathy, inferior calcaneal bursitis, calcaneal fracture, foreign bodies, circulatory problems, and obesity may contribute to pain in the calcaneous (Kosinski and Ramcharitar, 1994).

Bunions (Hallux Valgus) and Hammer (Claw) Toes. Bunions (hallux valgus) are misaligned great toe joints that can become tender and swollen (Ferrari, Higgins, and Prior, 2004). The first joint of the large metatarsal slants outward, with the tip angling toward the other toes. Bunions tend to run in families, but shoes that are too narrow in the forefoot and toe, particularly high heels, can aggravate this tendency. Figure 16-1 shows an example of hallux valgus.

Hammer or claw toes appear bent into a clawlike position. Hammer or claw toes are most often seen in the second metatarsal, when a bunion slants the large metatarsal toward and under it. The condition usually indicates muscle imbalance but is aggravated by ill-fitting shoes or socks that cramp the toes (Camasta, 1996). Figure 16-1 shows an example of hammer or claw toes.

Neuromas. Neuromas are enlarged, benign growths of nerves, most commonly occurring between the third and fourth toes, caused by bones or other tissue rubbing against and irritating the nerves (Larson et al, 2005; Thomson, Gibson, and Martin, 2004; Wu, 1996). Patients frequently describe the feeling of "walking on a marble." Abnormal bone structure or pressure from ill-fitting shoes also can create the condition. Neuromas result in pain, burning, tingling, or numbness between the toes and in the ball of the foot.

Charcot's Arthropathy. Charcot's arthropathy is a fairly rare, but serious, condition caused by the disruption or disintegration of some of the foot and ankle joints (Armstrong and Lavery, 1998). This results in redness, swelling, and deformity and may be misinterpreted as cellulitis. This condition is frequently associated with diabetes and discussed in greater detail in Chapter 16.

Lesions and Skin Alterations

Lesions and skin alterations can be superficial or deep and potentially lead to significant infection. Brief descriptions of selected lesions and skin alterations are presented in Box 17-1 and Figure 17-4.

Corns and Calluses. Corns and calluses are thickened, hyperkeratotic lesions composed of protective layers of compacted, dead skin cells and caused by repeated friction and pressure from skin rubbing against bony areas or against an irregularity in a shoe (Freeman, 2002; George, 1993; Mann and Mann, 2004). Corns ordinarily form on toes whereas calluses usually form on the plantar aspect of the foot. These lesions are the body's response to long-term, low-level insult. This protective mechanism provides extra strength to skin by causing thickening, which in turn causes more pressure. Eventually an ulcer may result, either under or through the area. This is especially problematic in the person with loss of protective sensation, who will remain unaware of pain or pressure as the process goes forward.

Plantar Warts. A wart, caused by a virus that enters the skin through a small cut or opening, initially presents as a small black dot (punctate hemorrhage) surrounded by or under a callus located on the plantar surface of the foot. The small, circular lesion appears raised and silver in color (Stulberg and Hutchinson, 2003).

Tinea Pedis (Athlete's Foot). Tinea pedis (Plate 7f) is a superficial fungal infection that starts between the toes or on the plantar aspect of the foot (Crawford, 2004; Gupta et al, 2003). Symptoms include dry, scaly skin, itching, inflammation, and blisters that range from mild, asymptomatic infection to a highly inflamed skin, intense itching, and pain with large weeping vesicles and deep fissures between the toes and on the plantar surfaces (Gupta et al, 2003). Predisposing factors include vascular disease and sports participation (Roseeuw, 1999). Symptoms may be less pronounced in elderly individuals and individuals with altered sensation. The moccasin type of tinea pedis, often mistaken for dry skin on the plantar

---

BOX 17-1 Brief Descriptions of Selected Foot Lesions and Skin Alterations

Corns
Thickened hyperkeratotic lesions that ordinarily form on toes; composed of protective layers of compacted, dead skin cells resulting from repeated friction and pressure (Figure 17-4, A).

Callus
Thickened hyperkeratotic skin usually on the plantar aspect of the foot; composed of protective layers of compacted, dead skin cells resulting from repeated friction and pressure (Figure 17-4, B).

Plantar Warts
A small, circular, raised lesion caused by a virus that enters the skin through a small cut or opening; presents initially as a small black dot (punctate hemorrhage), surrounded by or under a callus and located on the plantar surface of the foot

Tinea Pedis (Athlete's Foot)
A fungal infection that starts between the toes or on the plantar aspect of the foot; characterized by dry scaling, itching, inflammation, and blisters that range from a mild, symptom-free infection to a highly inflamed skin, intense itching, and pain with large, weeping vesicles and deep fissures between the toes and on the plantar surfaces (Plate 7F)

Xerosis
Dry skin; clinically characterized by raised or uplifted skin edges (scaling), desquamation (flaking), chapping, and pruritus.

Fissures
Linear cracks and breaks extending from epidermis to dermis (Plate 7F)

Maceration
Overhydration of the skin characterized by a white, "waterlogged" appearance

Blisters
Fluid-filled lesions that are caused by pressure, friction, or viral, fungal, or bacterial infection
Blisters greater than 1 cm in diameter are termed *bullae* (Plate 6 I). Blisters less than 1 cm in diameter are termed *vesicles* (Plate 6H).

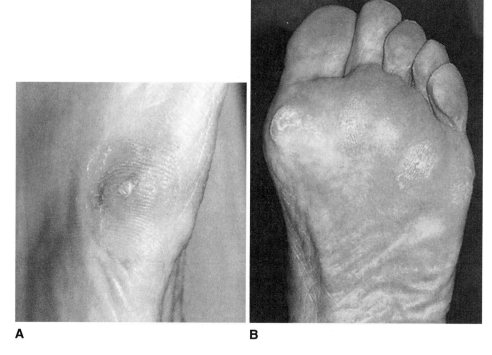

A   **B**

Fig. 17-4 Selected lesions and skin alterations. **A,** Corn. **B,** Callus. (From Seidel Henry M et al: *Mosby's Guide to Physical Examination*, ed 5, St Louis, Mosby, 2003.)

surface of the foot, does not respond to emollient application. Tinea pedis may also be combined with a secondary bacterial infection (Erbagci, 2004; Gupta, Skinner and Cooper, 2003).

Xerosis and Fissures. Xerosis, or dry skin, is a consequence of the skin's loss of natural moisturizing factors. The loss of moisture from the stratum corneum and intercellular matrix leads to xerosis. Clinically, xerosis appears rough, uneven, and cracked. Raised or uplifted skin edges (scaling), desquamation (flaking), chapping, and pruritus may be present. A person who has a decrease or loss of function of the sweat glands on the plantar surface of the foot will experience xerosis of the feet. Xerosis often leads to fissures: linear cracks and breaks from the epidermis to the dermis. Fissures can serve as a portal of entry for bacteria. Consequently, fissures are associated with an increased risk of cellulitis and foot ulceration (Pham et al, 2002).

Maceration. Maceration is overhydration of the skin that is characterized by a white, "waterlogged" appearance. The prolonged presence of moisture on the skin will precipitate maceration. Such overhydration of the stratum corneum weakens the collagen, promotes overgrowth of bacterial and fungal species of skin flora, and decreases the skin's ability to resist trauma. Maceration is prevented by keeping the skin dry and protected (Gupta, Skinner, and Cooper, 2003).

Blisters and Ulcerations. Blisters, elevated fluid-filled lesions, are caused by pressure, friction, and viral, fungal, or bacterial infections. A blister greater than 1 cm in diameter is referred to as a bulla whereas the blister that measures less than 1 cm in diameter is called a vesicle. An ulcer is a partial- or full-thickness wound, which develop from a variety of causes (i.e., mechanical, vascular, etc.).

Nail Disorders

Selected nail disorders are briefly described in Box 17-2 and Figure 17-5. Two common nail disorders (onychocryptosis and onychomycosis) are described here in greater detail.

BOX 17-2 Brief Descriptions of Selected Nail Disorders

Onychocryptosis (Ingrown Nail)
Penetration of a segment of the nail plate into the nail sulcus (groove) and subcutaneous tissue (Figure 17-5, *B*)

Paronychia
Infection of the tissues around the base of the nail (paronychium) (Figure 17-5, *A*)

Onychogryposis (Ram's Horn Nail)
Large, deformed, hypertrophic nail that has been permitted to grow without trimming or debridement

Onychomycosis
Fungal infection of the nail; characterized by discolored, thickened, and brittle nails
Psoriasis, lichen planus, allergic and irritant contact dermatitis, dyshidrosis, and atopic dermatitis, may mimic onychomycosis

Onychophosis
A deformity of the nail plate or bed that results in incurvated and involuted toenails that exert significant pressure on the nail grooves

Onychia
Inflammation of the cells that grow the nail (matrix), which causes a loosening of the nail plate
Frequently occurs on the great toe, leading to erythema and edema

Onychatrophia
Atrophy of the nails, causing them to become softer, thinner, and smaller or to fall off

Onycho(o) = "the nails"

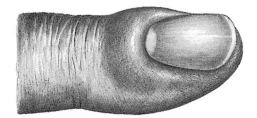

A   Paronychia

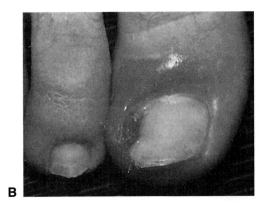

B

Fig. 17-5 Selected nail disorders. **A,** Paronychia. **B,** Onychocryptosis (ingrown nail). (A, From Seidel Henry M et al: *Mosby's Guide to Physical Examination*, ed 6, St Louis, Mosby, 2006. B, From White GM: *Color atlas of regional dermatology*, St Louis, 1994, Mosby.)

Onychocryptosis (Ingrown Nail). Onychocryptosis (more commonly known as an ingrown toenail) results from a segment of the nail plate penetrating the nail sulcus and subcutaneous tissue. Onychocryptosis is characterized by acute inflammation and pain, which can evolve into infection, (i.e., paronychia, cellulitis), ulceration, and possibly necrosis (Black, 1995; Rockwell, 2001; Yates and Concannon, 2002). Improper nail trimming, shoe pressure, injury, fungus infection, heredity, and poor foot structure precipitate ingrown toenails

(DeLauro and DeLauro, 2004). Ingrown nails can also be caused by onychogryposis (ram's horn nail), which is a large, deformed, hypertrophic nail that has been permitted to grow without trimming or debridement (Borovoy et al, 1983).

Onychomycosis (Fungal Infection of the Nail). Onychomycosis, a dermatophytic infection invading the nail bed, is a painless condition that occurs in conjunction with trauma to the nail. The infectious agent must be present on the susceptible host. Individuals most susceptible to onychomycosis include the elderly, individuals with chronically moist feet (such as athletes), and individuals with a compromised immune function. The dermatophytes invade the nail when protective functions are damaged. The nail is a food source for the organism, which causes nails to become discolored, thickened, and brittle. Pain can develop when the long, thick nails crowd shoes and cause conditions such as paronychia, subungual hemorrhage, and cellulitis. Nail conditions that may mimic onychomycosis include psoriasis, lichen planus, allergic and irritant contact dermatitis, dyshidrosis, atopic dermatitis, and bacterial and candidal infections (Scher et al, 2003).

ASSESSMENT

Components of an initial evaluation for the patient with actual or potential foot alterations are listed in Box 17-3.

Health History

Because of the interrelatedness of foot and nail health with general health, a health history is essential (see Box 17-3). Specific information should be elicited about routine care of the foot, any history of foot and nail problems, and how these problems were treated either personally or by a health care provider. Duration and types and effects of prior treatments, including prescription and over-the-counter medications, should be assessed (Piraccini, 2004; Sprecher, 2005). There is a lack of standardized quality of life questionnaires for foot diseases; however, it is important to solicit quality of life information from the patient (Drake et al, 1999; Garrow, Silman, and Macfarlane, 2004; Garrow et al, 2000; Katsambas et al, 2005; Kuyvenhoven et al, 2002; Vileikyte et al, 2003).

Physical Assessment

Perfusion and Sensation. Because so many patients with foot disorders have concomitant lower-extremity disease, perfusion and sensation must be assessed. The following discussion will present the unique assessment parameters for the foot and nail. Assessment parameters for perfusion (i.e., edema, skin color and temperature, nail blanching, capillary refill time, and venous fill time) and sensation are discussed in Chapters 15 and 16 respectively.

Functional Ability. A functional ability assessment includes gait, mobility, musculoskeletal function, balance, strength-hand dexterity, and visual cognition. *Cognition* is relevant for foot care with respect to the patient's ability to participate in self-management and communicate pain. *Strength-hand dexterity* can be partially assessed by observing the patient as he or she removes footwear and attempts to reach and inspect all areas of the foot, including the plantar surface.

Gait, mobility, and balance can be assessed with a screening tool called "get-up-and-go" (GUG). The GUG requires that the subject rise from a chair, walk 3 meters, turn around, return to the chair and sit down (Mathias, Nayak, and Isaacs, 1986). Originally, this test was graded on a 5-point scale with 1 as normal and 5 as severely abnormal, but this involved subjectivity in administering the scale. Hence the test was modified to include the time taken to complete the test: the "timed get-up-and-go" (TGUG) or "timed up-and-go" test

---

BOX 17-3 Components of an Initial Evaluation of a Patient with a Foot Disorder

History
- General: vision, strength, dexterity, mobility
- Blood glucose readings for the past month
- Personal or family history: skin, hair, or nail disease (especially rashes), lichen planus, (Plate 6B), psoriasis
- Specific history of foot problems: foot malformations, lesions, skin alterations, nail disorders, changes in sensation, foot/angle strength
- Prior treatments and medications (including over-the-counter) used to treat nail and foot problems

Physical Assessment
- Functional ability: gait, mobility, balance, hand strength and dexterity, visual cognition
- Health habits: smoking, exercise, hygiene, nutrition, and weight management
- Circulation: pulses, blanching, capillary refill, microvascular function (laser Doppler flowmetry), ankle-brachial index or toe-brachial index, temperature, hair growth
- Foot sensation: monofilament testing, vibration
- Skin alterations of the foot
- Foot lesions
- Foot malformations
- Nail disorders

Risk Assessment
- Ulceration risk
- Amputation risk

Equipment
- Footwear (including socks)
- Mobility aides (canes, walkers)

(Chen et al, 2003; Podsiadlo and Richardson, 1991). Adults without balance problems generally are able to complete the test in less than 10 seconds. Those dependent in most ADLs and mobility skills, according to the Barthel index (Mahoney and Barthel, 1965), take more than 30 seconds. The time taken to complete the task may vary with the use of an assistive device, and if the device is changed, test times cannot be compared. A final variation is the "expanded timed get-up-and-go" (ETGUG) test, in which a multimemory stopwatch is used to record the times of each component of the task. This procedure may better isolate functional deficits (Wall et al, 2000). State-of-the-art, computerized quantitative gait analysis is available and can be a useful adjunct to visual impressions of a patient's gait impairment. However, the complexity and expense of the testing generally restrict its use to part of a surgical decision making process when all conservative treatments have been exhausted (Banta, 2001; Davis et al, 1999).

A good test for balance is to stand on one foot with arms out to the side and eyes closed. Parameters for maintaining balance should be at least as follows:

- 15 seconds if less than 30 years old
- 12 seconds if 30 to 40 years old
- 10 seconds if 40 to 50 years old
- 7 seconds if over 50 years old

Improvements in balance can be achieved with exercise (American Orthopaedic Foot and Ankle Society, 2003).

Musculoskeletal function of the foot involves assessment of range of motion, deformities, and strength. The tops and bottoms of the feet, areas between the toes, and toenails must be inspected for deformities including corns, calluses, macerations, bunions, claw toes, misshapen or Charcot deformities, and any swelling of the legs or feet. Passive range of motion of the first metatarsophalangeal joint and the subtalar joint should be assessed. The maximal range of motion is determined from the maximal *inversion* to the maximal *eversion* of the foot for the subtalar joint (Figure 17-1 and Figure 17-6). If available, a goniometer can be used to quantify the arc or range of motion (Sauseng, Kastenbauer, and Irsigler, 2002) (Figure 17-7).

The clinician can also assess this by comparing both feet as the patient walks a few steps on the toes and then the heels. If the patient has difficulty with balance, cannot walk, or both, the clinician should have the patient sit on an exam table or the side of a bed. With the clinician's hands under the patient's foot, the patient is instructed to "press down on the gas pedal." Next, the clinician's hand is positioned on the top of the patient's foot and with the clinician's thumbs underneath, the patient is instructed to "pull the toes

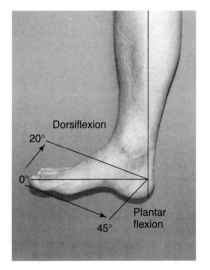
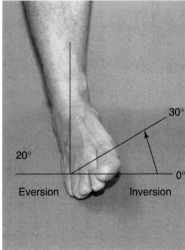
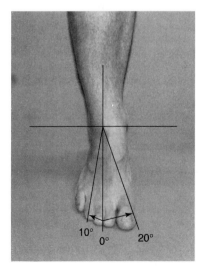

Fig. 17-6 Range of motion of the foot and ankle. (From Seidel Henry M et al: *Mosby's Guide to Physical Examination*, ed 6, St Louis, Mosby, 2006.)

TABLE 17-1 Foot Flexibility Exercises

	EXERCISE	INSTRUCTIONS	RECOMMENDATIONS
	Toe raise, toe point, toe curls	Hold each position for 5 seconds and repeat 10 times	Individuals with hammer toes or toe cramps
	Toe squeeze	Use cigarette filters or small corks. Place them between your toes and hold a squeeze for 5 seconds. Do this 10 times.	Individuals with hammer toes and toe cramps
	Big toe pulls	Place a thick rubber band around big toes and pull the big toes away from each other and toward the small toes. Hold for 5 seconds and repeat 10 times.	Individuals with bunions or toe cramps
	Toe pulls	Put a thick rubber band around all of your toes and spread them. Hold this position for 5 seconds and repeat 10 times.	Especially good for individuals with bunions, hammer toes, or toe cramps
	Golf ball roll	Roll a golf ball under the ball of your foot for two minutes—great massage for the bottom of the foot.	Individuals with plantar fasciitis (heel pain), arch strain, or foot cramps
	Towel curls	Place a small towel on the floor and curl it toward you, using only your toes. You can increase the resistance by putting a weight on the end of the towel. Relax and repeat this exercise 5 times.	Individuals with hammer toes, toe cramps, and pain in the ball of the foot
	Marble pick-up	Place 20 marbles on the floor. Pick up one marble at a time with your toes and put it in a small bowl. Do this exercise until you have picked up all 20 marbles.	Individuals with pain in the ball of the foot, hammer toes, and toe cramps
	Sand walking	Any chance you get, take off your shoes and walk in the sand at the beach. This not only massages your feet, but strengthens your toes	Good for general foot conditioning, watch out for glass!

From American Orthopaedic Foot and Ankle Society: *Foot fitness for life*, 2003, http://www.footcaremd.com/fc_a_footfitness03.html. Accessed April 21, 2005.

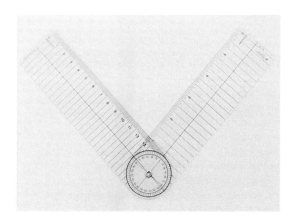

Fig. 17-7 Goniometer.

BOX 17-4 Cuticle and Nail Care

Cuticle and Nail Care
- Patients with very thick or ingrown nails require a referral to a foot care professional.
- Avoid excess manipulation of the cuticle, which may lead to infections.
- Excessively thick or loose cuticle can be removed through gentle trimming.
- Define the free nail border by assessing the tissue behind the toenails, using the beveled edge of an orangewood stick.
- Observe for the presence of hyponychium that has hypertrophied, hypergranulation tissue, ingrowing corners of the nail borders, hyperkeratosis, or other abnormal findings.
- Note the length and thickness and any accumulation of debris.
- Gently remove any loose debris from under the nail.

Basic Nail Trimming
- The best time to trim nails is after a bath or shower, when the nails are softer.
- Cutting the skin is to be avoided. Openings in the skin are avenues for bacteria or other infectious agents.
- Toenails should be trimmed straight across, no lower than $1/16$ to $1/8$ inch from the end of the toe, to prevent ingrown toenails.
- Smoothing the nail should be performed with an emery board.

toward the nose," while gentle pressure downward is being applied by the clinician. Any differences in strength between ankles should be noted. Any reports of a change in ankle strength in the past 6 months should also be recorded.

To assess toe flexibility, the patient can be instructed to pick up a marble or a small dishtowel with the toes (Table 17-1). To test ankle flexibility, the patient is instructed to stand on a stairs and hang his or her heel off a stair and let the heel go below the level of the stair. If this causes pain, the exercise should be stopped. The heel should be able to go below the level of the stair without causing strain in the calf. Some strain can be improved with flexibility exercises.

Foot and Nail. The foot should be inspected for the presence of malformations and impaired skin integrity (Box 17-1, Chapter 16, Table 16-3 and Figure 16-1). Properly or improperly trimmed nails and the condition of the nail should be documented (Box 17-2 and Box 17-4). Foot pain assessment includes location, duration, and intensity of pain to differentiate between different types of pain such as with plantar fasciitis (heel pain), metatarsalgia (forefoot pain), Achilles tendonitis (frequent jumping injury), or tarsal tunnel syndrome (repetitive motion injury) (Chang et al, 1994; Hayda et al, 1994; Hirose and McGarvey, 2004; Hsi, Kang, and Lee, 2005; Labib et al, 2002; Mondelli, Morana and Padua, 2004; Wilder and Sethi, 2004).

Clothing and Equipment

Footwear and Socks/Stockings. Skin breakdown is frequently caused by improper or ill-fitting footwear (Pinzur et al, 2001; Tyrrell, 2002). If a patient lacks sensation in the feet, he or she may buy shoes that are too tight and will trigger the formation of bunions, corns, or ulcers. The inside of the shoes should be checked for wrinkled lining, protruding tacks, or foreign objects. The clinician and patient should discuss the importance of wearing slippers or shoes rather than going barefoot at home. Interventions related to appropriate footwear will be discussed later in this chapter.

Mobility Aids (e.g., Canes, Walkers). Canes, crutches, walkers, wheelchairs, and other mobility aids

TABLE 17-2 Risk Determination and Management Strategies

	RISK CATEGORIES	MANAGEMENT STRATEGIES
0	Has a disease that leads to insensitivity	Examine feet at each leads to visit (at least 4 times/year)
		Foot clinic visit once a year
	Has protective sensation	Patient education
	Has not had a plantar ulcer	Proper shoe fit, correct styles
1	Does not have protective sensation	Examine feet at each visit (at least 4 times/year)
	Has not had a plantar ulcer	Foot clinic visit every 6 months
	Does not have a foot deformity	Patient education
		Well-fitted shoes, possibly in-depth, protective, accommodative orthoses
2	Does not have protective sensation	Examine feet at each visit (at least 4 times/year)
	Has not had a plantar ulcer	Foot clinic visit every 3 to 4 months
	Does have a foot deformity	Patient education
		In-depth shoes, possibly heat-moldable or custom-made
		Total contact orthoses
		Rocker soles
3	Does not have protective sensation	Examine feet at each visit (at least 4 times/year)
	Has a history of plantar ulcer	Foot clinic visit every 1 to 2 months
		Patient education
		In-depth shoes, possibly heat-moldable or custom-made
		Total contact orthoses
		Rocker soles (customized), extended steel shank
		Custom-made healing sandal

From Yetzer EA: Incorporating foot care education into diabetic foot screening, *Rehab Nurs* 29(3):80, 2004.

should be inspected for proper fit, signs of wear, breakage, or loose parts. The locking mechanism for folding walkers and canes should be inspected. Cane and crutch hand grips and tips should not be excessively worn. Patients need sufficient strength to operate the brakes on wheeled walkers that are provided with such systems, and the brakes should be tested to assure proper functioning. All fasteners (screws, nuts, and bolts) should be checked regularly to ensure that they are securely tightened.

Risk for Ulceration

Assessment must include factors that place a patient at risk for ulceration; history or of plantar ulcer, presence or absence of foot deformity, presence or absence of protective sensations, and presence of diseases that lead to decreased sensation. Based on these risk factors, a risk assessment tool with corresponding management strategies was developed by Gillis W. Long Hansen's Disease Center (Table 17-2).

Risk categories range from 0 (no risk) to 3 (greatest risk). Level of risk will determine the patient's management category (Yetzer, 2004). Chapter 16, Tables 16-1 and 16-2 show similar systems for identifying risk of ulceration and management strategies for patients with diabetes.

INTERVENTIONS
Offloading and Padding

Bony structures of the foot, such as prominent metatarsal heads, or toe deformities are at risk for mechanical trauma from the seams in socks and shoes. The cause of the pressure must be identified and eliminated if possible. Offloading techniques include total contact casting, removable splints and casts, customized shoes, pads, and inserts (Table 17-3 and Chapter 16, Figure 16-8).

Pressure can be redistributed, hyperkeratotic lesions reduced, and repetitive stress and friction eliminated with over-the-counter or custom-molded padding and

TABLE 17-3 Techniques for Offloading the Foot

METHOD	CHARACTERISTICS	METHOD	CHARACTERISTICS
Bed rest	Total non–weight-bearing		Requires at least weekly dressing changes
	Patient adherence is difficult	Felted foam pads	Simple to make
	Presents quality of life issues		Inexpensive
	Promotes hyperglycemia		Easy to use with dressings
	Promotes patient debilitation		Requires every 3 to 4 days replacement
	Increases risk of posterior heel pressures	Crest pads (adjunct for hammer or claw toes)	Simple to make
Total Contact Cast	Forces adherence		Commercially available
	Allows for limited ambulation		Inexpensive
	Requires specialized skill to make		May be used for wound prevention
	Not advisable for infected or highly exudative wounds		Requires frequent replacement
Walking splints/ removable casts	Allows for daily wound surveillance and care	Interdigital pads	Commercially available
	Requires strict patient adherence		May be used for wound prevention
Wedge-soled shoe	Commercially available		Ineffective if shoes are too narrow
	Can be customized		
	May cause balance problems	Lamb's wool	Commercially available
Healing shoe with large toe box and	Provides offloading to specific wound location		Inexpensive
customized inserts	Requires specialized equipment		May cause toe constriction
	Requires specialized skill to make	Padded socks	Commercially available
Adhesive felt pad	Simple to make		May be cause of foot pressure and/or toe constriction if shoe fit does not allow for increased padding
	Inexpensive		
	Easy to use with dressings		

WOCN Society: *Guideline for management of wounds in patients with lower-extremity neuropathic disease,* WOCN Clinical Practice Guideline Series #3, Glenview IL, 2004, Author.

inserts (WOCN Society, 2004; Freeman, 2002; Myerly and Stavosky, 1997; Saye, 1994). To manage diminished fat pads on the plantar surface of the foot, a normal change with aging, nonadherent silicone pads can be held in place with socks, thereby forming a cushion over areas such as prominent metatarsal heads. Many of the available commercial pads have an aggressive adhesive and should be avoided, especially with elderly or sensitive skin. Tubular pads are available that can be fit over toes to pad at-risk areas, either on the tips of toes or between toes where intradigital calluses may form. Lamb's wool can be woven between all toes or placed between at-risk toes. The wool provides inherent moisturizing through the lanolin while also absorbing perspiration and excess moisture (Kelechi and Lukacs, 1991; Ozdemir et al, 2004).

Hygiene and Routine Skin Care

Routine skin care includes hygiene and moisturizing to keep the foot free from xerosis, maceration, fissures, lesions, and ulceration (Bryant, 1995; Springett and White, 2002). Individuals who require assistance with nail care may also require assistance with foot hygiene. Routine skin care should include all of the following:

1. Inspect feet (especially between toes) daily
2. Moisturize daily

3. Schedule individual bathing routine to minimize drying effects
4. Use mild skin cleansers and lukewarm water
5. Dry feet completely (especially between toes)

Foot Odor. Foot odor is caused by excessive perspiration from the more than 250,000 sweat glands in the foot (American Podiatric Medical Association, 2005). Bacteria living in shoes and socks metabolize the sweat to form isovaleric acid, which is responsible for foot odor. In addition to washing the feet and changing shoes and socks even more frequently than daily, the feet can be dusted with nonmedicated baby powder or foot powder; an antibacterial ointment may also help. Soaking the feet in strong black tea for 30 minutes a day for a week controls foot odor in that the tannic acid in the tea kills the bacteria and closes the pores, keeping feet dry longer (American Academy of Orthopaedic Surgeons, 2002). The tea solution can be made by boiling two tea bags in a pint of water for 15 minutes and adding 2 quarts of cool water. Severe cases of foot odor may be caused by inherited hyperhidrosis (excessive perspiration). In severe cases the nerve controlling the sweat glands in the feet may be surgically severed, but there may be compensatory sweating in other areas of the body after surgery.

Cuticle and Nail Care

General tips for basic cuticle and nail care are presented in Box 17-4. About half of the foot care professional's activity is nail debridement. The following discussion will present the unique assessment parameters for the foot and nails. Nail debridement can be accomplished with manual nippers or with a mechanical rotary tool (Pinzur et al, 2001; Saye, 1994).

Manual Nippers. When using nippers, begin at one edge of the nail and take small nips along the border or top edge, nipping smoothly while working across the entire nail border. There is much debate regarding the best methods for debriding toenails (straight across versus rounding, or following the shape or contour of the top of the toe). If patients have problems with the corners curving and causing pain and thickening of the skin at the distal aspect of the nail groove, it is recommended that the corners be slightly rounded. Others who have puffy or a thick type of skin folds might require nails that are cut straight across so that the corners grow up out of the grooves.

Do not cut deeply into the corners, but do not leave sharp edges. Debride the nail until the desired length is achieved. Cut thickened, discolored, or unhealthy nails last to prevent the transmission of infection. Smooth each nail with the nail file, again beginning with healthy nails to prevent transmission of infection.

Mechanical Rotary Tool. The Dremel drill (cordless or plug-in) is a standard tool used for nail debridement (Maeda, Mizuno, and Ichikawa, 1990). A procedure for nail debridement with the use of a mechanical rotary tool is shown in Box 17-5.

Hazards. One concern with the use of the Dremel drill is the generation of nail dust that is dispersed in the air, is inhaled by the patient as well as the clinician, and settles on surfaces throughout the room. This aerosol nail dust, particularly that from onychomycotic toenails, can lead to conjunctivitis, rhinitis, asthma, coughing, hypersensitivity, and impaired lung function

---

BOX 17-5 Example of Nail Debridement with the Use of a Mechanical Rotary Tool

1. Before using a Dremel drill, patients should be informed that they will feel a vibration while the nail is being debrided.
2. Don appropriate personal protective equipment.
3. Support the toe between the index finger and thumb of the nondominant hand to prevent it from moving during debridement. The other toes should be held away from the bur during the procedure.
4. Set the speed of the grinder to 10,000 or 15,000 RPM.
5. Debride the nail by slowly and gently applying pressure as the grinder is moved from the proximal to distal portion of the plate.
6. Keep the nail plate visible at all times. Frequently stop grinding to wipe dust away with a cloth (do not blow).
7. Stop grinding when the nail is thin or when the dust becomes very fine and is not visibly produced during debridement.
8. DO NOT GRIND THROUGH THE NAIL PLATE! The soft underlying layers of the plate can be abraded. A subungual wound to the nail bed can result.
9. Avoid surrounding tissue that can become abraded.

(Abramson and Wilton, 1992a, 1992b; Gatley, 1991; Ward, 1995). These hazards have resulted in a great deal of controversy within the nursing community about the appropriateness of using drill types of mechanical nail avulsion and debridement tools (AllNurses.com, 2003-2005).

Drill selection. A variety of vacuum drills are available (i.e., Jan-L, Haswe, Ortho-fex, Osada, Suda). Some of the vacuum drills remove the large particles and still broadcast the small particles. Room air circulators with high-efficiency particulate arresting (HEPA) air filters that remove particles down to approximately 0.3 microns are helpful. Water spray drills are available as well. Tungsten carbide burs and bits are preferable in that they run cold, do not abrade the skin, produce big chunks rather than dust, and last longer. Ruby carvers and diamond bits are also preferable to steel. Using good-quality nippers to remove most of the fungal nail before using the drill for finishing and smoothing can minimize the generation of dust.

Cleaning and sterilization of equipment. Equipment that comes in contact with the patient must be kept clean and sanitized. Fungal spores can be difficult to eradicate. Cold soaking solutions must be antifungal. There are many ingredients which can accomplish this including glutaraldehyde, phenol, sodium hypochlorite, sodium bromide, and iodophors (McDonnell and Russell, 1999). Take care to read the label thoroughly to ensure that equipment is soaked for the recommended length of time. Equipment may also be sterilized in an autoclave. Alcohol does not kill fungus and should not be used in the cleansing of nail equipment. Properly cleansing equipment between patients is the single most important task in reducing or eliminating spread of infection.

Personal protective equipment (PPE). The clinician must consider personal safety when performing foot and nail care (Cope, 1998; Davis, Kugler, and Nixon, 1991; Mullins and Lee, 1998; Ward, 1995). Wearing gloves is a basic standard precaution that protects the wearer from infectious organisms commonly associated with foot care including fungus, bacteria, and viruses. While care is taken to avoid bloodshed, it is always a possibility. A mask is important when debriding with a mechanical rotary tool, especially if no vacuum device is used. Inhalation of micronized dust particles can cause lung irritation over time. The mask will muffle the voice and make it difficult for the patient to hear questions or instructions. The mask also hides your lips and might create difficulties for individuals who rely on lip reading to assist with hearing. A lab coat or apron will help to protect clothing. The clinician should wear easily washable clothing and may want to avoid solid or dark-colored clothing. Safety goggles protect eyes from flying debris. It is important that eye protection be properly fitted to avoid sliding and fogging. A hair covering such as a surgical cap may reduce dust and nail debris catching in the hair and ears.

Back safety. Another important aspect of personal safety is protecting the health of the clinician's back. Clinicians often get into awkward positions to provide the necessary care to the patient's feet. Positioning patients for both their comfort and the clinician's can be difficult. A comfortable, positionable, and height-adjustable chair is important to preserve back health. Depending on the setting, specialized seating and positioning devices may not be available. Having the patient lie down on the bed or exam table with the clinician working at the foot is effective if the height of the bed is adjustable. Sitting in a chair facing the patient's chair and having the patient's foot in the clinician's lap also works well for patients who can get the foot up and keep it there. Other individuals may prefer to have the affected leg lower, thus making it necessary for the clinician to sit on a small stool. Clinicians find creative ways to position themselves to meet the needs of clients in wheelchairs and those with other mobility limitations. It is important for the clinician to change position frequently, especially if performing nail care on many clients throughout the day. Standing and incorporating some backward bending to stretch back muscles can help to reduce back discomfort.

Care of Foot Malformations

Bunions and Hammer Toes. Steps can be taken to minimize the discomfort of bunions, but surgery is frequently required to correct the problem. When hammer toes are present, surgery may be necessary to realign the toes to their proper position. In the elderly, properly fitting shoes may eliminate pressure and avoid surgery (Chung, 1983).

Heel Spurs. Treatments for heel spurs range from exercise (such as the "alphabet exercise" where the patient moves the ankle in multiple planes of motion by drawing both lowercase and uppercase letters of the alphabet with the foot), to application of ice and use of antiinflammatory medication (e.g., nonsteroidal anti-inflammatory drugs [NSAIDs] or cortisone injections), and over-the-counter heel cups or custom-made orthotics.

Neuromas. Conservative treatment of neuromas can include padding, taping, orthotic devices, and cortisone injections, but surgical removal of the growth is sometimes necessary.

Treatment of Skin and Alterations

Callus and Corns. Callus and corns should be trimmed and assessed for underlying ulceration. However, since corns and callus are caused by repetitive stress, interventions should begin with eliminating the cause with appropriate footwear, padding, and offloading. A pumice stone can be lightly rubbed across calluses after a bath to help keep them under control, or a mechanical rotary tool can be used to thin excessively hard/thick calluses (Pitei, Foster, and Edmonds, 1999). This is done by slowly and gently moving the bur in one direction over the surface of the callus while avoid abrading the surrounding skin. The callus must not be removed below the level of healthy tissue. Acid-containing liquid corn removers can injure the foot's healthy skin and should be avoided, particularly in those with other underlying foot problems.

Xerosis and Fissures. Moisturizing, the central strategy in the prevention and treatment of xerosis, will retard water loss from the epidermis (Engelke et al, 1997; Loden, 2003; Luggen, 2003). Most moisturizers require application twice a day to be effective; however, there are a few "super" moisturizers that only need to be applied once a day to effectively prevent and treat xerosis. Moisturizers work best if they are applied immediately after bathing, to help the skin retain water (Loden, 2003).

Available emollient preparations contain a variety of active ingredients, including lanolin, glycerin, urea, and lactic acid. The latter two ingredients are natural moisturizers and have the added benefit of exfoliating the outer layers of the stratum corneum, to promote new growth of skin. Products with these ingredients can be obtained over the counter. If the percent of urea is over 10%, a prescription is required. A high concentration of urea is not always necessary and can cause a burning sensation when applied. One prospective, randomized, controlled double-blind study reported a statistically significant reduction of fissures when an over-the-counter product containing 10% urea and 4% lactic acid was used with 40 patients with diabetes (Pham et al, 2002).

Plantar Warts. Plantar warts can be difficult to treat and often need repeated treatments for positive results. Patients frequently use a variety of over-the-counter treatments. Should these be unsuccessful, over-the-counter 2% sodium salicylate patches may be applied, or duct tape occlusion therapy may be attempted. A piece of duct tape is placed on a lesion for 6 days; when it is removed, the wart is soaked in water and debrided with a pumice stone or emery board. Thereafter the cycle may be repeated. Up to 73% of warts are reported to be responsive to this form of treatment (Focht, Spicer, and Fairchok, 2002; Summers and Kaminski, 2003). Otherwise, the lesions may be removed by more traditional electrocautery or freezing techniques (Andrews, 2004; Stulberg and Hutchinson, 2003). Callused extensions may be pared for comfort (Pitei, Foster, and Edmonds, 1999). Sodium salicylate solution can be applied by iontophoresis (electrical current) to weight-bearing surfaces to decrease the pain and scarring associated with freezing and electrocautery, and to decrease the fixation problems associated with medicated patches (Soroko et al, 2002).

Plantar warts can be difficult to cure, and localized treatments are the standard of care (Allam et al, 2004; Schroeter et al, 2005; Stulberg and Hutchinson, 2003; Tandeter and Tandeter, 2005; Tucker, Ali, and Ransdell, 2003). In addition to over-the-counter salicylic acid patches, liquid nitrogen treatments also often require repeated application for effect; they can also be painful.

A new antiviral medication, 5% imiquimod cream (Aldara, 3M), that is currently approved by the Food and Drug Administration (FDA) for the treatment of external genital and perianal warts is unique in that it is systemically absorbed through the skin. Imiquimod cream reduces the DNA of human papilloma virus. This product is used under occlusion, meaning that the medication is applied and then covered with a plastic occlusive wrap. However, the use of imiquimod cream on the foot or for any warts other than external genital warts is considered "off label" use. Referral to a primary care provider or dermatologist is recommended for those with impaired sensation, mobility, dexterity, or vision.

Blisters (bullae). Treatment of blisters depends on etiology. Eliminating the cause of friction is imperative to allow a blister to heal. If the cause is friction or pressure, treatment will involve offloading and proper footwear. If the cause of the bulla is infection, the source of infections must be determined so the appropriate antifungal, antibiotic, or antiviral agent can be initiated. In general, blisters should be protected and left intact (Brennan, 2002; Knapik et al, 1995; Read, 2001). If a blister inadvertently becomes opened, wash with a gentle cleanser and cover with nonadherent dressing. Monitor for signs and symptoms of infection.

Tinea Pedis (Athletes Foot). Tinea pedis may clear readily with topical application of a fungicidal cream such as terbenifine (Tan and Joseph, 2004). Tinea pedis of long standing may respond well to oral antifungal treatment.

Toenail Conditions

Onychocryptosis (ingrown toenail). Treatment includes relieving the offending structures, which may clear the problem without use of antibiotics. Paraffin tulle gauze, or other suitable dressing, may be applied to the toenail bed afterwards. Removal of the first dressing can be painful and pain relief strategies are indicated (King, 2003a, 2003b). If inflammation of the paronychium (paronychia) evolves into infection, antibiotics are warranted. Severely ingrown toenails may have to be surgically treated by nail avulsion (Andreassi et al, 2004; Kuru et al, 2004). Appropriate nail trimming will prevent reoccurrence.

Onychomycosis (fungal infection of the nail). When onychomycosis causes painful ambulation or decreased function, a medical intervention is warranted. In the absence of painful ambulation or decreased function, treatment of onychomycosis is generally considered cosmetic and not reimbursed.

Topical and oral treatments are available for onychomycosis. Topical treatments have variable results. Ciclopirox (Penlac), an FDA-approved topical nail lacquer, is applied daily to the nail and surrounding skin and removed once weekly for 48 weeks (Baran and Kaoukhov, 2005; Sidou and Soto, 2004; Tan and

Joseph, 2004). Nails should be trimmed when the lacquer is off. Unfortunately, this product is often ineffective, even after many months. Topical applications of tea tree oil or menthol-containing petroleum jellies have shown improvement when used for at least 1 year (Ramsewak et al, 2003; Syed et al, 1999). These treatments have low risk of side effects (Bruynzeel, 1999).

Systemic antifungal agents have become more popular with the release of terbinafine and itraconazole (Baran and Kaoukhov, 2005). These agents are much less toxic to the liver, have a high affinity for the nail matrix, and are administered over a shorter period of time as compared to 12 months for griseofulvin (which also has a high toxicity profile) (Bell-Syer et al, 2002). Diagnosis of onychomycosis should be confirmed before usage since many nail diseases mimic fungal infections (Cohen and Scher, 1992). New nail growth can appear free of infection, but the nail will continue to appear diseased for up to 1 year, until the entire nail has grown out. Baseline hepatic function should be assessed and monitored throughout the course of treatment. Treatment for toenails can be costly, and is often not covered by insurance.

An important aspect of treating onychomycosis is to minimize the chance of recurrence. Shoes should be discarded or thoroughly cleansed at treatment onset. Ensure proper hygiene and apply clean socks daily. If the foot is reexposed to the fungal infection at any time after systemic treatment, infection can recur.

Blisters and ulceration. The etiology of foot ulceration is multifactorial (Boyko et al, 1999). The combination of high plantar pressures and sensory deficit is mainly responsible for ulcer development in the patient with a neuropathy. While the forefoot is the most common location for neuropathic ulcers, both rearfoot and forefoot pressures are increased in the diabetic neuropathic foot (Caselli et al, 2002; Frykberg et al, 1998; Pham et al, 2000; Stess, Jensen, and Mirmiran, 1997). A drop of the forefoot (equinus deformity) develops in the latest stages of peripheral neuropathy and may play a role in the etiology of foot ulceration.

Differential diagnosis is crucial before the treatment of foot ulcers. For example, friction and pressure can lead to bulla formation and subsequent ulceration; however, other conditions like fungal infection can also cause bulla formation.

Appropriate Footwear

A proper shoe fit involves more than just length and width measurements; the person's style of arch may require particular attention. Footprints can be read by placing the foot into a bucket of water, and making a footprint on a piece of brown paper (Figure 17-8). A footprint that is very wide in the middle is indicative of flat feet. The foot rolls excessively to the inside (overpronation), leading to arch strain and pain on the inside of the knee. Molded leather arch supports are available over the counter. Athletic shoe styles are designed with "control" features that aid in the prevention of the rolling-in motion. If arch supports or sports shoes are ineffective, a foot specialist can fabricate a custom-molded orthotic shoe insert.

If there is little or no connection in the footprint between the heel and forefoot, the person has a high

arch (underpronation). The foot rolls too much to the outside, with a lot of weight landing on the outside edge of the foot, making the ankle more susceptible to ankle sprains and stress fractures. "Stability" athletic shoes are built with extra cushioning. If prone to ankle sprains, the individual should wear high-top athletic shoes that cover the foot and ankle snugly to minimize damage from twists (American Orthopaedic Foot and Ankle Society, 2003).

Patients should inspect their old, well-worn shoes. Different wear patterns may be indicative of underlying foot problems (Figure 17-9). Wear on the ball of the foot may indicate that the heel tendon is tight. Heel-raising exercises can help stretch this tendon. Wear on the inner sole indicates overpronation (flat feet), and inner liners or orthotic supports may help. Toe-shaped ridges on the upper toe box may indicate that the shoes are too small, or that hammer toes are developing. Outer sole wear indicates a high arch, and orthotics may help. A bulge and wear to the side of the great toe may indicate that the shoe is too narrow or that a bunion is present. Unridged wear on the upper toe box generally indicates that the front of the shoe is too low (American Orthopaedic Foot and Ankle Society, 2003).

The American Orthopaedic Foot and Ankle Society, in collaboration with the National Shoe Retailers Association and Pedorthic Footwear Association, proposes several tips for appropriate footwear selection shown in Box 17-6. Additional suggestions include the following:

- Have the person stand next to his or her shoes and check whether the shoe is shaped like the feet, or are there areas of constriction?
- Examine the inside of the shoe by hand to check for seams, tacks, or rough places.
- Instruct the individual to purchase new shoes later in the day, when feet tend to be at their largest.
- Replace worn-out shoes as soon as possible.
- Select and wear the shoe appropriate for the activity (e.g., steel-toed boots for farm work, running shoes for running).
- The same pair of shoes should not be worn every day.
- Avoid walking barefoot, because the feet are more susceptible to injury and infection.
- Apply sunblock to the feet when wearing sandals or at the beach.

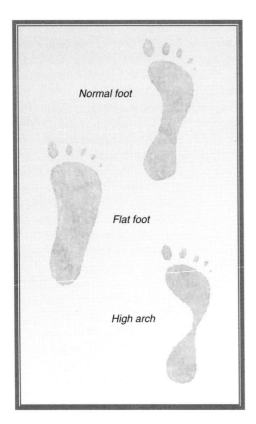

Fig. 17-8 Reading your footprint. (Modified from American Orthopaedic Foot and Ankle Society: *Foot fitness for life*, 2003, http://www.footcaremd.com/fc_a_footfitness03.html.)

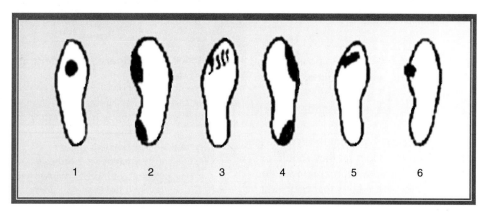

Fig. 17-9 Shoe wear patterns. **1,** Wear on the ball of the foot. **2,** Wear on the inner sole. **3,** Toe-shaped ridges on the upper toe box. **4,** Outer sole wear. **5,** Bulge and wear to the side of the big toe. **6,** Wear on the upper and above the toes. (Modified from American Orthopaedic Foot and Ankle Society: *Foot fitness for life,* 2003, http://www.footcaremd.com/fc_a_footfitness03.html.)

BOX 17-6 Tips for Appropriate Footwear Selection

Shoe Size
- Sizes vary among shoe brands and styles.
- Don't select shoes by the size marked inside the shoe.

Measurement
- Have your feet measured regularly.
- The size of your feet changes as you grow older.
- Have BOTH feet measured (most people have one foot larger than the other).

Fitting
- Fit to the largest foot
- Fit at the end of the day when your feet are their largest.
- Stand during the fitting process, and check that there is adequate space (3/8 inch to 1/2 inch) for your longest toe at the end of each shoe.
- Make sure the ball of your foot fits comfortably into the widest part (ball pocket of the shoe).
- Judge the shoe by how it fits on your foot.
- Select a shoe that conforms as nearly as possible to the shape of your foot.
- Don't purchase shoes that feel too tight, expecting them to "stretch" to fit.
- Your heel should fit comfortably in the shoe with a minimum amount of slippage.
- Walk in the shoe to make sure it fits and feels right.

Shoe Type
- A healthy shoe is a shoe that is shaped like your foot. That generally means a shoe that has a roomy and rounded or square toe box (the area of the shoe over the toes).
- The shoe should be made of a buttery-soft material that has some give like glove leather.
- Flat shoes (with a heel height of 1 inch or less) are the healthiest shoes for your feet. If you must wear a high heel, keep to a heel height of 2 inches or less, limit wearing them to 3 hours at a time, and take them off coming to and from work, dinner, or church.
- Look for soles that are shock-absorbing and skid-resistant, such as rubber rather than smooth leather.
- Avoid shoes that have seams over areas of pain such as a bunion.
- Avoid shoes with heavy rubber soles that curl over the top of the toe area (such as seen on some running shoes), since they can catch on carpets and cause an accidental fall.
- Lace-up rather than slip-on shoes provide a more secure fit and can accommodate insoles, orthotic devices, and braces.

Established in a collaboration between the American Orthopaedic Foot and Ankle Society, the National Shoe Retailers Association, and the Pedorthic Footwear Association (*Am Orthop Foot Ankle Soc,* 2003).

When purchasing shoes for someone who is unable to go to the store to try shoes on, a tracing of the foot may be made while the person is standing. When the new shoe is held over the tracing, the entire tracing should be covered.

A deep toe box is important to prevent their rubbing the tops of the toes. To break shoes in, they should be worn 10 to 20 minutes twice a day. Upon removal, the skin should be checked for any redness that may indicate possible sites for mechanical trauma such as pressure points, friction, and repetitive stress. Patients should be discouraged from going barefoot, even at home (Mazur, 2002). Socks with holes or that have been darned should be discarded, and the tops of the socks should not be so tight that they restrict circulation. White or light socks can show signs of drainage, which is often the first sign of ulceration.

Referral

Numerous specialists are potentially needed in the process of providing adequate foot and nail care. It is always important to identify the need for appropriate referrals (i.e., primary care provider, podiatry, orthopedics, dermatology, endocrinology, vascular surgery, general surgery, physical therapy, occupational therapy, pedorthist/orthotist, home health, pain management, diabetes education, smoking cessation, case/care manager or social worker, or wound care). Results of the foot screening must be communicated to the appropriate health care provider, along with the patient's foot ulceration risk and a record of the educational materials given to the patient and family (Dorgan et al, 1995; Patout et al, 2001; Plummer and Albert, 1995).

Patient and Caregiver Education

Assessment Findings. Involving patients in their own care decreases foot complications (Harwell et al, 2001; Lavery and Gazewood, 2000). It is critical to explain the importance of the specific assessments in terms of monitoring the health of the foot and nail to the patient and family to motivate a genuine desire to learn these new skills and adopt new self care skills. Any unusual findings of the foot screening should be discussed with the patient and the family. The patient and the family also need a thorough understanding of the patient's foot ulceration risk category and their role in preventing skin breakdown and amputation.

BOX 17-7 Components of Patient and Family Education
··

- Foot care (hygiene, skin care, inspection, nail care)
- Anatomy and pathophysiology affecting the foot
- Age-specific foot changes
- Ulcer and amputation risk
- Lifestyle choices that affect foot health (exercise, smoking, nutrition, and weight management)
- Plans for prevention of foot disorders
- Proper footwear
- Problems that should be reported
- Plan for follow up

Foot Care Instructions. Box 17-7 lists the components of patient and family education. Patients should be taught that they can protect the health of their feet by maintaining a normal weight to lessen changes due to osteoporosis (Harwell et al, 2001; Richbourg, 1998). Additional foot care instructions can be found in Chapter 16 Box 16-3 and Appendix D.

Home Remedies. Unsupervised home remedies for foot ailments should be avoided. Self-treatment has the potential of turning a minor problem into a major one. Persons with diabetes, poor circulation, or heart problems should not treat their own feet because they are more prone to infection. It is vital that individuals with diabetes see a foot care specialist at least once a year for a checkup.

Report Changes. The following situations should prompt an appointment with a health professional (American Orthopaedic Foot and Ankle Society, 2003; Gemmell, Hayes, and Conway, 2005; van Os et al, 2005).

- Foot or ankle pain that is intense
- Foot or ankle pain that persists for more than 72 hours
- Lower-extremity pain that increases with exercise or ambulation, rest, or elevation
- Swelling of one leg or foot that persists for more than 24 hours
- Sudden progression of a foot deformity
- Unilateral flattening of the foot arch
- Infection
- Loss of sensation
- A blister or ulcer on the foot that developed without the patient feeling it
- A blister or ulcer that on the foot that is not healing

SUMMARY

Foot and nail disorders are predominantly a reflection of the patient's overall health status. By conducting a regular and routine foot and nail assessment in conjunction with a routine skin assessment, preventive interventions can be identified that will avoid the discomfort and secondary complications that arise from foot and nail disorders. Routine foot care should be integrated into everyday practice, thus keeping the skin healthy and intact and minimizing the risk of trauma or malformation (Bryant and Beinlich, 1999; Howell and Thirlaway, 2004; Kelechi, 1996; Kelechi and Lukacs, 1996; Kosinski and Ramcharitar, 1994; Lukacs & Kelechi, 1993).

SELF ASSESSMENT EXERCISE

1. Which of the following is NOT important information in gathering the patient's pertinent health history?
   a. Arthritis status
   b. Smoking habits
   c. Vision problems
   d. Shoulder pain
   e. Nasal polyps
2. In assessing vascular function in the foot, which of the following is NOT diagnostically useful?
   a. A progressive decrease in temperature from the knee to the foot
   b. Femoral bruit
   c. Capillary refill time
   d. Doppler flowmetry
   e. Ankle-brachial pressure index
3. In instructing the patient and caregiver on proper shoe fit, which of the following is important to emphasize?
   a. Shoes should be selected based on the printed shoe size provided by the manufacturer.
   b. Shoes should be tested for fit early in the morning before the patient is too fatigued to adequately assess how it feels.
   c. Shoes should be fitted while the patient is sitting with the foot elevated on a slanted shoe-fitting stool.
   d. Shoes with heavy rubber soles that curl over the top of the toe area should be avoided.
   e. Shoes should be made of heavy, stiff leather to provide maximum support.
4. In treating warts on the foot, particularly in younger individuals, which of the following is NOT recommended?
   a. Over-the-counter salicylic acid patches
   b. Electrocautery

   c. Liquid nitrogen
   d. Duct tape
   e. Capsaicin ointment
5. Onychomycosis is which of the following?
   a. A bacterial infection
   b. Commonly painful
   c. Considered by most insurance companies to be a cosmetic issue, and its treatment is not covered unless it decreases ambulation
   d. Treatable with bleach solution soakings in persons with weak or frail skin
   e. Untreatable by systemic antifungals (terbinafine and itraconazole) because of high liver toxicity profiles
6. Options for toenail debridement should NOT include the use of which of the following?
   a. Manual nippers
   b. Mechanical rotary tools fitted with tungsten carbide burs
   c. Salicylate solutions
   d. Personal protective equipment to reduce exposure to dust
   e. Goggles
7. Which of the following causes foot odor?
   a. Fungi
   b. Isovaleric acid
   c. Foot powders
   d. Acetic acid
   e. Inherited hypohydrosis
8. Natural, age-specific changes of the foot do NOT include which of the following?
   a. Bunions
   b. Widening of the foot
   c. Flattening of the foot
   d. Loss of range of motion
   e. Thinning of the heel fat pad
9. Which of the following problems need NOT concern a patient?
   a. Foot pain that persists for more than 72 hours
   b. Foot pain that increases with elevation of the legs
   c. Swelling of one leg or foot that persists less than 8 hours
   d. Any loss of sensation
   e. Any sudden progression of a foot deformity
10. What causes maceration between the toes?
    a. Inflammation
    b. Allergy
    c. Excessively dry skin
    d. Excessively moist skin
    e. Systemic antifungal medications

REFERENCES

Abramson C, Wilton J: Inhalation of nail dust from onychomycotic toenails. Part I. Characterization of particles, 1984 *J Am Podiatr Med Assn* 82:111, 1992a.

Abramson C, Wilton J: Nail dust aerosols from onychomycotic toenails. Part II. Clinical and serologic aspects., 1984, *J Am Podiatr Med Assn* 82:116, 1992b.

Adler AI et al: Lower-extremity amputation in diabetes. The independent effects of peripheral vascular disease, sensory neuropathy, and foot ulcers. *Diabetes Care* 22:1029, 1999.

Aldridge T: Diagnosing heel pain in adults, *Am Fam Physician* 70:332, 2004.

Allam JP et al: Successful treatment of therapy-resistant plantar verrucae vulgares with systemic interferon-beta, *J Dermatol* 31:582, 2004.

AllNurses.com: *Foot care training*, 2003-2005, http://allnurses.com/forums/archive/index.php/t-41101.html; Accessed July 6, 2005.

American Academy of Orthopaedic Surgeons: *Smelly (malodorous) feet*, 2002, http://orthoinfo.aaos.org/fact/thr_report.cfm?Thread_ID=360&topcategory=Foot; Accessed April 25, 2005.

American Orthopaedic Foot and Ankle Society: *Foot fitness for life*, 2003, http://www.footcaremd.com/fc_a_footfitness03.html. Accessed April 21, 2005.

American Podiatric Medical Association: *General foot health. A biological masterpiece, but subject to many ills*, 2005, http://www.apma.org/s_apma/doc.asp?CID=317&DID=9406&rcss=print&print=yes; Accessed April 21, 2005.

Andreassi A et al: Segmental phenolization for the treatment of ingrowing toenails: a review of 6 years experience, *J Dermatol Treatment* 15:179, 2004.

Andrews MD: Cryosurgery for common skin conditions, *Am Fam Physician* 69:2365, 2004.

Armstrong DG, Lavery LA: Acute Charcot's arthropathy of the foot and ankle, *Phys Ther* 78:74, 1998.

Banta JV: The evolution of gait analysis: a treatment decision-making tool, *Connecticut Med* 65:323, 2001.

Baran R, Kaoukhov A: Topical antifungal drugs for the treatment of onychomycosis: an overview of current strategies for monotherapy and combination therapy, *J Eur Acad Dermatol Venereol JEADV*, 19:21, 2005.

Baran R, Kechijian P: Understanding nail disorders, *Eur J Dermatol EJD* 11:159, 2001.

Bell-Syer SE et al: Oral treatments for fungal infections of the skin of the foot, *Cochrane Database System Rev* 2 CD003584, 2002.

Benvenuti F et al: Foot pain and disability in older persons: an epidemiologic survey, *J Am Geriatr Soc* 43:479, 1995.

Black JR: Paronychia, *Clin Podiatr Med Surg* 12:183, 1995.

Borovoy M et al: Laser surgery in podiatric medicine—present and future, *J Foot Surg* 22:353, 1983.

Boyko EJ et al: A prospective study of risk factors for diabetic foot ulcer. The Seattle Diabetic Foot Study, *Diabetes Care* 22:1036, 1999.

Brennan FH: Managing blisters in competitive athletes, *Curr Sports Med Rep* 1:319, 2002.

Brod M: Quality of life issues in patients with diabetes and lower extremity ulcers: patients and care givers, *Qual Life Res* 7:365, 1998.

Bruynzeel DP: Contact dermatitis due to tea tree oil, *Trop Med Int Health* 4:630, 1999.

Bryant JL: Preventive foot care program: a nursing perspective, *Ostomy Wound Manage* 41:28, 1995.

Bryant JL, Beinlich NR: Foot care: focus on the elderly, *Orthop Nurs Natl Assn Orthop Nurses* 18:53, 1999.

Camasta CA: Hallux limitus and hallux rigidus. Clinical examination, radiographic findings, and natural history, *Clin Podiatr Med Surg* 13:423, 1996.

Cameron B: Making diabetes management routine, *Am J Nurs* 102(2):26, 2002.

Caselli A et al: The forefoot-to-rearfoot plantar pressure ratio is increased in severe diabetic neuropathy and can predict foot ulceration, *Diabetes Care* 25:1066, 2002.

Chang AH et al: Multistep measurement of plantar pressure alterations using metatarsal pads, *Foot Ankle Int* 15:654, 1994.

Chen J et al: Prevalence of lower extremity pain and its association with functionality and quality of life in elderly women in Australia, *J Rheumatol* 30, 2689, 2003.

Chung S: Foot care. A health care maintenance program, *J Gerontol Nurs* 9:213, 1983.

Cohen PR, Scher RK; Geriatric nail disorders: diagnosis and treatment, *J Am Acad Dermatol* 26:521, 1992.

Cope R: Prevention of exposure to bloodborne pathogens, *Clin Podiatr Med Surg* 15:347, 1998.

Crawford F: Athlete's foot, *Clin Evidence* 12:2266, 2004.

Davis JM, Kugler G, Nixon BP: Eye injury in a podiatrist, *J Am Podiatr Med Assn* 81:661, 1991.

Davis RB III et al: Clinical gait analysis and its role in treatment decision-making, *Medscape Gen Med* 1:e1, 1999.

DeLauro NM, DeLauro TM: Onychocryptosis, *Clin Podiatr Med Surg* 21:617, 2004.

Dorgan M et al: Performing foot screening for diabetic patients, *Am J Nurs* 91(11):32, 1995.

Drake LA et al: The impact of onychomycosis on quality of life: development of an international onychomycosis-specific questionnaire to measure patient quality of life, *J Am Acad Dermatol* 41:189, 1999.

Engelke M et al: Effects of xerosis and ageing on epidermal proliferation and differentiation, *Br J Dermatol* 137:219, 1997.

Erbagci Z: Topical therapy for dermatophytoses: should corticosteroids be included? *Am J Clin Dermatol* 5:375, 2004.

Ferrari J, Higgins JP, Prior TD: Interventions for treating hallux valgus (abductovalgus) and bunions, *Cochrane Database Syst Rev* 1:2004, CD000964.

Focht DR 3rd, Spicer C, Fairchok MP: The efficacy of duct tape vs cryotherapy in the treatment of verruca vulgaris (the common wart), *Arch Pediatr Adolesc Med* 156:971, 2002.

Fort Worth Orthopaedics Musculoskeletal Institute: *Foot anatomy*, http://www.fwortho.com/service/serv_foot_illus.htm; Accessed April 25, 2005.

Freeman DB: Corns and calluses resulting from mechanical hyperkeratosis, *Am Fam Physician* 65:2277, 2002.

Frykberg RG et al: Role of neuropathy and high foot pressures in diabetic foot ulceration, *Diabetes Care* 21:1714, 1998.

Garrow AP, Silman AJ, Macfarlane GJ: The Cheshire Foot Pain and Disability Survey: a population survey assessing prevalence and associations, *Pain* 110:378, 2004.

Garrow AP et al: Development and validation of a questionnaire to assess disabling foot pain, *Pain* 85:107, 2000.

Gatley M: Human nail dust: hazard to chiropodists or merely nuisance? *J Soc Occupat Med* 41:121, 1991.

Gemmell H, Hayes B, Conway M: A theoretical model for treatment of soft tissue injuries: treatment of an ankle sprain in a college tennis player, *J Manipulat Physiol Therapeut* 28:285, 2005.

George DH: Management of hyperkeratotic lesions in the elderly patient, *Clin Podiatr Med Surg* 10:69, 1993.

Gupta AK, Skinner AR, Cooper EA: Interdigital tinea pedis (dermatophytosis simplex and complex) and treatment with ciclopirox 0.77% gel, *Int J Dermatol* 42(Suppl 1):23, 2003.

Gupta AK et al: Treatments of tinea pedis, *Dermatol Clin* 21:431, 2003.

Harwell T et al: Foot care practices, services and perceptions of risk among Medicare beneficiaries with diabetes at high and low risk for future foot complications, *Foot Ankle Int* 22:734, 2001.

Hayda R et al: Effect of metatarsal pads and their positioning: a quantitative assessment. *Foot Ankle Int* 15:561, 1994.

Hirose CB, McGarvey WC: Peripheral nerve entrapments, *Foot Ankle Clin* 9:255, 2004.

Howell M, Thirlaway S: Integrating foot care into the everyday clinical practice of nurses, *Br J Nurs* 13:470, 2004.

Hsi WL, Kang JH, Lee XX: Optimum position of metatarsal pad in metatarsalgia for pressure relief, *Am J Phys Med Rehab Assn Acad Physiatr* 84:514, 2005.

Jolly GP, Zgonis T, Hendrix CL: Neurogenic heel pain, *Clin Podiatr Med Surg* 22:101, 2005.

Katsambas A et al: The effects of foot disease on quality of life: results of the Achilles Project, *J Eur Acad Dermatol Venereol JEADV* 19:191, 2005.

Kelechi T: Foot care in the home: nursing and agency responsibilities, *Home Healthc Nurs* 14:721, 1996.

Kelechi T, Lukacs K: Nursing foot care for the aged, *J Gerontol Nurs* 17:40, 1991.

Kelechi T, Lukacs K: Intrapreneurial nursing: the comprehensive lower extremity assessment form, *Clin Nurse Specialist CNS* 10:266, 1996.

King B: Pain at first dressing change after toenail avulsion. 1: The experience of nurses, patients and an observer, *J Wound Care* 12:5, 2003a.

King B: Pain at first dressing change after toenail avulsion. 2: Findings and discussion of the data analysis, *J Wound Care* 12:69, 2003b.

Knapik JJ et al: Friction blisters. Pathophysiology, prevention and treatment, *Sports Med (Auckland, N.Z.)* 20:136, 1995.

Kosinski M, Ramcharitar S: In-office management of common geriatric foot problems, *Geriatrics* 49:43, 1994.

Kuru I et al: Factors affecting recurrence rate of ingrown toenail treated with marginal toenail ablation. *Foot Ankle Int* 25:410, 2004.

Kuyvenhoven MM et al: The foot function index with verbal rating scales (FFI-5pt): A clinimetric evaluation and comparison with the original FFI. *The Journal of Rheumatology*, 29, 1023-1028, 2002.

Labib SA et al: Heel pain triad (HPT): the combination of plantar fasciitis, posterior tibial tendon dysfunction and tarsal tunnel syndrome, *Foot Ankle Int* 23:212, 2002.

La Porta GA, La Fata PC: Pathologic conditions of the plantar fascia, *Clin Podiatr Med Surg* 22:1, 2005.

Larson EE et al: Accurate nomenclature for forefoot nerve entrapment: a historical perspective, *J Am Podiatr Med Assn* 95:298, 2005.

Lavery L, Gazewood J: Assessing the feet of patients with diabetes, *J Fam Pract* 49(11 Suppl):S9, 2000.

Lemont H, Ammirati KM, Usen N: Plantar fasciitis: a degenerative process (fasciosis) without inflammation, *J Am Podiatr Med Assn* 93:234, 2003.

Leveille SG et al: Foot pain and disability in older women, *Am J Epidemiol* 148:657, 1998.

Loden M: Role of topical emollients and moisturizers in the treatment of dry skin barrier disorders, *Am J Clin Dermatol* 4:771, 2003.

Lukacs KS, Kelechi TJ: An intrapreneurial approach to foot care, *Clin Nurse Specialist CNS* 7:326, 1993.

Luggen AS: Wrinkles and beyond. Skin problems in older adults, *Adv Nurse Pract* 11:55, 2003.

Maeda N, Mizuno N, Ichikawa K: Nail abrasion: a new treatment for ingrown toe-nails, *J Dermatol* 17:746, 1990.

Mahoney FI, Barthel D: W. Functional evaluation: the Barthel index, *Maryland State Med J* 14:61, 1965.

Mann RA, Mann JA: Keratotic disorders of the plantar skin, *Instr Course Lectures* 53:287, 2004.

Mathias S, Nayak US, Isaacs B: Balance in elderly patients: the "get-up and go" test, *Arch Phys Med Rehab* 67:387, 1986.

Mazur ML: Barefoot in the dark. When neuropathy is in the picture, walking barefoot should never be an option, *Diabetes Forecast* 55:73, 2002.

McDonnell G, Russell D: Antiseptics and disinfectants: activity, action, and resistance, *Clin Microbiol Rev* 12:147, 1999.

Menz HB, Pod B, Lord SR: The contribution of foot problems to mobility impairment and falls in community-dwelling older people, *J Am Geriatr Soc* 49:1651, 2001.

Mondelli M, Morana P, Padua L: An electrophysiological severity scale in tarsal tunnel syndrome, *Acta Neurol Scand* 109:284, 2004.

Mullins N, Lee HH: Occupational exposure to HIV, hepatitis B, hepatitis C, and tuberculosis, *Clin Podiatr Med Surg* 15:363, 1998.

Myerly SM, Stavosky JW: An alternative method for reducing plantar pressures in neuropathic ulcers, *Adv Wound Care J Prevent Healing* 10:26, 1997.

Ozdemir H et al: Effects of changes in heel fat pad thickness and elasticity on heel pain, *J Am Podiatr Med Assn* 94:47, 2004.

Patout CA Jr et al: A decision pathway for the staged management of foot problems in diabetes mellitus, *Arch Phys Med Rehab* 82:1724, 2001.

Pelican P, Barbieri E, Blair S: Toe the line: a nurse-run well foot care clinic, *J Gerontol* 16(12):6, 1990.

Pham H et al: Screening techniques to identify people at high risk for diabetic foot ulceration: a prospective multicenter trial, *Diabetes Care* 23:606, 2000.

Pham HT et al: A prospective, randomized, controlled double-blind study of a moisturizer for xerosis of the feet in patients with diabetes, *Ostomy Wound Manage* 48(5):30, 2002.

Pinzur M et al: Development of a nurse-provided health system strategy for diabetic foot care, *Foot Ankle Int* 22:744, 2001.

Piraccini BM et al: Drug-induced nail abnormalities, *Expert Opin Drug Safety* 3:57, 2004.

Pitei DL, Foster A, Edmonds M: The effect of regular callus removal on foot pressure, *Foot Ankle Surg Am Coll Foot Ankle Surg* 38:251, 1999.

Plummer ES, Albert SG: Foot care assessment in patients with diabetes: a screening algorithm for patient education and referral, *Diabetes Educator* 21:47, 1995.

Podsiadlo D, Richardson S: The timed "up & go": a test of basic functional mobility for frail elderly persons, *J Am Geriatr Soc* 39:142, 1991.

Price P, Harding K: The impact of foot complications on health-related quality of life in patients with diabetes, *J Cutan Med Surg* 4:45, 2000.

Ramsewak RS et al: In vitro antagonistic activity of monoterpenes and their mixtures against 'toe nail fungus' pathogens, *Phytother Res PTR* 17:376, 2003.

Read S: Treatment of a heel blister caused by pressure and friction, *Br J Nurs* 10:10, 2001.

Resnick B: Dermatologic problems in the elderly, *Lippincott's Prim Care Pract* 1:14, 1997.

Richbourg MJ: Preventing amputations in patients with end stage renal disease: whatever happened to foot care? *ANNA J Am Nephrol Nurs Assn* 25:13, 1998.

Rockwell PG: Acute and chronic paronychia, *Am Fam Physician* 63:1113, 2001.

Roseeuw D: Achilles foot screening project: preliminary results of patients screened by dermatologists, *J Eur Acad Dermatol Venereol JEADV* 12(Suppl 1):S6, discussion S17, 1999.

Sauseng S, Kastenbauer T, Irsigler K: Limited joint mobility in selected hand and foot joints in patients with type 1 diabetes mellitus: a methodology comparison, *Diabetes, Nutr Metabol* 15:1, 2002.

Saye DE: The foot: ulcer and toenail debridement and pressure relief padding, *Ostomy Wound Manage* 40:14, 1994.

Scher RK et al: Brittle nail syndrome: treatment options and the role of the nurse, *Dermatol Nurs Dermatol Nurs Assn* 15:15, 2003.

Schroeter CA et al: Photodynamic therapy: new treatment for therapy-resistant plantar warts, *Dermatol Surg* 31:71, 2005.

Seidel HM et al, editors: Blood vessels. In *Mosby's Guide to Physical Examination*, ed 5, St Louis, 2003, Mosby, Elsevier Science

Sidou F, Soto P: A randomized comparison of nail surface remanence of three nail lacquers, containing amorolfine 5%, ciclopirox 8% or tioconazole 28%, in healthy volunteers, *Int J Tissue Reactions* 26(1-2):17, 2004.

Soroko YT et al: Treatment of plantar verrucae using 2% sodium salicylate iontophoresis, *Phys Ther* 82:1184, 2002.

Sprecher E: Genetic hair and nail disorders, *Clin Dermatol* 23:47, 2005.

Springett K, White RJ: Skin changes in the "at risk" foot and their treatment, *Br J Community Nurs* Dec:25, 2002.

Stess RM, Jensen SR, Mirmiran R: The role of dynamic plantar pressures in diabetic foot ulcers, *Diabetes Care* 20:855, 1997.

Stulberg DL, Hutchinson AG: Molluscum contagiosum and warts, *Am Fam Physician* 67:1233, 2003.

Summers JB, Kaminski J: Is duct tape occlusion therapy an effective treatment of warts? *Am Fam Physician* 68:1912, 2003.

Syed TA et al: Treatment of toenail onychomycosis with 2% butenafine and 5% *Melaleuca alternifolia* (tea tree) oil in cream, *Tropical Med Int Health TM IH,* 4:284, 1999.

Tan JS, Joseph WS: Common fungal infections of the feet in patients with diabetes mellitus, *Drugs Aging* 21:101, 2004.

Tandeter H, Tandeter ER: Treatment of plantar warts with oral valacyclovir, *Am J Med* 118:689, 2005.

Thomson CE, Gibson JN, Martin D: Interventions for the treatment of Morton's neuroma, *Cochrane Database Syst Rev* 3:2004 CD003118.

Tucker SB, Ali A, Ransdell BL: Plantar wart treatment with combination imiquimod and salicylic acid pads, *J Drugs Dermatol JDD* 2:124, 2003.

Turner C, Quine S: Nurses' knowledge, assessment skills, experience, and confidence in toenail management of elderly people. Why are nurses and nursing assistants reluctant to cut toenails? *Geriatr Nurs (New York, NY)* 17:273, 1996.

Tyrrell W: The causes and management of foot ulceration, *Nurs Standard* 16(30):52, 2002.

van Os AG et al: Comparison of conventional treatment and supervised rehabilitation for treatment of acute lateral ankle sprains: a systematic review of the literature, *J Orthop Sports Phys Ther* 35:95, 2005.

Vileikyte L et al: The development and validation of a neuropathy- and foot ulcer-specific quality of life instrument, *Diabetes Care* 26:2549, 2003.

Wall JC et al: The timed get-up-and-go test revisited: measurement of the component tasks, *J Rehab Res Devel* 37:109, 2000.

Ward PE: Atopy and reaction to nail dust inhalation, *Clin Podiatr Med Surg* 12:275, 1995.

Wilder RP, Sethi S: Overuse injuries: tendinopathies, stress fractures, compartment syndrome, and shin splints, *Clin Sports Med (Auckland NZ)* 23:55, 2004.

Williams J: We make foot exams a priority, *RN* 64(5):40, 2001.

WOCN Society: *Guideline for management of wounds in patients with lower-extremity neuropathic disease,* WOCN Clinical Practice Guideline Series #3, Glenview IL, 2004, Author.

Wu KK: Morton's interdigital neuroma: a clinical review of its etiology, treatment, and results, *Foot Ankle Surg Am Coll Foot Ankle Surg* 35:112, discussion 187, 1996.

Yates YJ, Concannon MJ: Fungal infections of the perionychium, *Hand Clin* 18:631, 2002.

Yetzer EA: Incorporating foot care education into diabetic foot screening, *Rehab Nurs* 29(3):80, 2004.

Younes NA, Albsoul AM, Awad H: Diabetic heel ulcers: a major risk factor for lower extremity amputation, *Ostomy Wound Manage* 50:50, 2004.

OBJECTIVES

1. Identify the three phases of burn care and discuss the goals of each phase.
2. Discuss the causes of burns including thermal, chemical, and electrical injuries.
3. Identify how the three zones of tissue damage relate to the depth of the burn wound.
4. Compare and contrast the severity of the burn trauma using the following terminology: superficial, superficial partial-thickness, deep partial-thickness and full-thickness burns.
5. Describe three common methods used to calculate the total body surface area of a burn.
6. Describe the advantages and disadvantages of at least four topical burn care products or dressings.
7. Describe the indications and techniques for escharotomy, fasciotomy, tangential excision, and skin grafting.
8. Distinguish among indicators for managing the patient with a burn in the outpatient setting, the inpatient setting and a specialized burn care facility.
9. Identify three principles of managing burn wounds in an outpatient setting.

Patients with massive tissue loss present the wound care professional with unique, complex care needs. In addition to topical wound care needs, the patient is at risk for numerous systemic complications associated with the absence of large amounts of epidermis and/or dermis (i.e., edema, wound infection, etc.). This chapter focuses on burn injury. However, the techniques used to assess the severity and extent of tissue damage and the principles of fluid resuscitation, infection control, and topical management are similar to those in other types of massive tissue loss. Calciphylaxis, necrotizing fasciitis, epidermolysis bullosa (EB), staphylococcal scalded skin syndrome (SSSS), toxic epidermal necrolysis (TENS), and graft versus host disease (GVHD) can precipitate massive tissue loss and are briefly discussed in Chapter 6.

Care of the patient with a burn is a complex process that requires a multidisciplinary team consisting of physicians, nurses, physical and occupational therapists, a pharmacist, a nutrition specialist, a case manager, and social workers. Additional management by the intensive care team, plastic surgeon, ophthalmology, psychiatric services, and child life specialists is frequently required to identify the needs of the individual patient with a burn. All burn team members must be knowledgeable about the concepts of wound care, wound healing, and pathophysiology. Team members must also be aware of the psychologic impact of acute injury, the phases of recovery from a burn injury, and the long-term rehabilitation needs of the patient.

EPIDEMIOLOGY

It is estimated that each year there are over 1 million burn injuries in the United States, with over 700,000 annual emergency department visits and over 45,000 hospital admissions. Annual fire and burn deaths are estimated at 4500 (Burn Foundation, 2000). The majority of these injuries involve burns of less than 10% of the total body surface area (TBSA). Flame burns and scalds from hot liquids account for about 75% of reported cases; almost one half of these burn injuries occur in the home (American Burn Association, 2002).

The National Burn Repository 2002 Report (American Burn Association, 2000), which includes data on over 73,000 burn cases from 46 U.S. and 3 Canadian burn centers, further identifies characteristics of burn-injured patients. Nearly 70% of all burn victims are male, with 37% of all burn injuries occurring in children 1 to 5 years of age. A second peak incidence occurs in the age range of adolescent through 39 years

361

of age. The mortality rate for these patients is from 5% to 6%.

PATHOPHYSIOLOGY

Major burn injuries affect all body systems; an understanding of the systemic response is essential for treatment. Burn care is divided into three overlapping phases of recovery: emergent, acute/wound care, and rehabilitation. The *emergent phase* is the first 72 hours after injury. Care during this period centers on emergency management and stabilization, fluid replacement, and beginning wound management. Complications of the emergent phase include pulmonary insufficiency, acute renal failure, and compartment syndrome to burned extremities.

The *acute/wound care phase* begins when stabilization of the patient has been achieved; goals of this period include healing partial-thickness wounds, grafting full-thickness wounds, and preventing complications. Wound management during the acute phase consists of debridement, daily wound care, and surgical interventions for wound closure. Complications that can occur during this period include wound infection, sepsis, pulmonary insufficiency, and multiorgan failure.

The *rehabilitation phase* begins when wound healing is complete and focuses on restoring or maximizing the patient's functional capacity. This phase may last several years and deals with functional and cosmetic problems associated with contractures and scar tissue formation.

TYPES OF BURN INJURY

Burns result from many sources: thermal, chemical, electrical, and radiation. Although management principles are similar for all types of burn injury, discussion will include special considerations for each type of injury and identification of at-risk populations.

Thermal

Thermal burns are the most common cause of burn injuries and result from exposure to flames, contact with hot liquids or hot objects, or radiation. The severity of injury is related to the temperature and duration of contact. When exposure is sudden and short, it is often referred to as a *flash* burn. Although all individuals are at risk for thermal injury, patterns of risk for the causes of thermal burns have been identified.

Flame burns are generally more common in older children and adults. Adolescents often participate in risky behavior, exploring their environment without adult supervision (Ying and Ho, 2001). With 20% to 30% of serious burn injuries in the adult occurring in the workplace, the workplace poses a significant risk to flame injuries for adults (Quinney et al, 2002).

Two thirds of childhood burn injuries are *scalds,* secondary to accidents in the home or deliberate abuse (Deitch and Rutan, 2000), with 75% of all scald burn victims being less than 3 years of age (Corrarino, Walsh, and Nadel, 2001). *Contact* injuries are common in young children, since infants and toddlers do not have the motor skills that facilitate withdrawal from a heat source (Helvig, 1993).

In the elderly, 70% of burn injuries occur in the home, and one half of these are scalds. The elderly have several predisposing factors associated with age that put them at particular risk for burn injury including reduced reaction times, decreased dexterity, decreased mobility, inaccurate risk assessment, and impaired senses (Redlick et al, 2002). Adults at work are also at risk for contact burns; exposure to hot objects or substances are the second leading cause of burn injury in the workplace (Hunt et al, 2000).

Flame. Flame burns commonly involve exposure to fire, with ignition of clothing. Outdoor trash and brush fires, frequently including the use of an accelerant, are a major cause of injury (Wibbenmeyer et al, 2003). House fires are also a significant cause of flame burn injury, and are associated with the additional risk of smoke inhalation injury. In 1998, an estimated 381,500 residential structure fires resulted in 3,250 nonfirefighter deaths, 17,175 injuries, and over $4 billion in property loss (American Academy of Pediatrics, 2000).

Contact. Contact burns are caused by hot liquids (referred to as scalds) or hot objects. Scalds are the most frequent cause of nonfatal burn injuries (Corrarino, Walsh, and Nadel, 2001). Most scald burns occur in the kitchen or bathroom of the home and involve hot water or cooking spills. Temperatures of up to 45° C (113° F) may be tolerated for relatively long periods of time without injury, but higher temperatures cause damage more quickly. As little as 10 seconds of exposure to water at 70° C can result in full-thickness injury in adults (Carrougher, 1997;

Jordan and Harrington, 1997). It takes less heat or a shorter duration of exposure to cause a deep burn in a child. At the temperature of most home water heaters (60° C, or 140° F) it takes as little as 5 seconds to produce tissue destruction in a child, and only 1 second in an infant (Helvig, 1993).

Contact burns can occur in the home or the workplace, and frequently occur on the hands, face, and upper body as the object is touched. Common causes of contact burns include space heaters, clothing and curling irons, cookware, and hot machinery and containers (Hunt et al, 2000; Wibbenmeyer et al, 2003).

Radiation

Radiation injuries occur secondary to exposure to particles or waves from sources such as air transmission, inhalation, ingestion, or direct contact. Radiation injuries are rare. The National Burn Repository Report (2002) notes that radiation injures represent less than 0.5% of burn center admissions. These injuries can range from minor to deadly. Severity of injury and prognosis is related to the type of radiation, rads absorbed, and duration of exposure (Supple, 2004).

Chemical

Chemical burns account for 2% to 6% of burn unit admissions, with approximately 60,000 people seeking medical treatment each year for chemical injuries. The most common causes of chemical injury are alkalis, acids, and organic compounds. Alkalis and acids can be found in products in the home and the workplace. Chemical injuries are often smaller in area than thermal burns, but are more likely to be full-thickness in depth (Winfree and Barillo, 1997). The severity of chemical burns is related to the agent of exposure, the duration of contact, and the agent's concentration, volume, and mechanism of action (American Burn Association, 2001). Tissue damage continues after initial exposure, until the chemical can be removed or inactivated (diluted) with irrigation. Initial treatment consists of removal of saturated clothing, brushing off dry chemicals, and copious irrigation with water (Winfree and Barillo, 1997). Health care providers must protect themselves from exposure by employing universal precautions, including eye protection, while caring for the chemical injured patient. In general, neutralization of the agent with another chemical is not recommended unless the exact mechanism is known, since the reaction may generate more heat and result in further tissue destruction (American Burn Association, 2001).

Alkalis. Alkalis are commonly found in oven and drain cleaners, fertilizers, heavy industrial cleaners, and in cement and concrete. Alkalis damage tissue by liquefaction necrosis and protein denaturation, which allows for deeper spread of the chemical into tissues and a more severe injury (Winfree and Barillo, 1997). Alkalis are the most frequent cause of chemical injuries to the eye. Since alkalis bind to tissue proteins, treatment consists of prolonged continuous irrigation to dilute the chemical and prevent progression of the injury. The majority of patients with chemical injury to the eye will be seen with swelling and/or spasms of the eyelids. It is important to maintain irrigation while not causing additional injury. This can be accomplished by placing catheters in the medial sulcus for irrigation with normal saline. An ophthalmologist should be consulted as soon as possible for all chemical injuries to the eye (American Burn Association, 2001).

Acids. Acids may be found in bathroom cleansers, rust removers, acidifiers for home swimming pools, and industrial drain cleaners. Acids damage tissue by coagulation necrosis and protein precipitation, which usually limits the depth and spread of tissue damage. One exception to this is hydrofluoric acid, which has uses in industry such as glass etching and cleaning semiconductors, and in the home as a rust remover. Hydrofluoric acid is a weak acid, but the fluoride ion penetrates the tissues rapidly and deeply and binds magnesium and calcium, which can produce cardiac arrhythmias from hypomagnesemia or hypocalcemia (Winfree and Barillo, 1997). Low concentrations may cause severe pain, which can be delayed 6 to 18 hours after injury. High concentrations cause immediate pain and tissue necrosis. Hydrofluoric acid burns are treated initially with copious irrigation, followed by topical calcium gluconate gel to neutralize the fluoride. Severe pain, failure to improve with topical calcium application, or evidence of deep tissue necrosis indicates the need for subcutaneous injection or intravenously administered calcium gluconate infusion (directly into the injured site) to bind the fluoride in an insoluble complex. The burn surgeon, with the assistance of interventional radiology, performs this procedure. Important interventions include monitoring cardiac activity and ionized calcium levels. Early excision of even small hydrofluoric acid injuries may be life-saving (American Burn Association, 2001).

Organic Compounds. Organic compounds such as phenols and petroleum products (gasoline, diesel fuel, and creosote) can be responsible for systemic toxicity, as well as contact chemical burns. Organic compounds cause cutaneous damage as a result of their fat solvent action and, once absorbed, can produce toxic effects on the pulmonary, renal, and hepatic systems (American Burn Association, 2001). Phenol, an organic acid frequently used in disinfectants and chemical solvents, damages tissue by causing coagulation necrosis of dermal proteins. Initial treatment consists of copious water irrigation, followed by cleansing with 50% polyethylene glycol, which increases the solubility of the phenol and allows more rapid removal of the compound (Winfree and Barillo, 1997).

Tar. Tar burns are generally discussed with chemical burns, although the bitumen compound itself is not absorbed and is not toxic. Tar burns are essentially contact burns, and emergency treatment consists of cooling the molten material with water to stop the burning process. Removal of the tar is not an emergency once it is cooled; this may be accomplished by covering the tar with a petroleum-based ointment to promote emulsification and removal of the tar (American Burn Association, 2001).

Electrical

Electrical injuries account for 4% to 6% of burn center admissions. It is estimated that there are as many as 50,000 injuries and 1000 deaths each year in the United States from electrical causes. Lightning, which accounts for more annual deaths than any other natural hazard in the United States, claims 300 to 600 lives per year (American Burn Association, 2005).

Classification of electrical injuries is divided into four categories: high voltage (more than 1000 V), low voltage (less than 1000 V), lightning strikes, and electric arc without the passage of current through the body. Because of the mechanism of injury, these patients are at risk for concomitant blunt trauma, soft tissue injuries, and thermal (flame or flash) burns. The highest incidence of injuries are work-related and high voltage, with the primary victims being young men (Arnoldo et al, 2004). Adolescents aged 11 to 18 are also at risk for high-voltage injury, primarily from touching power lines while engaging in risk-taking behavior. Children less than 6 years of age account for one third of electrical injuries. Generally these are of low voltage and involve injuries related to chewing on electrical cords or placing objects into electrical outlets (American Burn Association, 2005).

The Process of Electrical Injury. Tissue injury from contact with electricity results from electrical energy being converted into thermal or heat energy (American Burn Association, 2001). The extent of injury to the body when it becomes part of an electrical current is determined by (1) strength and type of the current, (2) pathway of flow, (3) local tissue resistance and (4) duration of the exposure.

Alternating current (AC) is involved in most electrical injuries and is produced by the reversal of electron flow every half cycle; the electricity flows back and forth from the power source to the contact point on the patient. This alternating flow can cause cardiac arrhythmias, respiratory arrest, loss of consciousness, and skeletal muscle tetany, so that the victim cannot release the grip on the source of the current (Luce, 2000). Direct current (DC) is found in lightning, batteries, on ships, in some mass transit systems, and in arc welding equipment (Winfree and Barillo, 1997). DC flows in one direction and injuries have more pronounced entrance and exit sites.

Body tissue resistance is an integral part of the pathophysiology of electrical injury. Various tissues of the body have different resistance to current flow. Once electrical contact is made with the skin and resistance is overcome, the body acts as a volume conductor, and current flows through the body part (Luce, 2000). Heat will dissipate through the skin, leaving nonviable tissue under intact skin. Bone has a very high resistance because it is dense. Current will flow along the surface of the bone and generate heat, thus damaging adjacent deep muscle while superficial muscle remains viable.

Damage from electrical contact is normally more severe in the extremities than in the trunk because of the smaller surface area and the combined effects of current passage, heat generation, and compression of vital structures (Lim, Rehmar, and Elmore, 1998). Edema can develop in fascial compartments, causing pressure and decreased blood flow to the muscle. If this compartment pressure is not relieved, muscle necrosis will occur. Symptoms of increasing pressure include (1) severe pain with flexion or extension of the muscles within the compartment, (2) numbness or tingling in a hand or foot, and (3) decreased or absent pulses. Decompression by escharotomy or fasciotomy may be necessary within several hours of the injury (American Burn Association, 2001). Of the different types of burn injuries, victims of high-voltage electrical injuries have a greater incidence of deep muscle necrosis, fasciotomy, and limb amputation (Arnoldo et al, 2004).

Electrical arc injuries occur when the current arcs, or jumps an air gap between two conductors, thus superheating the air (as high as 4000° C). Common arcing sites on the body are the flexion creases of the extremities. Flash and flame burns are produced when the arc ignites the patient's clothing or causes an explosion sufficient to cause a blunt trauma. The resulting small surface burns can conceal a tremendous amount of underlying soft tissue damage (Luce, 2000). Arc injuries may also occur without actual current flow into the body, in which case they are classified and treated as any flame/flash burn (Arnoldo et al, 2004).

Unique Complications. Electrical injury is associated with unique complications that may be immediate or delayed. As a result of the effects of electrical current on the conduction mechanism of the heart, cardiac arrhythmias, including ventricular fibrillation and cardiac standstill, may be encountered. Similarly, injury of the respiratory center and intense spasms of the respiratory muscles may cause respiratory arrest at the time of injury.

Because of the massive muscle and red blood cell destruction and subsequent release of myoglobin and hemoglobin into the bloodstream, patients are at risk for developing acute renal failure (acute tubular necrosis). These large molecules are more soluble in an alkaline urine, so brisk fluid resuscitation, which includes the addition of sodium bicarbonate, causing urine to be produced at a rate of 100 to 200 ml/hour in an adult patient, must be maintained from the onset of resuscitation (American Burn Association, 2001). Standard fluid resuscitation formulas do not apply to the electrically injured patient, since the surface extent of the injury is usually far less than the actual deep tissue damage (Luce, 2000).

Neurologic complications of electrical injuries have been reported to be as high as 67% (Grube et al, 1990). Immediate neurologic symptoms include a decreased level of consciousness, paraplegia or quadriplegia, or focal paralysis, which usually resolves within a matter of days (Wittman, 1994). Delayed symptoms may appear within the first few days following injury or take years to evolve; they include headaches, seizure activity, and impairment in attention, memory, or concentration. The incidence of peripheral mononeuropathies and polyneuropathies is as high as 25% in long-term follow-up (Arnoldo et al, 2004). Those patients with a history of electrical injury involving the head are at high risk for development of cataracts and other ocular disorders, sometimes more than a year after injury (Luce, 2000).

INHALATION INJURY

Inhalation injury is the most common accompanying injury seen in patients with burn injuries. The National Burn Repository Report (American Burn Association, 2002) found that inhalation injury is present in approximately 10% of patients admitted to burn centers; these patients have a mortality rate approaching 30%. There are three distinguishable types of airway inhalation injury: carbon monoxide poisoning, inhalation injury to the upper airway, and inhalation injury to the lower airway.

Carbon Monoxide Poisoning

Carbon monoxide poisoning and/or asphyxiation are responsible for most fatalities at fire scenes. Carboxyhemoglobin levels of 50% to 70% or more are often found in such patients. Carbon monoxide binds to hemoglobin with an affinity 200 times greater than oxygen. When sufficient hemoglobin is bound to carbon monoxide, tissue hypoxia occurs. The most immediate threat is to "hypoxia-sensitive" tissues, such as the brain. Levels of 40% to 60% carboxyhemoglobin cause obtundation and loss of consciousness. The half-life of carbon monoxide in the blood is about 4 hours on room air. Half-life is decreased to 1 hour on 100% oxygen. Early administration of 100% oxygen should be initiated as soon as possible (American Burn Association, 2001).

Upper-Airway Inhalation Injury

Upper-airway injuries are heat-related. Most respiratory-tract absorption of heat, and heat-related tissue damage, occurs above the level of the glottis. As with other burn injuries, tissue edema can occur very rapidly and cause airway obstruction. The patient with burns to the face, singed nasal and facial hair, edema of the tongue or pharynx, and increased respiratory rate should be monitored closely for airway obstruction due to edema. Intubation with mechanical ventilation may be necessary to provide adequate oxygenation until the edema resolves.

Lower-Airway Inhalation Injury

Lower-airway injuries are chemical in nature and are related to the inhalation of noxious chemicals that are products of combustion (Monafo, 1996). Health care providers must have a high degree of suspicion of lower-airway injury in patients with a history of flame-related injury in an enclosed space or a loss of consciousness at the scene. The airway mucosa becomes inflamed and usually contains carbon particles. Clinical evolution can be delayed from 1 to 3 days after exposure as the mucosa sloughs and secretions accumulate to obstruct the airway and cause atelectasis; patients develop pulmonary failure and pneumonia (Gordon and Goodwin, 1997). Treatment requires ventilatory support, meticulous pulmonary toilet, and general critical care management.

PHASES OF HEALING AND THE BURN PROCESS

Burn wounds go through the phases of wound healing as described in detail in Chapters 4 and 5. Arachodonic acid metabolites, oxidants, histamine, serotonin, kinins, and other vasoactive amines are released by damaged and ischemic cells into the burn wound and produce increased local and systemic hyperpermeability of the capillaries (Jordan and Harrington, 1997). The release of fluids through the hyperpermeable capillaries and the increased capillary pressure combine to create local or systemic edema. Capillary permeability returns to normal roughly 18 to 24 hours after injury.

For a small burn (total burn size is less than 15% to 20% TBSA), the development of edema is immediate, rapid, and usually limited to the wound site, and peaks within 8 to 12 hours (Ahrns, 1999). Intravascular fluid losses associated with these small burns can be managed with oral replacement at 150% of calculated maintenance rate. Intravenous supplementation can be used if the patient has difficulties meeting the oral intake goal.

Large burns reach maximum edema within 12 to 24 hours. Inflammatory mediators released from the damaged site cause the increased capillary permeability to occur not only at the site of injury but throughout the body (Ahrns, 2004). The outcome is a dramatic outpouring of fluids, electrolytes, and protein into the interstitial space. Hypovolemic shock develops during the emergent phase in patients with a burn wound of at least 15% to 20% TBSA unless interventions are started (Lim, Rehmar, and Elmore, 1998).

Loss of skin integrity also causes increased fluid and heat loss through the wound. Evaporative fluid loss caused by loss of the integrity of the skin is 4 to 20 times the normal rate, which contributes to hypovolemia; this fluid loss continues until all the wounds are closed. Hypothermia should be prevented rigorously throughout the phases of recovery. Hypothermia is a known contributor to coagulopathy in that it inhibits enzyme reactions of the coagulation cascade. The patient with burn injury has been shown to have an increased thermal neutral point, so that exposure to low temperatures results in an increase in the patient's metabolic rate (Jordan and Harrington, 1997). Restoration and maintenance of intravascular volume with fluid similar to that which is lost in the tissues becomes an essential aspect of burn management.

Excessive scarring is a key concern in the management of the patient with a burn injury. Altered regulation of the reparative process, such as excessive collagen deposition or the wound failing to become covered with epithelium, can lead to abnormal healing. Wounds that remain unhealed have a continuation of inflammation, which tends to stimulate more collagen synthesis and angiogenesis. Although the development of hypertrophic scarring is not fully understood, any factor that causes a persistent inflammatory process probably contributes to excessive scarring. Early wound closure, mechanical splinting for stretch and position, and diligent range of motion (ROM) exercise of the site are essential components of burn wound care (Greenhalgh and Staley, 1994; Jordan and Harrington, 1997).

Maturation of the scar tissue and grafted areas continues throughout the rehabilitation period.

During this phase, the wound tissue develops greater tensile strength as collagen deposits form scar tissue. The scar eventually becomes less erythematous, flattens, and appears to "mature." The final phase of maturation is reached when the wound normalizes in color and stops changing in form (Greenhalgh and Staley, 1994).

EVALUATION OF THE BURN INJURY

Zone of Tissue Damage

Determining burn depth can be difficult for even the most experienced burn care provider. Immediately following injury, burns may appear shallow but declare themselves to be deeper by the third day after the burn occurred (Gibran and Heimbach, 2000). The zone of tissue damage describes the extent of the injury from the deepest or most severely damaged area to the superficial or outermost area. The three zones of tissue damage are zone of coagulation, zone of stasis, and zone of hyperemia (Jackson, 1953).

The *zone of coagulation* is the area of greatest damage, is closest to the heat source, and is characterized by coagulation of the cells. Cellular damage from heat results in protein denaturation. If the damage in this zone extends through the entire dermis, a full-thickness injury has occurred. If the zone of coagulation is above the level of the dermal appendages, healing by reepithelialization will occur.

The *zone of stasis* surrounds the zone of coagulation and involves the vascular system in the area. Thrombosis and vasoconstriction cause transient dermal ischemia. Circulation will return, and tissue health will be restored, if the area is adequately perfused and protected from further damage such as infection, dessication, and mechanical stresses during transfers and repositioning.

The *zone of hyperemia* is the outermost area, and usually no cellular death occurs because this area is only minimally damaged. Cells in this zone recover in 7 to 10 days. The area is reddened because of vasodilatation and inflammation. The zone of hyperemia is similar to a superficial partial-thickness burn.

Severity of the Burn Wound

Treatment of the burn wound is based on the depth, extent, and severity of the injury. The depth of the injury is based on the number of cells injured or destroyed and on the functional capacity of the level of the skin. The traditional classification of burns as first-, second-, and third-degree has been replaced by the designations of superficial, superficial partial-thickness, deep partial-thickness, and full-thickness injury.

Superficial burns involve the epidermis only and heal without scar formation, pigmentation changes, or contractures. Symptoms include the classic signs of inflammation: pain, swelling, heat, and redness. The area blanches with pressure and is dry and painful. This type of burn occurs from overexposure to sunlight, a brief scalding with hot liquids, or a minor flash. After a few days, the outer layer of injured cells peels away, revealing healed new skin.

Superficial partial-thickness burns involve the epidermis, with portions of the burn extending into the dermis. It is characterized by blister formation and weeping; the wound is moist. Dermal structures such as nails, hair follicles, nerve endings, and sweat and sebaceous glands are intact and functional. These burns are associated with a great deal of pain since the wound is sensitive to air movement and temperatures. The basal layer of the dermis is intact, and after debridement of any blisters or allowing the fluid to resorb, healing occurs rapidly by epidermal regeneration, usually within about 2 weeks and with little scar formation.

Deep partial-thickness burns involve the epidermis and deeper areas of the dermis. These burns appear red with waxy white patches and, although blisters may be present, the wound bed is generally drier than seen with more superficial injuries. It may be difficult to distinguish deep partial-thickness burns from full-thickness burns, particularly with full-thickness scald injuries that may initially appear as a deep cherry red. Deep partial-thickness burns require a longer time to heal, and there may be scarring and disruption of the appearance and function of nails, glands, and hair. The injury to the dermis is partial, so healing by primary intention can occur. Factors such as wound infection and decreased blood flow can convert a deep partial-thickness burn to a full-thickness burn. Table 18-1 identifies risk factors for wound conversion.

Full-thickness burns result in the destruction of the epidermis and entire dermis. Healing will only occur at the wound margins and by skin grafting. The heat-coagulated blood vessels leave the tissue avascular, so the appearance of the burned tissue is a waxy white to a gray color. If the burn extends into the fat or has

TABLE 18-1 **Risk Factors for Conversion of Deep Partial- to Full-Thickness Burns**

LOCAL FACTORS	SYSTEMIC FACTORS
Impaired blood flow	Hypovolemia
Increased inflammation	Septicemia
Infection	Malnutrition
Open (nonhealed) wound	Excess catabolism
Surface exudate build-up	Chronic illness
Mechanical trauma	
Dressing changes	
Shearing	
Pressure	
Chemical trauma	
Topical agents	

been exposed to a prolonged flame source, it looks brown or black with a leathery and charred appearance. A full-thickness burn lacks pain sensation because of death of the nerves; a sign often used to distinguish a full-thickness burn from a partial-thickness burn. It is important to note that most burns are not uniform in depth; pain can be felt in the outer zones and varies with each burn and with each individual.

Another category of the full-thickness burn, often referred to as *fourth-degree burns,* results from an incineration type of exposure and electrical burns in which the heat is sufficient to destroy tissues below the skin. The damage includes fascia, muscle, or bone. This type of burn will require skin grafting and often local or regional flaps to cover the area definitively.

Lund-Browder Chart									
Area	0-1 Years	1-4 Years	5-9 Years	10-14 Years	15 Years	Adult	% 2nd	% 3rd	% TOTAL
Head	19	17	13	11	9	7			
Neck	2	2	2	2	2	2			
Ant. Trunk	13	13	13	13	13	13			
Post. Trunk	13	13	13	13	13	13			
R. Buttock	2.5	2.5	2.5	2.5	2.5	2.5			
L. Buttock	2.5	2.5	2.5	2.5	2.5	2.5			
Genitalia	1	1	1	1	1	1			
R.U. Arm	4	4	4	4	4	4			
L.U. Arm	4	4	4	4	4	4			
R.L. Arm	3	3	3	3	3	3			
L.L. Arm	3	3	3	3	3	3			
R. Hand	2.5	2.5	2.5	2.5	2.5	2.5			
L. Hand	2.5	2.5	2.5	2.5	2.5	2.5			
R. Thigh	5.5	6.5	8	8.5	9	9.5			
L. Thigh	5.5	6.5	8	8.5	9	9.5			
R.L. Leg	5	5	5.5	6	6.5	7			
L.L. Leg	5	5	5.5	6	6.5	7			
R. Foot	3.5	3.5	3.5	3.5	3.5	3.5			
L. Foot	3.5	3.5	3.5	3.5	3.5	3.5			

From the Medical University of South Carolina Children's Hospital Pediatric Burn Intake Form. (Charleston, SC)

Fig. 18-1 Lund-Browder chart for estimation of burn size. (From the Medical University of South Carolina Children's Hospital Pediatric Burn Intake Form, Charleston, SC.)

Calculation of Body Surface Area Burned

There are three methods to determine the extent of a burn injury: the Lund-Browder chart (Figure 18-1), the rule of nines (Figure 18-2), and the hand method. The Lund-Browder chart is the preferred method because it is the most accurate for patients of all ages (Mertens, Jenkins, and Warden, 1997). Areas of the body that are burned are identified as having partial- or full-thickness burns; superficial burns are not included in the calculation of total body surface area burned (TBSAB). The Lund-Browder chart is completed at admission to determine fluid requirements and repeated after 72 hours to recalculate any areas that may have extended.

The rule of nines is based on each anatomic region (of which there are 11), representing 9% (or multiples of 9%) of the TBSAB. The rule of nines must be modified for use in children, as it does not accurately reflect body surface area in children less than 15 years of age (Deitch and Rutan, 2000). The rule of nines method can serve as a quick guideline for transport and fluid resuscitation needs. With either method, areas of partial- and full-thickness burn are identified and added together to calculate the total percent of the body burned. The TBSAB is expressed as a percentage and helps estimate the extent of the injury for diagnosis, treatment, prognosis, and statistical analysis.

The hand method of determining the extent of a burn injury is useful for estimating small, scattered burns. The patient's hand, including the fingers, represents approximately 1% of his or her total body surface area (American Burn Association, 2001).

Referral Criteria

The American Burn Association has categorized burns as minor, moderate, and major (Table 18-2) and defined the criteria for burn center referral (Box 18-1). Patients with major burn injuries or those that meet the criteria identified in Box 18-1 and require treatment in a specialized center. A burn center is a facility with a burn physician as director and a highly trained, multidisciplinary staff dedicated to caring for the patient with burns (American Burn Association, 2001).

INITIAL INTERVENTIONS

As with any trauma victim, the initial assessment of the patient with a burn injury includes a primary and secondary survey. The primary survey includes

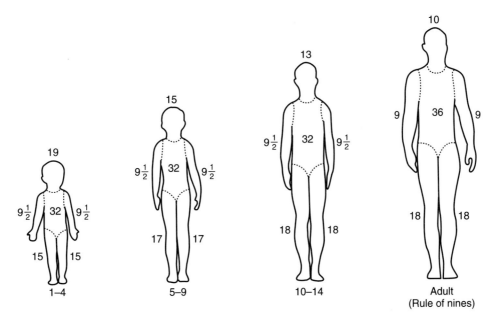

Fig. 18-2 Rule of nines calculations from infancy through adulthood.

TABLE 18-2 American Burn Association (ABA) Categories of Burn Injury

MINOR BURNS	MODERATE BURNS	MAJOR BURNS
Adults: 15% TBSA Children and elderly: 10% TBSA Less than 2% TBSA full-thickness burns not involving cosmetic or functional risk or impairment of the face, ears, eyes, feet, hands, or perineum	Adults: 15% to 25% TBSA, mixed partial-/full-thickness Children under 10 years of age or adults over 40 years of age: 10% to 20% TBSA Less than 10% TBSA full-thickness burns not involving cosmetic or functional risk or impairment of the face, ears, eyes, feet, hands, or perineum	All patients: more than 25% TBSA Children or adults over 40 years of age: 20% TBSA More than 10% TBSA full-thickness burns All burns of face, eyes, ears, hands, or perineum, especially if functional or cosmetic impairment exists All high-voltage electrical burns All burns with inhalation injury or major trauma Poor-risk patients

TBSA, Total body surface area.

BOX 18-1 American Burn Association (ABA) Criteria for Burn Center Referral (2001)

- More than 10% TBSA partial-thickness burns
- All full-thickness burns
- Burns that involve the face, hands, feet, genitalia, perineum, or major joints
- Electrical burns, including lightning injury
- Chemical burns
- Inhalation injury
- Presence of preexisting medical disorders that could complicate management, prolong recovery, or affect mortality
- Patients with concomitant trauma in which the burn poses the greatest risk of morbidity or mortality
- Burned children in hospitals without qualified personnel or equipment to care for children
- Patients who will require special social, emotional, or long-term rehabilitative intervention

Advanced Burn Life Support, as outlined by the American College of Surgeons Committee on Trauma (American Burn Association, 2001). The guidelines include the ABCDEF assessment: *a*irway, *b*reathing, *c*irculation, *d*isability, *e*xposure and evaluation, and *f*luid resuscitation.

The secondary survey is initiated after immediate resuscitative measures are established and includes a complete physical assessment and a medical history. Because care is based on the mechanism, location, and severity of the injury, every attempt should be made to obtain as much information as possible regarding the incident, such as if the injury occurred in an enclosed space, if chemicals were involved, and if the victim lost consciousness. Aspects of the patient's medical history such as preexisting disease, medications, allergies, alcohol or drug use, and immunization status influence management decisions (American Burn Association, 2001).

EMERGENT PHASE
Stabilization

The first 24 hours is devoted to fluid resuscitation, ventilatory management, and establishing the hemodynamic stability of the patient. During this phase, priorities involve estimating the depth and extent of the wound in order to calculate the severity of the injury and fluid resuscitation needs. Identification of the agent causing a chemical burn is also a priority, since specific treatments may be initiated. Early identification of full-thickness, circumferential wounds are important because full-thickness burn wounds require frequent assessment to determine if an emergent escharotomy or fasciotomy is needed.

Wound Intervention

The usual burn wound care given during this period follows patient stabilization and involves cleansing the areas with a nonirritating detergent and rinsing with warm water. The environment should be warmed to prevent hypothermia. Loose necrotic or devitalized tissue is lightly debrided, and large, intact bullae (over 2 cm) are opened. Small, frequent doses of intravenous analgesics are provided for pain control. Full-thickness wounds are usually dressed with a topical antimicrobial agent; systemic prophylactic antibiotics are not routinely used without identification of specific organisms (Jordan and Harrington, 1997). Patient weight and photographs of the burn wounds may be obtained at this time. Burn team members perform their initial assessments of the patient and plan interventions to promote healing and prevent complications.

Systemic Support

Fluid Resuscitation. Hypovolemia occurs during the first 24 to 48 hours after injury. Fluid and serum protein from the vascular compartment shift into the interstitial spaces, causing edema, blisters, weeping of fluid, and a decrease in circulating blood volume. To prevent hypovolemic shock and to maintain adequate cardiac output and renal and tissue perfusion, the fluid must be replaced. The amount of fluid for replacement depends on the extent and depth of the burn, and the patient's age and medical history. Many fluid resuscitation formulas exist, and most are based on the percent of TBSAB, body weight, or a combination of both (Table 18-3). While various methods of estimating fluid needs following burn injuries have been used, no single fluid formula has proven to be superior in limiting edema. All burn resuscitation formulas are a guide for estimating initial fluid needs. Each patient will react uniquely and may require more or less fluid than calculated by formula.

The goal of resuscitation is to maintain adequate vital organ perfusion, using the least amount of fluid necessary. According to The Advanced Burn Life Support (American Burn Association, 2001) lactated Ringer's (LR) solution is the preferred first-line fluid

for burn resuscitation because the composition and osmolality of LR most closely resembles normal body physiologic fluids (Ahrns, 2004). After the first 24 hours the consensus calls for the administration of a colloid-containing fluid (albumin diluted to physiologic concentration in normal saline) at 0.3 to 0.5 ml × body weight (kg) × %TBSAB of resuscitation is determined by routine and frequent surveillance of urinary output, mental status, peripheral temperature, systolic blood pressure, heart rate, and base deficit (Sheridan, 2002). Invasive hemodynamic monitoring (central venous pressure or pulmonary arterial pressure) is usually only required when the patient fails to respond to fluid resuscitation (Pessina and Ellis, 1997). The emergent period ends when the capillary permeability begins to normalize and the patient begins to diurese the large volume of fluid used for resuscitation, usually around the fourth day following injury. Maintenance fluids are then initiated and should be based on 1500 ml/m^2/day to replace insensible losses through the burn wounds.

Pulmonary. The physiologic effects of inhalation injury have been discussed previously, with an emphasis on early recognition and initiation of treatment. The uninjured pulmonary system also responds to cutaneous burn injury. The patient with burns over a large body surface area (BSA) develops edema to both burned and nonburned areas. The lungs are particularly susceptible to edema formation. Pulmonary edema results from increased capillary pressure combined with vasoconstriction of the microcirculation, overresuscitation and hypoproteinemia (Demling et al, 1979; Rutan RL, 1998).

Cardiovascular. The cardiovascular system is affected throughout the phases of burn recovery. In the emergent phase, there is an increased capillary permeability, decreased plasma volume, and decreased cardiac output. Decreases in circulating blood volume can result in tachycardia, hypotension, and decreases in central venous pressure and urine output. The depression of cardiac output seen immediately following burn injury, even before a decrease in blood volume can be detected, suggests that this effect results from neurogenic and humoral influence rather than from hypovolemia (Supple, 2004).

Vascular changes during burn injury also alter fluid and electrolyte balance. Alterations in electrolytes in

TABLE 18-3 Examples of Fluid Resuscitation Formulas for Patients with Burn Wounds

FORMULA	DESCRIPTION
Consensus formula	**First 24 hours, administer the following:** Adults: LR 2-4 ml/kg/% TBSAB Children: LR 3-4 ml/kg/% TBSAB Half of total given over first 8 hr after injury remaining half given over next 16 hr **Second 24 hours, administer the following:** Adults: colloid-containing fluid 0.3-0.5 ml/kg/TBSAB; electrolyte-free solution to maintain adequate urine output Children: colloid-containing fluid 0.3-0.5 ml/kg/TBSAB; half-normal saline to maintain adequate urine output
Parkland (Baxter) formula	**First 24 hours, administer the following:** LR 4 ml/kg/% TBSAB Half of total given over first 8 hours after injury remaining half given over next 16 hours **Second 24 hours, administer the following:** Dextrose in water, plus K+ to maintain normal electrolyte balance Colloid-containing fluid at 20%-60% of calculated plasma volume (0.35-0.5 ml/kg/% TBSAB)
Modified Brooke formula	**First 24 hours, administer the following:** Adults: LR 2 ml/kg/% TBSAB Children: LR 3 ml/kg/% TBSAB Half of total given over first 8 hours after injury remaining half given over next 16 hours **Second 24 hours, administer the following:** 5% albumin 0.3-0.5 ml/kg/% TBSAB to maintain urine output at 0.5-1.0 ml/kg/hour
Hypertonic saline/sodium (HSS) (Monafo)	Na+ 250 mEq/L Volume infused to maintain urine output 0.5 ml/kg/% TBSAB
Modified HSS (Warden)	For less than 40% TBSAB: **First 8 hours, administer the following:** 180 mEq/L Na+ (Mix 50 mEq/L NaHCO$_3$ in LR) Begin rate at 4 ml/kg/% TBSAB, adjust to maintain urine output of 30-50 ml/hr **At 8 hours after burn, administer the following:** LR at rate to maintain urine output of 30-50 ml/hr
Shriners: Galveston (Pediatric patients)	**First 24 hours, administer the following:** LR with 1.25% salt-poor human albumin 5000 ml/m^2 BSA burn, plus 2000 ml/m^2 BSA maintenance Half of total given over first 8 hr after injury remaining half given over next 16 hr

LR, Lactated Ringer's; *TBSA(B)*; total body surface area burned; *BSA*, body surface area.
Adapted from Ahrns KS and Harkins DR: Initial resuscitation after burn injury: therapies, strategies, and controversies, *AACN Clin Issues* 10(1):51, 1999.

the emergent and acute phases are common and must be monitored and treated accordingly. Hyperkalemia may be seen early in resuscitation as a result of the release of potassium from damaged cells and acidosis. Hypokalemia may also occur emergently secondary to hemodilution. During the acute phase, alterations in sodium, magnesium, calcium, and phosphorus must be monitored; loss of these electrolytes can occur through the open burn wound (Supple, 2004).

Renal. Acute renal failure immediately after the burn injury is thought to be secondary to the decrease in renal perfusion from hypovolemia. Additional excessive fluid losses from large burn wounds cause a shift of fluid to the interstitial space, further depleting circulating volume (Chrysopoulo et al, 1999). If fluid resuscitation is inadequate, hypovolemia will progress and acute renal failure will occur. With adequate resuscitation, renal blood flow and cardiac output increases and extravascular fluid is resorbed. Most burn centers recommend a urine output during the resuscitative phase of 30 ml to 50 ml/hour in adults and 1 ml/kg/hour in children weighing less than 30 kg (American Burn Association, 2001).

Neuroendocrine. The body responds to a thermal injury with a classic hemodynamic response. There is an almost immediate fall in cardiac output, metabolic rate, oxygen consumption, and blood pressure, along with ongoing fluid imbalance and cellular shock, for 3 to 7 days. This is followed by a slow increase to a hypermetabolic state with elevated catecholamine, glucocorticoid, and glucagon levels and a decrease in insulin. The increase in metabolic rate causes an increase in protein catabolism, gluconeogenesis, and lipolysis. This response is characterized by increased heat loss, negative nitrogen balance, and weight loss (Carrougher, 1997). Aggressive nutritional support is essential; requirements will decrease as the wound heals. The severity and duration of the hypermetabolic activity is directly proportional to the extent of injury. The peak occurs in the first 2 weeks and slowly returns to normal with closure of the wound.

Gastrointestinal. After burn injury, catecholamines can decrease peristalsis and absorption in the intestinal tract, resulting in paralytic ileus and decreased nutrient absorption. Decreased tissue perfusion and increased gastric secretions put the patient at risk for developing Curling's stress ulcer (Supple, 2004). Intestinal mucosal atrophy, caused by ischemia, affects the gastrointestinal system's ability to function as a bacterial barrier (Rutan, 1998). Early initiation of enteral feeding after burn injury can be safe and successful (Raff, Hartmann, and Germann, 1997), and has been shown to reduce caloric deficits (Gottschlich et al, 2002), prevent stress ulcers (Raff, Germann, and Hartmann, 1997), increase intestinal blood flow, preserve gastrointestinal function, and minimize bacterial translocation from the gut as a result of mucosal atrophy (Andel et al, 2001). In addition, early initiation of treatment with antacids, as well as measurement of gastric pH and subsequent treatment, has reduced the incidence of stress ulcers in the patient with a burn injury (Supple, 2004).

Nutrition. It is imperative that the patient with a burn injury receives adequate nutrition to meet the increased metabolic demands and energy needs for recovery. The enteral route is always preferred to provide nutritional support. Providing nutritional support by the parenteral route has no clear advantage and is used only in those patients with prolonged ileus or selected patients on mechanical ventilation (Tassiopoulos, 1999). Patients with burn injuries of 20% or greater TBSA will experience the hypermetabolic response and require nutritional support for optimal recovery. The patient's nutritional status and body composition at the time of injury may not provide sufficient body stores and nutrients to support wound healing and recovery (Mertens, Jenkins, and Warden, 1997). There are numerous formulas used to calculate the energy and protein required by the patient with a burn injury; most give consideration to the patient's age, preburn body weight, and the extent and depth of the burn. The patient with a burn injury loses a number of vitamins and trace elements in increased quantities, in particular vitamins A and C and zinc which require daily replacement (Tassiopoulos, 1999).

Pain and Anxiety Management. There are several sources of pain for the patient with a burn, resulting from the body's response to the injury or from the treatment regime. The wound itself and inflammation and edema formation are ongoing sources of pain. Frequent dressing changes and debridement, insertion of intravenous lines, blood draws, and other invasive monitoring procedures, physical and occupational therapy, and surgical procedures are all sources of pain and contribute to anxiety (Byers et al, 2001). Pain and anxiety may lead to prolongation of the stress response following injury, which could potentially delay wound healing and lengthen recovery time (Monafo, 1995).

Initially, during the hypermetabolic phase, opioids such as morphine sulfate are best administered in small, repetitive doses. Patient-controlled analgesia (PCA) devices are effective in the delivery of opioids and allow the patient a sense of control. Supplemental pain control measures (morphine, benzodiazepines, acetaminophen with codeine, acetaminophen, and nonnarcotic medications such as nonsteroidal antiinflammatory drugs) are necessary to control background or procedural pain (Davis and Sheely-Adolphson, 1997). Aspirin and NSAIDs are avoided during the acute phase because of the adverse effect on the coagulation system and propensity for gastric ulceration.

Anxiolytic agents are commonly given to augment pain medication in addition to diversionary activities, imagery, and relaxation, particularly during dressing changes (Davis and Sheely-Adolphson, 1997). Self-reported pain, pain rating tools and anxiety scores are of great value to the burn team since they indicate the degree of relief achieved with administered medications from the patient's perspective (Weinberg et al, 2000).

Surgical Interventions

Escharotomy. Deep partial-thickness or full-thickness burns that are circumferential, or nearly circumferential, to an extremity may require an escharotomy to relieve pressure. Edema and eschar formation can obstruct venous return and lead to decreased arterial blood flow. Early identification of extremities at risk and serial examination are essential. Wound dressings must be selected that will facilitate frequent examination. Parameters to monitor include temperature, pliability, voluntary motion, pain with passive motion, changes in the quality of pulses, and delayed capillary refill. Use of an ultrasonic flowmeter is the most reliable means to assess arterial blood flow. In most situations, frequent clinical assessments are sufficient to determine the need for escharotomy or fasciotomy, thus eliminating the need to insert pressure-monitoring catheters through contaminated wounds, which is associated with the risk of seeding compartments (Sheridan, 2002).

The escharotomy is a linear incision through the full-thickness wound dividing the eschar. The incision is only as deep as necessary to split the eschar and should not result in excessive bleeding or exposure of additional subcutaneous tissue to bacterial invasion. Full-thickness eschar lacks nerve endings, so pain is minimal, although small doses of narcotics are given intravenously to control anxiety and background pain. This procedure can be done at the bedside with a sterile field and scalpel or electrocautery to control the small amount of bleeding that occurs (Jordan and Harrington, 1997). Midmedial and midlateral incisions are designed to completely section the eschar while preventing injury to underlying superficial structures. Those structures most at risk during escharotomy are the brachial artery in the upper arm, the ulnar nerve at the elbow, the superficial peroneal nerve at the knee, and the neurovascular bundles and extensors of the digits (Sheridan, 2002). The escharotomy incision wounds are dressed with a topical agent and packed.

Similarly, deep circumferential burns to the chest and/or abdomen may restrict the expansion needed for breathing and adequate ventilation. Frequent assessment of the adequacy of chest expansion, quality of respirations, oxygenation, and mental status of the patient is essential. Circumferential chest burns require an escharotomy placed in the anterior axillary line bilaterally. If there is significant extension of the burn onto the adjacent abdominal wall, the incisions should be extended to this area and connected by a transverse incision along the costal margin (American Burn Association, 2001).

Fasciotomy. When the burn injury extends to the muscle, such as with a high-voltage electrical injury or skeletal trauma, edema develops beneath the fascia and muscle compartment, which precipitates tissue ischemia and nerve damage. A fasciotomy, or surgical incision of the fascia, is then necessary. This procedure is conducted in the operating room under general anesthesia.

ACUTE/WOUND CARE PHASE

Care of the burn wound is a priority of the acute/wound care phase. Goals of this phase are to heal partial-thickness wounds, graft full-thickness wounds, and prevent complications.

Topical Wound Management

The goals of burn wound care as identified by Honari (2004) include the following:

1. Control the growth of microorganisms.
2. Reduce the potential for invasive wound infection.
3. Prevent the wound from becoming a source of sepsis.
4. Prevent wound conversion (see Table 18-1).
5. Prepare the area for definitive closure.
6. Optimize healing, function, and cosmetic result.

Injured and nonviable tissues are mediums for microorganism growth. Wound cleansing and debridement, in conjunction with the appropriate topical agent, dressing, or skin replacement, is required to prevent infection and to promote wound healing. The burn team must consider many factors when planning and implementing wound care.

Initially, wound care is dependent on the location, extent, and depth of the wound. There can be significant differences in the management of burn injuries based on location, such as joint involvement, small BSA burns as opposed to large BSA burns, and partial as opposed to full-thickness burns. Other factors that will guide wound management include age of the patient, successful pain and anxiety management, and the ability of the patient and/or caregiver to participate in daily wound care.

Daily wound care in the burn center is accomplished in the hydrotherapy room, where burn team members perform gentle cleansing, debridement, and wound assessments. The patient is medicated for pain and anxiety before this procedure so it is an ideal time for physical and occupational therapy to perform ROM exercises and functional evaluations. Diversionary activities such as music or videos are often employed to assist with patient coping. For the child with burns, the child life specialist is invaluable in providing developmentally appropriate activities while role modeling supportive behaviors to caregivers.

Wound Care Based on Depth of Burn. *Superficial* burns such as sunburn or mild scalds should be cleansed and treated with a soothing lotion. Comfort measures are individualized and may include loose clothing, cool to lukewarm bathing, and use of pain medications such as acetaminophen.

Partial-thickness burns form blisters at the dermal-epidermal junction. Small blisters to the palms, fingers, or soles of the feet may be left intact if they do not limit range of motion. Larger blisters (over 2 cm) should be debrided (Honari, 2004).

Superficial partial-thickness burns, appropriately treated, will heal within 2 weeks. Biologic or biosynthetic dressings are ideal for these wounds. These dressings are applied immediately following initial debridement and can often be left in place until the wound is completely healed under the dressing. In addition, these dressings act as temporary skin replacements that provide wound closure, decreased pain, do not require dressing changes, and do not slow healing (Delatte et al, 2001). Topical antimicrobials are also appropriate for superficial partial-thickness wounds, but some may require daily or twice-daily dressing changes with pain and anxiety management.

Deep partial-thickness burns extend into the reticular layer of the dermis and regeneration is therefore slower. It may be appropriate to use biologic or biosynthetic dressings on small deep partial-thickness wounds, but larger wounds will most likely require topical antimicrobial application and frequent dressing changes. Large deep dermal burns are frequently excised and grafted to maximize wound closure and healing (Honari, 2004).

Full-thickness burns extend through the dermis and into subcutaneous tissue and, unless very small in size, will require surgical excision and closure of the wounds with skin grafts. Preoperatively, full-thickness burns are usually treated with daily or twice-daily dressing changes with topical antimicrobial application to control the growth of microorganisms and prepare the wound for grafting.

Topical Antibiotics. Silver sulfadiazine (Silvadene, Aventis Pharmaceuticals, Bridgewater, NJ; Thermazene, Kendall Company, Mansfield, MA) is probably the most frequently used topical antimicrobial for burn care. It is active against both gram-positive and gram-negative organisms and fungus. Silver sulfadizene is available as a 1% cream, is easy to apply without pain on application, and has a relatively low toxicity. It is used primarily as a prophylactic antibacterial on partial- and full-thickness burns (Honari, 2004). Silver sulfadiazine can cause a transient leukopenia, which resolves after the first week even with continued use.

Mafenide acetate (Sulfamylon, Bertek Pharmaceuticals, Morgantown, WV) is an 11.1% suspension cream. It has a broad spectrum of activity against most gram-positive and gram-negative organisms, including *Pseudomonas aeruginosa*, but minimal fungal activity. Mafenide penetrates burn eschar well, so it is useful for both partial- and full-thickness burns where infection is suspected (Honari, 2004) and for full-thickness burns with poor vascular supply, such as on the cartilaginous structures of the ears (Jordan and Harrington, 1997). Mafenide is a potent carbonic anhydrase inhibitor. Metabolic acidosis is a frequent side effect when used on burns greater than 25% TBSA. Other adverse effects can include pain on application to partial-thickness burns and a maculopapular rash. A 5% solution is now available and approved for use as a prophylactic agent applied as a soak to fresh autografts (Maggi et al, 1999).

Some burn centers rotate the use of silver sulfadiazene and mafenide acetate cream with each dressing change. This alternating therapy provides the advantages of both agents while minimizing side effects (McManus, 1996).

Bacitracin, neomycin, and polymyxin are topical antibiotic agents used to treat superficial partial-thickness burns, primarily because these agents are nontoxic, moisturizing, and can be used without secondary dressings. These ointments can be reapplied 1 to 5 times daily, so they are useful with facial and perineal burns. They are not effective against most gram-positive organisms and are moderately effective against gram-negative organisms (Honari, 2004).

Mupirocin (Bactroban™ GlaxoSmithKline, Research Triangle Park, NC) is an oil-based antimicrobial agent. It is active against a wide range of gram-positive bacteria including methicillin-resistant *Staphylococcus aureus* (MRSA) and some gram-negative organisms.

Silver Nitrate Solution. Silver nitrate 0.5% solution is an effective antimicrobial agent that provides a broad spectrum of coverage including *Staphylococcus*, *P. aeruginosa*, and fungus. It is painless upon application, has no hypersensitivity or resistance, but has little eschar penetrating capacity. Silver nitrate is a hypotonic solution and pulls electrolytes from the tissue through the open wound, stains, and requires extensive dressings with remoistening every 2 to 4 hours. For these reasons it is rarely used except when allergic

responses are experienced with other topical agents (Jordan and Harrington, 1997).

Antimicrobial Dressings. Topical elemental antimicrobial dressings (those containing ionic silver) provide a broad-spectrum of antimicrobial and bactericidal coverage, including vancomycin-resistant *Enterococcus*, MRSA, *P. aeruginosa*, and *Candida*. Because it may be left intact on the wound for up to 7 days, Acticoat™ (Smith and Nephew, Largo, FL), is an ideal antimicrobial dressing for partial-thickness burns, donor sites, and other areas where mechanical disturbance should be prevented, such as adjacent to fresh autografts. Acticoat is moistened before application and covered with a gauze dressing for 24 hours, at which time the outer dressing is removed or left opened to air(Honari, 2004). Ionic silver dressings are available in many forms and discussed in Chapter 19. However, because many dressings are contraindicated for some burns, it is essential to check the manufacturer's information for indications and contraindications.

Xeroform™ (The Kendall Company, Mansfield, MA) is 3% bismuth tribromophenate in a petrolatum blend on fine-mesh gauze. Xeroform is used for superficial and partial-thickness wounds such as donor sites, graft sites, and healing burns. Xeroform does not have an absorbent layer, so if drainage is present, a secondary gauze dressing must be placed over the xeroform (Honari, 2004).

Biosynthetic Dressings. Biosynthetic dressings are temporary dressings consisting of biologic and synthetic components. The biologic components are usually animal in origin, and the synthetic ingredients may be polymers or chemical elements (Honari, 2004). Temporary dressings offer many advantages when used as a primary dressing on burn wounds, including protection from bacterial contamination, decreased heat and water loss from the wound, decreased pain as sensory nerve terminals are covered, increased compliance with therapy and activities of daily living (ADLs), elimination of daily dressing changes, and ease of instructing the patient and/or family on home care (Delatte et al, 2001).

Biobrane™ (Bertek Pharmaceuticals, Morgantown, WV) is a biosynthetic wound dressing constructed of a silicone film with a nylon fabric partially embedded into the film. Bovine collagen is incorporated in both silicone and nylon components (Smith, 1995). Uses for Biobrane with burn injuries include (1) management of superficial partial-thickness wounds, (2) as a donor site dressing, and (3) on excised wounds that do not have eschar. Biobrane readily conforms to surface irregularities so it can be placed to the joints, the face, and the trunk. This adherence and flexibility is advantageous to the child with burns since it promotes an early return to ADLs, particularly for the child who does not like to be restricted by bulky dressings (Bishop, 1995). Biobrane is also available as a preformed glove for use on partial-thickness burns to the hand.

BGC Matrix™ (Brennan Medical, St. Paul, MN) combines beta glucan with collagen in a meshed reinforced wound dressing. Beta glucan, a complex carbohydrate derived from oats, is known to stimulate macrophages. BGC Matrix is useful in the management of partial-thickness wounds and donor sites. As the BGC Matrix dressing becomes dry and well-adhered to the wound, the dressing becomes quite stiff, which limits its use over joints and on the face and neck; these same properties make it ideal as a donor site dressing, since it does not easily become dislodged from the donor site as the patient resumes activity (Delatte et al, 2001).

For partial-thickness burns, both Biobrane and BGC Matrix dressings are placed on the clean wound immediately after initial debridement, and are held in position with SteriStrips. Fluff dressings and gauze wraps are applied for moderate compression, and the entire area is secured with elastic wrap bandaging and/or splinting to immobilize the area. These dressings are left intact for 24 to 48 hours, at which time, if the dressing is well adhered to the burn surface, it may remain on the wound until healing is complete.

Biologic Dressings. Biologic dressings can be used after wound debridement as primary dressings for partial-thickness burns and as temporary dressings to full-thickness wounds after burn excision when no donor sites are available for harvesting of autografts.

Allograft (homograft) is harvested from human donors and is available either fresh or cryopreserved. Allograft is considered to be the gold standard for coverage of open wounds when there are no available donor sites. Its beneficial properties, against which all other temporary dressings are measured, include

prevention of wound dessication, promotion of granulation tissue growth, decreased water and heat loss from the wound, prevention of a loss of exudative protein and red cells, limited bacterial proliferation, decreased wound pain, protection of exposed tendons, vessels, and nerves, and enhanced healing of partial-thickness burns (Pruitt, 1997). However, the allograft will eventually be rejected; some burn centers report rejection in as little as 5 to 9 days. In addition, allografts are associated with limited supply, variable quality, and the potential for disease transmission (Hansbrough et al, 1997).

Xenograft (heterograft, pigskin) is used primarily as a dressing for partial-thickness burns that are not expected to require skin grafting. Xenograft is easier to obtain but is not as effective as allograft when used as a temporary dressing to excised wounds because it does not establish vessel-to-vessel connections. The xenograft is rejected and undergoes vascular necrosis and sloughs, which creates more subgraft bacteria compared with allograft (Pruitt, 1997). Dressing application and care for partial-thickness burn application is similar to that of biosynthetic dressings.

Skin Substitutes. TransCyte (Smith and Nephew, Largo, FL) is a human cell–derived tissue-engineered product that is used as a temporary dressing for partial-thickness burns and as a biologic wound covering on full-thickness excised wounds while awaiting donor site availability. TransCyte™ consists of neonatal fibroblasts being isolated and grown aseptically on the nylon mesh of Biobrane. The end result is a dermal matrix consisting of collagens, fibronectin, tenascin, glycosaminoglycans, and multiple growth factors (Noordenbos, Dore, and Hansbrough, 1999). TransCyte™ has been compared favorably to allograft for its use on excised burn wounds, with several advantages such as easier removability, less bleeding at the time of removal, and no possibility of disease transmission (Hansbrough et al, 1997).

Integra™ (Integra LifeSciences Corporation, Plainsboro, NJ) is a bilayered product consisting of a dermal replacement layer made of porous matrix bovine collagen fibers and a glycosaminoglycan. This matrix allows for infiltration of fibroblasts, macrophages, lymphocytes, and capillaries from the wound bed. The outer layer temporarily serves as the epidermis and is silastic. Once adequately vascularized, a neodermis is formed, generally in 2 to 3 weeks. At this time, the outer silastic layer is removed and replaced with ultra-thin epidermal autografts (Ryan et al, 2002). Integra is indicated in the patient (1 with burns that cover a large surface area, 2 with burns that are full-thickness with minimal donor site availability, or 3) whose condition prevents autografting. Integra is applied in the operating room after burn excision. It is customarily meshed 1:1 (see the section later in this chapter on autografting for a discussion of meshing ratios) but not expanded, the meshing allows for better conforming to the wound bed and penetration of topical antimicrobials, and prevents fluid accumulation (Honari, 2004). General care of Integra is similar to that for meshed autografts.

Alloderm (LifeCell, The Woodlands, TX) is a commercially available, cryopreserved cadaver allograft that has been processed to remove all epidermal and dermal cells. The structure and biochemical information needed to direct normal revascularization and cell repopulation are preserved. The dermal matrix serves as a scaffold for normal tissue regeneration (Honari, 2004). Alloderm is acellular, and therefore immunologically inert. Alloderm must be placed concomitantly with thin autografts, so it is rarely used in those patients with limited donor site availability.

Surgical Procedures

Burn Excision. Early excision and closure of burn wounds by grafting in patients with major burn injuries has shortened hospital stays and decreased the incidence of infectious complications (Gray et al, 1982). The goal of burn excision is to remove the nonviable skin as soon as possible to reduce the risk of bacterial colonization and decrease the metabolic response to the burn injury (Wilson, 2000). Initial burn wound excision usually occurs at the earliest feasible opportunity following patient stabilization, generally within 3 to 4 days. For full-thickness burns that have extensive BSA involvement, excision and grafting may be staged to allow for healing and reharvesting of donor sites. Closure of the wounds at the time of excision is either permanent (autografts) or temporary with the use of biologic or biosynthetic dressings or skin substitutes (Box 18-2).

Tangential excision is a surgical technique in which sequential layers of eschar are removed with a knife or

---

BOX 18-2 Wound Coverings

Permanent Wound Coverings (Autografts)

Split-thickness skin graft (STSG): Sheet graft—thin, intact layer of skin (epidermis and portion of dermis); used for small burns or cosmetic areas

Split-thickness skin graft (STSG): Meshed graft—thin, intact layer of skin (epidermis and portion of dermis) meshed to provide expansion to cover a larger surface area

Full-thickness skin graft (FTSG): Entire thickness of skin to level of subcutaneous tissue (epidermis and entire dermis); used for small burns and in reconstructive surgery

Cultured epidermal autograft (CEA): Patient's own keratinocytes laboratory grown into sheets of epidermal cells (no dermis); used when availability of donor sites is limited

Temporary Wound Coverings

Allograft/homograft: human cadaver skin harvested from donors after death; becomes vascularized but is eventually rejected; fresh or cryopreserved

Xenograft/heterograft: porcine skin harvested after slaughter; cryopreserved or lyophilized for storage; develops collagen bond; not vascularized

Biosynthetics: Biobrane, BGC Matrix; useful as primary dressings for partial-thickness burns

Skin substitutes:

Integra: permanent dermal replacement (neodermis); grafted with ultra-thin autografts

TransCyte: permanent dermal matrix made from fibroblasts of neonatal foreskin

Alloderm: processed acellular cadaver allograft; grafted with thin autografts

---

dermatome until viable dermis or subcutaneous fat is exposed; the depth of the excision is determined by the appearance of punctuate bleeding indicating healthy tissue (Mozingo, 1998). This technique preserves surrounding healthy tissue and natural body contours. Blood loss may be considerable during tangential excision and must be minimized by the use of pads or dressings soaked in a topical epinephrine solution (1:10,000) and placed to the wounds immediately after excision. Elevation and wrapping extremities with elastic compression bandages also assist in obtaining hemostasis (Mozingo, 1998).

Fascial excision is removal of the eschar and underlying subcutaneous tissue with sharp scalpel dissection or electrocautery down to the level of the muscle fascia. This technique is usually reserved for those patients with very deep or extensive, life-threatening, full-thickness burns. Fascial excision provides a reliable wound bed for skin grafts, and there is less blood loss than with tangential excision. Disadvantages of fascial excision include poorer cosmetic result, loss of superficial nerves, and a high incidence of distal edema when the excision is circumferential (Mozingo, 1998).

Autografting. Prompt burn wound excision and autografting shorten the hospital stay and accelerate recovery and rehabilitation. Total overall wound size is the most important factor in determining the need for early operative management since this correlates with the physiologic threat represented by the injury (Sheridan, 2002). Patients with small deep partial- to full-thickness burns rarely develop sepsis; topical wound management for the first week allows time for the wound to fully evolve so that physical examination can determine true burn depth. Patients with larger injuries generally have a better recovery if their wounds are excised and closed early. Each patient must be assessed individually, but in general, if the burn is over 30% TBSA, autografting requires staged procedures, since the operative process of excision and harvesting skin involves blood loss, is physiologically stressful, and donor sites need time to heal before reuse.

Autograft, or a graft of the patient's own skin, is the most desirable method for burn wound closure because it is permanent and will not be rejected. *Split-thickness skin grafts (STSGs)* are the most commonly used autografts. The skin is harvested using a guarded dermatome, which controls the thickness of the graft, usually 0.008 to 0.0012 inches thick, and includes the epidermis and a thin layer of dermis. STSGs may be used as sheets or meshed to provide expansion (Mozingo, 1998). Sheet grafts provide a better functional and cosmetic result and are commonly used on the face, hands, feet, neck, and joints. One disadvantage of sheet grafts is that a collection of serous drainage or blood beneath the graft can lift the graft from the wound bed, causing loss. For this reason, dressings are usually not applied over sheet grafts so that frequent assessment can identify the presence of excess fluid or hematoma, which can then be removed by aspiration or rolling of a cotton-tipped applicator to the surface of the graft to remove collected fluid.

For large burn areas, the skin graft is meshed to allow more coverage with fewer donor sites. After the skin is harvested, it is placed on a plastic template and guided through a mechanical meshing device. Expansion ratios range from 1.5:1 to 9:1. Expansion ratios of 4:1 or greater require a longer time for interstices of the graft to close and are more prone to hypertrophic scar formation (Jordan and Harrington, 1997). The meshed graft is secured with staples or sutures and then covered with a nonadherent inner layer to prevent shearing. Fluff gauze moistened with a topical antimicrobial such as 5% Sulfamylon™ or triple antibiotic solution is then placed to prevent desiccation. If the graft is to an extremity or joint, splints are fitted at this time to maintain position of function while engraftment occurs.

The postoperative dressing is typically left in place for 5 to 7 days before removal, at which time the graft is inspected and re-dressed. The dressing is then changed daily until the graft is sufficiently stable to remain open to air, usually about 2 weeks. Physical and occupational therapy can be resumed after 5 to 7 days, starting with passive ROM exercises and progressing at an individual rate depending on the area grafted and the patient's condition. Splinting continues to areas at risk for contractures, but usually at this stage the patient has a rotating schedule of splinting as opposed to active use of the involved area.

An STSG donor site is similar to a superficial partial-thickness burn; healing occurs by epithelial migration from the epidermal appendages in 10 to 14 days. Numerous donor site dressings are available: fine mesh gauze or gauze impregnated with petrolatum or antimicrobials, polyurethane film, hydrocolloid and alginate dressings, or biosynthetic dressings. Choice of dressing depends on the preference of the burn center, location and size of the donor site, and the donor site proximity to other wounds. Healing of donor sites in a timely manner is especially important in those patients with large BSA burns who will need reharvesting to obtain full wound coverage. Consideration should be given in these patients to the use of subcutaneous administration of human growth hormone or the testosterone analog oxandrolone, both of which have been shown to significantly decrease weight and nitrogen loss and increase healing rates (Demling, 1999).

Full-thickness skin grafts (FTSGs) are obtained by surgically excising the entire thickness of the donor skin to the level of the subcutaneous tissue, resulting in grafts 0.025 to 0.030 inches thick. Transfer of the entire dermal layer is accomplished, which makes the graft durable and less prone to contracture. FTSGs are limited in use to small full-thickness burns and are used most frequently in reconstructive surgery. The FTSG donor site creates a full-thickness wound, which is usually closed by primary suturing or split-thickness grafting (Mozingo, 1998).

Cultured epidermal autografts (CEAs) (Epicell™ Genzyme Tissue Repair, Cambridge, MA) are sheets of proliferative, cultured autologous keratinocytes, ranging from 2 to 8 cell layers thick, attached to a petrolatum gauze backing. Autologous keratinocytes are human cells harvested from the healthy tissue of the patient; these cells are then processed to isolate and propagate specific cell types for transplantation in the form of CEAs. Each CEA is approximately 30 cm^2 in size. After initial biopsy, expansion of the epidermal cells to form CEAs takes 3 to 4 weeks. CEA may be considered for obtaining permanent coverage in those patients with large body surface area burns with limited donor site availability.

Reports of success rate have been highly variable, with factors such as mechanical trauma and local colonization or wound bed infection contributing to poor "take" of CEAs or subsequent graft loss. It has been reported that the percentage of take, or the amount of CEA that is permanent, is best when early excision of eschar followed by temporary coverage of the wound with allograft is performed while awaiting CEA placement (Rheinwald, 1992), with an average take of 72% when the allograft is completely removed before CEA placement. More consistent results, with an average take rate of 90%, were obtained when CEAs were grafted onto the allodermis left behind after only the superficial part of the engrafted allograft was removed. Some burn centers prefer to use thin, widely meshed autografts in conjunction with CEAs, particularly to those areas prone to mechanical stress.

Upon placement, CEAs are secured with staples and then dressed with a single layer of mesh gauze, which will remain in place for 7 to 10 days. Absorbent gauze dressings are used as a secondary outer dressing and are changed daily to prevent accumulation of fluid and bacteria. Topical antimicrobials may be applied, but care must be taken to employ agents that will not harm the CEA. During the 7- to 10-day period following CEA application, mechanical trauma and friction to the grafted sites must be prevented; all physical therapy is on hold during this time. Initial evaluation is performed at the end of the 7- to 10-day period, at which time daily care will be similar to that of autografts.

INFECTIOUS COMPLICATIONS

Patients with burn injuries are at considerable risk for infection from several different sources. Throughout recovery, there is a decreased immune response. The burn wound, being moist and rich in denatured proteins, provides an ideal environment for the growth of microorganisms. In addition, the burn wound and its care are primary sources for transmission of microorganisms throughout the body and to the environment. Other protective barriers to infection are also altered, including the respiratory, gastrointestinal, and genitourinary mucosal surfaces and the conjunctiva. The use of invasive devices such as endotracheal tubes, central and peripheral intravenous lines, and indwelling urinary catheters also weakens normal defenses and allows accumulation of exudates at insertion sites (Greenfield and McManus, 1997).

The most common organisms responsible for infection in the patient with a burn injury are grampositive. Bacteremia and pneumonia are most often caused by *S. aureus*. Group A *Staphylococcus* infections represent a threat to skin graft survival, particularly in pediatric patients, as they have a high incidence of nasopharyngeal colonization. Other gram-positive microorganisms of concern are Group A beta hemolytic *Streptococcus* and *Enterococcus* species. Both *S. aureus* and *Enterococcus* have increasing levels of antibiotic resistance. *P. aeruginosa* continues to be the primary gram-negative pathogen of concern in those burn centers that do not routinely practice early wound excision and grafting. *P. aeruginosa* is typically a later-developing infection in the patient with a burn injury and is becoming less frequent, and with a later onset, as a result of aggressive wound closure techniques.

Gram-negative bacteremia has been associated with mortality up to 50% higher than that predicted on the basis of the severity of the burn injury (Greenfield and McManus, 1997).

Nonbacterial sources of infection include yeast, fungus, and virus (e.g., herpes). *Candida* wound infections are uncommon the patient with a burn injury, although they are still the most common nonbacterial wound colonizers. Candidal infections are seen most frequently in those patients with large burns who receive broad-spectrum antibiotics for treatment of other infections. Systemic amphotericin B may be required to treat *Candida* infections. Fungi, in particular *Aspergillus* species, are commonly found on burn wounds. Fungi can be found almost everywhere in the environment, including the air, nonsterile wound supplies, and laundry items. Fungal infections are treated with a topical antifungal agent, systemic amphotericin B, and surgical excision of the infected tissue (Greenfield and McManus, 1997). A viral infection in the patient with a burn injury is usually localized. Herpetic infections most commonly occur in healing or recently healed partial-thickness burns. Acyclovir is the treatment of choice.

Prevention of burn wound infection is accomplished by the use of topical antimicrobials, meticulous dressing change and wound care techniques (including hand-washing), and continuous surveillance for changes in wound appearance or breakdown, exudate, and odor. Consequences of burn wound infection include conversion of partial-thickness wounds to full-thickness wounds, increased nutritional requirements, delays in healing, and increased scar and contracture formation (Greenfield and McManus, 1997). The usual systemic signs of infection are unreliable in the patient with a burn injury because a hypermetabolic state is present in all patients with a major injury. Assessment parameters for burn wound infection are summarized in Table 18-4.

Seeding of microorganisms from a colonized wound, invasive devices, or urinary tract infections may cause bacteremia, or bloodstream infections, in the patient

TABLE 18-4 Signs and Symptoms of Burn Wound Infection

	LOCAL CHANGES	SYSTEMIC CHANGES	LABORATORY FINDINGS
NONINVASIVE	• Change in color • Graft loss • Localized erythema or cellulitis at wound margins • Purulent or odorous drainage • Epithelial breakdown of healed areas	• Temperature above 101° F	• Leukocytes greater than 10,000
INVASIVE	• Conversion of partial-thickness wound to full-thickness wound • Breakdown of previously healed areas • Accelerated eschar separation • Tenderness, edema, erythema at wound margin • New necrotic areas	• Hemodynamic changes: tachycardia, hypotension • Oliguria • Paralytic ileus • Changes in level of consciousness	• Leukopenia less than 5000 • Leukocytosis greater than 10,000 • Elevated blood glucose • Positive blood cultures • Positive wound biopsy • Thrombocytopenia

Adapted from Greenfield E, MacManus AT: Infectious complications: prevention and strategies for their control, *Nurs Clin North Am* 32(2):297, 1997.

with a burn injury. Bacteremia is diagnosed on the basis of two successive positive blood cultures in which the organism is identified; supportive therapy and systemic antibiotics are initiated. A urinary tract infection is most frequently seen in patients with an indwelling catheter and is diagnosed by a positive urine culture. Treatment includes systemic antibiotics and removal of the catheter as soon as possible. The patient with a burn is also at risk for developing pneumonia because of the inhalation injury, mechanical ventilation, and prolonged immobility. Treatment of pneumonia includes systemic antibiotics based on culture and sensitivity results and aggressive pulmonary toilet (Greenfield and McManus, 1997).

PSYCHOLOGICAL CONSEQUENCES OF BURN INJURY

Patients with burn injuries sustain both physical and psychologic trauma as they recover. Adcock, Boeve, and Patterson (1998) identify common reactions and treatment options for the emergent, acute/wound care, and rehabilitative phases of burn recovery. The emergent phase is particularly emotionally stressful for the patient and family.

Delirium

Severely burned patients are treated in an intensive care unit (ICU) setting. A common reaction in this phase is delirium, which can result from pain medication and sedation, fluid and electrolyte imbalances, metabolic disorders, and postoperative states. Symptoms include disorientation, psychomotor agitation, disruptions in the sleep-wake cycle, and emotional lability. Symptoms vary in length, but typically are limited to the ICU setting. Treatment includes (1) control of the environment to minimize disorientation by decreasing noise, appropriate lighting, and grouping necessary treatments, (2) staff role modeling of supportive behaviors to the family, and (3) treatment with haloperidol or other antipsychotic drugs.

Grief and Depression

During the acute/wound care phase, patients have stabilized physically and become aware of the ramifications of their injury. Grief is a natural response to the burn injury and is related to changes in functional ability, body image, and separation from family.

Lengthy hospitalizations, medical setbacks, the patient's level of pain at rest, and stress of family conflicts can precipitate depression. Early resumption of ADLs and socialization with family and friends can often mitigate grief.

Anxiety

Anxiety is common early in the hospitalization and tends to decrease with time. Acute Stress Disorder (ASD) can occur after a traumatic event such as a burn injury. A diagnosis of ASD requires that the individual has developed symptoms of dissociation, avoidance, anxiety, reexperiencing the traumatic event, and increased arousal in response to the trauma. By definition, the diagnosis of ASD is appropriate only for symptoms that occur within 1 month of the event (Ehde et al, 2000). Symptoms of these psychologic problems that are often seen during this phase include sleep disorders and nightmares, behavioral regression, and interpersonal difficulties such as hostility, anger, and dependence. A combination of short-term counseling or supportive therapy, behavior modification strategies, and pharmacologic treatments are the most common psychologic interventions during this phase.

The rehabilitation phase deals with social reintegration and functional improvements. The first year after hospital discharge is usually the most difficult for the patient with a burn injury. Most patients slowly regain a sense of competence and realize the practical limitations imposed by any functional impairments. Common problems reported during the first year are related to vocational and emotional adjustments. Problems in long-term adjustment that persist past 1 year often involve low self-esteem and quality of life issues (Adcock, Boeve, and Patterson, 1998).

Post-traumatic stress disorder (PTSD) is an anxiety disorder that may develop after a person has experienced a traumatic event such as a burn injury. PTSD is characterized by persistent symptoms of reexperiencing the trauma, persistent avoidance of stimuli associated with the trauma and numbing of general responsiveness, and persistent symptoms of increased arousal. A diagnosis of PTSD requires that these symptoms persist for a minimum of 1 month and cause notable distress or impairment in functioning (Ehde et al, 2000).

Pediatric Considerations

Although children experience the same physical stress as adults during burn recovery, their behavioral responses can be quite different and are related to their stage of development. Behavioral responses typically include anxiety, agitation, anger, conditioned fear, and regression. Causes of psychologic and emotional distress include separation anxiety, repeated painful procedures, and loss of control and independence. The pediatric burn care team should incorporate into their plans of care interventions that enhance a feeling of security for children while providing for familiarity and interpersonal rapport (Adcock, Boeve, and Patterson, 1998). Specific interventions include the following:

1. Encouraging parents and family to be present during hospitalization
2. Role modeling supportive behaviors
3. Isolating painful procedures to a particular place and identifying the child's room as a "safe zone"
4. Allowing older children some control and choices regarding wound care and therapy
5. Preparation before and assistance with coping during painful procedures
6. Making appropriate resources available to children who may show long-term adjustment issues

Abuse and Neglect

Approximately 10% of child abuse cases involve burning, and up to 20% of pediatric burn admissions involve abuse or neglect (Ruth et al, 2003). Burn care providers, particularly nurses who often act as primary advocates for patients, must have an understanding of the assessment and interventional processes related to suspected abuse and neglect cases. Knowledge of individual institutions' protocols governing the management of these cases is imperative to maintaining patient safety and obtaining optimal outcomes. Primary responsibility for initial assessments, communications with law enforcement, and initiation of specific interventions may involve nursing or medical staff, specialized teams for abuse and neglect, and social services (Doctor, 1998). Similar considerations are also applicable to those adult patients who have been deliberately injured. Criteria for those burn injuries that are suspicious for abuse or

---

BOX 18-3 Non-Accidental Burn Criteria

- Multiple hematomas or scars in various stages of healing
- Concurrent injuries or evidence of neglect such as malnutrition
- History of prior hospitalization for "accidental" trauma
- Unexplained delay between the time of injury and first attempt to obtain medical attention
- Burns appearing older than the alleged time of the accident
- An account of the accident not compatible with the age and ability of the patient
- Responsible adults alleging that there were no witnesses to the "accident" and that the child was merely discovered to have been burned
- Relatives other than the parents bring the injured child to the hospital
- The burn being attributed to the action of a sibling or other child (this can in fact happen)
- The injured child being excessively withdrawn, submissive, or overly polite, or not crying during painful procedures
- Scalds on hands or feet, often symmetric, appearing to be full-thickness in depth, suggesting extremities forcibly immersed and held in hot liquid
- Isolated burns of the buttocks that in children could hardly be produced by accidental means

---

neglect were identified by Stone (1970), and are listed in Box 18-3 (Stone, 1970).

DISCHARGE PLANNING

Discharge planning is a complex process that requires the involvement of the entire multidisciplinary burn team. Rutan (1998) identifies essential characteristics of a discharge plan for the patient with a burn injury:

1. Oriented to the patient
2. Begins upon admission
3. Individualized for each patient
4. Well documented
5. Acknowledges that education of the patient and family is a key component

The main goal of treatment throughout all phases of recovery is a functional return of the patient to preburn lifestyle, or as close to it as is reasonably possible. The patient with a burn injury is identified as a candidate for discharge when wound healing is progressing; nutritional intake is adequate to support continued healing; pain, itching, and infection are controlled with medications by mouth; and the patient and/or caregiver have demonstrated competence in wound care and exercises. The discharge process is similar for major and minor burns and should incorporate five major areas of patient/caregiver education: (1) wound management, (2) pain and itch relief, (3) exercises, (4) scar maturation, and (5) emotional support for the patient and family.

An individualized plan of care that addresses age-specific needs is necessary for each patient with a burn injury (Rutan, 1998). The discharge goal for pediatric patients is social reintegration. Appropriate objectives to be met prior to discharge include the following:

1. The child will achieve an age-appropriate level of functioning.
2. The child and caregiver will understand the processes of injury and recovery.
3. The child will begin to integrate a new body image.

Many burn centers offer school reentry programs, which provide psychologic and social support for the child and education about the burn recovery process for teachers and classmates. Camps for the child with burns, staffed by burn care professionals, provide the opportunity for the child to meet and socialize with other children with burns. The camp is a safe environment for self-esteem–building activities.

Goals for discharge planning for the adult patient with a burn injury are often focused on returning to work. Employment equates with life satisfaction, provides an identity, and allows for financial independence. Collaboration with a vocational rehabilitation counselor is often necessary for a successful outcome.

The discharge plan for the elderly patient with a burn injury must take into consideration that the injury may have been a result of a chronic degenerative or physical process. Family members or other caregivers who can assist with wound care and activities of daily living are of particular importance to the elderly (Rutan, 1998).

REHABILITATION PHASE

The rehabilitation phase of recovery begins when wound healing is complete. The goal of this phase is to restore or maximize the patient's functional capacity. This phase may last several weeks to several years, depending on the extent and severity of the burn injury. Several complications of burn injuries begin during wound healing in the acute/wound care phase and may manifest after wound healing is complete in the rehabilitation phase: excessive scarring, contracture development, and itching.

Excessive Scarring

The skin's response to a burn injury is scar formation, the result of which may be barely noticeable or may lead to significant functional impairment and cosmetic disfigurement. Excessive scarring is more common in those patients who have deep partial- and full-thickness burns, since these wounds take a longer time to heal and are at greater risk for infection. Other factors that may be related to excessive scarring include the patient's age, pigmentation, family history, and location of the scar (Pessina and Ellis, 1997).

Excessive scarring can take the form of a *hypertrophic scar* or a *keloid*. Hypertrophic scars are red, raised, and lack elasticity, and they are painful and itchy. Hypertrophic scars remain within the boundary of the original injury, are more frequently seen after burn injury, and tend to show regression with time. Keloids appear as firm, fibrous nodules that extend beyond the original wound margin and are often hyperpigmented. Keloids have a higher incidence in people with darker pigmentations. Both hypertrophic scars and keloids demonstrate increased deposition of collagen, predominantly types I and III (Mafong and Ashinoff, 2000).

Treatment of hypertrophic scars includes several different modalities employed until the scar matures in 6 months to 2 years, as evidenced by the scar appearing avascular, flat, and soft (Staley and Richard, 1997). The use of garments to generate compression on an area of hypertrophic scarring has been in use by burn centers for more than 20 years, although the exact mechanism of action is not known. Pressure does decrease scar blood flow and may provide force that helps developing collagen to organize (Pessina and Ellis, 1997). Pressure garments may be prefabricated or custom-fit. To get the maximum benefit, the patient is instructed to wear the garments 23 hours/day. Gel sheeting is often used in conjunction with pressure garments, particularly in those areas of the body where it is difficult to get consistent pressure. Either hydrogel or silicone sheeting can be used; these fitted sheets are thought to soften the scar by maintaining scar hydration and reducing tension on the scar. Scar massage is another noninvasive approach that may be beneficial to stretch scars, although it is generally most helpful in preventing contractures.

Intralesional corticosteroid injections inhibit fibroblast growth and enhance collagen breakdown in the scar; the clinical result is a softer and flatter scar. Common side effects include hypopigmentation, atrophy, telangiectasia, and recurrence of the scar. Recommended treatment is between 10 and 40 mg/ml of triamcinolone acetonide with a dose limit to 20 mg per month. Topical steroid application poses less risk, but has been found to be ineffective (Mafong and Ashinoff, 2000). Surgical excision is a second-line therapy for hypertrophic scars, because recurrence rates have been reported at 50% to 100%. Surgery is most beneficial in the treatment of small scars over joints, which inhibit full range of motion; excision allows for reorientation and less tension on the new wound. The use of lasers has recently demonstrated successful long-term treatment of hypertrophic scars. The pulse-dye laser (PDL) appears to be the most promising, providing a high response rate and fewer recurrences (Mafong and Ashinoff, 2000).

Treatment of hypertrophic scarring can last several months to years. Compliance with the treatment plan may be difficult to achieve since patients find pressure garments uncomfortable, hot, and confining. It is important to instruct patients and caregivers that any treatment of hypertrophic scars is aimed at minimizing the scars. Complete normalization of the skin to preburn appearance and texture may not be possible.

Contractures

Scar contracture is the primary cause of functional deficits in the patient with a burn. A contracture is essentially a shortening of a scar over a joint surface, limiting joint mobility (Leman and Ricks, 1994). During the acute/wound care phase of recovery, the patient with a burn can experience intense pain, which inhibits movement. The patient tends to assume a comfortable position, usually flexed, which may predispose the new collagen fibers in wounds to fuse together in a shortened length (Johnson, 1994). Early splinting, ROM exercises, positioning, and use of pressure garments with flexible inserts over joint surfaces aid in the development of parallel fibers and maintaining soft-tissue length (Helm and Fisher, 1998). When a contracture does develop, serial casting and dynamic splints that exert a constant stretch on the joint can help reverse the problem. Some contractures will require surgical release to restore functional mobility (Leman and Ricks, 1994).

The location, extent, and depth of the injury are factors that affect the presence and extent of burn scar contractures. Specific "anticontracure" positions are used to align the extremities, neck, and trunk (Figure 18-3) (Ward, 1998). The burn physical and occupational therapists instruct other burn team members and patients/caregivers on appropriate positioning and splint use. Splints may be worn continuously, such as after grafting to maintain the area in the position of function, or scheduled with several hours off to encourage active range of motion. All splints must be checked frequently by nursing and caregivers for appropriate fit by assessing for areas of pressure and signs of neurologic complications, such as numbness and tingling.

Itching

Patients recovering from burn injuries experience itching from a variety of sources. Histamines released during the inflammatory phase of healing cause itch, particularly in large surface area burns that take longer to heal. Infection also prolongs healing time and causes excess collagen to be produced in the wound, leading to hypertrophic scarring and an increased amount of itch. Itching can also be a side effect of morphine administration, which is often used to manage burn pain (Matheson, Clayton, and Muller, 2001). Itching in a burn wound usually begins at the time of wound closure, and then peaks at about 2 to 6 months afterwards. Current standard of care for itching is a combination of oral antihistamines, skin moisturizers, pressure garments (thought to decrease histamine release), and the addition of opioids and sedatives. These interventions are effective in less than 20% of patients with burns who have severe itch (Demling and DeSanti, 2001). A recent study by Demling and DeSanti (2001) found that topical doxepin, a potent histamine receptor antagonist, was effective in

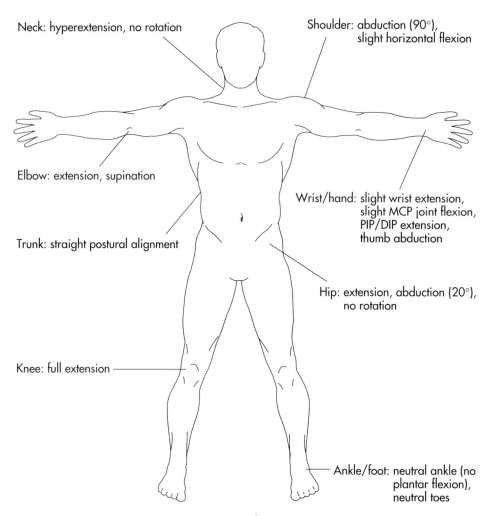

Fig. 18-3 Anticontracture positions of choice for patient with burns. From Ward RS. Physical rehabilitation. In Carrougher GJ, editor: *Burn care and therapy,* St. Louis, 1998, Mosby.

controlling severe pruritus in patients with burns that did not respond to standard treatment measures.

OUTPATIENT BURN MANAGEMENT

The American Burn Association injury severity grading system classifies burns as minor, moderate, or severe. Many minor and moderate burn injuries are now treated on an outpatient basis only. Patients with moderate and major burns are being discharged sooner than ever. Nationally, the number of burn admissions has remained fairly stable for a number of years, but

outpatient visits to burn clinics have been increasing. Factors influencing the shift to outpatient care include a desire to decrease health care costs, reduction in the risk of nosocomial infections, psychologic benefits of home care, increasing numbers of outpatient surgical procedures, direct referrals to burn clinics for care (Moss, 2004) and new developments in wound dressings.

The goals for the patient with a burn who is treated in the outpatient setting include wound protection, timely wound healing, adequate pain control, and rapid rehabilitation with return to school or work (Moss, 2004). The multidisciplinary burn team as previously described performs initial evaluation of the patient with a burn in the clinic setting. Assessment includes history of injury, medical history, psychosocial and economic assessments, and an evaluation of the location, extent, depth, and severity of the burn injury.

Patients with minor burn injuries may require hospitalization. Hospital admission in the case of a minor burn is contingent upon the presence of factors that will influence patient safety or the ability to heal as identified in the assessment. Potential reasons to admit a patient with a burn injury for inpatient care include suspicion that the injury was not accidental, presence of chronic disease that would prolong wound healing, lack of resources to provide daily care or return to clinic, the location of the burn impairing ability to provide self-care and perform ADLs, or wound care/therapy needs being such that pain cannot adequately be controlled with oral medication (Moss, 2004).

Wound care in the outpatient setting begins with gentle cleansing with mild soap and water to remove devitalized skin and debris. Appropriate pain medication by mouth is generally used for small burns seen in the clinic setting. If extensive debridement is required, additional medications for pain and anxiety will be needed, and this is best performed in the more controlled setting of the emergency department or inpatient burn unit. There remains some controversy over whether to shave the hair surrounding a wound or to unroof intact blisters (Moss, 2004).

Individual assessments regarding extent and depth of the wound and the size, location, and fragility of the blisters will dictate treatment. Wound care and dressings should be kept as simple as possible while still keeping the wound clean, moist, and protected. In addition to selecting a dressing that meets the needs of the wound, priorities include patient comfort, mobility, and activity. Evaluation of the risk for functional impairment is also performed at this time by physical or occupational therapy, and the appropriate splinting or exercises are implemented.

Patient and/or caregiver education is vital to successful outpatient management. Explanations regarding the depth of the wound and demonstration of appropriate wound care technique and dressing application should be given in conjunction with written instructions. Instructions should include information specific to the wound, signs and symptoms of infection, therapy schedule, activity restrictions, nutrition, pain management, and how to contact the burn team for assistance (Moss, 2004). Principles of minor burn wound management must be reviewed with the patient and family and should include (1) elevation to decrease edema to face and extremity burns, (2) wrapping fingers and toes individually, and (3) frequent gentle cleansing with reapplication of topical agents to perineal burns.

Initial follow-up visits may range in frequency from daily to weekly, based on factors identified in the initial assessment and including the extent and depth of the burn and the ability of the patient or caregiver to adequately perform daily care and monitor the wound. Once healing occurs, intermittent visits continue until the scar maturation process has ended, as evidenced by a mature scar that is soft, supple, of normal color, and without contractures, and no additional changes in the scar are expected (Moss, 2004). As the wound heals, patients are instructed on side effects of burn injury that may occur: excessive scarring, itching, sleep disturbances, discomfort associated with pressure garments, splinting and exercise, and color and texture changes to the skin. Newly healed burn wounds are more sensitive to ultraviolet light, so the need for protection in the form of a sunscreen with a sun protection factor (SPF) of 30 and covering the area with clothing should be incorporated into the teaching plan. Appropriate referrals for support and counseling should be made in a timely manner for those patients experiencing distress related to psychologic symptoms.

SUMMARY

Whether involved in the care of a patient with massive tissue loss or a minor burn, the wound care specialist must be familiar with the principles of initial assessment, management based on the type and severity of injury, and prevention of complications. Knowledge of the phases of recovery and the associated therapeutic and psychosocial needs of the patient contributes to optimal outcomes.

SELF-ASSESSMENT EXERCISE

1. What are the phases of wound healing that occur in burns?
2. What types of burns occur in the home?
3. Which zone of tissue damage experiences the most damage?
4. What actions will prevent further damage to the zone of stasis?
   a. Prevention of infection
   b. Protection from drying and exposure
   c. Turning or moving to relieve pressure
   d. All the above
5. The treatment of a burn wound is based on the _____, _____, and _____ of the burn.
6. Which is the most accurate method to calculate TBSA?
   a. Lund and Browder chart
   b. Rule of nines
   c. Palm method
   d. Harris-Benedict formula
7. The inflammatory response releases agents that affect which of the following?
   a. Urine output, blood pressure, respirations
   b. Vasoconstriction, fluid balance, metabolism
   c. Sodium retention, metabolism, temperature control
   d. Urine output, vasoconstriction, temperature control
8. Which of the following is the most accurate method to assess resuscitation adequacy?
   a. Preburn body weight
   b. Blood pressure
   c. Cardiac output
   d. Urine output
9. Early excision should occur between which days after injury?
   a. 1 and 2
   b. 3 and 5
   c. 5 and 8
   d. 9 and 12
10. Facial burns are best grafted with which of the following?
    a. 2:1 meshed graft
    b. Sheet graft
    c. Allograft
    d. Xenograft
11. Why are positioning and splinting done?
    a. To prevent contractures
    b. To provide comfort
    c. To reduce pain
    d. To prevent keloids
12. Which is the most common type of organism responsible for infection in the patient with a burn?
    a. Gram-positive bacteria
    b. Gram-negative bacteria
    c. Fungus
    d. Virus
13. How are minor burns identified?
    a. 10% to 15% TBSA deep partial-thickness in an adult
    b. 5% to 10% TBSA partial-thickness in a child
    c. 2% TBSA full-thickness in an adult not involving the eyes, ears, face, or genitalia
    d. All the above

REFERENCES

Adcock RJ, Boeve S, Patterson DR: Psychologic and emotional recovery. In Carrougher GJ, editor: *Burn care and therapy*, St. Louis, 1998, Mosby.

Ahrns KS: Initial resuscitation after burn injury: therapies, strategies, and controversies, *AACN Clin Issues* 10(1):46, 1999.

Ahrns KS: Trends in burn resuscitation: shifting the focus from fluids to adequate endpoint monitoring, edema control, and adjuvant therapies, *Crit Care Nurs Clin North Am* 16(1):75, 2004.

American Academy of Pediatrics: Reducing the number of deaths and injuries from residential fires, *Pediatrics* 105(6):1355, 2000.

American Burn Association: *Advanced burn life support course*, Chicago, 2001, Author.

American Burn Association: *National burn repository 2002 report*, Chicago, 2002, Author..

American Burn Association: *Look up and live: Prevention for electrical injuries, a campaign kit for burn awareness week 2005*, www.ameriburn.org/Preven/2005PreventionKit/ABA2005PreventionCampaign.pdf; Accessed July 1, 2005.

Andel H et al: Impact of early high caloric duodenal feeding on the oxygen balance of the splanchnic region after severe burn injury, *Burns* 27(4):389, 2001.

Arnoldo BD et al: Electrical injuries: a 20-year review, *J Burn Care Rehabil* 25(6):479, 2004.

Bishop JF: Pediatric considerations in the use of Biobrane in burn wound management, *J Burn Care Rehabil* 16(3 Pt 1):331; discussion 333, 1995.

Burn Foundation, Philadelphia, PA: *Burn incidence and treatment in the U.S.: 2000 Fact Sheet*, www.ameriburn.org/pub/BurnIncidenceFactSheet.htm, 2000.Accessed 3/28/05.

Byers JF et al: Burn patients' pain and anxiety experiences, *J Burn Care Rehabil* 22(2):144, 2001.

Carrougher GJ: Management of fluid and electrolyte balance in thermal injuries: implications for perioperative nursing practice, *Semin Perioper Nurs* 6(4):201, 1997.

Chrysopoulo MT et al: Acute renal dysfunction in severely burned adults, *J Trauma* 46(1):141, 1999.

Corrarino JE, Walsh PJ, Nadel E: Does teaching scald burn prevention to families of young children make a difference? A pilot study, *J Pediatr Nurs* 16(4):256, 2001.

Davis ST, Sheely-Adolphson P: Burn management. Psychosocial interventions: pharmacologic and psychologic modalities, *Nurs Clin North Am* 32(2):331, 1997.

Deitch EA, Rutan RL: The challenges of children: the first 48 hours, *J Burn Care Rehabil* 21(5):424, quiz 431, discussion 423, 2000.

Delatte SJ et al: Effectiveness of beta-glucan collagen for treatment of partial-thickness burns in children, *J Pediatr Surg* 36(1):113, 2001.

Demling RH: Comparison of the anabolic effects and complications of human growth hormone and the testosterone analog, oxandrolone, after severe burn injury, *Burns* 25(3):215, 1999.

Demling RH, DeSanti L: Topical Doxepin cream is effective in relieving severe pruritus caused by burn injury: a preliminary study, *Wounds* 13(6):210, 2001.

Demling RH et al: Effect of burn-induced hypoproteinemia on pulmonary transvascular fluid filtration rate, *Surgery* 85(3):339, 1979.

Doctor M: Abuse through burns. In Carrougher GJ, editor: *Burn care and therapy*, St. Louis, 1998, Mosby.

Ehde DM et al: Post-traumatic stress symptoms and distress 1 year after burn injury, *J Burn Care Rehabil* 21(2):105, 2000.

Flynn MB: Nutritional support for the burn-injured patient, *Crit Care Nurs Clin North Am* 16(1):139, 2004.

Gibran NS, Heimbach DM: Current status of burn wound pathophysiology, *Clin Plast Surg* 27(1):11, 2000.

Gordon M, Goodwin CW: Burn management. Initial assessment, management, and stabilization, *Nurs Clin North Am* 32(2):237, 1997.

Gottschlich MM et al: The 2002 Clinical Research Award. An evaluation of the safety of early vs delayed enteral support and effects on clinical, nutritional, and endocrine outcomes after severe burns, *J Burn Care Rehabil* 23(6):401, 2002.

Gray DT et al: Early surgical excision versus conventional therapy in patients with 20 to 40 percent burns. A comparative study, *Am J Surg* 144(1):76, 1982.

Greenfield E, McManus AT: Infectious complications: prevention and strategies for their control, *Nurs Clin North Am* 32(2):297, 1997.

Greenhalgh DG, Staley MJ: Burn wound healing. In Richard RL, Staley MJ, editors, *Burn care and rehabilitation principles and practice*, Philadelphia, 1994, FA Davis.

Grube BJ et al: Neurologic consequences of electrical burns, *J Trauma* 30(3):254, 1990.

Hansbrough JF et al: Clinical trials of a biosynthetic temporary skin replacement, Dermagraft-Transitional Covering, compared with cryopreserved human cadaver skin for temporary coverage of excised burn wounds, *J Burn Care Rehabil* 18(1 Pt 1):43, 1997.

Helm R, Fisher S: Rehabilitation of the patient with burns. In DeLisa H, editor: *Rehabilitation medicine: principles and practice*, ed 3, Philadelphia, 1998, JB Lippincott.

Helvig EI: Pediatric burn injuries, *AACN Clin Issues* 4(2):433, 1993.

Helvig EI: Development of burn outcomes and quality indicators. A project of the ABA Committee on Organization and Delivery of Burn Care, *J Burn Care Rehabil* 16(2 Pt 2):208, 1995.

Honari S: Topical therapies and antimicrobials in the management of burn wounds, *Crit Care Nurs Clin North Am* 16(1):1, 2004.

Hunt JP et al: Occupation-related burn injuries, *J Burn Care Rehabil* 21(4):327, 2000.

Jackson D: The diagnosis of the depth of burning, *J Br Surg* 40:588, 1953.

Johnson C: Pathologic manifestations of burn injury. In Richard RL, Staley MJ, editors, *Burn care and rehabilitation principles and practice*, Philadelphia, 1994, FA Davis.

Jordan BS, Harrington DT: Management of the burn wound, *Nurs Clin North Am* 32(2):251, 1997.

Leman CJ, Ricks N: Discharge planning and follow-up burn care. In Richard RL, Staley MJ, editors, *Burn care and rehabilitation principles and practice*, Philadelphia, 1994, FA Davis.

Lim JJ, Rehmar SG, Elmore P: Rapid response: care of burn victims, *Aaohn J*, 46(4):169; quiz 179, 1998.

Luce EA: Electrical burns, *Clin Plast Surg* 27(1):133, 2000.

Mafong EA, Ashinoff R: Treatment of hypertrophic scars and keloids: a review, *Aesthetic Surg J* 20(2):114, 2000.

Maggi SP et al: The efficacy of 5% sulfamylon solution for the treatment of contaminated explanted human meshed skin grafts, *Burns* 25(3):237, 1999.

Matheson JD, Clayton J, Muller MJ: The reduction of itch during burn wound healing, *J Burn Care Rehabil* 22(1):76; discussion 75, 2001.

McManus WF Jr: Thermal injuries. In Feliciano D, Moore EE, Mattox KL, editors: *Trauma*, Stamford, Conn, 1996, Appleton and Lange.

Mertens DM, Jenkins ME, Warden GD: Outpatient burn management, *Nurs Clin North Am* 32(2), 343, 1997.

Monafo WW: Physiology of pain, *J Burn Care Rehabil* 16(3 Pt 2):345, 1995.

Monafo WW: Initial management of burns, *N Engl J Med* 335(21):1581, 1996.

Moss LS: Outpatient management of the burn patient, *Crit Care Nurs Clin North Am* 16(1):109, 2004.

Mozingo DW: Surgical Management. In Carrougher GJ, editor: *Burn care and therapy*, St. Louis, 1998, Mosby.

Noordenbos J, Dore C, Hansbrough JF: Safety and efficacy of TransCyte for the treatment of partial-thickness burns, *J Burn Care Rehabil* 20(4):275, 1999.

Pessina MA, Ellis SM: Burn management. Rehabilitation, *Nurs Clin North Am* 32(2):365, 1997.

Pruitt BA Jr: The evolutionary development of biologic dressings and skin substitutes, *J Burn Care Rehabil* 18(1 Pt 2):S2, 1997.

Quinney B et al: Thermal burn fatalities in the workplace, United States, 1992 to 1999, *J Burn Care Rehabil* 23(5):305, 2002.

Raff T, Germann G, Hartmann B: The value of early enteral nutrition in the prophylaxis of stress ulceration in the severely burned patient, *Burns* 23(4):313, 1997.

Raff T, Hartmann B, Germann G: Early intragastric feeding of seriously burned and long-term ventilated patients: a review of 55 patients, *Burns* 23(1):19, 1997.

Redlick F et al: A survey of risk factors for burns in the elderly and prevention strategies, *J Burn Care Rehabil* 23(5):351; discussion 341, 2002.

Rheinwald JG: *The "allodermis" of homograft as a bed for cultured epidermal autografts* (Technical Bulletin), Cambridge, Mass, 1992, Genzyme Tissue Repair.

Rutan RL: Physiologic response to cutaneous burn injury. In Carrougher GJ, editor: *Burn care and therapy*, St. Louis, 1998, Mosby.

Rutan TC: Discharge planning. In Carrougher GJ, editor: *Burn care and therapy*, St. Louis, 1998, Mosby.

Ruth GD et al: Outcomes related to burn-related child abuse: a case series, *J Burn Care Rehabil* 24(5):318; discussion 317, 2003.

Ryan CM et al: Use of Integra artificial skin is associated with decreased length of stay for severely injured adult burn survivors, *J Burn Care Rehabil* 23(5):311, 2002.

Sheridan RL: Burns, *Crit Care Med* 30(11 Suppl):S500, 2002.

Smith DJ, Jr: Use of Biobrane in wound management, *J Burn Care Rehabil* 16(3):317, 1995.

Staley MJ, Richard RL: Use of pressure to treat hypertrophic burn scars, *Adv Wound Care* 10(3):44, 1997.

Stone N et al: Child abuse by burning. *Surg Clin North Am, 50*, 1419-1424, 1970.

Supple KG: Physiologic response to burn injury, *Crit Care Nurs Clin North Am* 16(1):119, 2004.

Tassiopoulos AK: Nutritional support of the patient with severe burn injury, *Nutrition* 15(11-12):956, 1999.

Upright J et al: American Burn Association committee on the organization and delivery of burn care: burn care outcomes and clinical indicators, *J Burn Care Rehabil* 17(2):17A, 1996.

Ward RS: Physical rehabilitation. In Carrougher GJ, editor: *Burn care and therapy*, St. Louis, 1998, Mosby.

Weinberg K et al: Pain and anxiety with burn dressing changes: patient self-report, *J Burn Care Rehabil* 21(2):155; discussion 157, 2000.

Wibbenmeyer LA et al: Population-based assessment of burn injury in southern Iowa: identification of children and young-adult at-risk groups and behaviors, *J Burn Care Rehabil* 24(4):192, 2003.

Wilson R: Massive tissue loss: burns. In Bryant RA, editor: *Acute and chronic wounds: nursing management,* ed 2, St. Louis: Mosby, 2000.

Winfree J, Barillo DJ: Burn management. Nonthermal injuries, *Nurs Clin North Am* 32(2):275, 1997.

Wittman MI: Electrical and chemical burns. In Richard RL, Staley MJ, editors, *Burn care and rehabilitation principles and practice,* Philadelphia, 1994, FA Davis.

Ying SY, Ho WS: Playing with fire—a significant cause of burn injury in children, *Burns* 27(1), 39, 2001.

19

Principles of Wound Management

BONNIE SUE ROLSTAD & LIZA G. OVINGTON

OBJECTIVES

1. Describe how the goal for the patient with a wound impacts on dressing selection.
2. Identify three principles of wound management.
3. Describe how the holistic approach to wound management correlates with the principles of wound management.
4. Describe the characteristics of a physiologic wound environment.
5. Identify at least five objectives in local wound management.
6. Define the terms occlusive, semiocclusive, moisture-retentive, primary dressings, secondary dressings, biologic dressings and synthetic dressings.
7. Discuss the relevance of wound care dressing performance parameters.
8. List two indications and one contraindication for each dressing category.
9. Describe the factors to consider when selecting a wound dressing.
10. Define cost-effectiveness in relation to local wound management.

Most often, the desired outcome when caring for the patient with a wound is for the wound to heal or wound closure. *Wound healing* has been defined as restoration of integrity to traumatized tissue or, more specifically, resurfacing, reconstitution and proportionate restoration of tensile strength of wounded skin (Deodhar and Rana, 1997).

In light of the fact that healing is dependent upon numerous factors such as the condition of the host, sufficient arterial perfusion, and nutritional status, complete wound healing is not always realistic. The goal for the patient with a wound may also be *palliation* (such as in the terminally ill patient when the wound correlates with "end of life" time frame) or *symptom*

management (such as with the patient for whom arterial revascularization is not feasible). Goals for wound healing should be used to guide decisions concerning wound management so that the interventions selected are realistic and appropriate for the patient's situation. When the goal is palliation and symptom control, expensive technologic treatment modalities and biologic dressings may be impractical. Unobtrusive, physiologic care may be the priority in these cases. Modification of the goal for the wound may be indicated when changes occur in the patient's condition.

Interim outcomes can also be established for the wound. These short-term markers help the patient and clinician to recognize wound improvement and serve to confirm that the patient's wound-healing response is following an appropriate trajectory. Examples are listed in Box 19-1. It should be noted that outcome measures and time frames are not standardized; these are examples only and should be modified before being applied to a specific clinical situation.

Before establishing the goal for the patient with a wound, a thorough patient assessment relative to the wound—the patient's ability to heal the wound—must

---

BOX 19-1 Examples of Interim Outcomes for Wound Management

- Resolution in extent of periwound erythema by 1 week
- 50% reduction in wound dimensions or depth of sinus tract in 2 weeks
- Reduction in volume of exudate
- 25% reduction in amount of necrotic tissue (or eschar) by 1 week
- Decrease in pain intensity during dressing change

be obtained. Wound etiology and the presence of cofactors that affect the healing response must be identified. Information should be obtained about the patient's health history, wound history, current and proposed care setting, living situation, caregiver status, financial situation, reimbursement issues, transportation concerns, work situation, and other individual issues (Gallagher et al, 2004; Morison, 2004; Pieper and DiNardo, 1998).

PRINCIPLES OF WOUND MANAGEMENT

Wounds do not occur as an isolated event within a patient. Consequently, the principles of effective wound management must incorporate a holistic approach that identifies and addresses all of the patient's physiologic needs (Box 19-2). Failure to address any one of these principles jeopardizes care and may result in an unhealed wound, complications, or recurrence.

BOX 19-2 Wound Management Principles

1. **Control or Eliminate Causative Factors**
   a. Pressure
   b. Shear
   c. Friction
   d. Moisture
   e. Circulatory impairment
   f. Neuropathy

2. **Provide Systemic Support to Reduce Existing and Potential Cofactors**
   a. Nutritional and fluid support
   b. Edema
   c. Control of systemic conditions affecting wound healing (i.e., blood glucose)

3. **Maintain Physiologic Local Wound Environment**
   a. Prevent and manage infection
   b. Cleanse wound
   c. Remove nonviable tissue (debridement)
   d. Maintain appropriate level of moisture
   e. Eliminate dead space
   f. Control odor
   g. Eliminate or minimize pain
   h. Protect periwound skin

Principle 1: Control or Eliminate Causative Factors

The first principle of management is to control or eliminate causative factors. Thus assessment focuses initially on determination of wound origin. A chronic wound has been referred to as a symptom because there are frequently numerous factors related to etiology as well as contributing factors (or cofactors) precipitating the wound. Addressing the cause of the wound must occur concurrently with local wound care. Diagnostic tests may be required to clearly establish the wound etiology, especially in the case of atypical or recalcitrant wounds (Seaman, 2000).

Having identified causative factors, steps must be taken to eliminate or control these factors. This may involve (but is not limited to) the following:

- Offloading to reduce pressure and repetitive stress as discussed in chapters 13, 15 and 16
- Reduce mechanical factors (that is, shear and friction) with interventions such as use of a turn sheet or trapeze, socks or heel protectors, a knee gatch when head of bed is elevated, and a light dusting of powder or cornstarch on sheets
- Use of sustained, external gradient compression therapy to reduce venous hypertension (Chapter 15)
- Measures to promote blood flow to ischemic areas, such as hydration, elimination of nicotine and caffeine, and avoidance of cold (Chapter 15)
- Patient education particularly regarding sources of potential trauma such as foot soaks and chemical callous removers

The importance of these familiar interventions cannot be emphasized too strongly. Failure to address causative factors will result in delayed healing or a nonhealing wound, despite appropriate systemic and topical therapy. There is no dressing available that can compensate for an uncorrected pathologic condition (Bolton et al, 1990).

Principle 2: Provide Systemic Support to Reduce Existing and Potential Cofactors

The complex phenomenon of tissue repair only transpires in the presence of adequate levels of oxygen, growth factors, cytokines, metalloproteases, and nutrients, and in the absence of deterrents. Thus assessment must include evaluation of the patient's cardiovascular and pulmonary function, nutritional and fluid status, and concomitant conditions that affect the wound-healing process. Assessment factors may include the following (WOCN Society, 2005):

- Cardiovascular and pulmonary function, such as blood pressure; pulse and respiratory rates; distal pulses; capillary refill; presence of absence of edema, pallor, temperature changes; and po_2
- Nutritional and fluid status, such as actual weight as compared with ideal weight; laboratory indicators of visceral protein status such as albumin, transferrin, and prealbumin; current total intake of calories and protein to include oral, enteral, and parenteral routes; clinical indicators of malnutrition such as joint edema, sparse hair, dry skin, and lethargy
- Conditions or factors known to deter wound healing, such as diabetes, corticosteroid administration, and immunosuppression

Having assessed the patient for needs related to the status of their general body systems, the wound care specialist must intervene to correct any deficiencies that negatively impact on wound healing potential. This may involve the following:

- Measures to support tissue oxygenation, such as hydration, elevation of edematous extremities, and administration of nasal oxygen to the patient with low po_2
- Measures to correct nutritional deficiencies, such as dietary or nutritional support consultation; provision of oral, enteral, or parenteral support; and provision of vitamin and mineral supplements
- Measures to control prolonged moisture on the skin from incontinence (urinary and fecal), such as bowel training or prompted voiding programs, external collection devices, and skin care
- Measures to control wound-healing deterrents, such as blood glucose control and administration of vitamin A for the patient on corticosteroids

Principle 3: Maintain a Physiologic Local Wound Environment

Topical wound management, the focus of this chapter, is the manipulation of the wound to positively influence the physiologic local wound environment. A *physiologic* wound environment is "characteristic of an organism's healthy or normal functioning." Therefore, a wound care dressing is used to mimic the skin so that a physiologic local wound environment is created that will promote adequate moisture level, temperature control, pH regulation, adequate local blood supply and control of bacterial burden. These various conditions create a milieu that is conducive to a successful and expedient journey from compromised skin to skin repair and restoration of function.

Adequate Moisture Level. A physiologic wound environment relative to moisture level involves promoting and maintaining a moist—not wet, not dry—wound surface using exogenous materials. These materials serve to maintain adequate moisture in the wound, absorb excess moisture present in the wound, or donate moisture to dry or desiccated tissues within the wound.

The human body is more than 65% water; the primary means of maintaining this level of moisture is located within the epidermis (Spruitt, 1972). The stratum corneum layer of the epidermis prevents loss of excessive amounts of water in the form of water vapor to the external environment. Therefore, hydration levels of healthy skin are maintained by an intact stratum corneum. When the stratum corneum has been removed or compromised, tissues or cells are subject to increased loss of water vapor and may desiccate and eventually die. Consequently, a physiologic wound environment is a local environment in which tissue hydration levels and therefore the viability of the wound tissue and various cells within the wound space (growth factors, platelets, etc.) (see Chapters 4 and 5) are maintained by something other than the stratum corneum. This substitute stratum corneum is the wound dressing and functions as a barrier to water vapor loss.

Donating (or providing) moisture to the wound is not the same thing as retaining moisture over time. Saline-moistened gauze may be used to provide moisture to a wound if changed or remoistened frequently; however, it cannot keep the wound continually moist on its own and is not considered moisture-retentive. Semiocclusive dressings such as films, foams, and hydrocolloids are able to keep a wound moist, even when no additional moisture is supplied, by "catching" and retaining moisture vapor that is being lost by the wound on a continual basis.

Tissues may subsequently become overly wet and the periwound skin macerated. Healthy tissues in the wound are moist, but not wet or dry. To manage high drainage levels, a dressing must also have a moisture absorptive capacity in addition to vapor transmission ability. The process of absorption physically moves drainage away from the wound's surface and edges and into the dressing material. At the other end of the hydration spectrum, wound tissue that is already dry may need to be actively rehydrated using dressing materials that donate water to the tissue.

Normal Temperature. The temperature of wound tissues should remain as close as possible to normal. All cellular functions are affected by temperature, including chemical reactions (e.g., metabolism, enzymatic catalysis, protein synthesis, and oxidation) and processes (e.g., phagocytosis, mitosis, and locomotion). Local hypothermia can impair both the healing process and the immune response; it can lead to increased risks of infection by causing vasoconstriction and by increasing hemoglobin's affinity for oxygen, both of which result in a decreased availability of oxygen to phagocytes. The consequence of hypothermia on phagocytes includes decreased phagocytic activity, decreased production of reactive oxygen products (Clardy, Edwards, and Gay, 1985), and impaired ability to migrate (Akriotis and Biggar, 1985; Wenisch et al, 1996). Reduced mitotic activity and decreased production of growth factors IL-1β and IL-2 have also been reported when surgical patients experience a reduction in core body temperature of 1° C (Beilin et al, 1998).

Local cooling can occur as a result of moisture-vapor loss from the exposed tissues. Wound management practices such as frequency of dressing change and wound cleansing technique (such as irrigation with refrigerated solutions) can also induce local hypothermia. Topical wound dressings that reduce moisture loss from wounded tissues and do not require frequent changes will diminish local cooling. The inherent insulating properties of occlusive and semi-occlusive wound dressings may be important contributors to their beneficial effects on wound healing.

Bacterial Balance. The importance of bacterial balance and interventions to attain bacterial balance are discussed in Chapters 9 and 10. Strategies for achieving a bacterial balance can be categorized as (1) the removal of nonviable tissue, (2) appropriate wound cleansing, (3) adherence to the appropriate level of infection control precautions (that is, standard precautions unless otherwise indicated), and (4) the use of antimicrobial dressings when indicated. For example, semiocclusive dressings reduce wound

infections by more than 50% as compared with traditional gauze dressings (Hutchinson, 1989, 1993). This supports the theory that semiocclusive dressings optimize the phagocytic efficiency of endogenous leukocytes by maintaining a moist wound environment and reduce airborne dispersal of bacteria during dressing changes (Lawrence, Lilly, and Kidson, 1992). In many cases semi-occlusive dressings serve as a mechanical barrier to the entry of exogenous bacteria (Mertz and Ovington, 1993). One study found that bacteria can penetrate up to 64 layers of gauze (Lawrence, 1994). The appropriate use of semi-occlusive wound dressings to achieve and maintain bacterial balance will be discussed later in this chapter.

pH. The relationship between pH and bacterial balance is described in Chapter 9. When the skin is broken the wound tissues become mildly alkaline as a result of respiratory alkalosis which subsequently increases the risk of bacterial invasion (Hermans, 1990) and impaired function of MMP's (Armstrong 2002; Ovington, 2002). The presence of urine, stool, or fistula drainage in a wound will affect the local pH as well. If the pH is too low, various cellular functions may decline or stop; the cells themselves may also die under conditions of very low or very high pH. Acetic acid, with a pH of 2.4 (1 M solution), is an effective antiseptic in controlling bacteria, especially anaerobes, but is also toxic to endogenous cells such as fibroblasts and white blood cells. Therefore, the pH of a physiologic wound environment should be similar to the pH of blood which is essentially neutral (7.4). The pH of the wound fluid beneath semiocclusive wound dressings facilitates maintenance of a mildly acidic to neutral pH repelling exogenous contaminants and exposure to air (Varghese et al, 1998; Wiseman, Rovee, and Alvarez, 1992).

OBJECTIVES TO ACHIEVE A PHYSIOLOGIC WOUND ENVIRONMENT

As described, a physiologic local wound environment is characterized by adequate moisture level, normal body temperature, bacterial balance, and neutral to mildly acidic pH. To maintain a physiologic local wound environment that optimizes healing, eight objectives must be addressed:

(1) Prevent and manage infection
(2) Cleanse the wound

TABLE 19-1 Objectives of a Physiologic Wound Environment

OBJECTIVES	INTERVENTIONS
(1) Prevent and manage infection	• Cover wound to protect from outside contaminants with dressings impermeable to bacteria with the most appropriate dressing or combination of dressings based on the wound assessment and the overall goals for the patient • Infection control precautions, no touch dressing application • Appropriate wound cleansing and debridement • Antimicrobials when indicated • Appropriate wound culture technique (see Chapter 9)
(2) Cleanse wound	• Normal saline with 4-15 (psi) of pressure/force to remove debris without harming healthy tissue
(3) Remove nonviable tissue	• Most appropriate debridement method or combination of debridement methods based on the patient's condition and wound assessment (see Chapter 10) • Method of debridement consistent with the overall goals for the patient • Select topical dressings that maintain moist wound environment to prevent tissue dessication (i.e., dressing that donates moisture when wound bed dry)
(4) Maintain appropriate level of moisture	• Dressing with a high MVTR will allow moisture to escape and evaporate to manage minimally exudative wounds • Moderate to heavily exudative wounds require absorptive dressings
(5) Eliminate dead space	• Absorbent or impregnated gauze or cavity dressings for large, deep wounds • Fluff packing material and loosely place into the wound with a cotton-tipped applicator • Ensure the packing material is in contact with the wound edges and can be easily retrieved
(6) Control odor	• Appropriate dressing change frequency • Cleanse with each dressing change • Debridement and antimicrobials as indicated • Charcoal dressings
(7) Eliminate or minimize pain	• Semiocclusive dressings • Nonadherent dressings • Dressings that require fewer changes • Pain control interventions as described in Chapter 25
(8) Protect wound and periwound skin	• Skin barriers (liquid, ointments or wafers) to protect the periwound skin from moisture and adhesives as described in Table 19-2d • Appropriate interval for dressing changes so that exudate does not pool on surrounding skin or undermine adhesive of wound dressing

MVTR, Moisture-vapor transmission rate.

(3) Remove nonviable tissue
(4) Maintain appropriate level of moisture
(5) Eliminate dead space
(6) Control odor
(7) Eliminate or minimize pain
(8) Protect the surrounding skin

These objectives guide decisions about topical dressing selection (Table 19-1).

WOUND CARE DRESSING PERFORMANCE PARAMETERS

The approach used to manage wounds has changed dramatically since the late 1880s but not as dramatically as since the early 1980s. Before 1980, gauze was the predominant dressing used for wound care; dressings fulfilled passive functions such as to "plug and conceal." Historically, passive dressing materials consisted of animal, vegetable, and mineral sources, including leaves, feathers, plant extracts, hot oil, waxes, papyrus, honey, fat, castor oil, gold, and gauze (Turner, 1997). Advances in our understanding of a physiologic wound environment has also signaled the demise of outdated, traditional wound treatments such as antacids, dry dressings, iodine packing, and heat lamps. Today, the standard of care in wound management is such that wound care products must address generally accepted performance parameters.

A fundamental performance parameter critical for all wound dressings to satisfy so that tissue dessication is prevented is providing a moist wound environment (tissue hyration). By satisfying this performance parameter alone, several objectives of a physiologic wound environment are attained: reduce pain, remove nonviable tissue and prevent infection.

Dressing materials are usually comprised of synthetic or natural polymers, and their ability to maintain tissue hydration can be characterized by a measurement known as moisture-vapor transmission rate (MVTR). MVTR and transepidermal water loss (TEWL) are similar quantities in that both refer to the quantity of water vapor that passes through a substance. In the absence of the stratum corneum, TEWL is increased by almost 200-fold (Rovee et al, 1972). Because TEWL through intact skin varies slightly by location on the body, this magnitude of difference may not be observed uniformly; however, investigators have reported differences in TEWL of intact as opposed to damaged skin at other anatomic sites, ranging from 50- to 100-fold (Bothwell et al, 1972).

Dressings transmit less moisture vapor than the average wound loses and thus facilitate moisture retention in the tissue as opposed to desiccation. In general, if the dressing material transmits less moisture vapor than the wound loses, the wound will remain moist. If the dressing material transmits more moisture vapor than the wound loses, the wound may dry out.

In addition to tissue hydration, general performance parameters of the *ideal* wound care product include healing or attainment of the highest possible function, infection control, pain relief or reduction, ease of use, and safety (Thomas, 1994). Each dressing should satisfy some objective of a physiologic wound environment (i.e., eliminate dead space) and thereby support healing. Infection control is attained by sterile packaging and some dressings provide a barrier to exogenous contaminants. The ideal dressing is not painful while in place or to apply and remove. The dressing should be easy for the caregiver to use so that sterility of the dressing is maintained, waste is minimized and the desired effect of the dressing is achieved.

Safety

Safety of wound care products is a performance parameter that is expected of all dressings and merits specific attention. Safety of wound care products is within the domain of the Food and Drug Administration (FDA); wound care products are classified as drugs, biologics, or devices. The number of wound care products is ever increasing, with at least 3852 wound care products on the market. Over 99% of all wound care products are classified as medical devices and registered with the FDA as a 510(k) device. Consequently, medical devices that are noncritical and substantially similar to devices manufactured before 1976 may be marketed without clinical testing by using a 510(k) (also known as a premarket notification or PMN) to the FDA. A PMN is also submitted when a device is introduced for the first time or a device has been significantly changed or modified (e.g., in the design, material, chemical composition, energy source, manufacturing process, or intended use) such that its safety or effectiveness could be affected.

Safety features of wound care dressings indicate that products are free from toxic chemicals and fibers (Collier, 1996; Flanagan, 1997) and that product biocompatibility has been tested and reported by the manufacturers. Safety should also demonstrate that the product does not increase the patient's risk of morbidity or mortality. The wound care specialist's role in safety includes correct use of the product as recommended by the manufacturer (including FDA-approved clinical indications) and proper education of the caregiver. It should also be remembered that while the use of more than one dressing in the wound may be warranted, there exists the potential for a negative interaction between the dressing ingredients, which could be harmful to the patient or nullify the effectiveness of individual products. Questions about dressing combinations should always be directed to the individual manufacturers.

The wound care specialist should be cautious of mixing different topical agents together for use in a wound because ingredients in one agent may interact with the ingredients in another. For example, the enzymatic activity of collagenase is adversely affected by certain detergents and heavy metal ions such as mercury and silver, which are used in some antiseptics, and is inactivated by povidone iodine. If the collagenase enzyme was combined with the use of a secondary cover dressing that releases silver ions, the silver ions would inactivate the enzyme, resulting in no enzymatic debridement and little or no antibacterial effect of the silver. Similarly, certain foams are degraded by hydrogen peroxide, and the two should not be used sequentially. It is of vital importance to thoroughly read product package inserts and instructions for use when two products are being used together or sequentially in the same wound.

WOUND CARE DRESSING CATEGORIES

In this section the categories of passive dressings that are used to manage wounds will be discussed. Table 19-2 is an example of a formulary for wound care products that summarizes much of this information. Guidelines for utilization as established by Part B Medicare are incorporated into the formulary. It is important to refer to manufacturer's product insert and clinical support data before using specific products. Examples of product brand names within this formulary are not intended as a product endorsement.

Several terms are used to refer to wound dressings; these terms are defined in Table 19-3. Wound dressings include both primary dressings and secondary dressings. The primary dressing is a therapeutic or protective covering applied directly to the wound bed to meet the needs of the wound. The secondary dressing serves a therapeutic or protective function, is used to increase the ability for the wound needs to be adequately met and/or secure the primary dressing. For example, a hydrocolloid dressing is the primary dressing when used over a shallow moderately exudative wound but will function as a secondary dressing when used over a wound filler that is applied to a wound with depth.

Most wound dressings today are semiocclusive rather than occlusive. *Semiocclusive* dressings provide a barrier function that protects the wound and periwound skin from microbial and physical insult. They also provide thermal insulation, odor control, compression, and delivery of antimicrobial agents. Moisture-retentive dressings (which emerged in the 1970s) are currently staples in the wound care portfolio and in the 1990s represented approximately 63% of the market of wound care dressings sold in the United States. (Ballard-Krishnan, van Rijswijk, and Polansky, 1994; Bux and Malhi, 1996.)

Common components in wound dressings include gauze, hydrogel (glycerin), foam (polymers), hydrocolloid, (carboxymethylcellulose), bovine or avian collagen, alginate, cellulose, cotton, or rayon and transparent dressing (polyurethane). Wound care dressings may be "single component dressings" containing, for example only alginate or hydrogel or hydrocolloid, or "multi-component dressings" in which an alginate may be combined with a hydrocolloid, for example. Wound care dressings containing multiple components are categorized according to the clinically predominant component (e.g., alginate, collagen, foam, gauze, hydrocolloid, hydrogel).

Alginate Dressings

Alginates are spun fibers of brown seaweed that act via an ion exchange mechanism to absorb serous fluid or exudate to form a hydrophilic gel that conforms to the shape of the wound. Specifically, the calcium ions present in the alginate are exchanged for sodium ions when it contacts any substance containing sodium, such as wound fluid. The resulting sodium alginate is a gel. Alginates are nonadhesive, nonocclusive primary dressings that are conformable to the wound architecture. These versatile dressings are available as sheets or rope and may be cut to the size of the wound or loosely packed into the wound (Plates 50 and 51).

Alginates are a primary dressing and require a secondary cover dressing such as a transparent film dressing, composite, foam or hydrocolloid. Because this dressing absorbs and holds exudate, a moist environment is created thus promoting granulation and epithelization as well as autolysis. When additional

Text continued on p. 410

TABLE 19-2a Formulary for Passive Local Wound Care Products

GENERIC CATEGORY	FUNCTION	DESCRIPTION	EXAMPLES	INDICATIONS	ADVANTAGES/ PRECAUTIONS	USAGE
ALGINATES OR OTHER FIBER GELLING DRESSINGS Plates 50-52	Absorption; Packing	Primary dressing derived from brown seaweed in rope or pad form, nonwoven pad or fibers composed of alginate salts. Gels as fluid is absorbed. Conformable moisture-retentive dressing which also insulate the wound.	AlgiSite M, Restore CalciCare, Sorbsan Aquacel Hydrofiber	Full thickness wound cavity, undermined area or tunnel. Moderate to heavy exudate; Contaminated and infected wounds. Odorous wounds with or without slough.	*Advantages* Absorbent, packing agent, easy to use and understand. *Precautions* Not recommended in non-draining wounds.	Loosely pack into a wound. Dressings may be layered into a deep wound. A secondary dressing is required to secure. Change up to once per day.
COMPOSITES	Absorption (minimal); Secure primary dressings	Composed of a impermeable barrier, an absorptive layer (other than an alginate, foam, hydrocolloid or hydrogel), a semi-adherent or nonadherent property for covering the wound and an adhesive border.	Alldress, Medipore Pad Soft Cloth Adhesive, TELFA Island Dressing	Partial and shallow full-thickness wounds. Minimal-heavy exudate (dressing dependent and when used in combination with another dressing such as an alginate).	*Advantages* Easy to use. Combines the advantages from more than one dressing group to address the characteristics of the wound. *Precautions* Dependent upon the type of composite dressing. Read the package labelling for specific information.	A paper-backing liner is removed and the dressing applied to the wound. Usual composite dressing change is up to 3 times per week, one wound cover per dressing change.

Category	Purpose	Description	Products	Indications	Advantages/Precautions	Application/Change
CONTACT LAYERS	Protect the wound base	A nonadherent, woven polyamide net that is placed in contact with the wound base. It allows passage of exudate from the wound to a secondary (usually gauze) dressing.	DERMANET, Mepitel Non-Adherent Silicone Dressing, Tegapore	Full thickness granular wounds; Minimal to heavy exudates, Donor sites/split-thickness skin grafts, In combination with negative pressure wound therapy.	*Advantages* For use with large or deep wounds to protect the wound base; antimicrobials may be applied under the dressing. *Precautions* Not recommended for use in shallow or dry wounds or in the presence of viscous exudate.	Applied to the wound base with a secondary absorbent dressing cover (i.e., gauze). Contact layer stays in place up to 7 days while the absorbent layers are changed as needed.
FOAM Plates 53-55	Absorption (minimal-heavy) Packing material	Semi-permeable hydrophilic foam, impermeable barrier- Thin and traditional thickness. Conformable, other characteristics are dependent on manufacturer (i.e., wafers, rolls, pillows, film covering, adhesive, surfactant impregnated or an odor absorbent charcoal layer.)	Alleyvn, PolyMem Lyofoam Tielle	Partial and full thickness wounds; Minimal to heavy exudate; Infected wounds; May be used in combination with other dressing materials (e.g, films, alginates, pastes, powders).	*Advantages* Nonadherent forms protect friable periwound skin. Conformable to shape around angular body contours. Used under compression in venous ulcers. *Precautions* Not recommended for desiccated wounds or those with sinuses (unless packing is added). Cavity Dressing pillows should not be cut.	Select a dressing approximately 2-3 cm larger than the wound. Dressing change may be up to 3 times per week. Usual dressing change for foam wound fillers is up to once per day.

Continued

TABLE 19-2a Formulary for Passive Local Wound Care Products—cont'd

GENERIC CATEGORY	FUNCTION	DESCRIPTION	EXAMPLES	INDICATIONS	ADVANTAGES/ PRECAUTIONS	USAGE
GAUZE	Absorption (minimal-heavy) Packing material	Woven or non-woven, Material may include cotton, rayon and/or polyester. Sterile and non-sterile. Bulk or 2-packs	Curity Gauze Sponge, Kerlix Super Sponge, NuGauze Packing Strips	Partial and full thickness wounds, Infected wounds, Wounds with cavities or tracts.	*Advantages* Packing large wounds. Use in combination with amorphous hydrogel or topical impregnated or contact layers. *Precautions* Adheres to wound tissue for nonselective debridement, may lint or shred if cut. Labor intensive approach. Wound may dry out.	Fluff the gauze and avoid pressure or tight packing. Monitor for dessication or saturation. Dressing change interval is dependent upon level of saturation.
IMPREGNATED GAUZE	Packing material Deliver antimicrobial, medications nutrients and moisture	Woven sponges that are impregnated with chemical compounds and agents (e.g. hypertonic or normal saline, petrolatum, zinc, iodoform)	Adaptic, Curasalt, Measalt,	Partial or full-thickness wounds. Infected wounds, Wound with cavities or tracts.	*Advantages* Dressing dependent. (Petrolatum makes the gauze nonadherent, hypertonic dry sponges provide absorption, antimicrobials decrease bioburden.) *Precautions* Dressing dependent.	Loose packing. Monitor for exudate to avoid maceration. Choose appropriate size and ingredients for dressing.

Continued

HYDROCOLLOID Plates 45-47	Absorption	Adhesive, absorptive, backing materials, impermeable barrier Variety of shapes, widths, sizes, contours and thicknesses.	DuoDerm Restore, Tegasorb.	Partial and full thickness wounds, Minimal-moderate exudates. May be used in combination with other dressing materials (e.g., pastes, alginates)	*Advantages* Barrier to external fluids, conformable, absorptive; may be used in combination with compression for venous ulcers. *Precautions* Not recommended for use in third-degree burns or wounds with heavy exudate, depth or friable periwound skin. May contribute to hypergranulation tissue.	Select a dressing with a minimum of 2-3cm overlap from the margin of the wound. May be cut to conform to difficult areas. Changed up to 3 times a week.
HYDROGEL Plates 56-58	Donates fluid to the wound	2 forms: fixed three-dimensional macro-structure sheets with or without adhesive or borders OR amorphous gel delivered from a tube or impregnated into strip packing materials. Composed of water or glycerine.	Curasol, *Amorphous* Hypergel, *Sheets* Elastogel, Vigilon. Intrasite gel	Partial and full-thickness wounds Dry to Minimal exudate. Necrotic wounds. Infected wounds. Used in combination with other dressing materials (e.g., gauze, films)	*Advantages* Promotes rapid autolysis, conforming. *Precautions* Not indicated for use in heavily exuding wounds. Some forms may be difficult for patients to use. Monitoring or periwound skin for maceration or candidiasis from inappropriate usage of product.	Sheets without adhesive border or wound fillers are changed up to once per day. Sheets with adhesive covers are changed up to 3 times per week.
SPECIALTY ABSORPTIVE DRESSINGS	Absorption	Highly absorptive layers of fibers such cellulose, cotton, or rayon. semi-adherent or nonadherent.	Surgipad combine dressing Tendersorb wet-pruf ABD pad Exu-Dry	Wounds with moderate to heavy exudate.	*Advantages* Absorbent, easy to use. *Precautions* Not recommended in non-draining wounds.	Non adhesive border dressings are usually changed daily. Adhesive border dressings are usually changed every other day.

TABLE 19-2a Formulary for Passive Local Wound Care Products—cont'd

GENERIC CATEGORY	FUNCTION	DESCRIPTION	EXAMPLES	INDICATIONS	ADVANTAGES/ PRECAUTIONS	USAGE
TRANSPARENT FILM Plates 42-44	Protects	Thin, transparent polyurethane adhesive film, impermeable	Op-Site, Polyskin II, Tegaderm film	Partial thickness minimally draining or closed wounds.	*Advantages* Promotes autolysis, use as a secondary dressing. *Precautions* Not recommended for infection	Allow 4-5 cm overlap from wound margin to the surrounding skin. Dressing may be left undisturbed up to 7 days.
WOUND FILLERS	Fill shallow wounds, Hydrate Absorb	Absorbent materials composed of starch copolymers in paste, powder or bead form. Requires a secondary dressing.	Biafine WDE, DuoDERM Sterile Hydroactive Paste, Multidex Maltodextrin Wound Dressing	Partial and shallow full thickness wounds, Minimal to moderate exudate, Necrotic wounds with moisture (promotes autolysis), Infected wounds	*Advantages* Absorbent, packing (filling) materials, may be used in combination with other dressings (i.e., film, hydrocolloid) to extend wear time. *Precautions* Not recommended for use in dry wounds, wound covered with eschar, deep wounds or those with tunnelling.	Applied to fill a shallow defect in a wound, A secondary dressing is then applied. Usual dressing change is up to once per day.
WOUND POUCHES Chapter 23 Figure 23-7	Contain heavy exudate and odor	Pouches adapted from ostomy care that have an integrated skin barrier to protect periwound skin and a drainage spout that can be connected to straight drainage. Odor proof pouch film.	Conva Tec Wound Manager Hollister Wound Drainage Collector	Highly exudative wound, Malodorous exudate	*Advantages* Pouch wear time is 4-7 days, skin protection and ease of use. *Precautions* These pouching systems are expensive, but effective. Education of the caregiver will minimize application errors and expenses.	Apply in similar fashion as an ostomy pouch and educate caregiver. Usual dressing change is up to 3 times per week.

TABLE 19-2b Formulary for Active Local Wound Care Products

GENERIC CATEGORY	FUNCTION	DESCRIPTION	EXAMPLES	INDICATIONS	ADVANTAGES/ PRECAUTIONS	USAGE
ANTIMICROBIALS Plate 59	Control or decrease bioburden	Topical antifungal and antibiotic agents available as ointments, impregnated gauzes, pads, island dressings and gels. (i.e., Silver, Iodine)	Iodosorb Gel, Excilon AMD Acticoat dressing	Partial and full thickness wounds; Odorous wounds with minimal to heavy exudate; Highly contaminated and infected wounds	*Advantages* Decreases microbial levels in the wound which may reduce healing time, easy to use and understand. *Precautions* See manufacture's insert as precautions for individual products vary. Not a substitute for systemic antibiotics.	Refer to package insert as each form has specific usage instructions.
COLLAGEN	Stimulate wound healing	Derived from bovine, porcine or avain sources. Available in nonadherent pouches or vials, gels loaded into syringes, pads, powders and freeze-dried sheets. Require a secondary dressing.	ColActive, PROMOAEGRAN Matrix hyCURE, FIBRACOL PLUS	Partial and full thickness wounds; Minimal to moderate exudate; Contaminate and infected wounds	*Advantages* May accelerate wound repair. Slight absorption; No adherence to the wound; Some forms may be left in the wound up to seven days; May be used with topical agents. *Precautions* Not indicated in 3rd degree burns or patients with sensitivities to bovine materials.	Refer to package insert as each form has specific usage instructions.

Continued

TABLE 19-2b Formulary for Active Local Wound Care Products—cont'd

GENERIC CATEGORY	FUNCTION	DESCRIPTION	EXAMPLES	INDICATIONS	ADVANTAGES/ PRECAUTIONS	USAGE
ENZYME DEBRIDING AGENTS	Chemical debridement	Proteolytic enzymes, fibrinolytic enzymes, collagenase and papain urea applied to wound to digest specific tissue.	Collagenase Santyl Ointment, Accuzyme (Papain-Urea-Chlorophyllin Copper)	Partial and full thickness wounds; Eschar or necrotic tissue in wound bed	*Advantages* Conservative debridement agents that are easy to understand and may be used in many care settings. *Precautions* Use with caution in patients with coagulation disorders. See package insert for instructions.	Gauze is used as a secondary dressing. When granulation tissue is present discontinue product use. Consult package insert for instructions.

TABLE 19-2c Other Wound Care Therapies

GENERIC CATEGORY	FUNCTION	EXAMPLE	DESCRIPTION	INDICATIONS	ADVANTAGES/ PRECAUTIONS	USAGE
NEGATIVE PRESSURE WOUND THERAPY (NPWT) See Figures 20-4 and 20-5	Subatmospheric pressure (aka negative pressure) Used to promote wound healing	Vaccum-Assisted Closure (V.A.C.®)	An open cell reticulated foam dressing is placed into the wound, sealed with semi-occlusive drape, and attached to sub-atmospheric pressure via an evacuation tube connected to a computerized pump.	Acute and chronic open wounds with depth. Partial and full thickness. Partial thickness burns.	*Advantages* Control for fluid and isolation of the wound is provided while dressing is in place. Suction also provides contraction to promote wound closure. *Precautions* Patients with active bleeding, clotting disorders and those on anticoagulants. See manufacture's package insert for indications and precautions.	Strict protocols are provided by the manufacturer on these products. Dressing changes are usually done every 2-3 days.
GROWTH FACTORS	Promote wound healing	Platelet derived Regranex (Becaplermin recombinant)	Short-chain proteins found naturally in the body, autologous or recombinant, heat sensitive, cause specific cell/s to proliferate	Diabetic, neuropathic and recalcitrant wounds, good vascularity, full thickness, clean granular wounds	*Advantages* Growth factor is delivered to the wound. *Precautions* Growth factors are contraindicated in patients with neoplasms.	Usually applied daily. Follow manufacturer instructions.

Continued

TABLE 19-2c Other Wound Care Therapies—cont'd

GENERIC CATEGORY	FUNCTION	EXAMPLE	DESCRIPTION	INDICATIONS	ADVANTAGES/ PRECAUTIONS	USAGE
TISSUE ENGINEERED SKIN (BIOSYNTHETIC DRESSINGS)	Temporary wound covering Promotes wound healing.	Biobrane, E-Z Derm Biosynthetic Dressing, Inerpan, (Sherwood Davis & Geck)	Biosynthetic dressings are composed of both man-made and biologic ingredients. The biologic components are typically animal in origin, and the man-made ingredients may be synthetic polymers or chemicals.	Depending on the specific product, these dressings may be used as temporary coverings for use before autografting or as dressings to optimize healing for burns, donor sites, or other wounds.	*Advantages* Temporary wound covering, permeability to topical antibiotics *Precautions* Specific to individual product, may include potential allergies to ingredients.	Usage is product specific.
TISSUE ENGINEERED SKIN	Promote wound healing.	Apligraf Dermagraft	Bioabsorbable matrix of collagen or suture material populated with living fibroblasts and/or keratinocytes from a human source.	Venous ulceration and full thickness neuropathic diabetic foot ulcers (that do not involve bone, muscle or tendon).	*Contraindication* Infected wounds, or on patients with known allergies to bovine collagen or hypersensitivity to the components of the shipping medium. *Precautions* Living cells are fragile and sensitive to extremes of temperature. They also have finite lifetime once shipped from the manufacturer.	Refer to manufacturer's guidelines for specific instructions.

TABLE 19-2d Formulary Periwound Skin Protection Products

GENERIC CATEGORY	FUNCTION	DESCRIPTION	EXAMPLES	INDICATIONS	ADVANTAGES/ PRECAUTIONS	USAGE
Skin Sealants Plates 48-49	Provides a transparent barrier of protection over vulnerable skin from the effects of moisture, mechanical or chemical skin injury	Liquid transparent film delivered by a wipe, wand or spray Contains a plasticizing agent such as copolymer; some products contain isopropyl alcohol	No Sting Skin Prep Protective Dressing, Cavilon No Sting Barrier Film, Skin Gel Wipes	Protect vulnerable periwound skin from wound exudate and moisture. • Protect skin from friction • Prevent skin stripping from adhesives	*Advantages* Fast and simple, dries quickly *Precautions* Non alcohol based products should be used when the skin is compromised.	Apply with each dressing change
Moisture Barrier Ointments	Provides a barrier of protection over vulnerable skin from the effects of mechanical or chemical skin injury	Petrolatum, dimethicone or zinc based ointments, delivered in tubes or single packets; Some products contain hydrophilic ingredients such as karaya or carboxymethyl cellulose for improved adherence to the skin	Caloseptine Ointment, Lantiseptic Skin Protectant, Proshield Plus Skin Protectant, Critic-Aid Clear Hydrophilic ointment	Protect vulnerable skin from moisture, wound exudate, urine, or feces.	*Advantages* Simple and fast *Precautions* Ointments impair the adhesion of wound dressings, some wound care treatments cannot be used with zinc.	Apply with each dressing change

Continued

TABLE 19-2d Formulary Periwound Skin Protection Products—cont'd

GENERIC CATEGORY	FUNCTION	DESCRIPTION	EXAMPLES	INDICATIONS	ADVANTAGES/ PRECAUTIONS	USAGE
Moisture Barrier Pastes Chapter 23 Figure 23-5	Provides a thick barrier of protection over vulnerable skin from the effects of mechanical or chemical skin injury	Zinc based thick paste, delivered in tubes or single packets; some products contain hydrophilic ingredients such as karaya or carboxymethyl cellulose for improved adherence	Critic-Aid Skin paste, Ilex Skin protectant paste Remedy Calazime protectant paste	Protect vulnerable skin from moisture, wound exudate, urine, or feces. Perianal, peri-rectal, or periwound denudement	*Advantages* More durable than ointments; generally will adhere to denuded skin. *Precautions* Paste impair adhesion of dressings, some wound care treatments cannot be used with zinc, difficult to remove.	Apply with each dressing change, no need to remove completely each time.

Product	Description	Composition/Form	Examples	Uses	Advantages/Precautions	Application
Solid Skin Barriers Chapter 23 Figure 23-5	Provides a solid adhesive moldable water-proof barrier for protection over vulnerable skin from the effects of mechanical or chemical skin injury	Solid adhesive Pectin, karaya, gelatine, carboxy-methyl cellulose, or combination based products; delivered in rings, strips or wafers of various sizes; also used with ostomy care	Stomahesive, Eakin, Premium skin barrier	Protect peri-wound skin from the effects of mechanical or chemical skin injury such as moisture, or wound exudate, and moisture anchor tape onto barrier instead of skin to prevent skin stripping	*Advantages* More durable than ointments, and pastes, waterproof, wear time can be several days, effective for anchoring tape and other adhesives *Precautions* Requires careful removal to prevent skin stripping from adhesive, may become loose and allow moisture underneath the barrier	Cut in strips or cut to fit around the wound, change PRN when loosens
Skin Barrier Powders Chapter 23 Figure 23-5	Absorbs and dries weepy denuded skin to improve the adherence of ointments, pastes and adhesive	Powder Pectin, karaya, gelatine, carboxymethyl cellulose, or combination based products; also used with ostomy care	Stomahesive Protective Powder, Karaya Powder, Premium Powder	Weepy denuded skin before applying ointments, pastes, or adhesive barriers to improve adherence	*Advantages* Easy to use *Precautions* Will impair adhesion if used on intact skin or if used in excess	Use as needed, remove excess after application. Discontinue when the skin is no longer denuded

TABLE 19-3 Definition of Terms

OCCLUSIVE	No liquids or gases (e.g., moisture-vapor, oxygen, and carbon dioxide) can be transmitted through the dressing material; e.g., Saran Wrap
SEMIOCCLUSIVE	No liquids, but variable levels of gases are transmitted through the dressing material; e.g., transparent film, hydrocolloid, foam
MOISTURE-RETENTIVE	A dressing that is able to consistently retain moisture at the wound site by interfering with the natural evaporative loss of moisture vapor; any semiocclusive dressing is by definition moisture-retentive
SYNTHETIC	Dressing that is composed of man-made materials, such as polymers
PASSIVE	Dressing that provides passive support for wound healing
ACTIVE	Product that actively manipulates the wound repair process
PRIMARY	A therapeutic or protective covering applied directly to wound bed to meet the needs of the wound
SECONDARY	A secondary dressing placed over a primary dressing that serves a therapeutic or protective function, is used to increase the ability for the wound needs to be adequately met and/or is used to secure the primary dressing
CONTACT LAYER	Dressing placed in direct contact with the wound and left in place while secondary dressing is changed

absorbency is needed, the alginate may be layered. As the volume of exudate decreases, the secondary cover dressing used can be replaced with a dressing with less absorbent characteristics.

Alginates may be changed as often as daily depending upon the volume of exudate. Some alginates become almost amorphous gels in the wound and will require irrigation with saline for removal, while others retain their structural integrity as they "gel" and can be lifted out of the wound (Plate 52).

Indications. Alginates are indicated for moderate to heavily exudative wounds with or without depth and with or without a clean granular wound bed.

Precautions. Alginates are contraindicated in third-degree burns and are not recommended for the dry or minimally exudative wound. If an alginate is used inappropriately with minimally draining wounds, the wound bed may become desiccated with alginate fibers imbedded in the wound. The alginate dressing should not be moistened prior to application. When packing deep tunnels or sinuses, ribbon gauze may be preferable since it is retrievable.

Collagen Dressings

Collagen dressings are usually formulated with Type I bovine (cowhides or tendon) or avian collagen or with Type III porcine collagen. Collagen products are nonadhesive, nonocclusive primary dressings available in a variety of formulations: particles encapsulated in nonadherent pouches or vials, gels loaded in a syringe, pads, and freeze-dried sheets. Collagens require a secondary cover dressing.

The formulation of collagen selected is based upon the wound size, wound architecture and volume of exudate. In a dry to minimally exudative wound, a gel may be applied $1/4$-inch thick. If the wound has depth, the gel is applied, and a saline-soaked gauze or other appropriate dressing is applied to fill the defect. In a moderate to heavily draining wound, collagen particle pouches or the collagen with alginate may be used. If the pad form is used, at least $1/4$ to $1/2$ inch between the pad and sides of the wound is needed to allow for expansion as exudate is absorbed. To increase product absorbency, collagen is also available in a formulation that contains 10% alginate. This collagen alginate dressing is cut to the size of the wound.

A new collagen product has been combined with oxidized regenerated cellulose (Promogran, Ethicon, Inc.). The collagen product chemically binds to members of the MMP family of enzymes rendering MMPs inactive. Thus the active levels of MMPs are brought back into the ranges found in healing wounds and growth factor proteins are protected from being degraded by the MMPs (Cullen, 2002; Ovington, 2002).

The frequency of change for a collagen dressing is determined by the formulation of the dressing selected and the amount of exudate from the wound. The manufacturer's instructions should be followed for proper utilization of these dressings.

Indications. Collagen can be used in the exudative shallow or deep wound but is best used when applied to a wound bed without necrotic tissue. This dressing may be particularly appropriate for recalcitrant wounds.

Precautions. Collagen dressings are contraindicated for use in third-degree burns and wounds that are dry or eschar-covered. While enzymatic purification renders the bovine material nonantigenic, most manufacturers cite sensitivity to bovine products as a contraindication for use.

Composites

Composite dressings are products combining physically distinct components into a single dressing that provides multiple functions. Composite dressings contain the following features: bacterial barrier; absorbent layer other than a foam, alginate, hydrocolloid, or hydrogel; either a semiadherent or nonadherent surface that contacts the wound; and an adhesive border. Composites look like Band-Aids of variable sizes. They may have semiocclusive or nonocclusive fabric covers.

Composite dressings should not be cut because the structure of the dressing design will be compromised. Composites should be sized to have at least 2.5 cm (1 inch) of dressing that extends onto intact surrounding skin. One dressing per dressing change is usually reimbursed with dressing-change intervals up to three times per week.

Indications. Composite dressings may be used alone or in combination with other dressings (e.g., alginate). In wounds with depth, a primary wound filler material is required to pack the wound before securing the dressing with a composite. Some forms are useful for nonocclusive dressing procedures.

Precautions. Composite dressings are contraindicated for use in third-degree burns. These dressings are not appropriate for use in heavily exudative wounds or as a primary dressing in full-thickness wounds.

Contact Layers

Contact layers are non-adherent single layer of woven or perforated polymer net sheets placed directly on an open wound bed to protect the wound tissue from direct contact with other agents or dressings applied to the wound. They are porous to allow wound fluid to pass through for absorption by an overlying dressing. The product stays in place during dressing changes, allows the passage of wound exudate through its mesh or perforations, and protects the wound bed from trauma.

Indications. These products are primary dressings for use in clean wounds without necrotic tissue. Generally contact layer material is applied as a liner over granular wound surfaces and overlaps onto surrounding skin. The material may or may not require taping to the skin. In deep wounds, gauze packing may also be required. A secondary dressing is then applied. Contact layers are usually changed once a week.

Precautions. Contact dressings are contraindicated for use in third-degree burns and infected wounds. Contact dressings are not recommended for shallow or small wounds, dry wounds or those with viscous exudate, and wounds with tunneling and extensive undermining.

Foam Dressings

Polyurethane foam dressings (open cell foam dressings) are sheets of foamed solutions of polymers that contain variably sized small open cells capable of holding wound exudate away from the wound bed. The moist environment is created by maintaining the exudate in the wound space.

Foam dressings are primary dressings and available in widely variable formulations (Plate 53). Most foam dressings are nonadhesive while a few do have an adhesive surface. Nonadhesive foam dressings are secured in position with a secondary dressing such as a transparent film dressing or a nonadhesive wrap such as roll gauze. The foam may be the traditional thickness (4 to 7 mm) or as thin as <1 mm. Generally, the thin foam dressing has an adhesive wound surface and an outer layer of a transparent film dressing which provides a waterproof barrier. The traditional thickness nonadhesive foam dressings may or may not have this outer layer of a transparent dressing; some have an adhesive border. Foams are available as wafers in variable sizes or rolls. Pads and circular, and tube-shaped foam cavity dressings which are composed of small pieces of absorbent foam contained in a bag of permeable material, are also available for packing wounds with depth.

The appropriate size of the foam dressing is one that extends onto the periwound skin at least 2.5 cm (1 inch). Foam other than cavity dressings may be cut or contoured to fit anatomic areas. Check manufacturer's instructions to determine which side of the dressing is applied to the wound surface. The usual dressing change for an open cell foam dressing is up to three times a week. Foam dressings used as wound fillers may be changed as often as once per day.

Indications. Because open cell foam is one of the most absorbent materials available, foam dressings are appropriate for moderate to heavy exudative wounds with or without a clean granular wound bed. Thin foams are indicated to protect intact skin and to manage superficial wounds with minimal exudate such as skin tears. The traditional thickness nonadhesive foam dressing is particularly useful for management of exudate under compression in venous ulcers and in any wound with friable or fragile periwound skin. Foam dressings may be used in combination with other dressings to enhance management of wound exudate (e.g., alginates, absorbent pastes or wound fillers).

Precautions. Foam dressings are contraindicated for use in third-degree burns. When applied to a dry or minimally exudative wound, the foam dressing may adhere to the wound surface and require irrigation to facilitate removal. Therefore, foam dressings are not recommended for the wound with little to no exudate. Foam dressings are also not indicated when tunneling is present. Some foam dressing formulations are not conformable to depth and may be difficult to use in anatomic areas that require contouring such as the gluteal fold. When a cavity foam dressing is used to fill deadspace, the size of the product should be determined carefully so that there is sufficient room in the wound for the cavity dressing to expand as it absorbs wound exudate. Some foam cavity dressings cannot be cut because the integrity of the dressing will be compromised.

Gauze

Gauze is available woven or nonwoven, as cotton or synthetic blends, sterile or nonsterile, in many forms (sponges, pads, ribbon, strips and rolls) and plain or impregnated. To increase its versatility and applicability, gauze may be impregnated by the manufacturer with substances such as iodinated agents, petrolatum, zinc paste, crystalline sodium chloride, chlorhexadine gluconate (CHG), bismuth tribromophenate (BTP), water, aqueous saline, hydrogel, or other agents. The ability of saline-moistened gauze dressings to keep a wound from drying out depends on the amount of exudate from the wound and the frequency with which the gauze is changed or moistened. It is possible to extend the ability of saline-moistened gauze to prevent loss of moisture by incorporating petrolatum-impregnated gauze into the dressing as an upper layer. The hydrophobic nature of petrolatum will block transmission of moisture through the upper dressing.

Indications. Indications for plain (or dry) nonimpregnated gauze in wound management are constrained by the fact that dry gauze does not promote a moist wound environment (unless the wound is heavily exudative). Nonwoven, nonimpregnated gauze is particularly useful for scrubbing, prepping, wiping, absorption, and protection; woven gauze is preferred for wicking, debridement, and packing. Impregnated gauze provides additional functions such as to hydrate the wound (e.g., hydrogel or aqueous saline impregnated), absorb exudate (e.g., dry, crystalline sodium chloride formulations), or deliver antimicrobial agents and nutrients. Unique fabrics are also formulated specifically to facilitate debridement.

Gauze dressings are particularly useful for packing deep wounds, undermining, and tunnels. Loose packing technique is always recommended. When numerous dressing changes are required daily, a more cost-effective type of dressing may be warranted that provides a higher degree of exudate absorption.

Precautions. Avoid wet to dry gauze debridement because it is not selective (i.e., removes viable and nonviable tissue) and is painful. Monitor the condition of periwound skin to avoid prolonged moisture exposure and subsequent maceration. Periwound skin protection may be warranted in the exudative wound and can be provided with an ointment or liquid or solid skin barrier.

Hydrocolloid Dressings

Hydrocolloid dressings are a formulation of elastomeric, adhesive, and gelling agents. The most common absorbent ingredient in the hydrocolloid is carboxymethylcellulose, which was adapted from ostomy skin barriers. Early versions of hydrocolloid dressings were described as being fully occlusive. Today most hydrocolloids are backed with a semiocclusive film layer, which renders them semiocclusive; that is impermeable to fluids and bacteria and semipermeable to gas and water vapor. The wound side of this dressing is adhesive and will adhere to a moist surface as well as dry skin but will not adhere to the moist wound bed.

As a primary dressing, the hydrocolloid is available as a wafer in several shapes and sizes; contoured dressing are also available that enhance adherence to anatomically challenging sites such as the sacrum, heel, knee, and elbow (Plate 45). Many hydrocolloid dressings have an adhesive border that extends beyond the actual hydrocolloid surface, which is designed to prevent shear and friction from causing the edges of the hydrocolloid to loosen and circumvent the need for additional tape along the borders of the dressing.

As wound fluid is absorbed, the hydrocolloid forms a viscous, colloidal gel in the wound bed thus enhancing the moist wound environment needed for granulation, epithelization and autolysis (Plate 46). This gel is easily irrigated out of the wound at dressing change. Hydrocolloid dressings are also formulated to contain an alginate, thus increasing the dressing's absorptive capacity.

When selecting the size of the hydrocolloid dressing, it should extend onto intact peri-wound skin at least 2.5 cm (1 inch). If the hydrocolloid is cut from a larger piece, the edges should be taped to avoid rolling or adhering to clothing or sheets. Because hydrocolloids are most effective at body temperature, it is recommended to hold the dressing in place with the hand for a short period of time (30 to 60 seconds) after application. These dressings are generally changed twice weekly or weekly although they can be changed as often as three times a week. Dressings should also be changed when the wound gel appears to have migrated beyond the margins of the wound onto periwound skin.

Indications. Traditional-thickness hydrocolloid dressings are indicated for minimal to moderate exudate in partial- and full-thickness wounds. The thin hydrocolloid absorbs minimal exudate but is more flexible with a lower profile. Therefore, thin hydrocolloid dressings are indicated for the partial thickness wound with minimal exudate or intact skin that needs protection against friction. Hydrocolloid dressings provide a great degree of conformability and flexibility useful for anatomical locations such as the elbow or sacrum. Hydrocolloid dressings may be used in combination with an absorbent powder (i.e., wound filler) or alginate.

Precautions. Hydrocolloid dressings are contraindicated for third-degree burns and are not recommended for the infected wound or dry eschar covered wound. Wounds that require monitoring more often than once or twice a week should not be treated with a hydrocolloid as the hydrocolloid will lose effectiveness if changed too often.

Hydrogel Dressings

Hydrogel dressings are glycerin- or water-based dressings that are primarily and uniquely designed to hydrate the wound. These extremely versatile dressings may also absorb a small amount of exudate. Hydrogel dressings are formulated as sheets or amorphous gel (Plate 56).

Hydrogel sheets are three-dimensional networks of cross-linked, hydrophilic polymers. The cross-linked polymer (polyethylene oxide, polyacrylamides, or polyvinylpyrrolidone) physically entraps water to form a solid sheet. While the hydrogel sheet may contain up to 96% water and the sheet may feel moist, water is not released when squeezed. Hydrogel sheet dressings can be adhesive or nonadhesive and are available in sterile and nonsterile versions with the nonsterile version considerably less expensive. Hydrogel sheets are available with or without a border adhesive of transparent film or closed cell foam. Gel sheets may be packaged with a polymer film on one or both sides of the sheet; one side is removed before placement on the wound bed. Hydrogel sheets have a cooling effect that can be further enhanced with refrigeration; a particularly effective intervention when a sustained "cooling sensation" is the priority (such as with a sunburn).

Hydrogel sheets that are composed primarily of water should be cut to the size of the wound, avoiding overlap (Plate 58) onto intact periwound skin to prevent maceration. The hydrogel sheet that is predominantly glycerin can be applied to the wound and overlap onto the periwound skin with minimal risk of periwound maceration. A skin barrier ointment or skin sealant (Plate 48) can be applied to the immediate periwound skin to further prevent maceration. The hydrogel sheet can be changed daily or up to three times a week; the amorphous hydrogel is usually changed daily.

Amorphous hydrogels are similar in formulation to the hydrogel sheet except that the polymer has not been cross-linked to form a sheet. The absence of cross-linking means that the amorphous hydrogel does not provide the same cooling effect noticed in the sheet hydrogel. These dressings vary widely in viscosity and are available in a foil package, tube, spray bottle or impregnated gauze or ribbon gauze strips.

To secure the nonadhesive hydrogel sheet and amorphous hydrogel, a secondary dressing is necessary. Secondary dressings that absorb exudate (i.e., foam dressings) should not be used in conjunction with the hydrogel since the dressing's absorptive capacity would negate the purpose of the hydrogel (that is, to donate moisture to the wound). The amorphous hydrogel is usually changed daily although the frequency of change is also dictated by the secondary dressing used.

Indications. All hydrogel dressings are indicated for the dry to minimally exudative wounds with or without a clean granular wound base. A feature unique to the hydrogel dressing is that it *donates* moisture to the wound; therefore it is commonly used to facilitate autolysis. Because the hydrogel dressing is available in a variety of formulations, the hydrogel dressing can be used in shallow wounds (sheet or amorphous), wounds with depth (impregnated gauze) and wounds with undermining or tunneling (impregnated gauze) (Plate 57). The nonadhesive formulations can be secured with roll gauze or mesh tubular dressings and are particularly useful for painful wounds, fungating lesions, thermal injuries and fragile periwound skin.

Precautions. Hydrogel dressings may be contraindicated for third-degree burns; the wound care clinician should check the manufacturer's package insert for further information.

Specialty Absorptive Dressings

Specialty absorptive dressings are unitized multi-layer dressings which provide (a) either a semi-adherent quality or nonadherent layer, and (b) highly absorptive layers of fibers such as absorbent cellulose, cotton, or rayon. These may or may not have an adhesive border. Specialty absorptive dressings are indicated for wounds with moderate to heavy exudate. Specialty absorptive dressings without an adhesive border are usually changed daily; those with an adhesive border are usually changed every other day.

Transparent Film Dressing

Transparent film dressings are polyurethane sheets coated on one side with an acrylic, hypoallergenic adhesive. The adhesive is inactivated by moisture and will not adhere to a moist surface, such as the wound bed or moist periwound skin. Distinguishing features of film dressings are the packaging, ease of use and application process. Film dressings are also available in a variety of sizes and features (Plate 42).

Film dressings have no absorbent capacity and are impermeable to fluids and bacteria. They are however, semipermeable to gas, such as oxygen and water vapor. The extent of semipermeability, measured as MVTR is variable. Traditional film dressings have a low MVTR that ranges from 400 to 800 $g/m^2/day$. A "high-permeability" film dressing has a MVTR of 3000 $g/m^2/day$ and higher and is specifically designed to be used over an intravenous site. High permeability film dressings will allow an excessive amount of moisture to escape if used over a wound and precipitate dessication. A collection of purulent-appearing fluid is typical when using a transparent film dressing (particularly in the presence of nonviable tissue) and should not be misinterpreted as indicative of an infection (Plate 44).

A film dressing should be selected that allows a 2.5-cm (1-inch) perimeter of intact surrounding skin. A liquid skin barrier may be applied to the peri-wound skin prior to dressing application to prevent skin stripping particularly in the presence of fragile skin. When removing the transparent film dressing, stretch the film in a direction parallel to the wound rather than pulling upward. The stretching action gently breaks the seal. Film dressings should be changed when the exudate extends beyond the edges of the wound onto periwound skin as seen in Plate 44. The typical dressing change is every three days.

Indications. Film dressings are indicated as a primary dressing for (1) prophylaxis on high-risk intact skin, (2) superficial wounds with minimal or no exudate and (3) eschar covered wounds when autolysis is indicated. Film dressings are commonly used as secondary dressings to other products such as alginates and foam.

Precautions. Transparent film dressings are contraindicated in third-degree burns. Film dressings should be avoided in arterial ulcers and infected wounds that require frequent monitoring. Since transparent films do not fill dead space, they should not be used as a primary dressing on wounds with depth, undermining or tunneling.

When a transparent dressing is being used to facilitate autolysis in an eschar covered wound, it must be monitored closely and possibly changed more frequently. During the autolysis process, the eschar will liquefy and the fluid that accumulates will potentially undermine the film's adhesive. As the eschar softens, liquefies and is removed, depth of the wound becomes apparent and alternative dressings will be indicated to fill deadspace and absorb exudate.

Wound Fillers

Wound fillers are available in hydrated forms (e.g., pastes, gels), dry forms (e.g., powder, granules, beads), or other forms such as rope, spiral, pillows, etc. As primary dressings, these products are used to fill deadspace as well as to absorb exudate and are indicated for shallow wounds with minimal to moderate exudate. Wound fillers may contain collagen, alginate or other gelling material, foam, hydrocolloid, or hydrogel. Because wound fillers are nonadherent, a secondary dressing (e.g., films, hydrocolloids, foams, composites, specialty absorptive dressings) will be required to secure the dressing and may also be used to increase absorptive capacity. The frequency of dressing change will be dictated by the type of secondary dressing selected and volume of exudate. Usual dressing change may be up to once per day. Wound fillers are contraindicated in third-degree burns and are not recommended in wounds with tunneling. Only hydrated forms of wound fillers are appropriate for dry wounds.

Antimicrobial Dressings

Recently, semiocclusive dressings that contain silver and iodine (Plate 59) have entered the market to assist with the management of infected or overcolonized wounds (see Chapter 10). The objective of these dressings is to provide a sustained release of the antiseptic agent at the wound surface to provide a long-lasting antimicrobial action in combination with maintenance of a physiological environment for healing.

Silver has been used widely as a topical agent because of its bactericidal properties. Silver is formulated as a cream (i.e., silver sulfadiazine) and more recently into a wide variety of semiocclusive dressings. Silver is a noble metal that possesses an antimicrobial effect when it is oxidized to silver ions. Silver sulfadiazine (2% to 7%), for example, has been shown to reduce bacterial density, vascular margination, and migration of inflammatory cells. Practitioners use dressings impregnated with silver since they demonstrate antimicrobial effects on broad-spectrum organisms. Silver released in a moist environment enhances the rate of reepithelialization by 40% in a meshed skin graft as compared to treatment with antibiotic solution. Silver-resistant pathogens exist and the potential mechanism of promoting resistance has been demonstrated (Brett, 2006). Therefore, judicious use of elemental antimicrobials is warranted. Use of silver dressings should be limited to a 2-4 week period, similar to the approach used with antibiotics.

Iodine has been complexed with a polymeric cadexomer starch vehicle to form a topical gel or paste (Iodosorb, Iodoflex; HealthPoint Ltd, Fort Worth, TX). The cadexomer moiety provides absorption of exudate from the wound, which results in a concomitant slow release of low concentrations of free iodine from the vehicle. Clinical studies in chronic wounds (venous ulcers, diabetic foot ulcers and pressure ulcers) have consistently shown that the cadexomer iodine product is effective at reducing bacterial counts in the wound. In addition, when compared to standard treatments (usually gauze and saline) and the cadexomer starch vehicle alone it appears to positively affect the healing process (Holloway, 1989; Laudanska, 1988).

Additional Topical Wound Care Categories

Additional categories of topical agents include growth factors, negative pressure wound therapy, pouching and skin substitutes. The description, indications for use and caveats to utilization are provided in Table 19-2 and in Chapters 4, 5, 18, 20 and 23.

SELECTING THE WOUND CARE DRESSING

Although dressings alone do not heal wounds, the correct selection and use of dressings can facilitate wound healing (Bolton et al, 1990). Dressing selection is based upon numerous parameters: wound assessment, wound history, dressing interactions, patient and caregiver needs and reimbursement issues.

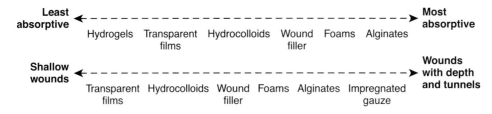

Fig. 19-1 Continuum of dressing selection with changing exudate and depth.

In addition, dressing selection is based on matching the attributes of the specific dressing (i.e., absorptive capabilities, adhesive versus nonadhesive) with the needs of the wound (Rolstad, 1997).

Wound Assessment Parameters

The essential question that guides decision-making in local wound care is, "What does the wound need to achieve a physiologic environment?" The answer is derived from a careful and accurate assessment and documentation of the wound status (Warriner, 2004). In addition, serial assessments indicate how the wound is responding to the treatment and progressing toward the planned goal. Ongoing reassessment and evaluation of healing may lead to changes in the local wound care dressing choice. For example, as exudate changes, the dressing may require a product with a different absorptive capacity. Over time, as nonviable tissue is removed from the wound base, a different type of dressing may be indicated to fill new depth and dead space to prevent abscess or premature closure. Figure 19-1 shows the continuum of passive dressing selection with changing exudate and depth. Several wound characteristics are influential when selecting topical therapy (Box 19-3). Once the patient and wound assessments are complete and the wound needs are identified, the wound care specialist must determine which wound care products can best meet those needs. (Table 19-4).

Etiology. The cause of the wound directly affects wound dressing treatment choices. For example, ulceration resulting from venous insufficiency requires compression and exudate management. Arterial ulcers (before revascularization) are generally nonexudative and as a result require dressings that provide moisture. Neuropathic ulcers commonly have tunnels, whereas

BOX 19-3 Parameters that Influence Topical Dressing Selection

- Wound Assessment
  - Etiology
  - Location of the wound
  - Extent of tissue loss (stage)
  - Wound size
  - Presence of undermining, sinus tracts, or tunnels
  - Condition of wound bed
  - Condition of wound edges
  - Volume of exudate
  - Condition of periwound skin
  - Bacterial burden
  - Odor
  - Wound pain
- Wound History
- Dressing Interactions
- Patient and Caregiver Needs
- Reimbursement Issues

pressure ulcers may have undermining; both require dressings to fill the defect or dead space.

Location of the Wound. Wound location, particularly the wound in areas that are difficult to manage, affects significantly the type of dressing selected. Digit dressings are useful for the toes and fingers. Dressings with a contour, such as a sacral shape, are more effective than square or rectangular dressings at the sacrum, coccyx, and heel. Elbows can pose application challenges, and flexible, conformable dressing materials are needed. Wounds in locations exposed to friction and shear from sheets, clothing, or braces require thin adhesive dressings with smooth backings.

Size and Extent of Tissue Loss (Stage). Wound size affects the selection of both dressing size

TABLE 19-4 Dressing Options Based on Key Wound Needs

MINIMAL ABSORPTION	MODERATE TO HEAVY ABSORPTION	DONATES MOISTURE	FILLS DEADSPACE	NON-ADHERENT
Thin Hydrocolloid	Hydrocolloid (standard thickness)	Hydrogels	Hydrogel (impregnated gauze)	Hydrogel
Thin Foam	Alginate	Gel formulations of select dressings such as collagen	Alginate	Alginate
Composite	Foam (standard thickness and cavity)		Foam cavity	Foam
	Specialty absorptive		Specialty absorptive	Specialty absorptive
	Wound filler		Wound filler	Wound Filler
	Gauze		Gauze	Gauze

and material. For example, a wafer or pad product form may be selected to cover the wound and extend at least 2.5 cm (1 inch) onto periwound skin to adequately secure the dressing. The extent of tissue loss influences wound dressing selection in that wound fillers or wound packing dressings will be needed to fill the dead space created by the tissue loss. For example, a hydrocolloid paste can fill a small amount of depth, whereas, a deeper wound may require an alginate or an impregnated gauze to adequately fill dead space (Walsh, 1996).

Condition of Wound Bed. When granulation is the primary tissue in the wound, a dressing selection that maintains a moist wound surface is usually ideal. The presence of slough or eschar in the wound will dictate the need for some form of debridement. Removal of necrotic tissue requires some form of debridement to decrease the bioburden in the wound and remove physical obstacles to wound closure. Moisture-retentive dressings promote autolysis through the maintenance of a moist wound-dressing interface. The type of dressing used to achieve or assist with debridement varies depending on the form of debridement selected. All of the dressing categories in the formulary except for dry gauze are moisture-retentive. The dressing selected is also based on volume of exudate and the architecture of the wound. For example, when the wound is minimally exudative and eschar-covered, one option for autolysis is to apply a hydrogel wafer dressing over the eschar, covered with a transparent dressing. Within 24 to 48 hours the eschar is typically rehydrated and loosening from the wound edges. At that time, the hydrogel may continue to be appropriate or another dressing may be indicated if depth to the wound is present or volume of exudate has increased.

Condition of Wound Edges. Tissue at the perimeter of the wound represents the wound edge. This area may be attached to the wound bed, unattached, or rolled downward into the wound. Attached wound edges are the ideal. Edges that are unattached or roll downward with epithelialization (referred to as a closed wound edge, or epibole) require extended healing times and often represent a nonhealing wound. Management of the unattached wound edges is similar to management of undermining; gentle packing is required. Removal of an epithelialized rolled wound edge is recommended and may be achieved by applying silver nitrate to the edge or by surgical excision.

Volume of Exudate. The volume and type of wound exudate represent a macroscopic index that is a critical point for local wound care decisions. The significance of volume of exudate in selecting a wound dressing is apparent in wound care decision trees and algorithms because it will be one of the first questions posed. Dressings designed for dry wounds hydrate the tissue. Conversely, exudative wounds require absorbent dressing materials. Several dressings are available that are designed to manage the full range of exudate volume, from minimal to heavy amounts (see Figure 19-1). Adequate containment of exudate is critical to manage increased bioburden in the wound, protect the periwound skin, control odor, and avoid overuse of wound care products. In addition, the prolonged presence of excessive amounts of moisture in the wound may increase the patient's risk for developing hyperplasia or hypergranulation tissue in the base of the wound (Plate 27). Methods of exudate management include moisture-vapor transmission such as with transparent dressings, and wicking such as with alginate or foam dressings.

Condition of Periwound Skin. The periwound skin can be intact, dry, cracked, macerated, erythematous, or infected (e.g., candidiasis). Each assessment influences the type of wound care products selected. For example, dry and cracked skin may require a moisturizer before applying the wound dressing. Intact skin, particularly vulnerable intact skin such as with the elderly, can be protected from adhesives and wound exudate with the use of skin protectants and liquid skin barriers.

Skin integrity is also affected by the technique used to apply and remove adhesives. When appropriate, less frequent dressing changes are preferred to prevent unnecessary exposure of the skin to adhesive removal. The presence of maceration indicates that wound exudate is not adequately contained or managed. Prolonged contact of wound fluid with the periwound skin also predisposes the patient to develop a fungal infection (most commonly candidiasis) or erythema at the periwound site. To correct this situation, either the type of dressing used should be modified to a more absorbent type (see Figure 19-2), or the frequency of dressing changes should be increased. A liquid skin barrier will also protect the periwound skin from damp or saturated wound dressings. Occasionally the patient will require an antifungal powder or lotion to treat a fungal infection, although milder cases may resolve spontaneously when the excessive wound exudate is managed effectively. Appropriate use of absorbent dressings or pouching to manage wound exudate reduces the incidence of periwound maceration, erythema, and candidiasis (Dealey, 1995).

Bacterial Burden. The presence of a wound infection or overcolonization (see Chapter 9) influences decisions concerning topical wound management. Therefore the wound should be assessed for signs and symptoms of an infection with each dressing change. When the wound is infected, a complete systemic assessment and appropriate treatment should be instituted.

Local dressings selected for use should have an indication for infected wounds listed on the product package insert. This does not apply to other wound care products such as cleansing agents and periwound skin-care products. Generally, occlusive dressings are not recommended for infected wounds, semiocclusive dressings should be monitored closely and changed more frequently than generally anticipated, and nonocclusive dressings are indicated as the most conservative topical wound care approach. Wound cleansing is necessary at each dressing change.

Antimicrobial nonprescription dressings are also available that have demonstrated, to a limited extent, evidence of clinical benefit (Bale, 1997; Bale and Jones, 1997; Mertz et al, 1994).

Odor. The presence of odor occurs to varying degrees in numerous wound care situations (Poteete, 1993). Odor is commonly associated with an infected wound. Highly colonized wounds, such as fungating lesions or pressure ulcers with necrotic debris, may also be malodorous. However, slight odors occur normally at dressing changes when wounds are occluded and are associated with the use of certain types of dressings (e.g., hydrocolloids). Also, odor may occur from dressing strike-through (i.e., leakage), poor hygiene, and inappropriate dressing use (e.g., extending dressing wear time beyond that which is recommended).

In the fungating wound, topical debridement, topical antibiotics, antimicrobial dressings, or odor-absorbent dressings are effective (Haughton and Young, 1995; Poteete, 1993). When leakage, hygiene, or inappropriate dressing selection and technique may be the problem, patient and caregiver education is needed.

Wound Pain. Pain at the wound site must be adequately described and objectively quantified before the wound care specialist can understand the origin of the pain and identify appropriate pain-control measures (Dallam et al, 1995). Chronic pain, such as with ischemia, requires maintenance pain-control measures; additional analgesics may be required during wound care procedures.

Pain at the wound site may be relieved or minimized by the use of moisture-retentive dressings; analgesics given before the dressing change may also be indicated.

However, pain that occurs during dressing changes should also prompt a re-evaluation of dressing change technique and wound care product choices (Szor and Bourguignon, 1999). Liquid skin barriers will protect skin from mechanical forces during dressing removal. Nonetheless, caregiver technique in the removal of tape (i.e., proper use of adhesives and supporting the tissue during dressing removal) has a dramatic effect on the patient's pain experience. Wound pain and control measures are discussed in more detail in Chapter 25.

Wound History

During the initial patient interview, it is valuable to obtain a history on the patient's wound that includes what dressings have been used thus far for the wound and the effect of those interventions. This information can then be used to identify dressings to avoid, dressings that may require extra encouragement for the patient to use again or dressings that will require additional periwound skin protection such as a skin barrier ointment, cream or liquid skin barrier.

In the presence of optimal care, if the wound has a history of senescence or recalcitrance that is not related to overcolonization, active wound therapies (i.e., growth factors, electrical stimulation and negative-pressure wound therapy [NPWT]) should be considered to manipulate the repair process. These therapies are represented in the formulary (Table 19-2) and discussed in greater detail in Chapters 5, 18 and 20.

Patient and Caregiver Needs

A holistic assessment of the patient requires identifying who is (or will be) providing care and in what care setting. Figure 19-2 demonstrates the numerous variables that impact product selection and potential outcomes of care. Clearly, the caregiver has a significant impact on the ability to achieve positive wound related outcomes. As the plan of care is being developed and dressing choices are being made, the availability, level of skill and care-related concerns of the caregiver will be important to ascertain and explore. A primary concern of the caregiver is ease of use.

The National Family Caregivers Association estimates that family caregivers provide approximately 75% of the home care in the United States (Turnbull, 1999). Hence, patient and caregiver familiarity with the process of wound cleansing and dressing changes,

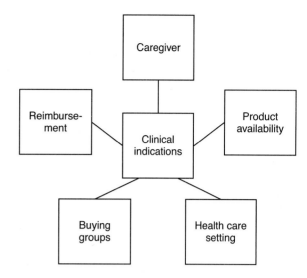

Fig. 19-2 Factors affecting wound care product selection and patient outcomes.

but also the implications of failing to follow the agreed upon plan of care. To enhance adherence with recommended wound care, products and procedures must be easy to understand and perform. Wound care products that require infrequent dressing changes with a limited number of steps in the application process and that use straightforward, simple procedures are most likely to be performed as instructed. For more discussion of facilitating cooperation and establishing a sustainable plan of care, see Chapter 26.

Reimbursement Issues

Reimbursement for supplies (and therefore access to product) is dependent on type of health care setting and how the setting is paid for services (see Chapter 27). When the patient needs to pay out-of-pocket for wound care supplies, the risk of nonadherence with the plan of care is increased. Therefore treatment decisions should be made while keeping in mind what is financially reasonable for the patient so that the patient is able to implement the plan of care (Turnbull, 1995).

WOUND CARE PROCEDURES

Procedures for application of specific dressing types can be found in Appendix B and D. Regardless of the type of wound or the wound dressing selected, there are fundamental procedures and techniques that must be followed: dressing removal, wound irrigation and cleansing, wound packing, dressing application, and securing the dressing. Standard precautions, as previously discussed, should be used with all procedures (Stotts et al, 1997), see also Appendixes.

Infection Control Measures

Bacterial bioburden in the wound may also be affected by the techniques used to apply and remove dressings and topical agents. Recent clinical guidelines for the treatment of pressure ulcers have advocated the use of clean dressings and clean technique over sterile technique, albeit with the caveat "until research proves otherwise." There is not much evidence that using sterile as opposed to clean techniques has a significant effect on wound healing outcomes (Bergstrom et al, 1994). There also appears to be a lack of agreement among wound care specialists as to what constitutes sterile technique as opposed to nonsterile technique (Faller, 1997).

A no-touch technique attempts to ensure that the processes used to care for the wound (dressing change and wound cleansing) will not add to the bioburden of the wound. The clean no-touch technique mandates the use of sterile primary and secondary dressings. Sterile cotton tipped applicators should be used to probe the wound and insert wound fillers, gauze or packing materials. Irrigant solution and the devices used to hold the solution as well as administer the irrigant should be sterile. Nonsterile gloves are used however the surface of the dressing that will contact the wound bed should not be touched.

Standard precautions (gloves, eye protection when splashes are possible, etc) should be routinely followed during wound care practices by the caregiver. Hand washing is the most effective and most frequently overlooked precaution (Pittet et al, 1999). Caregivers should wash their hands (1) before and after patient contact, (2) after contact with a source of microorganisms (body fluid and substances, mucous membranes, broken skin, or inanimate objects that are likely to be contaminated), and (3) after removing gloves. An easily overlooked opportunity for hand-washing is between care of a dirty and a clean body site; an

analogy could be made to the removal of the dirty wound dressing and application of a new dressing. Although it has not been researched specifically, two sets of gloves should be used. One set for dressing removal and wound cleansing and another set for dressing application. This is even more important in light of studies that suggest that at least 25% of the population and almost 40% of health care workers have nasal colonization by *S. aureus* (Crow, 1997), the most prevalent wound pathogen (Raz et al, 1996).

Dressing Removal

The goal of this procedure is to remove the dressing while protecting periwound skin and the wound base from trauma. Dressing changes are performed on a scheduled basis depending on the type of dressing in use; dressings that are oversaturated or leaking should be changed when that is detected. Universal precautions are indicated, and a clean technique is used. Adhesives are removed in the direction of hair growth. An edge of the dressing is gently rolled or lifted to obtain a starting edge. The tissue adjacent to the dressing is supported as the dressing is gently released from the skin. A moist gauze can be used to support the skin during removal to minimize the potential for stripping. If the dressing material is attached to the wound base, saline or a wound cleanser may be used to moisten the dressing and gently release it from the tissue. Disposal of dressing materials and contaminated gloves is performed in accordance with agency policies and procedures.

Wound Cleansing

Since bacteria cannot invade healthy tissue unless they first adhere or attach to it (Mertz and Ovington, 1993), wound-cleansing techniques that physically remove surface bacteria serve a preventive role. The physical removal of bacteria does not necessarily require the use of an antiseptic agent. Normal saline is an effective cleansing agent when delivered to the wound site with adequate force to agitate and wash away surface debris and devitalized tissue that may harbor bacteria. Irrigation is a common method of delivering the wound cleansing solution to the wound surface. Studies have shown that there is an optimal effective range of irrigation pressures that ensure adequate removal of surface debris (Rodeheaver et al, 1975). Pressures below

4 pounds per square inch (psi) are not sufficient to remove debris, and pressures above 15 psi risk driving the debris into the tissue rather than off of the surface. One easy way to ensure an irrigation pressure within this range is to use a 35 ml syringe and a 19-gauge needle, or angiocatheter (to avoid risk of needlestick).

Many studies have documented that the use of antiseptics (such as povidone iodine, Dakin's solution, acetic acid, or hydrogen peroxide) in open wounds are not only cytotoxic to bacteria but also to white blood cells and vital wound healing cells such as fibroblasts. This is because their primary mechanism of action is to destroy cell walls regardless of the identity of the cell. All of the aforementioned antiseptics have been shown to damage endogenous wound cells, and their use in open wounds should be weighed in light of this (Doughty, 1994; Hellewell et al, 1997; Lineweaver et al, 1985).

Often, commercial wound-cleansing solutions contain antimicrobial ingredients or other chemicals that can cause damage to wound cells. A recent evaluation of 10 commercial wound cleansers (both antimicrobial and nonantimicrobial) revealed that all inhibited the viability and phagocytic activity of polymorphonuclear leukocytes unless diluted 10- to 1000-fold (Hellewell et al, 1997). An earlier evaluation of commercial cleansers on the market in 1993 reported similar results (Foresman et al, 1993). The FDA does not regulate wound cleansers. The FDA designation of "wound cleansers" is intended primarily as a category of products to be used for minor, acute injuries as opposed to solutions for repeated use in chronic wounds.

Dressing Application

After dressing removal and wound cleansing, the surrounding skin is gently cleansed and dried. A skin sealant may be applied to the skin before dressing application to protect the skin. The selected dressing is then applied, according to manufacturer's instructions, without stretching the skin. In the gluteal fold, wafer dressings are folded in half before application to ensure that the adhesive seals into the anatomic contours. Applications of dressings at the heel or elbow may require cutting and shaping the dressing to customize the fit.

Wound Packing and Filling

The purpose of packing the wound is to fill dead space and avoid the potential of abscess formation by premature closure of the wound. Packing materials should be conformable to the base and sides of the wound. Assessment of the depth and undermining of tunneling is completed. When tunneling is present, strip gauze packing is used to fill narrow areas while allowing for dressing retrieval. For large, deep wounds, hydrating or absorbent-impregnated gauze is effective and usually requires fewer dressing changes than dry gauze. The packing material is fluffed and loosely placed into the wound with a cotton-tipped applicator so that the packing material is in contact with the wound edges and base. Gauze dressings may be necessary to act as an additional absorbent layer. A secondary cover dressing is then applied and secured. Overpacking of the wound should be avoided.

Securing the Dressing

When dressings are nonadhesive, a method of securing them is necessary to keep the dressing in place. Self-adhesive wraps, tape, Montgomery straps, gauze wraps, or tubular mesh dressings may be used. If the wound is located on the leg, a gauze wrap may be taped upon itself to avoid application of tape to the skin.

STANDARDIZATION AND DECISION MAKING TOOLS

Currently, there are more than 60 Health Care Finance Administration Common Procedure Coding System (HCPCS) codes for surgical dressings based on type and size. Although only about a dozen generic dressing categories exist (e.g., film, collagen, gauze), considerable performance and design variations occur within each category. For example, alginates are available in rope or pad form, in gelling or high-integrity form, with lateral or vertical absorption, and with high- or moderate-absorption capabilities.

At one time, decision making was simple because personal preference ruled. However, this was an expensive and nonstandardized approach, which is not compatible with today's capitated health care delivery system. In an attempt to simplify decisions, the "quick-fix, cookbook" approach with a "one size fits all" approach has been observed in some settings. In any case, standardization of products and wound treatments yields benefits, particularly when protocols and clinical pathways are established collaboratively based on (1) recent published guidelines, (2) a review of the literature for available research, or (3) best practice.

In general, wound care decisions concerning the type of dressings to be used (hydrogel, alginate, transparent film, etc.) should be based on wound characteristics, wound location, and the patient's situation. Specific brand product choices, however, are influenced by a variety of factors such as clinician familiarity and comfort with use. A 1994 survey of extended care facilities reported that product availability and reimbursement are more likely to influence dressing choice than the characteristics of the wound and patient condition (Ballard-Krishnan, van Rijswijk, and Polansky, 1994).

Attempts to standardize the process of product selection are increasingly common, and the desired objective is to reduce the clinician-to-clinician variability so that costs can be contained without compromising outcomes. Methods of decision analysis for wound care product selection translate research into clinical practice: algorithms, flow charts, collaborative pathways (also known as clinical pathways), and decision trees (Greer and Siezenis, 1989).

A key role of the wound care specialist is to standardize and organize wound care products available within their health care system with a product formulary (see Table 19-2) (Andrychuk, 1998; van Rijswik and Beitz, 1998). A wound care product formulary is set up similar to a drug formulary: generic categories, brand names, product description, dispensing units, indications for use, precautions, and instructions for use are included. Annual review of this formulary is recommended because wound care product research and development is ongoing and quickly paced (Salcido, 1999).

Decision-making tools are beneficial in that they can improve the accuracy of decisions making, guide treatment selection, and serve to educate the clinician concerning a particular disease entity (Letourneau and Jensen, 1998). The decision-making tools are usually accompanied by definition of terms to enhance clarity, and require policies, procedures and standing orders so that they can be put into effect by the specific caregiver. Figure 19-3 is an example of a local wound

management algorithm that incorporates principles and objectives of wound management to guide local wound product selection. Additional decision-making tools are located in the appendix.

EVALUATING OUTCOMES

Routinely, the wound care specialist must evaluate effectiveness of local wound treatments. At each patient contact, assessments are made to determine the patient's status and response to treatment. Examples of important questions include the following:

- Is the wound progressing toward the identified goal? If not, assess to ensure that care is being provided as recommended. Reevaluate macroscopic wound indices. If exudate has increased and autolysis is not in progress, is a more absorbent dressing required? Is the patient's condition deteriorating? Is the wound infected?
- Is the patient and/or caregiver able to perform the procedures correctly and on schedule? If not, review and demonstrate, and observe the caregiver doing procedures. Simplify the dressing and frequency of changes when possible.
- Is the nonhealing wound free of infection? If not, refer to Chapter 9.
- Is pain reduced? If not, reassess to ensure that a moist wound environment is being maintained as appropriate. Reassess whether the etiology of the wound has been reduced or eliminated. Confer with other team members to consider analgesia.
- If autolysis is in progress, is debriding occurring in a timely fashion? If not, consider sharp and surgical methods to augment autolysis.
- Is the topical therapy cost-effective? Cost-effectiveness is not sufficiently measured by the price of the dressing (frequently, the cost per unit for an interactive dressing is higher than that for dry gauze). It must instead reflect the cost of achieving a desired outcome. In this way, it is the cost of the outcome that is to be compared. When nursing time is factored in and healing rates are compared, moisture-retentive approaches have proven more cost-effective (Bolton, van Rijswijk, and Shaffer, 1996).

Four factors should be calculated into the cost of treatment for conservatively managed chronic wounds to achieve the desired outcome: (1) cost of all dressing materials, (2) nursing time, (3) treatment costs for

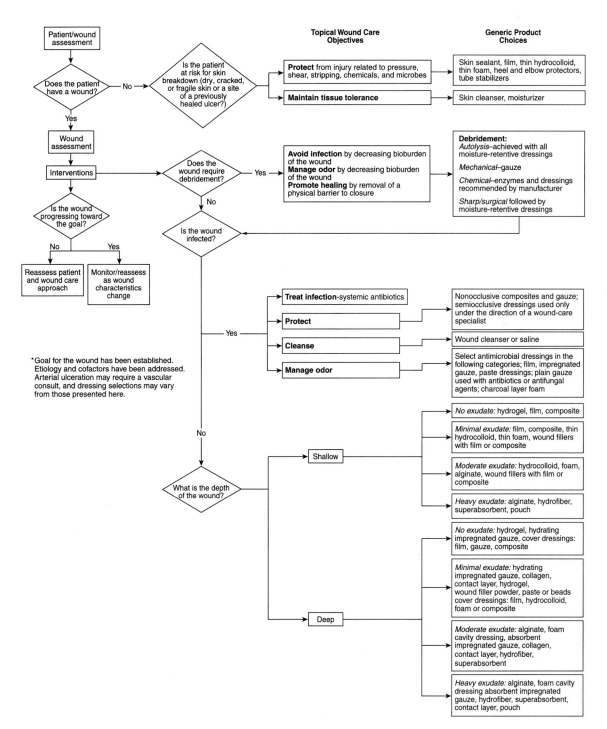

Fig. 19-3 Local wound management interventions algorithm. (Courtesy Bonnie Sue Rolstad, RN, MA, CWOCN, Copyright © 2000.)

complications, and (4) loss of work time and other related expenses (Bolton, van Rijswijk, and Shaffer, 1996; Hermans and Bolton, 1996).

On a per-patient basis, local wound management interventions should be planned with consideration for product reimbursement for the patient. Documentation, product selection, and the care setting affect how reimbursement occurs. Some wound care items are not reimbursed by Medicare (e.g., skin and wound cleansers, moisturizers) (Turnbull, 1995). If the patient is paying out-of-pocket for these supplies, wound care may be jeopardized.

Outcomes can also be tracked based upon the use of standardized protocols for an institution or wound care program (Bolton, 2004; McIsaac, 2005). The framework used by McIsaac measured how the use of best practice in a care system can be planned, implemented, and measured. One of the measures of this study was cost.

SUMMARY

The wounded skin is a complex pathophysiologic condition that necessitates a specific and intricate knowledge base, which includes assessments and interventions to achieve appropriate outcomes for the wound (Beitz, Fey, and O'Brien, 1999). Unfortunately, nonphysiologic approaches and inappropriate product use also remain commonplace (Ballard-Krishnan, van Rijswijk, and Polansky, 1994; Bux and Malhi, 1996).

A frequently stated axiom in wound care is, "All wounds are not the same." Consequently, many aspects of local wound management differ and numerous factors affect local wound treatment decisions. Therefore one treatment protocol is not appropriate for all wounds, and seldom does a wound progress to healing with only one type of dressing used; most wounds will require numerous modifications as wound characteristics change.

This chapter has reviewed a holistic approach to the patient and the maintenance of a physiologic wound environment. Even when the third principle of wound management is satisfied (to provide an optimum wound environment), realistic and appropriate goals for the patient with a wound can only be obtained when the first and second principles of wound management are also satisfied: to control or eliminate the causative factors and to provide systemic support of the patient.

Furthermore, understanding these principles of wound management prepares a wound care specialist to partner within interdisciplinary teams, to articulate underlying rationale, and to use a research-based approach to provide cost-effective care to the patient with a wound (Bowers, 1998; Powers, 1997).

SELF-ASSESSMENT EXERCISE

1. What are the three principles of wound management?
   a. Debridement, control of infection, and exudate management
   b. Establishment of a treatment goal, wound cleansing, and physiologic local wound care
   c. Assessment of the host, debridement, and physiologic local wound care
   d. Address the wound etiology, support the host, and maintain a physiologic local wound environment

2. Which of the following interventions indicates an attempt to control or eliminate the etiology of a venous ulcer?
   a. Resizing of shoe to include orthotics
   b. Applying an alginate and foam cover dressing
   c. Monitoring blood glucose levels
   d. Encouraging elevation of the leg 3 times daily

3. Which of the following statements is true of semiocclusive dressings?
   a. They are occlusive to liquids and gases.
   b. They are occlusive to liquids but transmit moisture vapor and gases.
   c. They are occlusive to gases and vapors but transmit liquids.
   d. They are inconsistent in their nonocclusive properties.

4. In the patient with a new approximated surgical wound, the primary wound care objective is which of the following?
   a. Absorption
   b. Hydration
   c. Cleansing
   d. Protection

5. On which of the following is dressing selection primarily based?
   a. Functions of the dressing
   b. Characteristics of the wound
   c. Product availability and cost
   d. Number of dressing changes required daily

6. In the patient with a highly exudative pressure ulcer, which category of dressings should be considered?

a. Hydrocolloids
b. Collagens
c. Transparent dressings
d. Alginates

7. Which of the following statements about wound care is TRUE?

a. Hydrocolloids absorb more exudate than alginate dressings.
b. Transparent dressings are contraindicated in the presence of eschar.
c. Wound fillers can be used to fill undermining and tunnels.
d. Silver-impregnated dressings are indicated when critical colonization is suspected.

8. List seven objectives for local wound management, and correlate each with a type of dressing that will assist in achieving that objective.

REFERENCES

Akriotis V, Biggar W: The effects of hypothermia on neutrophil function in vitro, *J Leukoc Biol* 37(1):51, 1985.

Andrychuk M: Pressure ulcers: causes, risk factors, assessment and intervention, *Orthop Nurs* 17(4):65, 1998.

Apelqvist J, Ragnarson Tennvall G: Cavity foot ulcers in diabetic patients: a comparative study of cadexomer iodine ointment and standard treatment. An economic analysis alongside a clinical trial, *Acta Derm Venereol* 76(3):231, 1996.

Armstrong DG, Jude EB: The role of matrix metalloproteases in wound healing, *J Am Podiatr Med Assn* 92(1):12, 2002.

Baker EA, Leaper DJ: Proteinases, their inhibitors, and cytokine profiles in acute wound fluid, *Wound Repair Regen* 8(5):392, 2000.

Bale S: Wound dressings. In Morison M et al: *Nursing management of chronic wounds*, ed 2, London, 1997, Mosby.

Bale S, Jones V: *Wound care nursing, a patient centered approach*, London, 1997, Bailliére Tindall.

Ballard-Krishnan S, van Rijswijk L, Polansky M: Pressure ulcers in extended care facilities: report of a survey, *J WOCN* 21(1):4, 1994.

Beilin B et al: Effects of mild perioperative hypothermia on cellular immune responses, *Anesthesiology* 89(5):1133, 1998.

Beitz JM, Fey J, O'Brien D: Perceived need for education vs. actual knowledge of pressure ulcer care in a hospital nursing staff, *Dermatol Nurs* 11(2):125, 1999.

Bergstrom N et al: *Treatment of pressure ulcers*: clinical practice guideline No. 15, Rockville, Md, 1994, US Department of Health and Human Services, Public Health Service, Agency for Health Care Policy and Research. AHCPR Pub No 95-0652.

Bolton L, van Rijswijk L, Shaffer F: Quality wound care equals cost-effective wound care: a clinical model, *Nurs Manage* 27(7):30, 1996.

Bolton L et al: Dressing's effect on wound healing, *Wounds* (2):126, 1990.

Bolton L et al: Wound healing outcomes using standardized care, *J WOCN* 31(3):65, 2004.

Bothwell J et al: The effect of climate on repair of cutaneous wounds in humans. In Maibach H, Rovee D, editors: *Epidermal wound healing*, Chicago, 1972, Yearbook Medical.

Bowers C: Development and implementation of evidence-based guidelines: a multisite demonstration project, *J WOCN* 25(4):187, 1998.

Brett DW: A discussion of silver as an antimicrobial agent: alleviating the confusion, *Ostomy/Wound Manage* 52(1):34, 2006.

Bux M, Malhi J: Assessing the use of dressings in practice, *J Wound Care* 5(7):305, 1996.

Chen W, Rogers A, Lydon M: Characterization of biologic properties of wound fluid collected during early stages of wound healing, *J Invest Dermatol* 99(5):559, 1992.

Clardy CW, Edwards KM, Gay JC: Increased susceptibility to infection in hypothermic children- possible role of acquired neutrophil dysfunction, *Pediatr Infect Dis J* 4(4):379, 1985.

Collier M: The principles of optimum wound management, *Nurs Standard* 10(43):47, 1996.

Cullen B: The role of oxidized regenerated cellulose/collagen in chronic wound repair. Part 2. *Ostomy Wound Manage* 48(6 Suppl):8, 2002 Review.

Dallam L et al: Pressure ulcer pain: assessment and quantification, *J WOCN* 22:211, 1995.

Dealey C: Common problems in wound care: caring for the skin around wounds, *Br J Nurs* 4(1):43, 1995.

Deodhar AK, Rana RE: Surgical physiology of wound healing: a review, *J Postgrad Med* [serial online] 1997 [cited 2006 Mar 15];43: 52-6. Available from: http://www.jpgmonline.com/article.asp?issn= 0022-3859;year=1997;volume=43;issue=2;spage=52;epage=6;aulast= Deodhar)

Doughty D: A rational approach to the use of topical antiseptics, *J WOCN* 21(6):223, 1994.

Faller N: *A survey exploring the ET nursing art of wound care: factors associated with clean versus sterile technique*, Amherst, 1997, University of Massachusetts. Unpublished doctoral dissertation.

Flanagan M: Wound cleansing. In Morison M et al, editors: *Nursing management of chronic wounds*, ed 2, London, 1997, Mosby.

Foresman PA et al: A relative toxicity index for wound cleansers, *Wounds* 5(5):226, 1993.

Greer JM, Siezenis LMLC: Methods of decision analysis: protocols, decision trees and algorithms in medicine, *World J Surg* (13)240, 1989.

Hansson C: The effects of cadexomer iodine in the treatment of venous leg ulcers compared with hydrocolloid dressing and paraffin gauze dressing, *Int J Dermatol* 37(5): 390, 1998.

Haughton W, Young T: Common problems in wound care: malodorous wounds, *Br J Nurs* 4(16):959, 1995.

Hellewell T et al: A cytotoxicity evaluation of antimicrobial and non-antimicrobial wound cleansers, *Wounds* 9(1):15, 1997.

Hermans M: Clinical and bacteriological advantages in the use of occlusive dressings. In Waldstrom T, editor: *Pathogenesis of wound and biomaterial-associated infections*, New York, 1990, Springer Verlag.

Hermans M, Bolton L: The influence of dressings on the costs of wound treatment, *Dermatol Nurs* 8(2):93, 1996.

Holloway GA et al. Multicenter trial of cadexomer iodine to treat venous stasis ulcer. *West J Med* 151(1):35, 1989.

Hutchinson J: Prevalence of wound infection under occlusive dressings, a collective survey of reported research, *Wounds* 1:123, 1989.

Hutchinson J: A prospective clinical trial of wound dressings to investigate the rate of infection under occlusion. In Hutchinson J: *Proceedings: advances in wound management*, London, 1993, MacMillan.

Kobza L, Scheurich A: The impact of telemedicine on outcomes of chronic wounds in the home care setting, *Ostomy Wound Manage* 46(10):48-53, 2000.

Laudanska H, Gustavson B: In-patient treatment of chronic varicose venous ulcers. A randomized trial of cadexomer iodine versus standard dressings, *J Int Med Res* 16(6):428, 1988.

Lawrence J, Lilly H, Kidson A: Wound dressings and airborne dispersal of bacteria, *Lancet* 339(8796):807, 1992.

Lawrence J: Dressings and wound infection, *Am J Surg* 167(1A):21S, 1994.

Letourneau S, Jensen L: Impact of a decision tree on chronic wound care, *J WOCN* 25:240, 1998.

Lineweaver W et al: Topical antimicrobial toxicity, *Arch Surg* 120(3):267, 1985.

McIsaac C: Managing wound care outcomes, *Ostomy Wound Manage* 51(4):54, 2005.

Merriam-Webster's Online Dictionary, http://www.m-w.com/cgi-bin/dictionary?book=Dictionary&va=physiologic; Accessed October 25, 2005.

Mertz P et al: Can antimicrobials be effective without impairing wound healing? the evaluation of a cadexomer iodine ointment, *Wounds* 6(6):184, 1994.

Mertz P, Ovington L: Wound healing microbiology, *Dermatol Clin* 11(4):739, 1993.

Morison, M: A framework for patient assessment and care planning. In Morison M, Ovington L, Wilkie K, editors: *Chronic wound care: a problem-based learning approach*, London, 2004, Mosby.

Nwomeh B, Yager D, Cohen I: Physiology of the chronic wound, *Clin Plast Surg* 25(3):341, 1998.

Ostomy/Wound Management (OWM) 2005 Buyers' Guide, 51(7) Malvern, PA, 2005, HMP Communications.

Ovington LG: Overview of matrix metalloprotease modulation and growth factor protection in wound healing. Part 1, *Ostomy Wound Manage* 48(6 Suppl):3, 2002.

Pieper B, DiNardo E: Reasons for nonattendance for the treatment of venous ulcers in an inner-city clinic, *J WOCN* 25(4):180, 1998.

Pittet D et al: Compliance with handwashing in a teaching hospital, *Ann Intern Med* 130(2):126, 1999.

Poteete V: Case study, eliminating odors from wounds, *Decubitus* 6(4):43, 1993.

Powers J: A multidisciplinary approach to occipital pressure ulcers related to cervical collars, *J Nurs Care Qual* 12(1):46, 1997.

Raz R et al: A 1-year trial of nasal mupirocin in the prevention of recurrent staphylococcal nasal colonization and skin infection, *Arch Intern Med* 156(10):1109, 1996.

Rodeheaver G et al: Wound cleansing by high-pressure irrigation, *Surg Gynecol Obstet* 141(3):357, 1975.

Rolstad B: Wound dressings: making the right match, *Nsg'97* 37(6):32hn 1, 1997.

Rovee D et al: Effects of local wound environment on epidermal healing. In Maibach H, Rovee D, editors: *Epidermal wound healing*, Chicago, 1972, Yearbook Medical.

Salcido R, editor: Resources in wound care: 1999 directory, *Adv Wound Care* 12(4):164, 1999.

Seaman S: Considerations for the global assessment and treatment of patients with recalcitrant wounds, *Ostomy Wound Manage* 46(1A Suppl):10S; quiz 30S, 2000.

Smiell JM et al: Efficacy and safety of recombinant human derived growth factor BB in patients with nonhealing lower extremity diabetic ulcers: A combined analysis of four randomized studies, *Wound Rep Regen* 7(5):335, 1999.

Soo C et al: Differential expression of matrix metalloproteinases and their tissue derived inhibitors in cutaneous wound repair, *Plast Reconstr Surg* 105(2):638, 2000.

Spruitt D: The water barrier and its repair. In Maebashi H, Rovee D, editors: *Epidermal wound healing*, Chicago, 1972, Yearbook Medical.

Stotts NA et al: Sterile versus clean technique in postoperative wound care of patients with open surgical wounds: a pilot study, *J WOCN* 24:10, 1997.

Szor JK, Bourguignon C: Description of pressure ulcer pain at rest and at dressing change, *J WOCN* 26:115, 1999.

Thomas S: *Handbook of wound dressings*, London, 1994, Macmillan.

Trengove NJ et al: Analysis of the acute and chronic wound environments: the role of proteases and their inhibitors, *Wound Rep Regen* 7(6):442, 1999.

Turnbull G: Weaving reimbursement of surgical dressings into the plan of treatment, *Ostomy Wound Manage* 41(7A Suppl):103S, 1995.

Turnbull G: The dollars and sense of patient teaching, *Ostomy Wound Manage* 45(3):16, 1999.

van Rijswijk L, Beitz J: The traditions and terminology of wound dressings: food for thought, *J WOCN* 25(3):116, 1998.

Varghese M et al: Local environment of chronic wounds under synthetic dressings, *Arch Dermatol* 122:52, 1998.

Wahl L, Wahl S: Inflammation. In Cohen IK, Diegelmann RF, Lindblad WJ, editors: *Wound healing: biochemical and clinical aspects*, Philadelphia, 1992, WB Saunders.

Walsh K: Decision-making in the care of cavity wounds, *Prof Nurse* 11(9):593, 1996.

Warriner RA: Wound Assessment. In Sheffield PJ, Smith A, Fife CE, editors: *Wound care practice*, Flagstaff, AZ, 2004Best.

Wenisch C et al: Mild intraoperative hypothermia reduces production of oxygen intermediates by polymorphonuclear leukocytes, *Anesth Analg* 82(4):810, 1996.

Wiseman D, Rovee D, Alvarez O: Wound dressings: design and use. In Cohen IK, Diegelmann RF, Lindblad WJ, editors: *Wound healing: biochemical and clinical aspects*, Philadelphia, 1992, WB Saunders.

Wound, Ostomy, and Continence Nurses (WOCN) Society: *Fact Sheets on Arterial Insufficiency; Peripheral Neuropathy; Venous Insufficiency*, http://www.wocn.org/publications/facts/; Accessed October 27, 2005.

Wysocki AB, Staiano-Coico L, Grinnell F: Wound fluid from chronic leg ulcers contains elevated levels of metalloproteinases MMP-2 and MMP-9, *J Invest Dermatol* 101(1):64, 1993.

Wysocki AB: Wound fluids and the pathogenesis of chronic wounds, *J WOCN* 23(6):283, 1996.

20 Devices and Technology in Wound Care

RITA A. FRANTZ, CRAIG L. BROUSSARD, SUSAN MENDEZ-EASTMAN, & RENEE CORDREY

OBJECTIVES

1. Describe the effects of at least four devices and technologies in wound management.
2. Describe the steps necessary to prepare a patient for at least three devices and technologies available for wound care.
3. List at least two indications and contraindications for each device and technology described in this chapter.
4. Explain how to reduce the risk of developing complications associated with at least four devices and technologies of wound management.

Several of the devices and technologies discussed in this chapter are used when the wound response to conventional therapies has been marginal. The level of evidence in terms of efficacy and effectiveness for many of these therapies is limited or has numerous design inadequacies. For example, treatment allocation may not be randomized, the standard treatment or control arm may be incomplete or poorly controlled, outcome measures may be inconsistent or obtained in a potentially biased fashion, and sample size is commonly too small to detect a difference. When viewed in the aggregate, however, these studies provide support for actual or potential enhancement of the wound-healing process.

Despite these limitations, the wound care specialist must be cognizant of these devices and technologies so that the biologic basis and plausibility for the modality is understood. The wound specialist should also be aware of the indications, contraindications, and side effects of these treatments. Although the wound care specialist may or may not actually perform the adjuvant therapy, he or she should understand the method used to apply these interventions.

HYPERBARIC OXYGENATION

Hyperbaric oxygenation is the systemic, intermittent administration of oxygen delivered under pressure. A hyperbaric environment exists when atmospheric pressure is greater than 1 atmosphere absolute (ATA) (Hammarlund, 1995). A medically significant hyperbaric exposure occurs when atmospheric pressure is increased to greater than 1.4 ATA or 10.2 pounds per square inch gauge pressure (psig) (UHMS, 1996). The typical hyperbaric oxygen treatment takes place at a pressure of 2.0 to 2.4 ATA, or 14.7 to 17.6 psig. For hyperbaric oxygenation to occur, the patient must breathe 100% oxygen while physically exposed to the hyperbaric environment (Shilling and Faiman, 1984). Topical application of oxygen is not hyperbaric oxygenation and has shown no significant benefit to wound healing. One case series, however, reported that the topical application of oxygen may assist in reepithelialization (Gordillo and Sen, 2003). Further study is needed to substantiate these findings. Oxygen under pressure functions as a pharmacologic agent in that it has a therapeutic dose, a toxic dose, side effects, contraindications, interactions with other drugs, and incompatibilities with other drugs (Heimbach, 1998). Just as wound care is not a subspecialty of hyperbaric oxygenation, neither is hyperbaric oxygenation a subspecialty of wound care. Hyperbaric treatment is indicated for conditions that are not wound-related (e.g., carbon monoxide poisoning, osteomyelitis, and decompression sickness).

Effects of Hyperbaric Oxygen

Effects of hyperbaric oxygen are twofold. The mechanical effect follows the physical law described by Boyle, which states that as barometric pressure increases, volume decreases. Therefore in the case of decompression sickness or air/gas embolism, hyperbaric treatment can be used to decrease the size of the embolism.

This physiologic effect follows the physical law described by Henry Law, which states that the amount of gas dissolved in a liquid is directly proportional to the partial pressure of the dissolved gas (Hammarlund, 1995; Sheffield, 1998b). The result is that oxygen tensions can be raised 10 to 13 times higher than oxygen breathed at ambient pressure (Hammarlund, 1995).

Hyperbaric Treatment in History

Much of what is know about the physical effects of hyperbaric treatment came from observations and studies of caisson workers and divers. The first description of a pressurization vessel dates to 1662, when Henshaw used bellows to increase and decrease pressures to treat respiratory problems. The nineteenth century saw the advent of caisson workers for bridge construction and the subsequent description of caisson's disease (or decompression sickness), bubble theory, and oxygen toxicity by Paul Bert in 1878 (Elliott, 1995). Eleven years later, Moir used recompression to treat decompression sickness in caisson workers building the Hudson River tunnel. The twentieth century also brought about extensive research and application of hyperbaric therapy for decompression sickness by the military.

Modern use of hyperbaric oxygenation began in 1955 to potentiate the effects of radiation on cancer patients (Kindwall, 1995a; Sheffield, 1998a). The National Academy of Science—National Research Council appointed a committee to review the physiologic basis for hyperbaric oxygenation in 1962 (UHMS, 1996). In 1966, this group published *Fundamentals of Hyperbaric Medicine,* which describes the physical and physiologic effects of hyperbaric oxygen; however, it does not address clinical conditions that were currently being given hyperbaric treatment (UHMS, 1996). The Undersea Medical Society (UMS) was founded in 1967 and was primarily devoted to diving and undersea medicine. The UMS became the Undersea Hyperbaric Medical Society (UHMS) in 1986. The UHMS is the primary, worldwide source of information on hyperbaric and diving medicine. The purpose of the UHMS is to "improve the scientific basis of hyperbaric oxygen therapy, [and] promote sound treatment protocols and standards of practice" (UHMS, 2004).

In addition to the UHMS, the American College of Hyperbaric Medicine offers certification and a method for physicians to set themselves apart as hyperbaric specialists (ACHM, 2004). The American Board of Medical Specialties does offer an examination for hyperbaric medicine that will require the completion of a fellowship in hyperbaric medicine once the grandfather period has expired in 2004. Nurses may obtain national certification in hyperbaric nursing through the Baromedical Nurses Association (BNA), an association that promotes the status and standards of baromedical nursing practice.

Indications for Hyperbaric Oxygenation

Hyperbaric oxygenation (HBO) should be considered an adjunct to wound treatment practices. Not all wounds benefit from hyperbaric treatment, nor are all wounds a candidate for it. Under no circumstance should patients be treated with hyperbaric oxygenation "just to see if it works." Patient selection should focus on the hypoxic nature of wounds. Wound hypoxia should be demonstrated with transcutaneous oxygen pressure (tcPo$_2$) monitoring. The origin of the wound must be considered. A pressure ulcer is best treated with pressure reduction, and a hypoxic wound is best treated by maximization of oxygen to the wound.

Frequently, caregivers question the efficacy of HBO for wounds. Many wound care providers complain that hyperbaric treatment does not work and is extremely expensive. A response to these statements would be that hyperbaric oxygenation is often the "last ditch effort" for problem wounds. These wounds may have responded extremely well had hyperbaric treatment been instituted earlier. Although it is understood that not all wounds heal, consideration for hyperbaric treatment should be given for those patients with lower-extremity wounds when it is known that these wounds may not heal. Hyperbaric treatment could mean the difference between a below- or above-the-knee amputation with appropriate circulatory assessment and preamputation preparation with hyperbaric oxygenation.

The UHMS is the primary source of investigative information related to hyperbaric medicine and diving

BOX 20-1 Indications for Hyperbaric Therapy

- *Air/gas embolism
- *Carbon monoxide poisoning
- *Decompression sickness
- Acute traumatic ischemia
- Compartment syndrome
- Crush injury
- Enhancement of healing in selected problem wounds
- Chronic refractory osteomyelitis
- Clostridial myositis and myonecrosis (gas gangrene)
- Compromised skin grafts and/or flaps
- Exceptional blood loss
- Intracranial abscess
- Necrotizing soft tissue infections
- Delayed radiation injury (soft tissue and bony necrosis)
- Thermal burns

*Primary therapy.
Source: Undersea and Hyperbaric Medical Society (UHMS), http://www.uhms.org/Indications/indications.htm, Accessed October 16, 2005.

BOX 20-2 Wound-Related Indications for Hyperbaric Therapy

- Thermal burns
- Acute traumatic ischemia
- Necrotizing infections
- Chronic refractory osteomyelitis
- Radiation tissue damage
- Compromised skin grafts and/or flaps
- Enhancement of healing in selected problem wounds, which fail to respond to established medical and surgical management:
  Diabetic foot ulcers
  Compromised amputation sites
  Nonhealing traumatic wounds
  Vascular insufficiency ulcers

Source: Undersea and Hyperbaric Medical Society (UHMS), http://www.uhms.org/Indications/indications.htm, Accessed October 16, 2005.

medicine worldwide. The UHMS continuously reviews scientific data on the therapeutic benefit of hyperbaric oxygenation and currently recognizes 13 pathologic conditions that are positively affected by hyperbaric oxygenation (Feldmeier, 2003). The UHMS sets forth treatment protocols and practice standards. The UHMS, as the global source of hyperbaric information, has designated the conditions or disease processes listed in Boxes 20-1 and 20-2 as an indication for hyperbaric therapy (Abramovich et al, 1997; Cianci and Sato, 1994; Elliott, 1995; Goad et al, 1984; Hirn, 1993; Hsu and Wang, 1996; Kindwall, 1995c, 1999; Lee et al, 1989; Ludwig, 1989; Mader, Ortiz, and Calhoun, 1996; Marx, 1995; Siriwanij, Vattanavongs, and Sitprija, 1997; Stegmen, 1998; Stephens, 1996; Tai et al, 1992; Zonis et al, 1995). Hyperbaric oxygenation is the primary therapy for arterial gas embolism, carbon monoxide poisoning, and decompression sickness. When used for any other indication, hyperbaric therapy must be integrated with the appropriate clinical and surgical treatments.

Wound indications for hyperbarics include crush injury, compartment syndrome, acute traumatic ischemia, clostridial myonecrosis and necrotizing infections, chronic refractory osteomyelitis, radiation tissue damage, compromised skin grafts and/or flaps, diabetic lower-extremity wounds, and select other problem wounds. The Wound, Ostomy and Continence Nurses (WOCN) Society recommends considering HBO in the treatment of patients with the following conditions:

- Limb-threatening diabetic wounds of the lower extremity (Wagner grades III and IV) (WOCN Society, 2004)
- Lower-extremity ischemic ulcers that are hypoxic as determined by a $tcPO_2$ level of less than 40 mm Hg and show improvement in periwound $tcPO_2$ levels to approximately 100% pure oxygen at normobaric pressures (WOCN Society, 2002)

Crush injury, compartment syndrome and acute traumatic ischemias benefit from hyperbarics because of the improved oxygen tension in tissue that is inadequately perfused because of a disruption of blood supply and edema associated with injury. Hyperbaric oxygen helps to decrease edema through its vasoconstrictive action. In addition, it helps to decrease reperfusion injury. The use of hyperbarics in these cases is emergent, and patients should be treated as early as possible for the best outcome.

Clostridial myonecrosis and necrotizing fasciitis are emergent conditions treated with hyperbaric oxygen and surgical excision. Clostridial myonecrosis is an anaerobic bacterial infection where clostridial toxins cause tissue death in advance of the bacteria. Hyperbaric oxygen helps to overcome the effects of the toxins and halts the progression of tissue destruction. Necrotizing fasciitis is an acute bacterial infectious process that may include anaerobic and aerobic bacteria that act synergistically to cause rapid tissue destruction. Hyperbarics, as an adjunct to surgical intervention, improves oxygenation and may have a direct effect on anaerobic bacteria as well as improving neutrophil activity.

Chronic osteomyelitis occurs when repeated attempts of standard interventions have failed. It is thought that hyperbaric oxygen improves available oxygen at the bone site to improve leukocyte killing ability through oxidative mechanisms. In addition, antibiotic activity may be enhanced. It is also thought that osteoclastic activity is improved and osteogenesis improved with the use of HBO.

Delayed radiation injury results from endarteritis and subsequent tissue hypoxia. There is typically a latent period of at least 6 months before the effects of delayed injury are seen. Injury may not be seen for many years and is often precipitated by injury or surgical procedures. HBO is used prophylactically before oromaxillary surgical procedures to prevent osteoradionecrosis. Soft-tissue radiation injuries including proctitis and cystitis can also be treated with hyperbaric oxygen. The rationale for the use of hyperbarics is the induction of neovascularization in the irradiated area.

Compromised grafts and flaps benefit from hyperbaric oxygenation through the increased diffusion distance of oxygen to support the ischemic graft or flap. In addition, it is now believed that graft and flap failure may have a component of reperfusion injury that is overcome with the administration of hyperbaric oxygen. Hyperbarics is not indicated in uncomplicated grafts or flaps, nor is it indicated in bioengineered tissues.

Diabetic lower-extremity wounds may benefit from hyperbaric oxygenation. As of April 2003, the Center for Medicare and Medicaid Services recognized diabetic lower-extremity wounds as a treatment indication for hyperbaric oxygen. In order to qualify for this indication, the person must have diabetes and a wound of the lower extremity resulting from diabetes that is Wagner grade III or higher. This wound must have failed to respond to standard wound care including assessment and correction of vascular insufficiency,

maximization of nutritional status, optimization of glycemic control, debridement of nonvital tissue, and maintenance of moist wound healing with the use of topical dressings. The wound must be appropriately offloaded, and infection should be resolving. If the wound has failed to show measurable signs of wound healing for at least 30 days of standard wound care, then HBO can be considered. The beneficial effect of HBO in the diabetic lower-extremity wound is in the maximization of oxygen delivery in what can be demonstrated as a hypoxic wound by transcutaneous oximetry (TCOM). Other data that supports the effectiveness of hyperbaric oxygen includes a TCOM measurement of 40 mm Hg that rises to more than 100 mm Hg while breathing 100% oxygen at 1 atmosphere absolute pressure. TCOM values of more than 400 mm Hg during a hyperbaric oxygen exposure is an indication that a successful outcome in the diabetic lower extremity wound is likely. TCOM values of less than 15 mm Hg when breathing room air and less than 100 mm Hg during a hyperbaric oxygen exposure are predictive of wound healing failure (Broussard, 2003; Feldmeier, 2003; Fife et al, 2002; Fife, 2004).

Hyperbaric oxygenation has been and is being used for other disease processes and conditions (Box 20-3). Although the UHMS does not currently recognize the use of hyperbaric treatment in these instances, research continues and is providing support (Asamoto et al, 2000; Baugh, 2000; Bern, Bern, and Singh,

---

BOX 20-3 Situations for Hyperbaric Therapy Under Investigation
••

Acute myocardial infarction
Acute cerebral vascular accident
Closed head injury
Spinal cord injury
Sickle cell crisis
Rheumatic diseases
Migraine/cluster headache
Multiple sclerosis
Radiation cystitis/proctitis
HIV/AIDS
Cerebral palsy

HIV/AIDS, Human immunodeficiency virus/acquired immunodeficiency syndrome.

2000; Carl et al, 1998; Gottlieb and Neubauer, 1988; Hughes, Schwarer, and Miller, 1998; Ishihara et al, 2001; Jordan, 1998; Kindwall, 1999; Laden, 1998; Mayer et al, 2001; Mychaskiw et al, 2001; Neubauer, 1998; Nighoghossian and Trouillas, 1997; Pascual, 1995; Reillo and Altieri, 1996; Sparacia, Sparacia, and Sansone, 1999; Wallace et al, 1995).

Contraindications

Rigorous assessment of the patient must be completed to rule out contraindications to hyperbaric therapy (Box 20-4). According to Boyle's law, any air-filled cavity must be assessed. Ears and sinus cavities must be assessed for the patient's ability to equalize pressure. A chest x-ray examination will rule out trapping of air in the lungs. Patients with a history of seizure activity should be assessed for seizure control. Hyperbaric treatment is absolutely contraindicated for patients who have a history of receiving bleomycin because this increases the risk for oxygen toxicity. Hyperbaric treatment is also contraindicated for patients receiving cis-platinum, sulfamylon, or disulfiram. Another absolute contraindication is untreated pneumothorax. Relative contraindications to hyperbaric treatment include pregnancy, known malignancy, emphysema, pneumonia,

---

BOX 20-4 Contraindications to Hyperbaric Oxygen Therapy

Absolute Contraindications
- Untreated pneumothorax
- History of bleomycin
- Adriamycin
- Disulfiram
- Cis-platinum
- Sulfamylon (mafenide acetate)

Relative Contraindications
- Pregnancy
- Upper respiratory infection
- Emphysema with CO_2 retention
- Hyperthermia
- Seizure disorder
- Spherocytosis
- History of spontaneous pneumothorax
- History of optic neuritis
- History of surgery for otosclerosis

BOX 20-5 Effects of Hyperbaric Oxygen in Wound Healing

Improved local tissue oxygenation
Improved cellular energy metabolism
Enhanced uptake of PDGF-BB
Promotion of collagen deposition
Promotion of neoangiogenesis
Enhanced epithelial cell migration
Decreased local tissue edema
Increased leukocyte-killing ability
Enhanced effectiveness of antibiotics

PDGF-BB, Platelet Derived Growth Factor—Beta Beta.

---

bronchitis, and hyperthermia (Foster, 1992; Heimbach, 1998; Kindwall, 1999b).

Effects on Wound Healing

The effects of HBO in wound healing are listed in Box 20-5. Disease states such as diabetes, peripheral vascular disease, compromised skin flaps or grafts, irradiation, and crush injury contribute to the development of chronic, problematic wounds. It is well documented in the literature that a relative state of hypoxia is needed for wound healing to occur; however, oxygen is also an essential precursor for select processes and has a multifaceted role in wound healing. Oxygen is required for energy metabolism, collagen synthesis, neovascularization, polymorphonuclear cell function, and antibacterial activity. Neither can cellular function and integrity be maintained, nor can cellular repair occur, without oxygen.

Hyperbaric oxygenation increases the capacity of blood to carry and deliver oxygen to tissues. This hyperoxygenation occurs because oxygen is administered under pressure to the patient. Consequently, hyperbaric treatment significantly enhances oxygen delivery to compromised tissues, increases oxygenation to the tissues, and may restore perfusion to compromised areas. The increased capacity of blood to carry oxygen assists in the restoration of cellular function. The volumetric levels of diffusion achieved with hyperbaric oxygenation are 2 to 3 times those obtained under normobaric conditions.

Increased oxygen enhances the uptake of growth factors. Collagen production is improved when oxygen tensions are increased above 40 mm Hg.

Increased oxygen at the wound site has an angiogenic effect promoting neovascularization and healing. Antibiotic activity is synergistically improved (especially the aminoglycosides) and leukocyte function is improved.

Another effect of hyperbaric oxygenation is vasoconstriction. Oxygen is a powerful vasoconstrictor and can be helpful in managing edema related to traumatic wounding or crush injuries. Although hyperbaric oxygen may seem injurious in that it decreases blood supply to an injured area, the increase in diffusion of oxygen more than compensates for the decrease in circulation associated with vasoconstriction. The effect of hyperbaric oxygenation is instantaneous in blood, with a subsequent plateau in soft tissues approximately 1 hour after exposure. The effect of hyperbaric oxygen declines steadily over 2 to 4 hours after exposure (Bonomo et al, 1998; Boykin, 1996; Davis and Hunt, 1988; Feldmeier, 2003; Hammarlund, 1995; Knighton and Fiegel, 1990; Mader et al, 1990; Sheffield, 1998b; Shilling and Faiman, 1984; Swanson, 1998; Zhao et al, 1994).

Treatment Protocol

Hyperbaric treatment protocols depend upon the specific disease process. Acceptable protocols for hyperbaric exposure have been outlined by the UHMS. However, this does not preclude physician preference and individualization to meet the patient's needs. Typically, a patient will receive a daily hyperbaric exposure 5 to 7 times per week. The treatment will last for 90 minutes at 2.0 to 2.5 ATA. The patient generally receives 40 to 60 treatments. Continuous assessment of the patient's progress assists the physician in determining when the maximum benefit from hyperbaric oxygen therapy has been reached (Feldmeier, 2003).

Patient Preparation and Safety. Two factors dictate that rigorous procedures are followed for patient preparation and patient safety. The first factor is the nature of hyperbarics (i.e., atmospheric pressure changes). Patient instruction should include air equalization techniques to prevent aural or sinus barotrauma. The patient should also be instructed not to hold his or her breath during ascent to prevent pneumothorax. The caregiver responsible for assessing the patient before treatment should assess breath sounds to prevent exposing a patient with compromised pulmonary status to the hyperbaric environment.

A random blood sugar measurement before the treatment should be obtained on all patients with diabetes, because hyperbaric oxygenation can significantly lower blood sugar levels. Vital signs are obtained to assess for hypertension and hyperthermia. Hyperbaric oxygenation is a potent vasoconstrictor and can predispose the patient to a hypertensive crisis; an oral temperature of greater that 102° F predisposes the patient to an oxygen toxicity seizure.

The second factor affecting patient preparation and safety is the pressurized high-oxygen environment. This is significant in any hyperbaric environment and is of extreme importance when the patient is pressurized in a 100% oxygen environment. Patients should be instructed not to use products that have a petroleum or alcohol base before going into the chamber. Box 20-6 provides a list of materials banned in the hyperbaric chamber. Cosmetic products such as hair spray, hair creams, lotions, Vaseline, deodorants, and perfumes must be removed before the treatment. Only cotton linens and clothing are allowed into the chamber to decrease spark potential. Prosthetics should be removed, including hearing aids. Although glasses, contacts lenses, and dentures are not absolutely contraindicated in the hyperbaric environment, they should be removed if the patient is at risk for seizure activity or has an altered mental condition (Hart, 1995;

BOX 20-6 Materials Banned in the Hyperbaric Chamber

• Cosmetic products, including the following:
    Hair spray
    Hair creams
    Lotions
    Deodorants
    Perfumes
    Lipstick
    Fingernail polish
• Petrolatum and products containing petrolatum
• Mineral oil and products containing mineral oil
• Dressing products containing synthetic fibers such as nylon
• Elastic products such as compression wraps
• Any device with a battery, such as hearing aids
• Dentures if at risk for seizure activity
• All jewelry

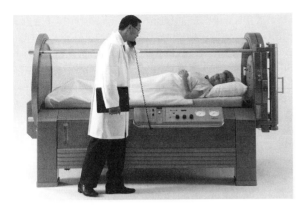

Fig. 20-1 HBO Sechrist 3200 Monoplace Chamber. (Courtesy Sechrist Industries, Anaheim, California.)

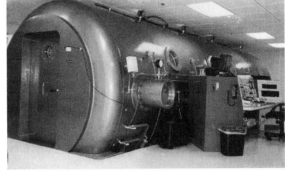

Fig. 20-2 HBO Gulf Coast Multiplace Chamber, outside view. (Courtesy Gulf Coast Hyperbarics, Inc., Panama City, Florida.)

Kindwall, 1995b, 1995e; Larson-Lohr and Norvell, 2002; UHMS, 2003; Weaver and Straas, 1991).

Hyperbaric Procedure. To achieve a hyperbaric state, the patient is placed into either a monoplace chamber or a multiplace chamber. The monoplace chamber (Figure 20-1) has rapidly become the predominant chamber seen in outpatient settings. A monoplace chamber is typically compressed with oxygen. These chambers have a maximum pressurization of 44 psi, or 3 ATA. The major advantage of using a monoplace chamber is that they are relatively inexpensive. The chamber may be placed anywhere that an adequate gas supply is available and can be housed in most areas without significant construction costs. Another advantage is that the monoplace chamber may be staffed by either a technician or nurse and a physician. Current reimbursement guidelines dictate that a physician must be present for the duration of a hyperbaric treatment.

Disadvantages of the monoplace chamber include the lack of direct patient contact it allows and the difficulty involved in monitoring the patient other than visually. Methods are available to monitor electrocardiogram (ECG), arterial blood pressure, pulmonary artery pressure, wedge pressure, central venous pressure, cuff blood pressure, temperature, and $tcPO_2$ monitoring. It is also possible to ventilate a patient in the monoplace chamber (Hart, 1999; Weaver and Straas, 1991).

The multiplace chamber (Figures 20-2 and 20-3) allows a caregiver to enter the chamber with the

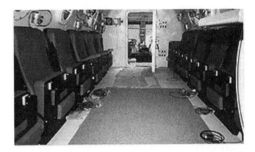

Fig. 20-3 HBO Gulf Coast Multiplace Chamber, inside view. (Courtesy Gulf Coast Hyperbarics, Inc., Panama City, Florida.)

patient. The caregiver, or tender, may be a technician, nurse, or physician. The multiplace chamber can accommodate multiple patients. The number of patients who can be treated simultaneously depends on the size of the chamber and whether the patients are ambulatory or chair- or bed-bound. The multiplace chamber can easily be equipped to handle the critically ill. The critically ill patient can be monitored the same as in the monoplace chamber. To breathe oxygen, the patient wears either a mask or a hood. The major disadvantages of the multiplace chamber include cost and housing of the chamber. The National Fire Protection Association (NFPA, 2002) sets forth structural requirements for a multiplace chamber. Another disadvantage of the multiplace chamber is that if a patient is unable to equalize pressure during pressurization, a multioccupant dive must be aborted. A final consideration of the multiplace chamber is staffing. The multiplace chamber requires a greater expenditure of staff than the monoplace chamber. The multiplace chamber is staffed with a chamber operator, tender, nurse, and physician (Kindwall, 1995e; NFPA, 2002; UHMS, 1994).

Side Effects. The most common side effect or complication of hyperbaric oxygenation is claustrophobia. Patients who experience claustrophobia should be reassured, and a tender should be present and in contact with the patient at all times. In the multiplace chamber the tender can offer direct physical comfort. In the monoplace chamber, the tender should maintain both visual and verbal contact with the patient. Benzodiazapenes offer relief of claustrophobia in most cases. Occasionally, a treatment is aborted and subsequent hyperbaric therapy is discontinued as a result of claustrophobia (Kindwall, 1995d).

Aural barotrauma, referred to as an "ear squeeze," will manifest as ear pain and may result in a hematoma to the tympanic membrane, hemorrhage in the middle ear, or tympanic rupture. If a patient experiences an ear squeeze, a myringotomy or placement of pressure equalization (PE) tubes may be necessary. Sinus barotrauma, or sinus squeeze, results in extreme sinus pain and may lead to hemorrhage of the sinus. The patient who comes for a hyperbaric treatment with a congested nasal passage may benefit from nasal decongestant sprays before the treatment. Oral decongestants may be indicated for a more long-term approach (Capes and Tomaszewski, 1996; Kidder, 1995; Vrabec, Clements, and Mader, 1998).

Visual acuity changes are not rare during hyperbaric therapy. Myopia may worsen after 20 or more hyperbaric exposures. Frequently, a patient who uses glasses to correct presbyopia will find that he or she is able to read without corrective lenses. The exact mechanism behind these visual changes is not known. The patient who experiences a visual change should be instructed not to change prescription eye wear for 2 to 3 months after hyperbaric treatment because the visual change is usually temporary (Maki, 1996).

A physiologic anomaly, breath holding, or cessation of respiration, can cause air to be trapped in the lungs. This trapped air can lead to a tension pneumothorax.

Should this occur in a multiplace chamber, the patient can be recompressed and the pneumothorax can be corrected within the chamber before decompression of the chamber. In a monoplace environment, the patient should be recompressed to treatment depth until supplies, equipment, and personnel are available. Once the team and supplies are assembled, the patient should be decompressed and treated immediately upon removal from the chamber.

Seizure activity from oxygen toxicity, although ominous in appearance, is self-limiting and benign. The patient in the monoplace environment should be maintained at pressure until seizure activity has stopped. If the patient is breathing oxygen by mask or hood, the oxygen should be stopped and the patient placed in air. Once the seizure has stopped, the patient can be removed from the chamber. Generally, no further precautions or anticonvulsant medications are necessary for subsequent treatments. Patients with a known history of seizure or who are predisposed to seizure activity would benefit from periodic, scheduled discontinuation of oxygen breathing (air breaks) during the treatment (Clark, 1995).

NEGATIVE-PRESSURE WOUND THERAPY

Negative-pressure wound therapy (NPWT) is a mechanical wound care treatment that uses controlled negative pressure to assist and accelerate wound healing. NPWT supports wound healing by evacuating wound fluids, stimulating granulation tissue formation, reducing the bacterial burden of a wound, and maintaining a moist wound environment. NPWT is achieved by placing open-cell reticulated foam dressing into the wound, achieving a seal with semiocclusive drape, and applying subatmospheric pressure via an evacuation tube connected to a computerized pump.

Mechanisms of Action

The mechanisms of action related to NPWT must be understood to support the rationale for its use in clinical practice. Known effects of NPWT fall into the following broad categories: fluid impact, wound perfusion, mechanical stretch, granulation tissue formation, and bioburden management.

Fluid Impact. One of the cornerstones of NPWT is the removal of fluid from a wound via suction, negative pressure. As the stagnant wound fluid is removed, harmful proinflammatory mediators are also removed. In addition to the removal of potentially infectious stagnant wound fluid, NPWT causes an interstitial gradient shift. This interstitial gradient shift is responsible for reduced edema, which leads to increased dermal perfusion (Morykwas, 1997a; Swartz, et al, 2001).

Banwell (1999) reported that interstitial fluid flow could modify the extracellular matrix components and alter organization of these products, including increased growth factor expression, cellular mitosis and decreased proteases. The benefits of decreased periwound edema (i.e., "third spacing") along with the cellular reorganization in the microenvironment of the wound are slowly becoming understood.

Perfusion. Data that supports quantitative effects of NPWT on wound perfusion include a porcine model, which responded to the application of NPWT, delivered at 125 mm Hg with a four-fold increase in blood flow (Morykwas et al, 1997b). The effects of NPWT on the vascular status of a wound is not completely understood but is likely due, in part, to interstitial fluid shifting, or edema resolution, which decompresses small vessels allowing more efficient blood flow. In addition to increased blood flow related to decompression, NPWT is also thought to enhance angiogenesis in the dermal vasculature via mechanical stretch that is theorized as mediated by enhancing vasomotor tone and vasoactive mediators. In another study, an immediate increase in blood flow was validated with transcutaneous ultrasonic Doppler velocity meter and laser Doppler imaging on the forearms of uninjured volunteers in response to NPWT (Banwell et al, 2003). The application of NPWT to burn wounds within 6 hours of injury has been reported to result in statistically significant increases in dermal blood flow (Banwell et al, 2002).

Mechanical Stretch. The mechanical stretch experienced by cells in the environment of negative pressure triggers an increased rate of cellular proliferation (i.e., neoangiogenesis and epithelialization) (Sumpio, 1987; Ryan and Barnhill, 1983). Another effect is uniform wound size reduction which results from equally distributed mechanical forces across the wound. Research conducted by Morykwas and colleagues (2003) suggests that gene activation may occur during wound healing and that by applying controlled stress, NPWT increases gene groups related to cellular proliferation and tissue growth.

Granulation Tissue Formation. One of the most obvious effects of NPWT is the stimulation of granulation tissue formation. Granulation tissue relies on the development of new capillary growth to develop a collagen matrix. Research quantifying this observation is limited to animal studies that indicate increased granulation tissue formation in pig wound models by 63% and 103.4% (continuous and intermittent therapy respectively) (Morykwas, 1997b).

Bioburden Management. Wound fluid is an excellent medium for bacterial growth. By removing stagnant wound fluid, the amount of bacterial colonization within a wound is decreased. This, along with increased circulation that results in higher nutrient and oxygen levels available to the wound, enhances resistance to infection. This process is beneficial to the process of wound healing because infection delays any phase of the wound-healing trajectory. The transparent dressing that secures NPWT to the wound also protects the wound from possible environmental bacterial assaults. Bacterial counts obtained from wound fluid in wounds with and without NPWT show a significant reduction in bacterial colonization in those receiving NPWT (Morykwas, 1997a). Microbiologic and Gram's staining of fluid from NPWT-treated wounds demonstrates large numbers of bacteria along with significant reduction in wound bioburden (Van Wicjck, 2002).

Indications

Because NPWT capitalizes on the body's own healing qualities to assist and accelerate wound healing, a patient must have an overall physiologic capacity to heal in order to be an appropriate candidate. Wounds must be free of necrotic tissue. Chronic wounds such as stages III and IV pressure ulcers, diabetic ulcers, acute and traumatic dehisced wounds, partial thickness burns, skin grafts, and muscle flaps are approved for NPWT.

Contraindications and Precautions

Contraindications and precautions for NPWT are listed in Box 20-7. Contraindications for NPWT include nonviable tissue within the wound bed, untreated osteomyelitis, nonenteric/unexplored fistulae, and malignancy

BOX 20-7 Contraindications and Precautions for Negative-Pressure Wound Therapy (NPWT)

Contraindications
• Malignancy in the wound
• Untreated osteomyelitis
• Nonenteric and unexplored fistula
• Necrotic tissue with eschar present
• Do not place V.A.C. dressing over exposed blood vessels or organs

Precautions
• Precautions should be taken for patients with the following:
   Active bleeding
   Anticoagulants
   Difficult wound hemostasis

Difficult wound hemostasis
• When placing V.A.C. Freedom dressings in close proximity to blood vessels or organs, take care to ensure that all vessels are adequately protected with overlying fascia, tissue or other protective barriers.
• Greater care should be taken with respect to weakened, irradiated, or sutured blood vessels or organs.
• Bone fragments or sharp edges could puncture protective barriers, vessels, or organs.
• Follow universal precautions
• Wound with enteric fistula requires special precautions to optimize V.A.C. therapy. Refer to V.A.C. *Therapy Clinical Guidelines* for detailed recommendations.

Source: http://www.kci1.com/products/VAC/vacfreedom/index.asp#indications; Accessed October 16, 2005.

in the wound. Response of tissue to mechanical forces is characterized by increased proliferation of cells. Malignant cells differ in genetic make-up and do not respond to the mechanical forces delivered in NPWT.

Precautions to consider when evaluating a patient for possible NPWT include unstable hemostasis. Active bleeding or use of anticoagulants does not render a patient inappropriate for negative-pressure wound therapy, but continued frequent assessment must be maintained and considered throughout the therapy. When vital organs are exposed, precautions such as the placement of mesh products over the organs to provide a protective interface layer should be deliberated.

NPWT has been successfully placed directly over the heart, the lung, the liver, the bowel, and the spleen (Morykwas et al, 1997b).

Application of NPWT

Once a patient has been deemed appropriate for treatment with NPWT and the device is applied, dressing changes are performed every 48 hours for most wounds, although many institutions have adopted a Monday-Wednesday-Friday schedule for ease of scheduling. The reticulated polyurethane dressings that are included with the FDA approved (Food and Drug Administration) device for NPWT are made of open cell foam to ensure equal distribution of the applied negative-pressure force to every surface of the wound communicating with the foam. The foam is trimmed to fit the entire surface of the wound, including sinus tracts and tunnels. Table 20-1 offers guidelines for foam selection.

There are numerous variations on the NPWT pump that offer varied sizes and functions such as a smaller (mini) unit or a unit that periodically instills fluids into a wound. A commonly used NPWT unit is pictured in Figure 20-4. Once the foam is placed and secured to the periwound skin with a clear adhesive drape, an opening is made (Figure 20-5) to accommodate an evacuation tube (Figure 20-6). This tubing will facilitate evacuation of wound fluid into a collection chamber located on the computerized vacuum pump. The distal end of the evacuation tubing is attached to a collection canister, completing a closed system from the wound to the collection canister.

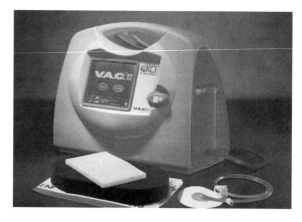
Fig. 20-4 The V.A.C. ATS System. (Courtesy KCI USA, Inc., San Antonio, Texas.)

TABLE 20-1 **Guidelines for NPWT Foam Selection**

POLYURETHANE FOAM	• Black, reticulated open-pored dressing that is effective in stimulating granulation tissue while supporting wound contraction • Hydrophobic properties of this foam repel moisture, which enhances exudate removal
POLYVINYL FOAM	• White, dense foam with a higher tensile strength compared to the polyurethane foam • Premoistened with sterile water and possesses overall nonadherent properties • Hydrophilic properties of this foam retain moisture • Indicated when granulation tissue formation must be controlled or when patient cannot tolerate the polyurethane foam

WOUND CHARACTERISTICS	INDICATED FOAM		
	Polyurethane Foam	Polyvinyl Foam	Either Foam
Deep, acute wounds with moderate granulation tissue present	■		
Deep pressure ulcers	■		
Flaps	■		
Painful wounds		■	
Tunneling, sinus tracts/undermining		■	
Deep trauma wounds			■
Wounds which require controlled growth of granulation tissue		■	
Diabetic ulcers			■
Dry wounds			■
Graft and bioengineered skin placement			■
Shallow chronic ulcers			■

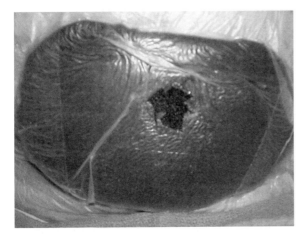

Fig. 20-5 NPWT foam is placed and secured. An opening is made to accommodate an evacuation tube. (Courtesy Susan Mendez-Eastman.)

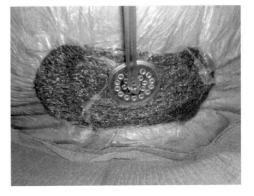

Fig. 20-6 NPWT Foam collapse. (Courtesy Susan Mendez-Eastman.)

TABLE 20-2 Recommended Therapy Guidelines for Treating Various Wound Types with NPWT

INITIAL CYCLE	SUBSEQUENT CYCLE	TARGET PRESSURE POLYURETHANE FOAM	TARGET PRESSURE POLYVINYL FOAM	DRESSING CHANGE INTERVAL
ACUTE AND TRAUMATIC WOUNDS AND PARTIAL THICKNESS BURNS				
Continuous first 48 hours	Intermittent for the duration of therapy	125 mm Hg	125-175 mm Hg (titrate up to accommodate excessive drainage)	Monday, Wednesday, Friday
SURGICAL WOUND DEHISCENCE				
Continuous throughout the duration of therapy		125 mm Hg	125-175 mm Hg (titrate up to accommodate excessive drainage)	Monday, Wednesday Friday
MESHED GRAFTS AND BIOENGINEERED TISSUES				
Continuous throughout the duration of therapy		75-125 mm Hg	125-175 mm Hg (titrate up to accommodate excessive drainage)	Remove dressing after 3-5 days
PRESSURE ULCERS				
Continuous first 48 hours	Intermittent for the duration of therapy	125 mm Hg	125-175 mm Hg (titrate up to accommodate excessive drainage)	Monday, Wednesday, Friday
CHRONIC WOUNDS				
Continuous first 48 hours	Intermittent for the duration of therapy	75-125 mm Hg	125-175 mm Hg (titrate up to accommodate excessive drainage)	Remove dressing after 3-5 days
FLAPS				
Continuous throughout the duration of therapy		75-125 mm Hg	125-175 mm Hg (titrate up to accommodate excessive drainage)	Remove dressing after 3-5 days

Once the dressing is in place and attached to the computerized NPWT unit, controlled negative pressure is applied. The target pressures for negative-pressure wound therapy vary from 75 mm Hg to 175 mm Hg, depending on the characteristics of the individual wound. The cycle of therapy, continuous or intermittent, is also based on research and general guidelines available from the manufacturers of NPWT units (Table 20-2). Continuous therapy maximizes removal of wound fluid and surrounding edema. Intermittent therapy usually runs on a cycle of 5 minutes of negative pressure followed by 2 minutes of no pressure, but it can be changed to reflect specific physician orders. The intermittent cycle capitalizes on the effects of mechanical stretch and repetitive release of biochemical messengers to the wound by alternating pressure and nonpressure. The parameters for negative pressure can be changed, if necessary, to accommodate excessive drainage or desiccation in the wound bed.

The wound is attached to the negative-pressure pump throughout the treatment. The evacuation tubing is long enough to allow limited movement around the pump. The tubing can also be clamped and disconnected for short periods of time. There are also portable NPWT devices on the market that fit into a waist pack and run on battery power for several hours. These allow the patient receiving NPWT to move freely and encourage increased activity as wound healing continues. If the negative pressure must be off for an extended amount of time, the NPWT dressing should be removed and replaced with a moisture-retentive dressing. Leaving the dressing assembly in a wound that is not receiving NPWT could lead to complications such as infection. The concept of controlled negative pressure for wound healing capitalizes on a dynamic system of events. If the dynamic nature of the therapy is stopped, the stagnant dressings beneath a semiocclusive film can become a hindrance to healing and may even cause damage to healthy tissue.

Monitoring of the dressing, the periwound site, the computerized pump and its parameters, and fluid collection are included in the daily maintenance of NPWT. The dressing assembly used in NPWT should be evaluated routinely for foam collapse and adherence (Figure 20-6). As with any therapy, the area visible around the dressing must be monitored for changes in character, such as erythema or warmth. The character and the amount of wound drainage in the collection canister must also be assessed at least daily and should be documented. Acute changes in wound characteristics should be reported to the physician. Wound measurement, tissue and fluid characterization, odor, pain, and the periwound site should be monitored and documented with each dressing change.

Dressing changes for NPWT are completed at the patient bedside using aseptic technique. Boxes 20-8 and 20-9 list guidelines for NPWT dressing application and removal. The disposable collection canister located on the computerized NPWT unit is changed weekly or as it is filled. The computerized pump has a digital display and alarms that indicate if the programmed pressure is not being maintained, the canister is full, or there is a blockage detected in the closed tubing system. If the NPWT pump alarm signals a leak, the dressing should be checked for leaks. Leaks in the transparent dressing can be patched with extra dressing or alternative transparent film. An airtight seal is necessary to maintain a negative-pressure environment. An alarm indicating that a blockage is detected should prompt the caregiver to release the clamps on the tubing assembly and to inspect the tubing assembly for a kink or a visible blockage within the tubing.

Pain has been reported in association with NPWT and may be triggered by the application of the suction or removal of the dressing (Hartnett, 1998). The use of analgesics at dressing changes can reduce the procedural pain (e.g., pain caused by dressing removal). Lowering the initial amount of negative pressure or the intensity in which the pressure is initially applied can also decrease pain. Increasing the amount of negative pressure slowly may allow the patient to tolerate the therapy, if pain is a factor. Additional strategies that can be used to address pain related to NPWT are listed in Box 20-10.

Use with Skin Grafts. When NPWT is used to enhance incorporation of a split-thickness mesh skin graft, it is placed over the graft intraoperatively. A nonadherent interface material must be laid on top of the graft before placement of polyurethane sponge. The placement of a nonadherent dressing protects the fragile graft from possible trauma during dressing removal and encourages capillary growth into the graft without an overgrowth of granulation tissue formation. Polyvinyl foam, which is premoistened and hydrophilic,

BOX 20-8 Recommendations for Applying the Negative-Pressure Wound Therapy Foam Dressing

1. Carefully remove the existing wound dressing and discard per institutional protocols.
2. Debride any eschar, hardened slough, or non-viable tissue.
3. Ensure adequate hemostasis.
4. Cleanse wound according to institutional protocols or physician order.
5. Cleanse and dry periwound tissue.
6. Prepare periwound tissue with a skin preparation product to enhance adherence of adhesive drape and assist in nontraumatic removal of adhesive drape.
7. Assess wound dimensions and pathology and select appropriate foam type and size.
8. Cut foam to the dimensions that will allow the foam to be placed gently into the wound.
   a. Do not cut the foam over the wound.
   b. Gently rub the freshly cut edges of the foam to remove any loose particles.
   c. Do not over pack the foam into the wound since this may cause damage to wound bed tissue.
9. Gently place the foam into the wound cavity, filling the entire wound base and sides, tunnels, and undermined areas.
   a. Count the number of pieces of foam and document the total number in the patient chart.
   b. Multiple pieces of foam can be used to adequately fill the wound.
   c. Ensure edges of multiple pieces of foam are in direct contact with each other to achieve even distribution of negative pressure.
10. Size and trim the adhesive drape to cover the foam dressing and overlap onto intact periwound tissue.
    a. Do not discard extra drape; you may need it later to patch any leaks.
11. Apply the tubing to the dressing.
    a. Cut a hole in the drape large enough to accommodate the specific tubing assembly.
    b. Using the attached tubing adhesive drape, or additional dressing drape, seal the tubing assembly on top of the dressing and ensure that it will not lie on bony prominences.

BOX 20-9 Recommendations for Removing the Negative-Pressure Wound Therapy Foam Dressing

1. Raise the tubing connections above the level of the therapy unit.
2. Engage clamp on the dressing tubing.
3. Separate canister tubing and dressing tubing at the connection junction.
4. Allow the therapy unit to pull any drainage in the canister tubing into the canister, then engage the clamp on the canister tubing.
5. Gently stretch drape horizontally and slowly pull up from the skin.
   a. Do not peel the drape.
6. Gently remove foam from the wound.
7. Discard dressing materials per institutional protocols.
8. Cleanse wound according to institutional protocols or physician order.

BOX 20-10 Troubleshooting: Pain Issues Related to the Use of Negative-Pressure Wound Therapy

The following interventions may be considered if a patient is experiencing pain related to negative-pressure wound therapy:
- Educate the patient as to what to expect before dressing changes or therapy initiation.
- Pressure setting can be adjusted downward to reduce pain.
- Use of the polyvinyl foam instead of the polyurethane foam.
- Using continuous-negative pressure throughout treatment course.
- Application of skin protection product before application of adhesive drape.
- Using a nonadherent meshed interface between the wound bed and the foam dressing.
- Allowing the patient to assist with dressing removal.
- Administration of prescribed topical or systemic analgesics before dressing removal.

can be placed directly on top of the skin graft. Anything that causes a graft to lose a snug fit against the vascular-rich bed of the wound places the graft at risk of failure. Split-thickness skin grafts often fail because of movement or an accumulation of fluid beneath the graft. NPWT assists with successful "take" of split-thickness mesh skin grafts by decreasing the ability of the graft to shift and evacuating fluid that may build up beneath the graft to cause a gap in the interfacing of the graft and vascular matrix of the wound bed. NPWT is used on split-thickness mesh skin grafts for 3 to 5 days following surgery. Upon removal of the dressing, the graft is evaluated for adherence. If the graft has a full take, NPWT is removed and discontinued. If there are areas of the graft that have not adhered, NPWT can be replaced for up to 3 additional days. If excess graft was harvested in surgery, it can be applied before NPWT replacement if needed. The addition of banked graft can be done at the bedside without the requirement of an additional surgical procedure. Continuous rather than intermittent therapy is used when placing NPWT over split-thickness meshed skin grafts.

ELECTRICAL STIMULATION

Electrical stimulation is a physical wound care modality that uses the transfer of electrical current to tissues to support wound healing. Devices used for wound healing applications consist of a source of electrical current, a minimum of two wires, or leads, and their corresponding electrodes (Figure 20-7). One lead is connected to the negative jack of the device and is the source of negatively charged electrons in an electrical circuit. This is referred to as the cathode. The other is connected to a positive jack on the device that serves as an electron depository for the flow of electrons in the electrical circuit. This is called the anode. Electrodes are attached to the patient end of the wires and placed on either the patient's wound bed or the adjacent skin. When the device is operating, a unidirectional current flows through this circuit causing positively charged ions (Na^+, K^+, and H^+) in the tissues and positively charged cells (activated neutrophils and fibroblasts) to migrate toward the cathode; negatively charged ions (Cl^-, HCO_3^-, and P^-) and negatively charged cells (epidermal, neutrophils, and macrophages) migrate toward the anode.

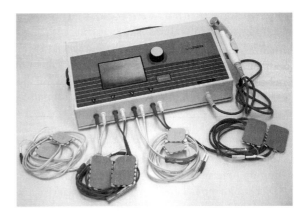

Fig. 20-7 Example of a high-voltage pulsed current electrical stimulation device. (Courtesy Rich-Mar Corporation, Inola, Oklahoma)

Physiologic effects of electrical stimulation will be described in this chapter and include the following:
- Galvanotaxic effect
- Stimulatory effects of cells
- Blood flow and tissue oxygenation
- Antibacterial effect

In an effort to examine the entire body of evidence on electrical stimulation and chronic wound healing, Gardner, Frantz, and Schmidt (1999) conducted a meta-analysis of 15 studies that assessed the efficacy of electrical stimulation. Studies included in the meta-analysis were limited to randomized, controlled trials (n = 9) and nonrandom, controlled trials (n = 6). Meta-analysis procedures were applied to a total of 24 electrical stimulation samples (n = 591 wounds) and 15 control samples wounds (n = 212). The calculated average rate of healing for the electrical stimulation samples was 22% per week compared to 9% for the control samples. The net effect of the electrical stimulation therapy was 13% per week, a 144% increase over the control rate. These data provide compelling evidence that electrical stimulation can produce a substantial improvement in the healing of chronic wounds.

Types of Electrical Stimulation

Although several electrotherapy modalities are cited in the literature, there are basically only two types of electrical current: direct current (DC) and alternating current (AC). However, alternating current is not being used in the treatment of wounds. The devices used to deliver the direct current are capable of delivering a current in a "pulsed" pattern. The term "pulsed," therefore, has been incorporated into the nomenclature of electrical stimulation (American Physical Therapy Association, 1990). This section will focus on the clinical application of direct current (DC) and pulsed current (PC).

To understand the basis of electrical stimulation as an adjunctive therapy for wounds, it is important to understand several terms. Table 20-3 provides a definition of terms relevant to electrical stimulation.

Direct Current. Direct current is characterized as a continuous, monophasic waveform (i.e., no pulses) in which the voltage does not vary with time. The parameters used to stimulate wound healing are typically 200 to 300 μA at a low voltage (less than 100 volts). The polarity that is selected determines the direction of current flow delivered to the wound tissue, with positively charged ions migrating toward the negative electrode (cathode) and negatively charged ions migrating toward the positive electrode (anode).

Wolcott and colleagues (1969) conducted one of the earliest clinical trials testing DC on human subjects with 75 ischemic skin ulcers previously resistant to healing. The specific current tested was low-intensity DC, which is DC with an amplitude of less than 1 mA.

TABLE 20-3 **Electrical Stimulation: Terms and Definitions**

TERMS	DEFINITIONS
Alternating current	Uninterrupted, bidirectional current flow
Amplitude	The maximum (peak) excursion of a voltage or current pulse
Amperage	Measure of the rate of flow of current; expressed as amperes (A), milliamperes (mA), or microamperes (μA)
Coulombs (C) or microcoulombs (μC)	Charge: a property of matter determined by the proportion of electrons (negatively charged particles) it contains; substance may be neutral, or positively or negatively charged; measured in units called coulombs
Current	Rate of flow of charged particles (ions or electrons); measured in units of amperes (A) or milliampere (mA)
Direct current	Uninterrupted, unidirectional current flow
Frequency	Number of pulses delivered per unit of time; also termed pulse rate. Frequency is the reciprocal of cycle time. Usually measured as pulses per second (pps), or Hertz (Hz). 0.1 Hz is on for 10 seconds, and a pulse of 1000 Hz is on for 1 millisecond.
Interpulse interval	Time between pulses when there is no voltage applied and no current flowing
Polarity	Property of possessing two oppositely charged electrodes in an electrical circuit (positive and negative); negative electrode (cathode) provides electrons in a circuit; positive electrode (anode) serves as depository to which electrons flow
Pulse duration	Time during which current is flowing
Voltage	Measure of force of the flow of electrons through a conductor (wound tissue) between two or more electrodes; created by difference of charges between two electrodes (one with excess in relation to the other); electrodes are polarized in comparison to each other (negative electrode and positive electrode)
Waveform	Graphic representation of current flow; may be monophasic (current that deviates from the isoelectric zero line in one direction and then returns to baseline) or biphasic (current that deviates above and below the isoelectric zero line); may be symmetric or asymmetric

They reported complete healing of 34 of the lesions with treatment, and the range of improvement in the remaining 41 ranged from 0% to 97%. Gault and Gatens (1976) subsequently reported similar results with the use of low-voltage continuous microamperage DC. Using six subjects with contralateral ulcerations as controls, their results showed a mean weekly healing rate of 30% for the treated group compared with 14.7% for the control group. Mean healing after 4 weeks was 74% in those treated with electrical stimulation and 27.3% in the controls. The benefits of DC were further substantiated by Carley and Wainapel (1985), who studied 30 subjects with chronic ulcerations who were paired according to age, diagnosis, and ulcer cause, location, and size. One member of the pair received low-voltage continuous microamperage DC therapy, whereas the other acted as the control. Results showed a 1.5 to 2.5 times faster healing rate for the treated group as compared with the controls. In each of these studies, treatment was initiated using the cathode as the active electrode and switching to the anode following a few days of therapy. A fourth study evaluated the effect of direct current on healing of venous ulcers (Assimacopoulos, 1968). Eight venous ulcers that had persisted from 8 months to 5 years were treated with 50 to 100 µA of DC, using the cathode applied to the wound tissue. All of the ulcers healed in an average of 30 days.

An important consideration in wounds being treated with DC is the potential for untoward skin irritation. Because the charged ions of Na^+ and Cl^- in the wound tissue move toward the cathode and anode, respectively, a chemical reaction occurs that produces caustic end products at the interface of electrode and tissue. In the case of the cathode, Na^+ reacts with H_2O to form NaOH and H_2, whereas the anode reacts with Cl^- and H_2O to form HCL and O_2. Even when DC is delivered at therapeutic doses, these products form at the electrode tissue interface, creating acid-base changes. If the dosage of DC is delivered at high amplitude over an extended period, the acid-base changes lead to tissue irritation that varies in intensity from erythema to blistering from electrochemical burning. This side effect can be diminished to some extent by using current amplitudes in the microamperage (µA) range.

Pulsed Current (PC). PC is characterized by a brief flow of unidirectional or bidirectional charged particles followed by a longer period of absent flow (American Physical Therapy Association, 1990). Electrodes placed on the tissues deliver the PC as a series of pulses, with each pulse separated by a period in which no current is flowing. PC can be visually constructed as a waveform that plots amplitude and time. Two types of waveforms are available as PC: monophasic and biphasic.

Direction of current (monophasic or biphasic). Figure 20-8 shows patterns of current for electrical stimulation waveforms. Monophasic PC is the movement of current in one direction away from the isoelectric zero line. Monophasic PC has been applied to clinical treatment of wounds using rectangular waveform (Feedar, Kloth, and Gentzkow, 1991; Gentzkow et al, 1991, 1993; Junger et al, 1997; Kjartansson et al, 1988; Weiss, Eaglstein, and Falanga, 1989) and twin-peaked waveform of high voltage (Akers and Gabrielson, 1984; Fitzgerald and Newsome, 1993; Griffin et al, 1991; Kloth and Feedar, 1988).

Biphasic PC is the movement of current in two directions on either side of the isoelectric zero line. Biphasic pulsed current is configured as charged particles moving above and below the isoelectric zero line in brief succession. The biphasic waveform may be *symmetrical or asymmetrical* with respect to the isoelectric zero line. The biphasic symmetrical waveform is characterized by an identical amplitude, duration, and rate of rise and decays of the current in relation to the isoelectric zero line. This creates a balanced electrical charge. In contrast, with the biphasic asymmetrical waveform, one or more of these elements of the current are unequal in relation to the isoelectric zero line. This produces waveforms that may be electrically balanced or unbalanced. Both biphasic symmetrical (Baker et al, 1996, 1997; Debreceni et al, 1995) and asymmetrical (Baker et al, 1996, 1997) waveforms have been studied as a modality for promoting wound healing.

Voltage of current. Although the various types of current require different stimulation parameters, the research evidence identifies a range of electrical charge that has supported positive wound-healing outcomes (Feedar, Kloth, and Gentzkow, 1991; Gentzkow et al, 1991, 1993; Griffin et al, 1991; Junger et al, 1997; Kloth and Feedar, 1988). This dosage of current, defined in microcoulombs (µC), is between 250 and 500 µC/sec.

The evolution of electrical stimulation devices lead to the evaluation of two different types of PC for

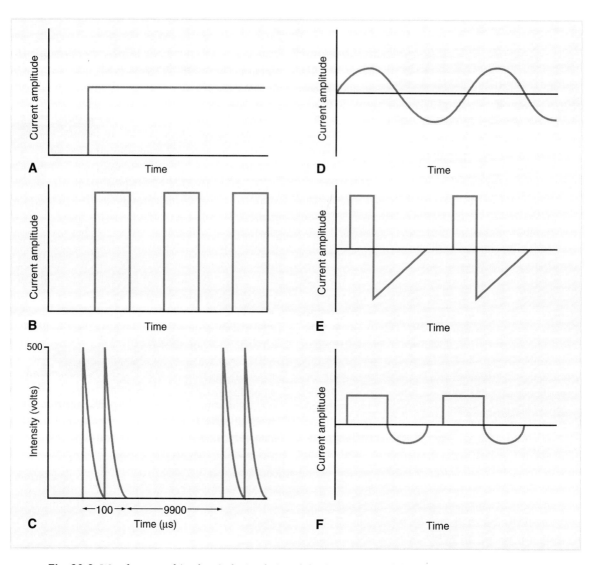

Fig. 20-8 Waveforms used in electrical stimulation. (**A**) Direct current; (**B**) Monophasic pulsed current; (**C**) Monophasic high voltage pulsed current; (**D**) Symmetric biphasic pulsed current (balanced); (**E**) Asymmetric biphasic pulsed current (balanced); (**F**) Asymmetric biphasic pulsed current (unbalanced). (Modified from Dyson M: Adjuvant therapies: ultrasound, laser therapy, electrical stimulation, hyperbaric oxygen and negative pressure therapy. In: Morison MJ, Ovington LG, editors: *Chronic wound care: a problem-based learning approach,* Edinburgh, Scotland, 2004, Mosby.)

treatment of chronic wounds: low-voltage amplitude and high-voltage amplitude. The low-voltage amplitude devices deliver PC with either a monophasic or biphasic waveform. Their pulse durations are relatively long and, consequently, low driving voltages (less than 150 V) are adequate. The high-voltage amplitude devices provide only monophasic PC. Their pulses are of short duration (10 to 20 microseconds),

and therefore these devices must have a high driving voltage (greater than 150 V). Each of these types of electrical stimulation devices has been examined in clinical studies of wound healing.

Low-voltage, monophasic pulsed current. One example of a low-voltage, monophasic PC is transcutaneous electrical nerve stimulation, or TENS. Clinical studies of low-voltage monophasic PC have been conducted with a variety of chronic wounds. However, they have used a relatively common set of treatment parameters consisting of a pulse duration of 140 to 150 microseconds, peak pulse amplitude of 30 to 35 mA, and pulse frequency of either 64 or 128 pulses per second (Feedar, Kloth, and Gentzkow, 1991; Gentzkow et al, 1991, 1993; Junger et al, 1997). These parameters created a collective pulse charge of 250 to 500 microcoulombs ($\mu C/sec$), producing a total "dose" of 0.89 to 1.78 coulombs (C) of electrical charge delivered to the wound each day.

In a randomized, controlled trial of 50 chronic wounds of different etiologies, Feedar, Kloth, and Gentzkow (1991) treated 26 ulcers twice daily for 30 minutes with pulsed cathodal stimulation at a frequency of 128 pulses per second and a peak amplitude of 29.2 mA. The negative polarity electrode was maintained until the ulcer was debrided and serosanguinous drainage appeared. Thereafter, the polarity was alternated between positive and negative every 3 days until the wound filled with granulation tissue. At this stage of healing, the frequency was decreased to 64 pulses per second while maintaining the same peak amplitude. The polarity of the treatment electrode was changed daily until the wound healed. The remaining 24 ulcers received a placebo control. The weekly rate of healing for the active treatment was 14% compared with 8.25% for the control group.

Using a similar protocol, Gentzkow and colleagues (1991) studied 37 subjects with 40 ulcers that were treated with low-voltage monophasic PC or a placebo for 30 minutes twice daily. At the end of the 4-week trial, the ulcers treated with the electrical stimulation showed a 49.8% decrease in surface area compared with a 23.4% decrease in size of the placebo treated ulcers (p = 0.042). The rate of healing of the actively stimulated group of ulcers was 12.5% per week compared with 5.8% per week for the placebo-treated group.

In a follow-up to their initial study, Gentzkow and colleagues (1993) conducted a prospective, baseline-controlled study in which all subjects received the same standardized, optimal wound treatment for 4 weeks (phase I). Those that did not show evidence of progress toward closure or appeared to deteriorate during the phase I control period were entered into phase II of the study. Sixty-one wounds on 51 patients were enrolled in phase 2, in which two 30-minute electrical stimulation treatments with low-voltage monophasic PC were added to standard wound care. Progress toward closure was measured as improvement in two or more wound characteristics or a change of at least one wound stage. Wounds were treated for a mean of 7.3 weeks, and 55 of the 61 wounds (82%) showed improvement in two or more wound characteristics, and 45 of 61 wounds improved by one or more wound stages.

The efficacy of low-voltage monophasic PC was investigated by another team of investigators in a multisite clinical trial (Wood et al, 1993). Although described as "pulsed low intensity direct current," the electrical stimulation used in this study was in reality a form of low-voltage monophasic pulsed current. The sample consisted of 71 patients with 74 stages 2 and 3 pressure ulcers. Forty-three ulcers were treated with an active device, and 31 ulcers received a placebo treatment 3 times a week, for 8 weeks, as part of a double-blinded protocol. Negative current was delivered initially via probe electrodes at 0.8 pulses per second to three different locations on opposite sides of the ulcer for 1 minute at 300 μA, followed by 3 minutes at each site at 600 μA. Of the 43 ulcers in the active treatment group, 25 had healed by the end of 8 weeks, whereas only one of the 31 ulcers in the placebo group healed. Although the low number of ulcers that healed in the placebo group raises questions regarding the effectiveness of the standard treatment used in the study, the response to the electrical stimulation is encouraging.

Low-voltage monophasic PC has been studied to a more limited extent for healing of venous leg ulcers. Junger and associates (1997) report treating 15 venous leg ulcers with low-voltage monophasic PC following failure to respond to standard compression therapy during a mean treatment duration of 79 months. Following treatment with electrical stimulation for an average of 38 days, the mean ulcer area had decreased from 16 to 6 cm^2, a change of 63% (p < 0.01).

Low-voltage, biphasic pulsed current. Studies of low-voltage, biphasic PC are limited to treatment of wounds in patients with impaired neurologic function secondary to spinal cord injury or diabetic neuropathy. In the study of patients with spinal cord injury, Baker and colleagues (1996) investigated the symmetric and the asymmetric biphasic waveform, as well as microcurrent stimulation. Subjects were randomly assigned to one of the three electrical stimulation treatment groups or the control group. Electrical stimulation was applied to a total of 185 pressure ulcers for 30 minutes daily. Analysis of the "good response" ulcer (n = 104) showed significantly better healing rates for those receiving stimulation with the asymmetric biphasic wave form compared with the control and microcurrent groups. However, healing rates for the symmetric biphasic–treated ulcers did not differ significantly from the other treatment groups.

A second study by Baker and colleagues (1997) applied the same treatment protocols in random fashion to 80 subjects with diabetic foot ulcers. Consistent with the findings of the earlier study, the healing rate for the asymmetric biphasic waveform group was significantly faster than for the control group (defined as the combined microcurrent stimulation and sham control groups). Healing of the symmetric biphasic-treated group failed to show a significant difference from the other treatment groups. Although these findings suggest that low-voltage, biphasic PC can augment healing when used in conjunction with standard wound care treatments, the contribution of the specific waveform characteristics (symmetric vs. asymmetric) remains unclear.

High-voltage pulsed current. Figure 20-7 shows an example of a high-voltage PC device. The effects of high-voltage PC on healing of chronic wounds have been investigated in both pressure ulcers and diabetic foot ulcers. Kloth and Feedar (1988) studied 16 subjects with stage IV pressure ulcers who were randomly assigned to receive either a high-voltage PC or a sham treatment in addition to standard wound care. The high-voltage PC was applied for 45 minutes, 5 days a week at 105 pulses per second and a current amplitude sufficient to produce a muscle contraction. This produced a charge of 342 μC/sec delivered to the ulcer tissue. The ulcers treated with the high-voltage PC had a mean healing rate of 44.8% with 100% healing in a mean period of 8 weeks. Those in the sham treatment group showed an increase in ulcer size of 29% over a period of 7.4 weeks.

Griffin and colleagues (1991) demonstrated acceleration of pressure ulcer healing in their study of high-voltage PC on 17 patients with spinal cord injury who had stages II, III, and IV pressure ulcers. Subjects were randomly assigned to receive either high-voltage PC or a placebo treatment for 1 hour per day for 20 consecutive days, using a cathode placed directly on the wound surface. The electrical stimulation was delivered at 100 pulses per second and 200 volts, which produced a charge of 500 μC/sec at the cathode. Findings revealed that ulcers treated with electrical stimulation showed a significant decrease in wound surface area as compared with the placebo-treated ulcers at day 5 ($p < 0.05$), day 15 ($p < 0.05$), and day 20 ($p < 0.05$).

The benefits of high-voltage PC in diabetic foot ulcer–healing were revealed in the work of Alon, Azaria, and Stein (1986) in a case series of 15 patients. Anodal stimulation was applied for 1 hour 3 times a week. Twelve of the 15 wounds achieved closure in a mean period of 2.6 months.

Physiologic Effects

The underlying physiologic effects of electrical stimulation are mediated by the endogenous bioelectric system in the human body and its response to positive and negative polarity. Several investigators have demonstrated the existence of transepithelial potentials on the surface of the skin (Barker et al, 1982; Cunliffe-Barnes, 1945; Illingsworth and Baker, 1980). These transepithelial potentials arise from Na^+ channels on the mucosal surface of the skin that allow Na^+ to diffuse from the area surrounding epidermal cells to the inside of the cells. As a result of the movement of Na^+ from the skin surface to the interior of epidermal cells, the exterior of the skin maintains a variable level of negative electrical charge (Foulds and Barker, 1983). Jaffe and Vanable (1984) demonstrated that when the epidermis is injured, current flows as ions are transmitted through the tissue fluid between the damaged regions of the epidermis. This "current of injury" has a positive polarity whereas the adjacent intact skin retains its negative polarity, producing a unidirectional force sufficient to attract reparative cells to the wound bed during the inflammatory and proliferative phases of healing (Vanable, 1989). Once reepithelialization has closed the wound, the current of injury disappears, suggesting that it does not play a role in the remodeling phase of healing. It is important to note that the flow of current out of the wound is blocked if the wound bed is allowed to desiccate and form a scab (Alvarez et al, 1983).

Galvanotaxic Effects. Positively and negatively charged cells are attracted toward an electric field of opposite polarity, a process termed galvanotaxis. Multiple in vitro studies have established that cells essential to tissue repair will migrate toward the anode or cathode created by an electric field within a tissue culture (Bourguignon and Bourguignon, 1987; Cooper and Schliwa, 1985; Eberhardt, Szczypiorski, and Korytowski, 1986; Erickson and Nuccitelli, 1984; Fukushima et al, 1953; Orida and Feldman, 1982; Stromberg, 1988; Yang, Onuma, and Hui, 1984). Preliminary evidence from in vivo studies has demonstrated that electrical stimulation creates a similar galvanotaxic response. Eberhardt, Szczypiorski, and Korytowski (1986) showed that treating wounds with electrical stimulation for 30 minutes increased the relative number of neutrophils in the wound exudate as compared to control wounds. Using the pig model, Mertz and associates (1993) treated experimentally-induced wounds with two 30-minute sessions of monophasic PC using varying polarity. They found that wounds treated initially with negative polarity (day 0) followed by positive polarity on days 1 to 7 showed 20% greater epithelialization as compared to wounds receiving only one type of polarity. In those wounds treated by alternating the polarity daily (negative one day; positive the next), epithelialization was limited by 45 percent. Although the influence of polarity on cell migration in *human* wounds remains to be elucidated more completely, these findings suggest that bioelectric signals play a role in facilitating the phases of healing.

Stimulatory Effects on Cells. Basic science studies have shown that electrical current has a stimulatory effect of on fibroblasts, a key cell in wound contraction and collagen synthesis. Using the pig model, Cruz, Bayron, and Suarez (1989) demonstrated that there are significantly more fibroblasts in burn wounds treated with electrical stimulation than in controls. Alvarez and others (1983), also employing the pig model, documented more fibroblasts and increased collagen synthesis in partial-thickness wounds. Castillo and colleagues (1995) replicated these findings when they used scanning electron microscopy to evaluate the effect of pulsed electrical stimulation on burn wounds in the rat model. They found significant increases in collagen density in those burn wounds treated with electrical current. The stimulatory effect of electrical current on fibroblasts, reported by Bourguignon and Bourguignon (1987), was observed when fibroblasts in culture increased DNA and protein (including collagen) synthesis in response to electrical stimulation. This effect was most noticeable near the negative electrode.

Blood Flow and Tissue Oxygen Effects. There is accumulating evidence that electrical stimulation exerts a positive influence on blood flow and localized tissue oxygen. Hecker, Carron, and Schwartz (1985) have shown that negative polarity increased blood flow in the upper extremity as measured by plethysmography. In a sample of patients diagnosed with Raynaud's disease and diabetic polyneuropathy, Kaada (1982) demonstrated that application of distant, low-frequency TENS produced pronounced and prolonged cutaneous vasodilation. Using skin temperature as a measurement of peripheral vasodilation, he found a rise in the temperature of ischemic extremities from 71.6° to 75.2° F (22° to 24° C), to 87.8° to 93.2° F (31° to 34° C). The latency from the stimulus onset to the abrupt rise in temperature averaged 15 to 30 minutes with a duration of response from 4 to 6 hours. Kaada (1983) subsequently reported successfully treating 10 patients with 19 leg ulcers, previously resistant to treatment, by applying a TENS device to the web space between the first and second metacarpals of the ipsilateral wrist. Using the burst mode, he delivered 15 to 30 mA of pulsed direct current by the cathode for 30 to 34 minutes 3 times a day. He proposed that the remote application of electrical stimulation enhanced microcirculation in the tissues of the ipsilateral lower extremity, as demonstrated by the increase in toe temperature and ulcer healing. Based on findings from subsequent basic research, he suggested that this improvement in tissue microcirculation was the result of activation of a central serotonergic link that inhibits sympathetic vasoconstriction (Kaada and Eielson, 1983a; Kaada and Eielson, 1983b; Kaada and Helle, 1984; Kaada et al, 1984).

Additional evidence of increased blood flow in wounds treated with electrical stimulation is provided by reports of increasing capillary density following implementation of this therapy. Fifteen venous leg ulcers, previously resistant to healing, were treated with monophasic PC for 30 minutes daily for an average of 38 days (Junger et al, 1997). Using light microscopy to measure capillary density, they found densities increased from a prestimulation baseline of 8.05 capillaries/mm^2 to 11.55 capillaries/mm^2 following stimulation (p < 0.039). Transcutaneous oxygen in the periwound skin was noted to increase from 13.5 to 24.7 mm Hg.

Although research on the effects of electrical stimulation on wound oxygenation has been minimal, preliminary studies demonstrate that cutaneous oxygen can be improved with electrical stimulation. In separate studies, investigators have shown that application of electrical stimulation improved cutaneous oxygen in the lower extremity of elderly patients, subjects with diabetes, and patients with spinal cord injuries (Gagnier et al, 1988; Peters et al, 1998). This work provides indirect evidence of the potential for electrical stimulation to increase wound oxygenation.

Antibacterial Effects. Preliminary evidence indicates that electrical stimulation has bacteriostatic and bactericidal effects on microorganism that are known to infect chronic wounds. Rowley, McKenna, and Chase (1974) demonstrated inhibition of *Pseudomonas aeroginosa* in infected ulcers of rabbit skin when negative polarity was used. They hypothesized that the inhibition was the result of electrochemical changes created by the current. In a study of 20 patients with burn wounds that had been unresponsive to conventional therapy for 3 months to 2 years, Fakhri and Amin (1987) showed a quantitatively lower level of organisms after treatment with DC stimulation for 10-minute intervals twice weekly. This decrease in bacterial count was accompanied by epithelialization of the wound margins within 3 days of beginning electrical stimulation. Although the mechanism underlying the bactericidal or bacteriostatic effect of DC remains unclear, the galvanotaxic effect on macrophages and neutrophils has been implicated (Eberhardt, Szczypiorski, and Korytowski, 1986; Orida and Feldman, 1982). These studies suggest that the anodal attraction of neutrophils to tissue with high bacterial levels may be a primary mode of action, rather than destruction of pathogens by electrolysis or elevation of the tissue pH. Although a limited number of studies have investigated the effects of PC, it appears that the voltage required to produce an antibacterial effect would create profound muscle contractions, and would therefore not be applicable in clinical practice (Guffey and

Asmussen, 1989; Kincaid and Lavoie, 1989; Szuminsky et al, 1994).

Application Method

The predominant type of electrical stimulation currently used for wound-healing applications is pulsed current. Regardless of the waveform of the PC selected for treatment, the electrodes are applied using one of two methods (Baker et al, 1996; Kloth and Feedar, 1988). The first method involves placing one electrode in direct contact with a clean, electrically conductive material (commonly a saline-moistened gauze dressing) that is positioned in the wound while the second electrode is placed on intact skin approximately 15 to 30 cm from the wound edge. With the second method the electrodes are positioned on the skin at the wound edges on opposite sides of the wound. The treatment protocol is similar, whether the device is a low-voltage or high-voltage stimulator. The pulse frequency is set to 100 pulses per second with a current or voltage sufficient to produce a comfortable tingling sensation or, in insensate skin, at a level just below the motor threshold (Feedar, Kloth, and Gentzkow, 1991; Gentzkow et al, 1991, 1993; Griffin et al, 1991; Kloth and Feedar, 1988). The polarity is determined by the status of the wound and the specific cells that are to be targeted for migration into the wound (Bourguignon and Bourguignon, 1987). Treatments are administered for 1 hour, 5 to 7 days a week, and are continued as long as the wound is progressing toward closure.

Indications and Contraindications

Guidelines disseminated by the Agency for Health Care Policy and Research (AHCPR), now called the Agency for Health Care Research and Quality (AHRQ), state that electrical stimulation is an acceptable complementary therapy for treating stage III and IV pressure ulcers when combined with a moist healing protocol (Bergstrom, 1994). The WOCN Society recommends the use of electrical stimulation to enhance the healing of recalcitrant stages III and IV pressure ulcers (WOCN, 2003).

Medicare will allow electrical stimulation therapy of chronic stage III or stage IV pressure ulcers, arterial ulcers, diabetic ulcers, and venous insufficiency ulcers if no measurable improvement is evidenced after at least 30 days of standard wound therapy (CMS, 2004).

Although national guidelines and regulatory bodies recommend electrical stimulation as an adjunctive treatment for some wounds, application in routine clinical practice is variable and inconsistent. Several factors continue to limit its transfer to mainstream practice.

1. The majority of clinicians who treat patients with wounds are unfamiliar with the therapy.
2. Many clinical settings do not have personnel with the necessary expertise to administer the treatment.
3. The FDA has not approved as yet any type of electrical stimulation device for wound healing. Consequently, devices cannot be marketed for this indication, although they can be marketed for other already approved indications, such as edema and pain, and subsequently used as an off-label treatment for wound healing.

As is the case with most therapies, certain contraindications apply to use of electrical stimulation (Box 20-11). It should not be used when basal or squamous cell carcinoma is suspected in the wound or surrounding tissue, or when osteomyelitis is present. Patients with electronic implants, such as pacemakers, should not be treated with electrical stimulation. Electrical stimulation is also contraindicated for use over the heart or when iodine or silver ion residues are present in the wound.

BOX 20-11 Contraindications and Precautions for Electrical Stimulation

- Placement of electrodes tangential to the heart
- Presence of a cardiac pacemaker
- Placement of electrodes along regions of the phrenic nerve
- Presence of malignancy
- Placement of electrodes over the carotid sinus
- Placement of electrodes over the laryngeal musculature
- Placement of electrodes over topical substances containing metal ions
- Exogenous iodine (EI) povidone iodine, and mercurochrome, unless thoroughly cleaned.
- Placement of electrodes over osteomyelitis

ULTRAVIOLET LIGHT

Ultraviolet light (UV) is a simple-to-use modality that may be a valuable tool in addressing wound bioburden, especially in this era of resistant organisms. Specialized lamps generate UV light. Hot quartz mercury vapor lamps produce UV-A and UV-B. These lamps require time to warm up and cool down. UV-C is created by cold quartz lamps. These are generally easier to use, and treatment may be started immediately, without a warm-up or cool-down period (Figure 20-9).

UV light consists of the portion of the electromagnetic spectrum that is at a higher frequency than visible light. The wavelength ranges from 320-400 nm for UV-A, 290-320 nm for UV-B, and 185-290 nm for UV-C. Ultraviolet light has long been used for many skin conditions, including psoriasis and acne vulgaris. In recent decades, that usage has declined with the advent of more topical and systemic treatments for those conditions, in addition to the increased awareness of the potential damage from UV radiation. However, UV-C has seen resurgence in the care of chronic wounds.

Physiologic Effects

UV light does not heat tissue. Instead, it is believed to alter cellular function, increase cell wall permeability through altering the shape of proteins, stimulate production of various chemicals such as prostaglandins and arachidonic acid, and increase the production of adenosine triphosphate (ATP) (Camp et al, 1978). The erythema that results increases local vasodilation,

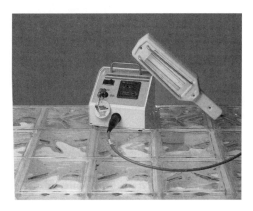

Fig. 20-9 Ultraviolet (UV) light. (Courtesy National Biological Corporation, Twinsburg, Ohio.)

tissue oxygenation, and histamine release. Erythema usually begins 2 to 4 hours after treatment and peaks at 12 hours, resolving within 24 hours. Several studies using high doses of UV showed benefits in wound healing (Freytes, Fernandez, and Fleming, 1965; Wills et al, 1983), but these older studies had a different standard of care for comparison than exists today. Therefore it is not known if UV will enhance wound healing in conjunction with advanced wound healing approaches. Nordback, Kulmala, and Jarvinen (1990) found equivalent closure times and tensile strength in animal wounds treated with UV and controls.

Each form of UV elicits different effects on tissue. UV-A and UV-B are nonionizing. They are both found environmentally, since they pass through the environment. UV-A produces a mild erythema, whereas UV-B elicits a stronger erythematous response while penetrating the epidermis. The impact of UV-A can be increased with the use or oral psoralens, a photosensitizing agent, before treatment. UV-A penetrates several millimeters into the skin, the deepest of the three forms. UV-B produces hyperplasia of the dermis and stratum corneum 3 days after treatment and has been used to be used to toughen scars (Parrish, Zaynoun, and Anderson, 1981).

UV-C is ionizing, though is not linked to skin cancers since it only penetrates the most superficial layers of the epidermis, which are sloughed often enough to prevent development of a neoplasm. Because the penetration is superficial to the melanocytes, the effect of UV-C is unrelated to skin tone. UV-C is recognized to be germicidal, which has come to be the primary use for UV treatment. Other evidence suggests that UV-C can increase epithelialization, increase epithelial cell turnover (Freytes, Fernandez, and Fleming, 1965), increase granulation tissue growth and tissue perfusion at lower doses (Ramsay and Challoner, 1976), and increase autolysis (Kloth, 1995; Spielholz and Kloth, 2000).

The bacteriocidal effects of UV have been recognized for over a century (Gates, 1928). UV-C has been demonstrated to kill methicillin-resistant *Staphylococcus aureus* (MRSA) and vancomycin-resistant enterococci (VRE) in vitro in 90 seconds (Conner-Kerr et al, 1998). The mechanism of action is theorized to be inhibition of DNA synthesis (Hall and Mount, 1981). Another in vitro study (Sheldon, Kokjohn, and Martin, 2005) found MRSA eradication with UV-C, with an even greater impact on *Pseudomonas.*

A case series by Thai and colleagues (2002) demonstrated reduced bacterial counts and more rapid healing with UV-C use, though treatment was not standardized and there was no control, limiting the ability to connect the UV to the improvements noted. Later, Thai and colleagues (2005) studied the effect of one 180-second UV-C treatment session on semi-quantitative swab culture results of 22 patients whose chronic ulcers contained high levels of bacteria and exhibited signs of infection. Types of wounds included pressure, venous, diabetic, and arterial etiology. Results showed a statistically significant reduction of predominant bacteria ($p = 0.001$, $n = 22$), and significant reductions of MRSA ($p < 0.05$) and *S. aureus* ($p < 0.01$).

Indications and Use

To benefit from the germicidal effects, UV-C is sometimes used in operating rooms to reduce surgical infections (Brown et al, 1996; Taylor, Bannister, and Leeming, 1995; Taylor and Chandler, 1997; Taylor, Leeming, and Bannister, 1993). Ultraviolet usage for chronic wounds involves UV-C for reducing bioburden. This application does not require determining a minimal erythematous dose (MED) since the wound base, not the periwound, is treated. There is limited evidence supporting periwound UV treatment for promoting wound closure.

The clinician should apply petrolatum to the periwound and drape the surrounding areas to prevent UV absorption. A common protocol is to keep the lamp 1 inch from the wound, perpendicular to the skin surface. Treatment is provided for 90 to 120 seconds. Treatment should be discontinued when the bioburden is adequately reduced.

Both the patient and the clinician must wear UV-blocking eye protection. Even if one does not look directly at the light, the waves may bounce off surfaces and reflect into the eye, causing damage. When using UV-A or UV-B, the MED must be determined before the initial treatment, and when there is any significant change in the patient's condition or skin tone, and with any change in the UV light bulb. Treatment intensity will likely have to be increased a small amount each day. Increasing time or decreasing distance from the skin may increase intensity.

Contraindications and Precautions

Safe and effective dosage of UV varies significantly between individuals. The impact of UV energy depends on its absorption by the tissue. Absorption is affected by the skin pigmentation, the distance from the light source, the intensity of the light source, the local skin thickness, the size of the treated area, and the angle of the light relative to the surface. The closer and more direct the light, the stronger the treatment. Lighter skin tones require shorter treatment times for UV-A and UV-B. Risks associated with UV therapy include tanning, burning, and premature skin aging. UV-C has a very low risk of causing burns.

Contraindications and precautions vary according to source and are listed in Box 20-12. Absolute contraindications include a history of skin cancer, systemic lupus erythematosus, fever, radiation therapy anywhere on the body within the previous 3 months, sarcoidosis, and treatment over the eye. Other conditions can be exacerbated by UV treatment, especially with UV-A or UV-B over large areas of the body. These conditions include pulmonary tuberculosis, cardiac disease, renal disease, hepatic disease, human immunodeficiency virus/acquired immunodeficiency syndrome (HIV/AIDS), hyperthyroidism, diabetes, and herpes simplex. Other conditions require the clinician to use caution when applying UV treatment, and may be considered relative precautions/contraindications. These conditions include acute eczema or dermatitis, radiation therapy more than 3 months earlier, and photosensitivity. The use of photosensitizing medication may shorten the treatment time or preclude treatment altogether. In addition to psoralens that are given to increase susceptibility to UV-A intentionally, tetracycline, sulfonamides, quinalones, gold medications for rheumatoid arthritis, thiazide diuretics, diphenhydramine, oral contraceptives, and phenothiazines may increase a person's sensitivity to UV. Treatment should not be administered if there is still erythema present from the last treatment (Michlovitz and Nolan, 2005; Cameron, 2003).

ULTRASOUND

Ultrasound (US) is a term used to describe sound waves greater than 20,000 Hertz (Hz), the upper limit of human hearing. Most clinical therapeutic applications

---

BOX 20-12 Contraindications and Precautions for Ultraviolet (UV) Light Therapy

Absolute Contraindications
- History of skin cancer
- Systemic lupus erythematosus
- Fever
- Radiation therapy anywhere on the body within the previous 3 months
- Sarcoidosis
- Treatment over the eye
- Presence of erythema from the last UV treatment

Conditions that Can Be Exacerbated by UV Treatment
(especially UV-A or UV-B over large areas of the body)
- Pulmonary tuberculosis
- Cardiac disease
- Renal disease
- Hepatic disease
- HIV/AIDS
- Hyperthyroidism
- Diabetes
- *Herpes simplex* infection

Use Caution When Applying UV Treatment
- Acute eczema or dermatitis
- Radiation therapy more than 3 months earlier
- Photosensitivity
- Use of photosensitizing medication (Box 20-13)
- May shorten the treatment time or preclude treatment altogether. Other than psoralens, which are given to increase susceptibility to UV-A intentionally, tetracycline, sulfonamides, quinalones, gold medications for rheumatoid arthritis, thiazide diuretics, diphenhydramine, oral contraceptives, and phenothiazines may also increase a person's sensitivity to ultraviolet.

HIV/AIDS, Human immunodeficiency virus/acquired immunodeficiency syndrome.

---

use a frequency of 1 MHz or 3.3 MHz. The user may elect to use a duty cycle. This results in a pulsing of the current, with periods of wave production followed by quiet periods. A 20% duty cycle is most commonly used, where the ultrasound is produced for 1 millisecond and is off for 4 milliseconds. Heat is produced but is dispersed so quickly that there is no temperature change

BOX 20-13 Examples of Photosensitizing Medications that May Increase Sensitivity to Ultraviolet

- Psoralens*
- Tetracycline
- Sulfonamides
- Quinalones
- Gold medications for rheumatoid arthritis
- Thiazide diuretics
- Diphenhydramine
- Oral contraceptives
- Phenothiazines

*NOTE: Psoralens are intentionally given to increase susceptibility to UV-A.

in the tissue. Ultrasound has been used to promote soft tissue healing for over 6 decades, primarily for orthopedic conditions. More recently, that use has extended into wound healing.

An ultrasound device consists of the control unit and the hand-held sound head, or transducer (Figure 20-10.) The user is able to control the intensity (amount of power used), whether those waves are continuous or pulsed, the duration of the treatment, and on some units, the wavelength. This device runs electricity through a crystal in the sound head, causing the crystal to vibrate. These vibrations create sound waves that pass through the sound head membrane and into the tissue, causing it to vibrate and heat up.

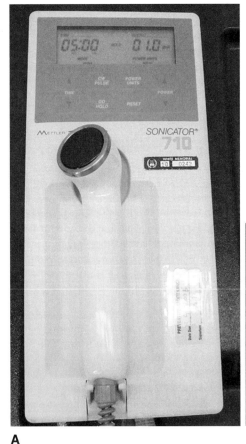

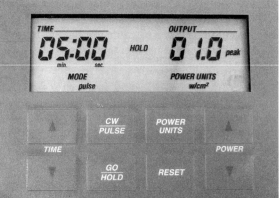

A   **B**

Fig. 20-10 A, An ultrasound device. **B,** Close-up of ultrasound parameter settings. (Courtesy Renee Cordrey.)

These waves elicit two types of effects: thermal and nonthermal.

Physiologic Effects

Nonthermal effects are attributed to cavitation, acoustic streaming, and microstreaming. Stable cavitation is the vibration of tiny bubbles in the interstitial spaces. With microstreaming, current eddies form around gas bubbles that are near vibrating particles. Acoustic streaming stimulates the movement of fluid within and between the cells. Some believe that using ultrasound in a water bath stimulates wound debridement through acoustic streaming of the water itself. These nonthermal effects occur with pulsed and continuous ultrasound. These forces stimulate an inflammatory response in wounds (Young and Dyson, 1990a).

The *thermal effects* of continuous ultrasound stimulate an increase in local circulation that disperses the heat and increases cell metabolism (Taskan et al, 1997). There are increases in the permeability of the cell membranes and skin, and increases in mast cell degranulation (Byl et al, 1992; Fyfe and Chahl, 1984), histamine release (Fyfe and Chahl, 1984), macrophage activity (Young and Dyson, 1990b), protein synthesis by fibroblasts, and angiogenesis (Young et al, 1990a) As a result, wounds may progress through the inflammatory phase more quickly (Demir et al, 2004), or acute inflammation may be reinitiated if healing has stalled. These effects are induced by continuous ultrasound.

Application and Method

There is no commonly used protocol for ultrasound. The literature has been inconsistent in techniques and results. In general, low-intensity ultrasound has ranged from 0.1 W/cm^2 to 0.3 W/cm^2, and medium-intensity US from 0.3-1.2 W/cm^2, and high-intensity US from 1.2-3.0 W/cm^2. Time of treatment has varied from 1 to 10 minutes, and transducer frequency has run between 0.3 MHz and 3 MHz. Frequency of treatment was between 1 and 5 days per week, and treatment duration ranged from 2 weeks through time until wound closure. Most of these studies used periwound techniques, though Peschen and colleagues (1997) used a water-immersion technique. Most used pulsed ultrasound, possibly because of the risks of thermal heating in a person with sensory or cognitive compromise. However, many studies do not offer full descriptions of parameters and technique, making application to clinical practice more difficult.

Research limitations with US studies are similar to the limitations previously described with other adjunctive therapies. In addition, treatment time and sound head movement pattern has not been modified appropriately to accommodate wound size and the effective radiating area (ERA) of the transducer. Ultrasound treatment is commonly combined with other modalities, which may also influence study results.

Several reviews have examined ultrasound research. Johannsen, Gam, and Tonny (1988) noted that the trends indicated that low-dose US was more effective than high-dose US, and that treating the wound edge had better results than treating the wound base, though the results were not statistically significant. Robertson and Baker (2001) identified eight randomized clinical trials addressing US. Seven were rejected because of inadequate controls, inadequate analysis, inadequate treatment details, insufficient sample size, or the use of multiple interventions.

Indications

In pressure ulcer research, the literature points to a lack of benefit. Two randomized, controlled trials (McDiarmid et al, 1985; ter Reit, Kessels, and Knipschild, 1996) demonstrated no difference in healing rates. A meta-analysis combining those two studies strengthened that conclusion with a stronger sample size (Flemming and Cullum, 2001). Though some trials did show a small improvement with the US group, the sample sizes were too small to reach statistical significance. Further, those gains are small enough to be of questionable clinical significance. Selkowitz and colleagues (2002) conducted a single-subject baseline-US-sham trial on a stage III coccyx ulcer, using low-intensity pulsed US. The baseline period had the greatest healing rate, and the sham the poorest, though that may be attributed to the natural variation in rates since a wound changes while it heals. The Cochrane Library review of US for pressure ulcers concluded that there was no evidence to support its efficacy (Baba-Akbari Sari et al, 2005).

Venous ulcer outcomes have been largely inconclusive, often with a lack of statistical significance, though they do trend towards effectiveness (Flemming and

Cullum, 2005; WOCN Society, 2005). Low-frequency ultrasound, at 30-60 kHz has shown some promise for venous insufficiency ulcers. Two studies (Peschen et al, 1997; Weichenthal et al, 1997) demonstrated increased wound closure with 30 kHz US at 0.1 W/cm². Several studies, using both high-intensity and low-intensity pulsed US, have found no significant difference in the percentage of wounds that closed during the treatment time compared to sham treatment (Ericksson, Lundeberg, and Malm, 1991; Luckstead and Coursey, 1995; Roche and West, 1984). Other studies showed improvement with US, but either lacked sufficient description of the baseline data to properly evaluate the results, had poor follow-up, or had significant differences between groups (e.g., wound size) that could lead to differences in the findings (Callam et al, 1986; Peschen et al, 1997; Dyson, Franks, and Suckling, 1976).

There is more research on surgically-induced wounds in laboratory animals. Taskan (1997) compared low-intensity pulsed US and sham US for 7 days on full-thickness wounds in mice. After a week of treatment, the new scar tissue of the US-treated mice showed a higher number of white blood cells, more fibroblasts, and higher collagen levels than that of the sham-treated mice. The US-treated scars also showed greater tensile strength on the twenty-fifth day after wound creation. Other work has found increases in macrophage and fibroblast activity (Young et al, 1990b), improved healing rates (El-Batouty et al, 1986), and increased tensile strength (Byl et al, 1992; Byl et al, 1993; Demir et al, 2004) after US treatments. Byl (1993) demonstrated that although both low-intensity and high-intensity US can improve tensile strength in the first week, low-intensity ultrasound was more effective at increasing tensile strength and collagen deposition beyond that period. Shamberger and colleagues (1981) found no effect on tensile strength, but an extremely low intensity was used (0.05-0.15 W/cm²) and a very high frequency, 5 MHz, which would be largely absorbed in the most superficial layers of tissue.

The better outcomes found in laboratory research are likely due to better-controlled situations and limited comorbidities, which are not always possible in a clinical setting. Additionally, induced wounds in animals are acute wounds, which are physiologically different than chronic wounds and would therefore respond differently to a given treatment. It has been shown that irradiated skin in animal models does not respond to ultrasound treatment (Lowe et al, 2001).

Contraindications and Precautions

The sound head must be kept in constant motion. If it stays in place for even 0.1 microseconds, standing waves and banding may occur. A standing wave happens when the sound wave reflects off tissue back onto itself. The resulting interference wave is twice as strong as the original wave, which increases tissue heating and potentially leads to burning. Banding is the separation of cells and plasma within the blood vessels. This action causes irreversible damage to the endothelial linings of the vessel walls.

Contraindications are related to the thermal and nonthermal effects of ultrasound. US must not be used over the eyes, the heart, the carotid sinuses, a pregnant uterus, or the exposed central nervous system (such as over a laminectomy site). The inflammatory and metabolic effects of US contraindicates its use in situations when they would be harmful, such as where there is active bleeding, active infection, over breast or other silicone implants, over malignancies, and in the presence of thrombophlebitis. US should not be used over pacemakers, active epiphyseal plates, the reproductive organs, or orthopedic cement or plastic components (because the increased reflection of the sound waves overheats local tissue). In a limb with arterial insufficiency a lower intensity nonthermal setting should be used, since heat dispersion is compromised and the increased metabolic demands cannot be met.

The clinician must exercise good judgment when deciding whether to use US. Ultrasound may often be used in the presence of a contraindication, if the treatment location is remote to the site of the contraindication. For example, US may be used on a foot wound despite the presence of a cardiac pacemaker or total hip replacement, or if the patient is pregnant, as the effects of US are localized. Caution should be used around superficial bones, since periosteum heats and burns easily from reflection off the bone. When using thermal US in a person with sensory or cognitive deficits the clinician should be especially vigilant, since the patient is not able to provide feedback relating to tissue heating. US may be used with caution in an area of acute inflammation if the benefits outweigh the risks of increasing inflammation.

MIST Ultrasound

Recently a new ultrasound technique has become available. MIST ultrasound (Celleration, Eden Prairie, MN), also called MUST (mist-ultra-sound transport) and UMT (ultrasound mist therapy), is a noncontact ultrasound method (Figures 20-11 and 20-12.) The device vaporizes saline or other fluids into microdroplets (60 microns) that are then propelled to the

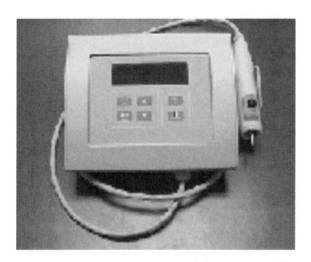

Fig. 20-11 The Ultrasound MIST® control unit. (Courtesy Celleration, Inc., Eden Prairie, Minnesota.)

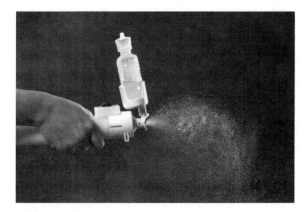

Fig. 20-12 The MIST® handset in action. (Courtesy Celleration, Inc., Eden Prairie, Minnesota.)

wound bed via 40-kHz US waves, at an intensity of 1.5 W/cm².

As this is a relatively new modality, published evidence is still sparse. One published in vivo study with diabetic mice (Thawer and Houghton, 2004) compared wounds treated with MIST and with sham MIST. They reported similar size after 10 days, but a greater concentration of collagen and blood vessels in the MIST-treated wounds. A recent randomized controlled trial on grade I and II diabetic foot ulcers (Ennis et al, 2005) found a higher percentage of closed wounds during the study period than did those in the sham treatment group.

There have been several poster presentations on the effects of MIST therapy. These unpublished studies have reported several benefits, including a reduction of bacterial load in vivo (Conner-Kerr et al, 2001) and in vitro (Kavros et al, 2002; Wagner et al, 2001), with demonstrated damage to the bacterial cell walls. The research did not include examination of the cell walls of the tissue, fibroblasts, macrophages, or other desirable cells. In an uncontrolled study, Lai and Pittelkow (2002), reported that MIST stimulated DNA synthesis for 2 days after an initial decrease for 4 hours and found no change in cell stress or apoptosis. Conner-Kerr and colleagues (2003) compared pulsed lavage with suction and MIST on acute animal wounds. Size decreases for both modalities were greater than the control group. The MIST-treated wounds demonstrated a greater concentration of blood vessels and thicker epidermal tissue in the healed wound. Conner-Kerr (2002) also reported faster closure of incisions in fibroblast cultures in specimens treated with MIST as opposed to the control samples. Another study (Liedl and Kavros, 2001) demonstrated an increase in tissue perfusion through laser Doppler flowmetry with both 1 MHz traditional ultrasound and with MIST ultrasound. There was no control or sham group.

SUMMARY

The use of devices and active technology to enhance and facilitate wound healing introduces exciting new interventions to augment the clinician's options in managing the patient with a chronic wound. Many of these therapies are provided in collaboration with nonnursing health care professionals. For example, physical therapists typically provide electrical stimulation, ultrasound and MIST therapies. However, these therapies do not replace appropriate topical wound care. Topical wound care during the use of these technologies must still strive to create an optimum wound environment. Finally, it is important to recognize that the treatment options presented in this chapter have mixed levels of research evidence concerning their efficacy and effectiveness in chronic wound management. HBO, electrical stimulation, and NPWT appear to have the higher levels of evidence of effectiveness. Nonetheless it is the clinician's responsibility to critically assess the status of the research before applying the intervention clinically. For example, many studies were limited to animal research, have small sample sizes, were not subjected to data analysis, or did not use a randomized, controlled research design. These interventions open a door to improved wound care and decreased healing time and, as a result, to support the patient's ability to achieve a sustainable plan of care. It is the wound care specialist's responsibility to stay informed, use these interventions wisely, and to use these interventions within a research project so that data can be obtained and the evidence for these interventions strengthened.

SELF-ASSESSMENT EXERCISE

1. Define hyperbaric oxygenation.
2. Which of the following statements about hyperoxygenation that occurs with hyperbaric treatment is true?
   a. Hyperoxygenation occurs because the hemoglobin molecule is saturated with oxygen molecules.
   b. Hyperoxygenation results from increasing the oxygen-carrying capacity of the plasma.
   c. It takes several treatments to achieve hyperoxygenation.
   d. It is possible for hyperoxygenation to be sustained for 8 to 10 hours after exposure.
3. All of the following personal care items are contraindicated during hyperbaric treatment EXCEPT:
   a. Hairspray
   b. Hearing aides
   c. Contact lenses
   d. Perfume
4. Wound care dressings with a petrolatum base should be removed during hyperbaric treatment: True or False?
5. The effects of electrical stimulation on wound healing are mediated by the influence of positive and negative polarity on which of the following?
   a. Necrotic tissue
   b. Exudate production
   c. Wound contraction
   d. Positively and negatively charged cells
6. Which of the following would impede current flow in injured tissue?
   a. Low tissue perfusion
   b. Desiccated wound bed
   c. High bacterial level
   d. Hydrocolloid dressings
7. Which of the following would contraindicate the use of electrical stimulation to promote wound healing?
   a. Malnourished patient
   b. Infected wound
   c. Poorly oxygenated wound
   d. Suspected basal cell carcinoma in wound
8. Which of the following wounds would benefit the most from the use of NPWT?
   a. A wound that requires controlled granulation tissue formation
   b. A superficial wound located on the anterior aspect of the leg
   c. A deep pressure ulcer located on the sacrum
   d. A painful wound located on the medial malleolus
9. Which of the following situations would be a contraindication for NPWT?
   a. A patient who is a paraplegic and has a stage IV pressure ulcer
   b. An obese patient with a venous stasis ulcer
   c. A patient with a large wound on the heel covered with black eschar
   d. A patient with a dehisced abdominal wound who is taking aspirin
10. Which form of ultraviolet radiation is most effective at reducing wound bioburden?
11. The minimal erythematous dose (MED) must be determined before wound base treatment with UV-C: True or False?
12. MIST therapy appears to have what benefits in wound healing?

REFERENCES

Abramovich A et al: Hyperbaric oxygen for carbon monoxide poisoning, *Harefuah* 132(1):21, 1997.

Akers TK, Gabrielson AL: The effect of high voltage galvanic stimulation on the rate of healing of decubitus ulcers, *Biomed Sci Instrument* 20:99, 1984.

Alon G, Azaria M, Stein H: Diabetic ulcer healing using high voltage TENS, *Phys Ther* 66:775, 1986 (abstract).

Alvarez OM et al: The healing of superficial skin wounds is stimulated by external electrical current, *J Invest Dermatol* 81(2):144, 1983.

American College of Hyperbaric Medicine: Certification, April 21, 2004, www.hyperbaric medicine.org; Accessed April 21, 2004.

American Physical Therapy Association: *Electrotherapeutic terminology in physical therapy: section on clinical electrophysiology*, Alexandria, Va., 1990, Author.

Asamoto S et al: Hyperbaric oxygen (HBO) therapy for acute traumatic cervical spinal cord injury, *Spinal Cord* 38(9):538, 2000.

Assimacopoulos D: Wound healing promotion by the use of negative electric current, *Am Surg* 34(6):423, 1968.

Baba-Akbari Sari A, Flemming K, Cullum NA, Wollina U. Therapeutic ultrasound for pressure ulcers. *The Cochrane Database of Systematic Reviews* 2000, Issue 4. Art. No.: CD001275. DOI: 10.1002/14651858.CD001275.

Baker L et al: Effect of electrical stimulation waveform on healing of ulcers in human beings with spinal cord injury, *Wound Rep Regen* 4(1):21, 1996.

Baker L et al: Effects of electrical stimulation on wound healing in patients with diabetic ulcers, *Diabet Care* 20(3):405, 1997.

Banwell P, Teot L: Topical negative pressure (TNP): the evolution of a novel wound therapy. *J Wound Care,* 12(1) January, 2003. Education Supplement.

Banwell PE et al: Dermal microvasculature flow in experimental partial thickness burns: the effect of topical sub-atmospheric pressure, *J Burn Care Rehabil* 21:s161, 2002.

Banwell PE: Topical negative pressure therapy in wound care, *J Wound Care* 8:2, 79-84, 1999.

Barker A, Jaffe L, Vanable J: The glabrous epidermis of cavies contains a powerful battery, *Am J Physiol* 11:R358, 1982.

Baugh MA: HIV: reactive oxygen species, enveloped viruses and hyperbaric oxygen, *Med Hypoth* 55(3):232, 2000.

Bergstrom N et al: *Treatment of pressure ulcers. Clinical practice guideline, No. 1.* Public Health Service, Agency for Health Care Policy and Research, Rockville, Md, 1994, U.S. Dept of Health and Human Services, AHCPR Publication No. 95–052.

Bern J, Bern S, Singh A: Use of hyperbaric oxygen chamber in the management of radiation-related complications of the anorectal region: report of two cases and review of the literature, *Dis Colon Rectum* 43(10):1435, 2000.

Bonomo SR et al: Hyperbaric oxygen as a signal transducer: upregulation of platelet derived growth factor-beta receptor in the presence of HBO and PDGF, *Undersea Hyper Med* 25: 211, 1998.

Bourguignon G, Bourguignon L: Electric stimulation of protein and DNA synthesis in human fibroblasts, *FASEB J* 1(5):398, 1987.

Boykin JV: Hyperbaric oxygen therapy: a physiological approach to selected problem wound healing, *Wounds* 8:183, 1996.

Broussard CL: Hyperbaric oxygenation and wound healing, *J WOCN* 30:210, 2003.

Brown IW Jr et al: Toward further reducing wound infections in cardiac operations, *Ann Thorac Surg* 62(6):1783, 1996.

Byl N et al: Low-dose ultrasound effects on wound healing: A controlled study with Yucatan pigs, *Arch Phys Med Rehabil* 73(7):656, 1992.

Byl N et al: Incisional wound healing: a controlled study of low and high dose ultrasound, *J Ortho Sports Ther* 18(5):619, 1993.

Callam M et al: Trial of ultrasound in the treatment of chronic leg ulceration. In Negus D, Jantet G, editors: *Phlebology '85*, London, 1986, Libbey.

Cameron MH: Physical Agents in Rehabilitation: From research to practice, ed 2, Philadelphia. 2003, Saunders.

Camp RD et al: Irradiation of human skin by short wavelength ultraviolet radiation (100–290 nm) (u.V.C): increased concentrations of arachidonic acid and prostaglandines E2 and F2alpha, *Br J Clin Pharmacol* 6(2):145, 1978.

Capes JP, Tomaszewski C: Prophylaxis against middle ear barotrauma in US hyperbaric oxygen therapy centers, *Am J Emerg Med* 14(7):645, 1996.

Carl UM et al: Treatment of radiation proctitis with hyperbaric oxygen: what is the optimal number of HBO treatments? *Strahlenther Onkol* 174(9):482, 1998.

Carley PJ, Wainapel SF: Electrotherapy for acceleration of wound healing: low intensity direct current, *Arch Phys Med Rehabil* 66(7):443, 1985.

Castillo E et al: The influence of pulsed electrical stimulation on the wound healing of burned rat skin, *Arch Med Res* 26(2):185, 1995.

Cianci P, Sato R: Adjunctive hyperbaric oxygen therapy in the treatment of thermal burns: a review, *Burns* 20(1):5, 1994.

Clark JM: Oxygen toxicity. In Kindwall EP, editor: *Hyperbaric medicine practice*, Flagstaff, Ariz, 1995, Best.

CMS Manual System Medical National Coverage Determination, 2004, http://www.cms.hhs.gov/manuals/pm_trans/R7NCD.pdf; Accessed October16, 2005.

Conner-Kerr T: In vitro study: effects of mist therapy and UVC on fibroblastic migration rates, *Symp Adv Wound Care*, poster presentation, 2002.

Conner-Kerr TA et al: The effects of ultraviolet radiation on antibiotic-resistant bacteria in vitro, *Ostomy Wound Manage* 44(10):50, 1998.

Conner-Kerr T et al: Effects of noncontact mist ultrasound therapy (must) on bacterial levels in a chronic wound bed, *Symp Adv Wound Care, poster presentation,* 2001.

Conner-Kerr T et al: Effects of pulsatile lavage with suction and mist ultrasound transport therapy on healing in acute porcine wounds, *Symp Adv Wound Care, poster presentation*, 2003.

Cooper MS, Schliwa M: Electrical and ionic controls of tissue cell locomotion in DC electric fields, *J Neurosci Res* 13:223, 1985.

Cruz N, Bayron F, Suarez A: Accelerated healing of full-thickness burns by the use of high-voltage pulsed galvanic stimulation in the pig, *Ann Plast Surg* 23(1):49, 1989.

Cunliffe-Barnes T: Healing rate of human skin determined by measurement of electric potential of experimental abrasions: study of treatment with petrolatum and with petrolatum containing yeast and liver extracts, *Am J Surg* 69(1):82, 1945.

Davis JC, Hunt TK: *Problem wounds: the role of oxygen*, Norwalk, CT, 1988, Appleton & Lange.

Debreceni L et al: Results of transcutaneous electrical stimulation (TENS) in cure of lower extremity arterial disease, *Angiology* 46 (7):613, 1995.

Demir H et al: Comparison of the effects of laser and ultrasound treatments on experimental wound healing in rats, *J Rehabil Res Dev* 41(5):721, 2004.

Dyson M: Adjuvant therapies: ultrasound, laser therapy, electrical stimulation, hyperbaric oxygen and negative pressure therapy. In: Morison MJ, Ovington LG, editors: *Chronic wound care: a problem-based learning Approach*, Edinburgh, Scotland, 2004, Mosby.

Dyson M, Franks C, Suckling J: Stimulation of healing of varicose ulcers by ultrasound, *Ultrasonics* 14:232, 1976.

Eberhardt A, Szczypiorski P, Korytowski G: Effect of transcutaneous electrostimulation on the cell composition of skin exudate, *Acta Physiol Pol* 37(1):41, 1986.

El-Batouty M et al: A. Comparative evaluation of the effects of ultrasonic and ultraviolet irradiation on tissue regeneration, *Scand J Rheumatol* 15:381, 1986.

Elliott DH: Decompression sickness. In Kindwall EP, editor: *Hyperbaric medicine practice*, Flagstaff, Ariz, 1995, Best.

Ennis WJ et al: Ultrasound therapy for recalcitrant diabetic foot ulcers: Results of a randomized, double-blind, controlled, multicenter study, *Ostomy Wound Manage* 51(8):24-39, 2005.

Erickson CS, Nuccitelli R: Embryonic fibroblast motility and orientation can be influenced by physiological electric fields, *J Cell Biol* 98:296, 1984.

Ericksson S, Lundeberg T, Malm M: A placebo controlled trial of ultrasound therapy in chronic leg ulceration, *Scand J Rehab Med* 23(4):211, 1991.

Fakhri O, Amin M: The effect of low-voltage electric therapy on the healing of resistant skin burns, *J Burn Care Res* 8(1):15, 1987.

Feedar J, Kloth L, Gentzkow G: Chronic dermal ulcer healing enhanced with monophasic pulsed electrical stimulation, *Phys Ther* 71(9):639, 1991.

Feldmeier JJ: Hyperbaric oxygen 2003: indications and results: The Hyperbaric Oxygen Therapy Committee Report, Kensington, MD, 2003, Undersea and Hyperbaric Medical Society.

Fife CE: Hyperbaric oxygen therapy applications in wound care. In Sheffield PJ, Smith APS, Fife CE, editors: *Wound care practice*, Flagstaff, Ariz, 2004, Best.

Fife CE et al: The predictive value of transcutaneous oxygen tension measurement in diabetic lower extremity ulcers treated with hyperbaric oxygen therapy: a retrospective analysis of 1144 patients, *Wound Rep Regen* 10:198, 2002.

Fitzgerald GK, Newsome D: Treatment of a large infected thoracic spine wound using high voltage pulsed monophasic current, *Phys Ther* 73(6):355, 1993.

Flemming K, Cullum N: Systematic reviews of wound care management: (5) beds; (6) compression; (7) laser therapy, therapeutic ultrasound, electrotherapy and electromagnetic therapy, *Health Tech Assess* 5(9):1, 2001.

Flemming K, Cullum N: Therapeutic ultrasound for venous leg ulcers, *Cochrane Database Syst Rev.* 2000;(4):CD001180.

Foster JH: Hyperbaric oxygen treatment contraindications and complications, *J Maxillofac Surg* 50:1081, 1992.

Foulds I, Barker A: Human skin battery potentials and their possible role in wound healing, *Br J Dermatol* 109:515, 1983.

Freytes HA, Fernandez B, Fleming WC: Ultraviolet light in the treatment of indolent ulcers, *South Med J* 58:223, 1965.

Fukushima K et al: Studies of galvanotaxis of human neutrophilic leukocytes and methods of its measurement, *Med J Osaka Univ* 4:195, 1953.

Fyfe M, Chahl L: Mast cell degranulation and increased vascular permeability induced by "therapeutic" ultrasound in the rat ankle joint, *Br J Exper Path* 65:671, 1984.

Gagnier KA et al: The effects of electrical stimulation on cutaneous oxygen supply in paraplegics, *Phys Ther* 68(5):835, 1988 (abstract).

Gardner S, Frantz RA, Schmidt FL: The effect of electrical stimulation on chronic wound healing: A meta-analysis, *Wound Rep Regen* 7(6):495, 1999.

Gates F: Discussion and correspondence on nuclear derivatives and the lethal action of ultraviolet light, *Science* 68:479, 1928.

Gault W, Gatens P: Use of low intensity direct current in management of ischemic skin ulcers, *Phys Ther* 56(3):265, 1976.

Gentzkow G et al: Improved healing of pressure ulcers using Dermapulse®, a new electrical stimulation device, *Wounds* 3(5):158, 1991.

Gentzkow GD et al: Healing of refractory stage III and IV pressure ulcers by a new electrical stimulation device, *Wounds* 5(3):160, 1993.

Goad RF et al: Diagnosis and treatment of decompression sickness. In Shilling CW, Carlston CB, Mathias RA, editors: *The physician's guide to diving medicine*, New York, 1984, Plenum Press.

Gordillo GM, Sen CK: Revisiting the essential role of oxygen in wound healing, *Am J Surg* 186(3):259, 2003.

Gottlieb SF, Neubauer RA: Multiple sclerosis: its etiology, pathogenesis, and therapeutics with emphasis on the controversial use of HBO, *J Hyperbaric Med* 3(3):43, 1988.

Griffin J et al: Efficacy of high voltage pulsed current for healing of pressure ulcers in patients with spinal cord injury, *Phys Ther* 71(6):433, 1991.

Guffey JS, Asmussen MD: In vitro bactericidal effects of high voltage pulsed current versus direct current against *Staphylococcus aureus*, *J Clin Electrophysiol* 1(1):5, 1989.

Hall JD, Mount DW: Mechanisms of DNA replication and mutagenesis in ultraviolet-irradiated bacteria and mammalian cells, *Prog Nucleic Acid Res Mol Biol* 25:53, 1981.

Hammarlund C: The physiologic effects of hyperbaric oxygen. In Kindwall EP, editor: *Hyperbaric medicine practice*, Flagstaff, Ariz, 1995, Best.

Hart GB: The monoplace chamber. In Kindwall EP, editor: *Hyperbaric medicine practice*, Flagstaff, Ariz, 1999, Best.

Hartnett JM: Use of vacuum-assisted wound closure in three chronic wounds, *J WOCN* 25:281, 1998.

Hecker B, Carron H, Schwartz D: Pulsed galvanic stimulation: effects of current frequency and polarity on blood flow in healthy subjects, *Arch Phys Med Rehabil* 66(6):369, 1985.

Heimbach RD: *Physiology and pharmacology of HBO2*. In Jefferson C. Davis Wound Care and Hyperbaric Medicine Center [Course], San Antonio, Tex, March 4, 1998, Hyperbaric Medicine Team Training, Southwest Texas Methodist Hospital and Nix Medical Center.

Hirn M: Hyperbaric oxygen in the treatment of gas gangrene and perineal necrotizing fasciitis: a clinical and experimental study, *Eur J Surg* 570(Suppl A9D):1, 1993.

Hsu LH, Wang JH: Treatment of carbon monoxide poisoning with hyperbaric oxygen, *Chung Hai I Hsueh Chih* 58(6):407, 1996.

Hughes AJ, Schwarer AP, Miller IL: Hyperbaric oxygen in the treatment of refractory haemorrhagic cystitis, *Bone Marrow Transpl* 22(6):585, 1998.

Illingsworth CM, Barker AT: Measurement of electrical currents emerging during the regeneration of amputated finger tips in children, *Clin Phys Physiol Meas* 1:87, 1980.

Ishihara H et al: Prediction of neurologic outcome in patients with spinal cord injury by using hyperbaric oxygen therapy, *J Orthop Sci* 6(5):385, 2001.

Jaffe L, Vanable J: Electric fields and wound healing, *Clin Dermatol* 2(3):34, 1984.

Johannsen F, Gam AN, Tonny K: Ultrasound therapy in chronic leg ulceration: a meta-analysis, *Wound Rep Regen* 6:121, 1988.

Jordan WC: The effectiveness of intermittent hyperbaric oxygen in relieving drug-induced HIV-associated neuropathy, *J Natl Med Assoc* 90(6):355, 1998.

Junger M et al: Treatment of venous ulcers with low-frequency pulsed current (Dermapulse): effect on cutaneous microcirculation [German], *Hautarzt* 48(12):879, 1997.

Kaada B: Vasodilation induced by transcutaneous nerve stimulation in peripheral ischemia (Raynaud's phenomenon and diabetic polyneuropathy), *Eur Heart J* 3(4):303, 1982.

Kaada B: Promoted healing of chronic ulceration by transcutaneous nerve stimulation (TNS), *VASA* 12(3):262, 1983.

Kaada B, Eielsen O: In search of mediators of skin vasodilation inducted by transcutaneous nerve stimulation: I. Failure to block the response by antagonists of endogenous vasodilators, *Genl Pharmacol* 14(6):623, 1983a.

Kaada B, Eielsen O: In search of mediators of skin vasodilation inducted by transcutaneous nerve stimulation: II. Serotonin implicated, *Genl Pharmacol* 14(6):635, 1983b.

Kaada B, Helle K: In search of mediators of skin vasodilation induced by transcutaneous nerve stimulation: IV. In vitro bioassay of the vasoinhibitory activity of sera from patients suffering from peripheral ischaemia, *Genl Pharmacol* 15(2):115, 1984.

Kaada B et al: Failure to influence the VIP level in the cerebrospinal fluid by transcutaneous nerve stimulation in humans, *Genl Pharmacol* 15(6):563, 1984.

Kavros SJ et al: The effect of ultrasound mist therapy on common bacterial wound pathogens, *Symp Adv Wound Care* 2002, Poster.

Kidder TM: Myringotomy. In Kindwall EP, editor: *Hyperbaric medicine practice*, Flagstaff, Ariz, 1995, Best.

Kincaid C, Lavoie K: Inhibition of bacterial growth in vitro following stimulation with high voltage, monophasic, pulsed current, *Phys Ther* 69(8):651, 1989.

Kindwall EP: A history of hyperbaric medicine. In Kindwall EP, editor: *Hyperbaric medicine practice*, Flagstaff, Ariz, 1995a, Best.

Kindwall EP: Contraindications and side effects to hyperbaric oxygen treatment. In Kindwall EP, editor: *Hyperbaric medicine practice*, Flagstaff, Ariz,, 1995b, Best.

Kindwall EP: Gas embolism. In Kindwall EP, editor: *Hyperbaric medicine practice*, Flagstaff, Ariz, 1995c, Best.

Kindwall EP: Management of complications in hyperbaric treatment. In Kindwall EP, editor: *Hyperbaric medicine practice*, Flagstaff, Ariz, 1995d, Best.

Kindwall EP: The multiplace chamber. In Kindwall EP, editor: *Hyperbaric medicine practice*, Flagstaff, Ariz, 1995e, Best.

Kindwall E: Contraindications and side effects to hyperbaric oxygen treatment. In Eric P, Kindwall EP, Whelan HT, editors, *Hyperbaric medicine practice*, Flagstaff, Ariz, 1999b, Best.

Kjartansson J: Transcutaneous electrical nerve stimulation (TENS) in ischemic tissue, *J Plast Reconstr Surg* 81(5):813, 1988.

Kloth L, Feedar J: Acceleration of wound healing with high voltage, monophasic, pulsed current, *Phys Ther* 68(4):503, 1988.

Kloth LC: Physical modalities in wound management: UVC, therapeutic heating and electrical stimulation, *Ostomy Wound Manage* 41(5):18, 1995.

Knighton DR, Fiegel VD: Oxygen as an antibiotic: the effect of inspired oxygen on infection, *Arch Surg* 125:97, 1990.

Laden G: HOT MI pilot study: hyperbaric oxygen and thrombolysis in myocardial infarction, *Am Heart J* 136(4 Pt 1): 749, 1998.

Lai JY, Pittelkow MR: In vitro study: physiological effects of ultrasound mist on fibroblasts, *Symp Adv Wound Care* 2002, Poster.

Larson-Lohr V, Norvell H, editors: *Hyperbaric nursing*, Flagstaff, Ariz, 2002, Best.

Lee HC et al: Hyperbaric oxygen therapy in clinical application: a report of a 12-year experience, *Chung Hua I Hsueh Tsa Chih (CHQ)* 43(5):301, 1989.

Liedl DA, Kavros SJ: The effect of mist ultra-sound transport technology on cutaneous microcirculatory blood flow, *Symp Adv Wound Care* 2001, Poster.

Lowe AS et al: Therapeutic ultrasound and wound closure: Lack of healing effect on x-ray irradiated wounds in murine skin, *Arch Phys Med Rehabil* 82(11):1507, 2001.

Luckstead A, Coursey RD: Consumer perceptions of pressure and force in psychiatric treatments, *Psychiatr Serv* 46:146, 1995.

Ludwig LM: The role of hyperbaric oxygen in current emergency medical care, *J Emerg Nurs* 15(3):229, 1989.

Mader JT et al: Hyperbaric oxygen as adjunctive therapy for osteomyelitis, *Inf Dis Clin North Am* 4: 433, 1990.

Mader JT, Ortiz M, Calhoun JH: Update on the diagnosis and management of osteomyelitis, *Clin Podiatr* 13(4):701, 1996.

Maki RD: Ophthalmic side effects of hyperbaric oxygen therapy, *Insight* 21(4):114, 1996.

Marx RE: Radiation injury to tissue. In Kindwall EP, editor: *Hyperbaric medicine practice*, Flagstaff, Ariz, 1995, Best.

Mayer R et al: Hyperbaric oxygen—an effective tool to treat radiation morbidity in prostate cancer, *Radiother Oncol* 61(2):151, 2001.

McDiarmid T et al: Ultrasound in the treatment of pressure sores, *Physiotherapy* 71:66, 1995.

Mertz PM et al: Electrical stimulation: Acceleration of soft tissue repair by varying the polarity, *Wounds* 5(3):153, 1993.

Michlovitz SL, Nolan TP Jr: *Modalities for therapeutic intervention*, ed 4, Philadelphia, 2005, FA Davis.

Morykwas MJ et al: Vacuum assisted closure: a new method for wound control and treatment: animal studies and basic foundation, *Ann Plast Surg* 38:553, 1997a.

Morykwas MJ et al: Vacuum-assisted closure: a new method for wound control and treatment: clinical experience, *Ann Plast Surg* 38:6,553, 1997b.

Morykwas LC et al: *Gene array analysis of stretched fibroblasts*, ETRS 13th Annual Meeting, Amsterdam, September, 2003.

Mychaskiw G et al: In vitro effects of hyperbaric oxygen on sickle cell morphology, *J Clin Anesth* 13(4):255, 2001.

National Fire Protection Association: *NFPA 99: standard for health care facilities*, Quincy, Mass, 2002, NFPA.

Neubauer R: Hyperbaric oxygen therapy beats carbon monoxide poisoning, decompression sickness, broken bones, gangrene, multiple sclerosis, severe burns, *Bottom Line/Health* 12(5):13, 1998.

Nighoghossian N, Trouillas P: Hyperbaric oxygen in the treatment of the acute ischemic stroke: an unsettled issue, *J Neurol Sci* 150(1):27, 1997.

Nordback I, Kulmala R, Jarvinen M: Effect of ultraviolet therapy on rat skin wound healing, *J Surg Res* 48(1):68, 1990.

Orida N, Feldman J: Directional protrusive pseudopodial activity and motility in macrophages induced by extracellular electric fields, *Cell Motil* 2:243, 1982.

Parrish JA, Zaynoun S, Anderson RR: Cumulative effects of repeated subthreshold doses of ultraviolet radiation, *J Invest Dermatol* 76(5): 356, 1981.

Pascual J: Hyperbaric oxygen and relief of migraine and cluster headache, *J Neurosci* 27(4):261, 1995.

Peschen M et al: Low-frequency ultrasound treatment of chronic venous leg ulcers in an outpatient therapy, *Acta Derm Venereol* 77(4):311, 1997.

Peters EJG et al: The benefit of electrical stimulation to enhance perfusion in persons with diabetes mellitus, *J Foot Ankle Surg* 37(5):396, 1998.

Ramsay CA, Challoner AV: Vascular changes in human skin after ultraviolet irradiation, *Br J Dermatol* 94(5):487, 1976.

Reillo MR, Altieri RJ: HIV antiviral effects of hyperbaric oxygen therapy, *J Assoc Nurses AIDS Care* 7(1):43, 1996.

Robertson W: Digby's receipts, *Ann Med History* 7(3):216, 1925.

Robertson VJ, Baker KG: A review of therapeutic ultrasound: Effectiveness studies, *Phys Ther* 81(7):1339, 2001.

Roche C, West J: A controlled trial investigating the effect of ultrasound on venous ulcers referred from general practitioners, *Physiotherapy* 70:475, 1984.

Rowley B, McKenna J, Chase G: The influence of electrical current on an infecting microorganism in wounds, *Ann NY Acad Sci* 238:543, 1974.

Ryan TJ, Barnhill RL: Physical factors and angiogenesis in development of the vascular system. Ciba Foundation Symposium 100. London: Pitman Books, 1983.

Selkowitz DM et al: Efficacy of pulsed low-intensity ultrasound in wound healing: A single-case design, *Ostomy Wound Manage* 48(4):40, 2002.

Shamberger R et al: The effect of ultrasonics and thermal treatment on wounds, *Plast Reconstr Surg* 68(6):860, 1981.

Sheffield PJ: *Physics of the hyperbaric environment*. In Jefferson C. Davis Wound Care and Hyperbaric Medicine Center [Course], March 1, San Antonio, Tex., 1998a, Hyperbaric Medicine Team Training, Southwest Texas Methodist Hospital and Nix Medical Center.

Sheffield PJ: *Hyperbaric medicine: a historical perspective*. In Jefferson C. Davis Wound Care and Hyperbaric Medicine Center [Course], March 1, San Antonio, Tex., 1998b, Hyperbaric Medicine Team Training, Southwest Texas Methodist Hospital and Nix Medical Center.

Sheldon JL, Kokjohn TA, Martin EL: The effects of salt concentration and growth phase on MRSA solar and germicidal ultraviolet radiation resistance, *Ostomy Wound Manage* 51(1):36, 2005.

Shilling CW, Faiman MD: Physics of diving and physical effects on divers. In Shilling CW, Carlston CB, Mathias RA, editors: *The physician's guide to diving medicine*, New York, 1984, Plenum Press.

Siriwanij T, Vattanavongs V, Sitprija V: Hyperbaric oxygen therapy in crush injury, *Nephron* 75(4):484, 1997 (letter).

Skagen K, Henriksen O: Changes in subcutaneous blood flow during locally applied negative pressure to the skin, *Acta Physiol Scand* 117(3:)411, 1983.

Sparacia B, Sparacia G, Sansone A: *H.B.O. and cerebral investigations in stroke*. University of Palermo Institute of Anesthesiology/Undersea and Hyperbaric Oxygen Therapy Section, Jan 15, 1999, www.mbox. unipa.it/; Accessed January 15, 1999.

Spielholz NI, Kloth LC: Electrical stimulation and pulsed electromagnetic energy: differences in opinion, *Ostomy Wound Manage* 46(5):8, 2000.

Stegmen DJ: *Decompression sickness*. In Jefferson C, Davis Wound Care and Hyperbaric Medicine Center [Course], March 3, San Antonio, Tex., 1998, Hyperbaric Medicine Team Training, Southwest Texas Methodist Hospital and Nix Medical Center.

Stephens MB: Gas gangrene: potential for hyperbaric oxygen therapy, *Postgrad Med* 99(4):217, 1996.

Stromberg BV: Effects of electrical currents on wound contraction, *Ann Plast Surg* 21(2):121, 1988.

Sumpio BE et al: Mechanical stress stimulates aortic endothelial cells to proliferate, *J Vasc Surg* 6:252, 1987.

Swanson K: The role of hyperbaric oxygen therapy in wound healing, *World Council Enterostom Ther J* 18(1):7, 1998.

Swartz M et al: Mechanical stress is communicated between different cell types to elicit matrix remodeling, *Proc Nat Acad Sci* 98(11):6180, 2001.

Szuminsky NJ et al: Effect of narrow, pulsed high voltages on bacterial viability, *Phys Ther* 74(7):660, 1994.

Tai YJ et al: The use of hyperbaric oxygen for preservation of free flaps, *Ann Plast Surg* 28(3):284, 1992.

Taskan I et al: A comparative study of the effect of ultrasound and electrostimulation on wound healing in rats, *Plast Reconstr Surg* 100(4):966, 1997.

Taylor GJ, Bannister GC, Leeming JP: Wound disinfection with ultraviolet radiation, *J Hosp Infect* 30(2):85, 1995.

Taylor GJ, Leeming JP, Bannister GC: Effect of antiseptics, ultraviolet light and lavage on airborne bacteria in a model wound, *J Bone Joint Surg Br* 75(5):724, 1993.

Taylor GJ, Chandler L: Ultraviolet light in the orthopaedic operating theatre, *Br J Theatre Nurs* 6(10):10, 1997.

ter Reit G, Kessels AG, Knipschild P: A randomized clinical trial of ultrasound in the treatment of pressure ulcers, *Phys Ther* 76(12):1301, 1996.

Thai TP et al: Ultraviolet light c in the treatment of chronic wounds with MRSA: A case study, *Ostomy Wound Manage* 48(11):52, 2002.

Thai TP et al: Effect of ultraviolet light C on bacterial colonization in chronic wounds, *Ostomy Wound Manage* 51(10):32, 2005.

Thawer HA, Houghton PE: Effects of ultrasound delivered through a mist of saline to wounds in mice with diabetes mellitus, *J Wound Care* 13(5):171, 2004.

Undersea and Hyperbaric Medical Society (UHMS): *Guidelines for clinical multiplace hyperbaric facilities*: Report of the Hyperbaric Chamber Safety Committee of the Undersea and Hyperbaric Medical Society, Kensington, Md, 1994, Author.

Undersea and Hyperbaric Medical Society (UHMS): *Hyperbaric oxygen therapy*: a committee report, Kensington, Md, 1996, Author.

Undersea and Hyperbaric Medical Society (UHMS): *Purpose*, March 1, 2004, www.uhms.org; Accessed March 1, 2004.

Vanable JW Jr: Integumentary potentials and wound healing. In Borgan RB, et al, editors: *Electric Fields in Vertebrate Repair*. New York: Alan R, Liss, 1989.

Van Wicjck R, Manicourt D, Feruzi-Lukina G: *Biological monitoring of wounds treated by negative pressure*, Nice, France, 2002, ETRS New Technologies Focus Group Meeting.

Vrabec JT, Clements KS, Mader JT: Short-term tympanostomy in conjunction with hyperbaric oxygen therapy, *Laryngoscope* 108(8):1124, 1998.

Wagner SA et al: The effect of mist ultrasound transport technology on common bacterial wound pathogens, *Symp Adv Wound Care* 2001, Poster.

Wallace DJ et al: Use of hyperbaric oxygen in rheumatic diseases: case report and critical analysis, *Lupus* 4(3):172, 1995.

Weaver LK, Straas MB, editors: Monoplace hyperbaric chamber safety guidelines: report to the Hyperbaric Chamber Safety Committee of the Undersea and Hyperbaric Medical Society, Kensington, Md, 1991, UHMS.

Weichenthal M et al: Low-frequency ultrasound treatment of chronic venous ulcers, *Wound Rep Regen* 5(1):18, 1997.

Weiss D, Eaglstein W, Falanga V: Exogenous electric current can reduce the formation of hypertrophic scars, *J Dermatol Surg Oncol* 15(12):1272, 1989.

Wills EE et al: A randomized placebo-controlled trial of ultraviolet light in the treatment of superficial pressure sores, *J Am Geriatr Soc* 31(3):131, 1983.

WOCN Society: *Guideline for management of patients with lower extremity arterial disease*, WOCN clinical practice guideline series #1, Glenview IL, 2002, Author.

WOCN Society: *Guideline for management of pressure ulcers*, WOCN clinical practice guideline series #2, Glenview IL, 2003, Author.

WOCN Society: *Guideline for management of patients with lower extremity neuropathic disease*, WOCN clinical practice guideline series #1, Glenview IL, 2004, Author.

WOCN Society: *Guideline for management of patients with lower extremity venous disease*, WOCN clinical practice guideline series #1, Glenview IL, 2005, Author.

Wolcott L et al: Accelerated healing of skin ulcer by electrotherapy: preliminary clinical results, *South Med J* 62(7):795, 1969.

Wood J et al: A multicenter study on the use of pulsed low-intensity direct current for healing chronic stage II and stage III decubitus ulcers, *Arch Dermatol* 129(8):199, 1993.

Yang W, Onuma EK, Hui S: Response of C3H/10T1/2 fibroblasts to an external steady electric field stimulation, *Exper Cell Res* 155:92, 1984.

Young S, Dyson M: Effect of therapeutic ultrasound on the healing of full-thickness excised lesions, *Ultrasonics* 28:175, 1990a.

Young S, Dyson M: Macrophage responsiveness to therapeutic ultrasound, *Ultrasound Med Biol* 16:809, 1990b.

Zhao LL et al: Effect of hyperbaric oxygen and growth factors on rabbit ear ischemic ulcers, *Arch Surg* 129:1043, 1994.

Zonis Z et al: Salvage of the severely injured limb in children: a multidisciplinary approach, *Pediatr Emerg Care* 11(3):176, 1995.

21 *The Role of Surgery in Wound Healing*

JOYCE M. BLACK & STEVEN B. BLACK

OBJECTIVES

1. List three factors considered in surgical decision making.
2. Discuss four methods of wound closure.
3. Identify urgent operative conditions.
4. Describe preoperative and postoperative interventions for patients undergoing surgical flaps.

Surgical intervention for chronic wounds is seldom the first choice, and commonly much local care of the wound has preceded any decision for surgery. However, there are some chronic wounds that deteriorate and require emergent operative management, as well as wounds that reach a point in the healing trajectory where surgery is indicated to aid wound closure. This chapter will address those wounds benefited by operative treatment, the decisions about operative care, and the care of the patient and wound before and after surgery.

HISTORY OF SURGERY FOR WOUNDS

Wounds have surely existed since the beginning of man, mostly the results of trauma. Various natural products were used for wound management over time. The Edwin Smith Papyrus, which was written over 5000 years ago and is the oldest known surgical treatise, has 142 different references to the management of sores and wounds. Surgical management of wounds is nearly as old. Hippocrates said, "He who wishes to be a surgeon should go to war." Indeed, his words highlight the relationship of surgical advances and war-related injury. Reconstructive surgery had its beginnings with traumatic injury, at a time when the nose was cut off as a form of punishment and during duals with swords. During the sixteenth century, noses were reconstructed

in Italy using the skin of the inner upper aspect. This flap is known as the Tagliacozzi flap. Today, surgery remains a very important aspect of wound care, and advances in surgical options continue to be made.

DEBRIDEMENT

As described in Chapter 10, debridement is the removal of devitalized and highly contaminated tissues with the goal of preserving viable tissues and critical anatomic structures such as tendon, nerve, vessels, and bone. Debridement is an example of the principle of creating a wound bed that is likely to heal either by acute wound-healing methods or by the attachment of surgically transferred tissues. A recurring criticism of sharp and surgical debridement is that they are non-selective, and thus viable as well as nonviable tissue is removed. Although this is true from a broad-brush perspective, most surgical debridements are done until the wound bed is clean and bleeding. Even though some layers of good tissue may be removed, it is more likely that a lot of devitalized tissue is removed. Using surgical or sharp debridement, the patient is spared weeks of other forms of debridement. Delaying debridement can lead to progressive necrosis from desiccation of the surface of the wound and continued multiplication of bacteria in the necrotic (avascular) portion of the wound bed. Techniques for wound debridement are discussed in Chapter 10.

SURGICAL DECISION MAKING

Assessment of the Patient

Sometimes it is easy to become fixated on the wound, but it is important to remember that the wound exists in a person and no two people are the same. The human body is designed to heal wounds. When healing is not occurring, the practitioner should determine what is impairing all body systems, as well as what is occurring in the wound that is preventing healing. A complete history and physical examination is required that looks for factors like cardiopulmonary disease, autoimmune disease, diabetes, vascular disease, nutritional status, and other systemic diseases that interfere with wound healing. As described in Chapter 4 wound healing can also be deterred by nicotine and medications, such as corticosteroids, and immunosuppressants. Surgery can be misconstrued as a "magic cure" for the wound, and it is important to remember that surgical wounds will not heal any better than the native wound if the patient's condition is not improved to support healing processes.

When deciding which patient should undergo a surgical wound closure, the patient's condition forms the primary aspect of the risk portion of the risk-benefit ratio. While it is always ideal to have a closed wound, the patient must be able to tolerate anesthesia, surgery, blood loss, and postoperative restrictions. An estimation of anesthetic risk, such as the American Society of Anesthesiologists (ASA) classifications, provides an objective measure of relative risk for surgery. The patient must also be able to tolerate pain and immobility following surgery.

Preexistent malnutrition must be corrected. A wound, including a surgical wound, cannot heal without adequate nutrition. A reasonable axiom is that if a patient developed a wound on any given amount of caloric and protein intake, that same wound cannot be healed without additional calories and protein.

A unique group of patients have emerged in the last few years: patients who have undergone gastric bypass. The creation of irreversible malabsorption for weight loss creates a situation in which some patients cannot consume adequate calories or vitamins to heal a wound. These patients will need parenteral, not enteral, support before and after surgery.

Assessment of the Wound

Planning surgery also requires an understanding of the wound in terms of causative factors and missing or needed tissue. Information concerning these two issues must guide the selection of the most appropriate surgical option.

Causative Factors for the Wound. What caused the wound? Is the wound acute or chronic? If the wound is chronic, what factors are contributing to the chronicity?

The wound complicated by an ischemic process will require improvement of blood flow to heal. Acute traumatic wounds may be missing fragments of skin, but with removal of these devitalized tissues and mobilization of surrounding skin, the laceration may be closed primarily. Chronic wounds are often due to several problems: most notably, pressure, infection, and malnutrition, all of which must be improved before healing can ensue.

Missing or Needed Tissue. When planning surgery for wound healing, it is important to fully understand exactly what tissues are missing in order to reconstruct the area. If a wound lacks only skin, replacing the skin (skin graft) may be a reasonable option, provided other patient conditions are well managed. However, simply putting skin on a wound without controlling infection or ischemia is a doomed enterprise. Frequently, tissue padding (i.e., subcutaneous tissue and muscle) is needed to protect a bony prominence from recurrent breakdown.

Selection of Wound Closure Method

Selecting a method of closure depends on a holistic assessment that considers the needs and goals of the patient. A common set of decision making steps (i.e., a reconstructive ladder) serves as a guide in plastic and reconstructive surgery (Figure 21-1). The simplest method that accomplishes the patient's goals is usually the first choice. In addition to the complexity of the surgery, consideration is also given to the donor site morbidity that would be created. For example, if a person lost a thumb, transplantation of the great toe to replace the thumb would be considered; however, the thumb would not be used to replace a great toe.

When considering donor site morbidity for pressure ulcer surgery, it is important to realize that tissues can be moved or donated only once. Therefore, the choice of what tissue is used is very important. Large wounds of the entire perineum in patients with paralysis may require removal of the leg and filleting the tissues to form an adequately-sized flap of muscle and skin to sufficiently close the wound. This situation is obviously a dramatic example of donor site morbidity.

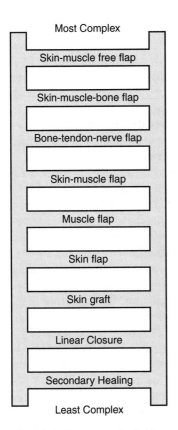

Most Complex

Skin-muscle free flap

Skin-muscle-bone flap

Bone-tendon-nerve flap

Skin-muscle flap

Muscle flap

Skin flap

Skin graft

Linear Closure

Secondary Healing

Least Complex

Fig. 21-1 Reconstructive ladder.

Wound closure methods include the following:
- Secondary healing
- Biosynthetic grafts
- Linear closure
- Skin grafts (autografts)
- Local flaps
- Distant (free) flaps

Secondary Healing. Letting a wound heal on its own with scar tissue is the simplest method of healing. Surgery to repair a small, clean stage II (partial-thickness) pressure ulcer would be rare. However, some partial thickness wounds (such as burns of the hands) create significant morbidity due to scars when left to heal on their own. Therefore skin grafting would be warranted. In addition, a chronically open and draining wound requires proper care of the etiologic factors, adequate nutrition, pressure relief and off loading, and local wound care to heal. Over prolonged periods the ongoing risk of infection from the open wound

BOX 21-1 **Examples of Surgical Tissue Flaps**
....
LOCAL FLAPS
Classified by anatomic structures:
- Skin flaps
- Fasciocutaneous
- Myocutaneous or musculocutaneous flaps

Classified by methods used to move the flap:
- Advancement flaps
- Rotation flaps
- Transposition flaps

Classified by methods of retaining perfusion:
- Random flaps
- Axial flaps

DISTANT (FREE) FLAPS

may prompt decisions for surgical closure. See other chapters in this text for information on secondary healing.

Biosynthetic Grafts. Composite materials that provide a scaffold for wound bed healing can be used to promote secondary healing of wounds. Materials that provide epidermal replacement can also be used to heal wounds. These products have some limited value, mainly in patients who are not candidates for autographs. Epidermal replacements are discussed in greater detail in Chapter 18.

Linear Closure. Bringing the edges of the wound together and securing the edges with suture, or linear closure, is a reasonable choice for surgical repair of traumatic wounds in which little tissue is missing. (Linear closure is the preferred term over primary closure, which only refers to timing of closure.)

Skin Grafts. Skin grafts (also called autografts) are sections of skin including the epidermis and a portion of the dermis that is removed from a donor site and transferred to cover a shallow and vascularized wound. The split-thickness skin grafts or STSG can be placed as entire pieces of skin or meshed to promote drainage of wound exudate and contouring to the skin surface. Skin grafts can also be full-thickness, but only where vascularity in the donor site is sufficient to heal full-thickness grafts. Skin grafts provide superficial coverage but do not replace deeper tissue layers, such as subcutaneous tissue and muscle; thus they are unable to provide the padding needed to protect bony prominences from recurrent breakdown. Skin grafts are commonly used to replace missing skin on venous stasis ulcers, burns, and so forth. While they are rarely, if ever, used in the surgical management of pressure ulcers, they may be used to close donor sites from flaps containing multiple layers of tissues.

Tissue Flaps. Tissue flaps involve the transfer of skin and underlying structures (such as subcutaneous tissue, fascia, and muscle) to fill a defect and pad it to resist pressure once healed. Flaps differ from skin grafts in that they carry their own blood supply with them. The native nutrient vessels are moved along with the flap, or reestablished (microsurgery) once the flap is transferred. Maintaining this blood supply is a crucial aspect of flap survival. Tissue flaps are either local or distant (free) flaps.

Local tissue flaps. Local flaps are most commonly used for pressure ulcers and are categorized by the anatomic structures they encompass, the method used to move the flap, or by the method used to perfuse the flap (Box 21-1).

Anatomic structures. Examples of tissue flaps classified by anatomic structures include skin flaps, fasciocutaneous flaps, and myocutaneous flaps.

Skin flaps, as the name states, are portions of skin moved from its usual location to cover a defect. Skin flaps are generally not used for pressure ulcer repair because they do not have enough padding or blood supply (provided by underlying muscle) to sustain pressure once the patient is sitting again.

Fasciocutaneous flaps include portions of the epidermis, dermis, and subcutaneous tissue supported by the underlying fascia. Fasciocutaneous flaps do provide padding and superficial coverage.

Myocutaneous (also called musculocutaneous) flaps involve rotation of all tissue layers (i.e., skin, subcutaneous tissue, fascia, and muscle). These flaps provide optimal coverage for a bony prominence and are therefore frequently used in the surgical reconstruction of a pressure ulcer. Myocutaneous flaps carry along with them the native arterial and venous blood supply to the muscle and its overlying skin. Because these flaps must survive on their original blood flow, they can only reach to certain areas. When pulled or stretched beyond their limits, blood vessels are also stretched and not able to perfuse the flap. Therefore postoperative monitoring of arterial inflow and venous outflow are important for flap survival.

Today the area of potential reach for each muscle flap is known. For example, the biceps femoris muscle (one of the lateral hamstring muscles) is supplied with blood via arteries from the profunda femoris. The flap has an arc of rotation that can cover defects of the ischium and groin.

Methods used to move the flap. Flaps can be classified according to the surgical technique used to transport them to the recipient site; these include advancement flaps, rotation flaps, and transposition flaps.

Advancement flaps involve elevation of the tissue to be transferred, undermining of the wound edges, and advancement of the tissue into the defect. Advancement flaps are useful in areas where there is significant redundant skin that can stretch.

Rotation flaps are used to fill defects adjacent to the donor tissue. A flap is outlined on three sides, the tissue is elevated, and the flap is rotated into the defect. The donor site may be closed surgically or may require a STSG for closure. Transposition flaps are rotation flaps that are moved across normal skin to fill a defect (as opposed to being directly adjacent to the defect).

Methods of retaining perfusion. Flap methods aimed at retaining perfusion include random flaps and axial flaps. All flaps of tissue carry with them a blood supply (unlike a skin graft). Random flaps depend on the dermal and subdermal vessels for their blood supply. Since these vessels are rather small, the blood supply to these flaps is somewhat tenuous. Axial flaps are designed to include an artery, which increases vascularity and the chances for flap survival. These vessels nourish the flap until new collateral capillary systems are established between the flap and the wound bed.

Distant (free) flaps. When tissue is not available locally, it can be brought in using a free flap. This type of operation is performed less commonly because it requires microvascular surgical techniques. In this approach, the donor tissue is completely removed from the donor site and transferred to the recipient site. The vessels are anastomosed by microvascular techniques to vessels near the wound. These types of flaps may be used to repair wounds of the lower third of the leg or the head and neck, and are sometimes used in breast reconstruction.

Tissue Expansion. An additional surgical option for wound closure is tissue expansion to stretch tissue including skin near the wound, which then can be move into the wound bed. Silastic expanders, or hollow pouches, are placed surgically into the subcutaneous or submuscular tissue layer in an area adjacent to the defect. Sterile fluid is injected into the expander at routine intervals until the pouch is fully expanded. This process induces expansion of the overlying tissue layers. When there is sufficient tissue to provide coverage of the defect, the expander is removed and the wound is closed.

NONOPERATIVE CONDITIONS

While it is important to know how to perform any given operation, it is equally important to know when not to operate. This discussion centers on the most common problems that rule out the use of surgical intervention; other conditions may also exist.

Pressure ulcers in the malnourished should not be repaired until the underlying malnutrition is controlled and the patient is anabolic again. If malnutrition is a volitional decision, then surgery should not be an option. If the reason the pressure ulcer did not heal was due to malnutrition, similarly the surgical wound will not heal for the same reasons.

Recalcitrant venous insufficiency ulcers require a bed of well-oxygenated granulation tissue to nourish a skin graft. If the edema cannot be controlled or the patient is unable to wear compression devices, a skin graft would not survive.

Calciphylaxis is due to ischemia in the skin from vascular calcification. It is most commonly seen in patients with renal failure, hypercalcemia, and hyperphosphatemia. Lesions usually develop on the legs and begin in areas of mottled skin that progress into painful, firm areas of necrosis. If surgery is considered at all, it is usually to debride the lesion to prevent sepsis. Unfortunately, until the underlying problems are controlled, the wounds will often reappear.

Stable eschar on the heel also presents a nonoperative condition. Stable eschar is dry, hard, and firmly attached to the underlying skin; any indications of an infection (induration, erythema, or pain) are absent. Stable eschar on the heels should be left intact: not debrided and not softened. Slowly, the eschar will release at the edges, as the underlying tissue heals. The loose eschar can then be trimmed. Moistening or softening the eschar encourages invasion of bacteria. Removal of the eschar exposes the fat pad, which can then desiccate and expose the calcaneous.

Operative closure of the ischemic wound is also contraindicated. Performing debridements on ischemic wounds will often make the wound larger with little hope of healing. Unless the arterial inflow can be reestablished, the wound is best left alone. Local wound care for ischemic wounds, such as arterial wounds, includes protection and coverage with dressing material that is easily removed.

Inability to adhere to postoperative care requirements can be a significant deterrent to healing a surgical wound. If the patient cannot remain off of a flap, consume adequate calories, and control fecal and/or urinary contamination of the incision, the skin graft or flap is likely to fail. It is important to keep in mind that there are only a given number of flap options to be used in a lifetime. Once a muscle is used, it cannot be used again. Therefore the decision to operate should be made only after the patient is adequately educated regarding the interventions necessary postoperatively to reduce complications and recurrence.

URGENT OPERATIVE CONDITIONS
Traumatic Wounds

Traumatic wounds come in all shapes and varieties; they also occur in patients of all ages and with many premorbid conditions. The surgical principles discussed previously again apply here. Patients with traumatic wounds need a thorough assessment to be certain that they do not have major vessel, nerve, or tendon injury (therefore the examination must be completed before the administration of local anesthetics). The wound is closed primarily when possible, without creating donor site morbidity, such as pulling the lower eyelid down and exposing the eye because the lid cannot close. Facial wounds require the use of small suture in order to avoid excess scar formation. The closure line should be clean and covered with a thin layer of antibiotic ointment until healed. Suture removal depends upon the body part being repaired (facial sutures are removed in 4 to 7 days, whereas suture in the lower leg or buttocks may require 2 weeks to support healing).

When patients are severely injured, the wound issues may come second in priority to tending to the airway, breathing, and circulation. Clean wounds should be dressed with normal saline gauze and, if possible, closed within 12 to 24 hours. After that time, they are considered contaminated. Operative closure should be a delayed primary closure, or the wound should be allowed to heal secondarily, with scar revision at a later date.

Abscess

An abscess is a local collection of pus and sometimes blood. Abscesses are incised and drained. The remaining cavity may require packing to prevent healing occurring at the surface before healing below.

Gangrene

Wet gangrene develops from a sudden interruption in blood supply such as with burns, freezing, hematoma, and injury that then becomes infected, or from primary infection of tissues from certain bacteria. Wet gangrene from any organism can quickly spread into surrounding tissues as a result of the bacteria destroying muscle and other tissues. The patient has pain and fever. The tissue becomes discolored, blistered, and boggy and may have crepitus if the wound is infected with gas-forming organisms such as *Clostridium perfringens (formerly known as Clostridium welchi)*. There is frequently no line of demarcation between normal and infected tissue. Anaerobic infections can develop into gas gangrene within 1 to 2 days, and if the patient develops bacteremia, there is 20% to 25% mortality. If recognized and treated early and aggressively, nearly 80% of patients will survive (Laor et al, 1995).

Surgery for wet gangrene includes radical removal of infected tissues or amputation. Hyperbaric oxygen therapy may also be used. Spreading gangrene is a surgical emergency. The wounds from these operations can be quite large and deep, with extensive areas of tissue loss.

In contrast, dry gangrene develops slowly from progressive loss of arterial supply, commonly in the extremities. A coagulative necrosis develops, and the tissue becomes black, dry, scaly, and greasy. There is a clear line of demarcation between viable and gangrenous tissue. The body will slowly slough the gangrenous tissue at the line of demarcation. Surgery may not be needed, unless the area becomes infected. Although the gangrene is not painful at this stage, it was likely quite painful earlier in the process because of ischemia, and adjacent compromised tissue may exhibit ischemic pain. Dry gangrene should be dressed with dry dressings and the tissue not moistened to prevent conversion to wet gangrene. Never soak an area of dry gangrene.

Necrotizing Fasciitis

Necrotizing fasciitis is a rapidly spreading, inflammatory infection of the deep fascia, with secondary necrosis of the subcutaneous tissues. The causative bacteria may be aerobic or anaerobic. Frequently, two synergistic bacteria that thrive in the tissues that have low levels of oxygen can be causative. Because of the common presence of gas-forming organisms, subcutaneous air is classically described in necrotizing fasciitis. Pain out of proportion to the physical findings is a hallmark sign. The infection spreads along the fascial plane. These infections can be difficult to recognize in their early stages, but they rapidly progress to septic shock and organ failure. Emergency aggressive surgical debridement is required to remove all the necrotic tissue. Empiric broad-spectrum intravenous antibiotics are used until culture findings are known; however, the shock does not improve until the involved tissue is debrided. Hyperbaric oxygen is an important adjunct to treatment where available.

PREOPERATIVE MANAGEMENT
Reducing Cofactors

When the wound team has the luxury of time, improving the patient's underlying condition is time well spent. This section will address methods to improve the preoperative condition of the patient, so as to improve the likelihood of success. There are many comorbid conditions that can delay healing of both chronic and acute surgical wounds. It is beyond the scope of this text to address all of them; rather, the common culprits behind nonhealing will be emphasized.

Arterial Inflow. Without adequate arterial blood inflow, wounds cannot heal. Arterial bypass surgery, stenting, or antiplatelet medications may improve arterial flow. In the interim, limbs impaired by lack of arterial flow should be protected from injury.

Bioburden. Infection is a common denominator to nonhealing. Wounds that have foul odor or a biofilm are likely infected or heavily colonized. Topical antibiotics and/or systemic antibiotics may be required. Of course, debridement may be advantageous.

Corticosteroids. Corticosteroids prevent inflammation, and since inflammation is critical for healing,

healing stalls in their presence. Many conditions, such as emphysema and rheumatoid arthritis, are treated with corticosteroids, and they often cannot be stopped. Sometimes vitamin A can be used to reverse the effects of corticosteroids, but one has to beware of hypervitaminosis A.

Diabetes. Diabetes, specifically blood glucose control, is an important issue in infection control. White blood cells become ineffective at phagocytosis when blood glucose is over 200 mg/dl. Diabetes also causes microvascular disease, which hinders healing in the feet. Although the mechanism is poorly understood, people with diabetes have a reduced ability to fight *Staphylococcus aureus* and fungal infections.

Malnutrition. One of the most common comorbid states hampering chronic wound healing is protein-calorie malnutrition. A wound simply will not heal in states of malnutrition, because the "building blocks" of cells and energy for cellular reproduction are not available. Malnutrition must be addressed before any operation. Patients who do not want to be "maintained artificially with life support through artificial feeding" can be encouraged to be tube fed to "jump start" their healing and restore strength. Dietitians should be involved to compute the appropriate calories and protein grams. A common problem is assuming that tube feeding or parenteral nutrition is meeting patient needs. In practice, these feedings are interrupted or slowed periodically for various reasons, so total calorie and protein intake still must be measured daily to ensure goals are met.

Nicotine. Nicotine is a vasoconstrictor, and if a patient smokes for 2 weeks before surgery or for 4 weeks after surgery, the resultant impairment in arterial flow will delay healing and increase the risk of infection. Programs to support smoking cessation should be offered. Health care providers must appreciate the addictive nature of nicotine, and the true intake of tobacco should be validated. Nicotine patches must not be used during times of wound healing; the sustained delivery of nicotine causes continuous vasoconstriction.

Spasms. Paraplegics, quadriplegics, and patients with other neurologic diseases have spasms that can lead to friction damage to or to pressure or pull on incisions. Spasm control is important to reduce tension on incision lines.

Wound Bed Preparation

Successful closure of any wound requires a clean, perfusing wound bed. Although the exact mechanism of action is unproven, it appears that suction reduces surrounding tissue edema allowing new, enriched blood to flow into the wound. Negative-pressure wound therapy (NPWT) is especially useful in speeding up the process of wound bed preparation for flaps, for treating dehisced wounds, or for preparing wounds for delayed linear closure (Fife et al, 2004).

OPERATIVE MANAGEMENT

Pressure ulcer excision and closure are commonly completed under general anesthesia, even in those patients with paralysis, to reduce spastic and reflexic muscle movement as well as to control their vasomotor instability. Blood loss is anticipated, and the patient has blood typed and cross-matched for intraoperative administration.

Sacral Ulcers. The sacrum is the most common location for pressure ulcers; large skin defects in the sacral area are not uncommon and can be associated with even larger areas of undermining. Fortunately, these ulcers are rarely deep. Ostectomy of the sacral prominence is necessary if bone is infected. Coverage is most commonly obtained with a large myocutaneous or fasciocutaneous flaps (Figure 21-2).

Greater Trochanteric Ulcers. Ulcers on the greater trochanter are seen in patients, many of whom have severe contractures and can only lie on their sides. The tensor fasciae latae (TFL) myocutaneous flap is the workhorse of ulcer covering in this region. It is most commonly designed as a transposition flap with a large resultant dog-ear (Figure 21-3). V-Y advancement (see following discussion of ischial ulcers for V-Y flap description) and rotation of the TFL flap often give an excellent functional and better esthetic result. Other flaps include the rectus femoris myocutaneous flap and random bipedicle or unipedicle fasciocutaneous flaps.

Ischial Ulcers. Ischial ulcers occur from prolonged erect sitting without changes in position. They are most common in paraplegics and quadriplegics. There is usually a small skin wound with a large cavity beneath the surface. The ischial tuberosity is the pressure point and is always involved, however ischial ostectomy is avoided if the bone is not infected, because the body

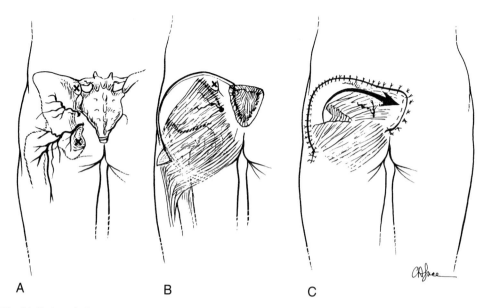

A   B   C

Fig. 21-2 Sacral ulcers can be closed with a gluteus maximus myocutaneous flap. **A,** The gluteus muscle is identified using landmarks (indicated by *X*) of the ischial tuberosity and the posterior iliac spine. **B,** The small segment of the muscle is rotated into the wound and is being fed by the superior gluteal artery. **C,** The muscle is divided and moved into the wound. The wound is closed primarily with a long incision to avoid tension. (Figure from Cohen S: Pressure sores. In McCarthy J: *Plastic surgery, Philadelphia,* 1990, Saunders.)

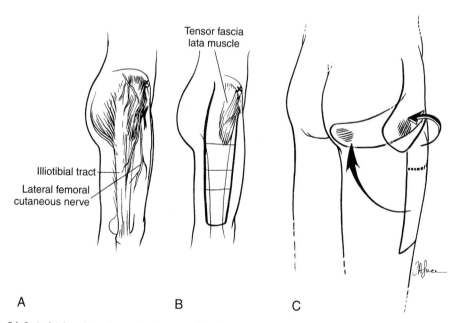

Tensor fascia lata muscle

Illiotibial tract

Lateral femoral cutaneous nerve

A   B   C

Fig. 21-3 Ischial and trochanteric ulcers can be closed using the tensor fascia latae flap. **A,** The muscle is found on the lateral thigh and fed by femoral circumflex artery, which enters at the superior anterior iliac spine. **B,** The advantage of the flap is the long muscle and skin cover. **C,** The arc of rotation can provide coverage for both ischial and trochanteric ulcers. (Figure from Cohen S: Pressure sores. In McCarthy J: *Plastic surgery, Philadelphia,* 1990, Saunders. Used with permission of WB Saunders.)

weight is then distributed onto the perineum and the resulting ulcers are very difficult to manage.

Many options for flaps exist, including the tensor fascia latae (see Figure 21-3). The hamstring V-Y myocutaneous flap may be used for patients with recurrent ulcerations in extremely large defects. This flap is particularly valuable for layer defects because thorough dissection yields 10 to 12 cm of advancement. It is called a V-Y flap because the flap is raised with V-shaped incisions and then closed as a Y. This flap is well vascularized by segmental perforators from the hamstrings originating from the deep femoral artery. However, because the origins and insertions of the muscles are severed, this flap cannot be used in an ambulatory patient. Additional myocutaneous flaps for ischial ulcer closure include the rectus abdominis flap and the gracilis flap.

The gluteus maximus muscle flap offers a large amount of well-vascularized tissue with which to fill the defect. Even in the patient with a spinal cord injury, significant muscle exists. Skin closure of the donor site can be obtained by linear closure in some cases or by a separate, inferiorly-based fasciocutaneous rotation flap.

Multiple Pressure Ulcers. Extensive ulcerations of the sacrum, trochanters, and ischium are not uncommon, particularly in paralyzed patients. Amputation of a lower limb and use of the skin and muscle from the thigh, called a total thigh flap, has sometimes been necessary to provide enough tissue to close these extensive multiple wounds. Before surgery, urologic evaluation is completed because of the frequency of urinary infection. Urinary diversion may be required. Fecal diversion (temporary colostomy) may also be necessary. Common complications after surgery include hemorrhage and infection. Prolonged immobilization on special pressure redistribution beds is needed postoperatively, or these flaps will fail.

POSTOPERATIVE MANAGEMENT
Skin Grafts

Survival of skin grafts depends on revascularization of the grafted skin. Initially the skin survives thanks to the plasma on the wound surface. Within 72 hours, new vessels should traverse the graft and change it to a pink color. The change in the color of the grafted skin signifies what is called a "take" and is often expressed as a percentage of take or adherence to the wound bed

that occurs through the ingrowth of new capillaries and fibrin bands. For example, a STSG is reported to have a 90% take after 72 hours when the first dressing is changed.

The two factors most commonly associated with skin graft failure are (1) failure to adequately immobilize the graft, which is critical to revascularization, and (2) infection. One of the most common clinical problems after lower-extremity skin grafting is the failure to prevent edema in the wound bed. The patient must keep the skin graft site elevated for at least 72 hours. All too often, the patient tries to get to the bathroom quickly or sit briefly on the edge of the bed, and the grafted site becomes engorged with blood despite stented dressings and wraps. Clear instructions are imperative.

NPWT is sometimes used over skin grafts to promote adherence. Although the actual mechanism of action is not known, it is likely that the NPWT immobilizes the graft and reduces edema in the wound bed. The graft must be meshed for the NPWT to be effective. The NPWT sponge cannot be placed directly on the graft, and constant suction *must* be applied for 72 hours. Any interruption of suction will likely disrupt the graft.

Once the graft has taken, the site is dry and prone to pruritus, dermatitis, or folliculitis. These conditions occur because sweat and oil glands are located in the deep dermis and are not transferred with partial-thickness skin grafts. Patients must be taught to develop lifelong strategies to protect and moisturize the skin.

The donor site for the STSG is a partial-thickness wound, which heals by reepithelialization. Donor sites require protection for healing. Usual covers for donor sites include transparent films, fine mesh gauze, Xeroform, and castor oil-balsam of Peru-trypsin ointment. The ointment was shown to lead to healing in an average of 11 days in a small study of 36 patients (Carson et al, 2003). In 1998, a review of healing rates, infection rates, and pain levels found that transparent film was the most efficacious cover for donor sites, leading to healing in an average of 9.47 days (Rakel et al, 1998).

Flaps

After surgery the patient is placed on a specialty bed, which provides pressure redistribution and eliminates shear (such as an air-fluidized bed). A minimum requirement is 3 weeks on a specialty bed. It is very important to not pull on the flap while turning the patient; the use of turning sheets is imperative. Drainage in the wound and undermined areas is removed with closed system suction drains until drainage is minimal, to reduce the risk of hematoma and infection.

Mobility and exposure to pressure is gradually increased, beginning 3 to 5 weeks after the procedure, with careful monitoring of skin and suture lines. It is important to provide chair or wheelchair padding after surgery to reduce the risk of ischemia. If the patient is wheelchair-dependent, the seat cushion should be assessed before use. Inadequate pressure redistribution may be the cause of the ulceration, and will recur without revision or replacement of the seat cushion.

Complications include flap necrosis due to spasm or stretch of the feeding blood vessels to the flap. The tissue appears pale and is cool or cold. The most common complication is recurrence of the ulcer. Early recurrences are due to mobilizing too much too early, which is frequently due to efforts to reduce hospital length-of-stay. Late recurrences are often due to failure to change the previous lifestyle behaviors that caused the first ulcer. It is crucial that support, equipment, and educational needs are addressed and in place before discharge to facilitate adaptation (Chapter 26) and prevent reoccurrence. Flaps are not as resilient as native tissue, and periods of time sitting on the flaps must be somewhat limited in duration *forever*. Once again, one must remember that there are only a few flap sites available for reconstruction of any given area; once they are all used, the prognosis is grim.

SUMMARY

Many surgical wound closure techniques are available. However, surgical closure of wounds is not a panacea and is not appropriate for all wounds or all patients. The success of surgical wound closures is contingent upon management of several issues such as the causative factors of the wound, the type of tissue missing and needed, the patient's general physiologic condition, the type of wound closure technique selected, preoperative nutritional status, postoperative care, and lifestyle behaviors.

SELF-ASSESSMENT EXERCISE

1. List four methods of wound closure.
2. List 3 ways to categorize local flaps.
3. Identify four urgent operative conditions.
4. Identify five cofactors that can delay healing of surgical wounds.
5. All of the following interventions are appropriate for postoperative management of the patient with a skin graft (STSG) EXCEPT:
   a. Elevate skin graft for 72 hours
   b. Negative pressure wound therapy (NPWT) to promote adherence
   c. Cleanse with Betadine twice a day
   d. Lifelong strategies to moisturize the skin

REFERENCES

Carson SN et al: Using a castor oil-balsam of Peru-trypsin ointment to assist in healing skin graft donor sites, *Ostomy Wound Manage* 49(6):60, 2003.

Fife CE et al: Healing dehisced surgical wounds with negative pressure wound therapy, *Ostomy Wound Manage* 50(4A):28, 2004.

Laor E et al: Outcome prediction in patients with Fournier's gangrene, *J Urol* Jul;154(1):89-92, 1995.

Rakel BA et al: Split-thickness skin graft donor site care: a quantitative synthesis of the research, *Appl Nurs Res* 11(4):174, 1998.

OBJECTIVES

1. Define the following terms; extravasation, infiltration, irritant and vesicant.
2. Identify two cytotoxic and two noncytotoxic agents that may cause tissue damage if extravasation occurs.
3. Describe the etiology and clinical manifestations of a fungating wound.
4. List two key goals and at least three potential interventions for the management of a fungating wound, extravasation, and radiation-induced skin damage.
5. Discuss the pathophysiologic basis for radiation-induced skin damage.
6. Differentiate between acute and late skin reactions to irradiation.
7. List two manifestations and two interventions for each stage of radiation skin reaction.
8. Identify key patient education information that will reduce the likelihood of acute radiation-induced skin reactions and prevent long-term complications in the irradiated field.

Alterations in skin integrity may also develop as a consequence of medical therapy given for pathologic conditions such as cancer. This chapter presents three commonly encountered oncologic complications that involve the skin. These can develop during the course of cancer therapy or months to years later. The risk factors, assessment, prevention, and treatment for each condition are described.

EXTRAVASATION

The role of the wound care specialist in the care of the patient with an extravasation is to provide consultation in the management of the wound resulting from the extravasation. Initial interventions required when an extravasation of a chemotherapeutic agent occurs are provided by the oncology staff as guided by national guidelines (ONS, 2001). Therefore it is not an expectation that the wound care specialist be familiar with each medication, irritant potential, or immediate post extravasation interventions specific to each medication. The wound care specialist, however, may be consulted for wound management once the tissue damage is evident. The following sections will address risk factors, prevention, assessment and treatment for extravasation injury to serve as a foundation and to facilitate informed treatment of the resulting skin injury.

Definition of Terms

Leakage of intravenous (IV) fluid into surrounding tissues may cause a tissue reaction that ranges from an inflammatory reaction and irritation to tissue necrosis (Schrijvers, 2003). In most situations, leakage of intravenous fluids or medications into surrounding tissues is innocuous. According to the Intravenous Nurses Society (1998), an *infiltration* is an inadvertent administration of a nonirritant solution into surrounding tissue which does not cause blistering or necrosis of the skin. When the solution however, causes an inflammatory reaction in the tissue, it is called an *extravasation*. Depending upon the severity of reaction, the fluid that causes an extravasation is referred to as either an irritant or a vesicant.

When an extravasation causes a local inflammatory reaction but does not cause tissue necrosis, the agent is called an *irritant*. Irritants produce pain, burning, or inflammation without necrosis when extravasated. These reactions occur at the injection site or along the vein (Schrijvers, 2003). Although these may cause erythema or tenderness, the symptoms are self-limiting, and there are no long-term sequelae.

In contract, when an extravasation results in blistering or tissue necrosis the fluid causing the extravasation is called a *vesicant*. The severity of injury caused by the vesicant is dependent upon several factors: 1) the specific drug administered, 2) its concentration, 3) the amount of drug extravasated, 4) the length of time that tissue is exposed to the drug, and 5) the anatomic site of the extravasation. Vesicants may be *noncytotoxic* solutions such as hyperosmolar solutions, vasopressor agents, and antibiotics (see Table 22-1). The tissue damage resulting from extravasation of noncytotoxic vesicants involves a defined space and is not progressive. It is important for the wound care specialist to be aware that the potential for significant local reactions caused by noncytotoxic agents exists, because these medications are administered to the patient population at large in a variety of health care settings.

Another subset of vesicant solutions is antineoplastic solutions and are referred to as, *cytotoxic vesicants*. Chemotherapeutic agents that leak into the tissue surrounding an IV site such as doxorubicin, daunorubicin, epirubicin, and mitomycin, can result in progressive and severe tissue destruction as well as significant pain. Not all chemotherapy agents however, are cytotoxic. In fact, less than half of the available antineoplastic drugs have a vesicant or irritant potential (Boyle and Engelking, 1995).

The incidence of extravasation of cytotoxic infusions ranges from as low as 0.1% to 6.5% to as high as 10% to 30% (How and Brown, 1998; Buck, 1998).

This widely discrepant incidence probably reflects the challenges in measuring extravasation incidence. According to Boyle and Engelking (1995) actual extravasation injuries are sporadic and underreported; the incidence of extravasation from vascular access devices is unknown.

Ulcer formation at the extravasation site of a cytotoxic agent may be delayed for several days or weeks as a result of diffusion of the drug into adjacent tissue. Subsequent tissue damage and the formation of slough will progress over several weeks and months and often require excision and skin grafting (Langer, Sehested, and Jensen, 2000).

Table 22-2 provides a list of cytotoxic agents and their potential for skin injury. It is important to note that the classification of antineoplastic agents is not flawless. For example, paclitaxel, normally classified as an irritant, may actually be a vesicant. In a case report, a patient experienced a delayed vesicant reaction to a paclitaxel extravasation that resulted in severe necrosis. No acute symptoms were reported at the time of extravasation. The site was erythematous and had areas of central necrosis requiring debridement and closure by a plastic surgeon (Herrington and Figueroa, 1997). Similarly, Kennedy and colleagues (2003) described a patient with an antecubital extravasation with a single dose of oxaliplatin. Formerly thought to be a nonvesicant, it caused significant muscle necrosis and fibrosis that did respond to conventional therapeutic modalities.

TABLE 22-1 **Noncytotoxic Vesicants**

ANTIBIOTICS	ELECTROLYTES	MISCELLANEOUS	VASOPRESSORS
Cephalothin	Calcium chloride	Acyclovir	Dopamine
Chloramephenicol	Calcium gluconate	Aminophylline	Epinephrine
Gentamicin	Potassium chloride	Dextrose 0.10%	Metaramenol
Nafcillin	Sodium bicarbonate	Diazepam	Norepinephrine
Oxacillin		Dobutamine	
Vancomycin		Mannitol	
		Phenytoin	
		Radiocontrast media	
		Total parenteral nutrition solutions (not intravenous lipids)	

TABLE 22-2 Cytotoxic Agents: Potential for Skin Injury

VESICANT	IRRITANT	MINIMAL	NONE
amsacrine	bortezomib	diethylstilbestrol	aldesleukin
carmustine	cisplatin	methotrexate	amifostine
dactinomycin	dacarbazine	mitoxantrone	asparaginase
daunorubicin	docetaxel	pemetrexed	BCG
doxorubicin	etoposide	porfimer	bleomycin
epirubicin	liposomal doxorubicin		buserelin
idarubicin	mesna (undiluted)		carboplatin
mechlorethamine	paclitaxel		cladribine
melphalan	porfimer		cyclophosphamide
mitomycin	teniposide		clodronate
plicamycin			cyproterone
streptozocin			cytarabine
vinblastine			dexrazoxane
vincristine			fludarabine
vinorelbine			fluorouracil
			fulvestrant
			gemcitabine
			goserelin
			ifosfamide
			interferon
			irinotecan
			leucovorin
			leuprolide
			mercaptopurine
			mesna (diluted)
			octreotide
			oxaliplatin
			pamidronate
			pentostatin
			raltitrexed
			rituximab
			trastuzumab

Source-Cancer Care Ontario, 2006.

Prevention of Extravasation

Recognizing patients at risk for extravasation, along with the risk profile of the medications, can signal the need for precautions that will decrease the occurrence of extravasation injuries. All departments in which cytotoxic agents are given must have written guidelines for handling cytotoxic agents, procedures to detect and treat acute extravasation, and an extravasation kit that holds all the necessary material and drugs to treat extravasation should it occur (Camp-Sorrell 1998; Hurst and Keith, 2005; ONS, 2001).

Factors that place a patient at risk for extravasation are grouped as patient factors, infusion site factors, and type of needle; risk factors are detailed in Box 22-1 (Buck, 1998; Ener, Meglathry, and Styler, 2004). Age, both young and old, is recognized as one of the most significant risk factors because of the condition of blood vessels and skin structure. Any condition that masks inflammation will mask the early warning signs of pending extravasation (i.e., pain and erythema) and therefore make the patient more vulnerable to extravasation. For example, it is difficult to identify erythema

BOX 22-1 Risk Factors for Extravasation Injury

Patient Factors

- Impaired ability to communicate pain (i.e., confusion, debilitation)
- Elderly
- Small blood vessels and immature skin structure (infants, neonates, premature babies, small children)
- Individuals with darker complexions (resulting from the difficulty in assessing early warning signs such as erythema)
- Inadequate veins

Infusion Site Factors

- Preexisting lymphatic impairment or obstruction (i.e., mastectomy, lymphedema)
- Site is located over a joint, tendon, nerve, or bony prominence
- Site is located within area exposed to prior radiation
- Peripheral neuropathy
- Recent venipuncture in the same vein
- Impaired vascularity (i.e., peripheral vascular disease)

Type of Needle

- Large cannula gauge (therefore smaller internal diameter of the needle)
- Steel needles

in darkly pigmented skin and pain in infants and individuals with paralysis or impaired communication.

Prevention of extravasation injuries includes a thorough assessment of the patient, the venous access, related risk factors, and knowledge of the vesicant potential of the drug. Vesicant agents should only be given through a newly established line. Infusions should be halted at the first sign of discomfort, altered infusion flow, lack of blood return, or a local reaction.

Assessment

During administration of irritants and vesicants, the injection site must be monitored closely for swelling, stinging, burning, bleb formation, pain, or redness. Induration, or obvious ulcer formation, is not an immediate manifestation, and visual inspection

cannot determine the potential for or extent of tissue impairment (Boyle and Engelking, 1995). Lack of blood return may suggest extravasation, but alone it is not always indicative of such. Because extravasation can occur without symptoms, periodic reassessment of the injection site after completion of the infusion is warranted. Table 22-3 lists the parameters that should be included when conducting an intravenous site skin assessment for possible extravasation or infiltration.

Extravasation must be distinguished from venous flare and infiltration. Venous flare involves the development of an erythematous streak along the course of the vein with pruritus, patchy erythema, and/or urticaria. Venous flare, a transient reaction, occurs in approximately 3% of cytotoxic agent infusions, does not have the serious sequelae of extravasations, and disappears within 30 minutes (ONS, 2001). As noted previously, infiltration and extravasation are separate processes. An infiltration scale is available in Table 22-4. The infiltration of any amount of blood product, irritant, or vesicant is classified as a grade 4 infiltration because of the potential for patient harm.

Interventions

Early intervention after extravasation can lessen the severity of tissue injury. It is estimated that one third of all extravasations will produce ulceration in the absence of therapy (Ener, Meglathry, and Styler, 2004). Treatment of extravasation of chemotherapy or biotherapy should be guided by the ONS guidelines available online through the National Guideline Clearinghouse (ONS, 2001). Interventions range from modalities such as thermal devices to alter the temperature of superficial skin, to manipulation of the pH of exposed tissue and injection of antidotes into the affected area to reverse the action of the infiltrated agent or to otherwise interfere with the process of cell destruction.

Once infiltration of a peripheral line is noted the following steps should be taken:

(1) Discontinue the infusion and disconnect the intravenous (IV) line, leaving the IV catheter or butterfly in place (Hadaway, 2004; ONS, 2001).

(2) Attempt to aspirate the residual drug from the catheter or butterfly by using a small (1- to 3-cc) syringe (Buck, 1998; ONS, 2001).

TABLE 22-3 Assessment of Extravasation versus Other Reactions

| ASSESSMENT PARAMETER | EXTRAVASATION | | SPASM/IRRITATION OF THE VEIN | FLARE REACTION |
	IMMEDIATE MANIFESTATIONS OF EXTRAVASATION	*DELAYED MANIFESTATIONS OF EXTRAVASATION*		
Pain	Severe pain or burning that lasts minutes or hours eventually subsides; usually occurs while the drug is being given around the needle site	Hours - 48	Aching and tightness along the vein	No pain
Redness	Blotchy redness around the needle site; it is not always present at the time of extravasation	Later occurrence	The full length of the vein may be reddened or darkened	Immediate blotches or streaks along the vein, which usually subside within 30 minutes with or without treatment
Ulceration	Develops insidiously; usually occurs 48-96 hours later	Late occurrence	Not usually	Not usually
Swelling	Severe swelling; usually occurs immediately	Hours - 48	Not likely	Not likely; wheals may appear along the vein line
Blood return	Inability to obtain blood return	Good blood return during drug administration	Usually	Usually
Other	Change in the quality of infusion	Local tingling and sensory deficits	Possible resistance felt in injection	Uricaria

Source-Cancer Care Ontario, 2006.

(3) Administer the appropriate antidote (if known) either through the catheter or subcutaneously (ONS, 2001).

(4) Elevate the affected limb to decrease swelling, palliate pain and increase net blood flow away from the area (ONS, 2001; Buck, 1998).

(5) Avoid even slight pressure on an extravasation site because this may spread the vesicant agent over a much broader area (ONS, 2001).

(6) Apply heat or cold to the site as indicated by national guidelines and institutional policy (ONS, 2001).

However, moist heat is contraindicated because it can precipitate maceration.

National guidelines and institutional policies should be followed to determine the appropriate type of compress (warm or cold) to use because it will vary according to the medication used. For example, cold compresses are preferred for all extravasations by cyto-toxic chemotherapy agents *except the vinca alkaloid medications* (vincristine, vinblastine or vinorelbine). Cold causes vasoconstriction and decrease fluid absorption. In contrast, cold has an adverse effect with

TABLE 22-4 Infiltration Scale

GRADE 0	GRADE 1	GRADE 2	GRADE 3	GRADE 4
No symptoms	Skin blanched Edema less than 1 inch Cool to touch with or without pain	Skin blanched Edema 1 to 6 inches Cool to touch with or without pain	Skin blanched, translucent Gross edema greater than 6 inches Mild to moderate pain Possible numbness	Skin blanched, translucent Skin tight, leaking Skin discolored, bruised, swollen Gross edema greater than 6 inches Deep pitting tissue edema Circulatory impairment Moderate to severe pain Infiltration of any amount of blood product, irritant, vesicant

From Intravenous Nurses Society: Intravenous nursing: standards of practice, *J Intraven Nurs* 21(1 suppl):S36, 1998.

the vinca alkalid extravasations (vincristine, vinblastine, and vinorelbine) and warming is preferred (Cancer Care Ontario, 2006). Intermittent application of cold as a compress is preferred, because continuous application of ice to the area may cause an increase in tissue necrosis. Since the optimal frequency and duration for the application of warm or cold compresses is not known, each intermittent application should be for as long as the patient can comfortably tolerate (ONS, 2001).

Further measures are outlined by the guidelines established by the Oncology Nursing Society (2001) that are specific to the infiltrate. In follow-up, the site should be monitored closely 24 hours later, at one week, two weeks and as indicated for pain, redness, swelling, ulceration, and necrosis. Depending upon the patient's overall health and immune status, if necrosis and ulceration develops, the wound care clinician may need to monitor the wound site more frequently. A referral to a plastic surgeon may be warranted if a large volume of vesicant was extravasated or the area and depth of tissue damage is significant (ONS, 2001). However, routine surgical excision is not warranted since not all vesicant extravasations will ulcerate (ONS, 2001; Heitmann, Durmus, and Infianni, 1998).

Documentation and close follow-up with appropriate consultations are highly recommended. Photographic documentation of the extravasation may also be mandated by institutional policy. It is

TABLE 22-5 Antidotes for Extravasation of Cytotoxic Agents

EXTRAVASATED DRUG	SUGGESTED ANTIDOTE
daunorubicin doxorubicin epirubicin idarubicin mitomycin	Dimethylsulfoxide (DMSO)
mechlorethamine	Sodium thiosulfate
vinblastine vincristine vinorelbine	Hyaluronidase injection (no longer available in Canada)

Source-Cancer Care Ontario, 2006.

important to record the date and time of the infusion, when extravasation was noted, the size and type of catheter, and the drug and amount administered, along with estimated amount of extravasated solution (Hadaway, 2004; ONS, 2001).

Antidotes. Since some antidotes may also be vesicants if extravasated, they should be used cautiously. In fact, most small extravasations (defined as less than 1 to 2 ml) do not result in serious problems or necessitate the use of antidotes (Cancer Care Ontario, 2006). Antidotes for extravasation of cytotoxic agents are listed in Table 22-5.

Antidotes for noncytotoxic agents include phentolamine and hyaluronidase. Phentolamine is an appropriate antidote for sympathomimetic agents such as dopamine. Phentolamine is an α-adenergic blocking agent that causes vasodilatation, thereby decreasing the local vasoconstriction and ischemia and subsequently restoring circulation. Hyaluronidase is an enzyme that degrades hyaluronic acid so that the extravasated fluid is better absorbed. Hyaluronidase is an antidote for several antibiotics, TPN, calcium, potassium and high concentration dextrose (Health Sciences Center, 2006).

Topical Wound Care. Topical care of extravasation wounds should be dictated by the characteristics of the wound. Key considerations include absorption of exudate, removal of nonviable tissue, prevention of infection, elimination of deadspace, and pain management. As the extent of the tissue damage is revealed, the characteristics of the wound will change and therefore the local wound care choices will need modification. Chapter 19 provides a framework for topical wound care treatment options based on wound characteristics. In the presence of painful necrosis, early surgical consultation is recommended. Surgical debridement may be indicated for extensive tissue damage or overwhelming infection.

Patient Education

Patient and family education is critical, especially when the patient is receiving ambulatory continuous infusion of a vesicant agent. The patient must be instructed that although the risk for extravasation can be minimized, it cannot be entirely eliminated. The patient should be taught to examine the needle site every 4 to 8 hours and to report any possible symptom of an extravasation immediately. Ambulatory infusion pumps with occlusion alarms should be used, and written instructions should be provided. Instructions should include whom to call 24 hours a day if extravasation is suspected (Wickham, Purl, and Welker, 1992). The legal implications of extravasation injuries are many, and the medical record should be strictly maintained and should reflect all of the steps taken to prevent and then manage the extravasation.

FUNGATING WOUNDS

Fungating wounds present a physical and emotional challenge to patients, families, and caregivers. Dowsett (2002) reports approximately 5% to 10% of patients with metastatic cancer will develop a fungating wound.

Etiology

Oral and breast cancers are the most frequent sites of direct extension of malignancy (Weiss and Rouke, 1999). Cancers of the head, neck, kidney, lung, ovary, colon, and penis may also be sites from which the lesions originate (Young, 1997). Unless the malignant cells are eradicated by single or combination anticancer treatments, the fungation will extend (Grocott, 2000a). Lymphoma, leukemia, and melanoma can also produce fungating skin lesions. The infiltration of the skin involves the spread of malignant cells along pathways that offer minimal resistance, such as tissue planes and blood and lymph capillaries, and through the perineural spaces (Collier, 1997).

Assessment

The fungating wound is an ulcerating malignant skin lesion and is defined by the British Columbia Cancer Agency (2001) as "a cancerous lesion involving the skin which is open and may be draining." These lesions may be a result of a primary cancer, a metastasis to the skin from a local tumor, or a tumor at a distant site. Because they are often diagnosed at a late stage and are likely to spread, fungating wounds carry a poor prognosis and have few treatment options (Haller, 2004).

Fungating wounds may present as a nodule or a lesion with a cauliflower-like appearance and have an increased tendency to bleed when disturbed. Lesions may ulcerate and form shallow craters with or without a sinus tract or fistula (Collier, 1997; Hallett, 1995). Fungating wounds often become infected with aerobic and anaerobic organisms that produce volatile fatty acids and other molecules with a pungent odor that can be a source of great embarrassment and distress to the patient, family, and caregivers. Common characteristics of fungating wounds are listed in Table 22-6.

Assessment should include not only the physical assessment but also a psychologic assessment of the patient's feelings and reactions to the wound and the disease. Isolation and social ostracism are possible if the lesions are visible and/or odor is apparent, especially at a time when the patient really needs to be close to his or her family and loved ones.

TABLE 22-6 **Characteristics of Fungating Wounds**
....

ASSESSMENT PARAMETER	DESCRIPTION
Appearance	Necrosis, slough, bleeding, ulceration
Odor	Sweet, foul (offensive)
Drainage/exudates	Clear, thick, thin; low, moderate, copious amount
Presence of infection	Increased drainage; fever, leukocytosis
Periwound skin	Erythemia, maceration, edema, tenderness, maculopapular rash
Size and shape of site	Interference with dressing application

Interventions

The goal of managing the malignant cutaneous wound is to promote quality of life and independence *as defined by the individual patient* (Goldberg, 1997; Haisfield-Wolfe and Rund, 1997, 1999). The patient, the family, and caregivers should all be involved in setting the principal aim of the treatment.

Support the Host. Treatment options for the fungating wound are aimed at the underlying pathology and include radiotherapy, chemotherapy, hormone therapy, surgery, cryotherapy, or laser therapy (NCI, 1999). However, treatment must be congruent with the goals and objectives as identified by the patient and family. The management of fungating wounds is most often palliative with the aim of controlling symptoms at the wound site and reducing the physical and psychologic effects of the wound on the patient's daily life (Grocott, 1997). In most situations, the quality of care given to patients with malignant fungating wounds is the most important factor in determining their quality of life (Williams, 1997).

Topical Wound Care. As with all wound care, a comprehensive wound assessment guides the selection of topical wound care options. However, the only appropriate topical wound care approach for this patient population is that which is based on the consideration of the patient's priorities and needs in tandem, combined with the wound assessment findings.

Chapter 19 is an important chapter to review to help with goal setting, objectives, and appropriate dressing selection. The wound care goals for the patient with a fungating wound may supercede the goals typically consistent with progressive wound repair and closure. In palliative care, wound healing is not a realistic goal. Quality of life issues are often emphasized and targeted to the areas of most concern to the patient and family. It is critical that documentation in the patient's record accurately reflects that wound healing is not consistent with the patient's goals. Table 22-7 provides options that specifically target common characteristics of the fungating wound, which include control of (1) wound pain, (2) bleeding, (3) odor, and (4) exudate (Collier, 1997; Grocott, 2000b; Williams, 1997; Young, 1997).

Pain management. Naylor (2002) describes a number of mechanisms that can cause fungating wounds to be painful, including the tumor causing pressure on nerves and blood vessels, or possible dermal exposure. A key source of pain is the trauma associated with dressing changes. Consequently, specific attention should be given to interventions that will control or minimize any discomfort associated with the dressing change process. For example, nonadhesive dressings may be more comfortable than adhesive dressings. Furthermore, dressings should be selected that allow for infrequent dressing changes (e.g., every other day) while still attaining the established objectives of the wound microenvironment. In addition, special attention should be directed to the periwound skin, which is often vulnerable to painful infection, epidermal stripping (Chapter 6), and maceration. Pain management options are discussed in more detail in Chapter 25.

Control of bleeding. The fungating wound has a tendency to bleed as a result of erosion of blood capillaries. Bleeding may aggravate pain. Infrequent dressing changes will reduce the potential for bleeding when used appropriately. Gentle, local pressure for 10 to 15 minutes can also be applied to stop bleeding (Goldberg, 1997; Haisfield-Wolfe and Rund, 1997, 1999) unless this proves uncomfortable to the patient. There are many different types of dressings available to assist in the control of bleeding (Collier, 1997). Absorbable hemostatic dressings and silver nitrate cautery sticks can be used to specifically control the bleeding on a case-by-case basis (see Table 22-7). Significant bleeding events may also require oral antifibrinolytics, radiotherapy, and embolization. Although vasoconstrictive effects can result in ischemia and consequently necrosis, topical adrenaline 1:1000 may be applied for emergent situations (Dowsett, 2002; Grocott, 1999).

Odor management. Odor is caused by bacteria that flourish in necrotic tissue. Subjective reporting by the patient should guide interventions (Collier, 1997). Odor can be controlled by reduction of bacteria (through debridement, antimicrobials, and hypertonic dressings) and by using deodorizers and containment devices. Many of these interventions can be used simultaneously to aggressively attack the problem of odor. Table 22-7 lists the available options.

Chloromycetin solution is an effective wound deodorant. Gauze is moistened with the chloromycetin solution and applied to the wound surface; it is generally changed twice daily so that the dressing will remain moist. Skin protection should be implemented to keep the solution from contacting the surrounding skin because chloromycetin will cause an irritant reaction on intact skin. Puri-Clens (Coloplast Corp.) may also be applied to wounds to control odor.

As an outer covering, charcoal-impregnated dressings can be used, either as a primary dressing (when the wound is not exudative) or as a secondary dressing (over a primary absorptive dressing), to suppress odor. These dressings are changed when they become moist (moisture inactivates the charcoal) and when the charcoal is saturated so that it is no longer effective. Charcoal dressings may require changes ranging from daily to every 2 or 3 days, depending on the extent of the odor.

Since necrotic tissue harbors bacteria and is therefore odiferous, conservative debridement may be considered for odor control (Young, 1997). There are a variety of debridement methods, each with its own indications and contraindications; they are discussed in detail in Chapter 10. However, when selecting a debridement option, it is important to consider the characteristics unique to the patient with a fungating wound. When the patient has neutropenia or immune-suppression, the wound bioburden may be sufficient to cause a wound infection. Without sufficient leukocytes, even autolysis is not a reasonable debridement option. Mechanical debridement may be contraindicated because of the tendency for these wounds to bleed. Finally, there are situations in which any type of debridement of the fungating lesion is contraindicated. For example, when the removal of necrotic tissue could reveal or damage underlying structures (e.g., pulmonary artery), dry eschar constitutes a protective covering.

Another measure to reduce bioburden, and consequently odor, is through the use of antimicrobials and antiseptics that are available in a variety of forms: gauze, creams, gels, and irrigants. Some silver antimicrobial dressings also contain charcoal to better control wound odor. Topical application of metronidazole as a gel or an irrigant has been reported effective in the reduction of odor from fungating wounds (BC Cancer Agency 2001; Finlay et al, 1996; Weiss and Rouke, 1999).

Exudate control. Assessment and management of the metabolic effects of the fluid losses from fungating wounds should be ongoing. Moderately or highly exudative wounds require dressings that are capable of absorbing high volumes of exudate. As with other wounds, dressings for fungating wounds should be changed when exudate is pooling over intact skin or when "strike-through" occurs. This time interval appears to be a function of the volume of exudate produced, volume of necrotic tissue present, and the patient's hydration status and activity level. Moderate to large amounts of exudate can be contained with foam dressings and alginates. Very heavily exudative wounds may require a superabsorbent pad in conjunction with an alginate dressing, a hydrofiber dressing, or maltodextrin powder. A contact-layer dressing can be used to line the wound so that absorbent dressings can be applied and removed without traumatizing the wound bed. Two-layer permeable vented dressings may also be used. With these dressings, the perforated nonadherent layer protects the wound surface and permits passage of exudate to an absorbent and permeable layer (Grocott, 1999).

Wound drainage pouches are available from most ostomy manufacturers. Pouching should be considered when dressings must be changed more often than 2 to 3 times daily, when the skin begins to show early signs of damage, when the patient's ability to ambulate is hampered, or when odor is uncontrolled. These products have various desirable features such as attached skin barriers, flexible adhesive surfaces, and an access window over the wound site. Many wound

TABLE 22-7 Interventions for the Fungating Wound

PAIN MANAGEMENT	CONTROL OF BLEEDING	ODOR MANAGEMENT	EXUDATE CONTROL
Nontraumatic dressings Contact-layer dressings Gel-, cream-, or ointment-impregnated (e.g., petrolatum gauze) dressings Nonadherent foams Dressings that require fewer changes and do not adhere to the wound	**Hemostatic dressings** Gel foam Alginates Silver nitrate sticks	**Wound cleansing** Ionic cleansers Antiseptics	**Exudate collection and containment** Foam, alginate and hydrofiber dressings Absorptive powders Wound drainage pouch
Periwound skin management Microporous tapes Nontape methods and wraps Skin sealants (alcohol-free) Barrier ointment/cream Hydrocolloid and pectin barrier wafers to anchor tape	**Nontraumatic dressing changes** Contact layer Gel-, cream-, or ointment-impregnated (e.g., petrolatum gauze) Nonadherent foams Dressings that require fewer changes and do not adhere to the wound	**Deodorizers** Charcoal dressings Chloromycetin solution	**Appropriate dressing** Change frequency if there is pooling on intact skin or strike-through of exudate
	Gentle local pressure	**Debridement** Hydrogel or enzymatic debriding agent indicated for eschar Wound fillers, alginates, foam indicated for exudative wound with slough	
		Reduction of bacterial burden Irrigation with ionic cleansers Antimicrobial dressings Absorptive dressings Sodium-impregnated gauze Oral antimicrobials Antimicrobial creams and gels (e.g., metronidozole)	

pouches also have an attached tubular drain spout that facilitates connecting the pouch to a drainage container so that the fluid does not pool over the wound site. These pouches have the added benefit of containing odor. Chapter 23 provides details about pouching draining wounds.

IRRADIATION TISSUE DAMAGE

Radiation therapy is an established, common treatment for cancer. Some estimate that as many as half of all patients with cancer will receive radiation therapy as a primary, adjunctive or palliative intervention. Although the techniques and technologies for radiotherapy have improved, skin reactions and complications continue to be problematic for patients (Lopez et al, 1998; Wells and MacBride, 2003), and the management of these skin reactions has been inconsistent with the goals of standardized care (Wickline, 2004).

Etiology/Pathology

Ionizing radiation generates free radicals and reactive oxygen intermediates that damage cellular components, including DNA. Unfortunately, the effects of radiation therapy are not restricted to malignant cells. Rapidly proliferating tissues such as intestinal mucosa, bone marrow, and skin are more susceptible to radiation. In skin, the rapidly dividing cells (keratinocytes, hair follicles, and sebaceous glands) are more sensitive to radiation (Hall and Cox, 1989). In addition, radiosensitization techniques enhance the effect of radiation on normal and malignant tissues (Camidge and Price, 2001).

The skin is particularly vulnerable to the effects of radiation since it is in a continuous state of cellular renewal.

Presentation

Clinically, irradiated skin looks dry because of sweat and sebaceous gland destruction. There is loss of elasticity because of atrophy and fibrosis, and telangiectasia and discoloration occur with loss of hair. When the skin receives a significant dose of radiation, a reaction will develop that evolves from erythema to dry desquamation to moist desquamation (Table 22-8). Additional skin complications include ulceration, necrosis, shedding or deformity of the nails, malignant tumors, and

TABLE 22-8 Radiation Skin Reaction: Stages and Treatment Goals

STAGE	DEFINITION	CLINICAL PRESENTATION
Stage I	Inflammation and slight edema	Pink and dusky coloration Mild edema Burning, itching, mild discomfort
Stage II	Dry desquamation	Partial loss of epidermis Dry, itching, scaling Hyperpigmentation
Stage III	Moist desquamation and blistering	Blister or vesicle formation Nerve exposure and pain Serous drainage
Stage IV	Epilation and suppression of sweat glands	Pigmentation changes Permanent hair loss Atrophy Ulceration

Adapted from Bruner DW, McGinn-Byer M: Ostomy care considerations for patients before and after radiation therapy, Progressions 5(3):18, 1993. And British Columbia (BC) Cancer Agency. Radiation skin reactions, 2006 available at http://www.bccancer.bc.ca/HPI/Cancer ManagementGuidelines/SupportiveCare/RadiationSkinReactions/default. htm accessed, March 20, 2006.

lymphedema caused by fibrosis of the lymph glands (Lopez, 1998).

The effects experienced by the normal tissues can be categorized as early or late. Acute reactions are an expected adverse effect of radiation and may occur 2 to 3 weeks after beginning therapy or when completing therapy (Strunk and Maher, 1993). Acute radiation therapy reactions are a function of the dose delivered, multiplied by the volume treated, over time exposed to radiation, rather than the total applied dose. Since acute radiation effects are cumulative, the greatest reactions occur toward the end of therapy. However, side effects are usually self-limiting, and most subside 1 to 3 months after therapy has ended (Bruner and McGinn-Byer, 1993).

Bruner and McGinn-Byer (1993) have described four stages of skin reactions to radiation therapy (see Table 22-8). Early skin manifestations can range from erythema to moist desquamation and blistering. Late skin changes include epilation and suppression of sweat glands.

Erythema is a red, macular rash, on warm-appearing skin that may feel sensitive and tight. It is an inflammatory response thought to be caused by dilation of the capillaries and increased vascular permeability. Edema may accompany erythema. A small study by Simonen et al (1998) describes erythema as developing in two phases, with the first peak within 10 days of initiating treatment and the second peak approximately 20 days after treatment, and intensifying as treatment progresses. Treatment effects such as erythema will be confined to the treatment area (Dunne-Daly, 1995).

Dry desquamation is red- or tanned-appearing skin that is dry, itchy, and peeling or flakey. This reaction is a result of the decreased ability of the basal cells of the epidermis to replace the surface-layer cells and the decreased ability of the sweat and sebaceous gland to produce sweat. This reaction could appear as early as 2 weeks into treatment (Dunne-Daly, 1995).

If the desquamation process continues, the dermis is eventually exposed and moist desquamation results. This reaction increases the risk of infection, discomfort, and pain, possibly requiring interruption of the treatment plan to allow for healing (NCI, 1999). This reaction could occur by the fourth week of treatment. It is possible to see a combination of erythema and dry and moist desquamation within a single treatment field (Wells and MacBride, 2003).

Late radiation therapy reactions are a function of the total dose and volume of the area irradiated. Late effects develop gradually over several months or years (Bruner and McGinn-Byer, 1993). A 10-year retrospective study reported irradiation-induced ulcers appeared after a mean latency period of 8 years and 7 months (Landthaler, Hagspiel, and Braun, 1995). The frequency of late reactions increased with total dose of irradiation and decreased with the increasing age of the patient. When ulceration and necrosis occur years after radiation therapy, they usually occur in conjunction with trauma or infection. These lesions can become very painful and difficult to manage (Dunne-Daly, 1995).

Another reaction to radiation is termed radiation recall. Radiation recall occurs when a patient develops a tissue reaction in a previously irradiated field following the administration of a chemotherapeutic agent. There can be a considerable time lapse between the radiation exposure and the recall-triggering reaction (Schweitzer et al, 1995).

Risk Factors

In a study conducted by Turesson et al (1996) patients treated with identical radiotherapy schedules show a substantial variation in the degree of acute and late normal tissue reactions. This makes it difficult to identify those at risk for severe radiation-induced skin reactions. Treatment schedule and total dosage in radiation therapy are based on the tumoricidal doses and the tolerance dose of the perifocal normal tissue.

According to Nachtrab and colleagues (1998), since large-scale variations occur between patients concerning side effects, one of the major goals of radiation research recently has been the development of a predictive in vitro assay. In a very small study, they found a radiation dose-dependent increase in micronucleus frequency. They concluded that the micronucleus test seemed to be a very promising tool in the evaluation of radiation sensitivity before therapy. However, larger studies are needed to confirm these findings and to optimize the methodology. Dubray, Delanian, and Lefaix (1997) attempted to develop biologic assays, which would potentially be able to predict the probability of increased normal tissue injury after irradiation in individual patients. Such a test would allow the adaptation of the treatment modalities to the radiobiologic behavior of normal tissues. To date, these expectations have not been met.

The quality of the irradiation and its modalities, including total dose, fractionation, and interfractional interval, appear to affect functional and cosmetic outcome the most. Risk factors that appear to influence the severity, onset, and duration of radiation skin reaction include age, general skin condition, and nutritional status. At risk for highest stages of reaction are those body areas within the treatment field including bony prominences and moist areas on the body such as skin folds, under the breast, the axillae, the neck, the perineum, and the groin (Fernando et al, 1996; Strohl, 1989; Wells and MacBride, 2003). In a study of 197 patients, Fernando and colleagues (1996) investigated the delivery method of radiotherapy and found that the semisupine positioning may enhance the skin reaction in patients who receive breast irradiation.

Patients receiving combination therapy are also at risk because the concomitant use of chemotherapy may sensitize the basal cells to radiation (Margolin et al, 1990; Thomas, Rowe, and Keats, 1997).

Care of Irradiated Skin

Care of irradiated skin focuses on prevention, hydration, and topical care of damaged skin (Table 22-9). The level of evidence related to the care of irradiated skin is primarily based on case series and expert opinion.

Care during and after radiation is aimed at minimizing patient discomfort, promoting healing, and reducing the physiologic effects of radiation (Dunne-Daly, 1995). Patients and caregivers are included in planning care and selection of goals and objectives. Intervention choices should be based on their ability to soothe the skin, promote patient comfort, and be compatible with ionizing radiation (Porock and Kristjanson, 1999).

Patient education concerning skin care is critical when preparing for radiation and during the course of

TABLE 22-9 Care of Irradiated Skin

Care objective for all patients with irradiated skin	Interventions

Prevent injury or trauma to treatment area	• Promote skin cleanliness and hydration.
	• Recommend loose non-binding clothing for comfort.
	• Prevent avoidable skin damage and infection.
	• Avoid irritants:
	  - topical products containing perfume, alcohol or astringents, deodorants
	  - Mechanical products such as jewelry, adhesives, and products which are difficult to remove
	• Use an electric razor for shaving if shaving is necessary.
	• Avoid extremes of heat (heating pads, hot tubs, sun lamps, etc.).
	• Avoid extremes of cold (ice packs).
	• Protect skin from direct sunlight and wind exposure.
	• Avoid swimming in chlorinated pools.
	• Avoid any skin products which interact negatively with radiation therapy treatment.

Care objectives for irradiated skin stage I and II skin reactions	Interventions
Promote cleanliness	• Use mild, non-alkaline, unscented skin cleanser • Apply cleanser with hand to body instead of washcloth and rinse well • Wash Hair mild, non-medicated shampoo • Sitz baths for perineal/rectal patients from beginning of treatment course • Use tepid water and pat skin dry or expose area to the air. Women may wish to use a perineal spray bottle following voiding.
Promote comfort	• Maintain skin hydration. Apply 2 or 3 times per day. • Gently apply lotion or cream with your clean hand following treatment. DO NOT rub skin. • Avoid petroleum **only** products (hydrophobic) and products containing Alphahydroxy acids (AHA)

Data from British Columbia (BC) Cancer Agency. Radiation skin reactions, 2006 available at http://www.bccancer.bc.ca/HPI/Cancer ManagementGuidelines/SupportiveCare/RadiationSkinReactions/default.htm accessed, March 20, 2006 and Bruner DW, McGinn-Byer M: Ostomy care considerations for patients before and after radiation therapy, *Progressions* 5(3):18, 1993.

Continued

TABLE 22-9 Care of Irradiated Skin—cont'd

Care objective for irradiated skin stage I and II skin reactions—cont'd	Interventions
	• Alleviate burning itching and shearing with use of cornstarch or powders if the area is dry
	• Avoid cornstarch or powders in moist areas i.e., groins, under breasts
Reduce inflammation	• Alleviate pruritus and inflammation
	• Use corticosteroid creams sparingly
Prevent trauma to the treatment area	• Minimize friction and irritation
	• Use either moisturizers OR cornstarch. Do **not** use concurrently.
	• Discontinue use of ANY powder or cornstarch if area becomes moist.
	• Avoid talcum powders at all times

Care Objectives for irradiated skin stage III and IV skin reactions	Interventions
Promote Cleanliness	• Cleanse with tepid tap water or normal saline.
	• Normal saline compress
	• Sitz baths
Maintain principles of moist healing (see also chapter 19)	• Semiocclusive dressings
Manage pain (see also chapter 25)	• Cover open areas to protect nerve endings
	• Moist wound healing
	• Non-adherent dressings
	• Secure dressings with mesh or stockinet instead of tape
	• Use products that do not require frequent dressing changes
Prevention of infection	• Regular assessment for signs of infection: Possible yeast infection in moist skin folds. -Culture wound following cleansing with normal saline.
	• Antibacterial or antifungal products as indicated
	• Reduce bioburden-eliminate infection
	• Use dressings that appropriately manages exudate

the therapy (Figure 22-1). It is imperative that patients are advised about the potential effects of treatment (Campbell and Farrell, 1998; Holmes, 1997). Patients also need to be aware of the possibility that skin reactions can be magnified by chemotherapy, as in radiation recall. Patients should be educated to avoid the use of any product within the treatment field and to put nothing on the skin that has not had the prior approval of the health care team (Campbell and Farrell, 1998). Patients must be instructed that any area of the body that has received radiation treatment should be treated tenderly, and that potential irritants should be avoided for the remainder of their life.

Skin Sealants. Researchers have attempted to find a form of protection for the skin during radiation treatments. Goebel and colleagues (1997) tested a liquid adhesive which, when applied to the skin, polymerizes rapidly to form a clear, tough, flexible, and waterproof skin sealant. Prophylactic use of the skin sealant on a small number of patients to minimize radiation-induced desquamation was well tolerated. However the use

PATIENT INFORMATION -- IRRADIATED SKIN

HOW TO HELP REDUCE RISK OF SKIN IRRITATION IN TREATMENT AREAS

*Use mild soaps.

*Pat dry with soft towel (avoid rubbing).

*Do not use perfumes, deodorants, or makeup.

*Do not wear tight-fitting clothes or girdles.

*Avoid using heating pads and/or ice packs.

*Check with your nurse or physician about creams or lotions that are safe to put on your skin.

*Avoid sun exposure. Use cover-ups, hats, umbrella, etc. Ask your nurse or physician about sunblocks.

WOUND CARE (circle or highlight)

Mild to moderate discharge (leakage)   Moderate to excessive discharge (leakage)

Your treatment

Creams/lotions you *can* use: How often:

_____   _____

_____   _____

_____   _____

Type of dressing

_____

_____

_____

Dressing change schedule

_____

_____

If you have questions call _____ **at** _____
                                (Contact person)   (Phone number)

Fig. 22-1

of skin sealants during radiation therapy is not an approved indication by the manufacturers.

Emulsions and Creams. A hypotonic oil-in-water emulsion (Biafine RE [Kinetic Concepts, Inc]) is advertised for use as prophylaxis and for management of both wet and dry desquamation in radiotherapy patients. For prophylaxis, erythema, and dry desquamation, a small amount of Biafine RE is recommended to be gently massaged on and around the irradiated area 3 times per day, 7 days per week. For moist desquamation, the recommendation is a thick layer (¼ to ½ inch of Biafine RE) on and around the affected area, covered with a moist or petroleum gauze, and secured with tape as necessary. The dressing should be renewed every 24 hours. Although there are ongoing clinical studies, none have as yet shown the efficacy of this regimen; there are many advertisements and statements by the distributor after 20 years of use in France in the management of radiodermatitis.

Topical corticosteroid creams (Cortaid, Topicort, hydrocortisone cream 1%) are sometimes used for the itching in erythematous and dry desquamation areas. Caution should be used with these preparations because corticosteroids reduce itching by inducing vasoconstriction to the area. In addition, corticosteroids can cause atrophy of dermal collagen, resulting in a thinning of the skin and increased susceptibility to infection (Dunne-Daly, 1995). Corticosteroid creams may mask superficial infection (Wells and MacBride, 2003) and delay wound healing.

Sucralfate cream has received some attention, since oral sucralfate is used to protect mucous membranes during radiotherapy and chemotherapy (Wickline, 2004). Small studies have indicated faster skin recovery time and lesser than expected skin reactions but more research is needed with more varied and larger patient populations (Delaney et al, 1997; Maiche et al, 1994).

Moist Wound Healing. Transparent film dressings, hydrogels, foams, alginates and hydrocolloid dressings have been used in the successful treatment of radiation-damaged skin, and studies have reported increased comfort with use of these dressings (Margolin et al, 1990; Shell, Stanutz, and Grimm, 1986; Strunk and Maher, 1993). The dressing chosen will depend on the characteristics of the skin breakdown. For example, transparent film dressings absorb little exudate and

would be indicated primarily for dry desquamation. In contrast, hydrocolloids can be used with minimal to moderate amounts of exudate such as what occurs with moist desquamation. Given the fact that irradiated skin is characterized by a loss of elasticity, atrophy and fibrosis, nonadhesive wound dressings are generally preferred to minimize trauma to irradiated skin, avoid skin tears and prevent pain upon dressing removal. See Chapter 19 for more information about wound care dressings.

Adjunctive, Interactive, and Surgical Intervention. Hyperbaric oxygen (HBO), growth factors, and biologic skin substitutes have been used in the treatment of radiation-induced necrotic wounds (Neovius, Lind and Lind, 1997; Williams et al, 1992). Interactive and adjunctive therapies are presented in detail in Chapter 20. The treatment of some of these wounds will involve surgical debridement with removal of all poor-quality tissue and timely reconstruction with well-vascularized soft tissue flaps (Lopez et al, 1998).

PRIMARY MALIGNANT AND MALIGNANT TRANSFORMATION WOUNDS

Malignancies can develop on the skin as a wound (the primary malignant wound) and wounds of any etiology can develop a malignancy (malignant transformation wounds). In general, when malignancies present as ulcers they often go misdiagnosed for a long time because practitioners mistake them for nonmalignant ulcers. An increase in the frequency of skin cancers and the malignant transformation of wounds is anticipated as the population of people with a transplant and/or who are immunosuppressed increases (Snyder, Stillman, and Weiss, 2003; Trent and Kirsner, 2003).

Examples of primary malignant wounds include Kaposi's sarcoma, lymphoma, melanoma, basal cell carcinoma, and squamous cell carcinoma. Primary malignant wounds have a rapid onset and develop in many locations of the skin, frequently on sun-exposed areas that have not had prior radiotherapy (Snyder, Stillman, and Weiss, 2003).

Of chronic wounds, 1.7% will undergo malignant degeneration, most commonly squamous cell carcinoma. This malignant transformation has been observed in venous ulcers, burns, pressure ulcers, and scar tissue. Marjolin's ulcers present as flat indolent lesions with indurated and elevated margins. They have a malodorous exudate and can be mistaken for infection. Marjolin's ulcers can be found in a variety of wounds and have also been reported in sinus tracts secondary to osteomylitis and fistulas (Kirsner et al, 1996).

Any clinical cause for suspicion such as raised borders, unusual wound base, unexplained pain, changes in shape or color, previous history, or family history of skin cancer requires referral for biopsy. Ulcers or lesions that do not respond to optimal therapy also warrant a referral for biopsy (Snyder, Stillman, and Weiss, 2003). Biopsy technique is critical to cancer detection. It is recommended that wounds are biopsied in multiple sites (i.e., at 12, 6, 3, and 9 o'clock positions) and multiple depths (e.g., 2, 4, and 6 mm). The biopsy sites should be recorded because if the wound does not respond as expected, rebiopsy is indicated (Snyder, 2006).

SUMMARY

Although the wound care specialist is not expected to be proficient in the overall care of the oncology patient, the management of potential skin complications associated with cancer requires the application of wound-healing principles. As with other chronic wounds, the goals for these types of wounds range from healing to palliation and symptom management. Collaboration with the oncology nurse, the chemotherapy nurse, and radiation oncology personnel will be valuable to establish guidelines for the prevention, early detection, and care of oncologic complications, such as extravasation, fungating lesions, and radiation skin damage.

SELF-ASSESSMENT EXERCISE

1. What is the key distinction between extravasation and infiltration?
   a. Extravasation occurs only with chemotherapeutic agents.
   b. Extravasation occurs only with vesicant solutions or agents.
   c. Infiltration involves less tissue than an extravasation.
   d. Infiltration can occur with any intravenous solution or agent.
2. Which of the following agents is known to precipitate significant local tissue reactions?
   a. Thiotepa
   b. Vinblastine
   c. Cyclophosphamide
   d. Bleoycin
3. Which of the following interventions is generally appropriate when an extravasation occurs?
   a. Apply a warm compress.
   b. Remove the intravenous needle immediately.
   c. Apply pressure to the extravasation site.
   d. Aspirate any remaining fluid in the catheter.
4. All of the following objectives are appropriate for the management of fungating wounds EXCEPT:
   a. Odor control
   b. Wound healing
   c. Exudate management
   d. Pain management
5. What is the primary objective of wound cleansing or debridement in the fungating wound?
   a. Reduce exudate production
   b. Promote a healing wound environment
   c. Control odor
   d. Provide pain relief
6. Which of the following characterizes a stage III radiation skin reaction?
   a. Dry desquamation
   b. Slight edema
   c. Epilation
   d. Blistering
7. Which of the following products should be avoided to minimize trauma to irradiated skin?
   a. Deodorants
   b. Emollients
   c. Hydrogels
   d. Skin sealants

REFERENCES

Bertelli G et al: Topical dimethylsulfoxide for the prevention of soft tissue injury after extravasation of vesicant cytotoxic drugs: a prospective clinical study, *J Clin Oncol* 13(11):2851, 1995.

Boyle DM, Engelking C: Vesicant extravasation: myths and realities, *Oncol Nurs Forum* 22(1):57, 1995.

British Columbia (BC) Cancer Agency: *Guidelines for the care of chronic ulcerating malignant skin lesions,* Cancer management manual, 2001, http://www.bccancer.bc.ca/HPI/CancerManagementGuidelines/ SupportiveCare/ChronicUlceratingMalignantSkinLesions/ CareofMalignantWounds.htm Accessed 5/17/05.

British Columbia (BC) Cancer Agency: Radiation skin reactions, 2006 available at http://www.bccancer.bc.ca/HPI/CancerManagement Guidelines/SupportiveCare/RadiationSkinReactions/default.htm accessed, March 20, 2006.

Bruner DW, McGinn-Byer M: Ostomy care considerations for patients before and after radiation therapy, *Progressions* 5(3):18, 1993.

Buck ML: Treatment of intravenous extravasations, *Pediatr Pharmacother* 4(1):1998.

Camp-Sorrell D: Developing extravasation protocols and monitoring outcomes, *J Intraven Nurs* 21(4):232, 1998.

Camidge R, Price A: Characterizing the phenomenon of radiation recall dermatitis, *Radiother Oncol* 59:237-245, 2001.

Campbell T, Farrell W: Palliative radiotherapy for advanced cancer symptoms, *Int J Palliat Nurs* 4(6):292, 1998.

Chen JL, Oshea M: Extravasation injury associated with low-dose dopamine, *Ann Pharmacother* 32(5):545, 1998.

Collier M: The assessment of patients with malignant fungating wounds: a holistic approach. Part 1, *Nurs Times* 93(44, suppl):1-4, 1997.

Delaney G et al: Sucralfate cream in the management of moist desquamation during radiotherapy, *Australas Radiol* 41:270, 1997.

Dowsett C: Malignant fungating wounds: assessment and management, *Br J Commun Nurs* 7(8):394, 2002.

Dubray B, Delanian S, Lefaix JL: Late effect of mammary radiotherapy on skin and subcutaneous tissues, *Cancer Radiother* 1(6):744, 1997.

Dunne-Daly CF: Skin and wound care in radiation oncology, *Cancer Nurs* 18(2):144, 1995.

Ener RA, Meglathry SB, Styler M: Extravasation of systemic hemato-oncological therapies, *Ann Oncol* 15:858, 2004.

Fernando IN et al: Factors affecting acute skin toxicity in patients having breast irradiation after conservative surgery, *Clin Oncol* 8(4):226, 1996.

Finlay IG et al: The effect of topical 0.75% metronidazole gel on malodorous cutaneous ulcers, *J Pain Symptom Manage* 11(3):158, 1996.

Goebel RH et al: *A new approach to the prevention of radiation-induced skin desquamation using a polymer adhesive skin sealant: final results of a prospective study,* Poster Presentation, San Antonio, Tex, 1997, Cancer Therapy and Research Center's Annual Breast Cancer Symposium.

Goldberg MT: Management of wound and pressure sores. In Berger A et al, editors: *Principles and practices of supportive oncology,* Philadelphia, JB, 1997, Lippincott.

Grocott P: Evaluation of a tool used to assess the management of fungating wounds, *J Wound Care* 6(9):421, 1997.

Grocott P: The management of fungating wounds, *J Wound Care* 8(5):232, 1999.

Grocott P: Palliative management of fungating, malignant wounds, *J Commun Nurs* 14(3):31, 2000a.

Grocott P: The palliative management of fungating, malignant wounds: a study focusing on patient's experiences of exuding wounds and investigating novel dressing systems, *J Wound Care* 9(1):4, 2000b.

Hadaway LC: Preventing and managing peripheral extravasation, *Nursing* 34(5):66, 2004.

Haisfield-Wolfe ME, Rund C: Malignant cutaneous wounds: A management protocol, *Ostomy Wound Manage* 43(1):56, 1997.

Haisfield-Wolfe ME, Baxendale-Cox LM: Staging of malignant cutaneous wounds: a pilot study, *Oncol Nurs Forum* 26(6):1055, 1999.

Hall E, Cox J: Physical and biological basis of radiation therapy. In Moss W, Cox J, editors: *Rationale, technique, results,* ed 6, St Louis, 1989, Mosby.

Haller SM: A large ulcerated fungating breast lesion, *Clin J Oncol Nurs* 8(1):76-78, 2004.

Hallett A: Fungating wounds, *Nurs Times* 27(91):88, 1995.

Hastings-Tolsma MT et al: Effect of warm and cold applications on the resolution of IV infiltrations, *Res Nurs Health* 16:171, 1993.

Health Sciences Center: Extravasation Injuries, Winnipeg, Manitoba, Canada. http://www.hsc.mb.ca/nursingpractice/january_01.htm. Accessed March, 18, 2006.

Heitmann C, Durmus C, Infianni G: Surgical management after doxorubicin and epirubicin extravasation, *J Hand Surg (Br)* 23(5):666, 1998.

Herrington JD, Figueroa JA: Severe necrosis due to paclitaxel extravasation, *Pharmacotherapy* 17(1):163, 1997.

Holmes S: The maintenance of health during radiotherapy: a nursing perspective, *J R Soc Health* 117(6):393, 1997.

How C, Brown J: Extravasation of cytotoxic chemotherapy from peripheral veins, *Eur J Oncol Nurs* 1(4):51, 1998.

Hurst, SM, Keith, BK: Innovative solutions: a collaborative effort of critical care oncology: the common ground of tubes and lines, *Dimens Crit Care Nurs* 24(1):37, 2005.

Intravenous Nurses Society (INS): Intravenous nursing: standards of practice, *J Intraven Nurs* 21(1 suppl):S36, 1998.

Kennedy JG et al: Vesicant characteristics of oxaliplatin following ante-cubital extravasation, *Clin Oncol* 15(5):237, 2003.

Kirsner RS et al: Squamous cell carcinoma arising in osteomyelitis and chronic wounds. Treatment with Mohs micrographic surgery vs amputation, *Dermatol Surg* 22(12):1015, 1996.

Landthaler M, Hagspiel HJ, Braun F: Late irradiation damage to skin caused by soft x-ray radiation therapy of cutaneous tumors, *Arch Dermatol* 131:182, 1995.

Langer SW, Sehested M, Jensen PB: Treatment of anthracycline extravasation with dexrazoxane, *Clin Cancer Res* 6:3680, 2000.

Lookingbill DP, Spangler N, Helm KF: Cutaneous metastases in patients with metastatic carcinoma: a retrospective study of 4020 patients, *J Am Acad Dermatol* 29(2 Part 1):228, 1993.

Lopez AP et al: What is your diagnosis? *Wounds* 10(4):132, 1998.

Maiche A, Isokangas O, Groha P: Skin protection by sucralfate cream during electron beam therapy, *Acta Oncologica* 33:201, 1994.

Margolin SG et al: Management of radiation-induced moist skin desquamation using hydrocolloid dressing, *Cancer Nurs* 13(2):71, 1990.

Moody M, Grocott P: Let us extend our knowledge base: assessment and management of fungating malignant wounds, *Prof Nurse* 8(9):586, 1993.

Nachtrab U et al: Radiation-induced micronucleus formation in human skin fibroblasts of patients showing severe and normal tissue damage after radiotherapy, *Int J Radiat Biol* 73(3):279, 1998.

National Cancer Institute: External radiation therapy: what to expect, 1999, http://www.cancer.gov/cancertopics/radiation-therapy-and-you/page5#4. Accessed May 18, 2005.

National Cancer Institute (NCI): *Pruritus* (PDQ), June 1997, http://www.nci.nih.gov/cancertopics/pdq/supportivecare/pruritus/Health Professional; Accessed May 18, 2005.

Naylor W: Assessment and management of pain in fungating wounds, *Br J Nurs* 10(22 Suppl):S33, 2001.

Neovius EB, Lind MG, Lind FG: Hyperbaric oxygen therapy for wound complications after surgery in the radiated head and neck: a review of the literature and a report of 15 consecutive patients, *Head Neck* 19:315, 1997.

Oncology Nursing Society: Chemotherapy and biotherapy: guidelines and recommendations for practice, 2001, National Guideline Clearinghouse. Available at http://www.guidelines.gov/summary/summary.aspx?doc_id=3209&nbr=002435&string=extravasation+AND+vesicant+AND+drugs; Accessed March 13, 2006. Mosby, Cancer Care Ontario | action cancer Ontario. Appendix 2 - Extravasation http://www.cancercare.on.ca/print/index_drugFormularyappendix2.htm pages 1-10 accessed March 17, 2006.

Porock D, Kristjanson L: Skin reactions during radiotherapy for breast cancer: the use and impact of topical agents and dressings, *Eur J Cancer Care* 8(3):143, 1999.

Schrijvers DL: Extravasation: a dreaded complication of chemotherapy, *Ann Oncol* 14 (Suppl iii):26, 2003.

Schwartz RA: Cutaneous metastatic disease, *J Am Acad Dermatol* 33:161, 1995.

Schweitzer VG et al: Radiation recall dermatitis and pneumonitis in a patient treated with paclitaxel, *Cancer* 1576(6):1069, 1995.

Shell JA, Stanutz F, Grimm J: Comparison of moisture vapour permeable (MVP) dressings to conventional dressings for management of radiation skin reactions, *Onc Nurs Forum* 13:11, 1986.

Simonen P, Hamilton C, Ferguson S et al: Do inflammatory processes contribute to radiation induced erythema observed in the skin of humans? *Radiother Oncol* 46(1):73, 1998.

Snyder RJ, Stillman RM, Weiss SD: Epidermoid cancers that masquerade as venous ulcer disease, *Ostomy Wound Manage* 49(4):63, 2003.

Snyder R: Skin cancers and chronic wounds. In Norman R, editor: *Handbook of geriatric dermatology,* Cambridge University Press, 2006 (in print).

Strohl RA: Radiation skin reactions, *Progressions* 1(3):3, 1989.

Strunk B, Maher K: Collaborative nurse management of multi-factorial moist desquamation in a patient undergoing radiotherapy, *J ET Nurs* 20(4):152, 1993.

Thomas S, Rowe HN, Keats J: The management of extravasation injury in neonates, Mid Glamorgan, Wales, 1997, World Wide Wounds, Surgical Materials Testing Laboratory, Brigend General Hospital, http://www.worldwidewounds.com/1997/October/Neonates/NeonatePaper.html; Accessed May 18, 2005.

Trent JT, Kirsner RS: Wounds and malignancy, *Adv Skin Wound Care* 16(1):31, 2003.

Turesson I et al: Prognostic factors for acute and late skin reactions in radiotherapy patients, *Int J Radiat Oncol Biol Phys* 36(5):1065, 1996.

Wells M, MacBride S: Radiation skin reactions. In Faithfull S, Wells M, editors: *Supportive care in radiotherapy,* New York, 2003, Churchill Livingstone.

Weiss PA, Rourke ME: Symptom management to enhance outcomes, *Oncology Nursing* Update 99(4):13, 1999.

Wickham R, Purl S, Welker D: Long-term central venous catheters: issues for care, *Semin Oncol Nurs* 8(2):133, 1992.

Wickline MM: Prevention and treatment of acute radiation dermatitis: a literature review, *Oncol Nurs Forum* 31(2):237, 2004.

Williams C: Management of fungating wounds, *Br J Community Nurs* 2(9):423, 1997.

Williams JA Jr et al: The treatment of pelvic soft tissue radiation necrosis with hyperbaric oxygen, *Am J Obstet Gynecol* 167:412, 1992.

Young T: The challenge of managing fungating wounds, *Community Nurse* 3(9):41, 1997.

Yucha CB, Hastings-Tolsma MT, Szevereny N: Effect of elevation on intravenous extravasations, *J Intraven Nurs* 17(5):231, 1994.

23 *Management of Drain Sites and Fistulas*

RUTH A. BRYANT & BONNIE SUE ROLSTAD

OBJECTIVES

1. Identify factors contributing to fistula formation.
2. List three complications that contribute to mortality from fistulas.
3. Describe three ways to classify fistulas.
4. Identify the six objectives of medical management for the patient with a fistula.
5. List factors known to impede spontaneous closure of fistula tracts.
6. Describe surgical procedures commonly used to close or bypass fistula tracts.
7. List eight goals for nursing management of the patient with a fistula.
8. Describe four essential assessments that guide the management of the patient with a fistula.
9. Explain the role of four different types of skin barriers, including their indications for use.
10. Identify features to be considered when selecting a fistula pouching system.
11. Briefly describe the "bridging" technique, and identify indications for its use.
12. Identify options for odor control in a wound managed with dressings and in a wound managed with pouching.

The presence of a draining fistula can be a frustrating and disheartening experience for the patient and family because it represents a major complication. It can also be a difficult experience for caregivers; however, management can be quite rewarding when effluent is successfully contained, odor is controlled, the patient is comfortable, and realistic resolution is attained. Management for this patient population requires astute assessment skills, knowledge of pathophysiology, competent technical skills, diligent follow-up, persistence, and knowledge of management alternatives.

The focus of this chapter is fistula management. Fistula management is more than skin protection and pouching. Therefore the first part of this chapter will present the medical and surgical aspects of managing a patient with a fistula. The second part of this chapter will address the nursing management (i.e., skin protection and pouching techniques) of the patient with a fistula. It should be noted that these techniques are also applicable to other types of wounds and drain sites that are not adequately contained by dressings.

EPIDEMIOLOGY AND ETIOLOGY

While there is a dearth of clear, representative epidemiologic data regarding fistula formation such as morbidity, mortality, and incidence, it is well established that gastrointestinal fistulas are very serious complications and are associated with high morbidity, high mortality, extended hospital stays, and increased costs. In general, fistulas develop in a wide array of complex patient conditions and are typically concentrated in large medical centers. The heterogeneous nature of this patient population leads to overreporting or underreporting of incidence, mortality, and so on. Nonetheless, the factors impacting on the prognosis of the patient with a fistula are well known.

Several factors are recognized as contributing to fistula formation:

- Malnutrition
- Sepsis
- Hypotension
- Vasopressor therapy
- Steroid therapy
- Technical difficulties with anastomosis
- Coexisting diseases such as inflammatory bowel disease, cancer or diverticulitis

Enterocutaneous fistulas (ECFs) develop either spontaneously or postoperatively. In many reports, 75% to 85% of ECFs are iatrogenic, occurring postoperatively, and representing a leak in the anastomosis. Risk factors for the development of postoperative ECF include reoperation requiring extensive lysis of adhesions, cancer, inflammatory bowel disease, emergency surgery where the bowel has not been adequately prepped, prior radiation therapy, and trauma surgery (Chamberlain, Kaufman, and Danforth, 1998; Minei and Champine, 1998; Sansoni and Irving, 1985). According to Wong, Annamaneni, and Buie (2004), postoperative fistulas that are caused by anastomotic breakdown are largely preventable by following basic surgical principles of anastomotic construction: (1) adequate blood supply, (2) lack of tension, and (3) good suture technique. Maykel and Fischer (2003) advocate specific prevention strategies when faced with emergency surgery: provide adequate intravenous fluids, ensure adequate circulatory support, keep the patient warm, and provide broad-spectrum antibiotics. In addition, when surgery is planned, they consider adequate nutritional preparation to be the most important step to prevent an anastomotic breakdown and identify the group at highest risk for this complication to be severely malnourished patients as manifested by a hydrated serum albumin level of less than 3 g/dl and a weight loss of 10% to 15% over a 4- to 6-month period.

Approximately 25% of fistulas will develop spontaneously and are associated with an intrinsic intestinal disease (cancer, radiation, diverticulitis, inflammatory bowel disease, appendicitis) or external trauma. Spontaneous fistulas are generally resistant to spontaneous closure. Patients who have been treated for a pelvic malignancy are particularly vulnerable for fistula formation because of the radiation damage to the rectum, the anal canal, and gynecologic organs (Rubin et al, 1989; Saclarides, 2002).

Irradiation triggers occlusive vasculitis, fibrosis, and impaired collagen synthesis—a process termed radiation-induced endarteritis. Unfortunately, because this endarteritis persists, complications may develop immediately after radiation or years later. Meissner (1999) reported that 17% of radiotherapy patients developed a fistula a mean of 3.4 years after receiving radiation therapy. Additional risk factors for irradiation-induced fistulas include coexisting processes such as atherosclerosis, hypertension, diabetes mellitus, advanced age, cigarette smoking, pelvic inflammatory disease, and previous pelvic surgery. Pelvic radiation doses that exceed 5000 cGy increase the incidence of bowel injury (Berry and Fischer, 1996; Hollington et al, 2004; Saclarides, 2002).

The three most common complications associated with fistulas are sepsis, malnutrition, and fluid and electrolyte imbalance. Hypertonic protein-rich fistula secretions contribute to fluid and electrolyte depletion and malnutrition because of loss of sodium bicarbonate and amino acids (Chamberlain, Kaufman, and Danforth, 1998; Moser and Roslyn, 1998). Sepsis occurs as a result of abscess and poor nutritional status thereby compromising the patient's immune response (Makhdoom et al, 2000).

Despite advances in antibiotic therapy, uncontrolled sepsis is the most common cause of death in patients with ECFs and accounts for mortality rates that range from 6% to 20% (Hollington et al, 2004; Maykel and Fischer, 2003; Wong, Annamaneni, and Buie, 2004).

TERMINOLOGY
Definitions

A fistula is an abnormal passage between two or more structures or spaces. This can involve a communication tract from one body cavity or hollow organ to another hollow organ or to the skin (Figures 23-1 to 23-3). Thus a gastrointestinal fistula is one that communicates between the lumen of the gastrointestinal tract

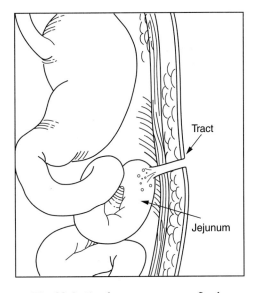

Fig. 23-1 Simple enterocutaneous fistula.

and another organ. An enterocutaneous fistula (ECF) is one that communicates specifically between the lumen of the gastrointestinal tract and the skin. A draining wound, surgically placed drain site, or wound dehiscence should not be misinterpreted as a fistula.

Classification

Several methods are used to classify the fistula. These classification schemes are useful in predicting the

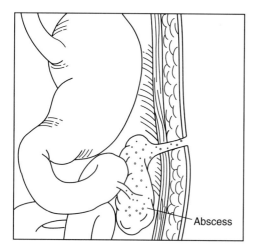

Fig. 23-2 Complex type 1 fistula with associated abscess.

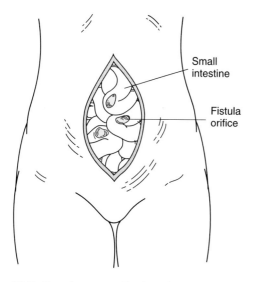

Fig. 23-3 Complex type 2 fistula with multiple openings associated with large abdominal wall defect.

BOX 23-1 Classification of Fistulas by Complexity

Simple
Short, direct tract
No associated abscess
No other organ involvement

Complex
Type 1
    Associated with abscess
    Multiple organ involvement

Type 2
    Opens into base of disrupted wound

morbidity rate, mortality rate, and potential for spontaneous closure (Wong, Annamaneni, and Buie, 2004).

From an anatomic perspective, the fistula may be simple or complex (Box 23-1). The simple fistula has a short, direct tract, no abscess, and no other organ involved, whereas the complex fistula is associated with an abscess, has multiple organ involvement, and may open into the base of a wound.

A fistula may be classified according to location; the internal fistula exists between internal structures whereas the external fistula communicates between an internal organ and the skin, vagina, or rectum. This is a more specific classification system in that the site of origin and site of termination are identified. Examples of such terminology are listed in Table 23-1.

Finally, a fistula may be classified according to volume of output (Table 23-2). High-output fistulas are most commonly defined as those producing more than 500 ml/24 hr; a moderate-output fistula is associated with 200 to 500 ml/24 hr, and a low-output fistula is one with less than 200 ml/24 hr (Dudrick, Maharaj, and McKelvey, 1999; Maykel and Fischer, 2003). The frequency of sepsis, malnutrition, and fluid and electrolyte imbalance is directly related to fistula output. Fistula output is a direct reflection of the fistula's site of origin. Distal large bowel fistulas typically have low output (under 200 ml/24 hr), whereas most proximal small bowel fistulas drain at least 1000 to 1500 ml/24 hr initially and are considered high-output. The high-output fistula is associated with severe malnutrition, significant fluid and electrolyte disturbance, higher

TABLE 23-1 **Fistula Terminology**

FROM	TO	NAME	INTERNAL/EXTERNAL
Pancreas	Colon	Pancreatico-colonic	Internal
Jejunum	Rectum	Jejunorectal	External
Intestine	Skin	Enterocutaneous	External
Intestine	Colon	Enterocolonic	Internal
Intestine	Bladder	Enterovesical	Internal
Intestine	Vagina	Enterovaginal	External
Colon	Skin	Colocutaneous	External
Colon	Colon	Colocolonic	Internal
Colon	Bladder	Colovesical	Internal
Rectum	Vagina	Rectovaginal	External
Bladder	Skin	Vesicocutaneous	External
Bladder	Vagina	Vesicovaginal	External

Modified from Irrgang S, Bryant R: Management of the enterocutaneous fistula, *J Enterostom Ther* 11:211, 1984.

TABLE 23-2 **Fistula Classification**

	DESIGNATION	CHARACTERISTICS
LOCATION	Internal	Tract contained within body
	External	Tract exits through skin
INVOLVED STRUCTURES	Colon	Colon
	Entero-	Small bowel
	Vesico-	Bladder
	Vaginal	Vagina
	Cutaneous	Skin
	Recto-	Rectum
VOLUME	High-output	Over 500 ml per 24 hours
	Moderate-output	200-500 ml per 24 hours
	Low-output	Under 200 ml per 24 hours

Modified from Boarini J, Bryant R, Irrgang S: Fistula management, *Semin Oncol Nurs* 2:287, 1986.

morbidity and mortality rates, and a lower spontaneous closure rate (Dudrick, Maharaj and McKelvey, 1999; Sitges-Serra, Jaurrieta, and Sitges-Creus, 1982; Wong, Annamaneni, and Buie, 2004).

MANIFESTATIONS

The passage of gastrointestinal secretions or urine through an unintentional opening onto the skin heralds the development of a cutaneous fistula. Manifestations of a fistula exiting through the vagina (i.e., rectovaginal or vesicovaginal) include passage of gas, feces, purulent material, or urine through the vagina: discharge that is extremely malodorous. Irradiation-induced

rectovaginal fistulas are often preceded by diarrhea, the passage of mucus and blood rectally, a sensation of rectal pressure, and a constant urge to defecate (Saclarides, 2002). Fistulas between the intestinal tract and the urinary bladder (such as the colovesical fistula) present with passage of gas or stool-stained urine through the urethra.

MEDICAL MANAGEMENT

The ultimate goal of the medical management of a fistula is to achieve spontaneous closure. Approximately 60% to 70% of all fistulas will close spontaneously when sepsis is controlled and nutrition support is adequate and appropriate (Berry and Fischer, 1996; Fischer, 1983; Rombeau and Rolandelli, 1987; Rose et al, 1986). Of the fistulas that heal spontaneously, 80% to 90% will do so within 5 weeks, given the patient is adequately nourished (Berry and Fischer, 1996; Maykel and Fischer, 2003). Factors known to correlate with spontaneous fistula closure include absence of sepsis, adequate nutritional support, low output, and the etiology of being a postoperative fistula (Campos et al, 1999). Approximately 90% of simple type 1 fistulas close spontaneously, whereas less than 10% of complex type 2 fistulas close spontaneously (Levy et al, 1989; Sitges-Serra, Jaurrieta, and Sitges-Creus, 1982). Only 8% to 26% of the spontaneous fistulas in patients with intrinsic disease such as Crohn's disease, cancer, or radiation heal spontaneously (Reber and Austin, 1989).

Achievement of the medical management goals requires patience, astute assessment skills, and the cooperation of many health care specialists. Medical management can be divided into nonsurgical treatment and surgical treatment. A comprehensive and effective interdisciplinary and multidisciplinary team approach is vital to achieve closure and reduce mortality and morbidity.

Medical Management: Nonsurgical Treatment

The nonsurgical treatment of fistulas requires a comprehensive plan of care with attention to the following six specific objectives:
1. Fluid and electrolyte replacement
2. Control of infection
3. Control of fistula output and skin protection
4. Nutritional support
5. Definition of fistula tract
6. Conservative management

Objective 1: Fluid and Electrolyte Replacement. From 5 to 9 liters of fluid rich in sodium, potassium, chloride, and bicarbonate are secreted into the gastrointestinal tract daily. The loss of fluid and electrolytes that accompanies the presentation of a high-output fistula may result in hypovolemia and circulatory failure. Such blood-volume imbalances must be corrected before initiating nutritional support or definition of the fistula tract. Adequate tissue perfusion and urine output must be maintained. Potential electrolyte imbalances should be anticipated and can be inferred from

our understanding of the usual electrolyte composition of gastrointestinal secretions.

Objective 2: Control of Infection. Sepsis is the major cause of death in patients with enteric fistulas, and these bacteria proliferate rapidly in the poorly vascularized tissue typically surrounding a fistula tract (Moser and Roslyn, 1998). Pooling of bowel contents as a result of the dehiscence of a suture line precipitates localized and then diffuse abdominal pain, ileus, fever and, ultimately, septic shock. The presence of systemic or local sepsis must be evaluated, typically with computed tomography (CT) scanning or ultrasound. Effective drainage can be accomplished by use of percutaneous radiographic techniques or surgery; the specific approach depends on abscess location, patient status, and available resources. Surgical laparotomy for control of sepsis should be limited to proximal diversion and drainage of the abscess; definitive repair of the fistula is undertaken at a later time. Abscess contents should be cultured (aerobic and anaerobic) and Gram's-stained to identify the causative organisms and sensitivities. Organisms are most commonly of bowel origin: coliform, bacteroides, and enterococci. Staphylococci may also be present. Antibiotics are only appropriate in the presence of an infection and in conjunction with adequate drainage of the abscess (Wong, Annamaneni, and Buie, 2004).

Objective 3: Control of Fistula Output and Skin Protection. Drainage of intestinal contents onto the skin will result in epidermal erosion and pain within only a few hours. Aggressive skin protection is essential and should be initiated at once. This will be discussed specifically later in this chapter under Nursing Management.

Intestinal output must be minimized. Conventional methods for achieving this goal is by giving the patient nothing by mouth and administering histamine (H_2) receptor antagonists. NPO (nothing by mouth) status decreases luminal contents, gastrointestinal stimulation, and pancreaticobiliary secretion. Administering H_2 antagonists such as cimetidine prevents stress ulcerations and decreases gastric, biliary, and pancreatic secretions. Despite reducing gastrointestinal secretions, H_2 receptors have not been shown to speed closing of the enterocutaneous fistula (Maykel and Fischer, 2003).

Although not a standard in routine fistula care, administration of somatostatin-14 has been shown to further decrease intestinal output in some situations. This naturally occurring hormone has extensive, well-known biologic effects that include inhibition of gastric, biliary, pancreatic, and salivary secretions, and reduced gastrointestinal motility, gastric emptying, and gall bladder emptying. When used in combination with total parenteral nutrition (TPN), a synergistic effect on reduced gastrointestinal secretions can be expected; fistula output reductions of at least 50% within 24 hours have been reported in addition to a significant reduction in the time to spontaneous closure of the fistula (Fagniez and Yahchouchy, 1999; Hesse, Ysebaert and de Hemptinne, 2001). The short half-life of 1 to 2 minutes requires that somatostatin-14 be administered through continuous intravenous infusion (250 mcg/hour). The analogue octreotide has a half-life of almost 2 hours, so it can be administered 3 times daily subcutaneously (300 mcg/day). Results from available prospective controlled studies and randomized controlled studies of octreotide have been mixed. Overall it appears to have similar but less dramatic reduction of output and closure rates (Makhdoom et al, 2000). The most encouraging results of octreotide are with postoperative, high-output small bowel fistulas in which fluid-, electrolyte-, and protein-store depletion is prevented. These medications are less effective with fistulas associated with intrinsic bowel diseases such as ulcerative colitis or Crohn's disease (Hild et al, 1986). Somatostatin or octreotide administration should be stopped if fistula output does not decrease in the first 48 hours of treatment or if there is no response after 2 to 3 weeks of treatment, respectively.

Maykel and Fischer (2003) recommend caution in using somatostatin. They report that because the use of somatostatin precipitates villous atrophy, the interruption of intestinal adaptation, and acute cholecystitis, somatostatin should not be used routinely in the treatment of the ECF.

Objective 4: Nutritional Support. Malnutrition is a significant complication that most patients with a fistula experience. Several factors contribute to the fistula patient's poor nutritional status. Often the patient is malnourished before the fistula develops.

Additional factors contributing to negative nitrogen balance include reduced protein intake, inefficient nutrient use, excessive losses of protein-rich fluids (especially from pancreatic and proximal jejunal fistulas), and the muscle protein breakdown (hypercatabolism) that occurs with sepsis.

Adequate nutritional support is achieved when the patient is maintained in a state of positive nitrogen balance and receives adequate vitamin and trace mineral replacement. The amount of calories and protein required will depend on the patient's preexisting status, sepsis, and fistula output. Caloric needs range from 30 to 40 kcal/kg/24 hr; the goal should be a calorie-nitrogen ratio of 150:1. Protein requirements are estimated at 1.5 to 1.75 g/kg/24 hr or 0.25 to 0.35 g of nitrogen/kg body weight/24 hr (Wong, Annamaneni, and Buie, 2004). It is important to initiate nutritional support without delay because the lean body mass is lost at a rate of 300 to 900 g per 24 hr depending upon degree of stress (Maykel and Fischer, 2003). Trace elements (e.g., copper, zinc, and magnesium), multivitamins, and vitamins (B, C, and K) must be supplemented (Maykel and Fischer, 2003; Wong, Annamaneni, and Buie, 2004). González-Pinto and Moreno Gónzález (2001) recommend twice the recommended daily allowance (RDA) for vitamins and trace minerals and up to 10 times the RDA for vitamin C.

The route of nutritional support is contingent upon the patient's ability to ingest sufficient quantities, the location of the fistula tract, the absorptive capacity of the bowel mucosa, and patient tolerance. Historically, the preferred route of nutritional support has been parenteral nutrition; accompanied by simultaneous "bowel rest," this has resulted in increased spontaneous closure rates and decreased mortality rates.

Recently an interest in the use of enteral nutrition has resurfaced because it is recognized that even small amounts of enteral nutrition will maintain the normal structural, immunologic, and hormonal integrity of the gastrointestinal tract and prevent translocation of bacteria. However, enteral nutrition requires approximately 4 feet of small intestine (Eckhauser et al, 2003; Maykel and Fischer, 2003). Enteral nutrition is appropriate when fistulas are located in the most proximal or distal portion of the gastrointestinal tract; however, the gastrointestinal tract must be functional and the patient cooperative. Many types of enteral solutions are available, and a dietician should be consulted to recommend the most appropriate solution and administration procedure so that gastrointestinal intolerance, such as diarrhea and abdominal distention, can be avoided.

Objective 5: Definition of Fistula Tract. After the patient is stabilized (fluid and electrolytes balanced and infection controlled), the fistula must be examined to ascertain (1) the origin of the fistulas tract, (2) the condition of adjacent bowel, (3) the presence of additional abscess pockets, and (4) the presence of distal obstruction or bowel discontinuity. Water-soluble contrast agents (e.g., Renografin, Hypaque, or Gastrografin) are preferred to visualize the fistula tract and are administered through a soft-tip catheter. A CT scan is indicated only when the patient is not responding to conservative treatment. If other organs are involved, additional tests such as a cystoscopy or intravenous pyelogram should be pursued (Wong, Annamaneni, and Buie, 2004).

Objective 6: Conservative Management. As already described, the majority of fistulas will heal spontaneously with patience, time, and conservative management (positive nitrogen balance with nutritional support, sepsis-free state). The challenge is trying to shorten the time to spontaneous healing, as well as increase the number of fistulas that heal spontaneously.

A relatively new technique for fistula closure is the insertion of clotting substances into the fistula tract. The concept of using fibrin for anastomosis of tissue was explored in the 1940s. Fibrin sealants (also referred to as fibrin glue) are composed of a concentrated allotment of fibrinogen/factor XIII/fibronectin and thrombin that congeals to form an insoluble fibrin clot when mixed with calcium chloride; this is a process that essentially replicates the last step of the coagulation cascade (Katkhouda, 2001). The mechanism of action is that the fibrin clue provides a "matrix" for the influx of various cells and collagen formation (Buchanan et al, 2003)

Fibrin sealant products can be created from the patient's own plasma (autologous) or from human plasma that has been collected and pooled from many donors (heterologous), after undergoing screening and viral testing. The fibrin glue is then applied endoscopically at the origin of the fistula to seal the fistula (Eleftheriadis et al, 1990; Hwang and Chen, 1996; Katkhouda, 2001; Lange et al, 1990). In a report by Eleftheriadis and colleagues (1990), no complications were noted and patients required an average of 2.4 applications. Hwang and Chen (1996) report no adverse reactions to fibrin glue; all 13 patients with a low-output ECF healed within 4 days and only two required a second infusion. While fibrin sealant products appear to have a role in the management of low-output fistulas (e.g., perirectal) the role of fibrin glue is yet to be determined relative to the complexity of the fistula and timing of the procedure.

Medical Management: Surgical Treatment

Immediate surgery is imperative when (1) a septic focus has been identified, (2) uncontrolled hemorrhage has developed, (3) bowel necrosis develops, or (4) an evisceration is present. However, closure of the fistula or excision of the fistula tract should not be attempted under these circumstances.

Surgical intervention to close the fistula will be required when impediments to spontaneous closure have been identified. Factors known to impede spontaneous closure are listed in Box 23-2. If the following factors are present and closure of the fistula is the ultimate goal for the patient, a surgical intervention will be necessary. Surgical procedures may also be indicated for palliation.

1. Presence of a foreign body close to the suture line
2. Compromised suture line (i.e., tension on the suture line, improper suturing technique, inadequate blood supply to the anastomosis)

BOX 23-2 Factors that Delay Spontaneous Fistula Closure

- Compromised suture line/anastomosis
- Distal obstruction
- Foreign body in fistula tract
- Epithelium-lined tract contiguous with the skin
- Presence of tumor or disease in site
- Previous irradiation to site
- Crohn's disease
- Presence of abscess or hematoma

3. Distal obstruction
4. Hematoma or abscess formation in the mesentery at the anastomotic site
5. Presence of tumor or disease in the area of anastomosis

The exact timing for surgical intervention is variable, depending on the patient's status. In general, operative interventions to close the fistula tract should be delayed until the patient is in optimum condition (i.e., positive nitrogen balance and control of infection are established). Given that the patient is nutritionally and metabolically stable, definitive surgery for a simple or complex type 1 fistula is appropriate when a persistently draining fistula is in a sepsis-free environment for 6 to 8 weeks. It is important that definitive surgery be delayed until the abdominal wall is soft and supple; tissues should return to a normal soft, pliable state, particularly in the presence of irradiated tissue (Gonzalez-Pinto and Gonzalez, 2001; Wong, Annamaneni, and Buie, 2004).

Complex type 2 fistulas invariably require definitive surgery; however, the timing of surgery is not well defined. Nutritional status, metabolic status, and immunocompetence should be normalized, and the obliterative peritonitis and the inflammation associated with chronic peritoneal contamination should be resolved (Wong, Annamaneni, and Buie, 2004). Judicious timing of surgery for complex type 2 fistulas is warranted. In one study, the time from fistula diagnosis to definitive operation ranged from 10 weeks to 13 months with a mean time of 4.2 months (Conter, Root, and Roslyn, 1988).

The surgical interventions available for the management of ECFs will either divert the gastrointestinal tract (without resection of the fistula) or provide definitive resection of the fistula tract. Factors such as location, size, and cause of the fistula, the patient's overall status, and the presence of irradiated tissue will influence the approach selected. However, Maykel and Fischer (2003) warn that the best results occur with resection of the fistula and end-to-end anastomosis, and that other surgical procedures represent a compromise.

Diversion techniques divert the fecal stream away from the fistula site; removal of the fistula is not accomplished. Resection of the fistula is not always appropriate or possible in the presence of extensive or recurrent malignancy, or when there is inadequate tissue perfusion in the vicinity of the fistula (secondary to numerous surgical resections, scar formation, uncontrolled diabetes, or prior irradiation).

Diversion can be achieved by creation of a stoma proximal to the fistula or by the making of an anastomosis (end-to-end or side-to-side) of the two segments of bowel on both sides of the fistula (such as an ileotransverse anastomosis when the fistula communicates with the right colon). This latter procedure may be referred to as an intestinal bypass in which the segment of bowel containing the fistula is completely isolated and separated from the fecal stream.

When closure of the fistula is the goal, resection of the fistula will be necessary. The advantage of this technique is that the diseased tissue is removed. An end-to-end anastomosis of the intestine with resection of the fistula tract is performed. To protect the anastomosis, diversion of the fecal stream through a temporary stoma may be indicated. If the distal part of the rectum is not suitable for anastomosis or the anal sphincters are not competent, a permanent stoma with a Hartmann's pouch may be the safest procedure.

Enteric fistulas communicating with the urinary tract will always require diversion of the fecal stream proximal to the fistula site to prevent urinary tract infections and pyelonephritis.

NURSING MANAGEMENT

The occurrence of an ECF is an unplanned event, a step backward in the recovery process (Phillips and Walton, 1992). Unlike the ostomy patient who has the benefit of a preoperative visit and ostomy site marking, the patient with a fistula is physically and psychologically unprepared for this outcome. The occurrence of a fistula lengthens recovery time, whether closure is spontaneous or occurs with surgical repair. This section focuses on the technical management of the patient with a fistula. However, these principles and techniques are applicable to other types of draining wounds and drain sites. Principles are presented so that management can be tailored to achieve effective solutions. However, the care plan must also include detailed attention to patient and family needs, involvement, education, and emotional support.

Technically, the patient with a fistula is one of the most challenging patients who wound and ostomy care providers encounter. Critical thinking skills are

---

BOX 23-3 Nursing Goals for Fistula Management

∙∙∙

Perifistular skin protection
Containment of effluent
Odor control
Patient comfort
Accurate measurement of effluent
Patient mobility
Ease of care
Cost containment

BOX 23-4 Fistula Assessment and Documentation Guide

∙∙∙

1. Source (e.g., small bowel, bladder, esophagus)
2. Characteristics of effluent
   a. Volume
   b. Odor? (If yes, describe)
   c. Consistency (e.g., liquid, semiformed, formed, gas)
   d. Composition
      (1) Color (e.g., clear, yellow, green, brown)
      (2) Active enzymes
      (3) Extremes in pH
3. Topography and size
   a. Number of sites
   b. Location(s)
   c. Length and width of each (include patterns)
   d. Openings (e.g., below skin level, at skin level, above skin level)
   e. Proximity to bony prominences, scars, abdominal creases, incision, drain(s), stoma
   f. Muscle tone surrounding opening (e.g., firm, soft, flaccid)
   g. Contours at the fistula opening (e.g., flat, shallow depth [$<1/16$ inch], moderate depth [$1/16$ to $1/4$ inch], or deep [$>1/4$ inch])
4. Perifistular skin integrity at each location (e.g., intact, macerated, erythematous, denuded or eroded, ulcerated, infected)

---

necessary to synthesize assessment data, product knowledge (advantages, disadvantages, effectiveness, and guidelines for use), patient needs, and physiology into realistic goals. Principles of wound care and principles of ostomy management are applied to the management of these clinical problems (WOCN Society, 1998). There is also an art involved in the techniques presented in this chapter. What to use, how much, and when can represent a delicate balance.

Goals

Effective nursing management of the ECF strives to achieve eight goals as listed in Box 23-3. Optimally, all the goals are achieved simultaneously; however, that is not always possible, and prioritizing is frequently necessary. For example, a pouching system may effectively contain output and odor as well as providing significant skin protection. However, complete mobility may not be possible, or the pouching system may be expensive. Interventions to achieve the above goals begin as soon as the patient is seen to have a fistula; they are not contingent upon medical diagnosis.

Four general perspectives are important when caring for a patient with a fistula (Rolstad and Wong, 2004):

1. Assess the pouching system and seal frequently, expect changes.
2. Build flexibility into the care plan.
3. Innovate, using the easiest, most practical approach first.
4. Recognize that care of the patient is frequently provided by inexperienced caregivers.

Assessment

The method selected to manage a fistula is guided by the assessment of four key fistula characteristics as outlined in Box 23-4. Since fistulas change in shape and contours over time, repeat assessment and monitoring are necessary, Modifications to the initial containment system are invariably necessary (Scardillo and Folkedahl, 1998; Wiltshire, 1996; Zwanziger, 1999).

Source. Initially, little information may be available regarding the origin of the fistula or the involved organs (if diagnostic studies have not yet been conducted). However, the probable origin of the fistula can be determined based on assessment of fistula output (volume, odor, consistency, and composition) (Table 23-3). This information provides insight into the patient's risk for altered skin integrity and provides decision points for selection of the management approach. For example, a fistula producing semiformed, odorous effluent is likely communicating with the left transverse or descending colon. Effluent from the transverse or descending

TABLE 23-3 Characteristics of Gastrointestinal Secretions

SOURCE	SECRETIONS	pH	24-HOUR VOLUME (cc)	COLOR	ELECTROLYTE CONCENTRATION			
					Na (mg)	K (mEq)	Cl (mg)	HCO_3 (mg)
Saliva	Ptyalin, maltase	6-7	1000-1200	Clear	20-80	16-23	24-44	20-60
Gastric juice	Pepsin, rennin (chymosin) lipase, hydrochloric acid	1-3.5	2000-3000	Clear/green	20-100	4-12	52-124	0
Pancreatic juice	Amylase, trypsin, chymotrypsin, lipase, sodium bicarbonate	8-8.3	700-1200	Clear/milky	120-150	2-7	54-95	70-110
Bile	Bile salts, phospholipids	7.8	500-700	Golden brown– greenish yellow	120-200	3-12	80-120	30-50
Duodenum Jejunum Ileum	Peptidase, trypsin, lipase, maltase, sucrase, lactase	7.8-8	2000-3000	Gold–dark gold	80-130	11-21	48-116	20-30
Colon		7.5-8.9	50-200	Brown	4	9	2	—

Na, Sodium; *K*, potassium; *Cl*, chloride; *HCO_3*, bicarbonate.

colon will be less damaging to the skin than the output from the ileum. Therefore, in this situation the primary goals of nursing management will be containment of effluent and odor.

Characteristics of Effluent. Characteristics of effluent that must be considered in fistula management include volume, odor, consistency, and composition. In general, the fistula with output volumes over 100 ml/24 hr requires a pouch or, in extreme situations, suction.

Odor is also a factor when selecting a management method. Just as a patient with a high-output fistula needs a pouching system, so might the patient with a malodorous output of only 10 to 20 ml/24 hr—even if just to contain odor. Odor may originate from numerous sources including exudate, necrotic or infected tissue, soiled dressings, dressing materials, and chemicals used in treatment.

Consistency of effluent is particularly important when using pouches, because it affects the type of drainage spout needed and subsequently the type of pouch selected. It will also influence whether additional skin barriers are necessary. Liquid effluent is much more corrosive than thick effluent and results in premature erosion of the skin barrier.

The color of effluent also acts as an indicator of fistula source (see Table 23-3). In the presence of effluent with active enzymes or extremes in pH, the perifistular skin will require aggressive protection. However, all perifistular skin should be monitored and protected from moisture, even when effluent composition does not include active enzymes. Until radiographic studies are performed, the enzymatic and pH composition of the effluent can be inferred from the volume and consistency of the drainage.

Cutaneous Opening. The size of the opening is determined by measuring the length and width in centimeters. A pattern is always useful, since a fistula is usually an irregular shape, and should be kept in the patient's room with supplies. The fistula opening may appear as a deep tunnel with the base not visible for assessment, or the base may be visible with the fistula exiting at a specific location. In some situations the fistula opening may exit above the skin level as mucosal or granulation tissue. Wound dressings may be warranted to pack the wound (e.g., alginates or foams) when the fistula is present in a deep wound base.

Abdominal Topography. Patient assessment is performed in a supine and a semi-Fowler's position. The cutaneous fistula locations are identified and documented. The area is then assessed for the presence of irregular skin surfaces that are created by scars or creases. This assessment indicates how flexible the adhesive in contact with the skin must be and whether filling agents, such as skin barrier paste or strips, are needed to level irregular surfaces (Plates 40 and 41). In addition, the number of cutaneous fistula openings, the location of each, and the proximity to bony prominence or other obstacles (i.e., retention sutures or stoma) are assessed and documented. These characteristics will help to determine what size and shape of adhesive surface is needed to secure the sites, yet avoid impinging on the prominence or protrusion. If two cutaneous sites are too far apart to be pouched in one system, two pouches may be necessary.

Muscle tone in the area and skin contours should also be assessed. Decreased abdominal muscle tone can be expected in the patient who lacks exercise, is overweight, and in the elderly or the infant. Aging affects subcutaneous tissue support. Muscle tone may be characterized as firm, soft, or flaccid.

It is also important to assess the level at which the fistula opening exits onto the skin. Contours of the skin surrounding the fistula opening may be classified as flat, shallow (less than $1/16$ inch), moderate depth

($1/16$ to $1/4$ inch), or deep (greater than $1/4$ inch) (Rolstad and Boarini, 1996). Fistulas emptying into deep, open wounds require more pouch adaptations than fistulas emptying flush with intact skin.

Perifistular Skin Integrity. Perifistular skin condition should be assessed and documented at each dressing or pouch change. Constant exposure of the epidermis to moisture, active enzymes, extremes in pH of fluids, and mechanical trauma frequently lead to breaks in skin integrity. Denudation of perifistular skin is a common complication in fistula patients and is often present when the patient is first seen with the fistula. Skin constantly bathed in fluid causes maceration, whereas effluent with enzymatic drainage or extremes in pH levels will create erythema and denuded or eroded perifistular skin.

Although it is best to visually inspect the skin, data can also be obtained from the nursing staff and patient to aid assessment. For example, when frequent dressing changes (every 4 hours) are reported, skin will deteriorate quickly as a result of chemical and mechanical injury. Patient reports of burning or stinging sensations around the fistula or wound commonly indicate denudation of the epidermis.

Patients with fistulas may also develop an infection in the perifistular skin as a result of entrapment of moisture against the skin. The origin of the infection is most commonly fungal and is characterized by an erythematous, papular rash with satellite lesions (Plate 41). Although less common, herpes zoster skin lesions may also occur. At times it may be difficult to distinguish between the erythema caused by such an infection and the erythema caused by chemical irritation from contact with the effluent.

Planning and Implementation

Four key questions should be asked when planning the approach to technical management of a fistula:

1. Is the output volume more than 100 ml/24 hr?
2. Is odor a problem?
3. Is the fistula opening less than 3 inches?
4. Is an access cap needed?

Figure 23-4 is an algorithm that incorporates these four questions to guide decision making for managing a fistula.

Fistulas can be managed with pouches, dressings, suction, or all three. When planning the specific fistula

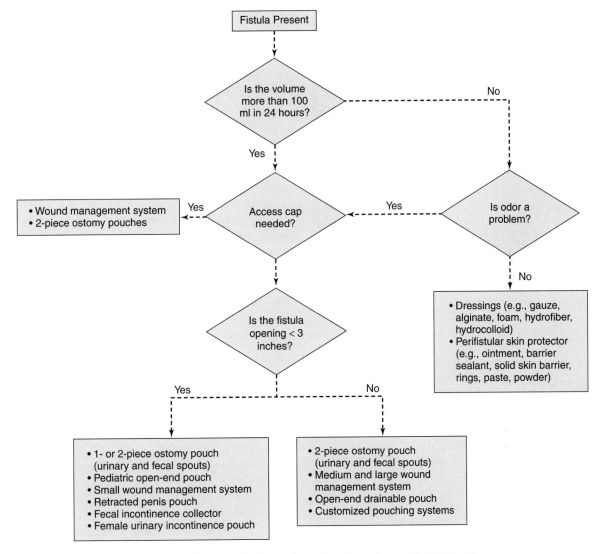

Fig. 23-4 Selecting a fistula pouch: an algorithm. (Designed by B. Rolstad.)

management approach, the four key questions discussed previously and the goals that have been identified by the health care team and patient must be considered. In most situations, the priority goals are containment of effluent, odor control, and perifistular skin protection. Initially some goals may be compromised, such as ease of care, patient mobility, and cost containment, because of the acuteness of the situation. This section presents

nursing interventions that facilitate attainment of each goal for the nursing management of fistulas.

Perifistular Skin Protection. The potential for skin breakdown is always present when a fistula exists regardless of the management option selected. Preventive strategies should be implemented early and be accompanied by frequent monitoring. Protective strategies include atraumatic adhesive removal and

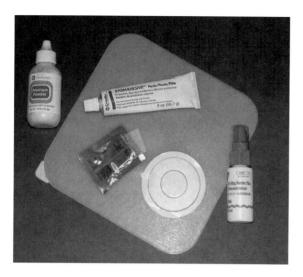

Fig. 23-5 Examples of skin barriers: wafer, paste, ring, powder, sealant.

protection of the skin from exposure to effluent. Dressings alone do not offer skin protection, thus the concurrent use of a skin barrier is often necessary. Skin barriers are available in various forms (Figure 23-5). Table 23-4 summarizes the characteristics and indications of each type.

If pouching is selected as the management approach, solid-wafer skin barriers are usually integrated into the pouching system during manufacturing. However, additional skin-barrier products may be required to caulk edges, fill creases, and/or add convexity.

At times, skin-barrier wafers and pastes need to be applied over an intact incision as a part of the management system. This is done to secure the system and prevent leakage of effluent from the fistula onto the incision.

Skin-barrier powders are used to absorb moisture from denuded skin and to create a dry surface.

TABLE 23-4 **Guide to the Use of Skin Barriers in Fistula Management**

TYPE OF SKIN BARRIER	CHARACTERISTICS	INDICATIONS
Solid wafers (4" × 4" or 8" × 8")	• Pectin-based wafers with an adhesive surface • Available as wafers or rings • Have moist tack • Have varied flexibility • May be cut into wedges, rings, or strips • Have varied durability to effluent • Changed only when they loosen from the perifistular edges or once every 7 days	• Provide skin protection, referred to as laying down a protective platform • Level irregular skin surfaces • Protect perifistular skin from effluent when dressings are used or skin is exposed • Gauze dressings are applied over the skin-barrier wafer and taped to the wafer rather than the skin • Level irregular skin surfaces • Protect perifistular skin from effluent when dressings are used or skin is exposed
Skin barrier rings	• Available in hydrocolloid and karaya formulations • Have moist tack • Have varied flexibility • Have varied durability to effluent • Hydrocolloid formulations • Recommended for fistula management	• Level irregular skin surfaces • Protect perifistular skin from effluent when dressings are used or skin is exposed

Adhesives or ointments can then be applied to the dry surface. For severely denuded skin, it may be necessary to create an "artificial scab" with the skin-barrier powder by alternating layers of the skin-barrier powder and a skin sealant or skin cement. The pouching system may then be applied directly over the artificial scab. To enhance adherence, it may be desirable to apply either skin cement or spray adhesive to the artificial scab and pouch adhesive surface. Skin-barrier powders should not be confused with talc or cornstarch, which do not provide skin protection.

In nonpouching management approaches, petroleum-based or zinc-based ointments are used to provide skin protection. These products are particularly useful in low-volume, odorless fistulas and are usually inexpensive. They are applied to perifistular skin, particularly the edges, and covered with dressings. Ointments are not intended for use under adhesives. Frequency of application is indicated on the product and may differ depending on the product formulation and use.

Containment of Effluent. Containment of effluent is accomplished with nonpouching and pouching approaches. The volume of effluent, presence of odor, abdominal contours, and care setting influence which approach is most effective.

Nonpouching options. Nonpouching options include dressings and barriers, drains, and suction techniques. The method chosen is greatly influenced by the volume of output.

Dressings and barriers. Nonpouching options are indicated when (1) fistula output is low (less than 100 ml/24 hr), (2) odor is not present, and (3) skin contours or the location of the fistula makes pouching impossible. Containment of effluent can be achieved with dressings intended for absorption, which include gauze (sponges or strip packing), alginates, foam, and combinations of dressings. Packing should only be done with dressing materials that may be retrieved from the wound. For example, a strip packing material may be gently packed into a low-volume drain site.

TABLE 23-4 Guide to the Use of Skin Barriers in Fistula Management—cont'd

TYPE OF SKIN BARRIER	CHARACTERISTICS	INDICATIONS
Paste (tube or strip forms)	• Commercial preparations contain alcohol, which can create burning sensation if skin is denuded • Extremely tacky; should be applied as a thin bead, smoothed into place with a damp gloved finger or tongue blade • Contains solvents; allow to dry briefly so that solvents can escape before other products are applied	• Level irregular skin surfaces • Protect exposed skin from effluent (i.e., with pouching) • Extend duration of solid wafer barrier when pouching
Powder	• Must be used lightly; may be used in combination with sealants to create an artificial scab	• Absorb moisture from superficial denudement before applying ointments or adhesives
Skin sealants	• Residual powder alters adhesion • Liquid, nonalcohol, and alcohol preparations • Nonalcohol skin sealants are indicated for use on denuded skin • Must be allowed to dry to permit solvents to dissipate • Available in various forms (wipes, gel, wands, roll-ons, and pump spray).	• May be used under adhesives to protect fragile skin during adhesive removal • Improve adherence of adhesives to skin (particularly oily skin) • Protect perifistular skin from effluent or maceration when dressings are used • Used in combination with skin barrier powders; creates an artificial scab

A 2-inch tail of dressing material is left outside the wound and will be used to retrieve the packing at dressing changes. Entrapment of effluent against the skin may cause maceration and breakdown; therefore skin barriers must be used in conjunction with the dressings to protect the perifistular skin (Table 23-4).

If, despite best efforts, perifistular skin becomes compromised or output volume exceeds 100 ml/24 hr, dressings become less effective and more time-intensive to manage. The application of additional dressings will not increase the absorbency of the dressing or lengthen the time between dressing changes. A good rule is that when dressings have to be changed more often than every 4 hours, a pouching system should be used. Conversely, when a fistula site has low volume, a small pouching system may be used so that the patient does not have to change the pouch more than once in 7 days. This approach provides convenience and protects perifistular skin.

Vaginal fistula drain device. Vaginal fistulas occasionally develop secondary to pelvic irradiation and create a challenging situation where the patient is incontinent of feces through the vagina. The uncontrolled passage of fecal material vaginally results in severe perivaginal skin denudation and discomfort. Aggressive nursing care is essential to prevent these complications.

Skin protection can be achieved with ointments and pads. Frequent dressing changes are necessary to avoid entrapment of caustic drainage contents against the skin. Unfortunately, ointments and pads for vaginal fistulas are less than optimal because they are labor-intensive, do not promote patient mobility, do not adequately contain the fecal contents, and fail to control odor. A female urinary incontinence pouch may be useful in these situations and may be connected to straight drainage. However, the difficult location and moist surface surrounding the vaginal orifice make application of an adhesive pouching system challenging.

A vaginal fistula drain device is another method of managing a vaginal fistula and does not require adhesives (Shield Health Care). This type of system can also be constructed with a Davol breast shield, Evenflo nipple shield, or vaginal diaphragm and a large Malecot catheter (Figure 23-6) (O'Connor, 1983). A cruciate incision is made through the nipple shield or diaphragm,

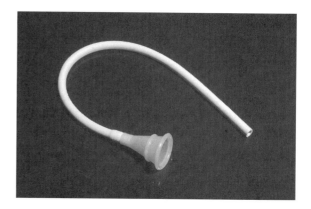

Fig. 23-6 Vaginal drain device; available commercially (Shield Health Care), or can be configured with Davol breast shield and large Malecot catheter.

through which the catheter is threaded. The shield or diaphragm serves to occlude the vagina so that the drainage is directed down the catheter.

The soft, cone-shaped device, shield, or diaphragm is inserted a short distance into the vagina. The discomfort that such manipulation of the labia and vagina can create for the patient can be minimized by lubrication of the device with a lidocaine (Xylocaine) lubricant. Tubing is attached to the device to channel the fistula contents into a straight drainage collection bag. The drainage tubing can be anchored to the patient's inner thigh.

A vaginal fistula drain device will remain in place effectively while the patient is reclining. As the patient becomes more ambulatory, the device may have a tendency to become dislodged; however, because the procedure is so easy, the patient can reinsert the vaginal drain as needed. Gentle irrigation of the tubing may be indicated if the tubing becomes occluded by fistula material. A vaginal fistula drain device may be a temporary or permanent management technique depending on the patient's status.

Closed suction systems. Closed suction systems continue to be a viable, reliable, and cost-effective method to manage high-output fistulas, especially when the fistula is located in a dehisced abdominal wound (Davis, Dere, and Hadley, 2000; Jones and Harbit, 2003; Kordasiewicz, 2004). Catheters attached to low, intermittent suction may be used when routine pouching is ineffective or overwhelmed by the volume of output (Beitz and Caldwell, 1998; Lange et al, 1989). However, suction does not provide complete containment of effluent; dressings and skin protection are still necessary. Effluent must be liquid if suction is to be effective; thick or particulate drainage will occlude the catheter. The wound is cleansed, and a layer of saline-moistened gauze is placed in the wound bed. The catheter is laid in the wound and directed toward the bottom of the setup. Another layer of moist gauze may be applied over the catheter, and a large transparent dressing may be applied as a secondary dressing (Hollis and Reyna, 1985; Jeter, Tintle, and Chariker, 1990). Skin-barrier paste is sometimes necessary to fill in irregular skin surfaces and to seal around the catheter as it exits from the transparent dressing. Suction tubing is then attached to the suction catheter and set at a low level of continuous suction. A hemovac can provide the suction for short periods to increase the patient's mobility. This dressing is usually changed every 1 to 2 days.

A catheter that is inserted into the fistula tract will act as a foreign body and may therefore interfere with healing and even increase fistula output (Welch, 1997). On the other hand, a catheter coiled in a defect above the orifice or in the open wound surrounding the fistula opening will not inhibit closure. Because firm tubes can injure fragile tissue, only soft, flexible suction catheters should be used with fistulas (Welch, 1997). Suction catheters should be considered a short-term intervention because of the limitations placed on patient mobility and the time-intensive nature of the care

Negative-pressure wound therapy. An evolution of the above-described technology is negative-pressure wound therapy (NPWT). This technique has demonstrated clinical wound healing benefits. The system incorporates a sponge and subatmostpheric pressure, which results in reduced periwound edema and mechanical stretching of cells. Mechanical stretching of cells is believed to stimulate the wound repair process. The use of NPWT is contraindicated for nonenteric (e.g., biliary and pancreatic) fistulas and for fistulas that have not been explored for involved organs, abscesses, distal obstruction, and so forth. NPWT has built-in sensors to alert caregivers to potential and actual breaches in the integrity of the system. Further information about the application and use of NPWT is presented in Chapter 20.

Pouching options. Volume and odor are the primary indications for pouching. Dressings are contraindicated when odor is problematic or the volume of effluent exceeds 100 ml/24 hr. However, patients with low-volume, nonodorous output may elect to pouch for convenience. The pouch may be changed once a week and is less expensive than dressings.

Numerous techniques have been reported in the literature for managing fistulas (Boarini, Bryant, and Irrgang, 1986; Davis, Dere and Hadley, 2000; Irrgang and Bryant, 1984; Jones and Harbit, 2003; Kordasiewicz, 2004; O'Brien, Landis-Erdman, and Erwin-Toth, 1998; Rolstad and Wong, 2004; Skingley, 1998; Smith, 1982, 1986). Ostomy pouches (fecal or urinary; adult or pediatric) can be used, as well as pouches specifically designed for managing complex wounds. Pouching preserves patient dignity by containing embarrassing odor and drainage. Pouching is an effective strategy for pain control because it requires less manipulation of the wound and protects the surrounding skin from painful denudement caused by caustic drainage. An effective pouching system also offers a sense of control to the nursing staff because effluent is contained and emptied at specific intervals. Pouch changes are then scheduled at convenient times **before** leakage occurs. By preventing the embarrassment of odor and leaking dressings, the patient's dignity is also supported. A routine pouch change procedure and fistula pouching tips are listed in Boxes 23-5 and 23-6 respectively.

Historically, frequent modifications of skin barriers, adhesives, and/or pouches were required to effectively manage the complicated fistula. Few alternatives were available to manage the fistula with a large cutaneous opening, irregular contours of the skin, and other unique situations. Materials used for pouches included garbage bags, colostomy irrigation sleeves, and sandwich bags. Today, however, manufactured wound-management systems are designed for the difficult-to-manage site. Solid-wafer skin barriers with new, durable formulations that provide longer wear time are integrated into most pouching systems. Cutting surfaces of the skin barriers are currently available to manage a broad range of fistula opening sizes, from the small opening of a starter hole to $9^{1}/_{2} \times 6$ inches. However, it remains essential to fill irregular skin surfaces so that a flat, stable surface is attained for the pouching system.

BOX 23-5 Sizable Pouch–Change Procedure: Fistula

1. Assemble equipment: pouch with attached skin barrier, pattern, skin-barrier paste, scissors, paper tape, closure clip, water, gauze, or tissue.
2. Prepare pouch.
   a. Trace pattern onto skin-barrier surface of pouch.
   b. Cut skin-barrier pouch to size of pattern.
   c. Remove protective backing or backings from pouch.
3. Remove and apply pouch.
   a. Remove pouch, using one hand to gently push the skin away from the adhesive.
   b. Discard pouch and save closure clip.
   c. Control any discharge with gauze or tissue.
   d. Clean skin with water and dry thoroughly.
   e. Apply paste around fistula or stoma. Fill in any uneven skin surfaces with paste or skin barrier strips. Use a damp finger or tongue blade to apply paste.
   f. Apply new pouch, centering wound site in opening.
   g. Tape edges of adhesive surface in a picture-frame effect with paper tape.
   h. Close bottom of pouch with clip.

BOX 23-6 Fistula Pouching Tips

Schedule the procedure, if possible, to allow education and participation from nursing staff and other caregivers.

Set up all equipment before starting the procedure; fistula function is unpredictable and may otherwise occur when adhesives are not completely set up.

Cut the opening in the pouch adhesive approximately $1/8^{th}$ inch larger than the fistula cutaneous opening. If periwound skin is exposed, a skin-barrier paste may be applied for protection. Apertures much larger than the actual fistula opening may be necessary with severe, deep depressions that create irregular skin surfaces. To prevent skin denudation, a skin-barrier paste is applied to the exposed skin (Plate 41).

Follow universal precautions with clean technique during procedures. The care of fistulas or drain sites is seldom a sterile procedure. Sterile products are an unnecessary expense and are not shown to control infection.

To remove adhesives from the skin, gently roll off adherent material with a dry gauze. Solvents may be used but must be cleansed thoroughly from the skin before adhesive application. Do not scrub or abrade the skin. It may be necessary to leave small amounts of residual paste or cement on the skin. This should not hinder pouch adhesion.

Cleanse the skin with tap water or a commercially available skin cleanser and gauze. Cleansers will emulsify fecal material and are primarily indicated when fistula drainage is adherent to surrounding skin. Cleansers should be nongreasy and rinsed thoroughly; use on denuded skin is discouraged. Dry thoroughly.

Position the pouch such in a manner that effluent will drain away from the fistula orifice. This will minimize pooling of corrosive effluent over the skin barrier, which ultimately erodes the skin barrier. The pouch can be angled off to the reclining patient's side, or drainage tubing can be attached to enable continuous drainage into a larger receptacle. Patients should be encouraged to monitor the pouch and recognize when it should be emptied.

Additionally, it may be necessary to select a pouching system that supports the perifistular tissue and stabilizes soft skin. In general, if the skin is soft or flaccid, a firm skin-barrier adhesive and possibly a belt may be indicated. In contrast, firm skin surrounding the fistula site will best be managed with a flexible, soft adhesive surface. Examples of soft, pliable materials include powder, skin-barrier paste, wafers, strips, and rings, whereas methods to achieve firm support may include firm rings, convexity in ostomy pouching systems, or a belt.

Features of a pouching system. Knowledge of available features of products is essential to make appropriate choices. Features include adhesive skin-barrier surface, pouch capacity, pouch material (film and outlet), and wound access (Box 23-7 and Figure 23-7).

Adhesive skin-barrier surface. When the cutaneous opening is less than 3 inches, a one- or two-piece ostomy pouch may be used. For fistulas greater than 3 inches, commercially available wound-management systems or modifications of larger pouches

BOX 23-7 Features of a Fistula Pouch

Adhesive Surface
- Integrated skin barrier
- Size and shape of cutting surface
- Sizable versus presized adhesive surface
- Presence or absence of starter hole
- Degree of flexibility of skin-barrier wafer

Pouch Capacity
- Volume (3- to 4-hours' capacity preferred)

Pouch Material
- Odorproof or odor-resistant pouch film
- Transparent versus opaque film
- Fecal outlet (clamp closure)
- Spout for liquids (urinary outlet)
- Wide drain for viscous material
- Wide tubular outlet can be converted to open-end drain

Wound Access
- Two-piece pouch
- Access window on wound-management system
- Wide tubular outlet can be converted to open-end drain

are warranted. In either case, the adhesive skin-barrier surface must be large enough to accommodate the fistula opening and generally allow for 1 to 2 inches of adhesive contact around the fistula. The adhesive surface should be applied in such a fashion as to avoid obstacles in the perifistular skin area, such as a bony prominence or drain site. If this is not possible, it may be necessary to find a pouch with a smaller adhesive surface.

Conversely, a large amount of adhesive contact (over 4 to 5 inches) with the surrounding skin is generally not necessary and may be detrimental. Movement-induced skin changes under the adhesive surface will precipitate leakage and disruption of the pouch seal.

Pouching systems may have a starter hole for cutting the opening into irregular shapes or may be presized (e.g., for round, regular shapes). Although starter holes are convenient for cutting, they restrict the positioning of the opening in the adhesive, since the opening includes the starter hole. In some situations the opening may have to be covered with a skin barrier so that

other locations on the adhesive may be cut to fit the size of the fistula.

A few pouches are available without an integrated skin-barrier wafer. In these situations, the fistula pattern must be used to cut a hole in the skin-barrier wafer and the pouch. The skin barrier is then attached to the pouch, and the system is applied directly to the skin.

Pouch capacity. The capacity of the pouch is predetermined by the size of the adhesive surface; typically pouches with larger adhesive surfaces have larger pouch capacities. Generally, a pouch with the capacity to contain 3 to 4 hours' worth of effluent is recommended so that the risk of leakage is minimized. A smaller-capacity pouch may be used if the caregivers or patient is willing to empty the pouch more frequently or if the pouch can be connected to straight drainage. Small-volume closed-end pouches may also be indicated for the patient with minimal malodorous output. This pouch would be changed and discarded once or twice a week.

Pouch outlet. Effluent consistency and volume dictate the type of outlet spout best for pouch management. Pouches are designed with either urinary (or liquid) outlets or fecal outlets (see Figure 23-7). The urinary outlet is indicated for liquid effluent and is convenient because it may be connected to straight drainage. When a urinary pouch is used for fistula care, the antireflux mechanism will obstruct flow; therefore the antireflux mechanism must be pulled apart. Fecal outlets (or open-end drains) are appropriate for thick, mushy effluent and are secured with a clamp.

The two-piece ostomy system, fecal incontinence collectors, and wound-management systems offer the benefit of having a urinary outlet that can be attached to a bedside bag. As the effluent thickens, the outlet can be trimmed off and secured with a clamp, transforming the pouch from a urinary to a fecal pouch without having to remove the pouch from the skin.

Most recently, two piece high-output pouches have been introduced to the market. These systems combine the desirable features of an ostomy system (i.e., presized adhesive surface and convexity) with outlets than can accommodate the varying consistency of effluent typical of a fistula.

Adaptations can be made to pouches to accommodate fistula consistency. For example, when formed output becomes liquid, urinary pouch–adapter latex

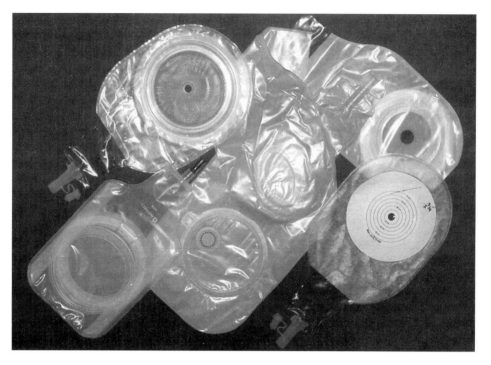

Fig. 23-7 Examples of pouches. Notice the variety in sizes for the adhesive surface, the outlet spouts, and the access windows.

drainage tubing can be attached to a fecal pouch. If the output begins to thicken or form particulate matter, wider respiratory tubing can be attached to the tail of an open-end drain (Box 23-8).

Wound access. At times, access to the fistula site may be desirable so that tubes can be advanced, the fistula can be assessed easily, or skin-barrier pastes can be reinforced. Access to the site without disruption of the pouch adhesive can be achieved with a two-piece pouch or with a pouch that has an attached "access window." When such access features are not available or have an inadequate adhesive surface size, wide open-end drains can be used. Cuffing the pouch film back can facilitate limited access to the fistula site.

Pouch film. Urinary drainage equipment and some fecal pouches may be more odor-resistant than odor-proof. More frequent pouch changes may be necessary to prevent the odor from permeating the pouch film, or more aggressive odor-management techniques (e.g., oral deodorizers) may be required. Pouching systems marketed as wound-management systems are

transparent to allow for visual inspection. Ostomy pouches adapted for fistula care provide choices in film color: transparent, opaque, or beige-tone.

Pouching system adaptations

Adhesives. Additional adhesive is available as cement, medical adhesive spray forms, and sheet form. Cements and sprays are applied according to the manufacturer's instructions; most require time to become tacky. They are used to enhance the tack of an existing adhesive and extend the adhesive surface on a pouch. Adhesives may also be warranted to improve the tack when several applications of skin-barrier powder are required in the presence of severe denudation. Occasionally, liquid adhesive may be used in combination with skin-barrier powders to protect exposed skin from caustic effluent. This procedure is similar to the artificial scab discussed previously.

Because fistulas vary in size and shape, and abdominal contours can be dramatic, large and unusually shaped pouch apertures may be necessary. Sheets of adhesives (or double-faced adhesive disks) can be used

BOX 23-8 Addition of Continuous Drainage Tube to Fecal Outlet Pouch

Equipment
- Fecal pouch or open-end drain
- Connector to fit the tubing and bedside system
- 5 inches of wide-lumen tubing or respiratory tubing
- Rubber band
- Bedside drainage system

Procedure
1. Cut the desired size for the fistula in the skin-barrier adhesive of a fecal pouch or open-end drain.
2. Insert the wide-lumen tubing or respiratory tubing into the drain spout.
3. Working at the adhesive surface, reach inside the pouch and pull the drain spout and tubing through the opening cut in the skin-barrier adhesive.
4. Wrap a rubber band securely around the tubing to secure.
5. From the bottom of the pouch, pull the tubing through so that the outlet spout is in its normal location. The tail of the pouch is now cuffed around the tubing inside the pouch.
6. Attach to bedside drainage system.

Note: If wide respiratory tubing is used, a condom catheter can be used to connect the pouch to bedside drainage

BOX 23-9 Procedure for Adding Adhesive Sheets to Enlarge Pouch Adhesive Surface

Equipment
- Pouch without floating collar
- Double-faced adhesive sheet or disk

Procedure
1. Remove protective paper from one side of adhesive sheet.
2. Attach this adhesive sheet adjacent to existing adhesive on pouch (edges may overlap slightly).
3. Trace desired opening size on protective paper, covering adhesive surface.
4. Cut to desired size.
5. Prepare solid skin-barrier wafer (usually 8×8 inches), attach to adhesive surface on pouch, and continue in usual fashion.

BOX 23-10 Procedure for Making a Temporary Fistula Pouch

Equipment
- Plastic bag
- Skin-barrier wafer
- Double-faced adhesive sheet or double-faced tape

Procedure
1. Remove protective paper from one side of adhesive sheet and apply to area of pouch where adhesive and barrier are intended to be (in the absence of adhesive sheets, substitute with overlapping strips of double-sided tape).
2. Remove other side of adhesive sheet or tape.
3. Attach skin-barrier wafer (top side toward exposed adhesive on pouch)
4. Cut the barrier of the pouch to the desired size.
5. Remove skin-barrier wafer protective paper backing.
6. Continue in the usual fashion.

to increase the adhesive surface on a pouch. Box 23-9 describes the procedure for adding an adhesive sheet to a pouch.

Another option is simply to create a pouch (Box 23-10). The advantage to this technique is that it offers immediate skin protection and containment of affluent with readily available supplies. While this is a temporary intervention, it allows the care provider time to design a management system and obtain commercially available products with the desirable features identified in the plan of care.

Saddlebagging. Another method that can be used to acquire a large adhesive surface is to attach two open-end drainable pouches (Figure 23-8). Pouch features that facilitate saddlebagging include no attached solid-wafer skin barrier, no floating collar, and no starter hole. A large solid-wafer skin barrier is then attached to the new combined adhesive surface, and

the pouch is prepared in the usual fashion. Box 23-11 describes the saddlebagging technique.

Bridging technique. The bridging technique is a procedure that can be used to isolate one area of a wound from another part of the wound. It has two primary indications for use:
1. Wounds may present with two distinct areas of "needs": one area of the wound has drainage and

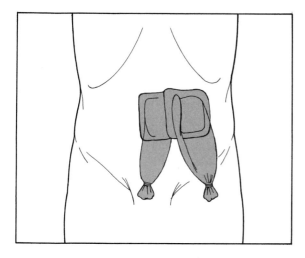

Fig. 23-8 Sketch of saddlebagging technique, where two open-ended drainable pouches are connected along the adhesive surface to create a large adhesive surface.

BOX 23-11 Saddlebagging Technique
....

Equipment
- Two open-end drains (without floating collar or attached skin barrier or starter hole)
- Solid-wafer skin barrier (8 × 8 inches)
- Skin-barrier paste

Procedure
1. Align pouches as final product is intended to appear on abdomen.
2. Peel protective backing away from adhesive along common edges of pouches approximately ½ to 1 inch.
3. Attach the two pouches along this ½- to 1-inch margin only.
4. Trace pattern of wound onto new adhesive surface (combined pouch adhesive surfaces).
5. Cut out pouch opening; do not cut into "seam" created by combining pouches.
6. Trace pattern onto solid-wafer skin barrier and cut out.
7. Remove protective paper backing from pouch adhesive surface and attach to solid-wafer skin barrier.
8. Prepare skin as indicated by wound contours and continue pouching procedure.

NOTE: Both pouches will fill with drainage and will require emptying.

requires containment, whereas another area requires moist wound healing or packing.

2. Very large wounds may be more manageable if the wound is "divided." Solid-wafer skin barriers are cut into small pieces to fill the wound at the selected bridge location and layered into place (Figure 23-9). A routine pouch or more complicated pouching system can then be applied over the bridge that now exists in the wound. Box 23-12 describes the steps involved in the bridging technique.

Catheter ports. When a catheter or tube is in place at a fistula site, leakage onto perifistular skin may occur. A pouching system with an attached catheter port may be used to collect the drainage. A catheter port is a nipple-shaped device that attaches to the external wall of a pouch. The catheter is disconnected, threaded through the pouch opening on the adhesive surface, and then threaded through the catheter port itself so the catheter can be reconnected to drainage. The pouch is then secured to the skin in the usual fashion. Detailed instructions from the manufacturer accompany the catheter port. With this technique, drainage around the catheter is collected in the pouch while the catheter continues to drain by suction or gravity (See Chapter 24, Figure 24-16).

Silicone molding. A silicone molding technique has been reported using a dental mold material to fashion an impression of the fistula opening and perifistular area in an attempt to create a smooth surface to which a pouch can be applied (Laing, 1977). When used, this procedure was reserved for the recessed fistula located in an open wound or the fistula surrounded by numerous irregular skin surfaces. However, the silicone mold procedure is less commonly used currently because of the advances in wound-management products (see Box 23-13).

Trough procedure. When fistulas are contained within the depressions of a wound in a manner such that a routine pouching system fails, this procedure may be useful. With the trough procedure, one or several strips of a transparent dressing are used to occlude the wound and trap effluent in the wound depression (Figure 23-10). A small opening is made in the transparent dressing at the most dependent aspect of the wound and an ostomy pouch is applied over this opening; no pattern is required.

To enhance adherence of the transparent dressing to the skin peripheral to the fistula or wound (and to

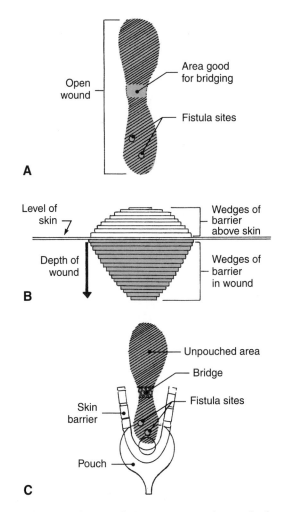

A

B

Open wound

Area good for bridging

Fistula sites

Level of skin

Depth of wound

Wedges of barrier above skin

Wedges of barrier in wound

Unpouched area

Bridge

Skin barrier

Fistula sites

Pouch

C

Fig. 23-9 Bridging technique. **A**, Area of wound where fistula sites are located and identified can be separated from remainder of wound. **B**, Cross-section view of tapered skin-barrier wedges used to fill the wound defect and to extend slightly above the level of the skin. **C**, Demonstration of how a pouch is applied over a bridge and fistula, leaving the area of the wound that is not draining available for more appropriate wound care.

protect perifistular skin), strips of a solid-wafer skin barrier should be applied. Directions for the trough procedure are listed in Box 23-14.

Control odor. In general, odor-control measures are indicated any time the patient and/or family perceives an odor to be objectionable, even if the odor seems almost imperceptible.

BOX 23-12 Bridging Technique

1. Assess wound and determine most appropriate location for "bridge." Be sure all sites from which drainage is produced are included in the side of wound to be pouched. For simplification of the bridging procedure, areas that are narrower or shallower should be selected.
2. Apply layered wedges of solid-wafer skin barrier and paste to create bridge. Wedges must be custom-cut to fit the dimensions of the wound at that level; usually the bottom wedge is narrowest, because the deepest part of the wound is typically the narrowest area. Each successive wedge is a little wider until the skin-barrier wafer wedges reach skin level.
3. Continue to layer solid-wafer barrier wedges above skin level, using progressively smaller and narrower wedges (to create a pressure-dressing effect).
4. Apply solid-wafer skin barrier to cover newly created bridge and extend onto intact skin. Paste may be needed to smooth "seams."
5. Continue with routine or complex pouching procedure as indicated.

NOTE: Skin barrier paste, adhesive spray, or cement may be used between wedges but are not routinely necessary.

The method of odor control depends on whether dressings or pouches are being used. Gauze dressings do not control odor; therefore charcoal-impregnated dressings may be needed over the gauze dressings. However, because charcoal becomes inactivated with moisture, these dressings should not come into contact with drainage materials. Charcoal dressings are most cost-effective with low-output fistulas, where the charcoal dressing remains intact for 24- to 48-hour periods. Pouches provide odor control. However, when the pouch is emptied, odor may be noticeable. Therefore, odor management must be a component of the care plan.

Odor is best controlled by use of a pouch to contain the effluent. A pouch may be the preferred management technique simply to contain the odor, regardless of the volume of output. Although most pouches have an odorproof film, the film's ability to contain odor varies. For example, many urinary pouches and

BOX 23-13 Silicone Mold

Equipment

Emesis basin
Tongue blade
Dow Corning Medical Grade Elastomer 382
Dow Corning Catalyst M and eye dropper
Red rubber catheter (optional)
Skin-barrier paste
Ostomy pouch with belt
Adhesives (silicone spray necessary to adhere to mold)

Preparation

1. Cleanse skin around the wound with water and pat dry.
2. Pour elastomer into dry emesis basin; usually 1 or 1½ ounces is enough for a moderate-sized cast.
3. Add 10 to 12 drops of Catalyst M for each ounce of elastomer.
4. Stir thoroughly with the tongue blade.
5. If necessary, place a suction catheter into fistula opening to contain drainage while the cast is setting.
6. When elastomer has slightly thickened, pour on patient's abdomen or in open wound around fistula orifice to a one-fourth inch thickness.
7. Allow mold to harden for 3 to 5 minutes in wound.
8. Gently lift mold out of wound.
9. Remove catheter from cast.
10. Trim edges of cast to form gently rounded surfaces.
11. Trim fistula opening in cast to be sure opening is adequate.

Application

1. Spread a smooth layer of skin-barrier paste on the back of the mold with a tongue blade, and allow it to set until it is firm to touch. Note: Silicone spray can be applied to this surface to increase adherence into or without the paste.
2. Place the mold into the wound. Seal the edges with the skin-barrier paste.
3. Apply tape on all edges of the mold.
4. Apply an ostomy pouch with belt tabs over the opening in the mold; attach belt.

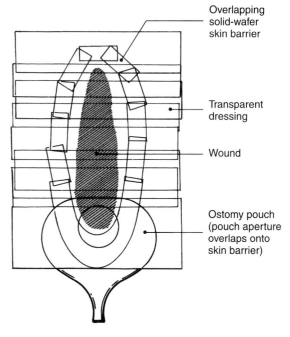

Overlapping solid-wafer skin barrier

Transparent dressing

Wound

Ostomy pouch (pouch aperture overlaps onto skin barrier)

Fig. 23-10 Sketch of trough procedure. Notice overlapping skin-barrier wafers and transparent dressing strips. Pouch opening must overlap onto the skin-barrier wafer at the inferior aspect of the wound.

urinary drainable systems are not odorproof, and so may become saturated with odor quickly.

To control odor one should (1) dispose of soiled linens and dressings from the room promptly, (2) use care in emptying pouches to prevent splashing effluent on the patient or on linens, (3) cleanse the tail of drainable fecal pouches after emptying, and (4) use deodorants appropriately.

Deodorants can be taken internally (orally) or used externally (in the pouch or as a room spray). Internal deodorants are in a tablet form but are generally discouraged in the presence of a pathologic condition such as a fistula. External deodorants are available in liquids, powders, and tablets and are placed in the pouch after each emptying. Room deodorants are particularly useful when emptying the pouch, changing the pouch, or changing dressings. The room deodorant selected should be one that eliminates odor rather than masks odor. With the many types of

BOX 23-14 Trough Procedure

1. Prepare skin and fill irregular skin surface as usual.
2. Apply overlapping strips of solid-wafer barrier along wound edges.
3. Apply skin-barrier paste to smooth "seams" (between barrier edges and along skin edges). NOTE: Inferior aspect of wound should be bordered with a solid piece of barrier instead of overlapping strips to prevent leakage.
4. Cut strips of a transparent dressing so that they are wide enough to cover wound and skin-barrier strips. Calculate length of strips so that strips overlap intact skin with 1- to 2-inch margins.
5. Reserve one strip of transparent dressing to be applied to the most inferior aspect of the wound.
6. Attach a drainable pouch (can be urinary or fecal) to this one strip of transparent dressing.
7. Cut hole in pouch or transparent-dressing adhesive surface so that it is lower than the inferior wound margins (it should clear the wound edges to provide adequate drainage).
8. Beginning at top of wound, apply transparent dressing in overlapping strips.
9. Attach the final strip of the transparent dressing (with the attached pouch) so that the bottom of the pouch opening is secured onto the skin-barrier wafer.

deodorants now available, patients, families, and caregivers should not have to tolerate the unfortunate odor that often accompanies fistulas.

Patient comfort. Areas to address to promote patient comfort include prevention and early treatment of perifistular skin irritation, pain control, and education to decrease anxiety. Leaking pouches, wet dressings on the skin, and odor in the patient's room all negatively affect morale. Medicating the patient before dressing or pouch changes may be indicated. Factors contributing to skin irritation include damp dressings, presence of caustic effluent in contact with the skin, and frequent tape application and removal. When selecting and evaluating a management technique, interventions appropriate to prevent unnecessary patient discomfort should be considered.

Accurate measurement of effluent. Accurate measurement of effluent from a fistula or drain site is critical to the success of fluid and electrolyte resuscitation

and nutritional support. As the patient becomes stabilized, accurate measurement of the effluent is less important. Pouching offers the most objective method of monitoring output, and suction is accurate only if the effluent does not leak around the catheters. Dressings can provide an estimate of volume if the dressings are weighed; however, this method is time-consuming, messy, and inconsistent from caregiver to caregiver.

Patient mobility. Consideration for optimizing the patient's activity should be of paramount importance when a fistula management method is being selected. Restrictions on physical activity predispose the patient to physical complications such as pneumonia, pressure ulcers, and thrombophlebitis, as well as to psychosocial complications such as depression and withdrawal. Because limitations on a patient's physical activity are sometimes necessary when suction or dressings are used to contain effluent, these interventions should be used only on a temporary basis. Pouches are less likely to restrict mobility.

Ease of use. Complex patient situations may necessitate unique pouching systems, which may be expensive and labor-intensive. Unfortunately, these unique adaptations often set up hurdles to the successfully participation of care providers. These complicated systems increase the chance of error in application and the time required of the caregiver. Therefore management may be complex initially and require the expertise of a certified ostomy nurse (COCN). As care progresses, the method of pouching should be simplified as much as possible to a more user-friendly system so it may be delegated. Several conveniences are available and should be considered as long as effectiveness is not compromised (Box 23-15).

Cost containment. Accountable, appropriate fistula management also requires selection of treatment options that are cost-effective. For example, a fistula pouch with a wound-access window is more costly than a sizable ostomy pouch, which would probably yield the same wear time. However, if use of a pouch with an access window prolongs wear time by providing access for wound care and paste application, it may be the most cost-effective option, even if it is changed every other day. Cost-containment implies attention not only to products and materials, but also to labor and time.

BOX 23-15 **User-Friendly Considerations in Fistula Care**
••

1. Whenever possible, use a presized pouch rather than sizable pouch.
2. Avoid suction when pouching is effective.
3. Fill skin defects with strip paste rather than tube paste in patients with manual dexterity problems.
4. Use pouching systems with convexity rather than creating convexity with layers of skin barriers.
5. Use one-piece rather than two-piece pouches.
6. Equipment should be selected that is easy to access in the community. Mail order of products is a convenience as long as orders are placed before the patient's supplies are depleted.

Evaluation

Accomplishment of Goals. The nurse should take time to reflect on the eight nursing management goals and evaluate how well these have been accomplished. Can steps be omitted? Is the skin intact? Is odor controlled? As the fistula stabilizes, the technical approach should be reevaluated and simplified as much as possible. One management system is seldom effective from the onset of the fistula until closure. For example, one fistula may be managed over its course with a pouch, dressings, or suction, or all three. While in the hospital, suction may be a workable option; however, mobility is compromised, and plans for home care are complicated. Therefore developing a pouching system that does not require suction would be an important simplification. Similarly, using products that are difficult to obtain is a complicating step and may be expensive. Planning to use an effective system that is easy and readily available is essential to facilitate the delivery of care.

Making Changes. It is important to expect change in fistula care and to modify interventions as needed. Seldom will the first pouch applied to a complex fistula be effective. Generally, modifications are necessary in the pouch pattern, size of adhesive surface, and use of skin-barrier pastes or wafer strips. It is best to make one change at a time so the effect of each modification can be accurately assessed. The addition of a belt may be warranted to add security to the pouch system, particularly on obese patients, or when the perifistular skin is mobile.

Close monitoring by the nurse must be provided for the duration of the fistula regardless of the health care setting. An inquisitive, analytic approach will facilitate identifying steps to improve the duration of the pouching system. For example, if the pouch leaks, is it between the skin and the barrier or the barrier and the pouch? Is the pouch being emptied when it is one third to one half full to prevent overfilling?

SUMMARY

Successful management of a patient with a fistula will require close monitoring and a plan of care that addresses the technical, educational, and emotional needs. Care often crosses many health care settings; settings with varying levels of expertise in the unique containment and skin protection vital to the patient's well being. In these situations, special arrangements must be made for appropriate follow-up for these complex patients.

SELF-ASSESSMENT EXERCISE

1. List at least four factors that may contribute to fistula development after a surgical procedure.
2. When might radiation-induced endarteritis cause fistulas?
   a. Only in the first month after irradiation
   b. Between 1 and 3 years after irradiation
   c. From 3 to 5 years after irradiation
   d. At any time after irradiation
3. List three complications that contribute to death from fistulas.
4. Define the term fistula.
5. A high-output fistula is defined as one that produces more than the following amount:
   a. 75 ml/24 hr
   b. 150 ml/24 hr
   c. 200 ml/24 hr
   d. 600 ml/24 hr
6. Define the involved structures for the following fistulas:
   a. Enterocutaneous
   b. Colocutaneous
   c. Vesicovaginal
   d. Rectovaginal
   e. Colovesical
7. List the four phases of medical management for the patient with a fistula.

8. Which of the following is the major cause of death in the patient with a fistula?
   a. Malnutrition
   b. Sepsis
   c. Operative complications
   d. Hypovolemia
9. List at least four factors known to delay spontaneous closure of fistulas.
10. List eight goals for nursing management of the patient with a fistula.
11. Which of the following is used to absorb moisture from irritated skin?
    a. Commercial skin-barrier pastes
    b. Adhesives
    c. Skin-barrier powders
    d. Skin sealants
12. Which of the following fistulas would be appropriately managed with gauze dressings?
    a. Volume of output 350 ml/24 hr
    b. Output noncorrosive and odorous
    c. Volume of output 50 ml/24 hr and noncorrosive
    d. Output with formed consistency and odorous
13. Explain when use of the bridging technique is indicated.
14. Identify options for odor control in wounds managed with dressings and wounds managed with pouches.
15. Skin-barrier paste is used with fistulas to achieve which of the following objectives?
    a. Absorb moisture from denuded skin
    b. Increase tack of pouch adhesives
    c. Level irregular skin surfaces
    d. Protect the skin from adhesives
16. The four most essential questions to ask when selecting a pouching system include which of the following?
    a. Volume, consistency, need for access, and ease of use
    b. Need for access, volume, odor, composition of effluent
    c. Opening size, odor, consistency, and ease of use
    d. Volume, opening size, odor, need for access

REFERENCES

Beitz JM, Caldwell D: Abdominal wound with enterocutaneous fistula: a case study, *J WOCN* 25(2):102, 1998.

Berry SM, Fischer JE: Classification and pathophysiology of enterocutaneous fistulas, *Surg Clin North Am* 76(5):1009, 1996.

Boarini J, Bryant R, Irrgang S: Fistula management, *Semin Oncol Nurs* 2:287, 1986.

Buchanan GN et al: Efficacy of fibrin sealant in the management of complex anal fistula, a prospective trial, *Dis Colon Rectum* 46:1167, 2003.

Campos ACL et al: A multivariate model to determine prognostic factors in gastrointestinal fistulas, *J Am Coll Surg* 188:483, 1999.

Chamberlain RS, Kaufman HL, Danforth DN: Enterocutaneous fistula in cancer patients: etiology, management, outcome and impact on further treatment, *Am Surg* 64(12):1204, 1998.

Conter RI, Root L, Roslyn JJ: Delayed reconstructive surgery for complex enterocutaneous fistulae, *Am Surgeon* 54:589, 1988.

Davis M, Dere K, Hadley G: Options for managing an open wound with draining enterocutaneous fistula, *J WOCN* 27(2):118-123, 2000.

Dudrick SJ, Maharaj AR, McKelvey AA. Artificial nutritional support in patients with gastrointestinal fistulas, *World J Surg* 23(6):570, 1999.

Eckhauser FE et al: Intra-abdominal abscesses and fistulae. In Yamada T et al, editors: *Textbook of gastroenterology*, Vol. II, ed 4, Philadelphia, 2003, Lippincott, Williams & Wilkins.

Eleftheriadis E et al: Early endoscopic fibrin sealing of high-output postoperative enterocutaneous fistulas, *Acta Chir Scand* 156:625, 1990.

Fagniez PL, Yahchouchy E: Use of somatostatin in the treatment of digestive fistulas, *Digestion* 60(suppl 3):65, 1999.

Fischer JE: The pathophysiology of enterocutaneous fistulas, *World J Surg* 7:446, 1983.

González-Pinto I, Moreno Gónzález E: Optimizing the treatment of upper gastrointestinal fistula, *Gut* 49(suppl IV):iv22, 2001.

Hesse U, Ysebaert D, de Hemptinne B: Role of somatostatin-14 and its analogues in the management of gastrointestinal fistulae: clinical data, *Gut* 49(suppl IV):iv11, 2001.

Hild P et al: Treatment of enterocutaneous fistulas and somatostatin, *Lancet* 2:626, 1986.

Hollington P et al: An 11-year experience of enterocutaneous fistulas, *Brit J Surg* 91:1646, 2004.

Hollis HW, Reyna TM: A practical approach to wound care in patients with complex enterocutaneous fistulas, *Surg Gynecol Obstet* 161:179, 1985.

Hwang TL, Chen MF: Short note: randomized trial of fibrin tissue glue for low-output enterocutaneous fistula, *Br J Surg* 83(1):112, 1996.

Irrgang S, Bryant R: Management of the enterocutaneous fistula, *J Enterostom Ther* 11:211, 1984.

Jeter KF, Tintle TE, Chariker M: Managing draining wounds and fistulae: new and established methods. In Krasner D, editor: *Chronic wound care: a clinical source book for healthcare professionals*, King of Prussia, Penn, 1990, Health Management.

Jones EG, Harbit M: Management of an ileostomy and mucous fistula located in a dehisced wound in a patient with morbid obesity, *J WOCN* 30(6):351, 2003.

Katkhouda N: The evolving role of fibrin sealants in surgery, Released on Medscape: March 16, 2001; accessed February 21, 2005. http://www.medscape.com/viewprogram/601?src=search

Kordasiewicz LM: Abdominal wound with fistula and large amount of drainage status after incarcerated hernia repair, *J WOCN* 31(3):150, 2004.

Laing BJ: Making silicone casts for enterocutaneous fistulas, *ET J* Fall: 11, 1977.

Lange MP et al: Management of multiple enterocutaneous fistulas, *Heart Lung* 18:386, 1989.

Lange V et al: Fistuloscopy. an adjuvant technique for sealing gastrointestinal fistulae, *Surg Endosc* 4:212, 1990.

Levy E et al: High-output external fistulae of the small bowel: management with continuous enteral nutrition, *Br J Surg* 76:676, 1989.

Magnotti LJ, Deitch EA: Digestion and absorption. In Rollandelli RH et al, editors: *Clinical nutrition: enteral and tube feeding*, ed 4, Philadelphia, 2005, Elsevier Saunders.

Makhdoom ZA, Komar MJ, Still CD: Nutrition and enterocutaneous fistulas, *J Clin Gastroenterol* 31(3):195, 2000.

Maykel JA, Fischer JE. Current management of intestinal fistulas. In: Cameron JL, editor: Advances in Surgery; St Louis, 2003, Mosby.

Meissner K: Late radiogenic small bowel damage: guidelines for the general surgeon, *Dig Surg* 16:169, 1999.

Minei JP, Champine J: Abdominal abscesses and gastrointestinal fistulas. In Feldman M., Sleisenger MH, Scharschmidt BF: *Sleisenger & Fordtrans's Gastrointestinal and Liver Disease. Pathophysiology/ Diagnosis/Management* (6ᵗʰ ed), Philadelphia, 1998, WB Saunders Company.

Moser AJ, Roslyn JJ: Enterocutaneous fistula. In Cameron JS, editor: *Current surgical therapy*, ed 6, St Louis, 1998, Mosby.

O'Brien B, Landis-Erdman J, Erwin-Toth P: Nursing management of multiple enterocutaneous fistulae located in the center of a large open abdominal wound: a case study, *Ostomy Wound Manage* 44(1):20, 1998.

O'Connor E: Vaginal fistulas: adaptation of management method for patients with radiation damage, *J Enterostom Ther* 10(6):229, 1983.

Phillips J, Walton M: Caring for patients with enterocutaneous fistulae, *Br J Nurs* 1(10):496, 1992.

Reber HS, Austin J: Abdominal abscesses and gastrointestinal fistulas. In Sleisenger M, Fortran J, editors: *Gastrointestinal disease pathophysiology diagnosis management*, vol 1, ed 4, Philadelphia, 1989, WB Saunders.

Rolstad B, Boarini J: Principles and techniques in the use of convexity, *Ostomy Wound Manage* 42(1):24, 1996.

Rolstad B, Wong WD: Nursing considerations in intestinal fistulas. In Cataldo PA, MacKeigan JM, editors: *Intestinal stomas: principles, techniques and management*, ed 2, New York, 2004, Marcel Dekker.

Rombeau J, Rolandelli R: Enteral and parenteral nutrition in patients with enteric fistulas and short bowel syndrome, *Surg Clin North Am* 67(3):551, 1987.

Rose D et al: One hundred and fourteen fistulas of the gastrointestinal tract treated with total parenteral nutrition, *Surg Gynecol Obstet* 163(4):345, 1986.

Rubin SC et al: Intestinal surgery in gynecologic oncology, *Gynecol Oncol* 34:30, 1989.

Saclarides TJ: Rectovaginal fistula, *Surg Clin N Am* 82:1261, 2002.

Sansoni B, Irving M: Small bowel fistulas, *World J Surg* 9:897, 1985.

Scardillo J, Folkedahl B: Management of a complex high-output fistula, *J WOCN* 25:217, 1998.

Sitges-Serra A, Jaurrieta E, Sitges-Creus A: Management of postoperative enterocutaneous fistulas: the roles of parenteral nutrition and surgery, *Br J Surg* 69:147, 1982.

Skingley S: The management of a faecal fistula, *Nurs Times* 94(16): 64, 1998.

Smith DB: Fistulas of the head and neck, *J Enterostom Ther* 9(5):20, 1982.

Smith DB: Multiple stomas, fistulas and draining wounds. In Smith DB, Johnson DR, editors: Ostomy care and the cancer patient: surgical and clinical considerations, New York, 1986, Grune & Stratton.

Welch JP: Duodenal, gastric, and biliary fistulas. In Zinner MJ, Schwartz SI, Ellis H, editors: *Maingot's abdominal operations*, vol 1, ed 10, Stamford, Conn, 1997, Appleton and Lange.

Wiltshire BL: Challenging enterocutaneous fistula: a case presentation, *J WOCN* 23(6):297, 1996.

Wong WD, Annamaneni RK, Buie WD: Management of intestinal fistulas. In Cataldo PA, MacKeigan JM, editors: *Intestinal stomas: principles, techniques, and management*, ed 2, New York, 2004, Marcel Dekker.

Wound Ostomy Continence Nursing (WOCN) Society: *Guidelines for management: caring for a patient with an ostomy*, Laguna Beach, Calif, 1998, Author.

Zwanziger PJ: Pouching a draining duodenal cutaneous fistula: a case study, *J WOCN* 26(1):25, 1999.

CHAPTER

24 — *Management of Gastrointestinal Feeding Tubes*

RUTH A. BRYANT

OBJECTIVES

1. Identify two primary reasons for use of gastrointestinal tubes.
2. Distinguish among the placement approaches for a gastrostomy and jejunostomy, including indications and overview of technique.
3. Discuss guidelines for feeding tube site selection.
4. Explain why tube stabilization is a priority in management of the patient with percutaneous tubes.
5. Describe at least two options for stabilization of gastrostomy or jejunostomy tubes.
6. For each complication listed, identify a prevention and management approach: peritubular leakage, tube migration, candidiasis, and tube occlusion.
7. Describe routine site care for the patient with a gastrointestinal tube.

Within the gastrointestinal (GI) tract, tubes are placed through a variety of techniques for the purposes of feeding, decompression, or drainage. Enteral nutrition offers many potential advantages over parenteral nutrition including lower rates of infectious and metabolic complications, decreased hospital length of stay, and reduced cost. Many of the benefits of enteral feeding are in part due to a preservation of gut integrity (Fish and Seidner, 2003).

Although first described in the thirteenth century, the planned surgical gastrostomy as a procedure was first proposed in 1837 and performed in 1849, with the first reported survival of the procedure performed by S. Jones in 1876 (Wu and Soper, 2004). Today the use of tubes is commonplace within the GI tract, as well as other organs and spaces, on a temporary or a long-term basis.

Malfunction of these tubes can result in skin erosion and irritation such that a referral to the wound care nurse becomes necessary. This chapter reviews the different types of gastrostomy and jejunostomy tubes, their purpose, procedures for placement, and nursing management. Potential complications are also presented. Other percutaneous tubes may also come to the attention of the wound care nurse, such as empyema tubes, biliary drainage tubes, and nephrostomy tubes. Although the principles for use and method of placement of such percutaneous tubes are beyond the scope of this textbook, principles of care (in terms of tube stabilization to prevent migration, movement, and peritubular skin irritation) are similar to those that are discussed in this chapter.

Effective nursing management of the patient with tubes placed percutaneously requires an understanding of the anatomy and physiology of the affected body system, the pathology involved, the rationale for tube placement, the method of tube insertion, and the anticipated length of time that the tube will be necessary. Although specific care procedures vary depending on the body system involved and the purpose of tube placement, management should always include routine care designed to maintain tube function and prevent peritubular complications, patient/caregiver education, and routine surveillance for tube dysfunction or complications. Comprehensive care is best provided with a collaborative team approach involving but not limited to the interventional radiologist, gastroenterologist, surgeon or internist, and nurse.

GASTROSTOMY AND JEJUNOSTOMY DEVICES

A gastrostomy is an opening into the stomach, and a jejunostomy is an opening into the jejunum. Such procedures may be used to provide decompression or enteral support for a patient unable to ingest adequate nutrients orally (DeChicco and Matarese, 2003).

Enteral support is generally appropriate through a nasogastric or nasoenteric feeding tube for short-term access (i.e., less than 3 to 4 weeks) in the patient who is at low risk for aspiration (Bloch and Mueller, 2004; DeChicco and Matarese, 2003; Wu and Soper, 2004). When the risk of aspiration exists, postpyloric placement of a tube is preferred. The patient's history and physical examination, barium studies, fluoroscopy, and

manometry are useful when evaluating the patient's risk for aspiration. Consultation with the neurologist and speech pathologist is also beneficial. Box 24-1 provides a list of risk factors for aspiration.

PLACEMENT APPROACHES

For over a century, gastrostomy placement required a surgical intervention involving anesthesia and the traditional preoperative preparation for abdominal surgery. Historically, a suture was placed around the base of the tube at skin level and then through the skin to immobilize the gastrostomy tube. Gastrostomy tubes were usually connected to suction for 12 to 24 hours to reduce tension on the suture line. Feedings were delayed until bowel sounds, tube patency, and proper placement of the tube was confirmed.

Today, a gastrostomy or jejunostomy is created by one of three approaches: surgical, endoscopic, or interventional radiologic. Open laparotomy is rarely performed owing to the success of the much less invasive endoscopic and laparoscopic techniques (Duh and McQuaid, 2000). Figure 24-1 presents an algorithm

BOX 24-1 **Risk Factors for Aspiration**
....

Altered mental status
Swallowing dysfunction
History of aspiration
Severe gastroesophageal reflux
Gastric outlet obstruction
Gastroparesis

From Gorman RC, Nance ML, Morris JB: Enteral feeding techniques. In Torosian MH: *Nutrition for the hospitalized patient: basic science and principles of practice,* New York, 1995, Marcel Dekker.

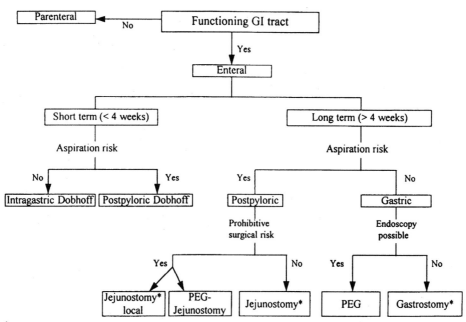

Fig. 24-1 Enteral access algorithm for selecting the most appropriate technique for an individual patient. (From Gorman RC, Morris JB: Minimally invasive access to the gastrointestinal tract. In Rombeau JL, Rolandelli RH: *Clinical nutrition: enteral and tube feeding,* ed 3, Philadelphia, 1997, WB Saunders.)

for determining the most appropriate means of enteral access.

Surgical Approaches

A surgically placed gastrostomy or jejunostomy tubes can be accomplished through an open surgical procedure or a laparoscopic procedure. Surgical placement is relatively expensive, requires anesthesia and the use of sterile dressings, and exposes the patient to many potential complications. The surgical approach is reserved for the patient with pharyngeal, esophageal, or gastric obstructions, upper GI tumors, or when abdominal surgery is already being performed for other purposes. Surgical placement is also performed when endoscopic placement has failed (Beyers, 2003).

Open Surgical Procedure. The most common open surgical procedures for gastrostomy tube placement are the Stamm, the Witzel, and the Janeway. The Stamm and the Witzel are the simplest procedures and are considered temporary; the Janeway is more of a long-term or permanent procedure (Bloch and Mueller, 2004; Gincherman and Torosian, 1996).

Stamm gastrostomy. Creation of a Stamm gastrostomy is begun by making a small incision in the left upper quadrant of the abdomen. Another small incision is made over and through the body of the stomach, through which a catheter (Foley, mushroom, Malecot, or gastrostomy replacement tube) is inserted (Figure 24-2). Several purse-string sutures are used to invaginate the stomach around the tube. The stomach is then fixed to the abdominal wall at the catheter site, and traditionally a nonabsorbable suture is used to secure the catheter to the skin. Although the Stamm gastrostomy is the simplest surgical technique to perform and remove, it is frequently difficult to manage and is plagued with complications such as peritubular leakage, wound infection, peritonitis, and tube dislodgement (Beyer, 2003).

Witzel gastrostomy. A Witzel gastrostomy is created similarly to the Stamm gastrostomy, with the additional construction of a 4- to 6-cm seromuscular tunnel of the stomach wall through which the gastrostomy tube is placed (Figure 24-3). The seromuscular tunnel is designed to reduce the risk of peritubular leakage particularly when the stomach is distended or the tube is removed.

Janeway gastrostomy. A Janeway gastrostomy is a surgically constructed, mucosa-lined gastric passageway that is brought out onto the abdominal surface as a permanent mucocutaneous stoma. Figure 24-4 illustrates how the Janeway gastrostomy is constructed. Postoperatively, an inflated balloon-tip catheter is placed

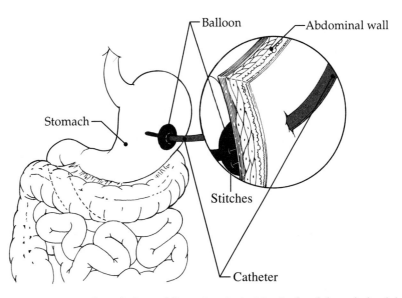

Fig. 24-2 Stamm gastrostomy tube technique–oblique view. An incision is placed through the abdominal wall into the stomach, through which a catheter is passed.

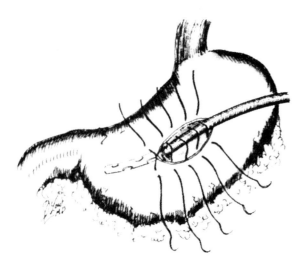

Fig. 24-3 The Witzel gastrostomy is similar to the Stamm gastrostomy with the addition of a 4- to 6-cm seromuscular tunnel of the stomach wall, through which the gastrostomy tube is placed. (From Patterson RS: Enteral nutrition delivery systems. In Grant JA, Kennedy-Caldwell C, editors: *Nutritional support nursing,* Philadelphia, 1988, Grune & Stratton.)

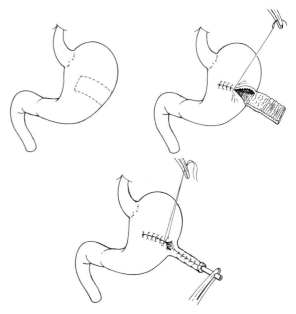

Fig. 24-4 Janeway gastrostomy. A surgically constructed, mucosa-lined gastric passageway that is brought out onto the abdominal surface as a permanent mucocutaneous stoma.

in the tract. Once the tract has matured (7 to 10 days), the tube is removed. A tube is inserted into the Janeway gastrostomy during each feeding and then removed. This type of permanent gastrostomy requires more operative time than the Stamm gastrostomy and results in many similar complications (Gorman, Nance, and Morris, 1995).

Witzel jejunostomy. The Witzel technique is the most common technique for surgically placed jejunostomy. The Witzel technique can be used to create a jejunostomy either at the conclusion of a surgical procedure or as an isolated procedure. The usual site is the left upper quadrant. A loop of jejunum 15 to 20 cm from the ligament of Treitz is brought up to the wound, and a circular purse-string suture is placed in the antimesenteric border. An incision through the center of the purse-string suture is made, and a 14-French (Fr) feeding catheter is inserted into the jejunal lumen and advanced. A serosal tunnel is constructed at the exit site in the jejunal wall, extending approximately 5 to 6 cm proximally. The catheter is brought to the skin through a separate incision and secured, typically

with sutures. The loop of intestine is anchored to the anterior abdominal wall (Wu and Soper, 2004).

Needle catheter jejunostomy. The needle jejunostomy is a simple procedure that is most often done at the conclusion of a surgical procedure when prolonged enteral support is anticipated. At approximately 30 to 40 cm distal to the ligament of Treitz, a 14- to 16-gauge needle is inserted into the jejunal wall. A feeding catheter is advanced through the needle 30 to 40 cm distally, and the needle is then withdrawn. A purse-string suture is then made around the tube to close the jejunal opening around the catheter. The loop of bowel is anchored to the anterior abdominal wall, and the catheter is secured to the skin (Figure 24-5) (Bland, Karakousis, and Copeland, 1995).

Laparoscopic Surgical Approach. The laparoscopic approach for insertion of the gastrostomy or jejunostomy is possible since the introduction of high-resolution video cameras and has the advantages of minimal invasion and few surgical side effects (Georgeson, 1997). This approach also provides the opportunity to selectively determine the site of the

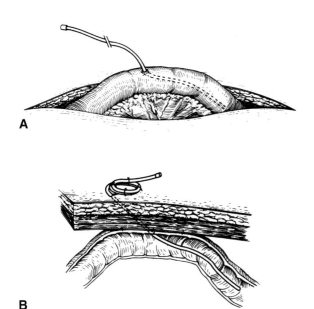

A

B

Fig. 24-5 Needle catheter jejunostomy. Technique for placement of a needle catheter jejunostomy. **A,** The catheter is inserted into the lumen of the jejunum for a distance of 40 to 50 cm and secured into place with a purse-string suture. **B,** The jejunum is secured to the anterior abdominal wall. The feeding catheter is removed postoperatively when the patient is tolerating oral feedings. (Reprinted with permission from Bland KI, Karakousis CP, Copeland EM: *Atlas of surgical oncology,* Philadelphia, 1995, WB Saunders.)

tube within the stomach (i.e., lesser-curvature gastrostomy rather than the more commonly selected greater-curvature), which may be important in the patient who is at high risk for reflux or aspiration. A key advantage to a laparoscopic approach is that the abdomen can be examined under direct vision without the need for a large surgical incision, so that biopsy specimens can be obtained if necessary or malignancy staging can be conducted (Coates and MacFadyen, 1996). This technique requires a smaller incision than the open surgical approach, and local or general anesthesia is still needed.

Laparoscopic gastrostomy. The indication for a laparoscopic gastrostomy for feeding is when the percutaneous endoscopic gastrostomy cannot be performed, such as with a morbidly obese patient. A small supraumbilical incision is made through which the camera port is placed, and a 5-mm port is placed in

the epigastrium. An atraumatic instrument is then used to grasp the stomach, and the site for the proposed gastrostomy is identified. An 18-gauge angiocatheter is passed through the anterior abdomen, at the site chosen for the gastrostomy, and into the stomach. The needle is then removed and a soft J-wire is passed into the stomach. Dilators (12 Fr and 14 Fr) are placed over this J-wire. A 16-Fr peel-away catheter is placed over the dilator, and a 16-Fr catheter is inserted through the sheath. The catheter is then positioned against the stomach wall by inflating the balloon or securing the internal bumper.

Laparoscopic jejunostomy. Specific indications for laparoscopic jejunostomy include concomitant laparoscopy for other problems, or difficult laparoscopic gastrostomy. As a minimally invasive procedure, reduced postoperative pain and shortened recuperative time are desirable advantages; general anesthesia is required. The procedure remains more expensive than percutaneous or surgical placement. Two methods described in Wu and Soper (2004) are briefly presented in this section.

The laparoscope is inserted through a small incision above the umbilicus. The proximal small bowel is identified, traced 25 cm distal to the ligament of Treitz, and the antimesenteric border is withdrawn into the umbilical wound. At this location in the small bowel, a Witzel tunnel is created or concentric purse-string sutures are placed and a 12-Fr catheter is inserted into the bowel. The bowel is secured to the fascia around the tube and returned to the abdominal cavity, and the fascia and skin are closed. The catheter is then tunneled subcutaneously to exit the skin at the site previously selected on the abdomen.

Another technique can be used in which T-fasteners are inserted through the skin into the bowel lumen to anchor and retract the bowel against the abdominal wall (Duh and McQuaid, 2000; Wu and Soper 2004). Once the bowel is anchored, a percutaneous jejunostomy tube can be placed directly through the abdominal wall (Figure 24-6).

Endoscopic Approach

The endoscopic approach to gastrostomy tube placement, known as the *percutaneous endoscopic gastrostomy* (PEG), was first described by Gauderer and colleagues in 1980 and has quickly become the procedure of choice. These devices can be placed under local anesthesia and conscious sedation outside the operating room, thus avoiding the complications associated with surgical procedures.

Contraindications to the PEG include inability to perform upper endoscopy, inability to illuminate the abdominal wall, ascites, esophageal obstruction, hepatomegaly, previous gastric resection, and uncorrectable coagulopathy (Bankhead and Rolandell, 2005).

Variations to the original technique exist; all involve a complete esophagogastroduodenoscopy, insufflation of air into the stomach, and transillumination of the stomach. After application of a topical pharyngeal anesthetic and sedation, an endoscope is passed into the stomach. Air is insufflated into the stomach, which distends the stomach against the anterior abdominal wall. The proposed gastrostomy site is then transilluminated. The endoscopy assistant indents the abdomen at the proposed gastrostomy site, which should be at least 2 cm below costal margin. At this point, several different techniques have been described to insert the PEG.

"Pull" (Ponsky) Technique. A small incision is made over the illuminated site, and a large-gauge angiocatheter is inserted into the stomach. The needle is then withdrawn, and 60 inches of suture is passed through the catheter into the stomach. With a biopsy snare, the endoscopist grasps the suture and pulls so that the endoscope is removed with the suture attached (Figure 24-7). The gastrostomy tube is attached to the

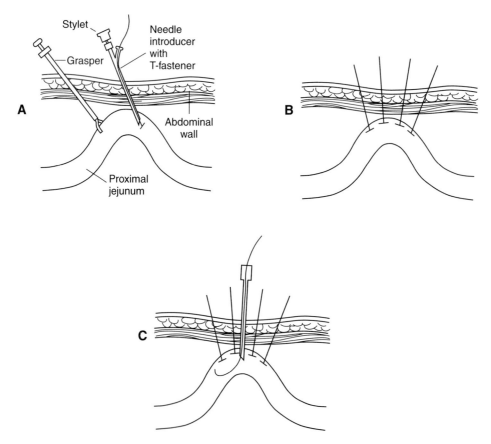

Fig. 24-6 Laparoscopic jejunostomy with T-fasteners, which are inserted through the skin into the bowel lumen to anchor and retract the bowel against the abdominal wall, before inserting a percutaneous jejunostomy tube directly through the abdominal wall.

suture; and by pulling on the suture at the abdominal gastrostomy site, the endoscopist draws the tube through the esophagus into the stomach and positions it snugly against the anterior stomach wall. To verify proper position of the PEG, an endoscope is passed again. Once placement is confirmed, the endoscope is removed and the PEG secured at the skin level.

"Over the Wire" (Sachs-Vine) Technique. With this technique, a long, flexible guidewire is inserted through the angiocatheter into the stomach. Again with use of the biopsy snare and endoscope, the wire is snared and pulled up through the esophagus and out the patient's mouth (Figure 24-8). The PEG tube is pushed over the guidewire and advanced through the esophagus to the stomach and positioned against the anterior stomach wall. As with the "pull" technique, PEG placement is checked with the endoscope, which is then removed, and the PEG is secured.

"Push" (Russel) Technique. Modifications to the Ponsky or Sachs-Vine technique of have been described in which the second passage of the endoscope is obviated.

Another technique is a modification of the push technique and involves passing a dilator with a peel-away introducer over the guidewire. The endoscopist confirms the position of the dilator, the dilator is removed, and a well-lubricated catheter is then placed through the introducer as the introducer is peeled away. The endoscopist verifies adequate placement of the catheter against the anterior stomach wall, and the endoscope is removed (Bankhead and Rolandell, 2005).

Percutaneous Endoscopic Jejunostomy (PEJ) Several innovative techniques have been described to obtain postpyloric enteral access through endoscopic placement of the percutaneous jejunostomy (PEJ). The two basic approaches, transpyloric PEJ and direct PEJ, are briefly described.

Transpyloric PEJ. Through a previously established gastrostomy, a small feeding tube with a weighted tip and an attached heavy suture tie are passed. Under endoscopic visualization, the suture is grasped with a biopsy forceps, and the suture and attached feeding tube are guided into the duodenum (Figure 24-9).

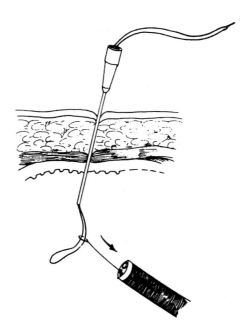

Fig. 24-7 Ponsky PEG (pull) technique. After installation of local anesthesia, a 10-mm transverse incision is made, through which a tapered cannula needle is introduced under direct endoscopic vision. A looped heavy suture is directed through the catheter into the stomach, secured with a polypectomy snare, and withdrawn from the patient's mouth.
(From Gorman RC, Morris JB: Minimally invasive access to the gastrointestinal tract. In Rombeau JL, Rolandelli RH: *Clinical nutrition: enteral and tube feeding,* ed 3, Philadelphia, 1997, WB Saunders.)

Continued

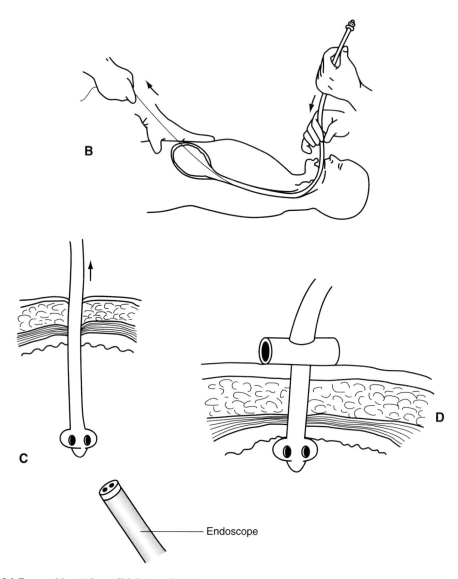

Endoscope

Fig. 24-7, cont'd B, The well-lubricated PEG catheter is now secured to the suture, and steady traction directed down the posterior pharynx into the esophagus. **C,** The endoscope is reintroduced, and under direct vision the catheter is pulled across the gastroesophageal junction and then approximated to the anterior gastric wall. It is imperative that the inner cross-bar gently approximates the mucosa without excess tension to avoid ischemic necrosis. The stomach is decompressed by aspiration, and the gastroscope is withdrawn. **D,** The outer cross-bar is gently approximated to the skin level and secured with two 0-0 Prolene sutures.

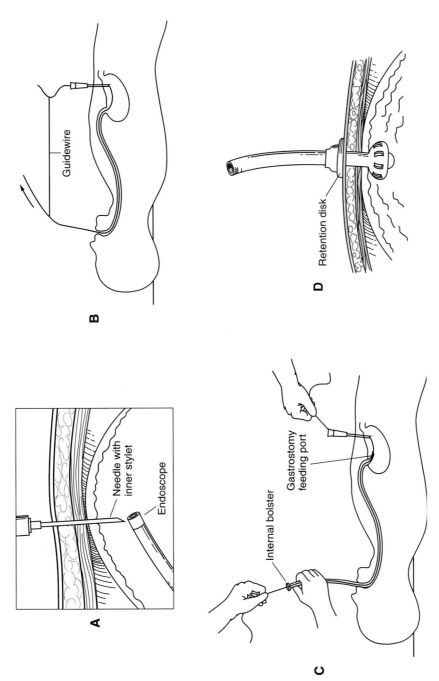

Fig. 24-8 Sachs-Vine technique for PEG insertion. **A,** Needle inserted through abdomen into stomach under visualization by endoscopist. **B,** Endoscope is withdrawn, pulling guidewire up through the esophagus, out the patient's mouth. **C,** PEG tube is pushed over the guidewire and advanced through the esophagus to the stomach. **D,** PEG positioned against the anterior stomach wall.

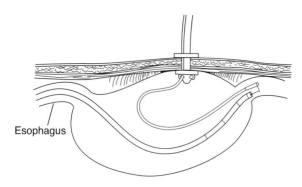

Esophagus

Fig. 24-9 Transpyloric PEJ. Endoscopist guides the weighted tip of feeding tube into the duodenum.

The endoscope is withdrawn. An excess amount of tubing is left within the stomach to allow peristalsis to pull the weighted tip past the ligament of Treitz.

The transpyloric PEJ is associated with considerable long-term complications, including (1) separation of inner PEJ tube from outer gastrostomy tube, (2) clogging of the small-diameter PEJ, and (3) kinking of the PEJ. Furthermore, the goal of reduced aspiration pneumonia has not been achieved, which may be the result of retrograde migration of the tube back into the stomach or impaired pyloric sphincter function triggered by the presence of the tube (Gorman and Morris, 1997).

Directed PEJ. A PEJ can be placed directly through the abdominal wall into the jejunum using a modification of the Ponsky PEG procedure. In this approach the endoscope is advanced past the pylorus approximately 20 cm distal to the ligament of Treitz, and the abdominal wall is transilluminated. Using a small-gauge needle, the jejunum is cannulated through the abdominal wall, a heavy thread is inserted, a biopsy forceps is used to grasp the thread, and it is withdrawn through the mouth. The thread is tied to a feeding tube (typically mushroom-tipped), which is then pulled into position under endoscopic observation.

Another direct PEJ technique involves a small incision in the upper quadrant. The endoscope is again inserted beyond the ligament of Treitz. The proximal end of the jejunum is clamped; in the small incision, a short segment of jejunum is eviscerated using the Witzel technique. The feeding tube is placed into the jejunum, the jejunum is returned to the abdominal

cavity, and the proximal and distal ends of the jejunum are secured to the abdominal wall.

The directed PEJ seems to alleviate the problems associated with the transpyloric placement (tube migration, clogging, and aspiration). Evidence for the long-term benefits, efficacy, and use of this procedure is still inconclusive.

Interventional Radiologic Approach

Percutaneous Gastrostomy via Radiologic Intervention. Recent advances have led to the development of a radiographic approach to percutaneous gastrostomy tube placement. Although not the first choice for enteral access, percutaneous tubes placed radiologically become an alternative when surgical or endoscopic procedures are not feasible.

In the radiographic approach the stomach is dilated with air and a needle is percutaneously inserted into the stomach. A J-wire is threaded into the stomach under fluoroscopic guidance, and the needle is then withdrawn. A 1-cm–long incision is made into the skin at the exit site of the wire. When entry into the stomach has been determined, the tract is slowly dilated and the permanent catheter is inserted. These catheters usually have a balloon, which is inflated and positioned snugly against the gastric wall. Stabilization at the skin surface is achieved by use of a suture or a tube stabilization device.

Percutaneous Jejunostomy via Radiologic Intervention. This technique first requires radiologic access to the stomach as described previously. A guidewire is then passed through the duodenum and into the jejunum. A balloon occluder catheter is inserted over the guidewire and placed in the jejunum. The balloon is inflated with air and water-soluble contrast so that the position can be checked by fluoroscopy. Still under fluoroscopic surveillance, an 18-gauge needle is inserted into the jejunum, and the balloon is punctured. A guidewire is passed into the tract, and the tract is dilated to approximately a 10-Fr size so that a feeding catheter can be inserted. The balloon occluder catheter is removed, and the feeding catheter secured to the skin.

Conversion of Gastrostomy to Gastrostomy-Jejunostomy Tube (G-J tube). Repeat aspirations may make it necessary to convert an existing gastrostomy tube to a gastrostomy-jejunostomy tube (G-J tube). This can be done using endoscopy or radiology with a combined G-J tube, or by inserting a smaller-diameter feeding tube through the gastrostomy tube. When a combined G-J tube is used, the gastrostomy tube is removed, and an angiocatheter and guidewire are inserted and advanced through the pylorus. The guidewire is further advanced distal to the ligament of Treitz, at which point the angiocatheter is removed. A G-J tube is then inserted over the guidewire and advanced into the jejunum; the guidewire is then removed. The gastrostomy internal bumper or balloon is secured snugly against the stomach mucosa. An external securing device (bumper, flange, or commercial device) is used to secure the tube against the skin. Three ports will be apparent: gastric (proximal port), duodenal or jejunal (distal port), and balloon port (Figure 24-10).

When a combined G-J tube is not available, a jejunal tube can be placed, and the external end of the jejunal tube can be threaded into a gastrostomy tube.

The gastrostomy tube is then advanced over the jejunal tube, and the internal gastrostomy bumper is positioned against the anterior stomach wall. Again, external stabilization of the tube to the skin is necessary.

Summary of Placement Techniques

The type of patient who typically requires these tubes is a major reason for the high morbidity rate. Patients commonly have multiple medical problems and are malnourished. For these reasons, the surgical approach to tube placement is quickly being replaced by the endoscopic or radiographic approach. Endoscopic techniques for enteral tube placement have a lower complication rate, are more cost-effective than surgical methods, and can be performed on an outpatient basis. These techniques require the ability to insert an endoscope. Laparoscopic and radiologic techniques are less frequently used but are options when endoscopy

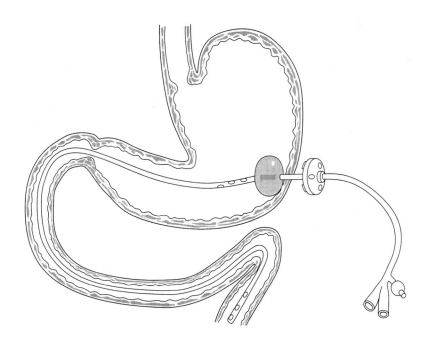

Fig. 24-10 Transgastric jejunal tube. This dual-lumen tube is placed surgically and allows for jejunal feedings while providing gastric decompression. (From Rombeau JL, Rolandelli RH: *Clinical nutrition: enteral and tube feeding,* ed 3, Philadelphia, 1997, WB Saunders.)

is not anatomically feasible or when surgery is too risky.

A key consideration for the type of tube placed is whether prepyloric or postpyloric delivery of enteral feedings is preferred (Welch, 1996). In the presence of significant gastroesophageal reflux, increased risk of aspiration, impaired gastric emptying, or primary disease of the stomach, a jejunostomy is preferred.

FEEDING TUBE FEATURES

The type of tube used for a gastrostomy or jejunostomy depends in part on the anatomic site in which the tube is placed and the reason for its placement. The features of the tube to consider include material composition, tube diameter, tip configurations, and number of ports.

Material Composition

Historically, gastrostomy and jejunostomy tubes were made from rubber, polyvinyl chloride, and latex, which are very stiff and uncomfortable. The softer and more pliable polyurethane and silicone tubes have been used most frequently because these materials are associated with less soft-tissue reaction and longer wear time. This is particularly advantageous to the older patient population because of the increased fragility of the GI mucosa (Lysen, 2003). Unfortunately, it is difficult to aspirate intestinal or gastric contents from silicone tubes because the walls of the tube collapse (Lysen, 2003).

Tube Diameter

The diameter of the outer lumen (OD) is referred to in French (Fr) units. A 1-Fr tube, for example, is 0.33 mm across. However, the internal diameter (ID) can actually vary for any outer-diameter French size depending on the material used. For example, silicone tubes have a thicker wall than polyurethane tubes; therefore their internal diameter will be smaller even though they are labeled with the same French size.

The risk of the tube becoming clogged is reduced as the internal diameter increases. However, when selecting a nasoenteric tube, for the patient's comfort, the smallest ID tube possible that allows the unimpeded flow of formula should be used. When administering enteral formulas containing fiber or viscous formulas, an 8-Fr tube or larger is recommended.

Gastrostomy tubes are most often 12 Fr, jejunostomy tubes should be 6 Fr and needle catheter jejunostomy tubes should be smaller than 8 Fr (Lysen, 2003).

Tip Configurations

Several tip configurations are illustrated in Figure 24-11. Foley catheters are commonly used as gastrostomy tubes. However, they are not specifically designed for this purpose. Consequently, the balloon of the Foley catheter is subject to decay from the gastric acid and requires periodic and regular replacement. In addition, Foley catheters do not have an external bumper and will migrate if an external tube stabilization device is not applied. Migration can cause gastric outlet obstruction by blocking the pylorus. Replacement gastrostomy tubes, which are silicone-based, are preferable.

Another tip available and used to a great extent on the PEG is the disc. This tip cannot be removed by simple extraction through the skin and must be cut off. The tip is passed through the GI tract or retrieved endoscopically. The PEG tip may also have a cross-bar or bulb tip, which cannot be extracted through the skin.

Tubes may also have a type of mushroom catheter known as a *pezzer tip*. These are rubber tubes with a stiff, round, pointed tip. The pezzer tip has only minimal tiny holes and unfortunately becomes easily plugged. This type of tip cannot be removed easily. The Malecot tube, also considered a mushroom catheter, has a bulbous tip with much larger openings. This type of tube can be more easily removed and is less likely to become obstructed.

Ports

Tubes with multiple ports are also available. Some gastrostomy tubes have 3 ports: balloon, feeding, and medication ports. A triple-lumen tube may be used when patients require both proximal decompression and enteral feeding. This tube actually has four outlets or ports: a gastric lumen for gastric suction, a proximal duodenal lumen for duodenal suction, a distal duodenal lumen for feeding, and a gastric balloon. To maintain proper tube placement, the gastric balloon is inflated with sterile water or air (depending on the manufacturer's specific recommendation), and a retaining disk or tube stabilization device is applied at skin level. These tubes may be confusing to the staff because they are placed in the anticipated location for a gastrostomy

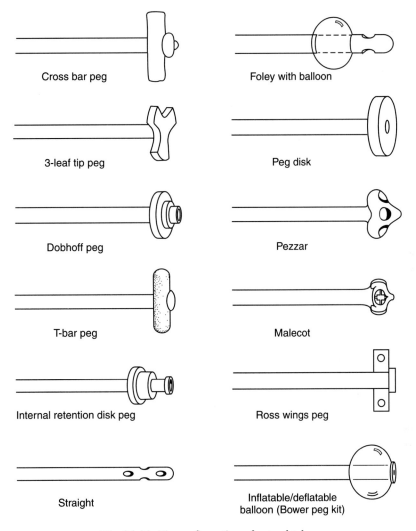

Cross bar peg

Foley with balloon

3-leaf tip peg

Peg disk

Dobhoff peg

Pezzar

T-bar peg

Malecot

Internal retention disk peg

Ross wings peg

Straight

Inflatable/deflatable
balloon (Bower peg kit)

Fig. 24-11 Tip configuration of enteral tubes.

tube but deliver feedings to the jejunum. Ports should be clearly labeled, and a diagram of the tube should be made available in the patient's care plan to provide clarity.

LOW-PROFILE GASTROSTOMY DEVICE (BUTTON)

A skin-level gastric conduit that is flush with the abdominal surface is known as a *gastrostomy button* (Foutch et al, 1989; Gauderer et al, 1988; Gauderer and

Stellato, 1986). The button was first developed for use in children who require long-term gastrostomy feedings. It is a short silicone tube with a flip-top opening, a one-way antireflux valve (to prevent leakage of stomach contents around the tube), and a radiopaque dome that fits snugly against the stomach wall (Figure 24-12). Some devices have special tubing that opens the reflux valve to permit decompression of the stomach.

To administer feedings, an adapter is passed through the one-way valve and connected to a feeding catheter.

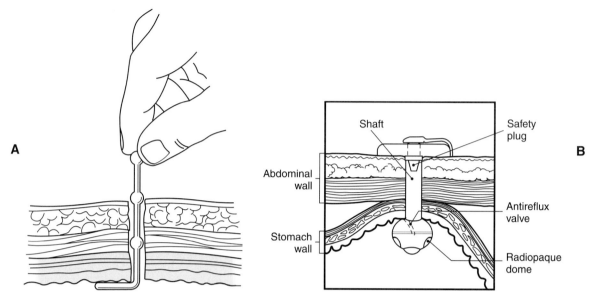

Fig. 24-12 Gastrostomy button. **A,** Correct gastrostomy button size is determined by using a device to measure the width of the abdominal wall. **B,** Gastrostomy feeding button in place.

When the feeding is completed, the tube is flushed with water, the adapter is removed, and the flip-top opening is closed.

A button can be inserted in a clinic setting in an established gastrostomy tract and does not require anesthesia. It may also be placed as the initial device in a one-step procedure (Georgeson, 1999). The device is available in different shaft lengths and diameters. Correct shaft length is critical to ensure the proper position of the dome of the button against the anterior stomach wall, hence preventing gastric reflux around the button. By insertion of a special measuring device into the tract, the appropriate shaft length is determined. An obturator is then inserted into the button to straighten the dome of the button, making insertion of the button into the tract possible. The button should be lubricated to facilitate insertion. Once it is in place, the obturator is removed and the flip-top opening closed. If the patient's weight changes, the device may have to be resized.

Disadvantages of the button include the potential for dysfunction of the antireflux valve with subsequent leakage and the need for replacement every 3 to 4 months. Studies and refinements of the device are ongoing; current reports demonstrate good success, few complications, and high user satisfaction.

NURSING MANAGEMENT OF ENTERIC TUBES

Optimal management for patients requiring long-term gastrostomy or jejunostomy tubes begins in the preplacement phase. Assessment of each patient should include the reason for the each tube alternative, risks and benefits associated with various treatment options, and the commitment of the patient or caregiver to long-term management. Preplacement information and instructions are critical to adequately prepare the patient and family for what they will be expected to do.

Nursing staff must also be prepared to care for the patient with an enteric tube. Much of the success of these tubes depends on proper care. Topics that must be addressed include preplacement site selection, site care, tube patency, tube stabilization, and management of complications. It is advisable to develop a competency checklist for the nursing staff who care for a significant number of patients with feeding tubes.

Preplacement Site Selection

Tube exit sites should be selected preoperatively to reduce the potential for complications and to facilitate self-care. Site selection is commonly based on vague guidelines such as "3 to 5 cm below the costal margin" and "avoidance of the costal margin." However, in the person who has a protuberant hernia or is malnourished or wheelchair-confined, this location may present a substantial problem such that it affects the integrity of the skin. Two techniques can be used to select a site preplacement, depending on whether the tube will be placed endoscopically or surgically (Hanlon, 1998).

Endoscopic Placement. When the tube is placed by the endoscopic approach, the location of the tube depends on transillumination. Therefore the specific site for the tube cannot actually be determined before the procedure. Nonetheless, by marking important abdominal landmarks (such as a skin crease, fold, or scar; the costal margin; belt line; prosthetic equipment; and hernia), the endoscopist can attempt to place the tube in a site that will avoid these landmarks. An indelible marker should be sufficient for these markings.

Surgical Placement. When the tube will be placed surgically, the technique used for preplacement site selection is the same as that used to mark a stoma site. The patient should be assessed standing, sitting, bending, and in the supine position. The objective is to find 1 inch of smooth skin surface that is free of creases, folds, and scars and avoids the beltline or bony structures. Again, a surgical marking pen can be used to place an X at the desired location. A transparent dressing may be applied over the marking when surgery is not scheduled for several days.

Site Care

Daily site care should include gentle cleansing with water; if desired, a mild soap can be used but should also be rinsed off. To clean under an external bumper or disc, a cotton-tipped applicator may be necessary. Diluted hydrogen peroxide is only used to clean accumulated crusty drainage at the insertion site and when soap and water are ineffective. Routine and regular use of hydrogen peroxide should be avoided because hyperplasia at the tube site is associated with frequent use of hydrogen peroxide. A moisture barrier may be used after cleansing around the tube to protect skin from drainage. Dressings under the external button are not recommended because they can trap moisture and allow movement of the tube. The external bumper of gastric tubes should be rotated 90 degrees once a day to keep the skin from ulcerating (O'Brien and Erwin-Toth, 1999). Jejunostomy tubes should NOT be rotated since they may become displaced.

Daily assessments should include the condition of the peritubular site and proper positioning of the stabilization device. The insertion site and surrounding tissue should be monitored for signs and symptoms of infection (i.e., erythema, induration, and pain). The external bumper should rest lightly against the skin. Soft tissue infections should be managed with culture-based antibiotics. Occlusive dressings for the tube site are generally unnecessary.

Tube Stabilization

The most common complications related to gastrostomy or jejunostomy placement are (1) leakage of gastric or jejunal contents around the tube onto the skin and (2) tube dislodgment. As many as half of all feeding tubes are dislodged by patients and their caregivers (O'Brien and Erwin-Toth, 1999). These complications are frequently attributed to the failure to adequately stabilize the tube. Therefore postplacement nursing management must include measures to stabilize the tube.

Adequate tube stabilization requires proper internal positioning and proper external (skin-level) positioning. To achieve proper internal positioning, a tube is used that has a balloon, bumper, mushroom, or disc tip. These devices are snugly positioned against the anterior wall of the stomach (Figure 24-13). When a balloon tip is used, it must be inflated with an adequate volume of sterile water or air (in accordance with the manufacturer's guidelines) to work properly (Lord, 1997). Although saline may be readily available, it should not be used for balloon inflation because saline can crystallize and cause the balloon to rupture. Because water and air will diffuse through the walls of the balloon, adequacy of inflation should be checked weekly and any time that peritubular leakage is noted. Tubes with balloon tips should not be used as jejunal tubes; an inflated balloon within the jejunum is sufficient to obstruct the jejunum.

Adequate skin-level stabilization of the tube is necessary to prevent (1) lateral movement in the tube

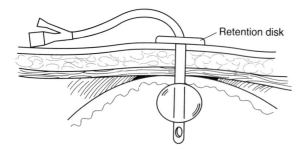

Fig. 24-13 Proper stabilization of gastrostomy tube. Tube is secured between anterior wall of stomach and abdomen by a properly inflated internal balloon and externally with a tube stabilization device. Side-to-side mobility of the tube and tube migration are thus prevented.

at skin level and (2) tube migration (in and out movements). Lateral movement of the tube contributes to leakage of gastric or intestinal contents onto the skin by eroding the tissue along the tract. Inflammation of the site can also develop from the presence of this chronic irritant. A stabilized tube should not allow lateral movement of the tube (Lord, 1997).

To maintain proper tube positioning in the stomach or small bowel, migration of the tube in and out of the tract must be prevented. Nonstabilized tubes are subject to migration as a result of gastric and intestinal motility and abdominal wall motion. The tube can actually migrate and obstruct the gastric outlet (causing gastric distention, nausea, and vomiting) and compromise tube function.

Historically, sutures have been used to stabilize tubes. Unfortunately, sutures can cause tearing of the skin, with subsequent inflammation and pain at the suture site. In addition, although sutures prevent tube migration, they do not eliminate lateral tube movement.

Baby-bottle nipples have been used to secure gastrostomy tubes. Typically the nipple is cut along one edge, wrapped around the tube, and secured with tape as the tube exits from the nipple. Although popular and readily available, this technique in isolation is not completely effective at preventing lateral movement or tube migration. Effective tube stabilization with a nipple can only be accomplished when it is used with tape to secure the nipple to the abdomen or with a skin-barrier flange. Box 24-2 describes these two methods of tube stabilization.

BOX 24-2 Methods of Tube Stabilization with Baby-Bottle Nipple

Use of Nipple with Skin-Barrier Wafer

1. Cut skin-barrier wafer to size of stomal opening at tube exit site.
2. Slit skin-barrier wafer along one edge so that wafer can be positioned around tube.
3. Remove protective paper backing and apply wafer to skin.
4. Slit nipple along one side and position around tube.
5. Secure nipple to wafer and tube with tape.

Use of Nipple with Skin-Barrier Flange and Convex Insert*

1. Cut opening in 1½-inch skin-barrier flange the size of stomal opening at tube exit site.
2. Peel off protective paper backing and apply barrier flange to skin.
3. Slit nipple along one side and position around tube so that the wide part of the nipple fits inside the flange.
4. Feeding the tube through the center of a convex insert (1¼-inch internal diameter), snap the convex insert into place inside the flange, securing the nipple. For ease of application, the convex insert can be applied so that the curve projects away from the patient's skin.
5. Tape nipple to tube. NOTE: A 1¼-inch skin-barrier flange can also be used. The wide end of the nipple will fit into the flange and is then secured with tape instead of a convex insert.

---

*NOTE: This procedure works best with Convatec SurFit flange and convex inserts.

Commercial external tube stabilization devices are also available (Figure 24-14). The commercial tube stabilization device is changed as needed; frequency is determined by the need to assess the tube site or provide site care. When frequent site care is required (as with newly placed tubes), a stabilization system that allows easy visualization of the site without removal of adhesives is desirable.

Many tubes are being created specifically as gastrostomy tubes complete with stabilization features inherent in the design, thereby eliminating the need for commercial external stabilization devices. For example, the

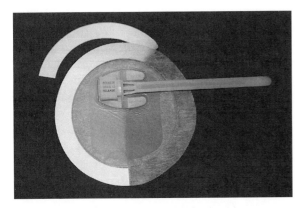

Fig. 24-14 Commercial external tube stabilization device.

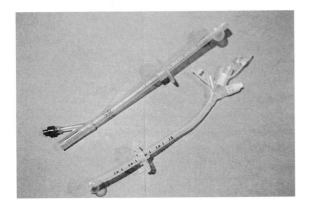

Fig. 24-15 Sample replacement gastrostomy tubes.

button has an internal dome, limited shaft length, and a flip-top cap to ensure stabilization of the tube. PEG tubes are designed with an internal bolster and an external bolster. The internal bolster can be a bumper, disc, or balloon that, when properly positioned, lies up against the anterior stomach wall. Exteriorly, on the abdominal surface, the bolster is a bumper or disc that can be adjusted to lie snugly against the abdominal wall. This stabilization is critical to prevent dislodgment of the tube, mobility, obstruction, and peritubular leakage. A few Silastic catheter–feeding tubes (with a balloon to secure the tube against the anterior stomach wall) have an adjustable external flange (Figure 24-15). Once the Silastic catheter is in position and the balloon is inflated, the flange is slid down against the skin, stabilizing the catheter without the use of adhesives.

Regardless of the type of stabilization device or bolsters used, adequate stabilization is critical to the success of the tubes. They secure the tube against the abdominal wall and against the anterior stomach wall. The tension between the internal and external securing devices should allow slight leeway from the skin to prevent necrosis of the skin or gastric mucosa (Lord, 1997). This leeway should be monitored daily because changes in abdominal girth, such as with ascites, can develop, which then predisposes the patient to a pressure point under the external stabilization device. Modifications should be made as necessary.

Tube Patency

All enteral feeding tubes require routine flushing. This easy procedure is key to the prevention of tube clogging (Bowers, 2000; Fish and Seidner, 2003; Lysen, 2003). In adults, the tube should be flushed with 20 to 30 ml of warm water every 4 to 6 hours during continuous feedings; with intermittent feedings the tube is flushed before and after the feeding. Tubes should always be flushed between each medication and after all medications are instilled; only liquid medications should be administered. When not in use, tubes should be flushed with 20 to 30 ml of warm water every 8 hours to maintain patency.

COMPLICATIONS

Although the placement and care of gastric or jejunal tubes may appear to be relatively simple, they are associated with numerous significant complications. Complications may be related to the surgical technique or the tube. Examples include tube dislodgement, skin erosion at the exit site, skin-site wound infection, bleeding, peritonitis, and bowel obstruction. The first time the wound care nurse sees a patient with an intestinal tube may be when a skin complication develops. Although the skin problem must be addressed, it is also necessary to investigate and correct the underlying problem precipitating the skin irritation.

Leakage

Leakage around the tube site warrants a thorough evaluation. Steps must be taken to correct any possible cause for the leakage. Replacing the tube with a larger size will not correct the problem. It is important to first check the adequacy of tube stabilization, appropriate balloon placement, adequate inflation of the balloon, and tube patency. The balloon should be deflated and reinflated with the amount of air or sterile water that is recommended by the manufacturer. Medications to reduce stomach acid may be warranted. When all attempts to halt the leakage fail, the tube may have to be replaced.

Skin Irritation

Skin irritation surrounding a tube is most commonly the result of chemical irritation (exposure to gastric or intestinal contents) or fungal infection. If all attempts to halt leakage fail, and tube replacement is not an option, methods to contain the drainage and protect the skin must be implemented. Hydrocolloids and absorbent dressings are not appropriate because they will trap drainage against the skin and cause chemical irritation.

To manage drainage around a tube site, an ostomy pouch and catheter port can be applied. By attaching a catheter port to the pouch, the tube can exit the wall of the pouch through the port, which allows for feeding, suction, or gravity drainage to continue. The ostomy pouch then contains peritubular drainage (Figure 24-16). Such a pouching system is cost-effective and allows collection, identification, and measurement of the drainage as well as skin protection. Instructions for containing peritubular leakage are outlined in Box 24-3. Frequency of pouch change is determined by the duration of the pouch seal; on average the pouch is changed every 4 to 7 days. If a urinary pouch is selected, it may be necessary to "pop" the antireflux mechanism within the pouch, particularly when drainage is thick or contains particulate matter.

Fungal infections such as candidiasis can result when moisture is trapped at the insertion site. Corrective measures include protecting the skin from moisture with skin sealants or ointments, or containing the moisture with appropriate dressings. Antifungal medications such as powders may be necessary when extensive candidiasis is present.

BOX 24-3 Pouching Procedure for Leakage Around Tube

1. Assemble pouch and catheter access device:
   a. Cut opening in barrier and pouch to accommodate tube site.
   b. Make small slit in anterior surface of pouch.
   c. Attach an access device to the anterior surface of the pouch.
   d. Tear paper backing on pouch or wafer but leave in place.
2. Prepare skin:
   a. Clean and dry skin.
   b. Treat any denuded skin (skin-barrier powder to denuded area; skin sealant if needed).
   c. Apply thin layer of skin-barrier paste to skin around insertion site, if needed.
3. Disconnect and plug tube.
4. Feed catheter through opening in pouch. Use water-soluble lubricant to pass tube, and use hemostat to pull tube through the pouch or barrier opening, the anterior wall of the pouch, and the access device.
5. Reconnect tube.
6. Ensure skin is dry; remove paper backing from wafer and secure pouch to skin.
7. Secure tube to stabilization device with tape.

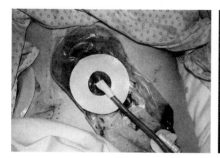 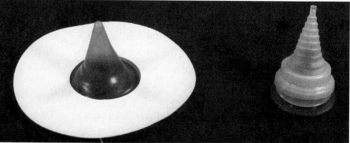

Fig. 24-16 Catheter access port attached to drainable ostomy pouch *(left)*. Two examples of a catheter access port *(right)*. (NuHope and Hollister, Inc.)

Allergic contact dermatitis can occur when a patient's skin is sensitive to anchoring devices, tapes, soaps, or other commercial products. Mechanical trauma and folliculitis can result from traumatic removal of tape or other products used to anchor the tube (O'Brien and Erwin-Toth, 1999). These issues are discussed further in Chapter 6.

Peristomal Hyperplasia. An overgrowth of granulation tissue at the tube exit site can develop and is commonly referred to as *hyperplasia* or *granulation tissue*. This overgrowth of granulation tissue seems to occur in response to chronic irritation of the tissue lining the tract. The source of the chronic irritation can be the type of tube material used (latex is more irritating than Silastic material), tube mobility (particularly the in-and-out movement of the tube), and the chronic presence of excessive moisture. Hyperplasia may or may not be uncomfortable. However, when allowed to persist, seepage from the overgrowth will develop and compromise the integrity of the external stabilization and skin integrity. Treatment should address the underlying causative factor for the hyperplasia. Once this is corrected, the hyperplasia should resolve. Occasionally debridement and cautery with silver nitrate sticks may be warranted. Because it can be painful for the patient, cautery with silver nitrate sticks should be done infrequently and only by an experienced care provider.

Tube Occlusion

The care plan should also incorporate measures to prevent or manage tube obstruction. Occlusion can result from administration of powdered or crushed medications in the feeding tube, viscous formulas, poor or inadequate flushing techniques, partially digested proteins, yeast, and aspiration of gastric or intestinal contents into the tube (Beyers, 2003; Frankel et al, 1998). Water should be used initially to dislodge an occlusion. This process can also assist in distinguishing a kinked tube from a clogged tube; kinked tubes allow slow passage of water, whereas clogged tubes do not allow any passage of water (Frankel et al, 1998). When irrigation with water fails, activated pancreatic enzymes should be instilled (Fish and Seidner, 2003). The use of cranberry juice, chymotrypsin, carbonated drinks, and meat tenderizers is discouraged because they tend to precipitate in the feeding solution within

the tube or cause adverse effects in patients with severe hepatic, renal, or coagulation abnormalities (Frankel et al, 1998; Metheny, Eisenberg, and McSweeney, 1988).

Declogging devices are also available. Some devices consist of a catheter that can be inserted into the feeding tube to which a syringe can be attached and a solution delivered to site of the occlusion. Some of these devices can be used to instill a mixture of pancreatic enzymes and sodium bicarbonate near the site of the clog. Devices that actually bore through the clog or brush the walls of the feeding tube are also available (Frankel et al, 1998). Box 24-4 provides a sample protocol for managing tube occlusion.

TUBE REMOVAL

Enteral tubes are removed when the patient is able to resume adequate nutrition orally and may need to be removed when hopelessly occluded, kinked, or malpositioned. The method of removal used will depend on the technique used to insert the tube and the type of tube tip used (Boxes 24-5 to 24-7). It is important to be familiar with the configuration of the tube in place and to have access to the manufacturer's information. Tube removal is a procedure that should be reserved for nurses who have successfully completed a formal competency check.

PATIENT EDUCATION

Patient education is a key nursing responsibility and is absolutely critical to the patient with a gastrostomy or jejunostomy tube. Since the hospitalization period after tube placement may be brief to nonexistent, detailed caregiver education is essential, and outpatient follow-up care is imperative. In some situations, percutaneous tube placement may be performed strictly on an outpatient basis. In either case, home health care will be important to facilitate patient and caregiver independence in the process, safety with the procedure, and monitoring for complications. Key content areas to be included in a patient teaching plan are listed in Box 24-8.

SUMMARY

Percutaneous tubes are contributing both to quantity and quality of life for many patients. Nurses play a vital role in providing tube stabilization, maintaining tube patency, providing surveillance for complications, and teaching the patient self-care.

BOX 24-4 Sample Protocol for Enteral Tube Occlusion

Method A

1. Attach 5-ml Luer-Lok syringe and attempt to flush the tube with warm water and moderate pressure.
2. If irrigation is unsuccessful, attach an "Intro-Reducer" and attempt to irrigate with warm water using a 20- to 60-ml syringe.
3. If unsuccessful, instill activated pancreatic enzyme mixture through "Intro-Reducer."

Method B

1. Attach a 30- to 60-ml syringe to the end of the enteral tube and aspirate as much fluid as possible. Discard the fluid.
2. Fill the syringe with 5 ml of warm water and attach it to the end of the enteral device. Instill the water under manual pressure for 1 minute, using a back-and-forth motion with the plunger to loosen the clot/obstruction.
3. Clamp the tube for 5 to 15 minutes.
4. Try to aspirate or flush the tube with warm water.
5. If the tube remains clogged, this procedure may be repeated with a pancrease and sodium bicarbonate solution (1 crushed Viokase tablet, or 1 teaspoon Viokase powder mixed with 1 non–enteric-coated sodium bicarbonate tablet, or 1/8 teaspoon baking soda dissolved in 5 ml warm water).

Adapted from Frankel EH et al: Methods of restoring patency to occluded feeding tubes, *Nutr Clin Pract* 13:129, 1998; Lord LM: Enteral access devices, *Nurs Clin North Am* 32(4):685, 1997.

BOX 24-5 Instructions for Removal of Original PEG Tube

Equipment needed

- Nonsterile gloves
- Gauze, 4 × 4

Procedure

1. Obtain permission from physician.
2. Using dominant hand, grasp PEG tubing above bumper and rotate it 360 degrees. If it does not rotate freely, stop and call physician. If it rotates freely, wrap it around your hand to maintain a firm grip.
3. Use other hand to stabilize the patient's abdomen around the site.
4. Exerting moderate force, pull on PEG tube until inner bumper comes through skin opening. There may be slight bleeding. If resistance is too great, stop and call physician.
5. Cover opening with gauze until ready to insert replacement gastrostomy tube. This should be inserted immediately to prevent closure of the tract.

NOTE: Original PEG tube must be at least 2 weeks past time of insertion before nurse should perform this procedure.

Courtesy Karen Huskey.

BOX 24-6 Instructions for Removal of Balloon Replacement Gastrostomy Tube

Equipment

- 20-ml Luer-Lok syringe
- 4 × 4 gauze
- Nonsterile gloves

Procedure

1. Connect 20-ml syringe to balloon port of tube and aspirate all water out of balloon. (NOTE: there may be less than 20 ml as a result of evaporation.)
2. Slowly withdraw the tube from abdominal site.
3. Cover opening with gauze until ready to reinsert replacement tube. The tube should be inserted immediately to prevent closure of the tract.

BOX 24-7 **Instructions for Insertion of Balloon Replacement Gastrostomy**

Equipment
- Replacement gastrostomy tube (G-tube) of correct size
- 60-ml syringe with male tip
- Lubricant (e.g., K-Y jelly)
- Stethoscope
- Nonsterile gloves
- 20 ml Luer-Lok syringe
- 20 ml sterile water

Procedure
1. Choose the replacement G-tube that is the same size as the previously used tube unless otherwise indicated.
2. Draw up 20 ml of sterile water into syringe. Do not use saline.
3. Insert syringe into the balloon port; fill balloon to assure proper inflation.
4. Withdraw water out of balloon and lubricate distal end of G-tube.
5. Gently insert G-tube into existing opening in abdomen. Tube should go in without resistance. If resistance is detected, pull back and attempt to insert again at a slightly different angle. If resistance is met again, stop and call physician.
6. Once G-tube is inserted into existing tract, gastric contents should return into the tube. To confirm proper placement, instill 30 ml of air into G-tube and auscultate for sound, which should be heard in the stomach (not the abdomen).
7. Once placement is confirmed, fill balloon with 20-ml water-filled syringe. (Check balloon port to determine the exact amount of water needed to fill balloon.)
8. After balloon is inflated, gently pull back on the tube until resistance is felt, then slide the external bumper or disc down until it rests lightly on the skin.
9. Rotate the catheter 360 degrees to confirm that tube has free rotation.
10. Cleanse skin around tube with soap and water; no dressing is necessary.

Courtesy Karen Huskey.

BOX 24-8 **Key Content for Patient Education**

1. Name of procedure
2. Purpose for tube insertion
3. Characteristics of normal tube function
4. Type of tube placed
5. Size of balloon (if present)
6. Tube stabilization (why it is important, how it is achieved)
7. Routine site care (daily)
8. Weekly balloon inflation checks (if present)
9. Signs and symptoms of complications, and appropriate response
10. Tube feeding schedule and procedure (when applicable)
11. Name of person to call with questions or problems
12. What to do if the tube falls out

SELF-ASSESSMENT EXERCISE

1. Identify two indications for the placement of a jejunostomy tube.
2. List the major content areas to be included in a teaching plan for the patient with a percutaneous enteral feeding tube.
3. Differentiate between the following:
   a. Janeway gastrostomy and Stamm gastrostomy
   b. PEG and gastrostomy button
   c. A Foley catheter and a gastrostomy replacement catheter
4. Discuss the indications for a radiologic approach to gastrostomy tube placement as compared with an endoscopic approach.
5. Identify advantages and disadvantages of a gastrostomy button.
6. Describe the process of selecting a site for the placement of a PEG.
7. Describe the significance of stabilization as it applies to percutaneous enteral feeding tubes.
8. List three options for stabilization of gastrostomy or jejunostomy tubes.
9. In managing peritubular gastrostomy leakage, what should be the initial goal?
   a. Determination of the cause for leakage
   b. Initiation of skin-protection measures
   c. Establishment of an appropriate pouching system
   d. Cauterization of tract with silver nitrate
10. Which of the following interventions is key to preventing an obstructed feeding tube?
    a. Flushing the enteral tube with activated pancreatic enzymes once daily
    b. Flushing the enteral tube with 20 ml of cranberry juice every 4 hours
    c. Flushing the enteral tube with 20 ml of warm water every 4 hours
    d. Flushing the enteral tube with 20 ml of carbonated beverage every 4 hours
11. To cleanse the jejunostomy site, the nurse should do which of the following?
    a. Use a skin cleanser 3 times daily
    b. Use a cotton-tipped applicator and warm water once daily
    c. Apply bacitracin ointment once daily
    d. Dab with diluted hydrogen peroxide once daily
12. The balloon on a PEG or replacement catheter is routinely filled with which of the following?
    a. Air
    b. Sterile water
    c. Normal saline
    d. Tap water

REFERENCES

Bankhead R, Rolandell R: Access to gastrointestinal tract. In Rolandelli RH, editor: *Enteral and tube feeding,* Philadelphia 2005, Elsevier Saunders.

Beyers PL: Complications of enteral nutrition. In DeChicco LE, Matarese MM, editors: *Nutrition support practice: a clinical guide,* Philadelphia, 2003, Saunders.

Bland KI, Karakousis CP, Copeland EM: *Atlas of surgical oncology,* Philadelphia, 1995, WB Saunders.

Bloch AS, Mueller C: Enteral and parenteral nutrition support. In Mahan LK, Escott-Stump S, editors: *Krause's food, nutrition, and diet therapy,* ed 11, Philadelphia, 2004, Elsevier.

Bowers S: All about tubes, *Nursing* 30(12):41, 2000.

Coates NE, MacFadyen BV Jr: Laparoscopic placement of enteral feeding tubes. In Latifi R, Dudrick SJ, editors: *Medical intelligence unit: current surgical nutrition,* Austin, Tex, 1996, RG Landes.

DeChicco RS, Matarese MM: Determining the nutrition support regimen. In DeChicco LE, Matarese MM, editors: *Nutrition support practice: a clinical guide,* Philadelphia, 2003, Saunders.

Duh QY, McQuaid K: Flexible endoscopy and enteral access. In Eubanks WS, Swanström LL and Soper HJ editors: *Mastery of endoscopic and laparoscopic surgery,* Philadelphia, 2000, Lippincott Williams & Wilkins.

Fish J, Seidner DL: Enteral nutrition support. In Hark L, Morrison G, editors: *Medical nutrition and disease: a case based approach,* Malden, Mass, 2003, Blackwell Science.

Foutch PG et al: The gastrostomy button: a prospective assessment of safety, success and spectrum of use, *Gastrointest Endosc* 35(1):41, 1989.

Frankel EH et al: Methods of restoring patency to occluded feeding tubes, *Nutr Clin Pract* 13:129, 1998.

Gauderer MWL, Ponsky JL: Gastrostomy without laparotomy: a percutaneous technique, *J Pediatr Surg* 15:872, 1980.

Gauderer MW, Stellato TA: Gastrostomies: evolution, techniques, indications and implications, *Curr Probl Surg* 23:657, 1986.

Gauderer MWL et al: Feeding gastrostomy button: experience and recommendations, *J Pediatr Surg* 23(1):24, 1988.

Georgeson KE: Laparoscopic versus open procedures for long-term enteral access, *Nutr Clin Pract* 12(1 Suppl):S7, 1997.

Georgeson KE: Laparoscopic gastrostomy. In Bax NMA et al, editors: *Endoscopic surgery in children,* New York, 1999, Springer.

Gincherman Y, Torosian M: Enteral nutrition: indications, methods of delivery and complications. In Latifi R, Dudrick SJ: *Current surgical nutrition,* New York, 1996, Chapman and Hall.

Gorman RC, Morris JB: Minimally invasive access to the gastrointestinal tract. In Rombeau JL, Rolandelli RH: *Clinical nutrition: enteral and tube feeding,* ed 3, Philadelphia, 1997, WB Saunders.

Gorman RC, Nance ML, Morris JB: Enteral feeding techniques. In Torosian MH editor: *Nutrition for the hospitalized patient: basic science and principles of practice,* New York, 1995, Marcel Dekker.

Hanlon MD: Preplacement marking for optional gastrointestinal and jejunostomy tube site locations to decrease complications and promote self-care, *Nutr Clin Pract* 13:167, 1998.

Lord LM: Enteral access devices, *Nurs Clin North Am* 32(4):685, 1997.

Lysen L: Enteral equipment. In DeChicco LE, Matarese MM, editors: *Nutrition support practice: a clinical guide,* Philadelphia, 2003, Saunders.

Metheny N, Eisenberg P, McSweeney M: Effect of feeding tube properties and three irrigants on clogging rates, *Nurs Res* 37(3):165, 1988.

O'Brien B, Erwin-Toth P: G-tube site care: a practical guide, *RN* 62(2):52, 1999.

Patterson RS: Enteral nutrition delivery systems. In Grant JA, Kennedy-Caldwell C, editors: *Nutritional support nursing,* Philadelphia, 1988, Grune & Stratton.

Rombeau JL et al: *Atlas of nutritional support techniques,* Boston, 1989, Little, Brown.

Welch SK: Certification of staff nurses to insert enteral feeding tubes using a research-based procedure, *Nutr Clin Pract* 11:21, 1996.

Wu JS, Soper NJ: Gastrostomy and jejunostomy. In Jones DB, Wu JS, Soper NJ, editors: *Laparoscopic surgery: principles and procedures,* ed 2, New York, 2004, Marcel Dekker, Inc.

25 *Managing Wound Pain*

·······································

DIANE L. KRASNER, DAG SHAPSHAK, & HARRIET W. HOPF

OBJECTIVES

1. Briefly discuss research and consensus documents related to wound pain.
2. List five standards developed by JCAHO for the assessment and management of pain in accredited health care settings.
3. Discuss the AHCPR recommendations related to pressure ulcer pain.
4. Describe the different types of pain experienced by patients with wounds.
5. Identify two ways to assess wound pain.
6. Define the Chronic Wound Pain Experience Model.
7. State three strategies for managing procedural wound pain.
8. State three strategies for managing nonprocedural wound pain.
9. Discuss the effects of wound pain on quality of life.
10. Describe the pharmacologic options for treating wound pain.

Over the past two decades there has been an explosion of interest in pain as evidenced by the proliferation of algologic (the study of pain or suffering, from Greek "algos") literature, regulatory mandates using pain as a quality of care indicator, and the diversity of pain management options. Similarly, there has been a growing interest in the phenomenon of wound pain (i.e., etiology, nature, physiologic, and psychologic impact and management). In December of 1994 the Agency for Health Care Policy and Research (AHCPR; currently known as the Agency for Healthcare Research and Quality [AHRQ]) published *Clinical Practice Guideline #15, Treatment of Pressure Ulcers* (Bergstrom et al, 1994). This guideline specifically addressed pressure ulcer pain, particularly as it relates to wound dressings and debridement, and stimulated interest in the subject. The panel noted that although there is only cursory mention of pressure ulcer pain in the literature, clinicians report anecdotally that patients experience pressure ulcer–related pain. Clinicians were urged to assess for pain (rather than assume that pain does not exist in nonverbal or unresponsive patients) and to undertake the clinical research that is needed to further develop an evidence-based practice in this area. The panel recommended three specific guidelines related to pressure ulcer pain:

1. Assess all patients for pain related to the pressure ulcer or its treatment.
2. Manage pain by eliminating or controlling the source of pain (e.g., covering wounds, adjusting support surfaces, repositioning). Provide analgesia as needed and appropriate.
3. Prevent or manage pain associated with debridement as needed.

Several consensus documents on general wound pain have also been published. The European Wound Management Association (EWMA) released a position document entitled *Pain at Wound Dressing Changes* in 2002. This document summarized the current knowledge of wound pain and trauma as a phenomenon, the theory of pain, and pain management interventions. Inspired by the EWMA position document and a publication by Reddy and colleagues (2003), the World Union of Wound Healing Societies (WUWHS) convened an international expert working group to develop a consensus opinion on dressing change–related wound pain. In 2004, the resulting consensus document *Minimizing Pain at Wound Dressing-Related Procedures* was released.

Recognizing pain as a major, yet largely avoidable, public health problem, the Joint Commission on Accreditation of Healthcare Organizations (JCAHO) has developed standards that create new expectations for the assessment and management of pain in accredited hospitals and other health care settings. Today, pain is considered the fifth vital sign. JCAHO standards have been endorsed by the American Pain Society (APS). Hospitals, home care agencies, nursing homes, behavioral health facilities, outpatient clinics and health plans are called upon to do the following:

- Recognize the right of patients to appropriate assessment and management of pain.
- Assess the existence and, if present, the nature and intensity of pain in all patients.
- Record the results of the assessment in a way that facilitates regular reassessment and follow-up.
- Determine and assure staff competency in pain assessment and management, and address pain assessment and management in the orientation of all new staff.
- Establish policies and procedures which support the appropriate prescription or ordering of effective pain medications.
- Educate patients and their families about effective pain management.
- Address patient needs for symptom management in the discharge planning process.

The JCAHO standards explicitly acknowledge that pain is a coexisting condition with a number of diseases and injuries, and requires explicit attention. According to JCAHO, unrelieved pain can slow recovery, create burdens for patients and their families, and increase costs to the health care system. Thus effective management of pain is a crucial component of good care (Hill, 2005).

DEFINITION OF PAIN

Pain is a complex subjective response with many dimensions: intensity, quality, physical and psychosocial impact, and personal meaning (Turk, 1993). McCaffery first defined pain in her pioneering research in this field: "[Pain is] whatever the experiencing person says it is and exists whenever he says it does" (1972). Today it is recognized that this definition poses a clinical dilemma since the individual who is unable to communicate, such as the patient with severe dementia, will not be able to verbalize his or her pain. However, the inability to communicate verbally does not negate the possibility that an individual is experiencing pain and is in need of appropriate pain-relieving treatment (EWMA, 2002; WUWHS, 2004). With McCaffery as co-chair, the International Association for the Study of Pain (IASP) and the APS subsequently redefined pain as "an unpleasant sensory and emotional experience associated with actual or potential tissue damage, or described in terms of such damage" (McCaffrey and Pasero, 1999). Table 25-1 provides additional pain-related terms and definitions.

TABLE 25-1 **Pain Terms and Definitions**

TERM	DEFINITION
Allodynia	Pain due to a stimulus that does not normally provoke pain
Analgesia	Absence of pain in response to stimulation that would normally be painful
Anesthesia	Absence of all sensory modalities
Anesthetic	Agent/agents that produce regional anesthesia (i.e., in one part of the body) or general anesthesia (loss of consciousness)
Causalgia	A syndrome of sustained burning pain, allodynia, and hyperpathia after a traumatic nerve lesion, often combined with vasomotor and sudomotor dysfunction and later trophic changes
Central pain	Pain associated with a lesion of the central nervous system
Dermatome	The sensory segmental supply to the skin and subcutaneous tissue
Dysesthesia	An unpleasant abnormal sensation, whether spontaneous or evoked. Special cases of dysesthesia include hyperalgesia and allodynia. Dysesthesia does not include *all* abnormal sensations, only those that are unpleasant (see *paresthesia*). Occasionally it is difficult for a patient to decide whether a sensation is pleasant or unpleasant

TABLE 25-1 Pain Terms and Definitions—cont'd

TERM	DEFINITION
Hyperalgesia	An increased response to a stimulus that is normally painful
Hyperesthesia	Increased sensitivity to stimulation, excluding special senses
Hyperpathia	A painful syndrome characterized by increased reaction to a stimulus, especially a repetitive stimulus, as well as an increased threshold
Neuralgia	Pain in distribution of nerve or nerves
Neuropathic pain	Any pain syndrome in which the predominating mechanism is a site of aberrant somatosensory processing (see entry below) in the peripheral or central nervous system. Some clinical neuroscientists restrict this definition to pain originating in peripheral nerves and nerve roots.
Neuropathy	A disturbance of function or pathologic change in a nerve; in one nerve, mononeuropathy; in several nerves, mononeuropathy multiplex; if symmetrical and bilateral, polyneuropathy
Nociceptor	A receptor preferentially sensitive to a noxious stimulus or to a stimulus that would become noxious if prolonged
Pain	An unpleasant sensory and emotional experience which we primarily associate with tissue damage or describe in terms of tissue damage, or both
Pain tolerance level	The greatest level of pain that a subject is prepared to tolerate. Because the pain tolerance level is the subjective experience of the individual, the same considerations limit the clinical value of *pain tolerance* level as *pain threshold*
Paresthesia	An abnormal sensation, whether spontaneous or evoked
Somatosensory	*Somatosensory input* refers to sensory signals from all tissues of the body including skin, viscera, muscles, and joints. However, *somatic* usually refers to input from body tissue other than viscera.
Suffering	A state of emotional distress associated with events that threaten the biologic and/or psychosocial integrity of the individual. Suffering often accompanies severe pain but can occur in its absence; hence *pain* and *suffering* are phenomenologically distinct.
Trigger point	A hypersensitive area or site in muscle or connective tissue usually associated with myofascial pain syndromes

Classification of Chronic Pain: Descriptions of Chronic Pain Syndromes and Definitions of Pain Terms, Second Edition, IASP Task Force on Taxonomy, From Merskey H, and Bogduk N (editors): IASP Press, Seattle, 1994.

PERCEPTIONS ABOUT PAIN

The patient's expectation of pain can be largely dependent upon his or her cultural and ethnic background, social support system, previous medical history, and prior pain experience. When a patient cannot communicate in the language of the care provider, effective management of his or her pain becomes more difficult and often leads to undertreatment. Commonly, inadequate analgesia is given because the provider's perception is that members of a certain ethnic groups have different pain tolerances (Lasch, 2002). However, studies indicate that when patients control their own analgesia (e.g., patient-controlled analgesia [PCA] pumps), patients self-administer similar doses for similar injuries independent of race or cultural background. Health care providers must be aware of obstacles such as language and cultural barriers and use more care and time in assessing and treating such patients. Interventions that alter a patient's expectation of pain may positively affect the pain experienced by that patient.

A long-held myth in wound care is that venous ulcers and pressure ulcers are not painful. Ironically, in a study of patients with venous ulcers, patients often did not request pain medication because they expected their wounds to be painful (Krasner, 1997). Therefore health care professionals often do not even assess for venous ulcer pain, which then contributes to the undertreatment of venous ulcer pain. In a study conducted by Dallam and colleagues (1995) involving 132 patients with pressure ulcers, 68% reported some type of wound pain, yet only 2% were given analgesics for pressure ulcer pain within 4 hours of pain measurement.

In a qualitative study of nurses providing care to patients with a pressure ulcer who experience pain, nurse generalists and advanced practice nurses were asked to reflect and write a story about the phenomenon of caring for the patient with wound pain (Krasner, 1996). Text analysis of the reflections from the 42 participants revealed three patterns of responses by the caregivers. By examining and understanding these patterns of response and the examples of behaviors relative to each response, valuable insight can be gained into the delivery of more sensitive care that is patient-focused rather than wound-focused.

The first pattern of response is described as "nursing expertly." With this type of response, the nurse uses a set of skills and behaviors that make a qualitative difference in the patient's care. Commonly employed skills include what is known as (1) read the pain (2) attend to the pain and (3) acknowledge the presence of or potential for pain, which is to also empathize with the patient. "Reading" the pain is a critical aspect of assessing for the presence of pain that extends beyond simply asking patients if they are experiencing pain. It is the recognition of signs associated with pain such as increased anxiety, sweating, bulging eyes, increased respirations, and exaggerated movement in bed. Unfortunately, when the patient is nonverbal, signs such as these are easily overlooked by the caregiver. Attending to the pain indicates that the nurse has taken steps to control pain with medications, positioning, distraction, and so on. Acknowledging the presence of pain or the potential for an intervention or procedure to trigger pain demonstrates empathy for the patient and creates an opportunity to (1) discuss the nature of the pain and (2) identify strategies to minimize or relieve the pain. Empathic care for the patient with pain is demonstrated by using a slower pace in performing procedures, conducting dressing changes in a gentle fashion, allowing short "breaks" during painful procedures, providing careful explanations for every step of the procedure, providing words of encouragement, and offering a menu of pain control interventions.

The second pattern of response reported in the study is to actually "deny the pain." In this type of response, the caregiver essentially fails to recognize or treat pain and leaves patients to deal with their pain alone. Ultimately, to "deny the pain" is associated with the care provider who is trying to cope with personally very uncomfortable situations such as a situation in which they feel powerless, a situation in which they feel as though nothing else can be done to ameliorate the patient's pain, or a situation in which the care provider perceives that the situation is "not the best" but acceptable and somewhat expected. Three key behaviors by the nurse are typical of this pattern of response. *Assuming pain does not exist* is in keeping with the erroneous but once commonly held belief that venous and pressure ulcers are not painful despite the twinges of pain or other verbal or nonverbal signs the patient would manifest. *Ignoring the patient's cries of pain* could be characteristic of situations such as when the patient continues to report the presence of pain with a dressing change or sharp debridement despite the analgesic given. *Avoidance of personal failure* is characteristic of the situation in which the nurse simply avoids interacting with the patient or limits the extent of contact with the patient because the patient continues to experience discomfort and all possible interventions for this patient have been exhausted.

The third and final pattern of response observed by this group of nurses was to "confront the challenge of pain" as exemplified by coping with the frustrations and "being with" the patient. A central benefit to this type of response by the nurse is the insight gained into the meaning of the pain experience to the patient. For example, the challenge of the pain may be triggered more by anxiety rather than pain. This insight can then be used to develop a more individualized plan of care.

CONSEQUENCES OF WOUND PAIN

Wound pain not only has a negative affect on quality of life, it leads to hypoxia that will impair wound healing and increase infection rates. Unfortunately, many patients with a wound suffer these negative consequences because undertreatment of patients with chronic wound pain is far too common.

Quality of Life

Chronic pain has been well documented to affect the patient's physical well-being, psychologic well-being, social concerns, and spiritual well-being. Patients experience lack of sleep, fatigue, anxiety, depression, and fear of future pain. Chronic pain also increases caregiver burden and greatly affects roles and relationships (Ferrell, 2005). Patients with wounds are at high risk for acute and chronic pain that tends to be moderately severe to severe in intensity. Uncontrolled pain is considered the most significant predictor of impaired quality of life (Dallam et al, 1995; Szor, 1999). Pressure ulcer pain, specifically, will also affect activities of daily living since the pain could limit the patient's mobility and ability to reposition, thus increasing the risk for the wound to deteriorate (Popescu and Salcido, 2004).

Specific to venous ulcer pain, Hofman and colleagues (1997) found that for 69% of the patients in their study, pain was "the worst thing about having an ulcer," disrupting sleep and negatively affecting quality of life. Previous studies reported similar findings in patients with venous ulcers (Phillips et al, 1994; Walshe, 1995). Using a Heideggerian hermeneutic phenomenology approach, Krasner (1997, 1998a, 1998b, 1998c) described the experience of patients with venous ulcer pain. The common pattern that emerged from the study was "carrying on despite the pain." Eight themes were identified (as listed in Box 25-1) that provide a glimpse

---

BOX 25-1 "Carrying on Despite the Pain": Eight Themes
....

- Patients expected pain with the ulcer
- Swelling was accompanied by pain
- Patients would avoid standing
- Painful debridement started the cycle of pain all over again
- Patients felt frustrated
- Pain interfered with their job
- Significant life changes were necessary
- Patients had difficulty finding satisfaction in new activities

---

at the impact of venous ulcer pain on quality of life and activities of daily living.

Physiologic

Wound pain that is inadequately treated can lead to poor wound healing and increased infection rates. These negative sequelae occur first because pain impedes the patient's ability to tolerate wound care, and secondly because pain may cause or worsen wound hypoxia. Poor pain control impedes the ability of the care provider to cleanse, dress, and debride the wound, all of which are required for healing. When pain is poorly controlled, patients frequently refuse debridement and cleansing and postpone needed dressing changes. These factors increase the risk of infection and allow wounds to stagnate.

Acute pain increases circulating catecholamines, including epinephrine (Derbyshire and Smith 1984; Halter, Pflug, and Porte, 1977), and leads to peripheral vasoconstriction and decreased perfusion of blood to the skin and extremities. This reduced perfusion lowers oxygen availability in the tissues (Akça et al, 1999).

As tissue oxygen decreases, leukocyte activity is progressively impaired so that bacteria have a greater likelihood of remaining viable and cause wound infections (Hopf et al, 1997b). To function properly (i.e., to remove cellular debris and kill bacteria in the wound), leukocytes require oxygen. A major mechanism by which leukocytes kill bacteria is oxidative bacterial killing. The membrane-bound enzyme phagosomal oxygenase or primary oxidase converts oxygen to superoxide, itself bactericidal. Superoxide is then converted to multiple other bactericidal oxidants within the phagosome, including hydrogen peroxide, hypochlorite (bleach), and hydroxyl radical (Allen et al, 1997; Babior, 1978; Hunt, 1988).

A hypoxic wound environment will further impair wound healing by disrupting fibroblast activity and angiogenesis. Collagen and new blood vessels must be manufactured at the wound edges for a wound to heal. However, fibroblasts require oxygen to replicate, migrate, function, and manufacture mature collagen (DeJong and Kemp, 1984; Hunt and Pai, 1972; Myllyla, Tuderman, and Kivirikko, 1977). Because angiogenesis is also oxygen-dependent, angiogenesis is slowed and delivery of oxygen to the fibroblasts is impaired (Knighton, Silver, and Hunt, 1981).

PAIN PHYSIOLOGY

Although pain is a subjective experience, objective physiologic mechanisms control how pain is initiated, transmitted, and perceived. The objective neural response to a painful stimulus (for example, at the wound) is called *nociception*. Nociception is defined as the detection of impending or actual tissue damage and is accomplished by specialized sensory nerve terminals (nociceptors) derived from A delta and C fibers. All nerve endings in the epidermis are considered nociceptors (Popescu and Salcido, 2004). When cells are damaged, chemicals are released, triggering the nerve fibers to transmit the pain impulses along nerve sheaths to the spinal cord. The spinal cord transmits the information to the brain, where it is centrally processed. Synaptic junctions in the spinal cord and brain will either attenuate or amplify the pain signal and thus affect how the pain signal's intensity will be perceived or interpreted.

In addition to the actual tissue injury that triggers the pain episode, psychologic, physical, emotional, and cultural factors, as well as the patient's expectations, collectively define an individual's pain experience. Thus the same type of injury in two different individuals often generates a very different pain experience in terms of severity, quality, and impact (Turk, 1993).

Reported pain may appear to be either less than expected or excessive given the degree of tissue injury. Distress out of proportion to the injury is often ascribed to anxiety as well as "catastrophizing." Catastrophizing has been defined as an exaggerated negative orientation to aversive stimuli that involves rumination about painful sensations, magnification of the threat value of the painful stimulus, and perceived inability to control pain (Sullivan, 1998a, 1998b, 1999).

Catastrophizing is significantly correlated with mood and personality variables, such as depression, fear of pain, coping strategies, and state and trait anxiety (Rosenstiel and Keefe, 1983; Sullivan, 1995). These variables have been shown to be one of the most important predictors of the pain experience. Preoperative levels of anxiety and catastrophizing can be predictive of postoperative pain intensity. Moderately anxious patients are at greater risk for developing greater postoperative pain (Granot and Ferber, 2005). Although these studies were performed in surgical patients and not patients with chronic wounds, the findings can likely be extrapolated to the wound patient as well.

Types of Wound Pain

Types of pain may vary by wound type and underlying etiology. For example, pain associated with lower-extremity wounds can be related to claudication, to nocturnal or rest pain from ischemia (arterial disease), increased edema (venous), or neuropathy (neuropathic). The types of pain typical of the lower-extremity ulcers (i.e., arterial, venous, and neuropathic) are described in detail in Chapters 15 and 16.

Before initiating pain management interventions (either pharmacologic or nonpharmacologic), the *type* of wound pain that is being experienced and the *source* of that pain must be determined. Interventions can then be tailored to the patient's needs and effective outcomes achieved. Pain experts categorize pain into two types: nociceptive and neuropathic.

Nociceptive (Acute) Pain. Nociceptive pain, also referred to as acute pain, is the normal processing of the pain impulse and serves to alert the individual to ongoing or impending injury. Acute pain is usually consistent with the degree of tissue injury; hence, greater tissue injury translates into greater pain sensation. Acute pain can be subclassified as procedural pain, operative pain, and cyclic or noncyclic pain, in which case severity of pain then depends not only on the degree of injury, but also on such factors as the site and circumstance of injury (APMP, 1992). Nociceptive pain is typically well localized, constant, and time-limited (the pain resolves when the painful procedure ends) and often has an aching or throbbing quality.

The persistence of severe, inadequately treated acute pain can lead to anatomic and physiologic changes in the nervous system (Woolf, 2000). The ability of neural tissue to change in response to repeated incoming stimuli, a property known as neuroplasticity, can lead to the development of chronic, disabling neuropathic pain (Cohen, Christo, and Moroz, 2004). Opioids are commonly used to manage nociceptive pain.

Neuropathic Pain. Neuropathic pain results from damaged or malfunctioning nerve fibers and may be visceral or somatic in origin. Nerves can be compressed by a tumor, strangulated by scar tissue, or inflamed by infection. Unlike acute pain, neuropathic pain is *not* an indication of impending tissue injury; rather, neuropathic pain is an indication that sensory nerves are malfunctioning. Common in chronic wounds, neuropathic pain is often described as burning; it may also have "electric shock–like" qualities. Typically, the pathologic process that initiated the neuropathic pain is not fully reversible. However, with appropriate management of the pathologic process, neuropathic pain can be reduced. Neuropathic pain often responds to antiseizure and antidepressant medications rather than opioids.

Numerous pathologic responses to pain may be seen and can result from inadequately treated pain, excessive inflammation, and other pathophysiologic processes. Chronic wound pain, such as with a pressure or venous ulcer, is commonly characterized by hyperalgesia (an increased response to a normally painful stimulus) and allodynia (pain due to a stimulus that normally does not provoke pain). In the presence of hyperalgesia, any touch to the wound surface or surrounding skin, regardless of how gentle, may be interpreted as painful. Allodynia is present when gentle cleansing of the periwound skin triggers a pain episode. Hyperalgesia and allodynia are responsible for the pain that is "out of proportion" to the stimulus (Popescu and Salcido, 2004). Thus routine dressing changes and periwound skin care become excruciating.

Visceral pain. Visceral pain stems from organs or the gastrointestinal tract. Visceral pain is often described as diffuse and gnawing or cramping and poorly localized (Hader and Guy, 2004). The neural signal crosses into the spinal cord at vagal ganglia as well as dorsal root ganglia. This type of pain is commonly seen in conjunction with injuries to internal organs such as with appendicitis, myocardial ischemia, pneumonia, or gastric ulcers (Hader and Guy, 2004).

Somatic pain. Somatic pain originates from the bone, joints, muscles, skin, and connective tissue. As with acute pain, somatic pain is also described as a throbbing, well-localized pain. The pain sensation from a wound is usually somatic and can be further subdivided as to the source of the pain.

Mixed-Category Pain. Occasionally, pain can be a complex mixture of nociceptive and neuropathic factors. Whereas initially the nervous system may malfunction, tissue injury results from this malfunction and triggers the release of inflammatory mediators. Venous ulcer pain has been reported to be a combination of nociceptive and neuropathic pain, a finding that has important ramifications for medicating for pain with polypharmacy (Krasner 1997, 1998a, 1998b, 1998c).

Causes of Wound Pain

In addition to identifying the type of pain present—nociceptive (acute) versus neuropathic—different factors have been identified that will trigger or cause the wound pain episode. Figure 25-1 further characterizes the types and causes of wound pain.

Intrinsic (Background) Wound Pain. Intrinsic wound pain, generally regarded as background pain, is often described as chronic and is frequently present even when the wound is undisturbed. Intrinsic wound pain stems from the development of feedback loops that can involve the afferent and efferent pathways of the nerves as they enter and exit the spinal cord. This is a type of persistent, underlying pain such as with a wound infection or an ischemic or neuropathic wound.

Incident Pain. Incident pain is the result of movement-related activities. This is also considered "break-through" pain. This kind of pain occurs, for example, with coughing or activity.

Procedural Pain. Procedural pain is pain associated with the acute manipulation of the wound to provide routine or basic interventions. Whether from removing a wound dressing or debridement, this pain is typically time-limited; therefore it may also interpreted as acute pain. For example, it occurs when applying compression stockings over a venous ulcer or getting dressed.

Operative Pain. Operative pain is the result of cutting tissue or prolonged manipulation (i.e., sharp debridement). A local or general anesthetic is necessary to manage operative pain (World Union of Wound Healing Societies, 2004).

ASSESSMENT OF PAIN

The goal for control of wound pain is to reduce or eliminate pain so the patient may resume and perform his or her activities; in cognitively impaired patients, the goal is to maximize their comfort and enhance their quality of life. A systematic and thorough assessment of wound pain is an essential first step so that appropriate interventions can be identified.

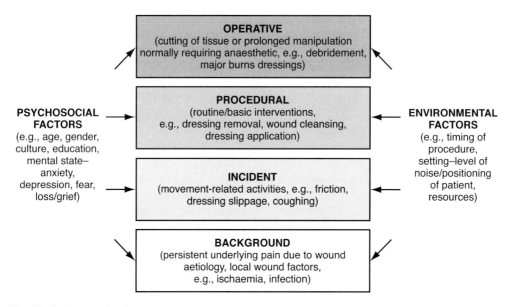

Fig. 25-1 Causes of pain. (From Classification of Chronic Pain: Descriptions of Chronic Pain Syndromes and Definitions of Pain Terms, Second Edition, IASP Task Force on Taxonomy, H Merskey and N Bogduk, IASP Press, Seattle, © 1994.)

As early as 1993, health care providers were advised to assess the person, not just the pain (Turk, 1993). This admonition becomes even more relevant in the cognitively impaired and nonverbal patient population because they are unable to verbalize the presence of pain. Furthermore, the patient's pain experience does not correlate with visible wound manifestations; there is no direct relationship between pathology and the intensity of pain (Turk, 1993). While superficial wounds with multiple exposed nerves may be intensely painful (because sensory nerve endings are most numerous in the dermis), some patients may not experience intense pain from these wounds. Conversely, subcutaneous tissue contains few sensory nerves, so that deep wounds with destruction of dermis would be expected to be less painful. In fact, necrotic and deep subcutaneous tissues can many times be debrided without significant analgesia, while debridement of wound edges, or debridement that disturbs the wound edges (as by pulling adherent eschar) may be extremely painful. Consequently, assessment of pain based upon wound depth is not appropriate and may be flawed; the wound pain experience is complex and dependent

on multiple factors. In general, wounds become less painful as they begin active healing. The mechanism is not clear but probably involves decreased inflammation, covering of exposed nerve endings, and decreased wound ischemia and hypoxia. Therefore pain intensity should decrease as wound healing occurs.

In practice, unfortunately, assessment and documentation of pain is inconsistent. Hollinworth (1995) reported inadequate pain management and poor accountability and inadequate or uninformed assessment, management, and documentation of pain at wound dressing changes. Nurses failed to assess pain verbally or to use pain assessment tools. Instead, there was reliance on nursing experience or nonverbal patient indicators to assess pain. In a cross-sectional quantitative study of 132 patients with pressure ulcer pain, Dallam and colleagues (1995) found that 59% reported having pain of some type; however, only 2% were given analgesics for the pain (within 4 hours of interview). In a study of venous ulcer healing and pain in current and former users of injected drugs, researchers found many of these patients were also denied adequate pain control based upon their history.

Researchers concluded that providers need to listen to patient concerns about pain medication, and with the patient, determine the best medication protocol (Pieper 1994; Pieper, Rossi, and Templin, 1998).

Therefore, pain assessment requires a pain history and the quantification of the severity of the pain for the verbal as well as the nonverbal or cognitively impaired patient (Feldt, 2000; Ferrell, Ferrell and Rivera, 1995; Jacox et al, 1994). Furthermore, because the condition of the wound greatly affects wound pain and the wound condition is frequently changing, pain assessment must be done regularly, with wound manipulations and dressing changes as well as on a routine daily basis. Finally, pain is assessed by type of pain; for example, nociceptive or neuropathic pain, and intrinsic pain (chronic noncyclic) or incident pain (acute cyclic). With this detailed assessment, appropriate pain-control measures can be identified.

Pain History

A pain history should include a description of the location and duration of the pain. This may be difficult to do when the patient is experiencing referred pain or when the pain is nonspecific. In addition, location and duration of pain should be characterized according to type of pain. Finally a one-time initial pain history should be obtained that addresses the following:

- Significant pain events and their effect on the patient (i.e., patients with fibromyalgia or other chronic pain syndromes tend to have a high tolerance to analgesic pain medications)
- Previously used methods and their effectiveness for pain control
- Patient's attitude toward the use of pain medications (including a history of substance abuse)
- Patient's typical coping response to stress or pain
- Family expectations and beliefs
- The way the patient describes and shows pain
- The patient's knowledge about and preferences for pain management methods and receiving information about pain management methods

Intensity of Pain Scales

Numerous techniques have been used to assess the intensity of pain as experienced by the patient, all of them obviously subjective measures. The AHCPR Acute Pain Management Guideline Panel states: "The single most reliable indicator of the existence and intensity of acute pain—and any resultant affective discomfort or distress—is the patient's self-report" (APMP, 1992).

Pain assessment tools are used to quantify the severity of pain and provide a means by which the effectiveness of pain control interventions can be measured. Intensity-of-pain scales range from simple visual analog scales to complex multidimensional, multipage instruments. For example, visual analog scales measure only one dimension of the pain phenomenon at a time (e.g., intensity, from "no pain" to "worst possible pain"), using words, numbers, faces, or other culturally congruent objects (e.g., coins and poker chips). Examples of these scales are provided in Figures 25-2 to 25-4. Visual analog scales are particularly useful in clinical practice for patients who are in active pain and do not have the capacity to complete a long, arduous questionnaire. Visual analog scales may also be used to measure pain distress and have been shown to be highly reliable instruments, even with the elderly (Herr and Mobily, 1991, 1993).

More complex pain assessment tools, such as the McGill Pain Questionnaire (Melzack, 1975; Wall and Melzack, 1994) and its modifications like the Dartmouth Pain Questionnaire (Corson and Schneider, 1984) measure a quality of the pain experience such as functional limitation or impact on quality of life, in addition to pain intensity. These descriptive scales are used primarily in specialized pain centers and for clinical research.

Pain Assessment Measures in the Nonverbal or Cognitively Impaired Patient

The cognitively impaired patient and the individual who cannot verbalize their pain are at risk for not having their pain identified and not having painful conditions treated. In fact, between 40% and 60% of long-term care residents do not use the analgesics and pain relief medications ordered for them (Horgas and Tsai, 1998; Kaasalainen et al, 1998a). Unfortunately instead of offering "as needed" analgesics to the patient periodically, clinicians often assume the patient must make a *request* for the "as needed" analgesic (Feldt, 2000). Of course, verbalization of pain or requesting pain medication is unlikely to occur in the nonverbal or cognitively impaired patient. In addition, the cognitively impaired individual has difficulty finding the

Simple Descriptive Pain Intensity Scale[1]

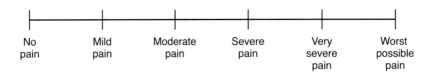

No pain   Mild pain   Moderate pain   Severe pain   Very severe pain   Worst possible pain

0-10 Numeric Pain Intensity Scale[1]

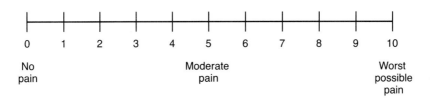

0 1 2 3 4 5 6 7 8 9 10

No pain   Moderate pain   Worst possible pain

Visual Analog Scale (VAS)[2]

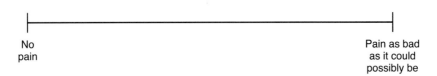

No pain   Pain as bad as it could possibly be

[1] If used as a graphic rating scale, a 10 cm baseline is recommended.

[2] A 10 cm baseline is recommended for VAS scales.

Fig. 25-2 Three examples of pain intensity scales as published by the AHCPR. (Bergstrom N et al: *Treatment of pressure ulcers*, Clinical Practice Guideline #15, Rockville, Md,, 1994, USDHHS, PHS, AHCPR Pub. No. 95-0622.)

words to describe discomfort or has impaired executive skills, limiting the ability to correlate a number on a pain scale with the sensation of pain or to interpret the "crying face" of the Wong-Baker Faces scale as an indication of "severe" pain (Kaasalainen et al, 1998b; Wynne, Ling and Remsburg, 2000).

However, cognitively impaired patients manifest several nonverbal behaviors that may be indicative of pain. These behaviors include grimacing, wincing, increased restlessness, rocking, rubbing or guarding of a body part, slowed movement, sighing and moaning, increased irritability, aggressive behaviors, increased resistance to personal care, social withdrawal, and changes in appetite or sleep patterns (Feldt, Warne, and Ryden, 1998; Weiner, Peterson, and Keefe, 1999).

Several observational pain assessment instruments are available; however, their ease of use, reliability, and validity are variable. The Discomfort Scale-Dementia of the Alzheimer's Type (DS-DAT) is a reliable tool but requires extensive training to achieve acceptable

Wong-Baker FACES Pain Rating Scale

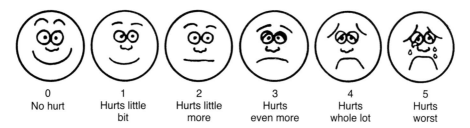

0	1	2	3	4	5
No hurt	Hurts little bit	Hurts little more	Hurts even more	Hurts whole lot	Hurts worst

Fig. 25-3 Wong-Baker Faces Pain Rating Scale.
Directions for use: Explain to the person that each face is for a person who feels happy because he or she has no pain (hurt), or feels sad because he or she has some or a lot of pain. Face 0 is very happy because he or she does not hurt at all. Face 1 hurts just a little bit. Face 2 hurts a little more. Face 3 hurts even more. Face 4 hurts a whole lot. Face 5 hurts as much as you can imagine, although you do not have to be crying to feel this bad. Ask the person to choose the face that best describes how he or she is feeling. Recommended for persons 3 years of age to older. (From Hockenberry MJ, Wilson D, Winkelstein ML: *Wong's Essentials of Pediatric Nursing*, ed 7, St. Louis, Mosby, 2005.)

Pain Rating Scales

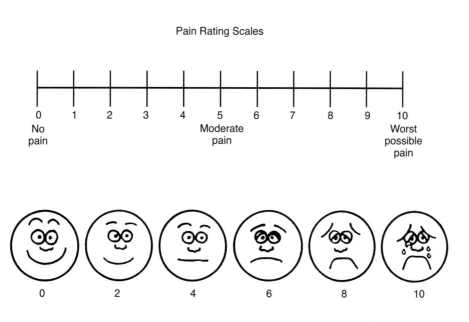

Point to each face using the words to describe the pain intensity. Ask the person to choose the face that best describes their own pain and record the appropriate number. Rating scale is recommended for persons age 3 years and older.

Fig. 25-4 Example of how a numerical pain rating scale with word anchors and the Wong-Baker faces scale can be combined onto one piece of paper so that the patient has a choice of pain rating scales. In this example, the numbers beneath the faces have been changed from a scale of 0 to 5 to a scale of 0 to 10 so that the recording of pain intensity is consistently on a 0 to 10 scale. (From Wong DL et al: *Whaley and Wong's nursing care of infants and children*, ed 6, St Louis, 1999, Mosby. Copyrighted by Mosby, Inc. Reprinted with permission.)

interrater reliability. The Pain Assessment in Advanced Dementia (PAINAD) is based on the DS-DAT and is an easy to use, easy to learn 5-item observational instrument (Warden, Hurley, and Volicer, 2003). The behavior items (breathing independent of vocalization, negative vocalization, facial expression, body language, and consolability) are rated from 0 to 2 based on specific descriptions for each score category. The total scores range from 0 to 10, with a higher score indicating severe pain. The PAINAD is provided in Table 25-2.

NONPHARMACOLOGIC PAIN CONTROL

Many pain control measures that are nonpharmacologic are essential when caring for a patient with a wound. A simple and effective intervention is to acknowledge a patient's pain and to make a commitment to the

TABLE 25-2   **Pain Assessment in Advanced Dementia (PAINAD) Scale**

ITEMS*	0	1	2	SCORE
Breathing independent of vocalization	Normal	Occasional labored breathing Short period of hyperventilation	Noisy labored breathing Long period of hyperventilation Cheyne-Stokes respirations	
Negative vocalization	None	Occasional moan or groan Low-level speech with a negative or disapproving quality	Repeated troubled calling out Loud moaning or groaning Crying	
Facial expression	Smiling or inexpressive	Sad Frightened Frown	Facial grimacing	
Body language	Relaxed	Tense Distressed pacing Fidgeting	Rigid Fists clenched Knees pulled up Pulling or pushing away Striking out	
Consolability	No need to console	Distracted or reassured by voice or touch	Unable to console, distract, or reassure	
				Total**

Breathing
1. Normal breathing is characterized by effortless, quiet, rhythmic (smooth) respirations.
2. Occasional labored breathing is characterized by episodic bursts of harsh, difficult, or wearing respirations.
3. Short period of hyperventilation is characterized by intervals of rapid, deep breaths lasting a short time.
4. Noisy labored breathing is characterized by negative sounding respirations on inspiration or expiration. They may be loud, gurgling, or wheezing. They appear strenuous or wearing.
5. Long period of hyperventilation is characterized by an excessive rate and depth of respirations lasting a considerable time.
6. Cheyne-Stokes respirations are characterized by rhythmic waxing and waning of breathing from very deep to shallow respirations with periods of apnea (cessation of breathing).

*See the description of each item below.
**Total scores range from 0 to 10 (based on a scale of 0 to 2 for five items), with a higher score indicating more severe pain (0 = "no pain" to 10 = "severe pain").

TABLE 25-2 Pain Assessment in Advanced Dementia (PAINAD) Scale—cont'd

Negative vocalization
1. None is characterized by speech or vocalization that has a neutral or pleasant quality.
2. Occasional moan or groan is characterized by mournful or murmuring sounds, wails, or laments. Groaning is characterized by louder than usual inarticulate involuntary sounds, often abruptly beginning and ending.
3. Low-level speech with a negative or disapproving quality is characterized by muttering, mumbling, whining, grumbling, or swearing in a low volume with a complaining, sarcastic, or caustic tone.
4. Repeated troubled calling out is characterized by phrases or words being used over and over in a tone that suggests anxiety, uneasiness, or distress.
5. Loud moaning or groaning is characterized by mournful or murmuring sounds, wails, or laments that are much louder than usual volume. Loud groaning is characterized by louder-than-usual inarticulate involuntary sounds, often abruptly beginning and ending.
6. Crying is characterized by an utterance of emotion accompanied by tears. There may be sobbing or quiet weeping.

Facial expression
1. Smiling is characterized by upturned corners of the mouth, brightening of the eyes, and a look of pleasure or contentment. Inexpressive refers to a neutral, at ease, relaxed, or blank look.
2. Sad is characterized by an unhappy, lonesome, sorrowful, or dejected look. There may be tears in the eyes.
3. Frightened is characterized by a look of fear, alarm, or heightened anxiety. Eyes appear wide open.
4. Frown is characterized by a downward turn of the corners of the mouth. Increased facial wrinkling in the forehead and around the mouth may appear.
5. Facial grimacing is characterized by a distorted, distressed look. The brow is more wrinkled as is the area around the mouth. Eyes may be squeezed shut.

Body language
1. Relaxed is characterized by a calm, restful, mellow appearance. The person seems to be taking it easy.
2. Tense is characterized by a strained, apprehensive, or worried appearance. The jaw may be clenched (exclude any contractures).
3. Distressed pacing is characterized by activity that seems unsettled. There may be a fearful, worried, or disturbed element present. The rate may be faster or slower.
4. Fidgeting is characterized by restless movement. Squirming about or wiggling in the chair may occur. The person might be hitching a chair across the room. Repetitive touching, tugging, or rubbing body parts can also be observed.
5. Rigid is characterized by stiffening of the body. The arms and/or legs are tight and inflexible. The trunk may appear straight and unyielding (exclude any contractures).
6. Fists clenched is characterized by tightly closed hands. They may be opened and closed repeatedly or held tightly shut.
7. Knees pulled up is characterized by flexing the legs and drawing the knees up toward the chest. An overall troubled appearance (exclude any contractures).
8. Pulling or pushing away is characterized by resistiveness upon approach or to care. The person is trying to escape by yanking or wrenching him- or herself free or shoving you away.
9. Striking out is characterized by hitting, kicking, grabbing, punching, biting, or other form of personal assault.

Consolability
1. No need to console is characterized by a sense of well-being. The person appears content.
2. Distracted or reassured by voice or touch is characterized by a disruption in the behavior when the person is spoken to or touched. The behavior stops during the period of interaction with no indication that the person is at all distressed.
3. Unable to console, distract, or reassure is characterized by the inability to soothe the person or stop a behavior with words or actions. No amount of comforting, verbal or physical, will alleviate the behavior.

patient to address the pain. Explaining the potential harmful effects of pain on healing, along with a careful explanation of how to manage pain, will help to shape the patient's expectations, as well as increase the individual's sense of control. Both of these strategies may reduce the pain experienced (APMP, 1992).

Additional interventions related to pain control begin with identifying the cause of the pain event. For example, wound manipulations or dressing changes can inflict procedural pain or cyclic acute pain. Appropriate and conscientious topical wound care can prevent or minimize considerable pain.

Wound Cleansing

Avoiding cytotoxic topical agents (such as antiseptics and antimicrobials), harsh chemicals, or highly concentrated agents for wound cleansing can significantly reduce wound pain. In general, the use of these agents should be avoided unless the wound warrants such intervention (e.g., a traumatic wound) and the patient has been adequately anesthetized (van Rijswijk, 1999).

Wound cleansing can be used as a strategy to reduce wound pain. The build-up of exudate in a wound bed can cause pressure and pain. Pain can be relieved by removing exudate with gentle flushing, low-pressure irrigation, or, in selected patients, cautious use of whirlpool.

Periwound Skin

Eroded or denuded wound margins can contribute significantly to the pain experienced by wound patients. The use of skin sealants on skin that is still intact can prevent painful denuding of skin or skin stripping. The use of ointments or skin barriers on open areas can prevent and/or minimize the pain secondary to damaged wound margins.

Debridement

Although many factors are considered when selecting a method of debridement, pain is a frequently neglected consideration. The AHCPR Treatment of Pressure Ulcers, Clinical Practice Guideline #15, states, "Regardless of the method [of debridement] selected, the need to assess and control pain should be considered" (1994). Wet-to-dry dressing changes for debridement (non-selective and painful) should be avoided. Using autolysis for debridement, when feasible and appropriate, can significantly reduce the pain associated with debridement.

Conservative or surgical sharp debridement provokes acute noncyclical pain, which leads patients to ask the clinician to stop unless additional analgesia or anesthesia is administered (Briggs, 2003; Enander Malmros, Nilsen, and Lillieborg, 1990; Evans and Gray, 2005; Hansson et al, 1993). When sharp debridement is indicated, pharmacologic interventions are an important consideration and are described in detail later in this chapter.

Inflammation and Edema

Inflammation and edema contribute to wound pain, so any measures that reduce inflammation and edema will likely also provide pain relief. This includes elevation of edematous extremities, appropriate edema-reducing dressings and devices (e.g., compression bandaging and sequential compression pumps), and systemic medications.

Support and Positioning

Binders, splints, body positioners, and other devices that stabilize a wound can significantly reduce pain, especially pain related to mobilization. Care must be taken to fit these devices properly so the wound dressing is appropriately accommodated and increased pressure on the wound does not result.

Positioning patients for comfort and off their wound can reduce pain at the wound site. If this is not possible, the judicious use of support surfaces can offer pain relief to bed- or chair-bound patients. Medicating patients before turning, repositioning, sitting up, or ambulation is logical but requires planning and coordination and therefore is too often omitted. Using lift sheets (to lift and move) instead of draw sheets (that drag) to move patients in bed prevents friction and shear that can cause painful injuries to the skin and deeper tissues. For many patients, splinting or immobilizing the wounded area (e.g., the use of an abdominal binder for a midline incision or wound) can offer significant comfort.

Certain medical devices, such as immobilizers and negative-pressure therapy devices, can become a source of pain. Various methods can be used to reduce that pain, including pressure relief and the use of nonadherent dressings at the device-wound interface.

Wound Dressings

There are many commercially available dressings designed for the care of wounds. These can vary from simple petroleum jelly–impregnated gauze to dressings that contain biologic factors thought to stimulate wound healing (e.g., lactate, protease inhibitors, growth factors, etc.). The main analgesic efficacy of these products appears to stem from their ability to keep the wound moist and protected from the environment, reduce inflammation, and stimulate healing. Moisture retentive dressings have been shown to have at least some capacity to reduce pain associated with wounds. Dressings can thus be selected for a particular patient with the aim of reducing pain. The most effective dressing will depend on patient factors such as the volume of exudate, maceration, or necrotic tissue. The major exception is that dry, wet-to-dry, or wet-to-damp dressings (plain gauze with or without water or saline, placed directly onto the wound surface) are generally the most painful. As it dehydrates, the gauze tends to become attached to the wound surface and, along with damaging new granulation tissue, is painful to remove. This is exaggerated even further because wet-to-damp or dry dressing must be changed 3 times per day, multiplying the trauma patients must endure.

The dressing change procedure, being cyclic in nature, is often dreaded by the patient with a wound. Box 25-2 lists several interventions to consider for pain control during dressing changes. It is important that dressings be selected that will, on removal, minimize the degree of sensory stimulus to the wound area. When removing a patient's dressing, every attempt should be made to avoid unnecessary stimulus to the wound such as drafts from open windows, prodding, and poking. Allowing patients to perform their own dressing changes if they are able, or to call "time-outs," can reduce the pain experienced by some. Whenever possible, timing the dressing change to occur at a time of day when the person is most "psyched" for it can be extremely beneficial. When an analgesic is given, the dressing change should be scheduled when the peak effect of the analgesic occurs (EWMA, 2002).

PHARMACOLOGIC INTERVENTIONS

The World Health Organization (WHO) Pain Clinical Ladder, a three-step analgesic ladder approach for the treatment of cancer pain, has also been used to guide

---

BOX 25-2 Interventions for Pain Reduction during Dressing Changes

- Minimize degree of sensory stimulus (e.g., drafts from open windows, or prodding and poking)
- Allow patient to perform their own dressing changes
- Allow "time-outs" during painful procedures
- Schedule dressing changes when the patient is feeling best
- Give an analgesic and then schedule the dressing change for when its peak effect occurs
- Soak dried dressings before removal
- Avoid use of cytotoxic cleansers
- Avoid aggressive packing
- Minimize the number of dressing changes
- Prevent periwound trauma
- Position and support wounded area for comfort
- Consider using low-adhesive or nonadhesive dressings
- Offer and utilize distraction techniques (e.g., headphones, TV, music, warm blanket)

---

the treatment of nonmalignant pain (Boxes 25-3, 25-4 and Figure 25-5). This approach uses a combination of pain control medications based on assessment of pain intensity. After reassessment, if pain persists, the ladder helps guide the clinician to add a medication or combination of medications to effectively control pain (McCaffery and Portenoy, 1999). Pharmacologic interventions can be topical, subcutaneous or perineural injectable, or systemic (McCaffery and Beebe, 1989; McCaffery and Portenoy, 1999).

Topical Medications

Topical analgesics are commonly used before debridement or before manipulation inside the wound margins, which includes wound packing or application of materials that contact the wound. These medications are usually in the form of a jelly, cream, or ointment, although liquid forms can also be used. They generally include lidocaine or another local anesthetic with sodium channel receptor blockade activity.

The most commonly used topical analgesics include 2% and 4% lidocaine jelly, which act on only the superficial layer of tissue and can inactivate exposed wound pain receptors. Topical anesthetics can

BOX 25-3 The WHO "Analgesic Ladder"

Step 1

Patients with mild to moderate pain should be treated with nonopioid analgesic, which should be combined with adjuvant drugs if indication for one exists.
For example: NSAIDs, acetylsalicylic acid, and acetaminophen

Step 2

Patients who have limited opioid exposure and are seen with moderate to severe pain, or who fail to achieve adequate relief after a trial of a nonopioid analgesic, should be treated with an opioid conventionally used for moderate pain.
For example: Step 1 medications plus codeine, tramadol, and so forth.

Step 3

Patients who are seen with severe pain or who fail to achieve adequate relief following appropriate administration of drugs on the second step of the analgesic ladder should receive an opioid conventionally used for severe pain.
For example: Step 1 medications and morphine (discontinue step 2 medications)
Note: Unrelieved pain should raise a red flag that attracts the clinician's attention.

WHO, World Health Organization; NSAIDs, nonsteroidal antiinflammatory drugs. Reference McCaffery M, Portenoy RK: Overview of three groups of analgesics. In McCaffrey M, Pasero C: *Pain clinical manual,* ed 2, St. Louis, 1999, pp: 115-117, Mosby.

BOX 25-4 Examples of Opioid, Nonopioid and Adjuvant Medications

Opioids
- Codeine
- Dolophine (Methadone)
- Fentanyl
- Hydromorphone (Dilaudid)
- Levorphanol
- Morphine
- Oxycodone (Percocet)
- Tramadol

Nonopioids
- Aspirin
- Acetaminophen
- Nonsteroidal antiinflammatory drugs (NSAIDS)

Adjuvant medications
- Trycyclic antidepressants
- Anticonvulsants
- Systemic local anesthetics
- Topical anesthetics

require greater than 15 to 30 minutes to reach optimal analgesic states. The strongest evidence base for effectiveness of topical analgesics in wound care is associated with a eutectic mixture of local anesthetics (EMLA cream). Instructions for use of EMLA cream can be found in Box 25-5 (Enander Malmros, Nilsen, and Lillieborg, 1990, Evans and Gray, 2005; Hansson et al, 1993; Holm, Andren, and Grafford, 1990).

Subcutaneous or Perineural Injectable Medications

Injectable medications (subcutaneous or perineural) frequently contain the same type of active drug that are found in the topical analgesic formulations (local

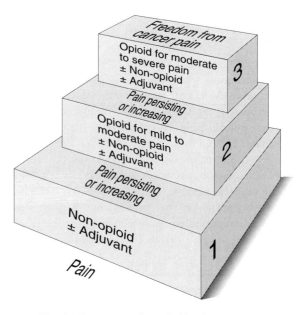

Fig. 25-5 WHO analgesic ladder for cancer pain.

BOX 25-5 **Application of Eutectic Mixture of Local Anesthetics (EMLA Cream)**

- 10 g EMLA can safely cover a surface area of approximately 100 cm².
- Apply directly to the wound.
- Cover with a plastic wrap for 20 minutes.
- If pain is not managed at 20 minutes then increase the time to 45 to 60 minutes.

Data from Evans E, Gray M: Do topical analgesics reduce pain associated with wound dressing changes? *J WOCN* 32(5):287, 2005.

anesthetics such as lidocaine). However, these medications are in solution and designed to be injected into the soft tissue. These medications include lidocaine or longer-acting agents (e.g., bupivacaine or tetracaine). Epinephrine can be added to these medications to cause vasoconstriction to increase the duration of action as well as to decrease bleeding. Epinephrine is contraindicated for use in distal areas such as hands and feet, because of the risk of necrosis from interruption of blood supply. Epinephrine is generally avoided in wounds because of the concern of impairing blood supply, although it may be useful in extremely vascular wounds. Injectable local anesthetics can be used for either field or regional blockade.

A **field blockade** is accomplished by injecting local anesthetic adjacent to or directly into the wound margins, encircling the entire area. It blocks transmission of pain signals that are carried in the superficial cutaneous nerves that supply the wound area. At times, it is less painful to inject within the wound edges. If tolerated, however, the block is generally more effective when the injection is made outside the wound margins. The inflammation in the wound may inactivate or reduce the activity of the local anesthetic.

A **regional** or **nerve block** is accomplished by injecting local anesthetic into an often singular, proximal location where the larger nerve bundles are contained. Examples of regional blocks would include digital blocks and ankle or wrist blocks. Regional blocks require more training but are useful in the management and debridement of wounds that either cross many dermatomes or cover a large area that is supplied by many separate proximal nerves, or in patients with severe periwound hyperalgesia.

Some nerve blocks can involve large nerve bundles near the spinal cord. An example of this is a percutaneous lumbar sympathetic block (LSB), which can be used for chronic lower extremity, wound pain. Trauma and inflammation may increase sympathetic tone and upregulate alpha receptors in the wound, leading to sympathetically maintained pain in lower-extremity ulcers (McLachlan et al, 1993). These procedures are usually performed using fluoroscopic x-ray guidance. For these blocks, the goal is not temporary relief but long-term blockade and thus often uses an alcohol-based medication to permanently inactivate nerve transmission of the painful area to the spinal cord (Hopf et al, 1997a).

All nerve blocks can be done safely in an outpatient clinic with properly trained personnel, monitoring appropriately for the degree of sedation required.

Systemic Medications

The goal of systemic medication administration as a pain control strategy is not to stop pain signal transmission from the wound, but to alter the response of the central nervous system to that pain signal. Whether the medication is given intravenously, subcutaneously, transcutaneously, or orally, there are many pain management choices when utilizing systemic pain control (Tables 25-3, 25-4, 25-5). These include nonsteroidal antiinflammatory drugs (NSAIDs), opioids (e.g., morphine, methadone, etc), oral lidocaine, acetaminophen, partial μ-receptor agonists (e.g., Tramadol), anticonvulsants (e.g., gabapentin [Neurontin]), antidepressants, and clonidine (a central α-2 adrenergic agonist that reduces sympathetic outflow) (Veith, Best, and Halter, 1984). These medications often act on different target locations to combat the perception of pain. For example, predominantly neuropathic pain is more responsive to antidepressants and anticonvulsants than to NSAIDs and opioids (WOCN Society, 2004). Some medications, like NSAIDs, can also act by secondary means to reduce pain; that is, aside from their direct analgesic properties, they reduce inflammation in the wound area, leading to a decrease in pain.

Combining several analgesic agents is often more successful than using a single agent. Drugs may act additively or synergistically. This may allow a reduction in the required dose of each agent, thus potentially

TABLE 25-3 Recommended Starting Doses (and Equivalence) for Opioid Treatment of Intrinsic Wound Pain

PO/PR (MG)	ANALGESIC	IV OR IM (mg)
30	Morphine	1-5/10/5-10
6	Hydromorphone (Dilaudid)	0.2-0.6/1.5
20	Methadone	10-20
Not recommended	Meperidine (Demerol)	10-30/100*
60	Codeine	30-60
5-10	Oxycodone (Percocet)	N/A

*Meperidine should not be used for analgesia because normeperidine, a metabolite, may accumulate. When high doses (1000 mg in a day or 600 mg/day for several days) are given, seizures are common. Meperidine also is more likely to cause dependence than other clinically used opioids.
Source: Acute Pain Management Guideline Panel. *Acute Pain Management: Operative or Medical Procedures and Trauma. Clinical Practice Guideline.* AHCPR Pub. No. 92-0032. Rockville, MD: Agency for Health Care Policy and Research, Public Health Service, U.S. Department of Health and Human Services. Feb., 1992.

TABLE 25-4 Agents Appropriate for Sedation/Analgesia for Procedures in Adults

AGENTS	DOSE (IV)	FREQUENCY
Diazepam	1-2 mg	q 3-10 min
Lorazepam	0.05 mg/kg (max = 4 mg)	one time
Midazolam	0.25-1 mg	q 1-5 min
Fentanyl	Loading dose up 1 mcg/kg then 12.5-50 mcg	q 5-10 min
Meperidine	12.5-25 mg	q 2-15 min
Morphine	1-3 mg	q 2-15 min
Droperidol	0.625-1.25 mg	q 5-10 min

reducing side effects, while providing equal or even superior analgesia (Hopf and Weitz, 1994). A patient with mixed nociceptive and neuropathic pain will require a combination of analgesics and antidepressants or anticonvulsants.

Because of their potency and reliable analgesic action, opioids are a mainstay of pain management both in the acute and chronic settings. One of the actions of opioids is to stimulate receptors in the central and peripheral nervous system that down-regulate both the afferent response to pain as well as central pain perception. Gabapentin (Neurontin) is an excellent drug for treating neuropathic pain, such as in patients with diabetic neuropathy. It is also often effective for wound pain, probably because of the neuropathic nature of much wound pain. The maximum recommended dose is 900 mg by mouth 3 times daily, but wound pain frequently responds to the lowest dose range of 100 to 200 mg 3 times daily. Side effects are few and minor.

Future research is necessary to confirm which strategies or groups of strategies optimize pain relief and for which type of pain. So, for example, applying a topical anesthetic compress before sharp debridement might be more effective for this type of acute noncyclic pain than taking an oral pain medication. Around-the-clock medications might be most effective for continuous chronic wound pain. Applying pain-reducing dressings or selecting pressure-reducing devices may prove to reduce acute cyclic pressure ulcer pain more effectively than pharmacologic measures. Dressing-related wound pain may be reduced if able patients were allowed to change their own dressings or to call "time-outs" during dressing changes.

Addiction Concerns

The degree of pain that a patient experiences and reports is often influenced by the fear of addiction.

TABLE 25-5 Pharmacological Interventions for Neuropathic Pain

TYPE OF PAIN	MEDICATION	TYPE OF PAIN	MEDICATION
Dysesthesia	Capsaicin cream topically applied TID to QID. May take 3 weeks to be effective Gabapentin Selective serotonin reuptake inhibitors (SSRIs) (e.g., fluoxetine, paroxetine) Serotonin and noradrenergic reuptake inhibitors (SSnaRI) (i.e., venlataxine) Dextromethorphan syrup Trycyclic antidepressants (e.g., imipramine, amitriptyline)	General neuropathic pain	Analgesics (e.g., lidoderm patch) Gabapentin Hemorrheologic agents (e.g., pentoxitylline (Trental) Diuretics (e.g., furesomide, metolazone, bumetanide). May diminish pain with reduction in vasodilitation. Platelet inhibitors, cilostazol (Pletal) Bisphosphonates (e.g., Pamidronate) Aldose reductase inhibitor (e.g., fidarestat, sorbinil) Anti-thromboembolitic therapy (e.g., heparin, warfarin, ASA, NSAIDS Clopodogrel (Plavix)
Paresthesia	Anticonvulsants (e.g., carbamazepine, Tegretol, phenytoin) Analgesics (i.e., Tramadol)		
Muscular Pain	Muscle relaxants (e.g., metataxalone lioresal, tizanidene by mouth)		

A common social and medical problem is drug and alcohol abuse. It can be especially difficult to treat painful wounds in such patients. Alcohol- and drug-addicted patients can exhibit tolerance to central nervous system (CNS) depressants and opioids, which could require increasing dosages of analgesic medications in these patients. In addition, liver and kidney disease associated with alcohol or other drug abuse may alter the metabolism and excretion of opioids and other analgesics. Together, tolerance and altered metabolism, along with variability in recent drug use by the patient and attitudes among health care providers toward addicted patients, make it difficult to design an effective analgesic regimen in these patients.

Furthermore, opioid-addicted patients may exhibit a tendency for hyperalgesia, in which they experience a greater intensity of pain than would be expected for a given wound. When treating these individuals, the fundamental principle of pain management is the same as it is for other patients: pain complaints should be taken seriously and treated aggressively (Cohen, Christo, and Moroz, 2004). Intravenous drug abusers will require higher doses of analgesics to obtain similar degrees of pain relief because of the development of opioid cross-tolerance. Working with the patient to control the pain is particularly important in caring for such patients.

Historically, patients have commonly been undertreated with opioid pain medications when opioids were indicated (Marks and Sachar, 1973; Owen, McMillan, and Rogowski, 1990). There are several reasons for this, including fear of respiratory depression, uncertainty as to dosing, and fear of causing addiction. Clinical experience will reduce uncertainty about dosing and side effects. The fear of addiction is unfounded; less than 0.1% of patients receiving opioids for acute pain become addicted (APMP, 1992). Patients frequently take inadequate doses of opioids because of the fear of addiction. They should be reassured and encouraged to use the drug appropriately. When the dose is inadequate because of side effects, different opioids should be tried, and adjunct agents added to reduce the required opioid dose.

Potential Complications of Medical Pain Management

Medications are rarely benign. Almost every drug has an associated set of potential side effects that can be inconvenient or harmful to the patient. While the Physician's Desk Reference lists every reported side effect for each medication, there are certain sets of complications that are commonly encountered in the setting of analgesic control. The most powerful systemic analgesic agents are opioids; they also have the most acutely serious side effects, including sedation and respiratory depression.

Whenever opioids are given, attention must be given to avoiding excess sedation and respiratory depression. This is particularly true when they are given to manage procedural pain. Most health care facilities recognize five categories of sedation (see Table 25-6). However, these categories are artificially drawn, since sedation is a continuum. Sedation is different from simple pain control; sedation implies that the medications are given to specifically facilitate the ability to perform a painful procedure. The use of analgesics or sedatives solely to provide analgesia and/or allay anxiety (such as during dressing changes) and with no intent of performing a procedure is **not** considered sedation. Nonetheless, such drugs must be used with caution,

since respiratory depression and sedation can be induced whenever these drugs are used. Box 25-6 provides prescribing principles for chronic pain management in the long-term care setting that have been developed by The American Geriatrics Society Panel on Persistent Pain in Older Persons (2002).

A patient receiving light sedation or more requires constant monitoring which, at a minimum, includes a cardiac monitor, pulse oximetry, and direct supervision by a provider not involved in performing the procedure. When a patient is being managed using sedation, the most serious common complication is respiratory depression; hence, it should only be performed in a setting that provides a medical practitioner who can provide a definitive airway and handle the complications of ventilatory and/or circulatory collapse. Whenever patients are given analgesics for procedural pain, consideration should be given to monitoring. Hospital guidelines should always be followed.

Less serious but common side effects of opioids include nausea, vomiting, constipation, urinary retention, and pruritus. All patients receiving opioids should be given stool softeners and counseled on ways to prevent constipation, including increased fluid and fiber intake. Antiemetic medications, changing to a different opioid, or limiting opioid dose by using nonopioid analgesics such as NSAIDs can manage nausea and vomiting. Pruritus can be managed with diphenhydramine or other antihistamines.

TABLE 25-6 Categories of Sedation

LEVEL	CATEGORY	DEFINITION
1	No sedation	
2	Minimal or light sedation	Patient responds normally to verbal commands. Ventilatory and cardiac functions unaffected.
3	Moderate or conscious sedation	Patient responds purposefully to verbal commands. The patient's spontaneous ventilation is adequate.
4	Deep sedation	Patient cannot be easily aroused. The patient can respond purposefully following repeated or painful stimulation. There is an increased probability of respiratory or hemodynamic compromise.
5	Anesthesia	Most often performed in the operating room. The patient is not arousable by painful stimulation.

BOX 25-6 Principles that Guide Chronic Wound Pain Management

Manage intrinsic (background) pain with medications provided on a routine schedule.

Manage break-through pain with fast-acting medications as required (PRN).

Consider the following regarding route of administration:

- Use the least invasive route first (i.e., administer medications orally, when feasible).
- Use topical patches or creams when oral medications are insufficient.

Analgesic dose should be titrated to an effective level starting with a low dose and advancing slowly.

Reassessment of background pain as well as procedural or incident pain should be ongoing and treatment individualized per patient need.

Monitor elderly closely for undesirable effects.

American Geriatrics Society Panel on Persistent Pain in Older Persons: The management of persistent pain in older persons, *J Am Geriatr Soc* 50(S6):1, 2002.

Side effects of NSAIDs include stomach pain, ulcers, and gastrointestinal bleeding; renal impairment; allergy, and platelet inhibition (Buckley, Brogden, and Ketorolac, 1990). Side effects of acetaminophen are few, but overdoses (more than 4 to 6 g per day) can result in acute fulminant liver failure. Care should be exercised in using opioid-acetaminophen combinations, especially those with relatively low-potency opioids and high doses of acetaminophen (500 mg per tab), such as Vicodin (hydrocodone-acetaminophen). Acetaminophen is a powerful adjunct, so it should be used when possible. For tolerant patients, it should be given separately as an around-the-clock drug to reduce the risk of liver injury. More potent opioids (e.g., oxycodone, hydromorphone [Dilaudid], morphine, or methadone) should be selected as well to reduce the number of doses required daily.

Side effects of antiepileptics and antidepressants include sedation, which usually resolves with continued use. These drugs can be started as a bedtime dose for several days to allow acclimatization.

Side effects of clonidine include sedation and dry mouth (acclimatization is rapid). It can also decrease blood pressure and heart rate, although it rarely causes hypotension or bradycardia. Clonidine is available as a transdermal patch, which allows constant plasma levels and improved compliance. Usually the lowest dose (a #1 or #2 patch) is sufficient. Clonidine may reduce opioid requirements in tolerant patients (Flacke et al, 1987). It often increases perfusion and oxygenation in patients with hypoxic wounds because of excess sympathetic tone or peripheral vascular disease, which may also reduce pain (Hopf and West, 1996).

WOUND PAIN MODELS

Many factors must be assessed to adequately manage wound pain: etiology, condition of the wound, topical wound care, type of pain, and source of wound pain. To assist the clinician in negotiating all these considerations so that pain is addressed through every aspect of the delivery of wound care, two models have been developed. The value of these models is that they go beyond simply listing all possible strategies for controlling wound pain. Rather, these models guide the clinician through a logical, systematic, and thorough assessment of the wound (i.e., etiology and the related interventions, topical wound condition and the related interventions, and type of pain) so that interventions can be selected based upon the patient's type of pain and source of pain.

The *Chronic Wound Pain Experience (CWPE) Model* (Krasner, 1995a, 1995b), was empirically and inductively derived, and can be used to assist with establishing a plan of care for pain control (Figure 25-6). The CWPE model introduces a new classification scheme tailored specifically to pain associated with wounds:

1. Noncyclic acute wound pain: a single episode of pain (i.e., that which occurs with sharp debridement)
2. Cyclic acute wound pain: acute wound pain that recurs as a result of repeated treatments (i.e., that which occurs with dressing changes)
3. Chronic wound pain: persistent, continuous pain that occurs without manipulation of the wound.

Each type of pain has a set of pain control options appropriate for that type of pain. The CWPE assumes that most patients with chronic wounds experience all three types of pain at some time, although not necessarily simultaneously. It is also recognizes that some

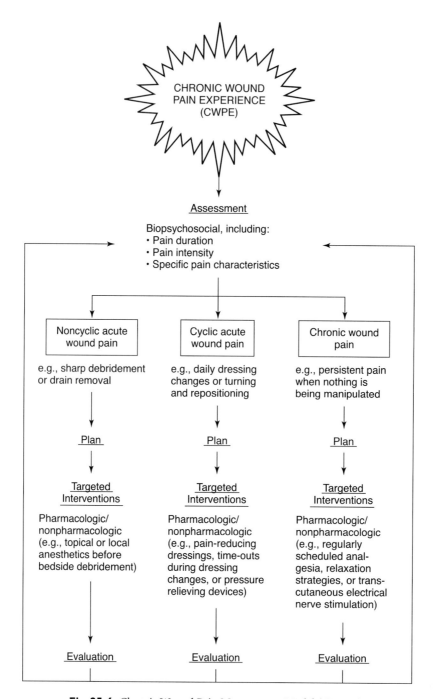

Fig. 25-6 Chronic Wound Pain Management Model (CWPM).

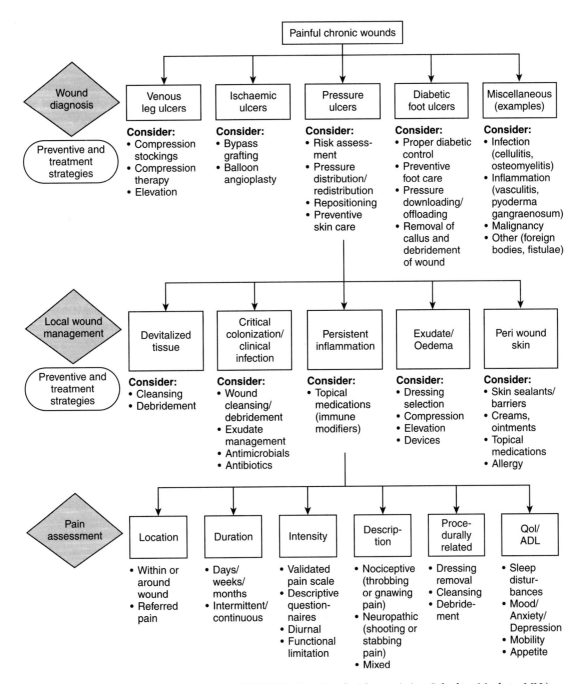

Fig. 25-7 Wound Pain Management Model (WPM). (Reprinted with permission Coloplast, Mankato, MN.)

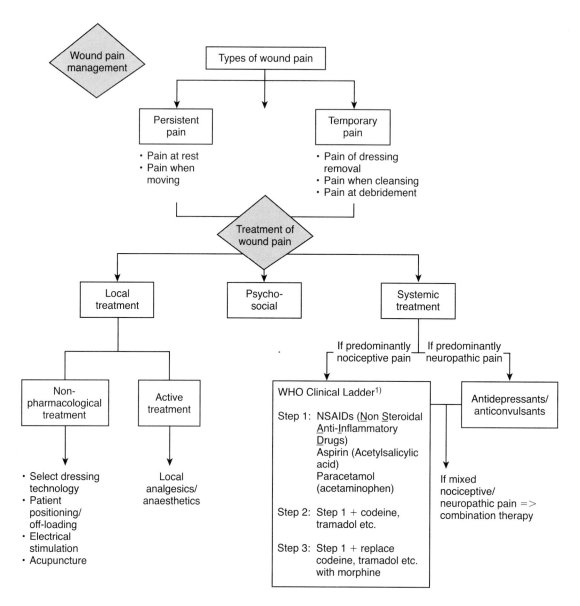

Fig. 25-7, cont'd Wound Pain Management Model (WPM). **Note:** Effective management of wound pain requires attention to many factors **BEFORE** initiating pharmacologic or nonpharmacologic interventions for pain control. Use this model to guide appropriate interventions that reduce pain associated with diagnosis or local wound management. After that a complete pain assessment and determination of type of wound pain can guide the treatment of wound pain.

patients may not experience or be able to indicate pain at all. Others may not experience one of the pain types because of the particular course of their treatment or disease (e.g., the patient who has never had sharp debridement may never experience noncyclic acute wound pain). Another assumption is that many commonly held beliefs about wound pain might lack validity (e.g., patients with diabetes do not experience wound pain in the presence of neuropathy).

The *Wound Pain Management Model (WPM)* was developed in 2003 by an international advisory panel of experts and designed to be a practical guide for the clinician (Figure 25-7). The WPM guides the clinician through four aspects of wound care: wound diagnosis, local wound management, pain assessment, and wound pain management. Using the WPM, the clinician is guided to determine the correct wound diagnosis; related prevention and treatment wound care strategies are then provided for each wound diagnosis. The next step in the WPM is to address local wound management needs. Based on five possible wound conditions (i.e., devitalized tissue, colonization/infection, inflammation, exudate/edema, and periwound skin), local wound management prevention and treatment strategies are listed. Next the clinician is guided to conduct a pain assessment including factors related to location, duration, intensity, description (type of pain), care procedures, and quality of life or activities of daily living. These are important preliminary steps in pain control so that their contribution to the pain event can be minimized or eliminated. Finally, the WPM addresses the treatment of wound pain incorporating local and systemic treatment options.

SUMMARY

Pain is a complex subjective response. For people with a painful acute or chronic wound, coping with the wound pain can be as challenging as coping with the wound itself. While pain has an impact on the patient's psychosocial status and activities of daily living, it also predisposes the patient to increased infection rates and exaggerated wound hypoxia.

In the current climate of outcome-focused healthcare, outcome measures such as "no pain" or "reduced pain" are reasonable, feasible, and warranted. These can be highly measurable target goals, or they can serve as intermediate goals on the way to healing outcomes.

Once the type of pain experience is identified, an appropriate plan of action for wound pain management can be established.

SELF-ASSESSMENT EXERCISE

1. Wound pain can affect which of the following dimensions?
   a. Productivity
   b. Quality of life
   c. Sleep
   d. All of the above
2. The AHCPR Pressure Ulcer Treatment Guideline recognizes the importance of which of the following?
   a. Routinely assessing for and treating pressure ulcer pain
   b. The routine use of the Faces pain rating scale
   c. The provider determining the patient's pain score
   d. Using a topical anesthetic cream before debridement
3. Which of the following dimensions of the Chronic Wound Pain Experience Model best describes the pain of conservative sharp debridement?
   a. Noncyclic acute wound pain
   b. Cyclic acute wound pain
   c. Chronic wound pain
   d. All of the above
4. According to the Chronic Wound Pain Experience Model, patients with wound pain may experience noncyclic acute wound pain, cyclic acute wound pain, and chronic wound pain at the same time: True or false?
5. Which of the following frequently causes procedural wound pain?
   a. Adhesive dressings
   b. Wet-to-moist gauze
   c. Debridement
   d. All of the above
6. Which of the following is included among best practices for managing wound pain?
   a. Assuming that the pain is bearable
   b. Medicating for pain after the procedure
   c. Using a combination of strategies
   d. Addressing nonprocedural pain before procedural pain
7. Decreasing swelling by compression in patients with venous ulcers has been shown in several recent studies to reduce venous ulcer pain: True or false?
8. List five interventions for pain reduction during dressing changes.

REFERENCES

Acute Pain Management Panel (APMP): *Acute pain management: operative or medical procedures and trauma. Clinical practice guideline,* Rockville, MD, 1992, USDHHS, PHS, AHCPR Pub. No. 92-0032.

Akça O et al: Postoperative pain and subcutaneous oxygen tension, *Lancet* 354(9172):41, 1999 (letter).

Allen DB et al: Wound hypoxia and acidosis limit neutrophil bacterial killing mechanisms, *Arch Surg* 132(9):991, 1997.

American Geriatrics Society Panel on Persistent Pain in Older Persons: The management of persistent pain in older persons, *J Am Geriatr Soc* 50(S6):1, 2002.

Babior BM: Oxygen-dependent microbial killing by phagocytes, *N Engl J Med* 198:659, 1978.

Bergstrom N et al: *Treatment of pressure ulcers,* Clinical Practice Guideline #15, Rockville, Md, 1994, USDHHS, PHS, AHCPR Pub. No. 95-0622.

Briggs M, Nelson EA: Topical agents or dressings for pain in venous leg ulcers, Cochrane Database Syst Rev, 2003, (2).

Buckley MM, Brogden RN. Ketorolac: A review of its pharmacodynamic and pharmacokinetic properties, and therapeutic potential, *Drugs* 39(1):86, 1990.

Cohen SP, Christo PJ, Moroz L: Pain management in trauma patients, *Am J Phys Med Rehabil* 83:142, 2004.

Corson J, Schneider M: The Dartmouth pain questionnaire: an adjunct to the McGill pain questionnaire, *Pain* 19:59, 1984.

Dallam L et al: Pressure ulcer pain: assessment and quantification, *J WOCN* 22(5):211, 1995.

DeJong L, Kemp A: Stoichiometry and kinetics of the prolyl 4-hydroxylase partial reaction, *Biochim Biophys Acta* 787(1):105, 1984.

Derbyshire D, Smith G: Sympathoadrenal responses to anaesthesia and surgery, *Br J Anaesth* 56:725, 1984.

Enander Malmros I, Nilsen T, Lillieborg S: Plasma concentrations and analgesic effect of EMLA (lidocaine/prilocaine) cream for the cleansing of leg ulcers, *Acta Derm Venereol* 70(3):227, 1990.

European Wound Management Association (EWMA): Position document: pain at wound dressing changes, 2002, Medical Education Partnership; http://www.ewma.org; Accessed September 25, 2005.

Evans E, Gray M: Do topical analgesics reduce pain associated with wound dressing changes? *J WOCN* 32(5):287, 2005.

Feldt KS, Warne MA, Ryden MB: Examining pain in aggressive cognitively impaired elders, *J Geront Nurs* 24(11):14, 1998.

Feldt KS: Improving assessment and treatment of pain in cognitively impaired nursing home residents, Ann Long-Term Care 8(9):36, 2000.

Ferrell B: Ethical perspectives on pain and suffering, *Pain Manage Nurs* 6(3):83, 2005.

Ferrell BA, Ferrell BR, Rivera L: Pain in cognitively impaired nursing home patients, *J Pain Symptom Manage* 10(8):191, 1995.

Flacke JW et al: Reduced narcotic requirement by clonidine with improved hemodynamic and adrenergic stability in patients undergoing coronary bypass surgery, *Anesthesiology* 67:11, 1987.

Granot M, Ferber SG: The roles of pain catastrophizing and anxiety in the prediction of postoperative pain intensity: a prospective study, *Clin J Pain* 21:439, 2005.

Hader CF, Guy J: Your hand in pain management, *Nurs Manage* 35(11):21, 2004.

Halter JB, Pflug AE, Porte D Jr: Mechanism of plasma catecholamine increases during surgical stress in man, *J Clin Endocrin and Metab* 45(5):936, 1977.

Hansson C et al: Repeated treatment with lidocaine/prilocaine cream (EMLA) as a topical anaesthetic for the cleansing of venous leg ulcers. A controlled study, *Acta Derm Venereol* 73(3):231, 1993.

Herr K, Mobily P: Pain assessment in the elderly: clinical considerations, *J Gerontol Nurs* 17(4):12, 1991.

Herr K, Mobily P: Comparison of selected pain assessment tools for use with the elderly, *Appl Nurs Res* 6(1):39, 1993.

Hill C: Joint Commission Focuses On Pain Management, 1999, http://www.jcaho.org/news+room/health+care+issues/jcaho+focuses+on+pain+management.htm; Accessed October 9, 2005.

Hofman D et al: Pain in venous leg ulcer, *J Wound Care* 6(5):222, 1997.

Hollinworth H: Nurses' assessment and management of pain at wound dressing changes, *J Wound Care* 4(2):77, 1995.

Holm J, Andren B, Grafford K: Pain control in the surgical debridement of leg ulcers by the use of a topical lidocaine-prilocaine cream, EMLA, Acta Derm Venereol Suppl (Stockh) 70:132, 1990.

Hopf H, Weitz S: Postoperative pain management, *Arch Surg* 129:128, 1994.

Hopf H et al: Clonidine increases tissue oxygen in patients with local tissue hypoxia in non-healing wounds, *Wound Rep Regen* 4(1):A129, 1996.

Hopf H et al: Percutaneous lumbar sympathetic block increases tissue oxygen in patients with local tissue hypoxia in non-healing wounds, *Anesth Analg* 84:S305, 1997a.

Hopf HW et al: Wound tissue oxygen tension predicts the risk of wound infection in surgical patients, *Arch Surg* 132(9):997; discussion 1005, 1997b.

Horgas AL, Tsai PF: Analgesic drug prescription and use in cognitively impaired nursing home residents, *Nurs Res* 47:235, 1998.

Hunt TK: The physiology of wound healing, *Ann Emerg Med* 17: 1265, 1988.

Hunt TK, Pai MP: The effect of varying ambient oxygen tensions on wound metabolism and collagen synthesis, *Surg Gynecol Obstet* 135:561, 1972.

Jacox A et al: *Management of cancer pain,* Clinical Practice Guideline #9, Rockville, Md, 1994, USDHHS, PHS, AHCPR Pub No. 94-0592.

Kaasalainen S et al: Pain and cognitive status in the institutionalized elderly: perceptions & interventions. J Gerontol Nurs. Aug;24(8): 24-31; quiz 50-1, 1998a.

Kaasalainen SJ et al: The assessment of pain in the cognitively impaired elderly: A literature review, *Perspectives* 22(2):2, 1998b.

Knighton D, Silver I, Hunt TK: Regulation of wound healing angiogenesis—effect of oxygen concentration, *Surgery* 90:262, 1981.

Krasner D: Carrying on despite the pain: living with painful venous ulcers: a Heideggerian hermeneutic analysis (doctoral dissertation), Ann Arbor, Mich, 1997, UMI.

Krasner D: The chronic wound pain experience: a conceptual model, *Ostomy Wound Manage* 41(3):20, 1995a.

Krasner D: Managing pain from pressure ulcers. In Pasaro C: Pain control, *Am J Nurs* 6:22, 1995b.

Krasner D: Chronic wound pain. In Krasner D, Kane D: *Chronic wound care: a clinical source book for healthcare professionals,* Wayne, Penn, 1998a, Health Management Publications.

Krasner D: Painful venous ulcers: themes and stories about living with the pain and suffering, *J WOCN* 25(3):158, 1998b.

Krasner D: Painful venous ulcers: themes and stories about their impact on quality of life, *Ostomy Wound Manage* 44(9):38, 1998c.

Krasner D: Using a gentler hand: reflections on patients with pressure ulcers who experience pain, *Ostomy Wound Manage* 42(3):20, 1996.

Lasch KE, Culture and pain, *Pain Clin Updates* 10(5), 2002. http://www.iasp-pain.org/PCU02-5.html

Marks R, Sachar E: Undertreatment of medical inpatients with narcotic analgesics, *Ann Intern Med* 78:173, 1973.

McCaffery M: *Nursing management of the patient with pain,* Philadelphia, 1972, JB Lippincott.

McCaffery M, Beebe A: *Pain: clinical manual for nursing practice,* St Louis, 1989, Mosby.

McCaffrey M, Pasero C: *Pain clinical manual,* ed 2, St Louis, 1999, Mosby.

McCarthy C, Cushnaghan J, Dieppe P: Osteoarthritis. In Wall P, Melzack R, editors: *Textbook of pain,* Edinburgh, 1994, Churchill Livingstone.

McCaffery M, Portenoy RK: Overview of three groups of analgesics. In McCaffrey M, Pasero C: *Pain clinical manual,* ed 2, St Louis, 1999, pp:115-117, Mosby.

McLachlan EM et al: Peripheral nerve injury triggers noradrenergic sprouting within dorsal root ganglia, *Nature* 363(6429):543, 1993.

Melzack R: The McGill pain questionnaire: major properties and scoring methods, *Pain* 1:277, 1975.

Myllyla R, Tuderman L, Kivirikko KI: Mechanism of the prolyl hydroxylase reaction. Part 2: Kinetic analysis of the reaction sequence, *Eur J Biochem* 80(2):349, 1977.

Owen H, McMillan V, Rogowski D. Postoperative pain therapy: a survey of patients' expectations and their experiences, *Pain* 41:303, 1990.

Phillips T et al: A study of the impact of leg ulcers on quality of life: financial, social and psychologic implications, *J Am Acad Dermatol* 31(1):49, 1994.

2006 Physicians' Desk Reference (PDR): Your Complete Print and Electronic Drug Information Solution. Thomson PDR pp. 1-3000, November 2005.

Pieper B: A retrospective analysis of venous ulcer healing in current and former drug users of injected drugs, *J WOCN* 23(6):291, 1994.

Pieper B, Rossi R, Templin T: Pain associated with venous ulcers in injecting drug users, *Ostomy Wound Manage* 44(11):54, 1998.

Popescu A, Salcido RS: Wound pain: a challenge for the patient and the wound care specialist, *Adv Skin Wound Care* 17(1):14, 2004.

Reddy M et al: Practical treatment of wound pain and trauma: a patient centered approach, *Ostomy Wound Manage* 49(4A Suppl):2, 2003.

Rosenstiel AK, Keefe FJ: The use of coping strategies in chronic low back pain patients: relationship to patient characteristics and current adjustment, *Pain* 17:33, 1983.

Sullivan MJL, Bishop S, Pivic J: The Pain Catastrophizing Scale: development and validation, *Psychol Assess* 7:524, 1995.

Sullivan MJL, Neish N: Catastrophizing, anxiety, and pain during dental hygiene treatment, *Comm Dent Oral Epidemiol* 37:243, 1998.

Sullivan MJL, Neish N: The effects of disclosure on pain during dental hygiene treatment: the moderating role of catastrophizing, *Pain* 79:155, 1999.

Sullivan MJL et al: Catastrophizing, pain, and disability in patients with soft-tissue injuries, *Pain* 77:253, 1998.

Szor JK, Bourguignon C: Description of pressure ulcer pain at rest and at dressing change, *J WOCN* 26(3):115, 1999.

Turk DC: Assess the person, not just the pain, *Pain Clinical Updates*, 1(3), 1993; http://www.iasp-pain.org.

van Rijswijk L: Wound pain. In McCaffery M, Pasero C: *Pain clinical manual*, ed 2, St Louis, Mosby, 1999.

Veith RC, Best JD, Halter JB: Dose-dependent suppression of norepinephrine appearance rate in plasma by clonidine in man, *J Clin Endocrinol Metab* 59:151, 1984.

Wall P, Melzack R: *Textbook of pain,* ed 2, Edinburgh, 1994, Churchill Livingstone.

Walsche C: Living with a venous leg ulcer: a descriptive study of patients' experiences, *J Adv Nurs* 22:1092, 1995.

Warden V, Hurley AC, Volicer L: Development and psychometric evaluation of the pain assessment in advanced dementia (PAINAD) scale, *J Am Med Dir Assoc* 4:9, 2003.

Weiner DK, Peterson B, Keefe EJ: Chronic pain-associated behaviors in the nursing home: resident versus caregiver perception, *Pain* 80: 577, 1999.

WOCN Society: *Guideline for management of wounds in patients with lower-extremity neuropathic disease,* WOCN Clinical Practice Guideline Series #3, Glenview IL, 2004, Author.

Woolf CJ, Salter MW: Neuronal plasticity: Increasing the gain in pain, *Science* 288:1765, 2000.

World Union of Wound Healing Societies: *Principles of best practice: minimising pain at wound dressing-related procedures. A consensus document*, London, 2004, MEP; http://www.wuwhs.org/pdf/consensus_eng.pdf.

Wynne CF, Ling SM, Remsburg R: Comparison of pain assessment instruments in cognitively intact and cognitively impaired nursing home residents, *Geriatr Nurs* 21:20, 2000.

26 *Facilitating Adaptation*

DENISE P. NIX & BEN PEIRCE

OBJECTIVES

1. Explain why the term noncompliance should not be used to describe patients.
2. List 10 potential barriers to achieving a sustainable plan.
3. List five factors to assess before developing an educational plan.
4. Explain the difference between short-term goals and long-term goals.
5. Summarize JCAHO standards statements for patient education.

A*daptation* is defined as "the dynamic, ongoing, life sustaining by which living organisms adjust to environmental changes" (Miller-Keane Dictionary, 2003) Because the patient with a wound requires a change in behavior for healing to occur and to prevent recurrence, facilitating adaptation becomes an essential function of the wound care specialist. Facilitating adaptation must be the underlying philosophic approach when establishing a plan of care.

Historically, the term *noncompliant* has been used to describe many of the patients who, for whatever reason, do not comply or adapt to interventions that a health care provider deems necessary. In a study by Hallett and colleagues (2000), 62 community nurses were interviewed about their perceptions of noncompliance. Descriptions of the noncompliant patient's behavior ranged from passive resistance and lack of motivation to overt refusal and deliberate interference with care. Patients, on the other hand, reported a lack of understanding of why or what they were supposed

to do, or an inability to perform prescribed interventions (Edwards, Moffatt, and Franks, 2002).

This gap in perception leads to obvious questions about the term *noncompliance*, which has been described as an arrogant term suggesting that the patient's job is to do what he or she is told to do by the health care provider (Rappl, 2004; van Rijswijk, 2004). In fact, it is not the wound care specialist's role to *make* the patient comply, adhere, or obey. Rather, the provider's role is to assist in the development of a **sustainable plan** designed to help achieve **mutually** agreed-upon goals.

SIGNIFICANCE

Today, the shift of health care in the America is toward finding ways to manage growth, because the cost of health care (as a percentage of our income) is increasing while, at the same time, our population is aging. One area of focus on the list of many health care experts is managing chronic disease. Chronic disease is known to increase with age, the aging population is growing, and current medical care of chronic diseases accounts for more than 75% of the nation's $1.4 trillion medical care costs (CDC, 2005). A significant part of these costs is related to repeated cycles of instability and hospitalization, and thus Centers for Medicare and Medicaid Services (CMS) is looking to community-based care that fosters patient independence to help manage chronic disease more effectively. Patients are being asked to assume greater responsibility for all aspects of their care. The consequences of failing to facilitate adaptation are severe and significant. These include wound deterioration, unplanned hospitalization, and reduced quality of life. Patient adaptation, involvement, and accountability affect outcomes in chronic disease management.

The authors gratefully acknowledge Barb Henry for assistance with manuscript preparation.

There is also considerable impact when adaptation does not occur. In the United States the economic costs related to medications being taken incorrectly, or not taken at all, add up to as much as $100 billion annually in health care and lost productivity, and up to $8.5 billion annually in preventable clinic visits and hospitalizations (Durso, 2001). The WOCN Society (2003) estimates that $2.2 to $3.6 billion is spent annually for the care of pressure ulcers. "Noncompliance" is cited as one of the causes of the 13% to 56% recurrence rate of pressure ulcers.

BARRIERS TO ADAPTATION

When planned interventions are not completed, the best question is not, "What's wrong with the patient?" Rather we should be asking, "What's wrong with the plan?" At this point, the patient and the wound management team must together reevaluate the goals to identify the actual or potential barriers to adaptation.

Ideally, this process should occur while developing the initial plan of care so that barrier can be minimized or eliminated at the onset. Potential or actual barriers and suggestions for minimizing the barriers are listed in Table 26-1 and described below.

Inappropriate Goals

The patient with a wound must make adaptations to accommodate to many situations because wound healing often involves the management of underlying disease. To understand the range of adaptations needed, it is essential to learn what impact the wound has on the patient's life. The goal of wound healing as a standard for all patients with a wound is unrealistic and often inappropriate. For example a patient who is malnourished and has exhausted all options for optimizing nutrition and does not care to receive enteral or elemental feedings will not achieve the goal of wound healing. Once the patient understands that the

TABLE 26-1 Barriers to Adaptation

BARRIER	INTERVENTION
Inappropriate goals	Collaborate with the patient; make sure goals are mutual
	Set goals based on best evidence
	Make sure goals are clearly understood
	Explain interventions needed to accomplish goals before the patient commits to the goal
	Adjust goals as needed for changes in assessment parameters
Depression	Collaborate with social services and physician for appropriate referrals
Cognitive impairment	Simplify procedures
	Choose products that are easy to use
	Use combination products to minimize steps
	Encourage use of memory aids
	Make an occupational therapy referral
	Clearly label supplies
	Dispense appropriate number of supplies
Impaired dexterity	Collaborate with occupational therapy
	Simplify procedures
	Choose products that are easy to use
	Use combination products to minimize steps
	Provide assistive devices
Impaired mobility	Assess transfer method
	Assess transportation method
	Provide assistive devices
	Clearly label supplies
	Dispense appropriate number of supplies

Continued

TABLE 26-1 Barriers to Adaptation—cont'd

BARRIER	INTERVENTION
Complicated regimens	Simplify procedures
	Choose products that are easy to use
	Use combination products to minimize steps
	Clearly label supplies
	Dispense appropriate number of supplies
Financial barriers	Collaborate with social services
Lack of	Identify payer and reimbursement sources
social/environmental	Learn prices of products and less expensive alternatives
resources	Learn resources and available funds available to patients with low income
	Financial guidance for prioritizing
Skepticism	Address concerns immediately
	Do not minimize concerns
	Recommend a second opinion
Unpleasant side effects	Educate regarding unpleasant side effects of therapy before setting mutual goals
of therapy	Provide alternative interventions (and goals as needed)
Regimens that interfere	Consider ADLs and lifestyle before developing the care plan
with activities of daily	Discuss potential interference with ADLs the intervention may cause
living (ADLs) and lifestyle	Provide alternative interventions (and goals as needed)
or are inconsistent with	
patient goals	

BOX 26-1 Questions to Help Determine
Why Goals Were Not Met

- Did the learner ever accept the goals, or were you teaching only what you believed to be important?
- What evidence do you have that the goals were appropriate?
- Were the goals clearly written and understood by teacher and learner?
- Were the goals broken into sufficient intermediate steps to provide guidance?

Data from Redman BK: *The Practice of Patient Education*, St Louis, 2001, Mosby Elsevier.

goal is not realistic, they may want to reconsider the tube feedings, or aim for a goal that keeps the patient home, avoids hospital admission, controls symptoms (e.g., odor, exudate), and enhances quality of life as defined by the patient. The wound care specialist must identify what the patient and family is willing to do to achieve their goals. Box 26-1 provides a list of questions to help determine why goals were not met (Redman, 2001).

Depression

The National Institute of Mental Health estimates that 18.8 million adults in America suffer from depression. This constitutes 9.5% of the population at any given time. Up to 80% of patients with depression are untreated or undiagnosed. Many patients with depression will not ask for help, have difficulty performing activities of daily living (ADLs), and may be unable to follow through with agreed-upon interventions (NIMH, 2001).

Cognitive Impairment

Cognitive impairment may be an obvious barrier to achieving a sustainable wound care plan; however, the presence of cognitive impairment can be subtle. It is important to review past medical records and talk with families so that cognitive deficits can be identified and the plan of care adjusted accordingly. In many settings, occupational therapy and speech therapy can assist in identifying cognitive deficits and can assist the wound care specialist in developing a plan of care that incorporates the unique learning needs of the patient.

Memory aids, for example, have shown effectiveness in medication compliance studies (Durso, 2001). For example, the chair-bound patient with skin breakdown potential might set a watch timer to serve as a reminder to do wheelchair push-ups to relieve pressure and prevent pressure ulcers.

Impaired Mobility

Impaired mobility appears to be another obvious barrier to achieving a sustainable plan of care. It is a direct barrier for the patient with a pressure ulcer and an indirect barrier for other patients, because it affects the patient's independence for activities essential for disease management and wound healing. The extent to which mobility affects a patient's life must be explored thoroughly before realistic goals and interventions can be put in place. Examples of topics to explore concerning mobility include the following:

1. Transportation/ambulation
   - Does the patient drive or rely on a friend, public transportation, or metro mobility (a transit service for people with disabilities)
   - Is the method of transportation safe for the patient and consistent with the plan of care?
   - If the patient travels sitting in a car, will the length of time sitting impair wound healing?
   - Can the patient ambulate in the home without a significant risk of falling?
   - Can the patient ambulate well enough to bathe him- or herself and prepare meals?
2. Transfer method
   - How does the patient transfer?
   - Will the method of transfer cause friction or shear to the wound?
   - Does the clinic have adequate support and equipment for safe transfer to the exam table if necessary?
3. Devices
   - Can the patient apply and remove the device independently?
   - Has the device been evaluated in place with the patient sitting in their regular wheelchair?
   - If the patient needs adaptive equipment, has the home been adapted to support the patient's independence (i.e., canes, crutches, and elevated toilet seats)?

Interventions that are implemented for wound management can actually impair mobility and lead to an ineffective plan of care. Examples of interventions that hinder mobility include:

1. Compression devices
   - Some compression devices limit ability to wear shoes and to exercise
2. Restricted sitting times
   - Limitations placed on sitting times can impair the patient's ability to work or to parent.
3. Devices for wound healing
   - Devices for wound healing can be difficult to handle and impair mobility.

Impaired Dexterity

A wound care specialist has the expertise and resources available to design a plan of care that accommodates to the individual with impaired dexterity. There are many combination dressings and products that eliminate the need for cutting tape. Return demonstrations are critical in these instances. Very often, the patient has learned to compensate for impaired dexterity and just needs an easy-to-apply product and some practice to master its use.

Complicated Regimens

Complicated regimens can lead to mistakes arising from confusion, or omission because of frustration. The potential for error is multiplied when complicated regimens are combined with other barriers such as cognitive deficits, impaired mobility, and impaired dexterity. The combination increases the chances of failure to perform prescribed interventions. The wound care specialist must work to make procedures as simple and understandable as possible. Interventions must be described in as few steps as possible. If multiple steps are required, using combination products can simplify the process (Nix and Ermer-Seltun, 2004). Dispensing appropriate amounts of supplies and clearly labeling them simplifies the procedure for the patient. Combining interventions with routines already established (e.g., mealtimes) will increase the likelihood of success.

Finances and Available Resources

Finances are a powerful risk factor. It is very important to be aware of the payer source and how much will be paid out of pocket. For persons who are elderly, chronically ill, or in a low-income bracket, as much as 31% of their total income may be going to health care.

Many patients cut corners in one aspect of their living (e.g., health care) to afford something else such as rent or food (Lantz, 2003).

As previously mentioned, many medications are not taken as prescribed; some 50% of prescriptions are written for medications that are never even picked up. Financial barriers are frequently sited as a cause for this (Durso, 2001). Wound care supplies can be very expensive. The wound care specialist must be aware of what prescribed interventions cost as well as less expensive alternatives. Many patients are experiencing great stress and may benefit from a discussion about how to prioritize their spending or apply for additional benefit.

The wound care specialist must understand the logistics of obtaining equipment to ensure patients receive proper care when they need it and do not get discharged without vital equipment being ready at the next care setting. Sometimes the resources simply are not there. This may be linked to finances or a lack of support from friends and family that can arise from distance or family dynamics. When shaping a plan of care it is essential to consider not only what is ideal, but also what is realistic; finances can be a powerful motivator. For example, a family member or patient who is not ready to learn a dressing change may become motivated and ready once it is learned how much he or she may have to pay out of pocket for home care.

Skepticism

Patients can become skeptical as they are inundated with information in today's society, from both sources that are credible and others that are misleading or inaccurate. There is a plethora of information on the Internet that can be quickly accessed by anyone. Some Internet sources are extremely helpful whereas others, if followed, can actually sabotage the plan of care. Criteria can be applied to assess the credibility of information on the Internet (see Chapter 1, Table 1-7). The wound care specialist should respectfully discuss this information with the patient. Becoming defensive or dismissing the patient's concerns will leave the patient feeling alienated. Interactions like this can damage the trust between patient and caregiver. The patient should have concerns addressed and be encouraged to obtain a second opinion, if desired.

Potential or Actual Side Affects

Studies have shown that people are less likely to adopt behaviors or implement interventions that have unpleasant side effects. Some examples concern nurses and handwashing, medications and nausea, and others. People make decisions and agree to interventions based on what they know. If they are uninformed about the side effects or do not understand what impact they may have, it is not surprising that the patient may choose to discontinue an activity or to not modify his or her behavior.

Knowledge Deficit

Knowledge deficits are probably the most common barriers associated with a failed plan of care. So and colleagues (2003) estimate that 50% of medical information is **lost** immediately after speaking with a health professional. The next section describes educational assessment and strategies. Because knowledge deficit is so closely linked to adaptation, strategies to facilitate adaptation should emphasize patient learning.

PATIENT LEARNING

Learning is defined as change in an individual caused by experience and does not include changes caused by development. The patient with a wound must learn new strategies and develop new motor skills and attitudes, which are learned in complex patterns, to promote new performance (Redman, 2001) that facilitates adaptation. Regulatory agencies such as the Joint Commission of Accreditation of HealthCare Organizations (JCAHO) have long recognized the importance of patient and family education. Box 26-2 summarizes a number of JCAHO standards for patient education (Canobbio, 2000).

Assessment

Patient education begins with an assessment of what the patient needs to know to achieve recovery and return of function. It must take into consideration all factors that influence the teaching-learning process with particular attention to experiences that influence the patient's ability, motivation, and readiness to learn (Box 26-3). Since education is a critical aspect of wound management, the educational assessment and plan will require a team approach as described in Chapter 2. For example, speech therapy and occupational therapy

BOX 26-2 Summary of JCAHO Standards Statements for Patient Education

- Provide the patient and family with information that will enhance their knowledge and skills necessary to promote recovery and improve functions.
- Encourage patient participation in decision making, and include the family in the teaching process.
- Use an educational program that begins with an assessment and addresses the identified learning needs, abilities, and preferences.
- Consider cultural, religious, physical and cognitive limitations, language, and financial barriers in education assessment.
- Educate patients about the safe and effective use of their medications according to their needs.
- Educate patients about the safe and effective use of equipment and supplies and means of obtaining them.
- Counsel patients as to foods and diets appropriate to illness as well as possible food-drug interactions.
- Provide patients leaving a facility with information on obtaining follow-up care and accessing community resources.

From Canobbio MM: *Mosby's handbook of patient teaching*, St Louis, 2000, Mosby Elsevier.

BOX 26-3 Educational Assessment Factors

- Age and developmental phase
- Cognitive abilities
- Physical ability
- Educational background
- Life experiences that may influence learning
- Cultural and religious practices
- Language skills
- Occupation
- Finances
- Type of health care coverage
- Support from family and friends
- Presence of pain

can provide vital assessment input for communication, language, and physical and cognitive limitations, as well as techniques to incorporate for successful teaching and learning.

Across Ages and Developmental Phases

In developing a plan of care for adults, whether the adult is adapting to his or her own wound management or caring for the wound of another person, the wound care specialist must incorporate basic principles of adult learning into the assessment of the patient. These principles were developed through research done in the 1970s to identify how adults learn. Malcolm Knowles' model (1970) is one of the most well known and is widely used today (Box 26-4). Stephen Covey's description of the three elements needed for an activity to become a habit (1990) is also relevant to adult learning (Figure 26-1).

If the adult is participating in the wound management of a child, features of development that are pertinent to helping children deal with procedures must be taken into consideration (Table 26-2).

BOX 26-4 Principles of Adult Learning

- Adults have a tendency toward self-direction. They have defined roles in life (work and family), and their self-concepts have generally progressed from dependence toward independence. Illness can sometimes cause regression towards dependence but most adults aspire to independence.
- Adult learning is affected by the individual's life experiences that can help or retard the process of learning. A chef, for example, might be easier to teach dressing changes to than an accountant, because a chef has worked with his or her hands on the job.
- Adults are not easily motivated to acquire new knowledge for its own sake. They require specific motivation to focus on learning, such as a problem they need to solve.
- Adults are most strongly motivated to learn what can be applied to their most pressing needs.

From Knowles MS: *The modern practice of adult education*, Englewood Cliffs, NJ, 1970, Prentice Hall/Cambridge.

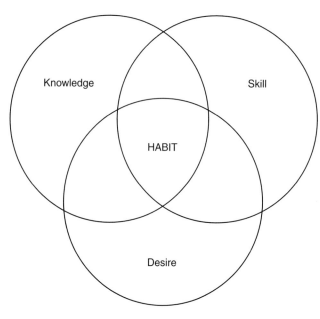

Fig. 26-1 Three elements needed for an activity to become a habit. (From Covey S: *The 7 habits of highly effective people*, New York, 1989, Simon and Schuster.)

- Mastering a new activity requires new knowledge, we need to know "what to do". (This is called the cognitive domain of learning.)

- Mastering a new activity requires new skill, we need to know "how to do it". (This is called the psychomotor domain of learning.)

- Mastering a new activity also requires desire, we need to "want to do it". (This relates to the attitude domain of learning.)

Across Settings

Although patient education has long been a cornerstone of health care practice, the shortening of stays have increased the need for a teaching plan that includes home care. Today's patient is assuming responsibility for aspects of care previously handled in the hospital. Therefore the wound care specialist must broaden the assessment of the patient's educational needs to include the current environment and the environment to which the patient will be transitioning to, and the available resources.

Providing ample time for patient teaching has always been a problem, but with shorter hospital stays, the wound care specialist must take even more care to develop a variety of strategies to ensure the patient's education needs are identified and that progress toward meeting these needs is communicated to providers in the next care setting. In acute care, the education plan begins at admission and must be incorporated into the routine care with the convenience of frequent daily encounters (Canobbio, 2000). Wound care education can be conducted in short sessions. For example, skin inspection could be taught during the patient's bath.

Protection of skin surrounding wounds and moist wound healing can be discussed during dressing changes. Each time a patient is repositioned, pressure ulcer prevention strategies should be taught.

Because of anxiety and discomfort, patients retain little of the instruction in the hospital. Therefore information should be limited to specific content, that is, skills and behaviors necessary to learn before discharge. What the patient needs to know to manage their condition and what can be learned in the limited time available should be prioritized to ensure critical information is mastered first. Early involvement of the family and other caregivers is essential if the patient's clinical condition is a barrier to the patient learning.

In preparing the patient for discharge and formulating the plan, the setting to which the patient will be transferred must be considered. If the patient will be discharged to home the environment must be deemed safe and suitable to carry out the necessary interventions for managing the patient's wounds and the underlying disease(s) (Canobbio, 2000). For example, if the patient's care plan includes limited sitting, does

TABLE 26-2 Features of Development that are Pertinent to Helping Children Deal with Procedures

	BIRTH-2 YEARS	2-7 YEARS	7-12 YEARS	ADOLESCENCE
How the child thinks and problem solves	• Sensory motor experience develops schema (well defined and repeated sequences of actions and perceptions). • Memory is obvious by 3-4 months • Begins using symbols for thought reasoning between about 18 and 24 months.	• Thinking is dominated by perceptions rather than logic. • Verbal communication important for learning. • Exploratory manipulations helps child learn. • Child watches, listens, ask questions (Why? How?). • Classifies similar things. • Perceptions limited to a single salient feature, so difficult for child to differentiate unessential from essential properties of an experience. • Uses memory to reconstruct past events. • Uses imagination to cope. • Egocentric point of view.	• Learns from interacting with peers and own experiences. • Able to understand viewpoints of others. • Able to see the relative nature of things (e.g., this hurts a little, that hurts a lot). • Uses deductive logic in respect to tangible (concrete) experiences (if this, then that). • Able to view things in context, for example, "The shot hurt, but it will make me better." • Evaluates painful intensive actions in terms of logical function rather than punishment. • Understands unseen body mechanics/functions. • Makes use of sensory and procedural information.	• Uses reason and logical thinking. • Interested in theoretically possible problems and questions. • Able to engage in self-reflection. • Learns from verbally presented ideas and arguments.
Major fears and worries	• Separation from parents • Anything unfamiliar, especially when not with a parent	• Separation from parents • Harm to body • Punishment for wrongdoing	• Body injury • Loss of body functions • Loss of control	• Uncertain about selves as persons • Concerned if body, thoughts, and feelings are "normal"
Understanding cause and effect	• By about 3 months, may associate an action with a result • In second year: magical thinking; belief that what is wished for happens	• Everything happens by intention • Misbehaviour is followed by punishment • Interprets unrelated events to be related	• Prior to about 9 years, children view their illness as a consequence of transgressions of rules • At about 9 years, children begin to understand that illness may have multiple causes	• Uses formal rules of logic and evidence to assess cause and effect.

Continued

From Pridham KF, Adelson F, Hansen MF: Helping children deal with procedures in a clinic setting: a developmental approach. *J Pediatr Nurs* 2: 13-22, 1987.

TABLE 26-2 Features of Development that are Pertinent to Helping Children Deal with Procedures—cont'd

	BIRTH-2 YEARS	2-7 YEARS	7-12 YEARS	ADOLESCENCE
Concept of time	• By about three months, shows anticipation for feedings • Can wait as a consequence of perceiving clues of a familiar and desired activity	• Organized around familiar activities of daily living. • By about age 4, has concept of time and day	• Has a concept of the past, future and present • Can understand time intervals between events and clock; time less dependent on activities or daily routine	• Can synthesize the past, present, and future in thinking
Intentions, goals, and plans	• By about 4 months, may show signs of intention/a sense of making an effort to get a result • In second year, child can make a choice of two options	• About age 4, begins to plan and anticipate actions in the near future; has objectives for activities	• Plans more elaborate projects that involve others to a greater extent	• By about age 15 makes plans for future • Can think in terms of tasks as well as responsibilities
Handling emotion	• By about 7 months, the child cries for attention or help • By about 9 months, begins to express fears (e.g., separation) in play	• Expresses emotion motorically and through play • Learns to label feelings • Needs trusted adult to reassure, set limits • Prevent loss of self control	• Greater capacity to express emotion in verbal terms. • Can use projective measures to describe fears (e.g., Explain how another child might feel or respond in a specific situation.)	• May use a range of modalities (i.e., verbal, written motoric activity) • Perhaps regressed ways of behaving. • Thoughts, feelings, and fears may be shared with peers
Relationship with parents/ clinicians	• Developing a sense of self/others • Latter half of first year, begins to sustain the memory of parent in parent's absence, at least for a short time • Depends on adult to know child's wants needs	• Likely to have had experience in relating needs and worries to adults • May not expect clinicians to understand feelings	• Tests limits set by others	• By mid adolescence, has begun to learn how to negotiate a relationship with adults
Self-evaluation	• Feelings about self derive from feeling tones communicated by others and perceived by the child	• Develops expectations of self; learns to inhibit own actions • Begins to use other children as models	• Evaluates self in terms of performance relative to peers and predetermined norms	• May consciously adopt a set of criteria to evaluate self

the patient have the resources necessary to transfer in and out of bed for short periods of sitting?

In the ambulatory care setting, waiting room time can be used to provide education through developed materials that prepare a patient to ask questions regarding disease, medications, diet, and dressings. Space can be provided for educational and audiovisual materials for the patient and family to review before and after their appointments.

Goals and Objectives

Identification and consideration of patient preferences and actions are central to evidence based decision-making (DiCenso, Guyatt, and Ciliska, 2005). Goals that are mutually agreed upon by the patient improve understanding and commitment by the patient to the plan of care. It is important that the wound care team and the patient are realistic when establishing goals for wound healing. Patient and family education is essential for realistic goals setting. Wound healing potential, for example, must be based on the most current evidence and communicated so the patient and family understand (e.g., a patient with peripheral vascular disease with an ankle-brachial index less than 0.5 requires revascularization for healing to occur; venous insufficiency requires compression for wound healing to occur; pressure ulcer healing is not realistic without pressure relief, nutrition support, and management of any urinary or fecal incontinence). When healing is no longer realistic the plan of care should be revised to focus on goals that support the patient's comfort and the need and desire for socialization.

Goals are prioritized into short- and long-term goals. Short-term goals focus on the most pressing issues such as pain control, infection prevention, and dressing changes. Long-term goals focus on disease management and fostering independence. Discharge goals vary by practice setting. Crucial decisions, such as the patient being able to return to their home and live alone, rest on the outcome of learning. The minimum performance necessary for the patient to function must be identified and progress toward this level must be communicated.

Instructional Methods

Measurable learning objectives must be established to support the goals. The wound care specialist should begin with basic lessons and progress according to the patient's ability. Table 26-3 provides a summary of instructor-centered, interactive, individualized, and

TABLE 26-3 **Summary of Instructional Methods**

INSTRUCTOR-CENTERED	INTERACTIVE	INDIVIDUALIZED	EXPERIMENTAL
Lecture	**Class Discussion**	**Programmed Instruction**	**Field or Clinical**
Passive students	Must have small class size	Most effective at lower learning levels	Occurs in natural setting during performance
Efficient for lower learning levels and large classes	May be time-consuming	Very structured	Active student involvement
	Encourages student involvement	Allows students to work at own pace	May be difficult for management and evaluation
		Extensive feedback for students	
Questioning	**Discussion Groups**	**Modularized Instruction**	**Laboratory**
Monitors student learning	Small class size	May be time-consuming	Requires careful planning and evaluation
Encourages student involvement	Student participation	Very flexible formats	Active student involvement in realistic setting
May cause anxiety for some	Effective for high cognitive and affective learning levels	Allows students to work at own pace	

Modified from Weston C, Cranton PA: Selecting instructional strategies, *J Higher Educ* 57(3): 259, 1986; In Redman, BK: *The practice of patient education,* St Louis, 2001, Mosby Elsevier.

Continued

TABLE 26-3 **Summary of Instructional Methods—cont'd**

INSTRUCTOR-CENTERED	INTERACTIVE	INDIVIDUALIZED	EXPERIMENTAL
Demonstration Illustrates an application of a skill or concept Students are passive	**Peer Teaching** Requires careful planning and monitoring Utilizes differences in student expertise Encourages student involvement	**Independent Projects** Most appropriate at higher learning levels May be time-consuming Active student involvement in learning	**Role-Playing** Effective in affective and psychomotor domains Provides "safe" experiences Active student participation
		Computerized Instruction May involve considerable instructor time or expense May be very flexible Allows student to work at own pace Student involvement in varying activities	**Simulations and Games** Provide practice of specific skills Produce anxiety for some Active student participation
			Drill Most appropriate at lower learning levels Provides active practice May not be motivating for some students

experiential instructional methods of teaching (Weston and Cranton, 1986).

Learning from printed materials is an economical use of time if they are well-designed to promote learning, and match the learner's reading and literacy levels. Approximately half the population in the United States struggle with basic reading skills. For many others, the materials available are written at a higher level than they can understand. The reading level of many individuals may be up to five grades below the grade they report to have completed (Redman, 2001). Graphic design techniques that increase readership, comprehension, and memory are summarized in Box 26-5 (Buxton, 1999). For low-literacy readers, increase the amount of white space and use question-and-answer or bullet (not paragraph) format (Massett, 1996). Photos and illustrations decrease the density of the text. Box 26-6 offers additional tips for authors of print materials. Appendix **D** includes examples of teaching materials.

Because different media provide different strengths, use of a variety of media methods is likely to lead to better outcomes than the use of a single medium (Redman, 2001). So and colleagues (2003) conducted a prospective, randomized study with 28 patients with burn injury to compare instructional methods with adherence to dressing changes and hypertrophic scar formation. The standard group received a written handout and verbal rationale for their dressing changes. The enhanced group received a written handout, verbal rationale for their dressing changes, and a video presentation about their burn care. Results revealed that the enhanced group had a statistically significant ($p < 0.001$) improved adherence to their care and less hypertrophic scar formation.

Evaluation and Discharge

As previously stated, crucial decisions, such as those about living safely alone, rest on the outcome of learning and the determination about whether the patient's

BOX 26-5 Graphic Design Techniques That Increase Readership, Comprehension, and Memory

To Direct Readers to the Message

Do

Use arrows, underlines, bold type, boxes, white space, and bullets to direct readers' eyes to the key messages.

Don't

Use italics, all capital letters, script, or screens of color over text.

Require reader to look in many directions on the page to read copy and find the message.

To Select an Easy-to-Read Typeface

Do

Use 10- to 14-point type size.

Use a typeface with serifs in the body copy (e.g., Times Roman).

Don't

Go below 10-point type size for good readers and 12-point for poor readers.

Mix typefaces or use more than three sizes of print on one page.

Use white letters on black background.

To Create Easy-to-Read Copy

Do

Use columns that are 40 to 50 characters wide, left-justified.

Use lots of white space.

Use highly contrasting colors for text and background such as black on white or cream.

Use the same dark color for headings and body copy or colors with similar intensity.

Don't

Break margins with illustrations or other graphics. If required, break only the right margin.

Use light or unusual ink colors such as red, green, or orange.

To Create Clear Visuals

Do

Convey one key message per visual. Print the message in a caption.

Make the message easy to grasp at a glance.

Use realistic drawings, photos, or humanlike figures.

Use visuals with which the audience can identify

Don't

Add any visuals simply to decorate the material.

Include any details or background in the visual that are not required to communicate the message.

Use highly stylized or abstract graphics.

Portray blood cells and other body parts as cartoon characters.

From Buxton T: Effective ways to improve health education materials, *J Health Educ* 30(1):47, 1999; In Redman, BK: *The practice of patient education*, St Louis, 2001, Mosby Elsevier.

BOX 26-6 Tips for Authors of Printed Teaching Materials

Photos and illustrations decrease the density of the text.

Make key messages easy to find.

Use the first paragraph to communicate the benefits the audience desires most and the actions to obtain them.

Provide true or fictional stories about people taking concrete actions and experiencing consequences that are interesting to the reader.

Describe, step by step, the action requested.

Provide pictures and words that evoke vivid imagery, which will be better remembered than abstract words.

Write text in second person (i.e., "you") to convey information personally relevant to readers.

Increase rehearsal of information by repeating it, highlighting it, or boxing it, and ask readers to perform specific activities.

Provide materials sensitive to the culture of those with whom they will be used, addressing their lifestyles and using cultural language and symbols.

From Redman, BK: *The practice of patient education*, St Louis, 2001, Mosby Elsevier.

essential needs can be met. Adequacy of learning must be evaluated in terms of meeting the final objectives and commonly accepted outcomes. Critical pathways (an example is provided in Appendix C) provide a structure of expected outcomes within particular time frames that guide all care, including patient education.

If established goals are not being met, barriers, goals, and interventions must be reassessed and adjusted. Sometimes changes are made in the care plan based on what the family and patient is willing or able to do to meet established goals. For example in the absence of a payer source, a family member may become willing to participate and learn a dressing change rather than pay out of pocket for someone else to do it.

Progress toward goals must be reported to the next care setting or follow-up source. Discharge information should include specific supplies needed for treatment, an available supply source, and step-by-step instructions with a generic list of products used with the example of what brand is currently in use.

SUMMARY

The three principles of wound management are (1) control or eliminate causative factors, (2) provide systemic support to reduce existing and potential cofactors, and (3) maintain a physiologic local wound environment. However, only with the participation and cooperation of the patient can these principles be followed. Regardless of the extent of the wound care specialist's level of expertise and regardless of the type of products or protocols used, wound healing will be delayed or nonexistent, and wounds associated with chronic conditions will often recur, if the patient experiences barriers to enacting the plan of care. Therefore, wound care services must be guided by an underlying philosophy, that the care provider partner with the patient to develop a sustainable plan of care based upon mutually agreed-upon goals. The wound care specialist is in a pivotal position to avoid discrediting the patient with guilt-ridden labels such as *noncompliance*. In contrast, it is the charge of the entire wound management team to facilitate the patient's adaptation to his or her condition and participation in the plan of care. When barriers to the patient's ability to adapt and become involved in care are identified and eliminated, the wound healing potential is maximized.

SELF-ASSESSMENT EXERCISES

1. Explain why noncompliance should not be used to describe patients.
2. List 10 potential barriers to achieving a sustainable plan.
3. List five factors to assess before developing an educational plan.
4. Explain the difference between short-term goals and long-term goals.

REFERENCES

Buxton T: Effective ways to improve health education materials, *J Health Educ* 30(1):47 1999.

Canobbio MM: *Mosby's handbook of patient teaching*, St Louis, 2000, Mosby Elsevier.

Centers for Disease Control and Prevention (CDC) 2005, http://www.cdc.gov/nccdphp/overview.htm; Accessed September 12, 2005.

Covey S: *The seven habits of highly effective people*, New York, 1990, Simon and Schuster.

DiCenso A, Guyatt G, Ciliska D: *Evidenced-based nursing: a guide to clinical practice*, St Louis, 2005, Elsevier Mosby.

Durso S: Technological advances for improving medication adherence in the elderly, *Ann Long-Term Care* 9(4):43, 2001.

Edwards LM, Moffatt CJ, Franks PJ: An exploration of patients' understanding of leg ulceration, *J Wound Care* 11(1):35, 2002.

Hallett CE, Austin L, Caress A, Luker KA: Community nurses' perceptions of patient 'compliance' in wound care: a discourse analysis, *J Adv Nurs*. 32(1): 115-123, 2000.

Knowles MS: *The modern practice of adult education*, Englewood Cliffs, NJ, 1970, Prentice Hall/Cambridge.

Lantz M: Economic noncompliance in the treatment of depression: when the patient can't afford prescription drugs, *Clin Geriatr* 11(09): 18-22, 2003.

Massett HA: Appropriateness of Hispanic print materials: a content analysis, *Health Education Res* 11:231, 1996.

Miller-Keane Encyclopedia and Dictionary of Medicine, Nursing and Allied Health, Philadelphia, Pennsylvania, 2003, Elsevier.

National Institute of Mental Health (NIMH): The number count: mental disorders in America, 2001, http//www.nimh.nih.gov/publicatr/numbers.cfm; Accessed May 23, 2005.

Nix D, Ermer-Seltun J: A review of perineal skin care protocols and skin barrier product use, *Ostomy Wound Manage* 50(12):59, 2004.

Pridham KF, Adelson F, Hansen MF: Helping children deal with procedures in a clinic setting: a developmental approach, *J Pediatr Nurs* 2(1):13, 1987.

Rappl L: Non-compliance: adding insult to injury, *Ostomy Wound Manage* 50(5):6, 2004.

Redman, BK: *The Practice of Patient Education*, St Louis, 2001, Mosby Elsevier.

So K et al: Effects of enhanced patient education on compliance with silicone gel sheeting and burn scar outcome: a randomized prospective study, *J Burn Care Rehabil* 24(6):411, 2003.

van Rijswijk L: Non-compliance no more, *Ostomy Wound Manage* 50(1):6, 2004.

Weston C, Cranton PA: Selecting instructional strategies, *J Higher Educ* 57(3):259, 1986.

Wound, Ostomy and Continence Nurses (WOCN) Society: *Guideline for management of pressure ulcers*, WOCN Clinical Practice Guideline Series #2, Glenview Ill, 2003, Author.

27 *Billing, Coding, and Reimbursement*

....

RUTH BRYANT, BEN PEIRCE, & KATHLEEN SCHAUM

OBJECTIVES

1. Discuss the impact of the U.S. Centers for Medicare and Medicaid Services on billing, coding, and reimbursement of wound care.
2. Describe the key features of the three current payment structures known as fee for service, prospective payment, and payment for performance.
3. Link four coding systems to their applicable care settings.
4. Define provider billing and "incident to billing," including who is allowed to use each method.

A successful wound care program is built not only on astute and efficient wound assessment and management skills but also on an understanding of the health care system's coverage and payment policies. Awareness of reimbursement billing guidelines and the terminology used (Table 27-1) will position the wound care specialist to meet the needs of more patients (CMS, 2005a) by utilizing resources in an evidence-based, justifiable manner that minimizes over-utilization while optimizing reimbursement to the facility or agency (Alterescu, 1997). Clinicians also earn the trust and respect of administration in their facility or agency when a concern for controlling the cost of care while maintaining program viability is evident.

The importance of being familiar with reimbursement guidelines has increased in the recent past because of regulatory changes at the Centers for Medicare and Medicaid Services (CMS). These changes have made the financial impact of clinical decisions more significant in every care setting (CMS, 2005a). While the changes have been painful for some clinicians and facilities, most were inevitable given the development of the U.S. health care system during the twentieth century.

HISTORICAL PERSPECTIVE

Throughout American history until the 1950s, health care was largely a self-paid system that had limited impact on the morbidity and mortality rates of society (Alterescu, 1997). People who could afford it had health care in their homes, mostly provided by a doctor at their bedside. Except for surgery, hospitals were largely a place for the poor to receive care near the end of life. This was the time in health care before many of the things routinely used today existed: infusion therapy, antibiotic therapy, invasive and noninvasive diagnostic testing and, of course, modern anesthesia and surgery.

By the 1960s, new technologies emerged that resulted in significant improvements in health care outcomes. As a result, there was marked growth in the number of facilities and clinicians that led to society's interest in health insurance to ensure access to care. A significant threshold was crossed in 1965 with the passage of the Social Security Act, which created the Health Care Financing Administration (HCFA), now known as the Centers for Medicare and Medicaid Services (CMS), and two national healthcare programs: Medicare and Medicaid. CMS is a federal agency administered by the Department of Health and Human Services and is divided into three primary lines or services as described in Table 27-2 (Turnbull, 2001).

The CMS, responsible for establishing the payment system for Medicare and Medicaid beneficiaries, pays over 50% of the health care dollars in the United States. Private insurers, health maintenance organizations (HMOs), and Veteran's Administration (VA) pay for the remaining health care services. Many of these programs set their coverage and payment policies to coincide with Medicare policies.

TABLE 27-1 Acronyms Used in Coding Billing and Reimbursement

ACRONYM	NAME
APC	Ambulatory Payment Classification
CMS	Centers for Medicare and Medicaid
CPT	Common Procedure Terminology
DMERC	Durable Medical Equipment Regional Carriers
DRG	Diagnosis-Related Groups
E&M	Evaluation and Management
HCFA	Health Care Financing Administration
HCPCS	Healthcare Common Procedure Coding System
HHRG	Home Health Resource Group
HMO	Health Maintenance Organizations
ICD	International Statistical Classification of Diseases
LCD	Local Coverage Determinations
OASIS	Outcome and Assessment Information Set
P4P	Payment for Performance
PPS	Payment Reimbursement System
RBRVS	Resource-Based Relative Value Scale
RUG	Resource Utilization Group
SADMERC	Statistical Analysis Durable Medical Equipment Regional Carrier
UPIN	Unique Provider Identification Number

MEDICARE

Medicare is an insurance program created for people aged 65 or older, for those of any age with permanent kidney failure, and for certain people under age 65 classified as disabled. Governed by federal statutes, regulations and national coverage policies, CMS contracts with commercial insurers to process claims. As illustrated in Figure 27-1, Medicare has three components:

- *Medicare Part A* is a hospital insurance program that covers care in inpatient hospitals including critical access hospitals and care in a skilled nursing facility (not custodial or long-term care). It also helps cover hospice care and some home healthcare. Medicare Part A has no premiums. Commercial insurance companies process Medicare Part A claims and are known as fiscal intermediaries.
- *Medicare Part B* is supplemental medical insurance and provides coverage for physician services, outpatient services, durable medical equipment, and other services not provided by Medicare Part A (e.g., services of an advanced practice nurse or physical therapist, and some home health care). Medicare Part B is available to all Medicare-eligible beneficiaries but they must pay a monthly premium, which is deducted from the social security check, and also pay an annual deductible. CMS contracts with four commercial carriers, each representing a region of the United States, to

TABLE 27-2 Centers for Medicare and Medicaid (CMS)

CMS DIVISION	RESPONSIBILITY
Center for Medicare Management	Administer and manage the traditional Medicare program
	Develop payment and coverage policy for Medicare providers
Center for Beneficiary Choice	Act as a resource for consumer information on Medicare, Medicare Select, Medicare + Choice (Medicare Advantage) and Medigap options
	Oversee and manage Medicare + Choice (Medicare Advantage) programs
	Conduct research and demonstration projects
	Perform claims appeal functions
Center for Medicaid and State Operations	Oversee health care programs administered by the states including the following:
	• Medicaid
	• State Children's Health Insurance Program (SCHIP)
	• Insurance regulation functions, survey and certification
	• Clinical Laboratory Improvement Act (CLIA)

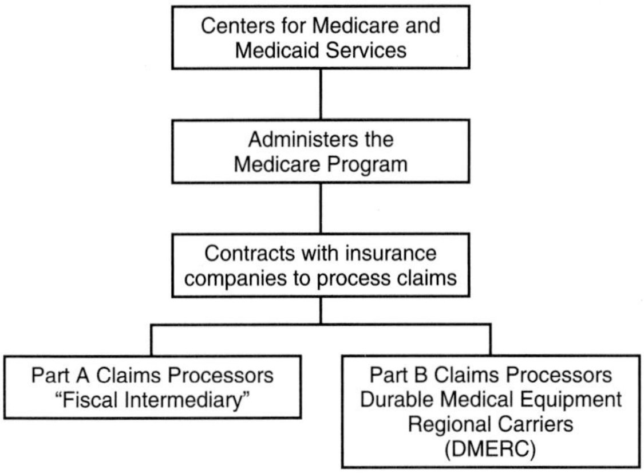

Fig. 27-1 Implementation of Medicare Policy. (Wound, Ostomy and Continence Nurses (WOCN) Society: *Professional practice manual*, ed 3, Mt. Laurel, NJ, 2005, Page 89.)

process durable medical equipment, prosthetics, orthotics, and supplies under the Medicare Part B program. These carriers are known as durable medical equipment regional carriers (DMERCs).

- *Medicare D* is a supplemental prescription drug program available to anyone with Medicare, regardless of their income. The participant pays a monthly premium and if they have limited income and resources, they may get this coverage for little or no cost. Coverage helps pay for prescription drugs. There are many different drug plans available in each state which are approved by Medicare, but administered by private companies.

MEDICAID

Authorized under Title XIX of the Social Security Act, Medicaid provides health services to individuals with low income and is administered jointly by federal and state programs. Within broad national guidelines, each state administers its own program and establishes its own eligibility and type, amount, duration, and scope of services. For this reason, Medicaid programs will vary greatly from state to state.

HISTORY OF MEDICARE PAYMENT SYSTEMS

Fee for Service

The initial structure for payment under the Medicare policy was a fee-for-service structure whereby services

were provided and bills were submitted and paid without questioning or scrutiny regarding treatment, effectiveness, or utilization of resources. This type of structure provided fertile ground for growth in the delivery of health care industry (i.e., technology advancement, research, and staffing). Under Medicare's fee-for-service reimbursement system, health care organizations tended toward maximizing service or utilization. Although clinicians providing care performed their jobs ethically, there were no incentives to ensure the services provided actually improved patient outcomes. The fee-for-service system encouraged providers to focus on providing costly interventions for acute problems and failed to encourage incentives for the early, proactive care needed to manage chronic diseases. In acute and subacute care, for example, the fee-for-service system fostered excess capacity in some profitable markets and shortages in others. In ambulatory and home health care, it fostered growth in utilization without measurable reductions in hospitalizations and emergent care; areas where community-based care was expected to significantly affect costs.

In spite of the benefits of these important advancements, within 20 years the cost of health care in America was growing more rapidly than incomes, and this growth failed to significantly improve the health of the average American (Foster, 2000). Hospital admissions for chronic disease, for example, had not decreased, and death and disability rates had failed to decrease as well. Congress was finally compelled to take action when demographers began publishing research that showed the age of the average America was increasing. This added additional pressure on projected future costs of Medicare and Medicaid. This growth in spending and lack of accountability eventually led Congress to pass legislation in the 1980s and 1990s that changed Medicare payment in every care setting (acute, subacute, out-patient, and home health) from a "fee-for-service" system to one of several forms of "prospective payment" (Twight, 1997).

Prospective Payment Systems (PPS)

In a prospective payment reimbursement system, health care organizations (and individual providers who bill for their services) are paid a predetermined amount to care for the patient regardless of what services are

TABLE 27-3 Type of Medicare Prospective Payment by Site of Service

SETTING/DEFINITION	MEDICARE PAYMENT SYSTEM	DRESSINGS	MEDICATIONS	BIOLOGICS	EQUIPMENT
Hospital	Diagnosis-Related Groups (DRGs) *Patients are classified into DRG groups based upon diagnosis, procedures performed, age, and discharge status. Each DRG is assigned a payment rate, which is adjusted geographically.*	Included (bundled)	Included (bundled)	Included (bundled)	Included (bundled)
Hospital-based wound care clinic Definition: receiving care for an acute or chronic wound in a hospital clinic	Ambulatory Payment Classification (APC) *Services and procedures are assigned to APC groups based upon resource utilization and clinical comparability. Each APC group is assigned a payment rate, which is adjusted geographically.*	Included (bundled) with each visit	Included (bundled) with each visit	Separately paid if assigned pass-through or new technology status or if assigned to a unique APC group	Patient purchases through a durable medical equipment (DME) supplier
Physician office Definition: receiving care for an acute or chronic wound in a physician's office or a nonhospital clinic	Resource-Based Relative Value Scale (RBRVS) *Services and procedures are assigned relative weights based on the resources (work, practice expenses, malpractice insurance). Each year a conversion factor is assigned that converts the relative weights into payment rates. The rates are then geographically adjusted.*	Included	Patient purchases through a pharmacy	Separately paid if assigned a HCPCS code that begins "J" and with if covered	Patient acquires through a DME supplier
Skilled Nursing Facility Medicare Part A	Resource Utilization Group (RUG)	Included (bundled)	Included (bundled)	Included (bundled)	Included (bundled)

Definition: receiving skilled nursing care after a related 3-day inpatient hospital stay. (Benefits last for 100 days as long as skilled care guidelines are met.)	*Resources needed to provide care for specific periods of time are assessed via a standard tool called the Minimum Data Set. The information derived from this tool sorts each patient into an RUG, which is assigned a unique payment rate and is geographically adjusted.*				Included
Nursing Facility Medicare nonskilled Part B or assisted living. Definition: resides in a nursing home and does not meet Part A guidelines or resides in an assisted living facility	Medicare Part B covers dressing supplies under the same guidelines as beneficiary residing at home.	Separately paid	Patient purchases through a pharmacy	Separately paid to either nursing facility or outside Part B entity	
Home health care. Definition: receiving any of the following: (1) part-time skilled nursing (2) PT or OT (3) Speech therapy (4) Home health aide services (5) Medical social services	Home Health Resource Group (HHRG) *The clinical, functional, and service resources needed for 60-day episodes of care are assessed via a standardized tool called the Outcome and Assessment Information Set (OASIS). The information derived from the OASIS groups each patient into an HHRG, which is assigned a unique payment rate and is geographically adjusted.*	Included	Patient purchases through a pharmacy	Patient acquires through a Part B entity	Provided by a Part B entity (DME supplier) if a covered item and medically necessary
Durable medical equipment supplier for patient (1) Residing at home and not receiving home health (2) Residing in a nursing home but not qualifying for Part A (3) Residing in assisted living facility	Durable Medical Equipment Regional Carrier (DMERC) Fee Schedule	Separately paid	Patient purchases through a pharmacy	Separately paid to Part B entity	Patient acquires through a DME supplier

provided or supplies are used. Table 27-3 lists the type of Medicare prospective payment (i.e., Home Health Resource Group [HHRG], Ambulatory Payment Classification [APC], etc.) by site of service.

The reimbursement amount varies by health care setting, but generally is determined by the average cost of services based on the diagnoses and/or patient assessment. Prospective payment systems encourage providers to analyze how they provide care to control costs and improve quality. This type of plan shifts the risk of unnecessary treatment from the payer to the provider. This change in reimbursement was challenging for many facilities and, as a result, they initially focused on cutting costs rather than on achieving the desired patient outcomes.

The Oasis Dataset and Coverage in Home Health Care. Medicare's payment to home health care agencies is based on a comprehensive patient assessment which includes several wound-related questions with credit for some diagnoses. Knowledgeable wound care specialists, therefore, can have a significant impact on the revenue earned by a home health care for a specific patient's 60-day episode. The comprehensive assessment, known as the Outcome and Assessment Information Set (OASIS), is completed by the registered nurse or physical therapist on admission, at recertification, and at discharge. The most extensive OASIS assessment is done on admission and contains 85 questions that cover the patient's clinical condition and functional status and includes several questions on services received. The payment received can range from $1100 to $5200 and is based on a subset of 23 OASIS questions, shown in Table 27-4, with some consideration for geographic location (Teenier and Peirce, 2003).

Because payment is directly affected by how several wound-related questions are answered, the Wound, Ostomy and Continence Nurses (WOCN) Society developed an OASIS Guidance Document that was accepted by CMS for clarification of how these questions could best be answered (WOCN Society, 2004). This document is available in Appendix E. There are additional resources available from the CMS website, www.cms.gov, under home health care.

Payment for Performance (P4P)

Another payment system, payment for performance, is being demonstrated in some settings as a supplement that may eventually replace the PPS. Ultimately, the goal of those who pay for health care is to pay for *outcomes* rather than procedures or interventions or diseases (Remington, 2005). The goals of improving quality and controlling costs are especially important since older members of society use more health care resources; over the next 30 years the population demographics are projected to continue their shift toward an older average age. To further encourage quality improvement, in 2005 CMS announced plans to add supplemental payment to providers across the continuum of care that excel at improving patient outcomes, a strategy to encourage and reward quality in the health care system (CMS, 2005b). Several demonstration projects for outcomes-based reimbursement have been initiated in the private and government sectors (Wright, 2004). For example, several large group physician practices began testing the financial incentives for improving care in a proactive and coordinated manner during 2005 (Twiss, Lang, and Rooney, 2005).

Predicated on the belief that current reimbursement programs have not curbed health care inflation or enhanced patient outcomes, P4P will provide incentives for excellent performance. P4P will attach reimbursement to performance indicators such as clinical and functional outcomes, resource utilization, or process-tracking measures. Thus this new proposed payment system is predicted to affect facility or agency processes, measurement, and outcomes (Twiss, Lang, and Rooney, 2005). The measure of success will be the agency or facility's ability to keep individuals healthy and in the least expensive health care setting (Wright, 2004). Payment reform through P4P is expected to improve quality of care by (1) reducing clinical practice variation, (2) reducing emergency room visits and unanticipated hospital admissions, (3) improving efficiency of care delivery, and (4) facilitating quicker and more efficient coordination among providers by using new information technologies.

CODING SYSTEMS

Billing involves submitting documentation for either a *service* or a *product* that has been provided and is anticipated to be covered by the payer. Actual payment for the service or product (i.e., reimbursement) is contingent upon following specific coverage policies

TABLE 27-4 OASIS Questions Affecting Home Health Care Reimbursement

	CLINICAL SEVERITY DOMAIN	
QUESTION	DESCRIPTION	VALUE
M0230/M0240	Primary home care diagnosis (or initial secondary diagnosis for selected ICD-9 diagnostic codes)	If orthopedic DG, add 11 to score If diabetes DG, add 17 to score If neurologic DG, add 20 to score
M0245	Payment diagnosis	Use if a V code is utilized in M0230/240 instead of a case mix diagnosis (noted above) that would attach additional points
M0250	IV/infusion/parenteral/enteral therapies	IV add 14; TPN add 20; enteral add 24
M0390	Vision alterations	add 6
M0420	Pain, more than daily	add 5
M0440	Wound/lesion	add 21 if also have burn/trauma primary diagnosis
M0450	Multiple pressure ulcers—2 or more stage 3 or 4	add 17
M0460	Most problematic pressure ulcer stage	If box (stage) 1 or 2, add 15 to score If box 3 or 4, add 36 to score
M0476	Stasis ulcer status	If box 2, add 14 to score If box 3, add 22 to score
M0488	Surgical wound status	If box 2, add 7 to score If box 3, add 15 to score
M0490	Dyspnea	If box 2, 3 or 4, add 5 to score
M0530	Urinary incontinence	If box 1 or 2, add 6 to score
M0540	Bowel incontinence	If box 2-5, add 9 to score
M0550	Bowel ostomy	If box 1 or 2, add 10 to score
M0610	Behavioral problems	If box 1-6, add 3 to score
	Scoring: Min = 0-7; Low = 8-19; Mod = 20-40; High = 41+	
	FUNCTIONAL STATUS DOMAIN	
M0650 (current) M0660 (current)	Dressing upper and lower body	Add 4 to score if M0650 = box 1, 2, or 3 OR M0660 = box 1, 2, or 3
M0670 (current)	Bathing	If box 2, 3, 4, or 5 add 8 to score
M0680 (current)	Toileting	If box 2-4, add 3 to score
M0690 (current)	Transferring	If box 1, add 3 to score If box 2-5, add to 6 score
M0700 (current)	Locomotion	If box 1 or 2, add 6 to score If box 3-5, add 9 to score
	Scoring: Min = 0-2; Low = 3-15; Mod = 16-23; High = 24-29; Max = 30+	
	SERVICE UTILIZATION DOMAIN	
M0175 line 1	NO hospital discharge past 14 days	If box 1 IS BLANK, add 1 to score
M0175 line 2-3	Inpatient rehab/SNF discharge past 14 days	If box 2 or 3, add 2 to score
M0825	10 or more therapy visits	If yes, add 4 to score
	Scoring: Min = 0-2; Low = 3; Mod = 4-6; High = 7	

ICD, International Statistical Classification of Diseases; *DG,* diagnostic group; *IV,* intravenous; *TPN,* total parenteral nutrition; *SNF,* skilled nursing facility.

BOX 27-1 Benefits to Billing When Reimbursement is Not Possible

- Provides data that can be used to justify current and additional staffing
- Tracks equipment, types of services, and procedures for cost center
- Documents volume of patients and diagnosis addressed

set forth by the payer. Therefore, billing does not ensure reimbursement.

Coding systems can be of great value even when billing does not lead to reimbursement (Box 27-1). Coding systems assist in quantifying and tracking the volume and range of services provided by the wound care specialist as well as the types of patients receiving these services. In addition, this process will provide evidence for additional services or staffing needs. Even if no new money is coming into the organization, the facility may transfer money from one department to another by tracking the billing codes thereby substantiating the services or products provided.

Established standardized coding systems are required to be used so that claims are processed in an orderly and consistent manner. Coding systems are used to classify products, services, and medical treatments; these classifications guide payment (i.e., coverage) to the health care provider and beneficiary. Code systems critical to the billing process are International Statistical Classification of Diseases (ICD), Common Procedure Terminology (CPT), and Healthcare Common Procedure Coding System (HCPCS) (pronounced "hick-picks"). Table 27-5 describes these coding systems and resources for each.

International Statistical Classification of Diseases (ICD)

The ICD is a detailed description of known diseases and injuries published by the World Health Organization (WHO) that is used worldwide for morbidity and mortality statistics. Every disease (or group of related diseases) is described with its diagnosis and is given a unique diagnosis code. Revised periodically, the current version used in the United States is the ICD-9-CM (CM standing for "Clinical Modification").

TABLE 27-5 Coding Systems and Resources Relevant to Wound Care

CODE	USE	RESOURCE MANUAL	EFFECTIVE DATES FOR REVISIONS
ICD	Classification system of patient diagnosis that support medical necessity for services, procedures, and products Describes disease/diagnosis and inpatient hospital procedures	ICD-9-CM International Statistical Classification of Diseases, 9th Revision, Clinical Modification	Effective October 1
CPT	Codes used to describe services and procedures performed by physicians and nonphysician practitioners Describes procedures, professional services and diagnostic tests	Current Procedural Terminology CPT	Effective January 1
HCPCS (level II) codes	Codes used to identify drugs, devices, biologics, and equipment used and ordered for patients	HCPCS Health Care Procedure Coding System National Level II Medicare Codes	Effective January 1

V Codes. The V codes (ICD-9 supplementary codes or codes which are non-classifiable to ICD-9 codes) identify encounters for reasons other than illness or injury, such as healthy patients receiving routine services (i.e., prophylactic vaccination), or for therapeutic encounters (i.e., cast change), for a problem that is not currently affecting the patient's condition (i.e., personal history of other diseases or hazards to health), and for preoperative evaluations. V codes can also describe the personal history of the patient and other conditions or problems that may be a focus of clinical attention or influence treatment.

CPT

The Common Procedure Terminology (CPT) codes, published annually by the American Medical Association (AMA), are a systematic listing and coding of procedures and services performed by physicians and nonphysician providers. The CPT code is a 5-digit code and provides a means for standardizing billing. New codes and changes to the CPT code criteria are issued annually. Hence, current codes should be used because they can affect billing and reimbursement. CPT codes are subdivided into specific procedures or general evaluation and management (E&M) visits.

E&M. The Evaluation and Management (E&M) codes are used for nonprocedural services (i.e., "visit" type services) such as dressing change, wound assessment, monitoring for resolution of complication, and patient teaching. These codes are categorized according to type of patient visit: new, established, initial inpatient consultation and follow-up inpatient consultation. For example, 99211 through 99215 designate established patient office visits. Visits are further categorized into levels according to the amount of time spent face-to-face with the patient or the complexity of the care and decision making provided based upon current criteria bullets. For example, the parameters for a level 1 E&M visit include a focused history and examination with a straightforward medical decision and self-limited or minor problem *or* 10 minutes of time with greater than 50% of the time spent in counseling or coordination of care. In contrast, the parameters for a level 5 E&M visit include a comprehensive history and examination, with complex medical decisions for a moderate to highly severe problem *or* 60 minutes of time with

greater than 50% of the time spent in counseling or coordination of care. CPT codes are essential to substantiate the need for the particular level of E&M code.

A superbill is utilized for the provider to document the corresponding CPT/E&M code and diagnosis or ICD-9 code. The superbill is then submitted to the coding and billing department so that a bill can be generated to the payer.

HCPCS. The Healthcare Common Procedure Coding System (HCPCS) was originally created for use under the Medicare program and is used today by virtually every payer in the United States. The HCPCS is divided into two levels referred to as level I and level II of the HCPCS. Level I of the HCPCS is the CPT code. Because CPT codes are established by the AMA and are limited to procedures and services performed by physicians (and nonphysician providers), they do not include medical equipment or services required by the patient.

HCPCS level II codes, developed in the 1980s, describe and identify health care equipment and supplies in the delivery of health care that are not identified by the HCPCS level I CPT codes. Among other items these include durable medical equipment, prosthetics, orthotics, medical supplies (DMEPOS), and ambulance services. A HCPCS code consists of one alphabet letter (A-V) and then 4 digits. Each code represents a category of similar items or services, not specific products or trade names. Suppliers are responsible to use one of the over 4000 categories of items or services to identify the items when submitting a claim form to the private or public health insurer.

HCPCS codes do not determine reimbursement (coverage or noncoverage) for an item or service. In fact, the existence of a HCPCS level II code does not guarantee reimbursement for that item. Each payer establishes "coverage and payment policies."

Carriers, fiscal intermediaries, DMERCS, and CMS write the coverage and payment policies for HCPCS level II codes. Also created by the CMS but under Title XVIII of the Social Security Act, the Statistical Analysis Durable Medical Equipment Regional Carrier (SADMERC) serves as a resource to DMERCs for further information on coding and reimbursement. Key components of the medical policy include coverage and payment rules, definitions, and utilization parameters (Appendix E) that guide the use of the HCPS codes.

BILLING FOR WOUND CARE PRODUCTS AND EQUIPMENT

Under the PPS payment system, some health care settings get reimbursed for services in a way that includes payment for procedures and treatments; that is, the payment is *capitated*. In those situations, separate billing for wound care products used by the Medicare beneficiary is not allowed. Table 27-3 describes the payment policy for wound care products by health care site.

Reimbursement for claims submitted to the DMERCs for Medicare Part B coverage of wound care products and equipment is guided by the Surgical Dressing Policy as established by the SADMERC and DMERCs. The surgical dressing LCD (Local Coverage Determinations) provides a definition of terms, allowable frequency of dressing change, and payment rules. A partial listing of the surgical dressing coding and payment policy is provided in Appendix E. The complete policy can be accessed online through the CMS and any of the four regional DMERCs. In addition, the manufacturer of each dressing can be contacted, and the HCPCS codes that have been verified by Medicare's SADMERC can be requested. When reviewing the coverage and payment policy, particular attention should be given to the nonmedical necessity coverage, definition of terms, and guidelines and payment rules. Additional guidance for wound care professionals to use in billing wound care supplies are provided as a hyperlink at the bottom of the Surgical Dressing LCDs. When the particular dressing used must be changed more often than allowed in the coverage policy, the wound care specialist or supplier must submit evidence of medical necessity to validate a deviation from policy before reimbursement will be allowed.

BILLING FOR WOUND CARE SERVICES

The ability to bill for services and receive payment for those services is dependent upon coverage policies of the carrier being billed, the health care setting, and the provider's educational background. Many issues overlap. Each insurance contractor will essentially have their own "rules" (coverage policies) about who can bill for services and how these bills are submitted. It is important to become familiar with these coverage policies since the wound care team is exploring

BOX 27-2 General Factors to Consider Related to Reimbursement

- The payment source drives reimbursement.
- Reimbursement is site-dependent.
- Reimbursement is credential-dependent
- Coding is a means of seeking reimbursement.
- Just because a code exists doesn't mean reimbursement will occur.
- All payment sources must be billed at the same rate.
- Private insurance and health maintenance organizations (HMOs) may be willing to negotiate reimbursement for nonphysician providers.
- Referral or prior authorization may be necessary for reimbursement to occur.
- Nonphysician providers (except the Advanced Practice Nurse) must bill Medicare as "incident to."
- Advanced practice providers may bill either "incident to" or directly with their own UPIN

reimbursement and billing options. For example, some payers will require a primary physician referral and/or prior authorization for reimbursement to occur. It is also important to keep in mind that unlike Medicare, many HMOs and private carriers are amenable to contracting for the services of a non-advanced practice wound care specialist. Box 27-2 lists general factors to consider and address when pursuing reimbursement.

In general it is best to consult with the different payers and billing/reimbursement specialists within the health care setting that is providing the wound care service to determine and explore billing and reimbursement options. They are an integral part of the wound management team. The services of the non-advanced practice wound care specialist are considered a part of "bundled care" when the individual is employed by the hospital, long-term care setting, or home care setting. However, in the outpatient care setting the advanced practice wound care specialist has the potential to bill for services as "incident to" or by utilizing their own unique provider identification number (UPIN).

"Incident to" Reimbursement

"Incident-to" refers to services provided that are an integral but incidental part of the physician's personal professional services to the patient (Gosfield, 2001). Nonphysician providers such as the wound care specialist can utilize this method. Incident-to rules require the following criteria to be met:

1. A nonphysician provider must be an employee of the physician or they are both employees of the same entity.
2. The initial visit must be performed by the physician, (i.e., the patient must be "established").
3. There must be direct personal supervision by the physician during treatment (i.e., physically present in same office suite and immediately available).
4. There must be evidence that indicates the physician has continuing active participation in the management of the treatment program.

While there are no Medicare requirements regarding qualifications of the nonphysician provider, state laws should be reviewed to determine if a requirement exists concerning licensure or national certification of the nonphysician provider. Essentially, the nonphysician provider is "invisible" on the claim form when submitted as "incident-to." Claims are paid at 100% of the physician fee schedule.

UPIN (Unique Provider Identification Number)

Billing with a UPIN is required for physician services and is an option for the qualified nonphysician advanced practice providers such as the nurse practitioner (NP). Each federal and private payer assigns a separate UPIN to the qualified physician and nonphysician providers. Using their own UPIN, the NP is reimbursed 85% of the fee schedule. Billing with a UPIN offers the NP the opportunity to bill for any services provided and authorized by state law, without regard to physician presence or the status of the patient as either new or established. Currently qualified providers are applying for a National Provider Identifier (NPI) that will be accepted by all payers.

Contracting for Services

A wound care specialist can always contract for services as an independent consultant with an HMO, insurance company, or in a health care setting (i.e., hospital, long-term care, or home healthcare agency).

In these instances the wound care specialist would bill the agency, facility, or carrier with whom they have a signed agreement in place.

COORDINATION OF CARE AND COVERAGE ACROSS CARE SETTINGS

Billing and reimbursement issues also have an impact on the patient's care when transferring from one health care setting to another as well as that health care facility or agency's ability to provide the type of care requested in a financially solvent manner. When left unaddressed, these issues will jeopardize the coordination of the patient's care across care settings. Issues that should be discussed and a planned coordinated approach developed are discussed in this section.

Learn and Follow the Medicare Coverage Guidelines

Medicare is the single largest payer for patients with wounds in all sites of service and tends to be the model other payers follow for determining coverage for supplies and services. Therefore the wound care specialist must learn to use the appropriate codes and follow the Medicare coverage guidelines that pertain to the services, procedures, medications, dressings, biologics and equipment that they provide and order for patients. Each year a designated member of the wound care program should review new coding books (Table 27-5), coverage policies that pertain to wound care (Box 27-3) and published guidance documents such as the WOCN fact sheets (2005) to identify additions, deletions, and changes that pertain to wound care practice.

BOX 27-3 Coverage Policies That Pertain to Wound Care

....

- Application of bilaminate skin substitutes
- Chronic wound care
- Debridement of ulcers and wounds
- Human skin equivalents
- Negative-pressure wound therapy
- Outpatient physical therapy
- Surgical dressings
- Unna's boots
- Profore boots
- Wound care

Ideally, coding experts or a reimbursement specialist should establish and monitor charges and coding. Also, they should assume the responsibilities of acquiring, maintaining, and reviewing Medicare coverage determinations, articles, and bulletins that pertain to the services, procedures, medications, dressings, biologics, and devices that are provided and ordered for patients with chronic wounds. Strategies for monitoring Medicare coverage determinations are listed in Box 27-4. Monitoring the website for new LCD and article drafts that are released for public comment can be a useful strategy to influence the final coverage

BOX 27-4 Strategies for Monitoring Medicare Coverage Determinations

- Identify Medicare Fiscal Intermediary (FI), Medicare Carrier, and/or Medicare Durable Medical Equipment Regional Carrier (DMERC) that processes the patient's Medicare claims.
- Monitor the Wound, Ostomy and Continence Nurses Society website reimbursement fact sheets for updated information.
- Visit the Medicare contractors' websites and search for all local coverage determinations (LCDs), articles, and bulletins pertaining to every professional in your practice, every service and procedure (CPT code) provided, and every drug, dressing, biologic, and piece of equipment (HCPCS code) used and ordered. Share those documents with your team of wound care professionals via a series of staff meetings, educational programs, and so on. Note that these coverage documents provide a tremendous amount of information including the following:
    - Medicare contractor name and type
    - Primary geographic jurisdiction
    - Effective dates of original determination and revisions
    - Indications and limitations of coverage and/or medical necessity
    - Coding information
    - ICD-9 codes that support/do not support medical necessity
    - Documentation requirements
    - Utilization guidelines
    - Revision history explanation
    - Related documents, such as articles

documents and share all coverage changes with the entire wound care team.

Identify a Facility's Primary Referral Sources

Identify a facility's primary referral sources for wounds and those to whom it typically refers patients with wounds. Clinicians will usually know who the primary referral sources are, but it is also prudent to review recent admissions and discharges to confirm this list. Meet proactively with the managers of these referral sources, and ask if the billing department can be included so that their needs are addressed as thoroughly as possible. During the discussion, identify any documentation needed to support their billing process and reduce their chances of a payment denial. Any attention paid to their reimbursement requirements shows an understanding of their needs and challenges. This discussion will often lead to discussions of a particularly complex case that challenges the resources of every provider involved.

Plan the Typical Pathway of a Patient through the Chain of Providers

When these complex cases emerge, it may be helpful to plan the typical pathway of a patient through the chain of providers and care settings. Discussing them as "typical" cases rather than taking up a specific one sometimes helps everyone involved see issues more objectively. Patients with chronic, wound-related diagnoses such as venous insufficiency or diabetic foot ulcers may go through several cycles of hospitalization, recovery, and rehabilitation each year. Establish common, long-term goals for these patients that will be consistently supported by providers in all care settings even if these patients are admitted to a facility for a short time. Once these long-term goals are established for a patient, communicate them and any progress made toward them to the next provider, so they can build on progress made by clinicians in the previous setting.

Review Wound Dressings Available in Each Care Setting and Agree on Equivalents

Review wound dressings available in each care setting and agree on equivalents so that physician provider orders reflect them and support a smooth patient transfer from one care setting to the next. It is important to understand that many facilities or agencies have established medical supply formularies, and using other products may not be practical unless planned well ahead of time.

Establish Accepted Methods of Communication

Establish accepted methods of communication of orders and patient assessments between providers to support efficient processes and reimbursement. It is important, for example, to provide comprehensive wound assessments to clinicians in the receiving care setting so that appropriate supplies and durable medical equipment can be prepared before the patient is transferred. CMS coverage for negative-pressure wound therapy, for example, in the home requires documentation of a wound assessment to be completed by a clinician in the care setting planning the transfer to continue the treatment uninterrupted in the home.

SUMMARY

Providers must understand a few basics to the billing and reimbursement process. This process will vary from setting to setting. One common goal of all settings is to provide cost-effective patient care. It should be stressed that the most cost-effective wound care may actually be achieved by using a more expensive product or procedure. Cost-effective care incorporates many-faceted procedures and products:

- They require the least disturbance to a healing wound bed.
- They require infrequent dressing changes and professional visits.
- They are readily available.
- They are easy for both the patient and the caregiver to use.
- Their use minimizes complications and the time to heal.

Understanding the current health care system and financial incentives can help the wound care specialist to demonstrate his or her valuable contribution by aligning activities with the goals of an organization. For example, the wound care specialist can standardize wound care products so that the organization is able to negotiate the best price for supplies based on increased volume, or identify at-risk patients for implementation of early interventions, thus reducing wound incidence rates. These examples (see also Chapter 1) are significant cost-saving strategies.

Understanding reimbursement can also improve relations with clinicians in other care settings. If a wound care specialist works in an out-patient wound clinic, for example, and understands that home health care agencies can no longer bill for supplies, he or she might contact the home health care agency before adding a costly new wound care product to their product list. By introducing the dressing through a discussion, out-patient clinicians can often convince the home health care agency that even though the new product is more expensive, it can reduce visits needed to change dressings and lower risks of emergency care to treat wound infections.

Obtaining accurate information on wound care reimbursement can be challenging but is well worth the effort. Wound care specialists knowledgeable in this area are able to be strong patient advocates while supporting high quality care.

SELF ASSESSMENT EXERCISE

1. Describe the difference between Medicare and Medicaid.
2. Describe the services provided by Medicare Part A, Medicare Part B and Medicare Part D.
3. A fee-for-service payment structure allows services to be provided and billed without scrutiny regarding treatment, effectiveness or utilization of resources: True or false?
4. Which of the following is true for payment for performance (P4P)?
   a. It was the payment structure used before PPS.
   b. It will eventually replace PPS.
   c. It involves payment only if the wound heals.
   d. None of the above.
5. Which of the following is true for level I Healthcare Common Procedure Coding System (HCPCS)?
   a. They are CPT codes.
   b. They are established by the AMA.
   c. They do not include medical equipment or services required by the patient.
   d. All of the above
6. Level II Healthcare Common Procedure Coding System (HCPCS) codes may not be used if level I HCPCS codes are already used: True or false?
7. List three methods for billing for services.

REFERENCES

Alterescu V: Managed care primer. In *Patient access to continence services: protecting it under managed care,* 1997, SUNA.

CMS: *Medicare general information, eligibility and entitlement manual,* http://www.cms.hhs.gov/manuals/101_general/ge101index.asp, 2005a; Accessed November 1, 2005a.

CMS Office of Public Affairs: *Fact sheet: Medicare "Pay For Performance (P4P)" Initiatives,* CMS Office of Public Affairs, 202-690-6145, January 31, 2005b.

Foster R: Trends in Medicare expenditures and financial status 1966-2000, *Health Care Financing Review* 22(1):35, 2000.

Gosfield AG: The ins and outs of "incident-to" reimbursement. *Fam Pract Manag.* Nov-Dec/8(10):23-7, 2001.

Remington L: Pay for performance is here. The link between outcomes, disease management and pay for performance. *Remington Report,* 13:2, 2005, www.remingtonreport.com; Accessed November 1, 2005.

Teenier P, Peirce B: OASIS: More than an assessment, *Extended Care Product News* 86(2):36, 2003.

Turnbull GB: Bits and pieces, *Ostomy Wound Manage* 47(8):9, 2001.

Twight C: Medicare's origin: the economics and politics of dependency, *CATO J, Interdisciplin J Pub Pol Anal* 16(3):309, 1997.

Twiss A, Lang C, Rooney H: Pay for performance preparedness, *Remington Report* 13:2, 2005; www.remingtonreport.com; Accessed November 1, 2005.

Wound, Ostomy and Continence Nurses (WOCN) Society: *OASIS Guidance document,* Glenview, Ill, 2004, Author.

Wound, Ostomy and Continence Nurses (WOCN) Society: *Professional practice manual,* ed 3, Mt. Laurel, NJ, 2005.

Wright K: The future of health care. Home is where the health is, *J WOCN* 31(6):315, 2004.

SELF-ASSESSMENT ANSWERS

CHAPTER 1

1. c
2. a
3. b
4. c

CHAPTER 2

1. A) Wound management is conceived as being the comprehensive holistic consideration of the patient so that all factors contributing to and affecting the wound are addressed as effectively as possible. Typically a physician oversees this level of care. In the United States, wound care nurses who are also nurse practitioners may function in the wound management oversight position. Many settings in the United States have certified wound care nurses who work collaboratively with designated physicians to manage patients with wounds.

B) Wound care is more reflective of topical therapy alone. Skills for wound care include wound assessment and appropriate product utilization for prevention and local care of wounds. A certified wound care nurse guides this particular aspect of treatment.

2. Advantages to a centralized multidisciplinary team of specialists include the following:
- Wound care, especially topical, is similar for all types of wounds.
- The staff will learn the nature of and treatment for all types of wounds.
- Treatment plans for different types of wounds will be standardized.
- Resources and the diagnostic and treatment armamentarium will be used optimally.
- The creation of a wound management specialty or service is facilitated.
- Wound treatments will gain credibility.
- Education and treatment will become more cost-effective.

3. Responsibilities of a multidisciplinary wound management committee or team include the following:
- Establish an individualized wound management plan for each patient.
- Review, update, and plan for follow-up for each patient at routine intervals.
- Standardize protocols for risk assessment
- Direct clinical trials of products using standard evaluation protocols
- Review quality assurance findings and patient care outcomes.
- Develop and implement strategies for quality improvement
- Support the development of patient education materials.
- Evaluate and disseminate outcome analysis results

4. Establishing a multidisciplinary wound management approach require the following:
- Characterization of the problem
- Definition of aims or goals
- Selection of a model or concept
- Integration of the concept in the national health care system
- Creation of the single elements of the organization (centers/teams)

5. Elements of a multidisciplinary wound management program include the following:
- Wound diagnosis
- Wound classification
- Wound treatment
- Follow-up for wounds
- Quality assurance
- Wound-healing research
- Education

CHAPTER 3

1. The skin serves as a protective barrier against the external environment and contributes to the maintenance of a homeostatic internal environment.

2. The key layers of the skin are epidermis, basement membrane, dermis, and hypodermis.

3. Cells in the stratum corneum are primarily epithelial cells, which are referred to as keratinocytes because they are almost completely filled with keratin, a fibrous protein.

4. c

5. Rete ridges are the epidermal protrusions of the basal layer that point downward into the dermis. They help to anchor the epidermis, thus providing structural integrity.

6. b

7. The two dermal proteins are collagen and elastin. Collagen is the protein that gives skin its tensile strength; key constituents are proline, glycine, hydroxyproline, and hydroxylysine. Collagen is secreted by dermal fibroblasts. Elastin provides the skin with elastic recoil; key constituents are proline and glycine (not hydroxyproline).

8. The six major functions of the skin are protection, thermoregulation, sensation, metabolism, immunity and communication

9.
- The keratinocytes of an intact stratum corneum provide a resistant barrier; the constant shedding of squames prevents entrenchment of microorganisms.
- The sebum secreted by the sebaceous glands maintains an acid pH (4 to 6.8), which inhibits growth of microorganisms.
- The normal skin flora provides bacterial interference to pathogens.
- The skin has an immune system: Langerhans' cells in the epidermis, and macrophages and mast cells in the dermis. Langerhans' cells are antigen-presenting cells, macrophages phagocytize bacteria, and mast cells contribute to the inflammatory response by release of histamine.

10. c

11. c

12. Premature infant skin is thin, poorly keratinized, and functions weakly as a barrier. Transepidermal water loss is high as are evaporative heat losses. Newborn skin and nails are thinner than those in the adult; with aging they will gradually increase in thickness. Newborn skin is not an effective barrier to transcutaneous water loss. Newborn dermis is 60% as thick as adult dermis; dermal fibers are finer than adult dermal fibers. Newborn dermis has a higher cellular component than adult skin. Rete ridges are weakly developed at birth. Capillary beds in the newborn dermis are disorganized.

13. In adolescent skin: hormonal stimulation increases the activity of sebaceous glands and hair follicles. In adult skin; dermis thickens; epidermal turnover time is increased; barrier function is reduced; number of active melanocytes is decreased; skin is dry; wrinkles; diminished sensory receptors; vitamin D production is decreased.

14. b

15. True

16. c

CHAPTER 4

1. Wounds involving only the epidermis and dermis heal relatively quickly because epithelial, endothelial, and connective tissue can be reproduced. Wounds extending through the dermis and involving deeper structures must heal by scar formation because the deep dermal structures, subcutaneous tissue, and muscle do not regenerate.

2. Wounds that are well approximated with minimal tissue defect are said to heal by primary intention. Wounds that are left open and allowed to heal by production of granulation tissue are said to heal by secondary intention. Wounds are described as healing by tertiary intention when there is a delay between injury and reapproximation of the wound edges.

3. Inflammatory response, epithelial proliferation and migration, and reestablishment and differentiation of epidermal layers are the major components of partial-thickness repair. If dermis is involved, connective tissue repair proceeds concurrently with reepithelialization.

4. A moist wound surface facilitates epidermal migration because epidermal cells can migrate only across a moist surface. In a dry wound, epidermal cells must tunnel down to a moist level and secrete collagenase to lift the scab away from the wound surface in order to migrate. Connective tissue repair begins earlier when the wound surface is kept moist because new connective tissue forms only in the presence of suitable exudate.

5. Inflammatory phase: hemostasis and inflammation. Proliferative phase: neoangiogenesis; matrix deposition/collagen synthesis; epithelialization; and, when a full-thickness wound is left to heal by secondary intention, contraction of wound edges. Maturation phase: matrix deposition and collagen lysis.

6. c

7. b

8. There is a limit to epidermal cell migration, and in full-thickness wounds epidermal cells are present only at the wound margins. In partial-thickness wounds, epidermal cells are present in the lining of hair follicles and sweat glands as well as at the wound periphery.

9. Chronic wounds are likely to begin with circulatory compromise as opposed to injury. Injury initiates hemostasis, which triggers the wound-healing cascade;

circulatory compromise does not trigger the wound-healing cascade. Chronic wounds also contain increased levels of protease produced by the prolonged presence and increased volume of proinflammatory cells.

10. Factors that affect wound healing include tissue perfusion and oxygenation, nutritional status, infection, diabetes mellitus, corticosteroid administration, immunosuppression, and aging. Systemic factors include renal or hepatic disease, malignancy, sepsis, hematopoietic abnormalities, and stress.

11. c

CHAPTER 5

1. selectins, integrins, and cell adhesion molecules
2. false
3. d

CHAPTER 6

1. Factors known to damage the skin include mechanical, chemical, vascular, allergic, infectious, immunologic, burn, and disease-related types.
2. b
3. a
4. Ulcers involve the loss of epidermis and dermis. Healing occurs by scar formation. Erosion involves partial loss of epidermis; tissue loss does not extend below the epidermis. Healing occurs without scarring.
5. Do not apply tape under tension; remove tape slowly by peeling skin away; use porous adhesives; use skin sealants, thin hydrocolloids, or solid-wafer barriers under adhesives; avoid use of tapes by using roll gauze or self-adherent tape; and use Montgomery straps.
6. Apply moisture-barrier ointments after each stool, apply rectal pouch if stooling occurs more than 3 times per 8 hours, and apply ointment pastes if moisture-barrier ointment is ineffective.
7. b
8. d
9. The two phases of an allergic contact dermatitis are sensitization phase and elicitation phase
10. c
11. d
12. TEN, SSSS, and GVHD can result in massive loss of epidermis.

CHAPTER 7

1. *Assessment* includes verification and interpretation of observations made. *Evaluation of healing* involves monitoring and assessment documented over time to reveal patterns and trends that indicate improvement or deterioration in the wound.

2. b
3. b
4. A partial-thickness wound is confined to the skin layers; damage does not penetrate below the dermis and may be limited to the epidermal layers only and heal primarily by reepithelialization. A full-thickness wound indicates that the epidermis and dermis into the subcutaneous tissue or beyond have been damaged; tissue loss extends below the dermis.
5. Indices of wound healing:
   - Etiology/type of skin damage
   - Factors that impede healing
   - Duration of wound
   - Anatomic location of wound
   - Extent of tissue loss (stage)
   - Characteristics of wound base
   - Type of tissue
   - Percentage of wound containing each type of tissue observed
   - Dimensions of wound in cm (length, width, tunneling, undermining)
   - Exudate (amount, type, odor)
   - Wound edges
   - Periwound skin
   - Presence or absence of signs of infection
   - Pain
6. Necrotic, nonviable, or devitalized tissue is tissue that has died and has therefore lost its physical properties and biological activity.
7. Eschar is black or brown necrotic, devitalized tissue; tissue can be loose or firm adherent, hard, soft or boggy.
8. Slough is soft, moist, avascular (necrotic/devitalized) tissue; it may be white, yellow, tan, or green; it may be loose or firmly adherent.

CHAPTER 8

1. a
2. b
3. a
4. a
5. d
6. d
7. b
8. d
9. c
10. d

CHAPTER 9

1. b
2. d
3. a

4. a
5. d
6. c
7. d
8. d
9. b

CHAPTER 10

1. d
2. c
3. Considerations in the use of enzymatic debridement include the following:
   - Enzymes are inactivated by heavy metal ions: chlorine, silver, and mercury
   - It is a slow method of debridement
   - It necessitates dressing changes once to 3 times daily
   - There is little evidence and few criteria available to guide selection of debriding enzyme, which is primarily based on clinician preference, cost, availability, and ease of use
   - Papain/urea agents can cause transient erythema and irritation on intact skin.
4. a
5. b

CHAPTER 11

1. a. Reduced supply of oxygen associated with poor peripheral perfusion is one factor associated with reduced acute wound healing. Reduction in supply of molecular oxygen impairs oxidative killing, effective phagocytosis and collagen production by fibroblasts.
   b. Elevated blood glucose levels is another factor. Hyperglycemia is associated with poor function of immune cells and reduced synthesis of collagen.
2. Observable characteristics of a healing acute surgical wound include absence of drainage and erythema, presence of well-approximated edge, steady decrease in discomfort at incision site, lack of drainage, erythema, dehiscence, excessive pain, and well-approximated edges. Joie, we do not state the characteristics of a healing incision besides the healing ridge ... can you put something in for this? Does this answer sound okay?
3. False
4. False
5. Nursing interventions to optimize wound-tissue perfusion include actively re-warm patient postoperatively, replace fluid, adequately control pain with medications and positioning, decrease exposure to cold, and reduce anxiety with patient education and/or medications
6. Palpable incisional induration is indicative of new collagen at postoperative days 4 to 8 and beyond.

7. Contributors to sympathetic nervous system activation include pain, cutting of afferent nerves, cold, hypovolemia, fear, and surprise
8. d
9. c

CHAPTER 12

1. Differences in the range within similar settings and between settings exist because (1) the data collector's ability to recognize damaged skin varies, (2) a standardized classification system is lacking (e.g., some studies define pressure ulcers as always having breaks in the skin, thus overlooking the potential for pressure damage with intact skin), (3) some institutions have a concentrated population of patients shown to be at increased risk for pressure development, and (4) studies vary in population, design, and expertise of researchers. According to the NPUAP, the prevalence of pressure ulcers in acute care hospitals is 3% to 14% and in nursing homes 15% to 25%. The literature reports a prevalence range of 25% to 40.4% for patients with spinal cord injury and 11.6% to 27.7% in the elderly.
2. A pressure ulcer is a localized area of tissue necrosis that develops when soft tissue is compressed between a bony prominence and an external surface for a period of time
3. a
4. Three factors that play a role in determining the negative effects of pressure are intensity of pressure, duration of pressure, and tissue tolerance
5. b
6. c
7. It is difficult to accurately assign a numerical value to capillary closing pressure because (1) capillary blood pressure is influenced by values such as arterial blood pressure and venous pressure, which vary from individual to individual, from one bony prominence to another, and from time to time; and (2) capillary closing pressure, which is commonly reported as 25 to 31 mm Hg, is based on studies in healthy adult males, whereas recent studies report capillary closing pressures as low as 12 mm Hg in the elderly.
8. c
9. When tissue interface pressures exceed capillary pressures, capillaries close and tissue hypoxia ensues; tissue hypoxia is tolerable for short periods, but prolonged ischemia results in tissue necrosis.
10. Amount and duration of pressure share an inverse relationship in producing tissue ischemia. It takes a long time for low pressure to create ischemia, whereas it takes a short time for high pressure to cause tissue ischemia.
11. d

12. b

13. Four variables that influence the extent of tissue damage associated with pressure are venous thrombus formation, endothelial cell damage, redistribution of blood supply in ischemic tissue, and altered lymphatic fluid flow in the area of pressure

14. Variables that contribute to cellular death in a pressure-damaged area are occlusion of capillaries, impaired perfusion through edematous tissue, and accumulation of metabolic wastes.

15. a

CHAPTER 13

1. Chair cushions, overlays, replacement mattresses, and bed systems are all forms of support surface devices.

2. The four functions of a support surface are pressure redistribution, temperature control, shear reduction and friction reduction

3. False

4. Limitations to the reliance of capillary closing values for support surface evaluation include the following:
- Capillary closing values are based on measurements of the fingertips of young healthy males.
- Lower capillary pressures have been reported in older patients.
- Skin-resting pressures do not ensure that blood flow through the capillaries is unimpeded.
- Pressure is 3 to 5 times greater at the bone than at the surface of the skin

5. Factors that guide the interpretation of the significance of interface tissue pressure readings include the following:
- The range of pressure readings obtained per site and the number of readings conducted per site should be reported instead of one single pressure reading per site.
- The procedure used to acquire the pressure reading should be described.
- The population tested should be described (i.e., healthy subjects as opposed to patients).
- Researchers should state how often equipment was recalibrated, because sensors are fragile and may malfunction.
- Factors known to affect the results of interface pressure measurements should be disclosed (transducer size and shape, the load shape and its interaction with the support material, the method of equilibrium detection, and the uniformity of the measurement technique).
- Uniformity of the measurement technique is necessary, because the skill of the person taking the readings may also make a difference.

6. False: a change in support surface may be necessary as the patient's overall condition and the skin or wound assessment change.

CHAPTER 14

1. a

2. True

3. Two factors that delay wound healing in obese patients are (1) blood supply to fatty tissue may be insufficient to provide an adequate amount of oxygen and nutrients; and (2) wound healing may be delayed if the patient has a diet that lacks essential vitamins and nutrients.

4. c

5. OHS is an acute respiratory condition wherein the weight of fatty tissue on the rib cage and chest prevents the chest wall from expanding fully. Because patients are unable to breathe in and out fully, ventilatory insufficiency can occur.

CHAPTER 15

1. c

2. b

3. c

4. d

5. The classic characteristics of an arterial ulcer include the following: small craters with well-defined borders, wound bed is pale or necrotic, there is minimal exudate from the wound, wound pain is present, and the wound is located distally, on pressure points of the feet, or in the area of trauma.

6. d

7. Venous blood in the lower leg creates a column of hydrostatic pressure (equal to about 90 mm Hg while standing). For venous blood to return to the heart, it must flow uphill against this pressure. The deep veins, intact one-way valves within the veins, and the contraction of skeletal muscles facilitate venous blood return. During ambulation, the calf muscle contracts and pumps blood out of the deep veins, and the one-way valves in the perforator system close to prevent backflow into the superficial veins; when the calf muscle relaxes, the valves in the perforators open to permit blood flow into the deep veins.

8. c

9. b

10. Elastic compression devices deliver a sustained pressure regardless of the patient's activity level (ambulatory or sedentary). Nonelastic compression devices work by compressing the calf muscle during ambulation. Compression devices provide a constant compression to the tissues and superficial veins; they also support the calf muscle during ambulation. The constant compression increases interstitial tissue pressure to reduce leakage of fluid from capillaries. By supporting superficial dilated veins, the diameter of vessels is decreased so that blood velocity is increased and sluggishness of blood flow is decreased, which diminishes the tendency for leukocyte margination and extravasation. The sedentary patient is usually best managed by elastic compression devices.

11. Chronic venous insufficiency and venous hypertension cause leakage of red blood cells and blood proteins into the tissues, which results in progressive dermal fibrosis. These fibrotic changes in the soft tissues result in progressive obstruction to lymphatic flow owing to distortion or obliteration of the lymphatic channels.

CHAPTER 16

1. Sensory neuropathy causes reduced sensitivity to pain and temperature changes, which results in increased susceptibility to injury. Motor neuropathy leads to a loss of innervation to the muscles, which causes foot deformities and changes in gait, which alter weight bearing and result in repetitive stress. These predispose the patient to callus formation and ulceration, unless weight is properly redistributed. Autonomic neuropathy causes a loss of sweating, which leads to chronically dry skin and predisposes the skin to cracking.

2. a
3. d
4. The following must be addressed in the management plan of a patient with a diabetic foot ulcer: causative factors, vascular status, presence of infection, presence of foreign body, degree of neuropathy, presence of necrotic tissue, presence of callus formation, glycemic control, nutritional status, and contributing systemic factors (e.g., smoking, obesity, visual impairment).
5. Routine precautions that one should include in the teaching of the patient with lower-extremity neuropathic disease include the following: daily washing with a mild soap; lubrication/moisturizing after bathing; daily skin inspection and prompt reporting of any skin lesion or callus formation; the fact that shoes must fit properly and that going barefoot is never appropriate; and professional care of toenails, corns, and callus.

CHAPTER 17

1. e
2. c
3. d
4. e
5. c
6. c
7. b
8. a
9. c
10. d

CHAPTER 18

1. The three phases of wound healing that occur in burns are inflammatory, proliferative, and maturation. The inflammatory response is characterized by vasodilation and increased capillary permeability; epidermal cells proliferate between meshed grafts and with partial-thickness wounds; and scar tissue formation and remodeling occur during the maturation phase.
2. All types of burns may occur in the home. Thermal burns occur with exposure to flames, scalds from cooking and hot water spills, and contact with hot objects. Electrical injury can occur when children chew on electrical cords or insert objects into electrical sockets. Chemical burns result from exposure to agents in the home such as rust removers and oven and drain cleaners.
3. The zone of coagulation is the area closest to the heat source and suffers the greatest amount of damage.
4. **(d)** The zone of stasis is an area of ischemia; restoration of circulation, prevention of further damage by infection, drying from exposure to air, rough handling during turning, or pressure will maintain tissue health in this zone.
5. The treatment of a burn wound is based on the *extent, depth,* and *severity* of the burn.
6. **(a)** The Lund and Bower chart is the most accurate for patients of all ages.
7. **(b)** The inflammatory response releases various vasoactive and chemotactic agents that affect vasoconstriction, fluid balance, and metabolism.
8. **(d)** The most accurate method to assess fluid resuscitation adequacy is a urine output of 30 to 50 ml/hr in adults or 1 to 2 ml/kg/hr in children.
9. **(b)** Early excision should occur as soon as possible after fluid resuscitation, before wounds can become colonized.
10. **(b)** Sheet grafts usually have a better cosmetic outcome for facial burns.
11. **(a)** Positioning and splinting are done for the prevention of contractures, which should begin with admission.
12. **(a)** Gram-positive bacteria are the most common type of organism responsible for infection in the patient with a burn.
13. **(d)** All of the answers are considered minor burns.

CHAPTER 19

1. d
2. d
3. b
4. d

5. b
6. d
7. d
8. Prevent and manage infection, cleanse wound, remove nonviable tissue (debridement), maintain appropriate level of moisture, eliminate dead space, control odor, eliminate or minimize pain, protect wound and periwound skin

CHAPTER 20

1. Hyperbaric oxygenation is the systemic, intermittent administration of oxygen delivered under pressure. A hyperbaric environment exists when atmospheric pressure is greater than 1 atmosphere absolute (ATA).
2. b.
3. c.
4. True.
5. d
6. b.
7. d.
8. b
9. c
10. UV-C
11. False
12. Reduction of bacterial load and wound size appear to be the benefits of MIST therapy.

CHAPTER 21

1. Methods of wound closure include secondary wound healing, biosynthetic graft, linear closure, skin graft, and flap creation.
2. The categorization of local flaps can be done according to anatomical structures they encompass, the method used to move the flap, or the method used to perfuse the flap.
3. Urgent operative conditions include traumatic wounds, abscess, wet gangrene, and necrotizing fasciitis.
4. Cofactors that can delay healing of surgical wounds include bioburden, administration of corticosteroids, diabetes, malnutrition, nicotine use, and spasms.
5. c

CHAPTER 22

1. b
2. b
3. d
4. b
5. c
6. d
7. a

CHAPTER 23

1. Factors that may contribute to fistula development after a surgical procedure include presence of foreign body close to suture line, tension on suture line, improper suturing technique, distal obstruction, hematoma or abscess formation in mesentery at anastomotic site, presence of tumor or disease in area of anastomosis, inadequate blood supply to anastomosis.
2. d
3. Three complications that contribute to death from fistulas are fluid and electrolyte imbalances, malnutrition, and sepsis.
4. A fistula is an abnormal passage between two or more structures or spaces.
5. b
6. **a.** An enterocutaneous fistula is between small bowel and skin.
    b. A colocutaneous fistula is between colon and skin.
    c. A vesicovaginal fistula is between bladder and vagina.
    d. A rectovaginal fistula is between rectum and vagina.
    e. A colovesical fistula is between colon and bladder.
7. Stabilization, investigation, conservative treatment, and definitive therapy are the four phases of medical management for the patient with a fistula.
8. c
9. Factors known to delay spontaneous closure of fistulas include complete disruption of bowel continuity, distal obstruction, foreign body in fistula tract, epithelium-lined tract contiguous with the skin, cancer in site, previous irradiation to site, Crohn's disease in site, and presence of large abscess.
10. Eight goals for nursing management of the patient with a fistula are skin protection, containment of drainage, odor control, patient comfort, accurate measurement of effluent, patient mobility, ease of use, and cost containment.
11. c
12. c
13. The bridging procedure should be used when it is helpful to isolate one area of a wound from another area of the wound. This may be needed for very large wounds or for wounds that have two distinct areas of "need."
14. Options for odor control in wounds managed with dressings: charcoal dressings can be secured over wound dressings; charcoal dressings must be kept dry. For wound managed with pouches, options include meticulous pouch hygiene, pouch deodorants, and room deodorants. Oral deodorants may be an option in either situation.
15. c
16. d

CHAPTER 24

1. Indications for the placement of a jejunostomy tube are drainage and decompression, and nutritional support when the patient is at risk for aspiration pneumonia.

2. The major content areas to be included in a teaching plan for the patient with a percutaneous enteral feeding tube are name and purpose of procedure, characteristics of normal tube function, why tube stabilization is important and how to ensure adequate stabilization, routine site care, signs and symptoms of complications (leakage, hyperplasia) and appropriate response, tube feeding schedule and procedure (when applicable), what to do if the tube falls out.

3. **a. Janeway:** Gastrostomy intended for long-term use, surgically constructed to provide mucosa-lined stoma, which can be intubated as needed.
   Stamm: Gastrostomy intended for short-term use; surgically placed; tube remains in place and must be stabilized with internal bolster or balloon and external stabilization device
   b. PEG: Nonsurgical endoscopic placement of gastrostomy tube; important to seat gastrostomy tube against gastric mucosa and externally against abdominal wall; has a lower complication rate than with surgery
   Gastrostomy button: Short silicone tube with flip-top opening and one-way valve, which prevents external reflux of stomach contents; feedings are administered after an adapter is passed through the one-way valve; insertion can be done as outpatient
   c. Foley catheter: Latex tube with balloon port; must be inflated to designated balloon size internally and have external tube stabilization device to properly anchor tube and prevent migration; balloon is degraded by gastric contents and needs to be replaced monthly
   Gastrostomy replacement catheter: Silastic catheter with balloon for internal anchoring against stomach wall and external bumper or flange for external stabilization

4. Radiologic approach to enteral feeding is appropriate when patient is not a surgical candidate and cannot have endoscopy safely performed because of obesity, ascites, and difficulty transilluminating the abdomen.

5. Advantages of a gastrostomy button: Low profile, prevents many complications associated with gastrostomy tubes (migration, leakage, inadvertent removal, tissue reaction), one-way valve allows feeding but provides continence
   Disadvantages of a gastrostomy button: Potential dysfunction of antireflux valve with leakage, need for replacement approximately every 3 to 4 months

6. To select a site for the placement of a PEG: Using a surgical marking pen, highlight on the abdomen any scars, the costal margin, hernias, beltline, creases, and folds.

7. Tube stabilization reduces tube migration, which can cause gastric outlet obstruction (with gastrostomy tubes), compromised tube function, and tract erosion, resulting in leakage and skin breakdown.

8. Options for stabilization of gastrostomy or jejunostomy tubes include use of commercial tube-stabilization devices, use of baby-bottle nipple placed around tube and secured to skin-barrier wafer, use of baby-bottle nipple placed around tube and secured with convex insert snapped over nipple and inside flange of skin-barrier wafer with flange, use of a gastrostomy replacement catheter that has attached external flange and internal balloon or bumper.

9. a
10. c
11. b
12. b

CHAPTER 25

1. d
2. a
3. a
4. True
5. 6
6. c
7. True
8. Interventions for pain reduction during dressing changes include the following: minimize the degree of sensory stimulus (e.g., drafts from open windows, or prodding and poking); allow patients to perform their own dressing changes; allow "time-outs" during painful procedures; schedule dressing changes when the patient is feeling best; give an analgesic and then schedule the dressing change when its peak effect occurs; soak dried dressings before removal; avoid use of cytotoxic cleansers; avoid aggressive packing; minimize the number of dressing changes; prevent periwound trauma; position and support wounded area for comfort; consider using low-adhesive or nonadhesive dressings; and offer and utilize distraction techniques (e.g., headphones, TV, music, warm blanket).

CHAPTER 26

1. Noncompliance suggests that the patient's role is to do what he or she is told to do by the health care provider. Achieving a **sustainable plan** relies on **mutually** agreed-upon goals.

2. Barriers to achieving a sustainable plan include the following: depression, cognitive impairment, impaired dexterity, impaired mobility, complicated regimens, financial barriers, lack of social/environmental resources,

skepticism, knowledge deficit, unpleasant side effects of therapy, regimens that interfere with ADLs and lifestyle, and therapy inconsistent with patient goals.

3. Factors to assess before developing an educational plan include learning readiness; physiologic needs; psychosocial needs; educational level; pain; and past learning, separating fact from fiction, building on past experiences, and so forth.

4. The difference between short term goals and long term goals are that short-term goals focus on the most pressing issues such as pain control and dressing changes, whereas long-term goals focus on disease management and fostering independence.

CHAPTER 27

1. Medicare is an insurance program created for people age 65 or older, for those of any age with permanent kidney failure, or for certain people under age 65 classified as disabled. Medicaid provides health services to individuals with low income.

2. *Medicare Part A* covers inpatient hospital care, care in a skilled nursing facility, hospice care, and care in small facilities that give limited outpatient services and are considered critical access hospitals in rural areas.
   - *Medicare Part B* is considered supplemental medical insurance and provides coverage for physician services, outpatient services, durable medical equipment, and others services not provided by Medicare Part A.
   - *Medicare Part D* is a supplemental prescription drug program. There are many different drug plans available in each state which are approved by Medicare, but administered by private companies.

3. True

4. b

5. d

6. False

7. Three methods for billing services are UPIN, incident-to, and contracting for services.

APPENDIX

B

POLICIES, PROCEDURES, AND DECISION MAKING TOOLS

B1—POLICIES PREVENTION OF SKIN BREAKDOWN

Policy

All patients will be assessed for risk of skin breakdown (Braden scale) at the first home care visit and with significant change in condition. Appropriate preventive interventions will be implemented.

Procedure

Risk Assessment

Risk assessment includes determining a person's risk for pressure ulcer development using the appropriate Braden scale. Pressure ulcer preventive interventions will target risk factors as determined by the pressure ulcer risk assessment.

- If over age 16, the Braden Scale will be used (See Appendix C).
- If under age of 16, the Braden Q Scale will be used (See Appendix C).

NOTE: Braden Scale for Predicting Pressure Score Risk (Braden Scale) is a standardized tool for determining level of risk for pressure ulcer development in adult patients. Level of risk is determined by the following scores:

15-18 = Mild risk
13-14 = Moderate risk
10-12 = High risk
9 or less =Very high risk.

Skin Inspection

A head-to-toe skin inspection will include palpation. During inspection, pressure points are examined closely for any of the following conditions:

- Alteration in skin moisture
- Change in texture, turgor
- Change in temperature compared to surrounding skin (warmer or cooler)
- Color changes, such as red, blue, or purplish hues
- Nonblanchable erythema
- Consistency, such as bogginess (soft) or induration (hard)
- Edema

- Open areas, blisters, rash, drainage
- Pain

NOTE: Blanching erythema is an early indicator of the need to redistribute pressure. Nonblanching erythema is suggestive that tissue damage has already occurred or is imminent, and indurated or boggy skin is a sign that deep tissue damage has likely occurred.

Preventive Interventions

1. Minimize or eliminate friction and shear

One or more of the following interventions and observations will be used to minimize or eliminate shear if it is identified as a risk factor:

- **Lift** body off the bed/chair rather than **dragging** as the patient is moved up in bed or chair.
- Avoid elevating head of the bed more than 30 degrees unless contraindicated. Sitting at a 90-degree angle when in the chair decreases shear/friction.
- Use transfer devices such as mechanical lifts, hover surgical mattress, slider boards, trapeze, surgical slip-sheets, and so on.
- Place a pad between skin surfaces that may rub together.
- Apply heel and elbow pads to reduce friction; they do not reduce pressure.
- Apply creams or lotions frequently to lower the surface tension on the skin and reduce friction.
- Apply a transparent film dressing, hydrocolloid dressing, or skin sealant to the bony prominences (such as elbows) to decrease friction.
- Keep skin well hydrated and moisturized.
- Lubricate or powder bedpans before placing under patient. Position the bedpan by rolling the patient on and off rather than pushing and pulling it in and out.
- Apply skin protectants and ointments to protect skin from moisture. Excessive moisture weakens dermal integrity and destroys the outer lipid layer. Therefore less mechanical force is needed to wound the skin and cause a physical opening.

2. Minimize pressure

Immobility is the most significant risk factor for pressure ulcer development. Patients who have any degree of immobility should be closely monitored for pressure ulcer development. One or more of the following interventions will be used if immobility is identified as a risk factor:

Patients in bed:

- Make frequent, small position changes.
- Use pillows or wedges to reduce pressure on bony prominences.
- At a minimum, turn every 2 hours.
- When lying on side do not position directly on trochanter (hip).
- Use pressure redistribution mattresses/surfaces.
- Free-float heels by placing a pillow under the calf muscle and keeping heels off all surfaces.

Patients in sitting position:

- Encourage patient to shift weight every 15 minutes (i.e., chair push-ups, if able to reposition self; have patient stand and reseat self if able; make small shift changes such as elevating legs).
- Reposition every hour if patient unable to reposition self.
- Utilize chair cushions for pressure redistribution.
- Use pressure support surfaces to redistribute (reduce/relieve) pressure as indicated.

All patients:

- Minimize/eliminate pressure from medical devices such as oxygen masks and tubing, catheters, cervical collars, casts, IV tubing, restraints.

3. Manage Moisture

Management of moisture from perspiration, wound drainage, and incontinence is an important aspect of pressure ulcer prevention. Moisture from incontinence may be a precursor to pressure ulcer development because of skin maceration and increased friction. Fecal incontinence is a greater risk factor for pressure ulcer development than urinary incontinence, because the stool contains bacteria and enzymes that are caustic to the skin. In the presence of both urinary and fecal incontinence, fecal enzymes convert urea to ammonia, raising the skin pH. With a more alkaline skin pH, the skin becomes more permeable to other irritants.

One or more of the following interventions will be used to minimize or eliminate moisture when it is identified as a risk factor:

- Contain wound drainage.
- Keep skin folds dry.
- Evaluate type of incontinence-urinary, fecal, or both.

- Implement toileting schedule or bowel/bladder program as appropriate.
- Check for incontinence a minimum of every 2 hours, and as needed.
- Cleanse skin gently at each time of soiling with pH balanced cleanser. Avoid excessive friction and scrubbing, which can further traumatize the skin. Cleansers with nonionic surfactants are more gentle on the skin than anionic surfactants in typical soaps.
- Use incontinence skin barriers (e.g., creams, ointments, film-forming skin protectants) as needed to protect and maintain intact skin, or to treat nonintact skin.
- Consider use of stool containment devices (e.g., fecal pouch, Flexi-seal, Zassi). Rectal tubes that are not FDA-approved will not be used.
- Assess for candidiasis, and treat as appropriate.

4. Maintain adequate nutrition/hydration

The patient who is malnourished and/or dehydrated is at an increased risk for pressure ulcer development. One or more of the following interventions will be used when nutrition is identified as a risk factor:

- Provide nutrition compatible with individual's wishes or condition.
- Encouraging hydration as well as high-protein and high-calorie supplements for the patient with multiple risk factors for pressure ulcers development.

5. Address sustainability of plan of care and goals

The ability of patients to participate in pressure ulcer prevention interventions may be affected by physical and behavioral factors. Noncompliance may be related to inability to participate, lifestyle issues, cultural differences, medical condition, physical condition, lack of trust, or knowledge gaps.

Possible activities to address:

- Provide education that increases patient/family knowledge of pressure ulcer risk and appropriate interventions.
- Identify barriers to patient participation and develop strategies to address those barriers.

Documentation

All assessments and skin inspection findings will be documented with in 24 hours of admission. A plan of care for prevention of skin breakdown will be documented?

Patient/Family Education

The patient, family, or caregivers will be educated in risk assessment and skin inspection technique. They will be informed of current status of risk assessment and skin inspection findings and be involved in planning interventions.

WOUND ASSESSMENT

Policy

All wounds will be assessed upon the first visit or occurrence. Wounds will be reassessed at least weekly and at the time of any significant change in the patient's condition or the wound condition. Pressure ulcers will be classified according to stage (see "Procedure"). All other wounds will be classified as either "partial-thickness" or "full-thickness" (of tissue loss). Assessments will include the following:

- Etiology (determine and document the causes or origins of the wound at time of the initial assessment, or as soon as possible thereafter)
- Anatomical location of the wound
- Centimeter measurements of wound length, width, depth, tunneling, and undermining
- Characteristics of wound bed, wound edges, surrounding skin, and exudate

Procedure

The following parameters will be documented:
A. Anatomical location of skin breakdown
B. Etiology (type) of skin breakdown
C. Classification of skin breakdown

Pressure-related classification (National Pressure Ulcer Advisory Panel)

Stage I: An observable pressure-related alteration of intact skin whose indicators as compared to an adjacent or opposite area on the body may include one or more of the following:

- Skin temperature (warmth or coolness)
- Tissue consistency (firm or boggy)
- Sensation (pain, itching)

Note that in skin of light pigment, the ulcer appears as a defined area of persistent redness, whereas in darker skin tones, the ulcer may appear with persistent hues of red, blue or purple.

Stage II: Partial-thickness skin loss involving epidermis, dermis or both. The ulcer is superficial and presents clinically as an abrasion, blister or shallow crater.

Stage III: Full-thickness skin loss involving damage to or necrosis of subcutaneous tissue that may extend down to, but not through, underlying fascia. The ulcer presents clinically as a deep crater with or without undermining adjacent tissue.

Stage IV: Full-thickness skin loss with extensive destruction, tissue necrosis, or damage to muscle, bone, or supporting structures (e.g., tendon, joint capsule). Undermining and sinus tracks also may be associated with Stage IV pressure ulcers.

Unstageable: When necrotic tissue is present, accurate staging is not possible until slough or eschar has been removed.

Reverse staging will not be used.

Non–pressure related classification

Non–pressure related wounds are classified by thickness. *Partial-thickness* and *full-thickness* are terms commonly used to classify wounds whose primary cause is something other than pressure. Examples of partial- and full-thickness wounds are skin tears, lacerations, surgical wounds, and vascular (venous and arterial) ulcers.

- **Partial-thickness:** wounds extend through the first layer of skin (the epidermis) and into, but not through, the second layer of skin (the dermis).
- **Full-thickness:** wounds extend through both the epidermis and dermis and may involve subcutaneous tissue, muscle, and possibly bone.

Approximated incisions

- Presence or absence of healing ridge during visits that occur within 4-9 postoperative days
- Presence of staples, sutures, or SteriStrips

D. Wound measurements in centimeters

Length and width

To ensure consistency, use the "clock" method for wound measurement: Visualize the wound as if it is the face of a clock. The top of the wound (at 12 o'clock position) is always toward the patient's head. Conversely, the bottom of the wound (at 6 o'clock position) is in the direction of the patient's feet. Therefore, length will be measured from 12 to 6 o'clock positions, using the head and feet as a guide. Width will be measured from side to side, or from 3 o'clock to 9 o'clock positions.

Depth

The depth of the wound can be described as the distance from the visible surface to the deepest point in the wound, perpendicular to the skin surface. To measure the depth of the wound, use a sterile, flexible, cotton-tipped applicator.

- Put on gloves and gently insert the applicator into the deepest portion of the wound.
- Grasp the applicator with the thumb and forefinger at the point level to the skin surface.
- Withdraw the applicator while maintaining the position of the thumb and forefinger.
- Measure (with a ruler marked in centimeters) from the tip of the applicator to that position.

Tunneling

Tunneling (also known as sinus tracts) is a passageway under the surface of the skin that is generally open at the skin level. However, most of the tunneling is not visible.

- Put on gloves and gently insert the sterile cotton-tipped applicator into the deepest extent of the tunnel.
- Pinch the applicator at the point where it meets the wound edge.
- Hold the pinched length of applicator next to a centimeter ruler to determine the depth of tunneling.
- Document the length and location of the tunnel using the "clock" method.

Undermining

Undermining is tissue destruction underlying intact skin. Both the direction and extent of undermining should be documented.

- Put on gloves and gently insert the sterile cotton-tipped applicator into the sites where undermining occurs.
- View the wound as though it is the face of a clock (as previously described). For example, the 12 o'clock position corresponds to the wound edge that aligns toward the patient's head.
- Progressing in a clockwise direction, gently probe to determine the extent of undermining (for example from 2 o'clock to 5 o'clock positions).
- Insert the cotton-tipped applicator into the deepest area of the undermining. Grasp the applicator with thumb and forefinger at the point where it is level to the skin surface.
- Withdraw the applicator while maintaining the position of thumb and forefinger. Measure (using a ruler marked in centimeters) from the tip of the applicator to that position.
- Document the extent and deepest measurement of undermining in a manner similar to the following example: *"Undermining from 2 o'clock to 5 o'clock positions. Deepest point is 2.5 cm at 3 o'clock position."*

E. Wound bed appearance (type and percentage of tissue in the wound bed)

F. Exudate/drainage

- Color
- Amount (percentage saturating dressing and type of dressing)

G. Periwound

- **All wounds**: assess and document condition of periwound skin condition (maceration, induration, erythema)
- **Lower extremity wounds**: assess and document edema and dorsalis pedis (DP) and posterior tibial (PT) pulses and sensation

H. Signs of infection

- New/increased slough
- Drainage excess, change in color/consistency
- Poor granulation tissue—friable, bright red, exuberant
- Redness, warmth, induration around the wound
- Sudden high glucose level in patient with diabetes
- Pain or tenderness
- Unusual odor
- Lack of improvement after 2 weeks of optimal management (including elimination or reduction of pressure ulcer risk factors as well as cofactors to impaired wound healing)

I. Pain

- Assess pain using a using a visual analogue scale or a faces rating scale

J. Patient/Family Education

The patient, family or caregivers will be educated regarding the following

- Signs and symptoms of infection
- Status or assessment of wound.
- Skin inspection and preventive interventions for skin breakdown*
- Pressure ulcer risk assessment findings*

---

*see policy for prevention of skin breakdown

WOUND MANAGEMENT

Policy

A wound treatment plan will be initiated for a patient at time of admission or upon development of a wound. The patient's treatment plan will be evaluated at least every 2 weeks thereafter and revised as necessary. The treatment plan will be based on the principles outlined below.

Procedure:

A. Establish realistic goals related to wound management in collaboration with the patient, family, caregivers and physician

- If wound healing is NOT a realistic goal, create a plan of care that will minimize pain, odor, and infection while optimizing quality of life.
- If wound healing IS a realistic goal, the following interventions should be incorporated into the care plan.

B. Control/eliminate causative factors

C. Optimize nutrition

- Complete a nutritional screening on admission per nutritional assessment policy and procedure
- Consult registered dietician (RD) per nutritional assessment policy and procedure
- Reassess and consider RD consult if wound does not improve within 1 week of optimal wound management

D. Prevent or manage pain

E. Remove devitalized tissue when appropriate

- In the presence of adequate perfusion, remove devitalized tissue through mechanical, autolytic, or enzymatic debridment.
- Heel ulcers with dry eschar need not be debrided if no signs of infection are present.
- Sharp debridement by a qualified professional should be conducted when indicated.

F. Cleanse wound

- Cleanse wound initially and at each dressing change.
- Use minimal mechanical force while cleaning a wound.
- Avoid cleaning wounds with abrasive or antiseptic agents. (Normal saline is most often appropriate.)

G. Provide a physiologic wound environment with appropriate dressings

- If blood supply to the wound site is adequate, keep the wound bed moist.
- If blood supply to wound site is NOT adequate, keep the wound clean and dry.
- Keep periwound skin dry and intact.
- Control exudate.
- Consider caregiver time.
- Eliminate dead space.
- Avoid overpacking the wound.
- Consider alternative therapies such as E-STIM, Ultrasound, V.A.C.,® and NPWT for treating stages III and IV pressure wounds or for recalcitrant stage II wounds that do not respond to optimal therapy.

H. Manage bacterial colonization and infection

- When treating multiple wounds on the same patient, attend to the most contaminated wound last.
- Clean technique may be used for chronic wounds and pressure ulcers.
- Perform cleansing and debridements of wounds as appropriate.
- Consider a 2-week trial of topical antibiotics or antimicrobials as a course of treatment for wounds that are not healing after 2 weeks of optimal care.
- Protect wounds from exogenous sources of contamination (e.g., feces).
- Immediately report signs of infection to the physician.

I. Assess and manage pain

- Assess pain using a using a visual analogue scale or a faces rating scale.

J. Patient/Family education

The patient, family or caregivers will be educated regarding the following:
- Signs and symptoms of infection
- Status or assessment of wound
- Skin inspection and preventive interventions for skin breakdown*
- Pressure ulcer risk assessment findings*

---

*see policy for prevention of skin breakdown

APPENDIX B2— PROCEDURES

Calcium Alginate

Brand _____

Location: _____

Frequency:_____

Purpose:

Promotes autolysis of necrotic tissue and absorbs exudate

Supplies (Circle):

a. Calcium alginate

b. Normal saline or hospital-approved wound cleanser to clean wounds

c. Tape

d. Gauze to dry peri-wound skin

e. Secondary dressing (ABD transparent dressing, border gauze)

f. Barrier ointment (zinc, Vaseline) or skin sealant

g. Sterile cotton-tip applicators (Q-tips)

h. Other: _____

Procedure:

1. Wash hands and apply gloves.

2. Remove and discard dressing. Remove gloves and wash hands thoroughly per hand washing policy. Apply new gloves, and put on appropriate personal protective equipment.

3. Cleanse with normal saline or hospital-approved wound cleanser.

4. Apply skin barrier to protect periwound skin from exudate.

5. Apply calcium alginate. If the wound has depth, gently fill wound space with alginate.

6. Cover with secondary dressings and secure as needed.

Gel/Ointment/Enzyme

Brand_____

Location: _____

Frequency:_____

Purpose:

Enzymes promote enzymatic debridement in a moist environment.

Ointments and gels facilitate autolysis.

Some ointments contain topical antimicrobials.

Supplies (Circle):

a. Gel/ointment/enzyme as applicable. (NOTE: most ointments and enzymes come from pharmacy.)

b. Normal saline or hospital-approved wound cleanser

c. Secondary dressing (4 × 4 cover sponge, ABD, border gauze)

d. Tape

e. Sterile gauze

f. Barrier ointment or skin sealant

g. Sterile cotton-tip applicators (Q-tips)

h. Other: _____

Procedure:

1. Wash hands and apply gloves.

2. Remove and discard dressing per facility policy. Remove gloves, wash hands, apply new gloves, and put on appropriate personal protective equipment.

3. Cleanse with normal saline or wound cleanser.

4. If needed, apply skin barrier around wound to protect patient's surrounding, intact periwound skin from moisture.

5. Apply thin layer of ointment to wound base or saturate into moist sterile gauze for packing into wounds with depth.

6. Cover with secondary dressings and secure as needed.

NOTE: Most enzymes require a moist environment to be effective

Hydrocolloid

Brand _____

Location: _____

Frequency:_____

Indication:

For noninfected, minimally exudative wounds

Purpose:

To promote autolysis of necrotic tissue

To provide protection to wound surface

To absorb exudate

Supplies (circle):

a. Hydrocolloid

b. Normal saline or hospital-approved wound cleanser

c. Gauze to dry around wound, and secondary dressing, i.e., 4 × 4 (1)

Procedure:

1. Wash hands and apply gloves.

2. Carefully remove and discard dressing per facility policy. Carefully remove gloves, wash hands, apply new gloves, and put on appropriate personal protective equipment.

3. Cleanse with normal saline or hospital-approved wound cleanser.

4. Apply hydrocolloid to wound base. Allow 1 additional inch of product to cover and protect surrounding, intact periwound skin.

5. Apply paper tape if needed to prevent dressing edges from rolling up.

Hydrogel Gauze Dressing

Brand: _____

Location:_____

Frequency: _____

Purpose:

To promote autolysis of necrotic tissue

To prevent tissue dehydration

Supplies (Circle all that apply):

a. Hydrogel product

b. Normal saline or hospital-approved wound cleanser to clean wounds

c. Tape

d. Gauze to dry around wound

e. Secondary dressing (ABD, 4 × 4 cover sponge, foam, border gauze)

f. Barrier ointment or skin sealant

g. Sterile cotton-tip applicators (Q-tips)

h. Other: _____

Procedure:

1. Wash hands and apply gloves.

2. Remove and discard dressing. Remove gloves, wash hands, apply new gloves, and put on appropriate personal protective equipment.

3. Cleanse with normal saline or wound cleanser.

4. Apply skin barrier to protect periwound skin from exudate.

5. Spread apart gel-impregnated sterile gauze and gently place or pack in wound base (or saturate gauze with hydrogel from a tube).

6. Follow with additional sterile gauze only if needed to fill depth of wound.

7. Cover with secondary dressing and secure as needed.

APPENDIX B3—DECISION MAKING TOOLS

INTERVENTIONS TO PREVENT SKIN BREAKDOWN BASED ON BRADEN SCORE FOR PRESSURE ULCER RISK

Interventions to Address Pressure as a Risk	Interventions to Address Risk Factors other than Pressure
At Risk (15-18)* • Frequent turning • Maximal remobilization • Protect heels • Manage moisture, nutrition, and friction and shear • Pressure-reduction support surface if bed- or chair-bound Note: If other major risk factors are present (advanced age, fever, poor dietary intake of protein, diastolic pressure below 60, hemodynamic instability) advance to next level of risk.	**Manage Moisture** • Use commercial moisture barrier • Use absorbent pads or diapers that wick and hold moisture • Address cause if possible • Offer bedpan/urinal and glass of water in conjunction with turning schedules
Moderate Risk (13-14)* • Turning schedule • Use foam wedges for 30 degrees lateral positioning • Pressure-reduction support surface • Maximal remobilization • Protect heels • Manage moisture, nutrition, and friction and shear Note: If other major risk factors present, advance to next level of risk	**Manage Nutrition** • Increase protein intake • Increase calorie intake to spare proteins • Supplement with multivitamin (should have vitamins A, C, and E) • Act quickly to alleviate deficits
High Risk (10-12) • Increase frequency of turning • Supplement with small shifts • Pressure reduction support surface • Use foam wedges for 30 degrees lateral positioning • Maximal remobilization • Protect heels • Manage moisture, nutrition, and friction and shear	**Manage Friction and Shear** • Elevate head of bed no more than 30 degrees • Use trapeze when indicated • Use lift sheet to move patient • Protect elbows and heels if exposed to friction
Very High Risk (9 or less) In addition to all of the above, use pressure-redistribution surface if patient has • intractable pain or, • severe pain exacerbated by turning, or • additional risk factors	**Additional General Care Issues** • No massage of reddened bony prominences • No donut type of devices • Maintain good hydration • Avoid drying the skin

*Low air loss beds do not substitute for turning schedules.

© Barbara Braden, 2001.

APPENDIX

C DOCUMENTATION TOOLS

CI—SCALES

NORTON SCALE

NORTON RISK ASSESSMENT SCALE

		Physical Condition		Mental Condition		Activity		Mobility		Incontinent		
		Good	4	Alert	4	Ambulant	4	Full	4	Not	4	TOTAL SCORE
		Fair	3	Apathetic	3	Walk/help	3	Sl. limited	3	Occasional	3	
		Poor	2	Confused	2	Chairbound	2	V. limited	2	Usually/Urine	2	
		Very Bad	1	Stupor	1	Bed	1	Immobile	1	Doubly	1	
Name	Date											

Frosm Norton D, McLaren R, Exton-Smith AN: *An investigation of geriatric nursing problems in hospital,* Churchill Livingstone, 1975, Edinburgh.

GOSNELL SCALE*

PRESSURE SORE RISK ASSESSMENT

I.D. _____

Age _____ Sex _____

Height _____ Weight _____

Date of Admission _____

Date of Discharge _____

Medical Diagnosis:

  Primary _____

  Secondary _____

Nursing Diagnosis:

  _____

  _____

Instructions: Complete all categories within 24 hours of admission and every other day thereafter. Refer to the accompanying guidelines for specific rating details.

DATE	Mental Status: 1. Alert 2. Apathetic 3. Confused 4. Stuporous 5. Unconscious	Continence: 1. Fully controlled 2. Usually controlled 3. Minimally controlled 4. Absence of control	Mobility: 1. Full 2. Slightly limited 3. Very limited 4. Immobile	Activity: 1. Ambulatory 2. Walks with assistance 3. Chairfast 4. Bedfast	Nutrition: 1. Good 2. Fair 3. Poor	TOTAL SCORE

		Vital Signs				24-Hour Fluid Balance		COLOR	GENERAL SKIN APPEARANCE				Interventions		
Date	T	P	R	BP	Diet	Intake	Output	1. Pallor 2. Mottled 3. Pink 4. Ashen 5. Ruddy 6. Cyanotic 7. Jaundice 8. Other	**Moisture** 1. Dry 2. Damp 3. Oily 4. Other	**Temperature** 1. Cold 2. Cool 3. Warm 4. Hot	**Texture** 1. Smooth 2. Rough 3. Thin/Transp 4. Scaly 5. Crusty 6. Other		No	Yes	Describe

PRESSURE SORE RISK ASSESSMENT MEDICATION PROFILE

Medication	Dosage	*Frequency	Route	Date Begun	Date Discon.
© 1988 Davina Gosnell					

*Suggested flow sheets for monitoring data.

GOSNELL SCALE

GUIDELINES FOR NUMERICAL RATING OF THE DEFINED CATEGORIES

Rating	1	2	3	4	5
Mental Status: An assessment of one's level of response to his environment	**Alert:** Oriented to time, place, and person Responsive to all stimuli, and understands explanations	**Apathetic:** Lethargic, forgetful, drowsy, passive, and dull Sluggish, depressed Able to obey simple commands. Possibly disoriented to time	**Confused:** Partial and/or intermittent disorientation to transpulmonary pressure Purposeless response to stimuli Restless, aggressive, irritable, and anxious and may require tranqualizers or sedatives.	**Stuporous:** Total disorientation Does not respond to name, simple commands, or verbal stimuli.	**Unconscious:** Nonresponsive to painful stimuli
Continence: The amount of bodily control of urination and defecation	**Fully Controlled:** Total control of urine and feces	**Usually Controlled:** Incontinent of urine and/or of feces not more often than once q 48 hrs OR has Foley catheter and is incontinent of feces	**Minimally Controlled:** Incontinent of urine or feces at least once q 24 hrs	**Absence of Control:** Consistently incontinent of both urine and feces	
Mobility: The amount and control of movement of one's body	**Full:** Able to control and move all extremities at will May require the use of a device but turns, lifts, pulls, balances, and attains sitting position at will	**Slightly Limited:** Able to control and move all extremeties but a degree of limitation is present Requires assistance of another person to turn, pull, balance, and/or attain a sitting position at will but self-initiates movement or request for help to move	**Very Limited:** Can assist another person who must initiate movement via turning, lifting, pulling, balancing, and/or attaining a sitting position (contractures, paralysis may be present.)	**Immobile:** Does not assist self in any way to change position Is unable to change position without assistance Is completely dependent on others for movement	
Activity: The ability of an individual to ambulate	**Ambulatory:** Is able to walk unassisted Rises from bed unassisted With the use of a device such as cane or walker is able to ambulate without the assistance of another person.	**Walks with help:** Able to ambulate with assistance of another person, braces, or crutches May have limitation of stairs	**Chairfast** Ambulates only to a chair, requires assistance to do so OR is confined to a wheelchair	**Bedfast:** Is confined to bed during entire 24 hours of the day	
Nutrition The process of food intake	Eats some food from each basic food category every day and the majority of each meal served OR is on tube feeding	Occasionally refuses a meal or frequently leaves at least half of a meal	Seldom eats a complete meal and only a few bites of food at a meal		

Vital Signs:	The temperature, pulse, respiration, and blood pressure to be taken and recorded at the time of every assessment rating
Skin appearance:	A description of observed skin characteristics: color, moisture, temperature, and texture
Diet:	Record the specific diet order
24-hour fluid balance:	The amount of fluid intake and output during the previous 24-hour period should be recorded
Interventions:	List all devices, measures and/or nursing care activity being used for the purpose of pressure sore prevention
Medications:	List name, dosage, frequency, and route for all prescribed medications. If a PRN order, list the pattern for the period since last assessment
Comments:	Use this space to add explanation or further detail regarding any of the previously recorded data, patient condition etc OR Describe anything which you believe to be of importance but not accounted for previously

BRADEN SCALE FOR PREDICTING PRESSURE SORE RISK

Patient's Name _____ Evaluator's Name _____ Date of Assessment

Category	1	2	3	4						
SENSORY PERCEPTION Ability to respond meaningfully to pressure-related discomfort	**1. Completely limited:** Unresponsive (does not moan, flinch, or grasp) to painful stimuli, due to diminished level of consciousness or sedation, OR limited ability to feel pain over most of body surface.	**2. Very Limited:** Responds only to painful stimuli. Cannot communicate discomfort except by moaning or restlessness, OR has a sensory impairment which limits the ability to feel pain or discomfort over 1/2 of body.	**3. Slightly Limited:** Responds to verbal commands but cannot always communicate discomfort or need to be turned, OR has some sensory impairment which limits ability to feel pain or discomfort in 1 or 2 extremities.	**4. No Impairment:** Responds to verbal commands. Has no sensory deficit which would limit ability to feel or voice pain or discomfort.						
MOISTURE Degree to which skin is exposed to moisture	**1. Constantly Moist:** Skin is kept moist almost constantly by perspiration, urine, etc. Dampness is detected every time patient is moved or turned.	**2. Moist:** Skin is often but not always moist. Linen must be changed at least once a shift.	**3. Occasionally Moist:** Skin is occasionally moist, requiring an extra linen change approximately once a day.	**4. Rarely Moist:** Skin is usually dry; linen requires changing only at routine intervals.						
ACTIVITY Degree of physical activity	**1. Bedfast:** Confined to bed	**2. Chairfast:** Ability to walk severely limited or nonexistent. Cannot bear own weight and/or must be assisted into chair or wheelchair.	**3. Walks Occasionally:** Walks occasionally during day but for very short distances, with or without assistance. Spends majority of each shift in bed or chair.	**4. Walks Frequently:** Walks outside the room at least twice a day and inside room at least once every 2 hours during waking hours.						
MOBILITY Ability to change and control body position	**1. Completely Immobile:** Does not make even slight changes in body or extremity position without assistance.	**2. Very Limited:** Makes occasional slight changes in body or extremity position but unable to make frequent or significant changes independently.	**3. Slightly Limited:** Makes frequent though slight changes in body or extremity position independently.	**4. No Limitations:** Makes major and frequent changes in position without assistance.						
NUTRITION Usual food intake pattern	**1. Very Poor:** Never eats a complete meal. Rarely eats more than 1/3 of any food offered. Eats 2 servings or less of protein (meat or dairy products) per day. Takes fluids poorly. Does not take a liquid dietary supplement, OR is NPO and/or maintained on clear liquids or IV's for more than 5 days.	**2. Probably Inadequate:** Rarely eats a complete meal and generally eats only about 1/2 of any food offered. Protein intake includes only 3 servings of meat or dairy products per day. Occasionally will take a dietary supplement, OR receives less than optimum amount of liquid diet or tube feeding.	**3. Adequate:** Eats over half of most meals. Eats a total of 4 servings of protein (meat, dairy products) each day. Occasionally will refuse a meal, but will usually take a supplement if offered, OR is on a tube feeding or TPN regimen, which probably meets most of nutritional needs.	**4. Excellent:** Eats most of every meal. Never refuses a meal. Usually eats a total of 4 or more servings of meat and dairy products. Occasionally eats between meals. Does not require supplementation.						
FRICTION AND SHEAR	**1. Problem:** Requires moderate to maximum assistance in moving. Complete lifting without sliding against sheets is impossible. Frequently slides down in bed or chair, requiring frequent repositioning with maximum assistance. Spasticity, contractures, or agitation leads to almost constant friction.	**2. Potential Problem:** Moves feebly or requires minimum assistance. During a move skin probably slides to some extent against sheets, chair, restraints, or other devices. Maintains relatively good position in chair or bed most of the time but occasionally slides down.	**3. No Apparent Problem:** Moves in bed and in chair independently and has sufficient muscle strength to lift up completely during move. Maintains good position in bed or chair at all times.							

Total Score

From *Nursing Research*, 2003 Jan/Feb, 52(1): 22-23

NUTRITIONAL ASSESSMENT

NESTLÉ NUTRITION SERVICES

Nestlé

Mini Nutritional Assessment
MNA®

Last name:	First name:	Sex:	Date:

Age:	Weight, kg:	Height, cm:	I.D. Number:

Complete the screen by filling in the boxes with the appropriate numbers.
Add the numbers for the screen. If score is 11 or less, continue with the assessment to gain a malnutrition Indicator Score.

Screening

A Has food intake declined over the past 3 months as a result of loss of appetite, digestive problems, chewing or swallowing difficulties?
0 = severe loss of appetite
1 = moderate loss of appetite
2 = no loss of appetite ? ☐

B Weight loss during the last 3 months
0 = weight loss greater than 3 kg (6.6 lbs)
1 = does not know
2 = weight loss between 1 and 3 kg (2.2 and 6.6 lbs)
3 = no weight loss ? ☐

C Mobility
0 = bed- or chair-bound
1 = able to get out of bed/chair but does not go out
2 = goes out ☐

D Has suffered psychologic stress or acute disease in the past 3 months
0 = yes   2 = no ☐

E Neuropsychologic problems
0 = severe dementia or depression
1 = mild dementia
2 = no psychologic problems ☐

F Body Mass Index (BMI) (weight in kg) / (height in m)^2
0 = BMI less than 19
1 = BMI 19 to less than 21
2 = BMI 21 to less than 23
3 = BMI 23 or greater ☐

Screening Score (subtotal max 14 points) ☐ ☐
12 points or greater Normal—not at risk—no need to complete assessment
11 points or below Possible malnutrition—continue assessment

Assessment

G Lives independently (not in a nursing home or hospital)
0 = no   1 = yes ☐

H Takes more than 3 prescription drugs per day
0 = yes   1 = no ☐

I Pressure sores or skin ulcers
0 = yes   1 = no ☐

Ref.: Guigoz Y, Vellas B and Garry P.J. 1994. Mini Nutritional Assessment: A practical assessment tool for grading the nutritional state of elderly patients. *Facts and Research in Gerontology.* Supplement #2:15-59.
Rubenstein LZ, Harker J, Guigoz Y and Vellas B. Comprehensive Geriatric Assessment (CGA) and the MNA: An Overview of CGA, Nutritional Assessment, and Development of a Shortened Version of the MNA. In: "Mini Nutritional Assessment (MNA): Research and Practice in the Elderly". Vellas B, Garry PJ and Guigoz Y, editors, Nestlé Nutrition Workshop Series. Clinical & Performance Programme, vol. 1. Karger, Bâle, in press.

With permission © Nestlé, 1994, Revision 1998. N67200 12/99 10M

J How many full meals does the patient eat daily?
0 = 1meal
1 = 2meals
2 = 3meals ☐

K Selected consumption markers for protein intake
• At least on serving of dairy products
(milk, cheese, yogurt) per day?   yes ☐   no ☐
• Two or more servings of legumes or eggs per week?   yes ☐   no ☐
• Meat, fish or poultry every day?   yes ☐   no ☐

0.0 = if 0 or 1 yes
0.5 = if 2 yes
1.0 = if 3 yes ☐.☐

L Consumes two or more servings of fruits or vegetables per day?
0 = no   1 = yes ☐

M How much fluid (water, juice, coffee, tea, milk...) is consumed per day?
0.0 = less than 3 cups
0.5 = 3 to 5 cups
1.0 = more than 5 cups ☐.☐

N Mode of feeding
0 = unable to eat without assistance
1 = self-fed with some difficulty
2 = self-fed without any problem ☐

O Self view of nutritional status
0 = views self as being malnourished
1 = is uncertain of nutritional state
2 = views self as having no nutritional problem ☐

P In comparison with other people of the same age, how does the patient consider his/her health status?
0.0 = not as good
0.5 = does not know
1.0 = as good
2.0 = better ☐

Q Midarm circumference (MAC) in cm
0.0 = MAC less than 21
0.5 = MAC 21 to 22
1.0 = Mac 22 or greater ☐.☐

R Calf circumference (CC) in cm
0 = CC less than 31   1 = CC 31 or greater ?   ☐.☐

Assessment (max. 16 points)   ☐☐.☐
Screening score   ☐☐
Total Assessment (max. 30 points)   ☐☐.☐

Malnutrition Indicator Score

17 to 23.5 points	at risk of malnutrition	☐
Less than 17 points	malnourished	☐

Subjective Global Assessment Scoring Sheet

Patient Name:_____Patient ID:_____Date:_____

	SGA Score		
	A	**B**	**C**

Part1: Medical History

1. **Weight Change**
   A. Overall change in past 6 months: _____kgs.
   B. Percent change: _____gain <5% loss
   _____5-10% loss
   _____> 10% loss
   C. Change in past 2 Weeks: _____increase
   _____no change
   _____decrease

2. **Dietary Intake**
   A. Overall change: _____no change
   _____change
   B. Duration: _____weeks
   C. Type of change:
   _____suboptimal solid diet _____full liquid diet
   _____hypocaloric liquid _____starvation

3. **Gastrointestinal Symptoms   (persisting for > 2 weeks)**
   _____none _____nauses   diarrhea _____ anorexia
   _____vomiting_____

4. **Functional Impairment   (nutritionally related)**
   A. Overall impairment: _____ none
   _____ moderate
   _____ severe
   B. Change in past 2 weeks: _____ improved
   _____ no change
   _____ regressed

Part2: Physical Examination

5. **Evidence of:**   Loss of subcutaneous fat
   Muscle wasting
   Edema
   Ascities (hemo only)

	SGA Score		
Normal	**Mild**	**Moderate**	**Severe**

Part3: SGA Rating (check one)

A. ☐ Well-Nourished   B. ☐ Mildly-Moderately Malnourished   C. ☐ Severely Malnourished

Reproduced from: Subjective Global Assessment: Covinsky KE, Martin GE, Beyth RJ, et al. The relationship between clinical assessments of nutritional status and adverse outcomes in older hospitalized medical patients. *J Am Geriatr Soc* 1999; 47:532-538.

SKIN ASSESSMENT

Skin the Vital Organ™

Assessment and Documentation Tool
Compliments of SWEEN® 24

Patient Information

Name_____

ID Number_____

Circle appropriate number and mark site(s) on adjacent body figure. *Definitions on back*

Skin Condition Code

1. Abrasion
2. Burn
3. Denudement
4. Ecchymosis
5. Exzema
6. Lesion-injury
    6a. Macule
    6b. Papule
    6c. Patch
    6d. Tumor
    6e. Pustule
    6f. Vesicle
7. Maceration
8. Nails—abnormal
9. Rash (redness or inflammation)
10. Scar
11. Skin tear
12. Tissue consistency—abnormal
13. Ulcer
14. Xerosis
15. Other

Comments: _____

_____

_____

Coloplast
Skin Health Division

Signature_____ Date_____

Reprinted with permission Coloplast, N MANKATO, Minnesota.

Skin Conditions Definitions and Codes

1. **Abrasion**–a surface layer of the skin abraded by friction[1]

2. **Burn**–skin injury resulting from exposure to heat, caustics, electricity, or some radiations; marked by varying degrees of skin destruction and hyperemia often with the formation of watery blisters and in severe cases charring of the skin

3. **Denudement**–removal of the epithelial covering from irritants such as urine and/or feces[1]

4. **Ecchymosis**–the escape of blood into the tissues from ruptured blood vessels marked by a livid black-and-blue or purple spot or area; often referred to as a bruise

5. **Eczema**–the most common type of dermatitis (inflammation of the skin) characterized by an episode of itching, redness and tiny bumps or blisters. When it develops into a long-term condition (chronic eczema), it leads to skin thickening, scaling, flaking, dryness and color changes

6. **Lesion**–a change or response to skin injury[2]

    6a. **Macule**–flat; discolored; nonpalpable; circumscribed

    6b. **Papule**–elevated; palpable firm; circumscribed

    6c. **Patch**–flat; discolored; nonpalpable; irregular in shape

    6d. **Tumor**–benign or malignant mass serving no physiologic function

    6e. **Pustule**–elevated; superficial similar to vesicle but filled with purulent fluid

    6f. **Vesicle**–elevated; circumscribed; superficial; filled with serous fluid

7. **Maceration**–an act or process of making the surface of the skin appear waterlogged[1]

8. **Nails (abnormal)**–any irregularity of the nail or surrounding area

9. **Rash**–a red or inflamed surface area of the skin, typically with little or no elevation[1]

10. **Scar**–a mark left (as in the skin) by the healing of injured tissue

11. **Skin Tear**–unintentional injury that causes damage to the epidermis and/or dermal layer of the skin[2]

12. **Tissue Consistency (abnormal)**–alteration of the skin such as, edema, hardness, or sponginess

13. **Ulcer**–a local defect or loss of tissue such as epidermis and dermis; may be concave and affect deeper structures; varies in etiology and size

14. **Xerosis**–abnormal dryness of the skin, a dermatosis that presents with dry skin and is the most frequent etiology of pruritus[3]

15. **Other**–any other noteworthy condition of the skin not otherwise categorized

Xerosis

Mild[†]

Moderate[†]

Severe

* As defined by *Merck Manual* 15th edition and the National Pressure Ulcer Advisory Panel.
References: 1. MEDLINEplus Health Information, Merriam-Webster. Available at: http://www2.merriam-webster.com/cgi-bin/mwmednlm. Accessed February 4, 2004. **2.** American Academy of Dermatology Public Resources. Available at: http://www.aad.org.pamphelts/eczema.html. Accessed February 4, 2004. **3.** DoctorUpdate. Available at: http://www.doctorupdate.net/du_toolkit/s_sorters/s1.html. Accessed February 4, 2004. †Photos provided by First Health Associates, Crestwood Care Centre, Chicago, IL

WOUND ASSESSMENT

TWO SAMPLE ITEMS FROM THE WOUND CHARACTERISTICS INSTRUMENT

Instructions: Circle the ONE NUMBER that best approximates your assessment of the wound:

Tissue-Floor of the Wound

Floor-tissue shine

(5)	(4)	(3)	(2)	(1)
(Glistening)		(Semi-glossy)		(Dull)

Floor-tissue moisture

(1)	(2)	(3)	(4)	(5)
(Dry)		(Moist)		(Wet)

Floor-tissue color

(5)	(4)	(3)	(2)	(1)
(Beefy red)		(Pink)		(Yellowish-brown)

Edge or Rim of the Wound (position of the wound where the open tissue meets the normal hair bearing skin)

Extension of external skin over the wound

(5)	(4)	(3)	(2)	(1)
(Appropriate to wound and moving inward)		(Undercut)	(Gnarled)	(No new growth apparent)

Color of majority of edge of the wound

(5)	(4)	(3)	(2)	(1)
(Dull, pale pink)				(No edge apparent)

Amount of new edge surrounding the wound

(=75% around the edge)	(5)
(>50%, but <75% around the edge)	(4)
(>25%, but <50% around the edge)	(3)
(Between 1% and 25% around the edge)	(2)
(No new edge apparent)	(1)

PRESSURE SORE STATUS TOOL

Instructions for use

General guidelines:

Fill out the attached rating sheet to assess a pressure sore's status after reading the definitions and methods of assessment described below. Evaluate once a week and whenever a change occurs in the wound. Rate according to each item by picking the response that best describes the wound and entering that score in the item score column for the appropriate date. When you have rated the pressure sore on all items, determine the total score by adding together the 13 item scores. The *higher* the total score, the more severe the pressure sore status. Plot total score on the Pressure Sore Status Continuum to determine progress.

Specific instructions:

1. SIZE: Use ruler to measure the longest and widest aspect of the wound surface in centimeters; multiply length $\times$ width.

2. DEPTH: Pick the depth, thickness, most appropriate to the wound using these additional descriptions:

  1 = Tissues damaged but no break in skin surface.

  2 = Superficial, abrasion, blister, or shallow crater. Even with, and/or elevated above, skin surface (e.g., hyperplasia).

  3 = Deep crater with or without undermining of adjacent tissue.

  4 = Visualization of tissue layers not possible due to necrosis.

  5 = Supporting structures include tendon, joint capsule.

3. EDGES: Use this guide:

Indistinct, diffuse	=	Unable to clearly distinguish wound outline.
Attached	=	Even or flush with wound base; *no* sides or walls present; flat.
Not attached	=	Sides or walls *are* present; floor or base of wound is deeper than edge.
Rolled under, thickened	=	Soft to firm and flexible to touch.
Hyperkeratosis	=	Callous-like tissue formation around wound and at edges.
Fibrotic, scarred	=	Hard, rigid to touch.

4. UNDERMINING: Assess by inserting a cotton-tipped applicator under the wound edge; advance it as far as it will go without using undue force; raise the tip of the applicator so it may be seen or felt on the surface of the skin; mark the surface with a pen; measure the distance from the mark on the skin to the edge of the wound. Continue process around the wound. Then use a transparent metric measuring guide with concentric circles divided into four (25%) pie-shaped quadrants to help determine percent of wound involved.

5. NECROTIC TISSUE TYPE: Pick the type of necrotic tissue that is *predominant* in the wound according to color, consistency, and adherence using this guide:

White/gray, nonviable tissue	=	May appear prior to wound opening; skin surface is white or gray.
Nonadherent, yellow slough	=	Thin, mucinous substance; scatterd throughout wound bed; easily separated from wound tissue.
Loosely adherent, yellow slough	=	Thick, stringy, clumps of debris; attached to wound tissue.
Adherent, soft, black eschar	=	Soggy tissue; strongly attached to tissue in center or base of wound.
Firmly adherent, hard/black eschar	=	Firm, crusty tissue; strongly attached to wound base *and* edges (like a hard scab).

6. NECROTIC TISSUE AMOUNT: Use a transparent metric measuring guide with concentric circles divided into four (25%) pie-shaped quadrants to help determine percent of wound involved.

7. EXUDATE TYPE: Some dressings interact with wound drainage to produce a gel or trap liquid. Before assessing exudate type, gently cleanse wound with normal saline or water. Pick the exudate type that is *predominant* in the wound according to color and consistency, using this guide:

Bloody	=	Thin, bright red.
Serosanguineous	=	Thin, watery, pale red to pink.
Serous	=	Thin, watery, clear.
Purulent	=	Thin or thick, opaque tan to yellow.
Foul purulent	=	Thick, opaque yellow to green with offensive odor.

PRESSURE SORE STATUS TOOL   (continued)

Instructions for use

8. EXUDATE AMOUNT: Use a transparent metric measuring guide with concentric circles divided into four (25%) pie-shaped quadrants to determine percent of dressing involved with exudate. Use this guide:

None	=	Wound tissues dry.
Scant	=	Wound tissues moist; no measurable exudate.
Small	=	Wound tissues wet; moisture evenly distributed in wound; drainage involves ≤25% of dressing.
Moderate	=	Wound tissues saturated; drainage may or may not be evenly distributed in wound; drainage involves >25% to ≤75% of dressing.
Large	=	Wound tissues bathed in fluid; drainage freely expressed; may or may not be evenly distributed in wound; drainage involves >75% of dressing.

9. SKIN COLOR SURROUNDING WOUND: Assess tissues within 4 cm of wound edge. Dark-skinned persons show the colors "bright red" and "dark red" as a deepening of normal ethnic skin color or a purple hue. As healing occurs in dark-skinned persons, the new skin is pink and may never darken.

10. PERIPHERAL TISSUE EDEMA: Assess tissues within 4 cm of wound edge. Nonpitting edema appears as skin that is shiny and taut. Identify pitting edema by firmly pressing a finger down into the tissues and waiting for 5 seconds; on release of pressure, tissues fail to resume previous position and an indentation appears. Crepitus is accumulation of air or gas in tissues. Use a transparent metric measuring guide to determine how far edema extends beyond wound.

11. PERIPHERAL TISSUE INDURATION: Assess tissues within 4 cm of wound edge. Induration is abnormal firmness of tissues with margins. Assess by gently pinching the tissues. Induration results in an inability to pinch the tissues. Use a transparent metric measuring guide with concentric circles divided into four (25%) pie-shaped quadrants to determine percent of wound and area involved.

12. GRANULATION TISSUE: Granulation tissue is the growth of small blood vessels and connective tissue to fill in full-thickness wounds. Tissue is healthy when bright, beefy red, shiny and granular with a velvety appearance. Poor vascular supply appears as pale pink or blanched to dull, dusky red color.

13. EPITHELIALIZATION: Epithelialization is the process of epidermal resurfacing and appears as pink or red skin. In partial-thickness wounds it occurs throughout the wound bed as well as from the wound edges. In full-thickness wounds it can occur from the edges only. Use a transparent metric measuring guide with concentric circles divided into four (25%) pie-shaped quadrants to help determine percent of wound involved and to measure the distance the epithelial tissue extends into the wound.

PRESSURE SORE STATUS TOOL   (continued)

NAME: _____

Complete the rating sheet to assess pressure sore status. Evaluate each item by picking the response that best describes the wound and entering the score in the item score column for the appropriate date.

LOCATION: Anatomic site. Circle, identify right **(R)** or left **(L)** and use "**X**" to mark site on body diagrams:

_____ Sacrum & coccyx   _____ Lateral ankle
_____ Trochanter   _____ Medial ankle
_____ Ischial tuberosity   _____ Heel   _____ Other site

SHAPE: Overall wound pattern; assess by observing perimeter and depth. Circle and *date* appropriate description:

_____ Irregular
_____ Round/oval   _____ Linear or elongated
_____ Square/rectangle   _____ Bowl/boat
                                 _____ Butterfly   _____ Other shape

Item	Assessment	Date	Date	Date
		Score	Score	Score
1. SIZE	1 = Length × width <4 sq cm 2 = Length × width 4-16 sq cm 3 = Length × width 16.1-36 sq cm 4 = Length × width 36.1-80 sq cm 5 = Length × width >80 sq cm			
2. DEPTH	1 = Nonblanchable erythema on intact skin 2 = Partial-thickness skin loss involving epidermis &/or dermis 3 = Full-thickness skin loss involving damage or necrosis of subcutaneous tissue; may extend down to but not through underlying fascia; &/or mixed partial- & full-thickness &/or tissue layers obscured by granulation tissue 4 = Obscured by necrosis 5 = Full-thickness skin loss with extensive destruction, tissue necrosis, or damage to muscle, bone, or supporting structures			
3. EDGES	1 = Indistinct, diffuse, none clearly visible 2 = Distinct, outline clearly visible, attached, even with wound base 3 = Well defined, not attached to wound base 4 = Well defined, not attached to base, rolled under, thickened 5 = Well defined, fibrotic, scarred or hyperkeratotic			
4. UNDERMINING	1 = Undermining <2 cm in any area 2 = Underming 2-4 cm involving <50% wound margins 3 = Underming 2-4 cm involving >50% wound margins 4 = Undermining >4 cm in any area 5 = Tunneling &/or sinus tract formation			
5. NECROTIC TISSUE TYPE	1 = None visible 2 = White/gray nonviable tissue &/or nonadherent yellow slough 3 = Loosely adherent yellow slough 4 = Adherent, soft, black eschar 5 = Firmly adherent, hard, black eschar			
6. NECROTIC TISSUE AMOUNT	1 = None visible 2 = <25% of wound bed covered 3 = 25% to 50% of wound covered 4 = >50% to <75% of wound covered 5 = 75% to 100% of wound covered			
7. EXUDATE TYPE	1 = None or bloody 2 = Serosanguineous: thin, watery, pale red/pink 3 = Serous: thin, watery, clear 4 = Purulent: thin or thick, opaque, tan/yellow 5 = Foul purulent: thick, opaque, yellow/green with odor			

Item	Assessment	Date	Date	Date
		Score	Score	Score
8. EXUDATE AMOUNT	1 = None 2 = Scant 3 = Small 4 = Moderate 5 = Large			
9. SKIN COLOR SURROUNDING WOUND	1 = Pink or normal for ethnic group 2 = Bright red &/or blanches to touch 3 = White or gray pallor or hypopigmented 4 = Dark red or purple &/or nonblanchable 5 = Black or hyperpigmented			
10. PERIPHERAL TISSUE EDEMA	1 = Minimal swelling around wound 2 = Nonpitting edema extends <4 cm around wound 3 = Nonpitting edema extends ≥4 cm around wound 4 = Pitting edema extends <4 cm around wound 5 = Crepitus &/or pitting edema extends ≥4 cm			
11. PERIPHERAL TISSUE INDURATION	1 = Minimal firmness around wound 2 = Induration <2 cm around wound 3 = Induration 2-4 cm extending <50% around wound 4 = Induration 2-4 cm extending ≥50% around wound 5 = Induration >4 cm in any area			
12. GRANULATION TISSUE	1 = Skin intact or partial-thickness wound 2 = Bright, beefy red; 75% to 100% of wound filled &/or tissue overgrowth 3 = Bright, beefy red; <75% & >25% of wound filled 4 = Pink &/or dull, dusky red &/or fills ≤25% of wound 5 = No granulation tissue present			
13. EPITHELIALIZATION	1 = 100% of wound covered, surface intact 2 = 75% to <100% of wound covered &/or epithelial tissue extends >0.5 cm into wound bed 3 = 50% to <75% of wound covered &/or epithelial tissue extends to <0.5 cm into wound bed 4 = 25% to <50% of wound covered 5 = <25% of wound covered			
TOTAL SCORE				
SIGNATURE				

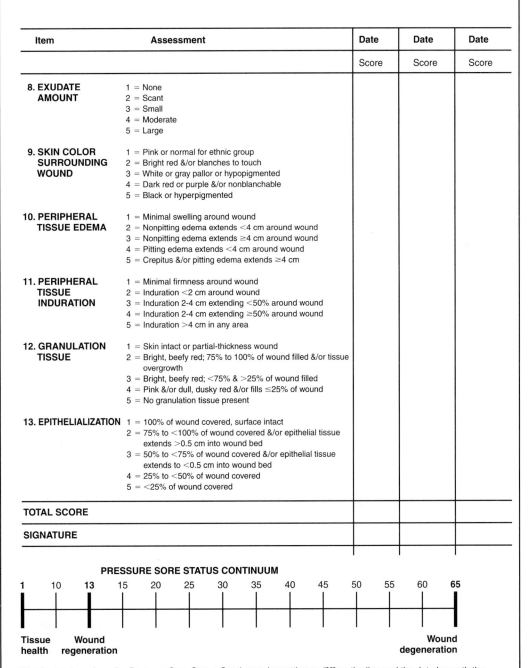

PRESSURE SORE STATUS CONTINUUM

1 10 **13** 15 20 25 30 35 40 45 50 55 60 **65**

Tissue health   Wound regeneration   Wound degeneration

Plot the total score on the Pressure Sore Status Continuum by putting an "**X**" on the line and the date beneath the line. Plot multiple scores with their dates to see at a glance regeneration or degeneration of the wound.

PUSH Tool 3.0

Patient Name: _____ Patient ID#: _____

Ulcer Location: _____ Date: _____

DIRECTIONS:
Observe and measure the pressure ulcer. Categorize the ulcer with respect to surface area, exudate, and type of wound tissue. Record a sub-score for each of these ulcer characteristics. Add the sub-scores to obtain the total score. A comparison of total scores measured over time provides an indication of the improvement or deterioration in pressure ulcer healing.

	0	1	2	3	4	5	
Length	0 cm²	<0.3 cm²	0.3-0.6 cm²	0.7-1.0 cm²	1.1-2.0 cm²	2.1-3.0 cm²	.
× Width	.	6 3.1-4.0 cm²	7 4.1-8.0 cm²	8 8.1-12.0 cm²	9 12.1-24.0 cm²	10 >24.0 cm²	**Sub-score**
Exudate Amount	0 None	1 Light	2 Moderate	3 Heavy	.	.	**Sub-score**
Tissue Type	0 Closed	1 Epithelial Tissue	2 Granulation Tissue	3 Slough	4 Necrotic Tissue	.	**Sub-score**
.	.	.	.	.	.		**Total Score**

Length × Width: Measure the greatest length (head to toe) and the greatest width (side to side) using a centimeter ruler. Multiply these two measurements (length width) to obtain an estimate of surface area in square centimeters (cm²). Caveat: Do not guess! Always use a centimeter ruler and always use the same method each time the ulcer is measured.

Exudate Amount: Estimate the amount of exudate (drainage) present after removal of the dressing and before applying any topical agent to the ulcer. Estimate the exudate (drainage) as none, light, moderate, or heavy.

Tissue Type: This refers to the types of tissue that are present in the wound (ulcer) bed. Score as a "4" if there is any necrotic tissue present. Score as a "3" if there is any amount of slough present and necrotic tissue is absent. Score as a "2" if the wound is clean and contains granulation tissue. A superficial wound that is reepithelializing is scored as a "1". When the wound is closed, score as a "0".

　　4 - Necrotic Tissue (Eschar): black, brown, or tan tissue that adheres firmly to the wound bed or ulcer edges and may be either firmer or softer than surrounding skin.
　　3 - Slough: yellow or white tissue that adheres to the ulcer bed in strings or thick clumps, or is mucinous.
　　2 - Granulation Tissue: pink or beefy red tissue with a shiny, moist, granular appearance.
　　1 - Epithelial Tissue: for superficial ulcers, new pink or shiny tissue (skin) that grows in from the edges or as islands on the ulcer surface.
　　0 - Closed/Resurfaced: the wound is completely covered with epithelium (new skin).

PRESSURE ULCER HEALING CHART
(use a separate page for each pressure ulcer)

Patient Name: _____ Patient ID#: _____

Ulcer Location: _____ Date: _____

Directions: Observe and measure pressure ulcers at regular intervals using the PUSH Tool. Date and record PUSH Sub-scale and Total Scores on the Pressure Ulcer Healing Record below.

	PRESSURE ULCER HEALING RECORD												
DATE													
Length× Width													
Exudate Amount													
Tissue Type													
Total Score													

Graph the PUSH Total Score on the Pressure Ulcer Healing Graph below.

PUSH Total Score	PRESSURE ULCER HEALING GRAPH												
17													
16													
15													
14													
13													
12													
11													
10													
9													
8													
7													
6													
5													
4													
3													
2													
1													
Healed 0													
DATE													

WOCN GUIDANCE ON OASIS SKIN AND WOUND STATUS M0 ITEMS

OVERVIEW AND BACKGROUND

As mandated by the Balanced Budget Act of 1997, Home Health Reimbursement shifted to a prospective payment system effective October 2000. Under this system, payment is based on the patient's clinical serverity, functional status, and therapy requirements. The system for wound classification uses terms such as "nonhealing", "partially granulating", and "fully granulating"; these terms lack universal definition and clinicians have verbalized concerns that they may be interpreting these terms incorrectly. The WOCN Society has therefore developed the following guidelines for classification of wounds. These items were developed by consensus among the WOCN's panel of content experts.

M0 445: Does the patient have a Pressure Ulcer?

M0 450: Current number of Pressure Ulcers at Each Stage

M0 460: Stage of Most Problematic (Observable) Pressure Ulcer

1	Stage I
2	Stage II
3	Stage III
4	Stage IV
NA	No observable pressure ulcer

Definitions:

Pressure Ulcer: Any lesion caused by unrelieved pressure resulting in damage of underlying tissue. Pressure ulcers are usually located over bony prominences and are staged to classify the degree of tissue damage observed.

Stage I: Non-blanchable erythema of intact skin, the heralding lesion of skin ulceration. In individuals with darker skin, discoloration of the skin, warmth, edema, induration, or hardness may also be indicators.

Stage II: Partial thickness skin loss involving epidermis, dermis, or both. The ulcer is superficial and presents as an abrasion, blister, or shallow crater.

Stage III: Full thickness skin loss involving damage to or necrosis of subcutaneous tissue that may extend down to, but not through, underlying fascia. The ulcer presents clinically as a deep crater with or without undermining of adjacent tissue.

Stage IV: Full thickness skin loss with extensive destruction, tissue necrosis, or damage to muscle, bone, or supporting

structures (e.g. tendon, joint capsule). Undermining and sinus tracts may also be associated with Stage IV pressure ulcers.

Non-observable: Wound is unable to be visualized due to an orthopedic device, dressing, etc. A pressure ulcer cannot be accurately staged until the deepest viable tissue layer is visible; *this means that wounds covered with eschar and/or slough cannot be staged, and should be documented as non-observable.*

M0 464: Status of Most Problematic (Observable) Pressure Ulcer

1	Fully granulating
2	Early/partial granulation
3	Not healing
NA	No observable pressure ulcer

- *Fully Granulating:* Wound bed filled with granulation tissue to the level of the surrounding skin or new epithelium; no dead space, no avascular tissue; no signs or symptoms of infection; wound edges are open.

- *Early/Partial Granulation:* ≥25% of the wound bed is covered with granulation tissue; there is minimal avascular tissue (i.e., <25% of the wound bed is covered with avascular tissue); may have dead space; no signs or symptoms of infection; wound edges open.

- *Non-Healing:* Wound with >25% avascular tissue OR signs/symptoms of infection OR clean but non-granulating wound bed OR closed/hyperkeratotic wound edges OR persistent failure to improve despite appropriate comprehensive wound management. Note: A new Stage 1 pressure ulcer is reported on OASIS as not healing.

M0 468: Does the patient have a stasis ulcer?

M0 470: Current number of Observable Stasis Ulcer(s)

M0 474: Does this patient have a least one Stasis Ulcer that cannot be observed?

M0 476: Status of the Most Problematic (Observable) Stasis Ulcer

1	Fully granulating
2	Early/partial granulation
3	Not healing
NA	No observable stasis ulcer

Definitions:

Full Granulating: Wound bed filled with granulation tissue to the level of the surrounding skin or new epithelium; no dead space, no avascular tissue; no signs or symptoms of infection; wound edges are open.

WOCN Society OASIS Guidance Document – Spring 2001
Wound, Ostomy and Continence Nurses Society • 4700 W. Lake Avenue • Glenview, IL 60025

- *Early/Partial Granulation:* ≥25% of the wound bed is covered with granulation tissue; there is minimal avascular tissue (i.e., <25% of the wound bed is covered with avascular tissue); may have dead space; no signs or symptoms of infection; wound edges open.
- *Non-Healing:* Wound with >25% avascular tissue OR signs/symptoms of infection OR clean but non-granulating wound bed OR closed/hyperkeratotic wound edges OR persistent failure to improve despite appropriate comprehensive wound management.

M0 482: **Does the patient have a Surgical Wound?**
M0 484: **Current number of (Observable) Surgical Wounds**
M0 486: **Does the patient have at least one Surgical Wound that cannot be observed due to the presence of a non-removable dressing?**
M0 488: **Status of the most problematic (Observable) Surgical Wound**

1 Fully granulating
2 Early/partial granulation
3 Not healing
NA No observable surgical wound

Description/Classification of Wounds Healing by Primary Intention (i.e., approximated incisions)
- *Fully granulating/healing:* Incision well-approximated with complete epithelialization of incision; no signs or symptoms of infection; healing ridge well defined.
- *Early/partial granulation:* Incision well-approximated but not completely epithelialized; no signs or symptoms of infection; healing ridge palpable but poorly defined.
- *Non-Healing:* Incisional separation OR incisional necrosis OR signs or symptoms of infection OR no palpable healing ridge.
- *Description/Classification of Wounds Healing by Secondary Intention* (i.e., healing of dehisced wound by granulation, contraction and epithelialization).
- *Fully Granulating:* Wound bed filled with granulation tissue to the level of the surrounding skin or new epithelium; no dead space, no avascular tissue; no signs or symptoms of infection; wound edges are open.
- *Early/Partial Granulation:* ≥25% of the wound bed is covered with granulation tissue; there is minimal avascular tissue (i.e., <25% of the wound bed is covered with avascular tissue); may have dead space; no signs or symptoms of infection; wound edges open.
- *Non-Healing:* Wound with ≥25% avascular tissue OR signs/symptoms of infection OR clean but non-granulating wound bed OR closed/hyperkeratotic wound edges OR persistent failure to improve despite comprehensive appropriate wound management.

GLOSSARY

Avascular: Lacking in blood supply; synonyms are dead, devitalized, necrotic, and nonviable. Specific types include slough and eschar.

Clean Wound: Wound free of devitalized tissue, purulent drainage, foreign material or debris.

Closed Wound Edges: Edges of top layers of epidermis have rolled down to cover lower edge of epidermis, including basement membrane, so that epithelial cells cannot migrate from wound edges; also described as epibole. Presents clinically as sealed edge of mature epithelium; may be hard/thickened; may be discolored (e.g., yellowish, gray, or white).

Dead Space: A defect or cavity.

Dehisced/Dehiscence: Separation of surgical incision; loss of approximation of wound edges.

Epidermis: Outermost layer of skin.

Epithelialization: Regeneration of epidermis across a wound surface.

Eschar: Block or brown necrotic, devitalized tissue; tissue can be loose or firmly adherent, hard, soft or soggy.

Full Thickness: Tissue damage involving total loss of epidermis and dermis and extending into the subcutaneous tissue and possibly into the muscle or bone.

Granulation Tissue: The pink/red, moist tissue comprised of new blood vessels, connective tissue, fibroblasts, and inflammatory cells, which fills an open wound when it starts to heal; typically appears deep pink or red with an irregular, "berry-like" surface.

Healing: A dynamic process involving synthesis of new tissue for repair of skin and soft tissue defects.

Healing Ridge: Palpatory finding indicative of new collagen synthesis. Palpation reveals induration beneath the skin that extends to approximately 1 cm on each side of the wound. Becomes evident between 5 and 9 days after wounding; typically persists till about 15 days post-wounding. This is an expected positive sign.

Hyperkeratosis: Hard, white/gray tissue surrounding the wound.

Infection: The presence of bacteria or other microorganisms in sufficient quantity to damage tissue or impair healing. Wounds can be classified as infected when the wound tissue contains 10^5 (100,000) or greater microorganisms per gram of tissue. Typical signs and symptoms of infection include purulent exudate, odor, erythema, warmth, tenderness, edema, pain, fever, and elevated white cell count. However, clinical signs of infection may not be present, especially in the immunocompromised patient or the patient with poor perfusion.

Necrotic Tissue: See avascular.

Non-Granulating: Absence of granulation tissue; wound surface appears smooth as opposed to granular. For example, in a wound that is clean but non-granulating, the wound surface appears smooth and red as opposed to berry-like.

Partial Thickness: Confined to the skin layers; damage does not penetrate below the dermis and may be limited to the epidermal layers only.

Sinus Tract: Course or path of tissue destruction occurring in any direction from the surface or edge of the wound; results in dead space with potential for abscess formation. Also sometimes called "tunneling". (Can be distinguished from undermining by fact that sinus tract involves a small portion of the wound edge whereas undermining involves a significant portion of the wound edge.)

Slough: Soft moist avascular (devitalized) tissue; may be white, yellow, tan, or green; may be loose or firmly adherent.

Tunneling: See sinus tract.

Undermining: Area of tissue destruction extending under intact skin along the periphery of a wound; commonly seen in shear injuries. Can be distinguished from sinus tract by fact that undermining involves a significant portion of the wound edge, whereas sinus tract involves only a small portion of the wound edge.

WOUND/SKIN ASSESSMENT FLOW SHEET

Date								
Wound location (see key below)								
Wound type								
P = Pressure V = Venous A = Arterial I = Incision O = Other								
Length in cm								
Width in cm								
Depth in cm								
Tunnel location (_____ o'clock position)								
Tunnel depth in cm								
Undermining location (_____-_____ o'clock positions)								
Undermining depth in cm								
Stage **Pressure ulcers only—do not reverse stage** I – Observable pressure related alteration. Examples include nonblanchable erythema of intact skin, purple, blue, boggy, firm II. Partial-thickness skin loss involving epidermis and/or dermis. The ulcer is superficial and presents clinically as an abrasion, blister, or shallow crater. III. Full-thickness skin loss involving damage or necrosis of subcutaneous tissue. IV. Full-thickness skin loss with extensive destruction, tissue necrosis or damage to muscle, bone, or tendon. X. Unable to stage because of necrotic tissue covering. **Etiology other than pressure** FT = Full-thickness OR PT = Partial-thickness								
% granulation								
% slough								
% other								
Amount of exudate L = Large S = Small, mild M = Moderate N = None								
Type of exudate s = serous Ss = serosanuinous P = Purulent								
Odor F = Foul M = Mild N = None								
Periwound skin E = Erythema M = Maceration I = Indurated N = Normal/Intact								
Right lower extremity pulses (see key below)								
Left lower extremity pulses (see key below)								
Right lower extremity edema (0, 1+, 2+, 3+, 4+)								
Left lower extremity edema (0, 1+, 2+, 3+, 4+)								
INITIALS								

SIGNATURE	INIT	SIGNATURE	INIT	SIGNATURE	INIT

Wound location key: 1. Sacrum; 2. Ischium a. left, b. right; 3. Trochanter a. left, b. right; 4. Heel a. left, b. right; 5. Medial malleolus a. left, b. right; 6. Lateral malleolus a. left, b. right; 7. Other

Lower extremity pulses: 1. dorsal pedal pulse palpable; 2. dorsal pedal pulse present with Doppler; 3. post-tibial pulse palpable; 4. post-tibial pulse present with Doppler

WOUND MANAGEMENT

MULTIDISCIPLINARY ACTION PLAN

Section VIII: Multidisciplinary Action Plan				
PHYSICIAN DOCUMENTATION REVIEWED BY ALL DISCIPLINES AS FOUNDATION OF PATIENT PLAN OF CARE.				
Discipline	Date	Learning/Discharge Need:	Plan and/or Action	Signature
Nursing				
Nutrition				
Respiratory				
Pharmacy				
Rehab Services OT, PT, ST				
Diabetic Education				
Wnd/ Ostomy Continence				
Discharge Planning				
Social Services				
Other				
Other				

MDC Dates: Attended by:

1. _____

2. _____

3. _____

4. _____

Home Care Clinical Pathway for Wound Management (nonpalliative)

VISIT SCHEDULE: PT: PRN RN: 3W1 2W4 1W4 HHA: 2W3 1W6

Outcome/Goals— Patient or caregiver will do the following:

- Describe and incorporate a diet that promotes healing
- List signs and symptoms of wound infection
- Describe when to notify physician
- Demonstrate competency in skin inspection
- Demonstrate ability to order wound care supplies
- Describe disease process and measures to manage and prevent reoccurrence
- Demonstrate competency in dressing changes by 1 week
- Demonstrate competency in preventive interventions for skin breakdown

RN VISIT	VISIT 1 WEEK 1	VISIT 2 WEEK 1	VISIT 3 WEEK 1	VISIT 4 WEEK 2	VISIT 5 WEEK 2	VISIT 6 WEEK 2	SUBSEQUENT VISITS
Nursing Assessment	• Total systems assessment per admission policy and procedure • Home safety, activity tolerance, pain, ADLs, and need for HHA • Nutrition and refer to RD per policy • Skin Inspection and pressure ulcer risk assessment * • Wound assessment** • Weekly wound measurements** • For lower extremity wounds: signs of impaired perfusion and neuropathy*	• Effects of medications • Skin inspection • Pressure ulcer risk assessment (if change in condition noted) • Wound assessment**	• Effects of medications • Skin inspection • Pressure ulcer risk assessment if change in condition noted • Wound assessment**	• Skin inspection and pressure ulcer risk assessment * • Wound assessment** • Weekly wound measurements** • If wound does not exhibit improvement within 1 week of optimal care, notify physician and reassess • Nutrition RD referral • Need for wound specialist • Lower-extremity assessment (if applicable) for signs of impaired perfusion and neuropathy*	• Effects of medications • Skin inspection • Pressure ulcer risk assessment (if change in condition noted) • Wound assessment**	• Effects of medications • Skin inspection • Pressure ulcer risk assessment (if change in condition noted) • Wound assessment**	• Skin inspection and pressure ulcer risk assessment * • Wound assessment** • Weekly wound measurements** • If wound does not exhibit improvement within 1 week of optimal care, notify physician and reassess • Nutrition RD referral • Need for wound specialist • Lower-extremity assessment (if applicable) for signs of impaired perfusion and neuropathy*

*Refer to Policy and Procedure for Prevention of Skin Breakdown **Refer to Policy and Procedure for Wound Assessment

continued

Home Care Clinical Pathway for Wound Management (nonpalliative)—cont'd

RN VISIT	VISIT 1 WEEK 1	VISIT 2 WEEK 1	VISIT 3 WEEK 1	VISIT 4 WEEK 2	VISIT 5 WEEK 2	VISIT 6 WEEK 2	SUBSEQUENT VISITS
	• Sustainability of the goals and plan of care (compliance)			• Cofactors that may impair wound healing (e.g., noncompliance, poor glucose control ineffective offloading, over colonization) • Sustainability/ appropriateness of the goals and plan of care			• Cofactors that may impair wound healing (e.g., noncompliance, poor glucose control, ineffective offloading, over colonization) • Sustainability/ appropriateness of the goals and plan of care
Teaching	• Goals and plan of care • Visit schedule • Medication regime • Basic principles of wound care • Skin safety and preventive interventions • Signs and symptoms of infection	• Med #1 • Optimize nutrition to promote healing • Recall previous teaching • Dressing change procedure • Skin inspection/ preventive interventions return demonstration	• Med #2 • When to notify physician • Recall previous teaching • Dressing change return demonstration	• Med #3 • Order wound supplies • Recall previous teaching • Skin inspection and preventive interventions return demonstration • Dressing change return demonstration	• Med #4 • Recall Previous Teaching • Importance of activity and exercise instruction	• Review all meds • Recall previous teaching • Recall visit #5 • discharge	• Client-specific teaching • Recall previous teaching

Teaching Aides	• Wound care video • Handout "Preventing Pressure Ulcers: A Patient's Guide"	• Handout "Your Guide to Better Nutritional Health" • Step-by-step instructions for dressing change	• Wound care video • Handout "Preventing Pressure Ulcers: A Patient's Guide" • Step-by-step instructions for dressing change	• Handout "Your Guide to Better Nutritional Health" • Wound care video • Handout "Preventing Pressure Ulcers: A Patient's Guide" • Step-by-step instructions for dressing change		• Written discharge instructions?	• Handout "Your Guide to Better Nutritional Health" • Wound care video • Handout "Preventing Pressure Ulcers: A Patient's Guide" • Step-by-step instructions for dressing change
Discharge Planning	• Assess environment, safety, home support, and learning needs • Assess need for PT/OT evaluations and refer as needed	• Assess needs and identify need for community resources • Assess recall #1 and compliance	• Assess recall #2 assess compliance or sustainability of the goals and plan • Assess home support • Assess need for WOCN referral and refer as needed • Assess need for RD referral and refer as needed	• Assess recall #3 assess compliance or sustainability of the goals and plan • Assess home support • Assess need for wound specialist referral and refer prn	• Assess recall #4 assess compliance or sustainability of the goals and plan • Assess home support • Refer to PT/OT as needed	• Discharge if medically stable—wound healed or CLT/CG demonstrate wound care and knowledge of teaching and prevention of further breakdown • Plan follow-up with physician	• Plan for physician follow-up • Continue to assess, recall, and support system

Variance Code A: Patient Related B: Situation Related C: Systems Related

OUTCOME/GOALS PATIENT OR CAREGIVER WILL	VISIT PROJECTED	VISIT MET	VARIANCE	VARIANCE REASON	INITIALS
Describe and incorporate a diet that promotes healing	2				
List signs and symptoms of wound infection	1				
Describe when to notify physician	2				
Demonstrate competency in skin inspection	1				
Demonstrate ability to order wound care supplies	4				
Describe disease process and measures to manage and prevent reoccurrence	4				
Demonstrate competency in dressing changes by 1 week	2				
Demonstrate competency in preventive interventions for skin breakdown	1				
Exhibit no new skin breakdown	ongoing				

Signature	Initials	Signature	Initials

ADLs, Activities of daily living; HHA, home health assessment; RD, registered dietician; PT, physical therapy; OT, occupational therapy; CLT/CG, Courtesy Queen of Peace Hospital, New Prague, Minnesota.

HOMECARE SERVICES
WOUND TRENDING RECORD

a. SURGICAL	d. DIABETIC / NEUROPATHIC	g. FISTULA	MED. REC.#
b PRESSURE	e. VENOUS / STASIS	h. DRAIN / TUBE	
c. TRAUMA	f. ARTERIAL	i. OTHER	PATIENT NAME:

Document at least 1 x week   Document on initial assessment, deterioration and recert

Document all other parameters with each dressing change.

Location: Check corresponding box	USE CORRESPONDING NUMBER(S) FROM LIST TO IDENTIFY LOCATION OF WOUND(S) ON FIGURE

1. □ Sacrum
2. □ Coccyx
3. □ (R) Heel
4. □ (L) Heel
5. □ (R) Ischium
6. □ (L) Ischium
7. □ (R) Trochanter
8. □ (L) Trochanter
9. □ (R) Malleolus
10. □ (L) Malleolus
11. □ Back
12. □ Occipital
13. □ (R) Shoulder
14. □ (L) Shoulder
15. □ (R) Ear
16. □ (L) Ear
17. □ (R) Foot
18. □ (L) Foot
19. □ (R) Leg
20. □ (L) Leg
21. □ (R) Arm
22. □ (L) Arm
23. □ (R) Hand
24. □ (L) Hand
25. □ Chest
26. □ Abdomen
27. □ Perineum
28. □ Nose
29. □ Other _____

Right Left   Left Right

Right Left   Left Right

SKILLED CARE COMPLETED		Wnd ___ Location: ___ Type: _____	Wnd ___ Location: ___ Type: _____
Wound #_____	**BRADEN PER POLICY**	Risk for pressure ulcers per Braden Scale: □ Mild (15-18 pts) □ Moderate (13-14 pts) □ High (10-12 pts) □ Very High (9 or below)	Risk for pressure ulcers per Braden Scale: □ Mild (15-18 pts) □ Moderate (13-14 pts) □ High (10-12 pts) □ Very High (9 or below)
	SIZE	L ___ cm x W ___ cm x D ___ cm	L ___ cm x W ___ cm x D ___ cm
Cleansed: _____	**STAGE** Do not reverse stage	ONLY STAGE PRESSURE ULCERS □ I □ II □ III □ IV □ Unstageable	ONLY STAGE PRESSURE ULCERS □ I □ II □ III □ IV □ Unstageable
Applied/packed: _____	**HEALING OUTCOMES**	□ Improved □ Healed □ Not Healed	□ Improved □ Healed □ Not Healed
Covered: _____	**WOUND PRODUCTS REMOVED**	□ Transparent dressing □ Nu-gauze____ □ Hydrocolloid □ 2x2's □ Hydrogel □ 4x4's □ Alginate □ Kerlix roll____ □ Foam □ ABD____ □ Silver dressing □ Other: ____ □ Enzyme □ N/A □ Antibiotic Ointment □ Impregnated gauze □ Unna boot	□ Transparent dressing □ Nu-gauze____ □ Hydrocolloid □ 2x2's □ Hydrogel □ 4x4's □ Alginate □ Kerlix roll____ □ Foam □ ABD____ □ Silver dressing □ Other: ____ □ Enzyme □ N/A □ Antibiotic Ointment □ Impregnated gauze □ Unna boot
Secured: _____			
Protected periwound skin: _____ _____ _____			
Wound #_____	**TRACTS/ UNDERMINING**	□ None □ Tracts □ Undermining Location _____ Size : _____	□ None □ Tracts □ Undermining Location _____ Size : _____
Cleansed: _____	**EXUDATE AMOUNT**	□ N/A □ 0% □ 25% □ 50% □ 75% □ 100%	□ N/A □ 0% □ 25% □ 50% □ 75% □ 100%
Applied/packed: _____	**EXUDATE TYPE & COLOR**	□ Serous □ Creamy □ Beige, Tan □ Sanguineous □ Yellow □ Green □ Serosanguineous □ N/A	□ Serous □ Creamy □ Beige, Tan □ Sanguineous □ Yellow □ Green □ Serosanguineous □ N/A
Covered: _____	**EXUDATE ODOR**	□ None □ Mild □ Foul □ N/A	□ None □ Mild □ Foul □ N/A
Secured: _____	**WOUND BED APPEARANCE**	□ Granular (Red): □ 0 □ 25 □ 50 □ 75 □ 100 □ Slough (Yellow): □ 0 □ 25 □ 50 □ 75 □ 100 □ Eschar (Black): □ 0 □ 25 □ 50 □ 75 □ 100	□ Granular (Red): □ 0 □ 25 □ 50 □ 75 □ 100 □ Slough (Yellow): □ 0 □ 25 □ 50 □ 75 □ 100 □ Eschar (Black): □ 0 □ 25 □ 50 □ 75 □ 100
Protected periwound skin: _____ _____ _____	**PERIWOUND / SURROUNDING SKIN**	□ Clear/Intact □ Erythema □ Discoloration □ Maceration □ Callous □ Induration □ Edema ____ □ Denuded	□ Clear/Intact □ Erythema □ Discoloration □ Maceration □ Callous □ Induration □ Edema ____ □ Denuded
PT / CGR Teaching □ N/A □ Pt □ Cgr verbalized understanding re: □ S/S of infection □Universal precautions □ Pt □ Cgr returned demo wnd care of: _____	**WOUND PAIN**	□ No □ Yes □ with w/c only □ **See VPR**	□No □ Yes □with w/c only □ **See VPR**
	PRESSURE REDUCING SURFACE DEVICE	□ Heel protection □ Alternating air overlay/ □ Elbow protection mattress □ Static air overlay / □ Low air loss, mattress zoned bed □ Foam overlay / □ Air fluidized bed mattress □ Gel overlay / □ Low air loss mattress overlay mattress □ N/A	□ Heel protection □ Alternating air overlay/ □ Elbow protection mattress □ Static air overlay / □ Low air loss, mattress zoned bed □ Foam overlay / □ Air fluidized bed mattress □ Gel overlay / □ Low air loss mattress overlay mattress □ N/A
Pt. Tolerated care:	**REFERRAL DIAGNOSTIC**	□ Nutrition consult □ Lab / blood work □ N/A	□ Nutrition consult □ Lab / blood work □ N/A

Signature / Title	Date	Time

GUIDELINES FOR COMPLETING WOUND TRENDING RECORD

RISK FOR SKIN BREAKDOWN – BRADEN SCALE (Circle)To be completed on Initial Assessment, whenever there is a change in the patient's status and with the re-certification											
SensoryPerception:		Moisture:		Activity:		Mobility:		Nutrition:		Friction & Sheer:	
Completely limited	1	Constantly moist	1	Bedfast	1	Immobile	1	Very Poor	1	Problem	1
Very Limited	2	Moist	2	Chairfast	2	Very limited	2	Prob. Inadequate	2	Potential problem	2
Slightly Limited	3	Occas. moist	3	Walks Occas.	3	Slightly limited	3	Adequate	3	No apparent prob.	3
No Impairment	4	Rarely moist	4	Walks Freq.	4	No limitations	4	Excellent	4		

Scores: Mild (15 – 18 pts)   Moderate (13-14 pts)   High (10 – 12 pts)   Very High (9 or below)   **TOTAL SCORE:** [   ]

If score is less than or equal to 18, implement potential for skin breakdown interventions.

STAGING (Stage Pressure Ulcers Only)   Stage on initial assessment, with deterioration and recert

Stage I :   An observable pressure related alteration of intact skin whose indicators as compared to the adjacent or opposite area on the body may include changes in one or more of the following: skin temperature (warmth or coolness); tissue consistency (firm or boggy) and / or sensation (pain, itching). In individuals with darker skin: discoloration of the skin (red, blue or purple hues), warmth, edema, induration, or hardness may also be indicated.

Stage II: Partial thickness skin loss involving epidermis, dermis or both. The ulcer is superficial and presents as an abrasion, blister or shallow crater.
Partial Thickness: Loss of epidermis and possible partial loss of dermis.

Stage III: Full thickness skin loss involving damage or necrosis of subcutaneous tissue that may extend down, but not through, underlying fascia. Ulcer presents clinically as a deep crater with or without under mining of adjacent tissue.
Full Thickness: Tissue destruction extending through the dermis to involve the subcutaneous layer and possible muscle and bone

Stage IV: Full thickness skin loss with extensive destruction, tissue necrosis, or damage to muscle, bone or supporting structures (e.g.: tendon or joint capsule). Undermining or sinus tracts may also be associated with Stage IV ulcers.

Unstageable
(Eschar)   Black or brown necrotic, devitalized tissue; tissue can be leathery and hard or soft and firmly adherent.
     DO NOT REVERSE STAGE

TRACTS / UNDERMINING:

Tracts: Normally presents as a narrow tunneling of tissue destruction that may extend down to the fascial layer including tendon, muscle and bone.

Undermining   Tissue destruction to underlying intact skin along wound margins.
Indicate undermining and tracts using clock face
i.e.   12-3 = 6 cm: 6-9 = 8 cm   11-12 = 3 cm

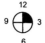   Measure Tracts and Undermining weekly

EXUDATE AMOUNT: Amount of exudate seen on primary or secondary dressings. Indicate percentage (as delineated under "wound bed" instructions).

EXUDATE TYPE:
    Serous: Clear and colorless exudate that contains serum and has a thin, watery consistency.
    Serosanguineous: Nonpurulent exudate that consists of both blood and serous fluid; usually clear and pink-tinged in appearance.
    Sanguineous: Red, bloody wound exudate.
    Creamy: Exudate with the consistency of cream = may be of any color. May represent normal findings or, when associated with other signs and symptoms of local infection, represents an abnormal finding.

EXUDATE COLOR:
    Beige, Tan, Whitish: Normal color when not associated with other local S/S of wound infection. Normally associated with certain products (eg., hydrocolloids, hydrogels, & Silvadene cream) and wound beds with slough.
    Yellow: May be normal or abnormal finding. Normal if associated with a clean, granular wound. Abnormal if associated with other local S/S of wound infection.
    Green: Always an abnormal finding. Characteristic color seen in wounds infected with pseudomona and other anaerobic microorganisms.

WOUND BED: Wound bed may consist of 1 or all types of the following tissues. Specify the percentage of wound bed surface area that each type of tissue occupies; percentages documented reflect the ranges below:
    0% = 0-5%   25% = 6-34%   50% = 35-65%   75% = 66-94%   100% = 95-100%
    Granulation: Soft tissue consisting of connective tissue and many new capillaries; typically appears beefy – red, shiny and "grainy."
    Slough: Necrotic tissue and cells separating from a wound bed; usually is yellow/beige, "stringy" and loose hanging.
    Eschar: Thick, leathery necrotic tissue; devitalized tissue.

PERIWOUND SKIN: Describe the appearance of skin immediately surrounding the wound by measuring and documenting the size of each characteristic:
    Erythema: Redness of the skin surface due to capillary congestion vasodilatation.
    Maceration: Softening of tissues by soaking in fluids. Dissolving of connective tissue components causing degenerative changes.
    Induration: Abnormal firmness of tissue with a definite margin. Marked by loss of elasticity and pliability.
    Denuded: Stripping or laying bare of any part; loss of superficial epidermis.
    Discoloration: An increase or Decrease in pigmentation not consistent with surrounding skin, may be purple, brown, etc.
    Callous: A firm, thickened area of tissue usually seen on the diabetic foot from repeated pressure or shear.
    Edema: Presence of abnormally large amounts of fluid in the interstitial space.

APPENDIX

D PATIENT EDUCATION

....

DRESSING GUIDELINES

STORING AND CARING FOR DRESSINGS

At home, dressing may be provided by _____, as order by your physician. Carefully follow the guidelines below on how to store, care for, and change dressings (if you should be instructed to do so):

- Store dressings in their original packages (or in other protective, closed plastic packages) in a clean, dry place. It the package becomes wet or soiled, discard it immediately.
- Wash your hands with soap and water before touching clean dressings.
- Take dressings from the box or package only when they will be used.
- Discard any dressings that become wet or dirty.

CHANGING DRESSINGS (See Basic Steps of Wound Care)

Ask your doctor or nurse to show you how to remove dressings and put on new ones. If possible, he or she should watch you change the dressing at least once.

Ask for written instructions if you need them. Discuss any problems or questions about changing dressings with the doctor or nurse.

Wash your hands with soap and water before and after each dressing change. Use each dressing only once. You should check to be sure the dressing stays in place when changing positions. After the used dressing is removed, place it in a sealed plastic bag before disposal. This will prevent the spread of germs that may be on dressings.

Basic Steps of Wound Care

Task	Steps
Prepare	1. Wash hands with soap and water. Get supplies together: _____ _____ 2. Move into a comfortable position with adequate lighting that allows maximum access to wound. 3. Protect bed linen and furniture with a plastic bag.
Remove Dressing	1. Place hand into a glove or a small plastic bag 2. Grasp old dressing with bag-covered hand and gently remove the dressing. 3. Turn the bag inside-out over the old dressing. 4. Close the bag tightly before throwing it away.
Cleanse Wound	1. Put on disposable plastic gloves. (Wear glasses or goggles and plastic apron if drainage might splash) _____ 2. Dry the skin surrounding the wound by patting with a soft, clean towel.
Observe Wound	1. Look at the wound carefully. As the wound heals, it will slowly become smaller and drain less. New tissue at the bottom of the wound is light red or pink and may look lumpy and glossy. Do not disturb this tissue. 2. Tell your nurse if the sore is larger, if the drainage increases, or if there are signs of infection.
Put on a New Dressing	1. Place a new dressing over the wound as follows: _____ _____ 2. After putting on the new dressing, remove gloves by pulling them inside-out. Soiled bandages and gloves should be placed in securely fastened plastic bags before you put them in the garbage can with your other trash.

Bergstrom, N., Allman, R.M., et al, *Clinical practice guideline, treatment of pressure ulcers,* Number XV, AHCPR Publication No. 95-0652 Rockville, MD. Agency for Health Care Policy & Research, Public Health Service, U.S. Department of Health and Human Services, December 1994.

IMPROVING APPETITE AND DRINKING MORE FLUIDS

Review your medical conditions with your physician, nurse or dietitian before changing your diet or drinking a lot more liquids.

- Ways to improve appetite and fluid intake:
  - Brush your teeth and use mouthwashes frequently.
  - Eat small, frequent meals.
  - Avoid empty calories.
  - Allow sufficient time between meals and eat slowly.
  - Plan a rest period before meals to prevent fatigue.
  - Add flavourings and spices if lack of taste is a problem (lemon juice, mint, cloves, basil, cinnamon,baco(bits).
  - Drink at least 2 quarts of liquid a day, if not on restrictions.
  - Keep an insulated glass filled with water near your chair or at your bedside for easy access.
  - Try popsicles—they are a good fluid source.
  - Low-salt clear soups and broths are also a good fluid source.

NUTRITIONAL GUIDELINES GOOD NUTRITION AND WOUNDS

- A balanced diet will help wounds heal and help prevent new wounds from forming.
- Protein, calories, vitamins, and minerals are all important to maintaining healthy skin.
- Review your medical conditions with your physician, dietitian, or nurse before changing your diet.
- Weigh yourself weekly. If your notice a sudden increase or decrease, you may need a special diet or supplements. Tell your nurse about any weight change.

Bergstrom, N., Allman, R.M., et al, *Clinical practice guideline treatment of pressure ulcers,* Number XV, AHCPR Publication No. 95-0652 Rockville, MD. Agency for Health Care Policy & Research, Public Health Service, U.S. Department of Health and Human Services, December 1994.

HELP US PROTECT YOUR SKIN FROM PRESSURE ULCERS

What is a Pressure Ulcer?

A pressure ulcer, sometimes called a bedsore, is an injury to the skin and underlying tissue caused by pressure.

Pressure ulcers usually occur over bony parts such as the tailbone, shoulders, elbows, hips, and heels. Pressure ulcers begin as reddened areas on the skin and can lead to pain, muscle damage and infection.

What Causes a Pressure Ulcer?

Pressure ulcers occur from pressure on the skin, squeezing tiny blood vessels which supply the skin with nutrients and oxygen. When the skin is starved of nutrients and oxygen, the tissue dies and a pressure ulcer (wound) forms.

Sliding down in a bed or chair can also cause pressure ulcers. This stretches or bends blood vessels, causing pressure ulcers. Rubbing or friction on the skin may contribute to pressure ulcers.

Are You at Risk?

If you have any of the following conditions you may be at risk for pressure ulcers:

- o Inability to change positions in the bed or chair
- o Loss of bowel and/or bladder control
- o Poor nutrition or hydration
- o Lowered mental awareness
- o Head of the bed is raised too high

How to Prevent Pressure Ulcers?

Take Care of Your Skin:

- Allow members of your health care team to inspect your skin at least once a day.
- If you notice abnormal areas, notify your nurse as soon as possible.
- Moisturize dry skin, but do not rub or massage skin over bony parts of your body.

Limit Pressure in bed:

- If you are in bed, reposition or asked to be repositioned every 2 hours.
- Try to keep the head of your bed as low as possible (unless other medical conditions do not permit it). If you need to raise the head of the bed for activities, try to raise it to the lowest point possible for a short period of time.
- Keep your heels off the bed, pillows should be placed under your legs from mid-calf to ankle but not behind your knees.

Reduce Friction:

- When shifting positions, or moving in bed, don't pull or drag yourself across the sheets. Also, don't push or pull with your heels.
- Avoid repetitive movements like rubbing your foot on sheets to scratch an itchy spot.

Limit Pressure in the chair:

- If you are in a chair for long periods of time, talk to your nurse about getting a chair cushion to redistribute pressure. Do not use doughnut-shaped cushions – they can cause injury to deep tissues.
- Reposition every 15 minutes while in the chair or ask to be repositioned every hour.

Safeguard Your Skin from Moisture:

- Clean your skin thoroughly (or ask for help) as soon as possible after soiling.
- Use absorbent pads that pull moisture away from your body.
- Apply cream or ointment to protect your skin from urine and/or stool.

THE DIABETIC FOOT

People with diabetes are at increased risk for developing foot sores. If untreated, a foot sore can get worse and may result in amputation. Proper foot care and appropriate shoes can prevent diabetic foot ulcers.

Q. What is a foot ulcer?

A. A foot ulcer is a breakdown in the skin and soft tissues of the feet. It can start as a small sore. It can grow into a deep hole.

Q. Why do diabetics get foot ulcers?

A. One complication of diabetes is peripheral neuropathy or damage to the nerves that sense pain, touch and temperature. A diabetic with neuropathy does not feel pain when a foot gets injured. So, stepping on a tack or a hot sidewalk may not cause pain. Because of this lack of feeling, a diabetic may not realize his or her foot is in trouble. Skin ulcers in those who have poor circulation and high blood sugar levels do not heal well. The sore can become infected and spread deeper into the foot.

Q. Is it possible to test for nerve damage or neuropathy in the diabetic foot?

A. Yes, a health care provider can test the sole of your foot with monofilament, a nylon fiber that bends when it is pushed against the foot. If you are unable to feel a monofilament, you may be at risk for developing foot ulcer.

Q. How can I prevent a foot ulcer?

A. You should examine your feet daily for skin breakdown or signs of infection (redness, increased warmth). Look for calluses. A callus means too much pressure is being applied to that part of your foot. If you can't see your feet because of poor vision, or can't reach your feet because of arthritis, you may need to ask a friend or relative to examine your feet. You should have a doctor, nurse, physician's assistant, or podiatrist examine your feet regularly. Contact your health care provider immediately if you think you have an infection or ulcer on your foot.

Q. Can I test myself for diabetic nerve damage?

A. Yes. You can order a free monofilament, and test the sensation in your feet regularly at home. To order a monofilament, call the Lower Extremity Amputation Program (LEAP) at 1-888-275-4772. This is a free service of the Department of Health and Human Services.

Q. What kind of shoes should I wear?

A. Properly fitted shoes can prevent diabetic foot ulcers. Your shoes should not be too tight. Stand on a piece of paper and draw an outline of your foot, then place your shoe on top of the outline. Properly fitted shoe should be roomy enough not to squeeze your foot into the shoe. The toe box of your shoes should be high enough so that the shoe does not rub on your toes. Athletic running or walking shoes can reduce pressure damage to the feet. If you are diabetic with neuropathy or have had a foot ulcer or an amputation, you should wear custom-made shoes with cushioned inserts.

Q. Where can I get custom-fitted shoes?

A. Your health care provider can direct you to a shoemaker specially trained to build shoes for diabetics. The shoe will be designed to fit your foot. Cushioned inserts are molded to the contours of your foot to reduce pressure damage to your foot when you walk. Custom-made shoes with inserts cost several hundred dollars. Most insurances will help pay for these shoes if you have a prescription from a health care provider accepted by your insurer. Since 1993, Medicare will pay for one pair of custom shoes and three customs inlays per calendar year for diabetics with neuropathy, callus, deformed feet, or poor circulation.

Q. Where can I find out more information about diabetic foot care?

A. The Lower Extremity Amputation Prevention Program (LEAP)
Bureau of Primary Health Care (BPHC)
Division of Programs for Special Populations
4350 East West Highways, 9th Floor
Bethesda, Maryland 20814
Phone: 1-888-ASK-HRSA(1-888-275-4772)
website: http://bphc.hrsa.gov./leap

From The AGS Foundation for Health in Aging, New York, NY. By Jean Thiefelder, MD, University of Nebraska Medical Center; Content Expert: Lynn Mack-Shipman, MD, University of Nebraska Medical Center

Pheripheral Arterial Disease

SYMPTOMS OF PAD

- Painful cramping of the leg or hip muscles during walking, in some cases severe enough to hinder walking, that stops during rest; or numbness, weakness, or a feeling or heaviness in the legs with no pain
- Burning or aching in the feet and toes while at rest and particularly while lying flat (this is a sign of more severe PAD)
- Cooling of the skin is specific areas of the legs or feet
- Color changes in the skin, particularly in the arms or legs
- Toe and foot sores that do not heal promptly

RISK FACTORS FOR PAD

- Smoking is the number one risk factor for PAD and will interfere with treatment of the disease. People with PAD should stop smoking completely because even one or two cigarettes daily can affect treatment.
- Diabetes is a significant risk factor for PAD. People with diabetes should keep strict control of their blood sugar to avoid serious problems resulting from PAD.
- Older age is a predictor for PAD—it occurs more frequently in those 60 years of age or older.
- People with a family history of heart disease are at greater risk for PAD.
- High blood pressure is a risk factor because it causes damage to the artery walls, which can lead to PAD.

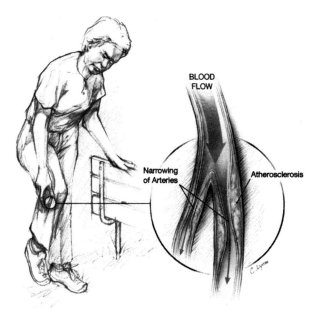

TREATMENT

- The buildup of plaque in arteries that occurs in PAD can often be stopped or even reversed. People with PAD should quit smoking, exercise regularly, and eat a healthy diet low in fat and salt. In more serious cases, medication, surgery, or both may be necessary to treat PAD. Your doctor can test you for PAD and recommend the best treatment.

MANAGEMENT OF VENOUS INSUFFICIENCY AND VENOUS ULCERS

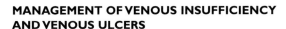

Description of Problem: The veins in the legs are responsible for returning blood to the heart. They have a hard job because they have to pump the blood "uphill". There are two things that help move the blood back to the heart: the calf muscle and one-way valves in the veins. This is how it works. When you walk or flex your foot, it causes the calf muscle to contract. When the calf muscle contracts, it squeezes the veins deep in your leg and helps to propel the blood back to the heart. The one-way valves help by preventing "backflow" of the blood.

Venous insufficiency occurs when there is damage to the valves, the calf muscle is not working, or there is a blockage in one of the veins. Any of these problems makes it hard to get the blood back to the heart. When the blood is not moving through the veins properly, the pressure builds up in the veins; this causes fluid and proteins and white blood cells to leak out of the veins into the tissues. The end result is swelling of your legs and damage to the tissues. When the tissues are damaged, very minor trauma can cause an ulcer.

From Stevens LM, Glass RM (ed), JAMMA, September 19, 2001 – Vol 286, No. 11.
Sources: American Heart Association, Centers for Disease Control and Prevention, National Institutes of Health, Society of Cardiovascular & Interventional Radiology, Vascular Disease Foundation, World Health Organization.

Risk Factors for Venous Insufficiency: You are more likely to have problems with your veins if you have had any of the following:

- Deep vein thrombosis (clot in the leg vein)
- Thrombophlebitis (inflammation of vein and blood clot in vein)
- Multiple pregnancies (especially if they are close together)
- Obesity
- Prolonged standing or sitting
- Inability to walk normally—any condition that causes you to walk with a "shuffle"
- Family history of varicose veins and venous insufficiency

Signs and Symptoms of Venous Insufficiency: You may have venous insufficiency and should be checked by a doctor if you notice any of the following:

- Swelling in the legs that gets worse when your legs are down and gets better when your legs are up
- Aching pain that gets worse when your legs are down and gets better when your legs are up
- Discoloration (bruised appearance) around your ankles and lower legs (caused by blood leaking into your tissues)
- Varicose veins
- Redness, scaling, and itching of your lower leg (dermatitis)
- Sores (ulcers) around your ankles or lower leg

Treatment for Venous Insufficiency and Venous Ulcers: There are several approaches to treatment of venous insufficiency and venous ulcers:

- Surgery is sometimes done to tie off the vein with the damaged valve.
- The *most common* approach to treatment is use of elastic stockings or compression wraps to eliminate the swelling and provide support for the veins. This approach is very effective but it requires diligent adherence to the treatment plan. The wraps are usually applied once or twice weekly by a nurse or doctor; they are frequently used until the swelling is under control. Once the swelling is under control and any ulcers are healing, you will probably be given a prescription for elastic stockings. The stockings must be correctly fitted and must be worn whenever you are out of bed. The nurse or fitter will teach you "tips" to help you get the stockings on correctly and will teach you how to care for them.
- You need to avoid standing in one position for long periods of time, and you need to avoid sitting with your legs down. Walking is actually very good for you, as long as your wraps or stockings are in place. When you are sitting or lying down, you should elevate your legs so they are higher than your heart. (This helps get the blood back to your heart and also helps to reduce the swelling.)
- Medications may be used to treat any infection or inflammation, and special dressings may be used to treat any ulcers.
- It is very important to realize that you will probably need to wear elastic stockings for the rest of your life, even after the ulcer is healed and the swelling is controlled. This is because the underlying problem is still there— you still have the venous insufficiency. Your nurse or doctor will tell you what type of stockings you need to wear and how often you need to replace them. (Most stockings need to be replaced every 3 to 6 months.) It is also important to realize that you need the *prescribed stockings*—regular support hose will not give you enough support and you will be at risk for more ulcers. The good news is that there are many types and colors of elastic stockings so you can still "look good" while protecting yourself from ulcers!

Courtesy Dorothy Doughty.

CODING AND REIMBURSEMENT

Requirements for Coverage and/or Medical Necessity

1) Wound care orders
   - Written, signed, and dated order by health care provider
   - The order must specify (a) the type of dressing (b) the size of the dressing (c) the number/amount to be used at one time (d) the frequency of dressing change, and (e) the expected duration of need.
   - A new order is needed every three months or if the quantity is increased.

2) Documentation
   - Documentation for medical necessity must include (a) number of surgical/debrided wounds being treated with a dressing, (b) type of wound (e.g., surgical wound, debrided wound, etc.), (c) whether the dressing is being used as a primary or secondary dressing.
   - Monthly documentation of wound status is required by a nurse, physician or other health care professional.
   - Evaluation is expected on a more frequent basis (e.g., weekly) in patients in a nursing facility or in patients with heavily draining or infected wounds.
   - Evaluation must include the type of each wound (e.g., surgical wound, pressure ulcer, burn, etc), its location, its size (length x width in cm.) and depth, the amount of drainage, and any other relevant information.

3) General information
   - Use of more than one type of wound filler or wound cover in a single wound is rarely medically necessary.
   - It may not be appropriate to use some combinations of a hydrating dressing on the same wound at the same time as an absorptive dressing (e.g., hydrogel and alginate).
   - Composite dressings, foam and hydrocolloid wound covers, and transparent film, when used as secondary dressings should not be changed more frequently than once a day. If more frequent changes are required, an alternative secondary dressing should be used.
   - Dressing size must be based on and appropriate to the size of the wound. For wound covers, the pad size is usually about 2 inches greater than the dimensions of the wound.

- No more than a one month's supply of dressings may be provided at one time.

Specific Coverage Guidelines for Individual Products

Alginate or other fiber gelling dressing (A6196-A6199):
- Covered for moderately to highly exudative full thickness wounds
- Not medically necessary on dry wounds or wounds covered with eschar.
- Dressing change frequency is up to once per day.
- One wound cover sheet of the approximate size of the wound or up to 2 units of wound filler (1 unit = 6 inches of alginate or other fiber gelling dressing rope) is usually used at each dressing change.
- Inappropriate to use alginates or other fiber gelling dressings in combination with hydrogels.

Composite dressing (A6200-A6205):
Dressing change frequency up to 3 times per week; one wound cover per dressing change.

Contact layer (A6206-A6208):
Used to line the entire wound; not intended to be changed with each dressing change. Dressing change frequency up to once per week.

Foam dressing (A6209-A6215):
- Used on full thickness wounds with moderate to heavy exudate.
- Dressing change frequency up to 3 times per week.
- Dressing change frequency for foam wound fillers is up to once per day.

Gauze, non-impregnated (A6216-A6221, A6402-A6404, A6407):
- Dressing change frequency up to 3 times per day for a dressing without a border and once per day for a dressing with a border.
- Not necessary to stack more than 2 gauze pads on top of each other.

Gauze, impregnated, with other than water, normal saline, hydrogel, or zinc paste (A6222-A6224, A6266):
Dressing change frequency up to once per day.

Gauze, impregnated, water or normal saline (A6228-A6230):

There is no medical necessity for these dressings; payment based on sterile non-impregnated gauze.

Hydrocolloid dressing (A6234-A6241):

Used on wounds with light to moderate exudate; dressing change frequency up to 3 times per week.

Hydrogel dressing (A6231-A6233, A6242-A6248):

- Used on full thickness wounds with minimal or no exudate
- Documentation needed to substantiate medical necessity in stage II ulcers (e.g., sacro-coccygeal area).
- Dressing change frequency up to once a day for dressing without adhesive border or hydrogel wound fillers; up to 3 times per week with an adhesive border.
- Appropriate amount to use must line the surface of the wound not to fill a cavity.
- Use of more than one type of hydrogel dressing (filler, cover, or impregnated gauze) on the same wound at the same time is not medically necessary.

Specialty absorptive dressing (A6251-A6256):

- Used for moderately or highly exudative wounds.
- Dressing change frequency up to once per day for a dressing without an adhesive border and up to every other day for a dressing with a border.

Transparent film (A6257-A6259):

- Used on open partial thickness wounds with minimal exudate or closed wounds.
- Dressing change frequency up to 3 times per week.

Wound filler, not elsewhere classified (A6261-A6262):

- Dressing change frequency up to 3 times per week.

Wound pouch (A6154):

- Dressing change frequency up to 3 times per week.

Tape (A4450,A4452):

- Reimbursed when needed to hold on a wound cover, elastic roll gauze or non-elastic roll gauze.
- Additional tape is usually not required when a wound cover with an adhesive border is used.
- Quantities of tape submitted must reasonably reflect the size of the wound cover being secured.
- Usual use for wound covers measuring 16 square inches or less is up to 2 units per dressing change; for wound covers measuring 16 to 48 square inches, up to 3 units per dressing change; for wound covers measuring greater than 48 square inches, up to 4 units per dressing change.

Supply Codes

CPT/HCPCS Codes

The appearance of a code in this section does not necessarily indicate coverage.

HCPCS MODIFIERS:

A1 – Dressing for one wound

A2 – Dressing for two wounds

A3 – Dressing for three wounds

A4 – Dressing for four wounds

A5 – Dressing for five wounds

A6 – Dressing for six wounds

A7 – Dressing for seven wounds

A8 – Dressing for eight wounds

A9 – Dressing for nine wounds

LT - Left side

RT – Right side

A4450 TAPE, NON-WATERPROOF, PER 18 SQUARE INCHES

A4452 TAPE, WATERPROOF, PER 18 SQUARE INCHES

A4462 ABDOMINAL DRESSING HOLDER, EACH

A4465 NON-ELASTIC BINDER FOR EXTREMITY

A6010 COLLAGEN BASED WOUND FILLER, DRY FORM, PER GRAM OF COLLAGEN

A6011 COLLAGEN BASED WOUND FILLER, GEL/PASTE, PER GRAM OF COLLAGEN

A6021 COLLAGEN DRESSING, PAD SIZE 16 SQ. IN. OR LESS, EACH

A6022 COLLAGEN DRESSING, PAD SIZE MORE THAN 16 SQ. IN. BUT LESS THAN OR EQUAL TO 48 SQ. IN., EACH

A6023 COLLAGEN DRESSING, PAD SIZE MORE THAN 48 SQ. IN., EACH

A6024 COLLAGEN DRESSING WOUND FILLER, PER 6 INCHES

A6025 GEL SHEET FOR DERMAL OR EPIDERMAL APPLICATION, (E.G., SILICONE, HYDROGEL, OTHER), EACH

A6154 WOUND POUCH, EACH

A6196 ALGINATE OR OTHER FIBER GELLING DRESSING, WOUND COVER, PAD SIZE 16 SQ. IN. OR LESS, EACH DRESSING

A6197 ALGINATE OR OTHER FIBER GELLING DRESSING, WOUND COVER, PAD SIZE MORE THAN 16 SQ. IN. BUT LESS THAN OR EQUAL TO 48 SQ. IN., EACH DRESSING

A6198 ALGINATE OR OTHER FIBER GELLING DRESSING, WOUND COVER, PAD SIZE MORE THAN 48 SQ. IN., EACH DRESSING

A6199 ALGINATE OR OTHER FIBER GELLING DRESSING, WOUND FILLER, PER 6 INCHES

A6200 COMPOSITE DRESSING, PAD SIZE 16 SQ. IN. OR LESS, WITHOUT ADHESIVE BORDER, EACH DRESSING

A6201 COMPOSITE DRESSING, PAD SIZE MORE THAN 16 SQ. IN. BUT LESS THAN OR EQUAL TO 48 SQ. IN., WITHOUT ADHESIVE BORDER, EACH DRESSING

A6202 COMPOSITE DRESSING, PAD SIZE MORE THAN 48 SQ. IN., WITHOUT ADHESIVE BORDER, EACH DRESSING

A6203 COMPOSITE DRESSING, PAD SIZE 16 SQ. IN. OR LESS, WITH ANY SIZE ADHESIVE BORDER, EACH DRESSING

A6204 COMPOSITE DRESSING, PAD SIZE MORE THAN 16 SQ. IN. BUT LESS THAN OR EQUAL TO 48 SQ. IN., WITH ANY SIZE ADHESIVE BORDER, EACH DRESSING

A6205 COMPOSITE DRESSING, PAD SIZE MORE THAN 48 SQ. IN., WITH ANY SIZE ADHESIVE BORDER, EACH DRESSING

A6206 CONTACT LAYER, 16 SQ. IN. OR LESS, EACH DRESSING

A6207 CONTACT LAYER, MORE THAN 16 SQ. IN. BUT LESS THAN OR EQUAL TO 48 SQ. IN., EACH DRESSING

A6208 CONTACT LAYER, MORE THAN 48 SQ. IN., EACH DRESSING

A6209 FOAM DRESSING, WOUND COVER, PAD SIZE 16 SQ. IN. OR LESS, WITHOUT ADHESIVE BORDER, EACH DRESSING

A6210 FOAM DRESSING, WOUND COVER, PAD SIZE MORE THAN 16 SQ. IN. BUT LESS THAN OR EQUAL TO 48 SQ. IN., WITHOUT ADHESIVE BORDER, EACH DRESSING

A6211 FOAM DRESSING, WOUND COVER, PAD SIZE MORE THAN 48 SQ. IN., WITHOUT ADHESIVE BORDER, EACH DRESSING

A6212 FOAM DRESSING, WOUND COVER, PAD SIZE 16 SQ. IN. OR LESS, WITH ANY SIZE ADHESIVE BORDER, EACH DRESSING

A6213 FOAM DRESSING, WOUND COVER, PAD SIZE MORE THAN 16 SQ. IN. BUT LESS THAN OR EQUAL TO 48 SQ. IN., WITH ANY SIZE ADHESIVE BORDER, EACH DRESSING

A6214 FOAM DRESSING, WOUND COVER, PAD SIZE MORE THAN 48 SQ. IN., WITH ANY SIZE ADHESIVE BORDER, EACH DRESSING

A6215 FOAM DRESSING, WOUND FILLER, PER GRAM

A6216 GAUZE, NON-IMPREGNATED, NON-STERILE, PAD SIZE 16 SQ. IN. OR LESS, WITHOUT ADHESIVE BORDER, EACH DRESSING

A6217 GAUZE, NON-IMPREGNATED, NON-STERILE, PAD SIZE MORE THAN 16 SQ. IN. BUT LESS THAN OR EQUAL TO 48 SQ. IN., WITHOUT ADHESIVE BORDER, EACH DRESSING

A6218 GAUZE, NON-IMPREGNATED, NON-STERILE, PAD SIZE MORE THAN 48 SQ. IN., WITHOUT ADHESIVE BORDER, EACH DRESSING

A6219 GAUZE, NON-IMPREGNATED, PAD SIZE 16 SQ. IN. OR LESS, WITH ANY SIZE ADHESIVE BORDER, EACH DRESSING

A6220 GAUZE, NON-IMPREGNATED, PAD SIZE MORE THAN 16 SQ. IN. BUT LESS THAN OR EQUAL TO 48 SQ. IN., WITH ANY SIZE ADHESIVE BORDER, EACH DRESSING

A6221 GAUZE, NON-IMPREGNATED, PAD SIZE MORE THAN 48 SQ. IN., WITH ANY SIZE ADHESIVE BORDER, EACH DRESSING

A6222 GAUZE, IMPREGNATED WITH OTHER THAN WATER, NORMAL SALINE, OR HYDROGEL, PAD SIZE 16 SQ. IN. OR LESS, WITHOUT ADHESIVE BORDER, EACH DRESSING

A6223 GAUZE, IMPREGNATED WITH OTHER THAN WATER, NORMAL SALINE, OR HYDROGEL, PAD SIZE MORE THAN 16 SQUARE INCHES, BUT LESS THAN OR EQUAL TO 48 SQUARE INCHES, WITHOUT ADHESIVE BORDER, EACH DRESSING

A6224 GAUZE, IMPREGNATED WITH OTHER THAN WATER, NORMAL SALINE, OR HYDROGEL, PAD SIZE MORE THAN 48 SQUARE INCHES, WITHOUT ADHESIVE BORDER, EACH DRESSING

A6228 GAUZE, IMPREGNATED, WATER OR NORMAL SALINE, PAD SIZE 16 SQ. IN. OR LESS, WITHOUT ADHESIVE BORDER, EACH DRESSING

A6229 GAUZE, IMPREGNATED, WATER OR NORMAL SALINE, PAD SIZE MORE THAT 16 SQ. IN. BUT LESS THAN OR EQUAL TO 48 SQ. IN., WITHOUT ADHESIVE BORDER, EACH DRESSING

A6230 GAUZE, IMPREGNATED, WATER OR NORMAL SALINE, PAD SIZE MORE THAN 48 SQ. IN., WITHOUT ADHESIVE BORDER, EACH DRESSING

A6231 GAUZE, IMPREGNATED, HYDROGEL, FOR DIRECT WOUND CONTACT, PAD SIZE 16 SQ. IN. OR LESS, EACH DRESSING

A6232 GAUZE, IMPREGNATED, HYDROGEL, FOR DIRECT WOUND CONTACT, PAD SIZE GREATER THAN 16 SQ. IN., BUT LESS THAN OR EQUAL TO 48 SQ. IN., EACH DRESSING

A6233 GAUZE, IMPREGNATED, HYDROGEL FOR DIRECT WOUND CONTACT, PAD SIZE MORE THAN 48 SQ. IN., EACH DRESSING

A6234 HYDROCOLLOID DRESSING, WOUND COVER, PAD SIZE 16 SQ. IN. OR LESS, WITHOUT ADHESIVE BORDER, EACH DRESSING

A6235 HYDROCOLLOID DRESSING, WOUND COVER, PAD SIZE MORE THAN 16 SQ. IN. BUT LESS THAN OR EQUAL TO 48 SQ. IN., WITHOUT ADHESIVE BORDER, EACH DRESSING

A6236 HYDROCOLLOID DRESSING, WOUND COVER, PAD SIZE MORE THAN 48 SQ. IN., WITHOUT ADHESIVE BORDER, EACH DRESSING

A6237 HYDROCOLLOID DRESSING, WOUND COVER, PAD SIZE 16 SQ. IN. OR LESS, WITH ANY SIZE ADHESIVE BORDER, EACH DRESSING

A6238 HYDROCOLLOID DRESSING, WOUND COVER, PAD SIZE MORE THAN 16 SQ. IN. BUT LESS THAN OR EQUAL TO 48 SQ. IN., WITH ANY SIZE ADHESIVE BORDER, EACH DRESSING

A6239 HYDROCOLLOID DRESSING, WOUND COVER, PAD SIZE MORE THAN 48 SQ. IN., WITH ANY SIZE ADHESIVE BORDER, EACH DRESSING

A6240 HYDROCOLLOID DRESSING, WOUND FILLER, PASTE, PER FLUID OUNCE

A6241 HYDROCOLLOID DRESSING, WOUND FILLER, DRY FORM, PER GRAM

A6242 HYDROGEL DRESSING, WOUND COVER, PAD SIZE 16 SQ. IN. OR LESS, WITHOUT ADHESIVE BORDER, EACH DRESSING

A6243 HYDROGEL DRESSING, WOUND COVER, PAD SIZE MORE THAN 16 SQ. IN. BUT LESS THAN OR EQUAL TO 48 SQ. IN., WITHOUT ADHESIVE BORDER, EACH DRESSING

A6244 HYDROGEL DRESSING, WOUND COVER, PAD SIZE MORE THAN 48 SQ. IN., WITHOUT ADHESIVE BORDER, EACH DRESSING

A6245 HYDROGEL DRESSING, WOUND COVER, PAD SIZE 16 SQ. IN. OR LESS, WITH ANY SIZE ADHESIVE BORDER, EACH DRESSING

A6246 HYDROGEL DRESSING, WOUND COVER, PAD SIZE MORE THAN 16 SQ. IN. BUT LESS THAN OR EQUAL TO 48 SQ. IN., WITH ANY SIZE ADHESIVE BORDER, EACH DRESSING

A6247 HYDROGEL DRESSING, WOUND COVER, PAD SIZE MORE THAN 48 SQ. IN., WITH ANY SIZE ADHESIVE BORDER, EACH DRESSING

A6248 HYDROGEL DRESSING, WOUND FILLER, GEL, PER FLUID OUNCE

A6250 SKIN SEALANTS, PROTECTANTS, MOISTURIZERS, OINTMENTS, ANY TYPE, ANY SIZE

A6251 SPECIALTY ABSORPTIVE DRESSING, WOUND COVER, PAD SIZE 16 SQ. IN. OR LESS, WITHOUT ADHESIVE BORDER, EACH DRESSING

A6252 SPECIALTY ABSORPTIVE DRESSING, WOUND COVER, PAD SIZE MORE THAN 16 SQ. IN. BUT LESS THAN OR EQUAL TO 48 SQ. IN., WITHOUT ADHESIVE BORDER, EACH DRESSING

A6253 SPECIALTY ABSORPTIVE DRESSING, WOUND COVER, PAD SIZE MORE THAN 48 SQ. IN., WITHOUT ADHESIVE BORDER, EACH DRESSING

A6254 SPECIALTY ABSORPTIVE DRESSING, WOUND COVER, PAD SIZE 16 SQ. IN. OR LESS, WITH ANY SIZE ADHESIVE BORDER, EACH DRESSING

A6255 SPECIALTY ABSORPTIVE DRESSING, WOUND COVER, PAD SIZE MORE THAN 16 SQ. IN. BUT LESS THAN OR EQUAL TO 48 SQ. IN., WITH ANY SIZE ADHESIVE BORDER, EACH DRESSING

A6256 SPECIALTY ABSORPTIVE DRESSING, WOUND COVER, PAD SIZE MORE THAN 48 SQ. IN., WITH ANY SIZE ADHESIVE BORDER, EACH DRESSING

A6257 TRANSPARENT FILM, 16 SQ. IN. OR LESS, EACH DRESSING

A6258 TRANSPARENT FILM, MORE THAN 16 SQ. IN. BUT LESS THAN OR EQUAL TO 48 SQ. IN., EACH DRESSING

A6259 TRANSPARENT FILM, MORE THAN 48 SQ. IN., EACH DRESSING

A6260 WOUND CLEANSERS, ANY TYPE, ANY SIZE

A6261 WOUND FILLER, GEL/PASTE, PER FLUID OUNCE, NOT ELSEWHERE CLASSIFIED

A6262 WOUND FILLER, DRY FORM, PER GRAM, NOT ELSEWHERE CLASSIFIED

A6266 GAUZE, IMPREGNATED, OTHER THAN WATER, NORMAL SALINE, OR ZINC PASTE, ANY WIDTH, PER LINEAR YARD

A6402 GAUZE, NON-IMPREGNATED, STERILE, PAD SIZE 16 SQ. IN. OR LESS, WITHOUT ADHESIVE BORDER, EACH DRESSING

A6403 GAUZE, NON-IMPREGNATED, STERILE, PAD SIZE MORE THAN 16 SQ. IN. LESS THAN OR EQUAL TO 48 SQ. IN., WITHOUT ADHESIVE BORDER, EACH DRESSING

A6404 GAUZE, NON-IMPREGNATED, STERILE, PAD SIZE MORE THAN 48 SQ. IN., WITHOUT ADHESIVE BORDER, EACH DRESSING

A6407 PACKING STRIPS, NON-IMPREGNATED, UP TO 2 INCHES IN WIDTH, PER LINEAR YARD.

GLOSSARY

abrasion Wearing away of the skin through some mechanical process (friction or trauma).

abscess Localized collection of pus in any part of the body.

advanced wound care dressings Refers to any of the newer dressings that are semiocclusive.

aerobe Microorganism that lives and grows in the presence of free oxygen.

allodynia Painful sensation or intolerance to normal objects touching the skin.

altered tissue perfusion Condition when oxygenated blood does not flow freely through the vessels to the tissue.

anaerobe Microorganism that lives and grows in the absence of free oxygen.

antibacterial Agent that inhibits the growth of bacteria.

antibiotic A natural substance that has the capacity to destroy or inhibit bacterial growth.

antimicrobial Agent that inhibits the growth of microbes.

antiseptic A chemical agent that prevents or inhibits microorganism growth.

apoptosis Programmed cell death initiated when activating molecules bind to their specific receptors on target cells; a mechanism to delete unwanted cells from the body.

arterial Pertaining to one or more arteries, which are vessels that carry oxygenated blood to the tissue.

arteriosclerosis Term applied to several pathologic conditions in which there is thickening, hardening, and loss of elasticity of the walls of blood vessels, especially arteries.

atrophie blanche Dermal sclerosis with dilated abnormal vasculature with ivory-white plaques on the ankle or foot and hemosiderin-pigmented borders.

autocrine stimulation The process of one cell acting on or stimulating specific cellular activities within itself.

autologous skin graft Graft of patient's own skin; also known as autograft.

autolysis Disintegration or liquefaction of tissue or of cells by the body's own mechanisms, such as leukocytes and enzymes.

avascular Lacking in blood supply.

bactericidal Agent that destroys bacteria.

bacteriostatic Agent that is capable of inhibiting the growth or multiplication of bacteria.

blanching Becoming white; maximum pallor.

callus A common, usually painless thickening of the skin at locations of pressure or friction.

cell migration Movement of cells in the repair process.

cellulitis Inflammation of tissue around a lesion, characterized by redness, swelling, and tenderness; signifies a spreading infectious process.

claudication Inadequate blood supply that produces severe pain in calf muscles during walking; subsides with rest.

collagen Main supportive protein of skin, tendon, bone, cartilage, and connective tissue.

colonized Presence of bacteria that cause no local or systemic signs or symptoms.

contamination The soiling by contact or introduction of organisms on to a wound.

contraction The pulling together of wound edges in the healing process.

crater Tissue defect extending at least to the subcutaneous layer.

crusted Dried secretions.

cytokine Substances other than growth factors that contribute to the regulation of cellular function and wound repair; examples include tumor necrosis factor-α and interferons.

debridement Removal of devitalized tissue.

debris Remains of broken-down or damaged cells or tissue.

decubitus A Latin word referring to the reclining position; a misnomer for a pressure sore; its plural is "decubitus ulcers."

dehiscence Separation of wound edges.

demarcation Line of separation between viable and non-viable tissue.

denude Loss of epidermis.

dependent pain Pain occurring when extremity is lower than the heart.

dermal Related to skin or dermis; synonym is "integumentary."

dermal wound Loss of skin integrity, which may be superficial or deep.

dermis Inner layer of skin in which hair follicles and sweat glands originate; involved in Stages II to IV pressure ulcers.

edema Presence of abnormally large amounts of fluid in the interstitial space.

endocrine stimulation The process of one cell acting on or stimulating specific cellular activities in distant cells.

enzymes Biochemical substances that are capable of breaking down necrotic tissue.

epibole Edges of top layers of epidermis have rolled down to cover lower edges of epidermis, including basement membrane, so that epithelial cells cannot migrate from wound edges; also described as closed wound edges.

epidermis Outer cellular layer of skin.

epithelialization Regeneration of the epidermis across a wound surface.

erosion Wearing away or gradual destruction of a surface caused by inflammation, injury, or other causes.

erythema Redness of the skin surface produced by vasodilatation.

eschar Thick, leathery necrotic tissue; devitalized tissue.

excoriation Linear scratches on skin.

exudate Accumulation of fluid in a wound; may contain serum, cellular debris, bacteria, and leukocytes.

fibroblast A cell or corpuscle from which connective tissue is developed.

filariasis a disease of the tropics that is caused by an infection with any of several round, thread-like parasitic worms; the most common is an infection with a parasite that lives in the lymph system.

fistula An abnormal passage from an internal organ to the body surface or between two internal organs.

friction Surface damage caused by skin rubbing against another surface.

full-thickness wound Tissue destruction extending through the dermis to involve the subcutaneous layer and possibly muscle and bone.

granulation Formation or growth of small blood vessels and connective tissue in a full-thickness wound.

growth factors Polypeptides that control growth and differentiation of cells (e.g., platelet-derived growth factor [PDGF], fibroblast growth factor [FGF], and epidermal growth factor [EGF]).

hydrophilic Attracting moisture.

hydrophobic Repelling moisture.

hyperemia Presence of excess blood in the vessels; engorgement.

hyperkeratosis Excess growth of keratin resulting in thickening of skin, typical appearance is white/gray in color and is firm to touch (e.g. callus).

induration Abnormal firmness of tissue with a definite margin.

infection Overgrowth of microorganisms capable of tissue destruction and invasion, accompanied by local or systemic symptoms.

inflammation Defensive reaction to tissue injury; involves increased blood flow and capillary permeability and facilitates physiologic cleanup of the wound; accompanied by increased heat, redness, swelling, and pain in the affected area.

insulation Maintenance of wound temperature close to body temperature.

intertriginous An area where apposing skin surfaces are in prolonged contact, such as in the groin or the axilla and under the breasts; friction and moisture entrapment are common complications.

intertrigo A mild inflammatory process that occurs on apposing skin surfaces as a result of friction and moisture; characterized by erythema, superficial linear erosions at the base of the skin fold, or circular erosion between the buttocks.

ischemia Deficiency of blood caused by functional constriction or obstruction of a blood vessel.

lesion A broad term referring to wounds or sores.

leukocytosis Increase in the number of leukocytes ($>10,000/mm^3$) in the blood.

maceration Softening of tissue by soaking in fluids.

macrophage type of white blood cell that regulates wound repair through the ability to destroy bacteria and devitalized tissue and produce a variety of growth factors.

MMP Matrix metalloproteinase; enzymatic compound capable of connective tissue degradation; classified as collagenases, gelatinases, and stromelysins.

moisture-retentive wound dressings General term that refers to any dressing that is capable of consistently retaining moisture at the wound site by interfering with the natural evaporative loss of moisture vapor.

MVTR Moisture-vapor transmission rate; measured in units of weight of moisture vapor per area of material per time period (e.g., $g/m^2/day$).

necrotic Dead; avascular.

neuropathy Neuropathic progression from functional to structural to nerve death.

nongranulating Absence of granulation tissue; wound surface appears smooth as opposed to granular (cobblestone, berrylike appearance).

occlusive wound dressings No liquids or gases can be transmitted through the dressing material.

osteomyelitis Inflammation of bone and marrow, usually caused by pathogens that enter the bone during an injury or surgery.

pallor Lack of natural color, paleness.

paracrine stimulation The process of one cell acting on or stimulating specific cellular activities within a neighboring cell.

paresthesia Abnormal neurologic sensations described as "pins and needles," "electric-like"; "numb, aching feet," or "as if my feet have been in ice water"; "knifelike" or shooting pains.

partial-thickness wound Loss of epidermis and possible partial loss of dermis.

pathogen Any disease-producing agent or microorganism.

periwound The area immediately around the wound.

phlebitis Inflammation of a vein.

physiologic wound environment In a wound, the presence of the physical, chemical, and biotic (living) factors that are characteristic of healthy intact skin; desirable to facilitate the natural process of wound healing.

pliable Supple, flexible.

pressure sore Area of localized tissue damage caused by ischemia because of pressure.

purpura Bleeding beneath the skin or mucous membranes; it causes black and blue spots (ecchymosis) or pinpoint bleeding.

pus Thick fluid indicative of infection containing leukocytes, bacteria, and cellular debris.

pyogenic Producing pus.

reactive hyperemia Extra blood in vessels occurring in response to a period of blocked blood flow.

scab Dried exudate covering superficial wounds.

semiocclusive wound dressings No liquids are transmitted through dressing naturally; variable levels of gases can be transmitted through dressing material; most dressings are semiocclusive.

senescent cells An age-related decrease in the proliferation potential in dermal fibroblasts; an occurrence observed in chronic wounds in which fibroblasts have an impaired responsiveness to growth hormone; a response that may be due to the increased number of senescent cells.

shear Trauma caused by tissue layers sliding against each other; results in disruption or angulation of blood vessels.

sinus tract Course or pathway that can extend in any direction from the wound surface; results in dead space with potential for abscess formation.

slough soft, moist avascular (necrotic/devitalized) tissue; it may be white, yellow, tan, or green; it may be loose, stringy, or firmly adherent.

stasis Stagnation of blood caused by venous congestion.

stemmer sign A thickened skin fold at the base of the second toe or second finger that is an early diagnostic sign for lymphedema. A positive result occurs when this tissue cannot be lifted; only grasped as a lump of tissue. In a negative result, it is possible to lift the tissue normally.

strip Remove epidermis by mechanical means; denude.

synthetic wound dressings Dressings that are composed of man-made materials, such as polymers, as opposed to naturally occurring materials, such as cotton.

TIMP Tissue inhibitor of matrix metalloproteinases; binds to the MMPs to render the MMP inactive.

trophic Changes that occur as a result of inadequate circulation, such as loss of hair, thinning of skin, and ridging of nails.

ulcer Open sore.

undermine Tissue destruction to underlying intact skin along wound margins.

unstageable pressure ulcer Covered with eschar or slough, which prohibits complete assessment of the wound.

varicosities Dilated tortuous superficial veins.

vasoconstriction Constriction of the blood vessels.

vasodilatation Dilatation of blood vessels, especially small arteries and arterioles; preferred spelling to "vasodilation."

venous insufficiency Deep or superficial veins become incompetent, permitting reverse flow and resulting in raised pressure in the superficial veins during ambulation.

venous Pertaining to the veins.

wound base Uppermost viable tissue layer of the wound; may be covered with slough or eschar.

wound margin Rim or border of wound.

wound repair Healing process; partial-thickness healing involves epithelialization; full-thickness healing involves contraction, granulation, and epithelialization.

xenograft Tissue from another species (such as a pig) used as a temporary graft.

Index

Page numbers followed by b indicate boxes, f, figures, t, tables.